HEALTH CARE
MANAGEMENT
AND THE LAW

LAW
Principles and Applications

HEALTH CARE MANAGEMENT

AND THE LAW

Principles and Applications

DONNA K. HAMMAKER
WITH SARAH J. TOMLINSON

DELMAR
CENGAGE Learning

Australia • Brazil • Japan • Korea • Mexico • Singapore • Spain • United Kingdom • United States

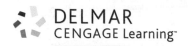

BP45

**Health Care Management and the Law:
Principles and Applications**
Donna K. Hammaker with Sarah J. Tomlinson

Vice President, Career and Professional
    Editorial: Dave Garza

Director of Learning Solutions: Matthew Kane

Senior Acquisitions Editor: Tari Broderick

Managing Editor: Marah Bellegarde

Product Manager: Natalie Pashoukos

Editorial Assistant: Ian Lewis

Vice President, Career and Professional
    Marketing: Jennifer Ann Baker

Marketing Director: Wendy Mapstone

Marketing Manager: Michele McTighe

Marketing Coordinator: Scott Chrysler

Production Director: Carolyn Miller

Production Manager: Andrew Crouth

Content Project Manager: Brooke Greenhouse

Senior Art Director: Jack Pendleton

For product information and technology assistance, contact us at
Professional & Career Group Customer Support, 1-800-648-7450

For permission to use material from this text or product, submit all requests
online at **cengage.com/permissions.**
Further permissions questions can be e-mailed to
permissionrequest@cengage.com

Library of Congress Control Number: 2010920214

ISBN-13: 978-1-4283-2004-8
ISBN-10: 1-4283-2004-0

Delmar
5 Maxwell Drive
Clifton Park, NY 12065-2919
USA

Cengage Learning products are represented in Canada by Nelson Education, Ltd.

For your lifelong learning solutions, visit **delmar.cengage.com**
Visit our corporate website at **cengage.com**

NOTICE TO THE READER
Publisher does not warrant or guarantee any of the products described herein or perform any independent analysis in connection with any of the product information contained herein. Publisher does not assume, and expressly disclaims, any obligation to obtain and Include information other than that provided to it by the manufacturer. The reader is expressly warned to consider and adopt all safety precautions that might be indicated by the activities described herein and to avoid all potential hazards. By following the instructions contained herein, the reader willingly assumes all risks in connection with such instructions. The publisher makes no representations or warranties of any kind, including but not limited to, the warranties of fitness for particular purpose or merchantability, nor are any such representations implied with respect to the material set forth herein, and the publisher takes no responsibility with respect to such material. The publisher shall not be liable for any special, consequential, or exemplary damages resulting, in whole or part, from the readers' use of, or reliance upon, this material.

Printed in the United States of America
1 2 3 4 5 13 12 11 10

1/21/11

CONTENTS

PART IV • AFFORDABLE HEALTH CARE 141

PART VI • STRATEGIC HEALTH CARE RESTRUCTURINGS 253

PART VIII • IMPROVING THE QUALITY OF HEALTH CARE 391

PART IX • OUR HEALTH CARE SYSTEM'S RESPONSE TO ILLNESS 441

PART X • END-OF-LIFE HEALTH CARE 529

PART XIII • CONCLUSION 729

PREFACE

> "With regard to excellence, it is not enough to know, but we must try to have and use it."
>
> —ARISTOTLE (384 B.C.-322 B.C.), GREEK PHILOSOPHER, FROM "NICHOMACHEAN ETHIC"

AUTHORS' VISION

Throughout this text are two strong recurring themes: namely, that there is a health care crisis in the U.S. and that the nation's health care laws must be reformed to create a system that works properly. The time for change is now. A related premise is that the convergence of many health care sectors is rapidly changing the laws governing provider competition and regulation. These changes require the American legal system to expand the boundaries of health care law as it recognizes what is best and what is essential in the U.S. health care system. Scientifically advanced U.S. medical institutions, with their elaborate systems of specialized knowledge, advanced technologies, and rules of behavior, contain some of the best elements of the American health care system.

While each industry segment faces unique legal challenges, more and more of these challenges overlap with established legal principles and the hard rules of law. Health care organizations are increasingly shifting legal strategies to stay ahead of the curve of emerging issues and government regulations. Providers are constructing new breakthroughs in health care delivery. Established pharmaceutical manufacturers are investing heavily in biotechnology and medical devices. Traditional medical-research-focused companies are venturing into the realm of commercialization. Together, they are seeking to reclaim some of the mislaid status of American medicine and return to the ideals of reason through modern science. All of this active change is taking place amid innovative U.S. reform initiatives and an increasing focus on global health. Health law should challenge these dynamic changes with a stern but fair message about limits.

This textbook does not distinguish between access to health care for resident citizens and resident noncitizens or more specifically, those in the U.S. without status, sometimes labeled undocumented, unauthorized, or illegal immigrants. Whether or not there is agreement on their right to do so, those without status access the American health care system, including its emergency rooms and public clinics. Therefore, it only made sense to include noncitizen residents in the discussion and the proposed solutions. This textbook assumes this segment of the U.S. population accesses health care to the same extent as U.S. citizens; therefore, all materials addressed in this textbook encompass resident citizens and noncitizens alike.

TEXT APPROACH

Real-World Knowledge

This text bridges research and practice, reflecting new, real-world knowledge of the health care industry and government agencies. The health law concepts in this text are practical; application of the concepts seeks to provide health care managers with sufficient knowledge of the law to become intelligent, critical thinkers in professional practice. Students are not being prepared to become health law attorneys; rather, they will gain a sense of when and why they should consult attorneys.

This is a practical health law text relevant to undergraduate students seeking the basic management skills required to work in health care organizations, as well as graduate students currently working in health care organizations as health industry administrators, physicians, nurses, pharmacists, therapists, scientists, and other administrative and clinical managers. This text is also relevant to those general health care consumers who are simply attempting to navigate the complex American health care system. Every attempt is made within the text to support health law and management theory with practical applications.

Depth and Breadth

This text does not overwhelm students with legal theory; instead, it covers basic legal principles and then focuses on practical applications of the law in the real world of health care delivery and practice. Challenging, current administrative and judicial decisions are presented. Students can customize their learning experiences by selecting from thirty-nine topic chapters or studying a specific topic in-depth, using the chapter bibliographies and multiple resources provided. There is a focus on interpretation, insight, and ideas; in other words, the focus is more on the meaning of the law, not only on what occurs pursuant to it.

Ethics Learning

The practice and theory of ethics is an underlying theme woven throughout this text. Students can develop and strengthen their skills in ethics through the examination of the difficult moral dilemmas presented. They can build a framework within which to think through the ethical implications of management decisions.

Best Practices

The text seeks to apply the best practices to the health care industry. Students are exposed to health care management models and their evolution in a law context, whether when seeking new models to overcome the failure of markets and governments to help millions of people suffering from HIV/AIDS and diseases rampant in third world countries, or when searching for ways to better understand the complex and quickly evolving biotechnology industry. Management, leadership, and the dynamics of competition in the U.S. health care industry are emphasized. Students learn about key elements that allow our U.S. health care culture to operate.

State-of-the-Art Research

This text is traditional legal scholarship written with state-of-the-art research methods, using searchable online databases that are revolutionizing research on health care management and the law, including foremost:

- Knowledge@Wharton (The Wharton School of the University of Pennsylvania)
- Medline/PubMed
- NLM (National Library of Medicine)
- OnlineWSJ (Wall Street Journal)
- OVRC (Opposing Viewpoints Research Center owned by Thomson Reuters, parent company of the Delmar Cengage imprint)
- ProQuest
- LexisNexis

The text reviews jurisprudence and seeks common themes as well as conflicts. Knowledge of the innovations transforming global health industry practices and public policy are clearly explained so that students' minds can be opened to new possibilities in order to apply what they learn.

Primary Research with Industry Experts

While background information was obtained from a comprehensive search of published literature and reports obtained from various government, business, and medical trade journals, this secondary research was supplemented with reviews by over thirty health industry experts. Their shared opinions and insights helped supplement the online databases with company, medical, and trade literature on current and future trends.

ORGANIZATION OF THIS TEXT

The goals of this text are to engage those students who will be leading and shaping twenty-first-century health care organizations and to raise questions about current health law issues such as:

- Emergence of the U.S. as a player in the global health care industry
- Innovative new approaches to the payer/provider model
- The future of tailored therapeutics

The text is divided into thirteen broad parts:

Part I, "Introduction," provides a brief familiarization with the U.S. health care system.

Chapter 1, *Processes for Thinking About the U.S. Health Care System*, describes how the greatest obstacle to transforming the U.S. health care system may be the nation's collective thinking.

Chapter 2, *Introduction to Health Law*, describes how the legal system functions through the separation of governmental powers that is central to the U.S. Constitution.

Part II, "Overview of Specific Health Laws," explains two commonly occurring health care legal issues.

Chapter 3, *Health Care Compliance Programs*, focuses on the prevention of health care fraud and abuse.

Chapter 4, *Antitrust and Regulation of Health Care Providers*, addresses how antitrust influences hospitals and managed care.

Part III, "Access to Health Care," addresses Americans' resolve to obtain the best health care system for as little investment as possible.

Chapter 5, *Access to and Reimbursement for Medically Necessary Health Care*, draws attention to the challenge of finding a way to provide access to basic medical care for all U.S. residents.

Chapter 6, *Medicaid and SCHIP Access to Medically Necessary Health Care*, draws attention to the challenge of finding a way to provide access to basic health care for U.S. residents at the bottom of the economic pyramid.

Chapter 7, *Medicare Reforms*, draws attention to the challenge of reforming Medicare, including Medicare's complex prescription drug plan.

Part IV, "Affordable Health Care," examines how to ensure that as parts of the U.S. health care system offer some of the best medical care of any place in the world to those who can afford it, the masses are not left behind.

Chapter 8, *Mutually Affordable Health Care*, examines whether nonprofit hospitals are required to provide mutually affordable health care in return for substantial tax exemptions.

Chapter 9, *Patient Rights and Responsibilities*, looks at patient rights, anti-managed-care legislation, and universal coverage.

Chapter 10, *Tort Reform and Reducing the Risk of Malpractice*, covers how malpractice occurs, as well as peer review processes and medical standards of care, tort reform, and the malpractice insurance crisis.

Part V, "Development of Human Capital," concentrates on staffing of U.S. health care organizations and the laws affecting health care employee management.

Chapter 11, *Human Resources Departments*, addresses two views of human resources in health organizations: first, as a strategic department that works directly with senior management to improve organizational effectiveness, and second, in its traditional role,

with involvement in many responsibilities now being outsourced.

Chapter 12, *Employers' Health Care Costs*, deals with growing efforts to trim employers' health care costs, with particular attention directed to the growing prevalence of smoking- and weight-related conditions.

Chapter 13, *Labor and Management Relations*, covers fundamental topics, such as unionization of physicians and nurses, as well as the newer concerns of nurse workload management and hiring of foreign physicians and nurses to meet unmet staffing needs.

Part VI, "Strategic Health Care Restructurings," describes how the health care and insurance industries are being pressured to move toward fewer restrictions on care instead of more.

Chapter 14, *Trends in Health Care Restructurings*, examines the movement of the U.S. health care system into integrated delivery systems that are multi-tiered based on the economic pyramid.

Chapter 15, *Integration Deals in the Health Care Sector*, looks at two sides of the restructuring coinage: mergers and acquisitions and bankruptcies.

Chapter 16, *Business Process Outsourcing*, addresses a rapidly expanding integration and outsourcing industry offering health care organizations services, such as finance, accounting, claims processing, adjudicating disputes, customer relationship management, and data analysis.

Part VII, "Producers of Medical Products," looks at the producers of medical products: pharmaceuticals, biotechnology, biopharmaceuticals, medical devices, and information technology.

Chapter 17, *Pharmaceuticals*, recognizes that while the industry is frequently criticized for charging high drug prices and making too much money, a realistic view of the pharmaceutical industry involves the costly interplay of high risks and long timelines for product development.

Chapter 18, *Biotechnology and Biopharmaceuticals*, explains the laws affecting gene therapy and other biological science fields, such as genomics, bioinformatics, and proteomics, that hold the potential for breakthroughs that might transform health care delivery.

Chapter 19, *Medical Devices*, describes how the use of implantable devices to treat heart disease, orthopedic complaints, and other conditions is growing rapidly via advancing technology, the continued prevalence of diseases from an aging and overweight population, and greater acceptance by physicians and patients of implantation as an alternative or complement to medication.

Chapter 20, *Health Information Technology*, examines how technology is reshaping the way hospitals, physicians, patients, and payers interact with one another.

Part VIII, "Improving the Quality of Health Care," covers four areas where broad agreement exists regarding what should be done to combat rising health care costs and improve the quality of medical treatment.

Chapter 21, *Disease Management*, describes the demand for greater transparency regarding how physicians effectively treat patients and the concomitant drive to develop clinical information technology databases and other processes to assist health care providers in making responsible medical treatment decisions.

Chapter 22, *Evidence-Based Medicine*, describes a discipline that has been around for a little more than a decade and is at the top of the list of industry improvements in the U.S. to help rein in health care costs and provide more reliable medical treatment.

Chapter 23, *Improving Patient Safety and Decreasing Medical Errors*, reviews programs targeting patient safety to prevent dangerous lapses in care, such as when providers fail to explain and monitor medical product use, deliver test results, or schedule follow-up care.

Part IX, "Our Health Care System's Response to Illness," takes a systematic look at mortality and other dimensions of ill health and death in the U.S., with a focus on the costs of living with a disease or disability.

Chapter 24, *Human Body Parts Industry*, describes a billion-dollar business intertwined with the U.S. health care system.

Chapter 25, *Organ Procurement and Transplantation*, explains the principles of organ procurement and transplantation and further describes the billion-dollar body parts industry.

Chapter 26, *HIV/AIDS Pandemic*, describes the devastating global HIV/AIDS epidemic, as attention increasingly focuses on U.S. companies holding patents and controlling prices for HIV/AIDS medications.

Chapter 27, *Mental Health*, focuses on the health care system's response to illness, and charts the costs of living with a chronic disease or disability.

Part X, "End-of-Life Health Care," is comprised of three chapters dealing with the "right-to-die" controversy.

Chapter 28, *Hospice Care*, covers a specialized and growing niche in the health care economy.

Chapter 29, *Mature Minor Rights to Refuse Life-Sustaining Medical Treatment*, focuses on the question of whether mature minors have the right to refuse life-sustaining medical treatment.

Chapter 30, *Care of the Critically Ill and Dying*, deals with the question of whether human beings have a right to die at a time and place of their own choosing.

Part XI, "Our Health Care System's Response to New Technologies," looks at emerging discoveries in regenerative and reproductive medicine and gene therapy with the potential to take health care in an entirely new direction.

Chapter 31, *Stem Cells and Regenerative Medicine*, looks at the potential of stem cell therapy and the controversy surrounding the use of embryonic stem cells.

Chapter 32, *Reprogenics and Assisted Reproductive Medicine*, discusses reprogenics, at the intersection of reproductive medicine and genetics, as well as synthetic biology, both of which are rapidly taking genetic techniques, ingredients, and diagnostic tools, and are engineering personalized medicines that have the potential to revolutionize the delivery of health care.

Part XII, "Additional Pressing Issues Facing Our Health Care System," is comprised of five chapters describing pivotal issues and real-world pitfalls students may confront.

Chapter 33, *Global Pandemics and Other Public Health Emergency Threats*, deals with community health and safety in the event of a pandemic or bioterrorist attack, and the appearance of novel or previously controlled or eradicated infectious agents, or biological toxins.

Chapter 34, *Health Care Issues for Women*, focuses on the disparate provision of medical care for procreation concerns, and addresses reproductive issues against the backdrop of how the newer forms of contraception and maternity care coverage are falling out of reach for more women in the U.S.

Chapter 35, *Clinical Trials*, provides an overview of the complex multistage pathways to FDA approval of the end results of medical product research and development.

Chapter 36, *Food Safety*, examines the debate between the food industry and public health advocates over junk food, advertising, and obesity.

Chapter 37, *Environmental Safety*, addresses the quandary of the modern U.S. health care system: mainly, that while it is the most expensive in the world, Americans are neither healthier nor do they live longer than residents in other countries.

Chapter 38, *Prevention of Child Abuse and Neglect*, examines survival-threatening physical abuse, psychological maltreatment, neglect, and sexual abuse of children and its challenges to provide the necessary health care services.

Part XIII, "Conclusion," provides a brief overview of how our health care system may be revised and refurbished, which is one of the most important issues the U.S. is confronting in terms of politics, economics, law, and ethics.

Chapter 39, *Future Prospects: Health Care Management and the Law*, summarizes the ideas in Chapters 1 through 38 of this text and provides an overview of the shifts required to develop policy frameworks for instituting changes in health care management and the law in each of the major health care sectors: life sciences, health care delivery, and medical products.

TEACHING AND LEARNING MATERIALS

Dramatic changes in the health care industry marketplace have pushed forward new questions about value creation. Because the global health care industry is a uniquely regulated environment, and there are genuine medical issues that place individual lives at risk, the integrity of this textbook is very important. This text will help instructors prepare their students for these real-world challenges.

The technology-enhanced learning tools accompanying this text are available in multiple formats to fit individual readers' learning preferences, and a range of instructional tools will meet virtually every instructor's needs.

Student Study Guide

Students are provided with a study guide as a resource to help them further learn how to apply management principles and health law concepts and to master terminology. This guide includes:

- **Chapter Outlines**
- **Review Questions** that assess students' knowledge
- **You Judge** cases currently being litigated or recently decided, sometimes in conflicting ways, by lower federal and state courts, Congress, and state legislatures. Students are given the opportunity to think through undecided health law issues and reach their own reasoned conclusions. Each of the broad issues in You Judge contains fierce ideological currents that students, as future executives in the health care industry, should fully understand.
- **Additional Web Links** that provide the opportunity to do further research on the health law topics presented in each chapter

Instructor Resources CD-ROM

The Instructor Resources CD-ROM is a robust computerized tool for instructional needs. This comprehensive and convenient CD-ROM contains:

- **Instructor's Manual** to enhance class discussion and measure student progress. It includes a wide variety of valuable resources to help instructors plan the course and implement activities by chapter. The availability of this manual in an electronic format increases its value as a teaching resource. It includes:
  - Learning objectives for each chapter
  - Suggested talking points for the Moral Dilemma questions from the text focus on what is being done, the correctness of assumptions and choices, and what might be done differently in future, similar situations
  - Suggested talking points for the You Judge cases in the study guide
  - Additional group and individual activities
  - Links to health law Web sites providing additional materials to research cited in the Law Notes and Chapter Bibliographies
- **PowerPoint Presentations** are available to visually enhance lectures and aid students in note taking.
- **ExamView® Computerized Testbank** contains short-answer, multiple-choice, and true/false questions for each chapter. This versatile program enables you to create your own tests and to write additional questions.
- **Comprehensive Syllabus Templates** have been developed to help instructors customize specific course titles.

WebTUTOR™

WebTutor™ will be available to accompany the book. An exciting online ancillary, it takes any course beyond classroom boundaries. WebTutor™ is a content-rich, Web-based teaching and learning aid that reinforces and helps clarify complex concepts. The WebCT™ and Blackboard™ platforms also provide rich communication tools for instructors and learners, including a course calendar, chat, e-mail, threaded discussions, Web links, and a whiteboard. Instructors will have the ability to moderate online collaboration within their classroom, allowing students to form communities of interest on health care topics and creating a "Public Square" environment to address management and health law solutions.

Online Companion

Visit the online companion for additional student and instructor resources, including:

- Instructor's Manual (password protected)
- Summaries of specific court decisions recently decided, as well as the full decisions
- Additional data-driven facts from the text

ABOUT THE AUTHORS

Donna K. Hammaker, a health law attorney, serves on the faculty at the Pennsylvania State University M.B.A. program in Biotechnology and Health Industry Management and at Immaculata University's School of Nursing. Director of the Health Care Management and the Law Institute, she has earned graduate degrees from Temple University School of Law and the Wharton School of the University of Pennsylvania and has done post-doctoral studies at the Hebrew University Faculty of Law and London School of Economics. She is a member of the Pennsylvania Bar, U.S. District Court, Eastern District of Pennsylvania, and the U.S. Court of Appeals Third Circuit. Hammaker was president and chief executive officer of Collegiate Health Care, the nation's first inter-university managed care organization.

Collaborating author Sarah J. Tomlinson is a new attorney clerking for the Honorable Roger N. Nanovic, II, President Judge of the Pennsylvania Court of Common Pleas, Carbon County. She earned her J.D. from Villanova University School of Law and her M.B.A. from the Pennsylvania State University. She is a member of the Pennsylvania Bar. While at Villanova, Tomlinson was published in and later served as Managing Editor of Student Works for the *Villanova Sports & Entertainment Law Journal*, as well as President of the International Law Society.

The authors are members of the National Health Lawyers Association, Society of Hospital Attorneys, American Association of Nurse Attorneys, and the Pennsylvania and American Bar Associations.

Interaction with the Authors

The standard for this text is excellence. Every instructor adopting this text must have an excellent experience with it, along with its ancillary teaching materials. Adopters of this text may e-mail the authors to ask questions regarding materials in this text, to offer suggestions, or to share teaching concerns. If we, as instructors of the next generation of health care managers, can help our students reclaim a supple awareness of the challenging principles of the American rule of law, our health care system may regain some of its earlier prestige. As Tocqueville maintained in his 1840 influential text about American law and society, *Democracy in America*, the greatest task of each generation is not to erase the past and reconstruct the present, but to recognize what was best in the past, what was essential, and to carry it forward. Our health care system will thrive again when the U.S. learns to acknowledge the force of this insight. However, if health law is seen as nothing but a collection of arbitrary rules and regulations ripe for re-engineering our health care system, and social forces are treated as legal obstacles to be overcome, rather than as shared boundaries to be reckoned with, the U.S. health care system will stay in its current crisis mode. Health law should not be a wholly owned subsidiary of any one ideology. Instead, health law should challenge all ideologies, with a firm understanding of the limits of law in a democracy.

Partners in Health

The authors are contributing a portion of their royalties to Partners in Health (PIH), a nonprofit founded by Dr. Paul Farmer that focuses on delivery of quality health care to those at the bottom of the economic pyramid. PIH is affiliated with Harvard Medical School and one of its teaching hospitals, the Brigham and Women's Hospital, as well as the François-Xavier Bagnoud Center for Health and Human Rights at the Harvard School of Public Health.

Donna K. Hammaker
and
Sarah J. Tomlinson
2010 January

ACKNOWLEDGEMENTS

This text has been reviewed by individuals chosen for their diverse perspectives of the health industry and technical expertise. Joseph L. Fink III, health law attorney and pharmacist, who is Professor of Pharmacy Law and Policy at the University of Kentucky College of Pharmacy, with joint faculty appointments as Professor of Health Services Management in the UK College of Public Health, Professor of Health Administration in the Martin School of Public Policy and Administration, and as Professor of Clinical Leadership and Management in the UK College of Health Sciences, and Victoria Ipri (http://www.theconfidentcopywriter.com/) reviewed and provided clear perspective on every chapter in the text. The authors are indebted to the following individuals for their review:

Ashby, Michele: Health Care Consultant
Anderson, Brent: Siemens Medical Services
Baddad, Naima: Octagon Research Solutions
Benelli, Kathy: Someday Isle
Benning, Shawn: Johnson & Johnson
Bezio, Timothy: ConvaTec, Inc.
Bilo, Michael: Pfizer
Burhans, Sara Baumler: Shire Pharmaceutical
Caranfa, Justin: Precision Therapeutics
Crowland, Keith: Kaiser Permanente Northwest
    Doody, Patrick: Aetna
Enright, Patty: ROI Performance Solutions
Epelbaum, Gleb: Johnson & Johnson
Everitt, Kevin: ICON Clinical Research
Fischer, Carol: AstraZeneca
Hopkins, Patrick: Genzyme
Huber, Veronique: Sanofi-Aventis
Johnson Camp, Sharlene: Johnson & Johnson
Knadig, Thomas: Health Care Management & Law
    Institute

Li, Fangbiao: Schering-Plough
Liu, Jeffrey: Abbott Laboratories
Mennor, Robert: Siemens Medical Services
Mullen, Eliose: United Food & Commercial Workers
    Union
Nelson, Ginny: Pennsylvania Hospital-Penn
    Medicine
Orfanakos, Jim: SAP America
Pentz, William: Cephalon
Reid, Melissa: GlaxoSmithKline
Rode, Jerry: Rolls-Royce NA
Sacco, Carolyn: Mpathy Medical
Spinks, Scott: Johnson & Johnson
Walton-Bongers, Cynthia: Penn State University-
    Great Valley/Drexel University
Weber, Michael: Merck
Wesoloskie, Wendy: Merck
Wright, Peter: ReMed
Wu, Jason: Graceway Pharmaceuticals

All the illustrations in this text were designed by Kimberly Virgilio of Virgilio Designs (http://www.virgiliodesigns .com/).

REVIEWERS

Jamie Clark, J.D.
Department of Health Sciences
Armstrong Atlantic University
Savannah, GA

Joseph L. Fink III, B.S.Pharm, J.D.
Professor
Department of Pharmacy Practice and Science
University of Kentucky
Lexington, KY

Craig D. Heckman, J.D.
Adjunct Graduate Faculty
Public Health Department
Western Kentucky University
Bowling Green, KY

Jerry W. Jackson, MHA, J.D.
Adjunct Professor
Health Science/Health Administration Program
California State University, Northridge
Northridge, CA

Nancy Kubasek, J.D.
Professor of Legal Studies
Bowling Green State University
Bowling Green, OH

Ruth L. Scheuer, DrPH, J.D.
Assistant Clinical Professor
Health Policy and Management
Mailman School of Public Health, Columbia University
New York, NY

J. Jean Thompson, MSHR, RHIA
Instructor
Health Information Management Department
East Central University
Ada, OK

William I. Weston, J.D., PhD
Dean
School of Legal Studies
Kaplan University
Ft. Lauderdale, FL

How To Use This Text

One of the strengths of this text is the consistent approach to topics in each chapter. Each chapter has been methodically developed for use at both the introductory and advanced levels by merely changing the amount of guidance provided. The same format is used in each chapter:

In Brief

provides a succinct overview of each chapter.

In Brief

This chapter describes how the greatest obstacle to transforming the U.S. health care system may be the nation's collective thinking. A simple idea in theory—that what is seen and acted upon is more a product of what is inside people's heads than what is out in the world—has far-reaching implications for the American approach to health care reform. The nation's mental models may create and limit opportunities.

Fact or Fiction

sections at the beginning of each chapter are short vignettes of in-depth articles pulled from the headlines or drawn from actual court cases pertinent to the chapter, demonstrating that society cannot always separate fact from fiction or always know what the law is.

Fact or Fiction

Gorillas in Our Field of Vision

What is it that makes mental models (relationships and concepts) of the American health care system so difficult to recognize and change?

Human memory and perception are very malleable and can be much more so than most people think. For instance, in one research study, recounted in the book, *The Power of Impossible Thinking*, subjects were asked to watch a video and count the number of times players with white shirts passed a basketball. Most of the subjects achieved a fairly accurate account of the passes, but less than half saw something more important: a person in a black gorilla costume walking right into the center of the action and then moving off. More than half the subjects were so involved in the counting task that they could not see the gorilla, an entire gorilla, right in front of their eyes!

It is sobering to consider. Mental models and attention create blinders that limit what the human brain sees. The question to keep in mind when thinking of the U.S. health care system is: are we failing to see the gorillas moving through our field of vision right now?

(See *Law Fact* at the end of this chapter for the answer.)

—Wind & Crook 2006

Law Fact

explains the outcome of the "Fact or Fiction" section that introduces every chapter and applies what is put forth and has been decided thus far in each chapter.

Law Fact

Gorillas in Our Field of Vision

What is it that makes mental models (relationships and concepts) of the American health care system so difficult to recognize and change?

The gorillas in our collective field of vision can be seen in neuroscience research. Neural activity due to sensory stimuli disappears in the cortex. The sensory stimuli cease to exist. We do not really see what we take in. Stimulation flows into our brains, evoking an internal pattern, which our brains use to represent the external situation. We think we see the real world, but we actually see what is already in our own minds.

—Wind & Crook (2006)

Moral Dilemmas

dispersed throughout each chapter offer students the opportunity to apply relevant court decisions on both sides of a health law issue to specific problems. Students are then asked to describe and analyze selected controversies. This is where students can reinforce practical insights gained in the chapter to assess or improve the outcome of timely issues facing the U.S. health care system.

Moral Dilemmas

1. What is inside people's heads when it comes to the health care industry that differs from reality in the health care industry?

2. What is it that makes mental models of the American health care system so difficult to recognize and change?

PRINCIPLES AND APPLICATIONS

is the heart of each chapter. It explains the basics of health law for students with little or no legal background—namely, the importance of health law, its basic principles, and how it applies to practical management applications. Specific examples and cases illustrate how health law principles are applied in the real world.

PRINCIPLES AND APPLICATIONS

The increasingly complex U.S. antitrust laws are commonly referred to as competition laws outside the U.S. (Bork, 1978, 2008). In theory, in a free enterprise system, the health care industry could direct its limited resources to the uses that would best satisfy patients with minimum intervention by the government. Of course, when the government pays for more than half of the health care provided in the U.S., with the remaining care regulated by government (McHugh, 2008), it is clear why the concept of free enterprise is totally theoretical in today's marketplace. Free enterprise in health care exists only in theory; it does not exist in reality.

When competition is stifled, the long arm of government antitrust enforcement should replace the invisible hand of the market as the regulator of dealings among health care providers and between providers and patients (Areeda & Hovenkamp, 2005). The court decisions described in this chapter contain some of the rules of the competitive game in which health care providers are the players, courts are the referees, and patients are the spectators.

In theory, in a competitive market comprised of integrated health care systems, the system that provided the best quality care for particular diseases would treat all the patients in a specific region diagnosed with certain diseases because no one else could obtain the treatment outcomes that this given health care system could. All the specialists in the region treating these diseases would be affiliated with this health care system because of its stellar patient care and reputation. Increased system specialization would drive efficiencies and medical costs downward. All the employers, health insurers, and other third-party payers would encourage patients in the region with certain diseases to utilize this health care system because of its treatment outcomes, innovative care, and prices for medical services (*see* Porter & Teisberg, 2006). None of this would violate any antitrust laws because no one else would be treating patients as well as this particular health care system.

After this health care system became the only provider in the region for treating specified diseases, antitrust law would prevent this system from artificially

LAW NOTES

at the conclusion of each chapter provide detailed endnotes citing the research supporting the "Principles and Applications" section in the main text. At times, the Law Notes expand upon the ideas described in the main text, explain important caveats, or offer additional examples of a compelling fact. The Law Notes are for those students who want to investigate certain topics in more depth.

LAW NOTES

1. The theoretical perspective of this chapter was developed by Wharton marketing professor Yoram ("Jerry") Wind and Colin Crook (*see generally* Wind & Crook, 2006; Wharton, 2005).
2. Mental models of the U.S. health care system are the images, assumptions, and stories people carry in their minds of themselves, other people in the health care industry, health care institutions (physician offices, hospitals, medical products companies), and every aspect of the nation's health care system. The nature of the mind exerts a significant effect on our perceptions of the U.S. health care system; people's view of health care is dependent both on the way the U.S. health care system is and on the way they are (*see generally* Metzger, 2005).
3. There is a sharp distinction between the mental model Americans have of the U.S. health care system and the model of how the system is serving their own personal medical needs. Americans believe the U.S. health care system needs reform, particularly when it comes to health insurance coverage and costs. At the same time, they are generally pleased with the quality of medical treatment, and are generally satisfied with the quality of their current health care and health insurance coverage; they like its choices and its intensive, high-quality technology approach to curing their ailments. On balance, Americans still favor maintaining their current mental models of health care, 59 percent to 41 percent. In a word, the American public seems to be calling for surgery on the current mental model of the U.S. health care system (essentially reforms to expand coverage to those who need it and actions to rein in costs), rather than an entire transplant operation to uproot the current system (*see* Saad, 2008).

COURT CASES

challenging, current administrative and judicial decisions are presented which focus on practical applications of the law in the real world of health care delivery and practice.

TERMINATION OF HOSPITAL PRIVILEGES BY PHYSICIAN-OWNERS OF SPECIALTY HOSPITAL

Arnett Physician Group, P.C. v. Greater Lafayette Health Services, Inc.
[Physicians Group v. General Hospital]
382 F.Supp.2d 1092 (U.S. District Court for the Northern District of Indiana 2005)

FACTS: The case involved contract disputes and negotiations between the Arnett Physician Group and its affiliated clinic, health plan, and HMO against the only existing general acute-care hospital in the Indiana community of Lafayette. The general hospital terminated Arnett's exclusive service contract and HMO agreement in response to the physicians' attempt to open their own specialty hospital. Twenty-one physicians subsequently left the Arnett Physician Group and became affiliated with the existing general hospital.

ISSUE: Did the general hospital unlawfully conspire with the physicians who left the Arnett Physician Group to join the hospital, and did the hospital violate antitrust law in denying the physicians who remained with Arnett access to the hospital's services?

HOLDING AND DECISION: No, staffing decisions at a single hospital cannot violate antitrust law.

ANALYSIS: The court held Arnett did not have antitrust standing resulting from a contract dispute with a single hospital. The hospital was found to have simply decided to substitute one exclusive radiology services provider for another. The hiring of physicians by the hospital did not amount to anticompetitive activity or confer antitrust standing. Further, there was no evidence connecting the hospital's termination of staff privileges by the Arnett Physician Group to their efforts to set up a competing acute-care hospital. A publicity campaign by the hospital against construction of a new hospital does not cause antitrust injury. Public expressions of opinion about competitors' plans cannot provide the basis for an antitrust claim and such conduct is clearly lawful.

RULE OF LAW: Antitrust laws protect competition, not competitors.

(*See generally* Miller).

PART I

INTRODUCTION

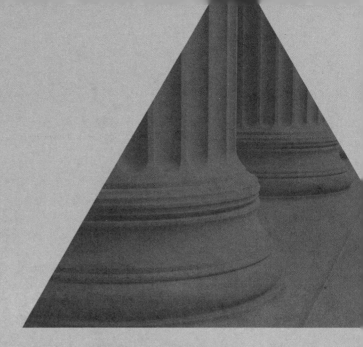

CHAPTER 1

PROCESSES FOR THINKING ABOUT THE U.S. HEALTH CARE SYSTEM

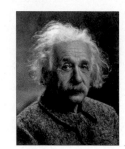

"How strange is the lot of us mortals? Each of us is here for a brief sojourn; for what purpose he knows not, though he sometimes thinks he senses it. But without deeper reflection one knows from daily life that one exists for other people—first of all for those upon whose smiles and well-being our own happiness is wholly dependent, and then for the many, unknown to us, to whose destinies we are bound by the ties of sympathy. A hundred times every day I remind myself that my inner and outer life are based on the labors of other men, living and dead, and that I must exert myself in order to give in the same measure as I have received and am still receiving . . ."

—ALBERT EINSTEIN (1879–1955), THEORETICAL PHYSICIST, FROM *THE WORLD AS I SEE IT* (1949)

IN BRIEF

This chapter describes how the greatest obstacle to transforming the U.S. health care system may be the nation's collective thinking. A simple idea in theory—that what is seen and acted upon is more a product of what is inside people's heads than what is out in the world—has far-reaching implications for the American approach to health care reform. The nation's mental models may create and limit opportunities.

FACT OR FICTION

GORILLAS IN OUR FIELD OF VISION

What is it that makes mental models (relationships and concepts) of the American health care system so difficult to recognize and change?

Human memory and perception are very malleable and can be much more so than most people think. For instance, in one research study, recounted in the book, *The Power of Impossible Thinking*, subjects were asked to watch a video and count the number of times players with white shirts passed a basketball. Most of the subjects achieved a fairly accurate account of the passes, but less than half saw something more important: a person in a black gorilla costume walking right into the center of the action and then moving off. More than half the subjects were so involved in the counting task that they could not see the gorilla, an entire gorilla, right in front of their eyes!

It is sobering to consider. Mental models and attention create blinders that limit what the human brain sees. The question to keep in mind when thinking of the U.S. health care system is: are we failing to see the gorillas moving through our field of vision right now?

—Wind & Crook 2006
(See *Law Fact* at the end of this chapter for the answer.)

PRINCIPLES AND APPLICATIONS[LN1]

The gorillas that we see (or fail to see) in our field of vision are determined by our mental models or the hypotheses in our minds as to what exists (subjects in shirts passing a basketball . . . or something more). Wind and Crook define mental models in terms of cognitive neuroscience. Mental models are internal patterns in the brain evoked by neural activity. Sensory stimuli flow into the cortex and evoke internal patterns, which the brain uses to represent the external situation. People think they see the real world, but they actually see the neural patterns or mental models (or structured relationships and concepts) already in their minds. People do not see the sensory stimuli they take in; they see the mental models evoked by their neural activity (*see generally* Freeman, 2000, 2001).[LN2]

The focus of this chapter and, indeed, this textbook, is how we can best cultivate an ability to see health care differently without casting aside all new ideas as preposterous, and without losing all perspective on the past and present. The goal is to embark on a journey toward discovering a better U.S. health care system by considering new ideas while retaining the best of the old and present ideas.

- What wisdom and opportunities can be found in seemingly out-of-the-ordinary ideas?
- What fresh perspectives can be discovered by exploring new medical technologies, new medical products, and new and different systems of delivering health care to different consumer segments?
- Where should these new ideas come from?
- Which perspectives should be retained in order to make sense of new ones?

The nation's collective thinking may be the obstacle to the impossible concept of an effective, efficient, high-quality health care system accessible to all U.S. residents. To transform the nation's health care organizations to achieve this quality health care for all citizens will require a transformation of the American consumer's idea of what constitutes health (Gattinella, 2009).

"NEW" APPROACH TO HEALTH CARE

Changing the nation's thinking about health care creates powerful opportunities for action. The health care industry plays a major role in the U.S. economy and, according to the Pacific Research Institute and by almost any objective account, a highly positive role.

The health care industry employs thirteen million Americans and accounts for one out of ten jobs in the U.S. (Pipes, 2009). Admitting blindness in completely understanding such a complex system could be the beginning of newfound wisdom; in other words, any reform of the U.S. health care system will first require acknowledging the gorilla in the room.

The debate about the right to health care, access, fairness, efficiency, and quality are the players in the white shirts. The gorilla is the $2.5 trillion in health care spending each year (Hartman, 2009). The total effective cost for health care includes costs from the:

- Federal budget
- State budgets
- Private, third-party health insurers
- Out-of-pocket costs covered by health care consumers

The federal budget funded 54 percent of the total health care spending in 2008, up from 45 percent in 2004 and 38 percent in 1970 (CBO, 2008). Clearly, health care costs are being shifted to the federal government. While private health insurance premiums increased to $775 billion in 2007 (Hartman, 2009), health care costs are increasingly being shifted to individuals. As high-deductible health insurance plans are taking more of the market share, out-of-pocket spending for health care increased to $268.6 billion in 2007 (Hartman, 2009).

Costs are obfuscated by cost-shifting from the government programs (Medicare and Medicaid) and the subsidizing of employer-provided insurance

under the federal tax code. These two hidden costs hide the true costs of health care as widely detailed by the health care consulting group, the Lewin Group (Pipes, 2009). As illustrated in Figure 1-1, health care costs were over 16 percent of the gross domestic product in 2008, according to the Office of the Actuary at the Centers for Medicare and Medicaid (CMS).

The gross domestic product was $13.33 trillion in 2008 (CIA, 2009). Obviously, this percentage cannot continue to grow indefinitely; the danger is that the current health care system, if left as it is, could resolve this cost problem by gradually denying coverage to more and more people.

Questions about funding and rapidly escalating costs indicate the U.S. health care system is not sustainable in its current form (Gorman, 2009). The Congressional Budget Office attributes the bulk of the escalating costs to the development of new treatments and other medical technologies (CBO, 2008). Today, people get joints replaced and have laparoscopic surgery to repair damage past generations simply "learned" to live with; health care costs are increasing because there are now more expensive

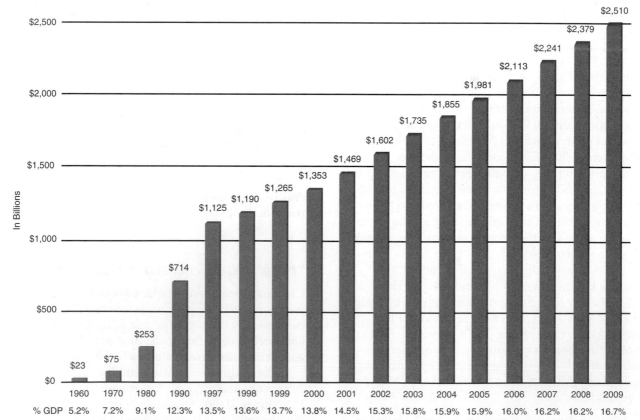

FIGURE 1-1: National Health Expenditures and Their Share of Gross Domestic Product

Delmar/Cengage Learning

Data retrieved from: Kaiser Family Foundation with data from the Centers for Medicare and Medicaid Services, Office of the Actuary, National Health Statistics Group (2009, January).

medical products and ways of using old products. On a per-capita basis, however, the U.S. spends about twice as much as most other industrialized economies without garnering any tangible benefits on health, infant mortality, or longevity.

- How does the American health care consumer make sense of data like this when:
  - 53 percent of American households cut back on health care because of cost concerns
  - 27 percent postpone needed medical care
  - 20 percent do not fill their prescriptions
  - 15 percent cut their pills in half or skip doses
  - 34 percent procrastinate about dental care

  (Kaiser, 2009)
- Is the U.S. health care system working as well as it could or do the mental models about what is going on need to be modified?

Data Driven

People often think the world is how they see it and that the facts are the facts as they know them. Each of these data-driven facts are explained in the remaining chapters of this textbook, along with citations to their sources of authority.

For further discussion, the online supplement contains over seventy data-driven facts, updated periodically, specific to each chapter.

Hypothesis Driven

Although individuals are data driven, they are also driven by hypotheses or their mental models. Consider:

- What do most people think about once they read these facts?
- Are there any underlying hypotheses behind these facts?

What is the meaning of these data-driven facts?
- About one-seventh of the American population has no health insurance, and most of them are earning middle-class incomes; this lack of coverage causes two deaths every hour.
- While tax-exempt hospitals receive over $12.6 billion in tax exemptions each year, they are not necessarily required to offer free or reduced-cost care to the uninsured or underinsured in return for their tax exemption.
- Top executives at the nation's health care systems are compensated with multimillion-dollar salaries and lavish benefits, seemingly without regard to performance, while top-performing lower wage employees are often not paid living wages.
- From the estimated $1.9 trillion employers spend on health care costs each year, over 60 percent of the costs go toward treating tobacco-related illnesses.
- Reprocessed medical devices are a cause for concern, as FDA standards are not always strictly adhered to, patients are not necessarily informed they are receiving a reprocessed device, and such devices are often obtained from unregulated sources, such as the Internet.
- Estimates indicate ninety million people in the U.S. live with a preventable chronic disease, the ongoing care for which amounts to 75 percent of the annual $2.5 trillion health care budget.
- Although evidence-based medicine can help pinpoint which treatments are best for which conditions, patients often still do not receive the best available treatment because health care professionals are not aware of the best treatment or have their own reasons for not using it:
  - Almost one-third of the surgeries performed on Medicare patients are unnecessary.
  - One-third of medical spending is devoted to services that do not improve health or the quality of care; it is essential that this $825 billion in ineffective spending, much of which may actually make things worse for patients, be acknowledged in health care reform efforts.
- The largest portion of hospital expenses are incurred in the last few weeks of life.
- Reproductive health care needs are not adequately met in the U.S., as evidenced by the high rate of teen pregnancies, unintended pregnancies and abortions, and the lack of access to birth control.
- The recent increase in weight-related chronic illnesses in the U.S. coincides with the change in American eating habits, with dietary intake consisting mostly of highly processed, prepackaged, and ready-made meals high in carbohydrates and sodium content; at the same time, fully one-third of the daily calories Americans eat are eaten outside the home at fast-food and chain restaurants.
- While the biggest burdens to the U.S. health care system are depression and violence, they receive scant attention in the health care reform debates; yet the cost of gun violence in the U.S. is equal to the cost of smoking, obesity, and other preventable health care illnesses combined.

- What is the explanation underlying these facts and what needs further investigation?
  - The U.S. spends more on health care than any other country in the world, yet ranks twenty-eighth in life expectancy: is this because it is the only industrialized nation in the world that does not provide medically necessary health care for all its residents, or could it be the open immigration and economic policies of the U.S.?
  - Should the U.S. bear the highest burden in the world for research and development of pharmaceutical drugs because it has one of the world's highest incomes per capita?
- Is there a single, coherent hypothesis that makes sense of all these assorted facts?
  - If the nation's health care laws and regulations are complex, exceedingly nuanced, and incomplete, does this regulatory complexity drive up health care costs and compliance overhead? If so, is this one reason why at least one-third of the U.S. health care costs are the result of management and administrative overhead expenses, or is this one-third ratio the norm for U.S. service industries in general?
  - Should the U.S. spend $770 billion every year to administer a heavily regulated private-based health care system, where the government covers more than half the costs?
- Should the nation's leaders examine the hypotheses underlying some of these facts as they undertake reform of the American health care system, or would they simply be reinventing the wheel based on prior reform efforts?
  - Should the nation grant hospitals over $12.6 billion in tax exemptions each year, while their executives are paid multimillion-dollar salaries and granted lavish benefits? Or are hospital administrators at the nation's leading tax-exempt health care systems being paid a rate comparable to executives in other sectors of the economy, and if so, is health care different?
- Is the U.S. being mindful of the process of transforming its health care system?
  - The U.S. has one of the highest infant mortality rates in the world; is this because reproductive services are not available to many women or because more babies survive high-risk pregnancies?
  - If evidence-based medicine is not being used by most health care providers, is this why one-third of the nation's medical spending is devoted to services that do not improve health or the quality of care, and may make things worse, or is this a faulty association?

- Should the U.S. rush to health care reform given the rapidly escalating costs of a stressed health care system?
  - If the U.S. decides to provide universal health care coverage, what would happen if tens of millions of people were suddenly added to the health care system? Would such a change greatly increase the need for primary care physicians, physician assistants, nurse practitioners, and advance practice nurses? Can this staffing need be met, even with imports of foreign health care professionals?

Mind Barriers

There is a need to continually examine the mental models that shape thinking on health care reform (*cf.* Wind & Crook, 2006). Americans may think the barriers to reform are too complex or that established interests are too entrenched to change, but often these barriers to creating the health care system this nation should have are simply in the nation's collective mind (*see* Wharton, 2005).

For example, consider rare diseases. Abbey Meyers' son suffered from Tourette Syndrome (TS) but was being helped by an experimental medication manufactured by McNeil Laboratories, a division of Johnson and Johnson. When McNeil dropped the drug because the patient population was too small to be profitable, Abbey Meyers became a consumer advocate. Her crusade: change the law to create incentives for the pharmaceutical industry to develop drugs for rare diseases. She founded the National Association for Rare Disease and, within two years, the FDA approved a drug for her son's TS. But Abbey Meyers did not stop crusading once her son's medical needs were met. She continued to pull together other health care consumers with rare diseases and, together, they made their voices heard. Congress responded to the group's call for new treatments with the Orphan Drug Act, giving pharmaceutical companies a seven-year monopoly for bringing new drugs for rare diseases to market (Anand, 2005).

The mental model of a modest sideline envisioned for the pharmaceutical industry has instead become a multibillion-dollar business. What changed? The impossible: companies discovered they could profit in small markets. The Orphan Drug Act became a powerful boost to the emerging biotechnology industry.

Today, more than half of the biopharmaceutical products manufactured by biotechnology companies are for rare diseases. Amgen and Genentech, two of the largest biotechnology companies in the world, were built on orphan drugs for rare diseases. What changed? The impossible: collective thinking about how to provide incentives to the pharmaceutical industry.

New mental models were created and orphan drugs to treat rare diseases suddenly became profitable.

Abbey Meyers never envisioned such monumental changes would arise from her simple efforts to obtain the right medication for her son's TS (Anand, 2005). Meyers proved the impossible was possible: The only barriers to achieving her goal were in McNeil's corporate mind.

- What are the potential blind spots in the U.S. health care system?
- What is holding back U.S. health care reform?
- How can the nation challenge the forces that block health care reform?
- What possibilities would be revealed if barriers to reform no longer existed, and how can the nation rid itself of obstacles and barriers to change?
- What are the challenges and risks of adopting new mental models of health care, and is the nation ready for them?

Moral Dilemmas

1. What is inside people's heads when it comes to the health care industry that differs from reality in the health care industry?

2. What is it that makes mental models of the American health care system so difficult to recognize and change?

Testing Reality

Instead of accepting the U.S. health care system as it is, extensive testing is needed to find out what the system really is and what is working. Areas to explore include:

- What incentives can be created to insure the uninsured and provide universal insurance coverage?
- How can the health care system motivate individuals to adopt behaviors that prevent most chronic diseases and illnesses?
- What will induce health care providers to use evidence-based medicine?

It is not impossible to create the right insurance incentives; the nation simply needs to change its thinking, like Abbey Meyers did when she needed a medication for her son. Perhaps, new hypotheses and a new mental model should be developed to achieve universal health care coverage with:

- Individual mandates
- Subsidies to ensure affordability
- Mechanisms to ensure insurance availability
- Management of risks that can prove profitable

NEUROLOGY OF INTERNAL PATTERNS

Neurology has shown that people do not really see what they take in. Readers of this chapter likely did not really see the data-driven facts at the start of this chapter. As stimulation flows into the brain, it evokes an internal pattern the brain uses to represent the external situation, so people are not aware that what they are actually seeing and thinking is what is already in their own minds (Wind & Crook, 2006).

Walter Freeman, a biologist, theoretical neuroscientist, and philosopher at the University of California at Berkeley, has conducted pioneering research on how brains generate meaning. Freeman discovered that the neural activity due to sensory stimuli disappears in the cortex. It disappears. Humans do not really see what they take in (Wharton, 2005). People do not always see the gorilla in the room.

When stimulation flows into the brain, it evokes in its place an internal pattern, which the brain uses to represent the external situation. Humans think they see the real world, but they actually see what is already in their minds (*see generally* Freeman).

- How can this textbook be used to come up with different ways of viewing health care?
- What chapters are overwhelming with information, and is it possible to zoom-out to look at the broader context?
- What chapters are limited by an overly broad perspective, and is it possible to zoom-in to examine the details more closely?
- Does this textbook cause indigestion from too much data or does it cause hunger because it does not provide enough information, and what needs to be done to respond to both sets of feelings?

Power of Internal Models

If humans are not aware of the power of their internal models, they may just accept what they think they see as reality. This misunderstanding of reality can be limiting, and sometimes even dangerous. (Wharton, 2005)

Humans tend to be comfortable and dependent upon their current mental models (Wind & Crook, 2006). Changing the U.S. health care system opens it up to uncertainty and risk, along with perhaps your job, or your provider or employer's way of doing business. Most people and organizations are risk averse, staying within their comfort zones, even if it causes increasing problems (Wind & Crook, 2006).

For instance, Merck stayed with the blockbuster marketing model for Vioxx, even when patients died from the drug. The biotechnology industry continues to sell its orphan drugs at exorbitantly high prices even as Congress debates changing the laws that enabled biotechnology to evolve into a multibillion-dollar business, using the same mental models the pharmaceutical industry used when a generic drug industry arose to challenge its pricing of drugs.

Filtered Thinking

Once people know their view of health care is shaped and filtered by their own thinking, they recognize the need to constantly test their mental models against the health care system this nation *should* have (*see* Wharton, 2005).

- Do the medical services most Americans think they have meet the expectations of what Americans want and need in health care?[LN3]
- Does the U.S. health care system meet the needs of most Americans, and do most Americans think it will continue to do so?
- Is the U.S. health care system worth the costs, and how might the health care system look without this limitation?
- How can the current health care system design new experiments to test the limits of mental models or gain new insights that might suggest new models for reform of the U.S. health care system?

TEST MENTAL MODELS

Individuals and organizations must constantly test their mental models instead of simply accepting what they think things are. This testing and re-testing will help determine what the facts are and what works.

Medical Innovation

For instance, the unmet medical needs facing the U.S. health care system are considerable:

- About 1,500 people die every day from cancer
- An estimated 4.5 million Americans have Alzheimer's disease, a number that has doubled since 1980
- There are approximately 400,000 multiple sclerosis patients and, every week, about two hundred more patients are diagnosed
- Thousands of patients today suffer from rare genetic disorders; most people have never even heard of these diseases, but they traumatize patients, and leave behind a trail of broken, frustrated families

(Mullen, 2005)

Yet, the system attributes the growth in health care costs to the development of new treatments and other medical technologies (CBO, 2008). How should the U.S. health care system reconcile the need

for medical innovation to treat cancer, Alzheimer's disease, multiple sclerosis, and rare genetic disorders with the need to reduce or slow cost growth? The unspoken hypothesis—that rationing or controlling spending on medical innovation is one way to control health care costs—shows the need to consider whether the nation's current mental models, which focus on spending, still fit in a world of rapid medical innovation.

Ideally, American medical innovation should not be limited because of costs. There has to be a way to remove this restraint. What possibilities might be obtainable if health care costs were no longer a limitation?

American consumers of health care will not stand for a decrease in the pace of adoption of new medical treatments or procedures or limiting the breadth of their application (Nichols, 2009). In all likelihood, the U.S. is not going to ration medical care as has been done in Europe. The U.S. will always allow Americans to buy what they want; however, they may be allowed to buy the most innovative treatments with their own money, especially care for preventable medical conditions.

Preventable Medical Conditions v. Treatable Conditions

What if the U.S. health care system focused on where $2.2 trillion in health care costs is being spent? According to the World Health Organization's Commission on the Social Determinants of Health, 50 percent of health status, or what makes individuals ill or well, is determined by health behavior (Solar & Irwin, 2007). This supports the research findings that most chronic illnesses are preventable (*see* Kelly et al., 2007; Marmont & Wilkenson, 2005).

As shown in Figure 1-2, of the $2.2 trillion spent annually on health care, 80 percent is devoted to the 10 percent that determines individuals' health status; less than 4 percent is devoted to improving health behavior and preventive medicine (Davis, 2007). At issue is whether the nation's priorities should be realigned so that 80 percent of the spending is directed to the 50 percent that determines health status. If the focus of health care were to change, some issues to consider might become:

- What medical conditions are preventable?
- When are they preventable?
- What level of health care will be provided for preventable medical conditions, so as to provide a financial incentive for people to change their behaviors to prevent chronic disease and illness in the first place?

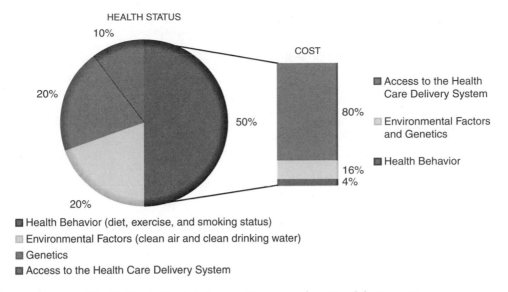

HEALTH STATUS
10%
20%
50%
20%

COST
80%
16%
4%

■ Access to the Health Care Delivery System

■ Environmental Factors and Genetics

■ Health Behavior

■ Health Behavior (diet, exercise, and smoking status)
■ Environmental Factors (clean air and clean drinking water)
■ Genetics
■ Access to the Health Care Delivery System

FIGURE 1-2: Attributes of Individual Health Status Compared to Health Care Costs

Delmar/Cengage Learning.

The hypotheses to modify health behaviors and prevent medical conditions from ever occurring are different from the mental model to access the health care delivery system to treat these same conditions.

WORLD OF CONSTANT CHANGE AND EVOLUTION

Debates in neuroscience focus on the brain as a computer versus an evolutionary-based biological system, and the influence of nature versus nurture in shaping thinking (Wind & Crook, 2006). The human brain constantly changes and evolves over time. Over one billion neurons continually die and regenerate. Several trillion synapses are continually destroyed and re-created. As illustrated in Figure 1-3, the human brain selects and reinforces or weakens certain synapses to forge the complex neural structures that determine thinking (Wind & Crook, 2006). Individuals reshape their neural models every day through their day-to-day experiences and thinking.

Individual Micro-Trends

This idea of reshaping the brain's neural models day-by-day brings the issue of micro-trends to the forefront. Forget about huge, sweeping universal changes in health care (mega-trends); the biggest trends today are micro: small, under-the-radar patterns of individual behaviors that take on real power when propelled by modern communications and an increasingly independent-minded population

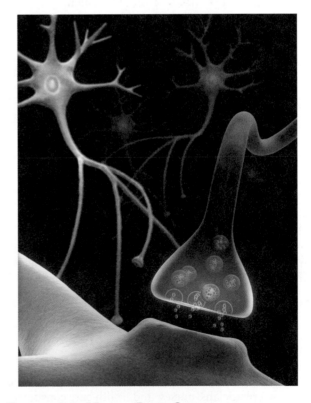

FIGURE 1-3: Human Brain Synapses

Copyright istockphoto.com.

(Penn & Zalesne, 2008). In the U.S., intense identity groups (micro-trends) can:

- Create new markets for risk management of health care costs
- Spark a social movement that focuses on behavioral change and preventive medicine
- Produce political change to bring about universal health care or more evidence-based medicine or financial incentives for observing healthy diet and exercise

The chapters in this textbook attempt to identify important health care trends in the law as they are happening. Small patterns of change and reform can be detected in state legislatures and in the appellate federal and state courts, and even sometimes in Congress.

Power of Thinking

Practical steps to understand, and perhaps change, thinking about the nation's health care system, include:

- Becoming explicitly aware of why people see the U.S. health care system the way they do and what that implies
- Testing the relevance of current mental models against the rapidly changing health care environment and seeing if they still fit or whether the models need to change and new ones need to be generated
- Developing a portfolio of models, which:
  - Minimizes the risk of switching models entirely
  - Allows the use of models that work best for particular situations
  - Prevents new models from becoming dogma, an absolute transformation, or revolution
- Overcoming the inhibitors to change and reform by reshaping the infrastructure that supports the old models and changing the thinking of others
- Quickly generating and acting upon new mental models by experimenting and continuing to assess and strengthen hypotheses and models

"ADAPTIVE DISCONNECTS"

Adaptive disconnects in the nation's health care system occur when everyone adapts their thinking at different rates. This is shown by Figure 1-4 and the:

- Differences in perspectives between health insurers and the insured
- Distinction between the goals and priorities of regulators and the regulated
- Divergence of views within health care delivery systems between administrative and clinical staff, and among physicians, nurses, and health care consumers
- Different perceptions of what should be done from varying disciplines in medical products companies, such as product development, finance, operations, and marketing

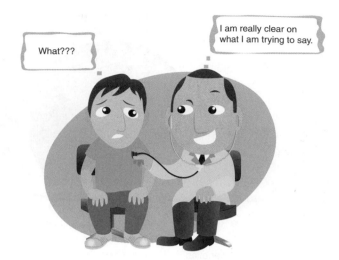

FIGURE 1-4: Adaptive Disconnects

Delmar/Cengage Learning.

- Variations between what is considered ethical and unethical, right and wrong, legal and illegal
- Differences in facts and opinions as to what health care reforms are needed or not needed

To arrive at real reform of the U.S. health care system, perhaps someone should seek out the most complex and sophisticated minds and put them in a room together, and have them ask each other the questions they are asking themselves. For instance, directing more than a billion dollars in federal funds for comparative effectiveness research to help determine whether medical treatments and devices are worth the money is much easier than coming up with new thinking about the need for these treatments in the first place.

Moral Dilemmas

1. What is holding back U.S. health care reform?

SUPPORT OF "OLD" MENTAL MODELS

It is not enough to simply change one's thinking about health care, however. The practical infrastructures and routines that support "old" mental models must be addressed. It is significantly more difficult to shift the nation's emphasis upstream from managing diseases to preventing them; this is not how the U.S. health care system is currently structured.

- What mental models does the U.S. health care system currently use?
- What other models could each of the health care sectors use?

- How does the choice of models shape each health care sector's position on issues and their decisions about it?

(*See generally* Wind & Crook, 2006)

Misaligned Incentives

Similarly, incentives in place in the nation's health care system are sometimes misaligned, making it difficult for new medical technologies to gain acceptance. While a new drug or technology might produce better outcomes than an existing treatment, there can be resistance to its adoption.

An example of this misalignment is the introduction of Gleevec, a drug produced by Novartis Pharmaceuticals, to fight chronic myeloid leukemia. While Gleevec is expensive (at about $25,000 per year), it can obviate the need for a $200,000 bone marrow transplant. The drug is potentially beneficial to patients, but economic calculations as to how much money a drug saves are not always made when it prevents patients from having surgery. (Pipes, 2009) The health care system does not always reflect economic benefits to individual patients.

- What mental models underlie the decisions and actions of Novartis and hospital transplant centers or insurers and leukemia patients?
- What are some varied models for diagnosing chronic myeloid leukemia, and how do they change the treatment options available?

ZOOMING-IN AND ZOOMING-OUT

In light of the immense complexity of the nation's health care industry, industry leaders must learn to both zoom-in and zoom-out. When examined in detail, parts of a system, like almost any phenomenon, will seem to be unstable, even fluctuating wildly.

For instance, it is important for the biotechnology industry to develop the ability to zoom-in and zoom-out in its thinking. Zooming-in focuses on details underlying core medical technologies. Zooming-out is a sense of how those technologies will play out in the larger health care environment, such as how society will pay for the advanced medical technologies being developed.

PROCESS OF MAKING SENSE OF THINGS

Neuroscience research studies how the brain works. Individuals must focus on what to do with the facts and data they receive and understand the process of making sense of things. While genetics provides the basis of who individuals are, experience strengthens and weakens genetic capabilities.

Understanding the Forces

Health care systems, like individuals, can focus on the forces that shape and reshape the mental models of their environment. For instance, $19 billion is being directed to health information technology by the federal government for implementation of a national health information network (Gattinella, 2009). To ensure a successful rollout, focus could be directed to:

- Education on how electronic health records (EHRs) have been shown to reduce medical errors and costs to counterbalance forces predicting turmoil from this effort to modernize the nation's inefficient, paper-clogged health system
- Influencing others (the end-users: primary care physicians, physician assistants, nurse practitioners, advance practice nurses, and nurses; the providers hospitals and medical products industries)
- Developing rewards and incentives for implementation

Studies by the National Center for Policy Analysis indicate that when EHRs are combined with the emerging field of genomics, a force will be unleashed that will throw open the door to personalized medicine, new medical treatments, and ultimately, more medical care (*see* Pipes, 2009). Thus, this advancement in technology is by no means the hoped-for fix for rising health care spending.

Moreover, EHRs and a national health information network could be powerfully disruptive for some lucrative sectors in the medical products industry, such as affecting so-called blockbuster drugs. A national HIT network would include EHRs that would allow health providers and others to track outcomes for drugs and devices, eventually resulting in the pharmaceutical and medical devices industries making fewer decisions about treatments. Much of the information physicians now use comes from studies paid for by the medical products industry. The more information is independently generated, analyzed, and distributed, the more the blockbuster model for drugs is in doubt.

- What impact will these changes have on the current commercial models for the pharmaceutical, biotechnology, and medical devices industries?
- What are the implications for drug development, and will the new model that emerges be sustainable?
- Will there be a market for blockbuster drugs in the future?

Information is a dual-edged sword in health care. Better information might blow apart some of the blockbuster markets in the pharmaceutical industry. It might also increase demand for other drugs in smaller, more focused markets. If so, will there be a future market for stand-alone medical products companies? All are hidden forces that shape the mental models of what a national health information network will accomplish with $19 billion from the nation's individual taxpayers.

"New" Approach to Decision-Making

There are several ways to change the nation's approach to decision-making about health care. First, the process for making sense of the nation's health care system should be understood in terms of mental models. Second, the difficulties in setting cost limits and seeing things differently must be recognized. Lastly, the neurology of internal patterns must be implicitly understood. Only then can the national framework for decision-making be transformed by:

- Recognizing issues
- Gathering the relevant facts
- Putting *all* the mental models on the table
- Evaluating alternative actions from various perspectives
- Testing *every* mental model
- Making decisions

- Testing the results of those decisions
- Repeating the process all over again

(*see* Wind & Crook, 2006)

PRACTICAL IMPLICATIONS OF THE "NEW" NEUROSCIENCE

The practical implications are limitless for the "new" neuroscience of mental models. There is great risk in changing old views of the nation's health care system, with its focus on models of managed cost. At the same time, there are great possibilities in the unprecedented opportunities to blend the best of the old and the new (Wind & Crook, 2006).

As you read the following chapters, always ask: What mental models underlie the court decisions and health care actions reported? What are some different models for looking at the same situations outlined in each chapter, and how do the mental models change the options available? Pay particular attention to how different mental models often define the battle lines on issues.

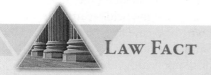 **LAW FACT**

GORILLAS IN OUR FIELD OF VISION

What is it that makes mental models (relationships and concepts) of the American health care system so difficult to recognize and change?

The gorillas in our collective field of vision can be seen in neuroscience research. Neural activity due to sensory stimuli disappears in the cortex. The sensory stimuli cease to exist. We do not really see what we take in. Stimulation flows into our brains, evoking an internal pattern, which our brains use to represent the external situation. We think we see the real world, but we actually see what is already in our own minds.

—Wind & Crook (2006)

CHAPTER SUMMARY

- Ideally, the development of a better U.S. health care system might be accomplished by considering new ideas, while retaining the best of the old and present ideas.
- The obstacle to an effective, efficient, high-quality health care system accessible to all U.S. residents may be the nation's collective thinking.
- Health care costs were over 16 percent of the gross national product in 2008; the more they increase, the more likely it may be that more people will be denied coverage.
- The U.S. spends about twice as much on health care as most other industrialized economies without garnering any tangible benefits on health, infant mortality, or longevity.
- Americans may think the barriers to reform are too complex, or that established interests are too entrenched to change, but often these barriers to creating an ideal health care system are simply in the nation's collective mind.
- People are not aware that what they are actually seeing and thinking is what is already in their own minds, due to the way the brain interprets new information.

- Many readers may not have fully absorbed the arguably shocking facts presented in this chapter because we tend to be unwilling to change our mental models.
- In order to improve health care in the U.S., individuals and organizations must constantly test their mental models instead of simply accepting what they think things are.
- The U.S. must find a way to reconcile the cost of health care with what health care consumers actually need; for example, it may not make sense to spend the most money on developing new and innovative medical technology when consumers cannot access existing technology.
- Instead of rationing health care across the board, Americans would likely prefer to ration it for preventable conditions or for highly innovative and overly expensive treatments.
- Another possible way to control costs would be to focus more heavily on preventive care and consumers' lifestyle behaviors, particularly smoking and weight control.
- Adaptive disconnects in the nation's health care system occur when everyone adapts their thinking at different rates.
- In light of the immense complexity of the nation's health care industry, participants must learn to see and understand both the minute details and the broader context in order to effect reformation.
- Neuroscience can be helpful in understanding how the brain works to create and preserve mental models and how to change the framework for decision-making in order to develop new mental models.

LAW NOTES

1. The theoretical perspective of this chapter was developed by Wharton marketing professor Yoram ("Jerry") Wind and Colin Crook (*see generally* Wind & Crook, 2006; Wharton, 2005).
2. Mental models of the U.S. health care system are the images, assumptions, and stories people carry in their minds of themselves, other people in the health care industry, health care institutions (physician offices, hospitals, medical products companies), and every aspect of the nation's health care system. The nature of the mind exerts a significant effect on our perceptions of the U.S. health care system; people's view of health care is dependent both on the way the U.S. health care system is and on the way they are (*see generally* Metzger, 2005).
3. There is a sharp distinction between the mental model Americans have of the U.S. health care system and the model of how the system is serving their own personal medical needs. Americans believe the U.S. health care system needs reform, particularly when it comes to health insurance coverage and costs. At the same time, they are generally pleased with the quality of medical treatment, and are generally satisfied with the quality of their current health care and health insurance coverage; they like its choices and its intensive, high-technology approach to curing their ailments. On balance, Americans still favor maintaining their current mental models of health care, 59 percent to 41 percent. In a word, the American public seems to be calling for surgery on the current mental model of the U.S. health care system (essentially reforms to expand coverage to those who need it and actions to rein in costs), rather than an entire transplant operation to uproot the current system (*see* Saad, 2008).

CHAPTER BIBLIOGRAPHY

Anand, G. (2005, November 15). Lucrative niches: How drugs for rare diseases became lifeline for companies: Federal law gives monopoly for seven years, fueling surge in bio-technology profits, a teen's $36,000 treatment. *Wall Street Journal*, p. A1.

CDC (Centers for Disease Control & Prevention). (2005). *The guide to community preventive services: What works to promote health. Task force on community preventive services*. Atlanta, GA: CDC.

CIA (Central Intelligence Agency). *World factbook*. (2009). Langley, VA: CIA.

Cochrane Collaboration. (2006). *Cochrane handbook for systematic reviews of systematic interventions*. Sydney, Australia: Cochran.

Davis, K. (2007). *Slowing the growth of U.S. health care expenditures. What are the options?* Prepared for the Commonwealth Fund/Alliance for Health Reform 2007 Bipartisan Congressional Health Policy Conference. New York, NY: Commonwealth Fund.

Freeman, W. (2001). *How brains make up their minds*. New York, NY: Columbia University Press.

___. (2000). *Neurodynamics: An exploration in mesoscopic brain dynamics (perspectives in neural computing)*. Philadelphia, PA: Springer (overview of Freeman's published works).

___. (1995). *Societies of brains. A study in the neuroscience of love and hate (The International Neural Networks Society)*. New York, NY: Routledge's Lawrence Erlbaum Taylor & Francis Group.

___. (1975). *Mass action in the nervous system: Examination of neurophysiological basis of adaptive behavior through the ego.* St. Louis, MO: Elsevier's Science & Technology Academic Press.

Gattinella, W., chief executive officer, president, and director of WebMD. (2009, February 20). Keynote Address at the 2009 Wharton Health Care Business Conference at the Park Hyatt at the Bellevue, Philadelphia, PA.

Gorman, K., managing partner and founder, Putman Associates. (2009, February 20). Remarks at the Panel discussion on health care policy: Will reform become reality? at the 2009 Wharton Health Care Business Conference, Philadelphia, PA.

Hartman, M. (2009). National health spending in 2007: Slower drug spending contributes to lowest rate of overall growth since 1998. *Health Affairs, 28* (1), 246-261.

Kaiser (Kaiser Family Foundation). (2009). *More than half of Americans say family skimped on medical care because of cost in past year; worries about affordability and availability of care rise.* Menlo Park, CA: Kaiser.

Kelly, M. P. et al. (2007). *The social determinants of health: Developing an evidence base for political action. Final Report to the World Health Organization, Commission on the Social Determinants of Health from the Measurement and Evidence Knowledge Network (MEKN).* London, England: National Institute for Health and Clinical Excellence and Santiago, Chili: Universidad del Desarrollo.

Marmont, M., & Wilkenson, R. (2005). *Social determinants of health.* New York, NY: Oxford University Press.

Metzger, M. B. (2005). Bridging the gaps: cognitive constraints on corporate control and ethics education. *University of Florida Journal of Law & Public Policy, 16*, 435-577.

Mullen, J. C. (2005, April 27). Gene therapy. *Wall Street Journal*, p. A17.

Nichols, L., director, health policy program, New American Foundation. (2009, February 20). Remarks at the Panel discussion on health care policy: Will reform become reality? at the 2009 Wharton Health Care Business Conference, Philadelphia, PA.

Penn, M., & Zalesne, E. K. (2008). *Microtrends: The small forces behind tomorrow's big changes.* New York, NY: Twelve Publishers of Hachette Book Group.

Pipes, S. (2009, March 6). Health reformers ignore facts. *Wall Street Journal*, p. A15.

Saad, L. (2008, December). *Americans rate national and personal healthcare differently: Public thinks U.S. healthcare system has problems, but own coverage is fine.* Washington, DC: Gallup. (reporting on a Gallup survey of over one thousand adults).

Solar, O., & Irwin, A. (2007). *Towards a conceptual framework for analysis and action on the social determinants of health.* Geneva, Switzerland: World Health Organization, Commission on Social Determinants of Health.

Wharton (Wharton School at the University of Pennsylvania). (2005, June 3). What's behind the 4-minute mile, Starbucks and the moon landing? the power of impossible thinking. *Knowledge @ Wharton.*

Wind, J., & Crook, C. (2006). *The power of impossible thinking: Transform the business of your life and the life of your business.* Philadelphia, PA: Wharton School Publishing.

CHAPTER 2

INTRODUCTION TO HEALTH LAW

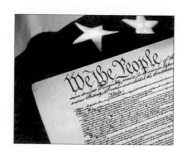

> "We the People of the United States, in Order to form a more perfect Union, establish Justice, insure domestic Tranquility, provide for the common defence, promote the general Welfare, and secure the Blessings of Liberty to ourselves and our Posterity, do ordain and establish this Constitution for the United States of America."
>
> —PREAMBLE, CONSTITUTION OF THE UNITED STATES OF AMERICA (1776)

IN BRIEF

This chapter describes how the U.S. legal system functions through the separation of governmental powers that is central to the U.S. Constitution. The role of "the People" and the agencies the federal government uses to administer and enforce U.S. health laws is reviewed. Crucial public health issues currently facing relevant federal agencies are outlined here and subsequently addressed in greater detail throughout this textbook.

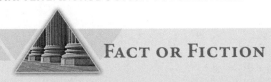

FACT OR FICTION

COMPREHENSIVE HEALTH CARE REFORM

Should the U.S. health care system overhaul be passed through Congress's budget reconciliation process?

Created in 1974, the omnibus budget reconciliation process allows federal legislation dealing with entitlement programs, such as health care reform, to be enacted by Congress on a simple majority vote after twenty hours of debate. This process precludes a filibuster in the Senate and makes it more difficult for individual U.S. Senators to amend legislation on the floor (Wawro & Schickler, 2007), which might unravel deals struck in congressional committees (GAO, 2006, 2007). Critics of budget reconciliation maintain the process is an attack on federalism, since the Senate has historically been the arena where states have significant influence. One issue being debated is whether the budget reconciliation process shifts too much power to congressional committees and away from members of Congress.

Under the principle of federalism, one of the founding principles of the U.S. Constitution, the federal and state governments should share the power to govern. The federal government has certain *expressed powers* (also called *enumerated powers*). The Constitution's Necessary-and-Proper Clause gives the federal government the *implied power* to pass any law "necessary and proper" for the execution of its express powers.

Opponents of universal health care believe the federal government has grown beyond the bounds permitted by its express powers. One fear is the federal government may be increasing too greatly in both its size and its influence on the everyday lives of Americans and in its expansion relative to the state governments. One side of this debate asserts the provision of universal health care by the federal government may exceed Congress's power, a power rightly belonging to the states. The other side maintains the states are legally subject to the dictates of the federal government when there is a national need to regulate an industry, such as the insurance industry that spans state borders.

It appears large majorities of Americans believe the U.S. Constitution implies everyone has a fundamental right to medically necessary health care (Kaiser, 2008a). If so, then the country may be ready for the federal government to comprehensively overhaul American health care. While major health care reform legislation will require significant intergovernmental mandates for decades to come, the current debate centers on whether there should be a social consensus in Congress for any reform, or whether health care reform is too important to be stalled by congressional protocol.

— 2 U.S.C.A. §§ 601-688, 900-907d (2009) (primary governing laws for the federal budget process).

(See *Law Fact* at the end of this chapter for the answer.)

PRINCIPLES AND APPLICATIONS

To understand health law, it helps to have a basic understanding of the:

- Declaration of Independence
- U.S. Constitution
- Bill of Rights (the first ten Amendments to the U.S. Constitution)
- Three separate but equal branches of government: judiciary, legislative, and executive
- Distribution of governmental powers between the federal and state governments
- Different types of laws: common, statutory, administrative, and constitutional

This chapter focuses on the facets of the American federal government with the most impact on health care as presented in the 2009 U.S. Government Manual and illustrated in Figure 2-1. Most of the fifty states have created similar organizations and government agencies. All budget and staffing information is from reports submitted to the Congressional Appropriation Committees for 2009.

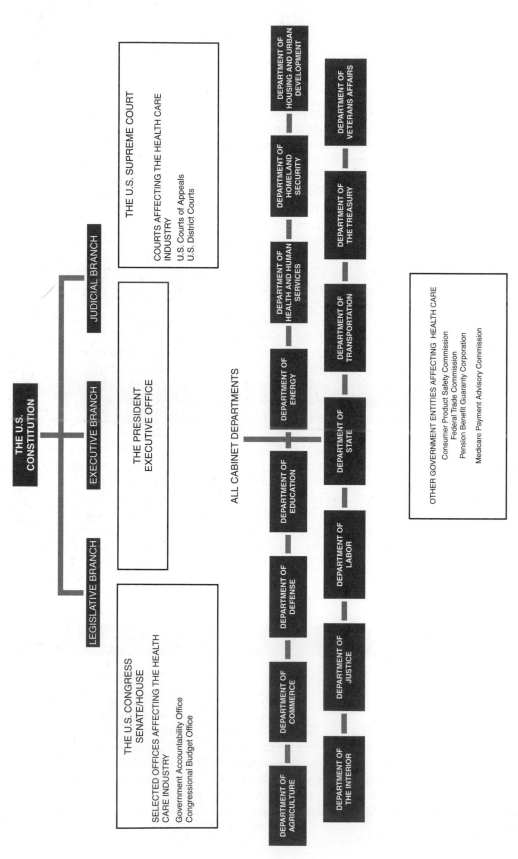

FIGURE 2-1: Organization of the Federal Government

Delmar/Cengage Learning

THE DECLARATION OF INDEPENDENCE

The Declaration of Independence is the nation's keystone document (Weinstein, 2007); its principles form the basis of the U.S. Constitution and the Bill of Rights. The unalienable rights concept, embodied in the Declaration, is the foundation of the fundamental rights of all Americans and the basis for the concept of limited government in the U.S.

> We hold these truths to be self-evident, that all men are created equal, that they are endowed by their Creator with certain unalienable Rights, that among these are Life, Liberty and the pursuit of Happiness. That to secure these rights, Governments are instituted among Men, deriving their just powers from the consent of the governed.
>
> —The Declaration of Independence, paragraphs 2-3 (1776)

The very idea that people have rights that precede and are superior to government is based on the self-evident truths articulated in the Declaration of Independence (Claremont Institute Center for Constitutional Jurisprudence, 2004).

U.S. CONSTITUTION AND BILL OF RIGHTS

The U.S. Constitution and Bill of Rights, along with the Declaration of Independence, are salient expressions of the unique character of American democracy (Rahdert, 2007). When the U.S. Constitution was sent to the states for ratification, several states insisted a Bill of Rights be added, but no such bill could list all of the rights intended to be protected. The failure to do so, however, raised the implication that only the enumerated rights were to be preserved in this emerging democracy. So the Ninth Amendment was ratified, stating unenumerated rights are protected in addition to the rights enumerated and protected in the Bill of Rights.

The Ninth Amendment states individuals have tacit rights, in addition to the rights explicit in the Bill of Rights. The legislative branch was given the authority to enumerate the unenumerated rights by using the power to set forth laws that would bring the rights to fruition through the executive branch and subject to review through the judicial branch. These creative powers are not unique to the Ninth Amendment; for example, the First Amendment's enumerated rights also require the three separate branches of government to balance and protect the rights to freedom of speech, property, and due process of law.

Underlying this separation of powers doctrine regarding enumerated and unenumerated rights is the Constitution's natural rights and common law foundations. When laws become removed from these foundations, the result is often divisive controversies, such as the right to life-sustaining drugs and the right to die debates, and even the right to health care debate itself. Confusion reigns until the balance is restored to its grounding in the consent of the governed.

JUDICIAL BRANCH

In any democracy, there are many sides to the evolving debate over rights. On one side of this ongoing debate is the judicial branch, with judges who sometimes become impatient (often justifiably) with the founding principles of the U.S. Constitution and who use their powers to create rights based on their self-conceptions of evolving social values. On the other side of this debate are judges who go overboard in recognizing only those rights specifically expressed in the Constitution. Both extreme sides of this democratic debate ignore the presumptions at the very foundation of the Constitution (Meyerson, 2008). These are the uniquely American beliefs in:

- Individual freedom
- Independence (limited government)
- Individual autonomy (personal responsibility)
- Liberty (representative democracy)
- Free markets

The Constitution no more authorizes the judicial branch to invent rights than it allows the judiciary to ignore rights meant to be protected when it addresses the most difficult, sometimes divisive, cases that arise. Nevertheless, the law must be ascertained and applied by the bench, rather than invented from behind it (Blackstone & Cooley, 2003). Generally the judicial branch gets it right, even if a case must go through several levels of appeal to arrive at the correct interpretation of the law.

Organization of the Judicial Branch

The judicial branch is divided into trial courts (courts of first instance) and appellate courts. Trial courts function with a judge and a jury. Juries make findings of fact while judges decide conclusions of law (jury trials), or judges make decisions of both fact and law (bench trials).

In the common law system, courts follow the adversarial system. Procedural law governs the rules by which courts operate: civil procedure for private disputes and criminal procedure for violation of criminal laws.

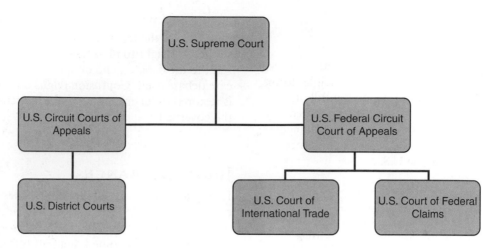

Figure 2-2: Organization of the Federal Court System

Delmar/Cengage Learning

Federal Courts

The federal courts, as illustrated in Figure 2-2, are comprised of:

- U.S. Supreme Court
- U.S. Courts of Appeals
- U.S. District Courts

Every health law case of *first impression* (known as *primae impressionis* in Latin) that has been decided by the U.S. Courts of Appeals within the last three years is summarized in the "Principles and Application" sections of this text. The health law cases decided by the U.S. Supreme Court within the past three years are also examined.

U.S. Supreme Court

Article III, § 1 of the U.S. Constitution provides that the " judicial Power of the United States, shall be vested in one supreme Court, and in such inferior Courts as the Congress may from time to time ordain and establish." The U.S. Supreme Court was created in accordance with this provision in 1790 and is comprised of the Chief Justice and such number of Associate Justices as may be determined by Congress, which in 2009 was eight, for a total of nine Justices (*see* 28 U.S.C.A. § 1 (2008)).

The President nominates the Justices with the advice and consent of the Senate. The term of the U.S. Supreme Court begins on the first Monday in October and lasts until the first Monday in October of the following year. Approximately eight thousand cases are filed with the Court in the course of a term; some one thousand applications are filed each year that can be acted upon by a single Justice (GovM, 2009).

While appellate jurisdiction has been conferred upon the U.S. Supreme Court by Congress, Congress has no authority to change the original jurisdiction of the Court as defined in Article III, § 2 of the U.S. Constitution (*see* 28 U.S.C.A. §§ 1251, 1253-1254, 1257-1259 (2009), and various special statutes). This means that the Supreme Court can only review certain kinds of cases and has no authority to review other kinds, and Congress cannot alter the Supreme Court's authority to hear certain kinds of cases.

U.S. Courts of Appeals

Ninety-four district courts are organized into twelve circuits, each of which has a U.S. Court of Appeals. Courts of appeal hear appeals from the district courts located within its regional circuit, as well as appeals from decisions of federal administrative agencies and the U.S. Tax Court.

Moral Dilemmas

1. Should Americans be concerned about the fact that the average tenure of U.S. Supreme Court Justices has increased to almost thirty years, when every other major court of its kind in the world has rejected life tenure and forty-nine out of fifty states have rejected it for their state supreme courts?

2. Is life tenure for a U.S. Supreme Court Justice a good idea or is it an eighteenth-century anachronism?

In addition, the U.S. Federal Circuit Court of Appeals hears appeals in specialized cases:

- Patent laws (such as disputes between providers of medical products)
- U.S. Court of International Trade (counterfeit medical products)
- U.S. Court of Federal Claims (vaccine injuries)

U.S. District Courts

The U.S. District Courts are the trial courts of the federal court system. Within limits set by Congress and the U.S. Constitution, the district courts hear civil and criminal federal cases.

Bankruptcy courts and the Vaccine Court are separate units of the district courts. Federal courts have exclusive jurisdiction over bankruptcy and vaccine cases, which means bankruptcy and vaccine cases cannot be filed in state courts. The Vaccine Court, with one chief special master and seven associate special masters, hears cases of children injured as a result of compulsory childhood vaccines and, like the bankruptcy courts, was established by Congress to bypass traditional civil tort litigation (*see* National Childhood Vaccine Injury Act of 1986, 42 U.S.C.A. §§ 300aa-2 *et seq.* (2009)). The Court of International Trade and the Court of Federal Claims have nationwide jurisdiction.

State Courts

The organization of each state's judiciary, illustrated in Figure 2-3, is patterned after the federal judicial system. As in the federal courts, every health law case of *first impression* that has been decided by the highest appellate state courts (state supreme courts) within the last three years is summarized in this text.

"The People" and the Judicial Branch

Americans have always been interested in questions related to "the People" and the judicial branch. With hundreds of ballot initiatives in almost every state, initiatives are becoming more a part of American political discourse than ever before, with spending on such polling approaching a half-billion dollars each election year (Perkins, 2007).

What role "the People" retain in the U.S. Constitutional order is not just a theoretical issue; the increasing number of popular referenda and ballot initiatives addressed to American voters has made it a debate with real consequences. The breadth of this debate is not limited to the topic of the right to gay marriage. "The People" may also play a role in deciding health care issues like:

- Abortion rights
- Physician-assisted death
- Right to health care
- Right to end-of-life medical treatments
- Right to medical marijuana
- Rights of adolescents
- Rights of women to the morning-after pill
- Smoking measures

Perhaps more important, the way ordinary Americans choose to live and die gives meaning to health law. Because the American legal system often takes its cue from tradition, it is critical to decide when the judicial branch should defer to customary practice, both when interpreting the U.S. Constitution and when applying legislation and the rules of law that govern most health care decisions in the U.S.

LEGISLATIVE BRANCH

Congress makes the controlling choices in policy debates and establishes the acknowledged standards of law (*see Panama Refining Co. v. Ryan*, 293 U.S. 388, 426 (U.S. Supreme Court 1935)). This principle of legislation is grounded in the notion of "democratic legitimacy" (Barnard, 2003). Democratic legitimacy is the concept, first coined by F. M. Barnard, professor emeritus at the University of Western Ontario, that political accountability is as important to the democratic ethic as political participation. Barnard argues that laws must be tempered by a sense of universal humanity. In a democracy, the people's role does not begin and end in the voting booth when members of Congress are elected to take legislative action on behalf of the public;

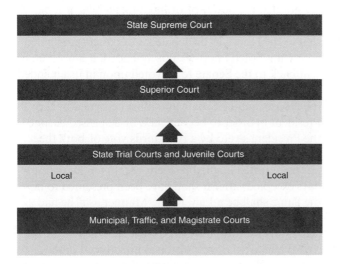

FIGURE 2-3: General Organization of State Court Systems

Delmar/Cengage Learning

legitimacy assumes ongoing public involvement and regular public deliberation regarding issues of national concern. Democratic legitimacy depends on the nature of the congressional debate that precedes decision-making as much as the actual vote to enact legislation. To be legitimate, laws adopted by the legislative branch should comply with well-reasoned and recognized rules and tradition. The legitimacy of laws is challenged, as need be, through the judicial branch.

These democratic principles extend equally to the executive and judicial branches when they execute and apply the laws emanating from the legislative branch. Execution of the legislative laws by the executive branch should be well-reasoned and in compliance with recognized standards. The judicial branch's interpretation of the policy choices made by both the legislative and executive branches should comply with well-reasoned rules that are consistent with the democratic traditions in the U.S. Constitution, which, in turn, reflects the Founders' beliefs in compassion and the universality of the human race (*see* Rehfeld, 2008).

Failure to comply with a health law does not necessarily indicate malicious intent. Compliance with the law is required simply because the legislative branch of government has determined it is the law. The law is the policy choice made by Congress based on what it, as the American people's representative, determines to be in the nation's best interests.

U.S. Congress

Congress was created by Article I, § 1, of the U.S. Constitution, providing that "All legislative Powers herein granted shall be vested in a Congress of the U.S., which shall consist of a Senate and House of Representatives."

The Senate is composed of one hundred Senators, two from each state elected by the people to serve for six-year terms. There are three classes of Senators; a new class is elected every two years. The House of Representatives is comprised of 435 members, a number determined by the population in each state. Representatives are elected by the people for two-year terms, all terms running for the same period.

Officers of Congress

The Vice President of the U.S. is the Presiding Officer of the Senate. The Presiding Officer of the House of Representatives, the Speaker, is elected by the House.

The positions of Senate majority and minority leader were created in the early 1900s and are elected at the beginning of each new Congress by a majority vote of the Senators in their political party. In cooperation with their party organizations, leaders are responsible for managing the flow of legislation. Leaders serve as ex officio members of their respective party's policymaking bodies and are aided by an assistant floor leader, or whip, and a party secretary. The House leadership is structured essentially the same as the Senate (GovM, 2009).

Congressional Committees

The work of preparing and considering legislation is done largely by congressional committees. There are sixteen standing committees in the Senate and nineteen in the House of Representatives. The House Science and Technology Standing Committee and the Senate Health, Education, Labor, and Pensions Standing Committee most affect health care.

In addition, there are select committees and various congressional commissions and joint committees composed of members of Congress. The Senate and House may also appoint special investigating committees. A vote of the entire Senate or House chooses the membership of the standing committees; members of other committees are appointed under provisions of the measure establishing them.

Delegated Enactment of Laws

Congress cannot transfer the power of making laws to any other hands, for it is a delegated power from the people; they who have it cannot pass it over to others (Locke, 2008). This principle is a fundamental democratic concern that significant policy decisions should be grounded in the consent of the governed.

Under the U.S. Constitution, the Senate and House are granted the power of originating all bills. If a bill originates and is approved in the Senate; the bill is then sent to the House to be debated and possibly amended before it is voted upon. If it is amended, it must then be sent back to the Senate to be voted upon in its amended form and vice versa. All bills must be passed by both the House and the Senate and must be signed by the President in order to become law, or be passed despite the President's veto by a two-thirds vote of both the House and Senate. Article I, § 7 states: "If any Bill shall not be returned by the President within ten Days (Sundays excepted) after it shall have been presented to him, the Same shall be a Law, in like Manner as if he had signed it, unless the Congress by their Adjournment prevent its Return, in which Case it shall not be a Law."

When a bill or resolution is introduced in the Senate or House, the usual procedure for its enactment into law is:

• Assignment to the House committee having jurisdiction:

- If favorably considered, it is reported to the House in its original form or with recommended amendments
  - If unfavorably considered, it is reported out or allowed to die in committee without action
- If the bill or resolution is passed by the House, it is messaged to the Senate and then referred to the Senate committee having jurisdiction:
  - In the Senate committee the bill or resolution, if favorably considered, may be reported in the form as received from the House, or with recommended amendments
  - The approved bill or resolution is reported to the Senate, and if passed, is returned to the House
  - Note: This entire procedure is reversed if the bill originates in the Senate. For instance, if a Senate bill is amended and then passed by the House, the amended House bill must be returned the Senate for approval.
- If the Senate or the House does not accept the amendments to a bill by the other body, a conference committee comprised of members of both bodies is usually appointed to effect a compromise
- If the bill or joint resolution is finally approved by both the Senate and the House, it is signed and presented to the President
- Once the President signs the bill or joint resolution, the measure becomes law

(GovM, 2009)

Government Accountability Office

The Government Accountability Office (GAO), established in 1921, is the investigative arm of Congress charged with examining all matters relating to the receipt and disbursement of public funds (*see* 31 U.S.C.A. § 702 (2004)). The GAO is an independent, nonpartisan agency that works for Congress and is often referred to as the congressional watchdog because it investigates how the federal government spends taxpayer dollars (GovM, 2009) (including the $2.3 trillion behind the bailouts in 2008 (Hilsenrath, 2008)).

The GAO gathers information to help Congress determine how effectively the executive branch is doing its job. The GAO's work routinely answers such basic questions as whether government health care programs are meeting their legislative objectives or providing effective service to the public. (GovM, 2009). For instance, the GAO challenged the medical inaccuracies in abstinence-only education programs as violating the Public Health Service Act's requirement that educational materials contain medically accurate information about condom effectiveness. The GAO's report on the thirteen most widely used abstinence-only education-funded curricula revealed eleven contained major errors and distortions of public health

information, including statements that condoms are not effective against HIV and other sexually transmitted diseases (STDs) (GAO, 2006).

The GAO supports congressional oversight by:

- Evaluating how well government policies and programs are working
- Auditing agency operations to determine whether federal funds are being spent efficiently, effectively, and appropriately
- Investigating allegations of illegal and improper activities

(GovM, 2009)

With virtually the entire federal government subject to its review (GovM, 2009), the GAO issues a steady stream of reports and testimonies by its officials. Its reports help Congress better understand newly emerging issues with far-reaching impacts. For instance, the GAO criticized the Office of the National Coordinator for Health Information Technology for its lack of progress on privacy issues and raised a host of concerns about the application of existing federal privacy laws to the emerging National Health Information Network (GAO, 2007).

Congressional Budget Office

The Congressional Budget Office (CBO), established in 1974, provides Congress with economic analyses of fiscal, budgetary, and program policy issues, as well as with information and estimates required for the congressional budget process (*see* 2 U.S.C.A. § 601 (2004)). This enables Congress to have an overview of the federal budget and to make overall decisions regarding spending and taxing levels and the deficit these levels incur.

One of the most controversial activities of CBO is its projection of costs and savings from proposed legislation. Congressional budget rules allow the rate of mandatory spending and tax spending to grow automatically. If the cost of health care grows, spending will automatically grow. Instead of limiting the growth of health care programs, Congress has limited itself in its ability to pass legislation that would increase spending, known as Pay-as-You-Go (PAYGO) (Westmoreland, 2008).

PAYGO restricts Congress to passing only legislation with a net estimated cost of zero, or projected to result in additional revenue for the government. If a new program would increase spending above the current level (a term that, incidentally, has never been defined), Congress would have to either reduce other programs or increase tax revenues. While total government borrowing, in the form of Treasury bonds and notes, could pass $1.5 trillion ($1,500,000,000,000) in the fiscal year ending September 2009 (49 percent of the gross national product), borrowed funds are not an offset for PAYGO. PAYGO estimates the official costs of legislation; a score that is too costly makes new programs harder to pass.

PAYGO assumes that the future effects of programs can be estimated. For instance, if legislation is proposed to make a new health service available under Medicare, the CBO estimates the increased costs of this proposal over the expected year-to-year automatic increases. In doing so, the CBO also offsets increases with any expected decreases. For instance, if legislation would require Medicare coverage for a drug, CBO's scorekeeping would include both the costs of the drug and any offsetting reductions in the need for hospital care (Westmoreland, 2008). There is debate, however, over whether any supposed offset reductions ever materialize.

EXECUTIVE BRANCH

Two issues face the executive branch: its unprecedented growth and its encroachment into the judicial and legislative branches of a federal system established on the principle of separate but equal branches of government.

Expansive Growth and Resultant Long-Term Fiscal Gap

The executive branch faces a long-term fiscal gap. Projected spending as a share of gross domestic product will double from roughly 20 percent to over 40 percent by 2045 (Walker, 2005), driven largely by health care and Social Security entitlements and interest payments. Meanwhile, the federal government continues to expand with social spending and political earmarking. Federal expenditures have increased from $1.8 trillion in 2000 to $2.8 trillion in 2007 ($2,800,000,000,000) (CBO, 2007). In 2008, outlays rose significantly over and above the $2.8 trillion in expenditures for unemployment insurance, food stamps, and other programs meant to be economic stabilizers (Hilsenrath, 2008).

Decline of Separate but Equal Governance

With the growth of the executive branch, agency-promulgated guidelines have become universal in the federal government. There is debate, however, over whether agency guidelines and nonbinding policy statements are resulting in a reduction in the shared but equal doctrine elsewhere in the federal governance system, particularly for the judicial branch. The actual impact of agency guidelines and their voluntary and cooperative enforcement procedures is often unspoken. Often the issuing agencies declare the guidelines to be nonbinding,

even for themselves. Notwithstanding this disclaimer, the health care industry and the judicial branch frequently rely upon agency guidelines in a precedent-like manner. The guidelines often become valued far more than the persuasive power of their ideas. This raises the more general concern as to whether the judicial branch is ceding its role as the check on the executive branch (Greene, 2006).

Such questions regarding the judiciary's role in the separation of powers are broadly analogous to those raised regarding Congress's role in the legislative process. Congress is often criticized for writing nonspecific legislation with delegation that arguably transfers legislative power to the executive and judicial branches (Lowi, 1969).

Moral Dilemmas

1. Should the independent federal regulatory agencies be truly independent and free of executive and legislative branch control?

Federal Departments and Agencies Affecting Health Care

Eleven departments exist in the executive branch they are part of the President's Cabinet and report to the President. The U.S. Department of Health and Human Services (HHS) has the most direct impact on health care particularly the Food and Drug Administration (FDA) and the Centers for Medicare and Medicaid Services (CMS).

U.S. Department of Health and Human Services

Budget:	$698 Billion
Employees:	67,000+

Funding for HHS is greater than all the other federal agencies combined. The size of the HHS departmental budget is also more than double the size of the budget of global retailer Wal-Mart. By comparison and in terms of revenue, HHS is equal to more than seven IBMs.

Created in 1798 as a Cabinet-level department, HHS is comprised of eleven agencies that report to the Secretary of HHS:

• Administration for Children and Families (ACF)
• Administration on Aging (AOA)

- Agency for Healthcare Research and Quality (AHRQ)
- Agency for Toxic Substances and Disease Registry (ATSDR)
- Centers for Disease Control and Prevention (CDC)
- Centers for Medicare and Medicaid Services (CMS)
- Food and Drug Administration (FDA)
- Health Resources and Services Administration (HRSA)
- Indian Health Service (IHS)
- National Institutes of Health (NIH)
- Substance Abuse and Mental Health Services Administration (SAMHSA)

As illustrated in Figure 2-4, seven of the eleven agencies are components of the U.S. Public Health Service: AHRQ, ATSDR, CDC, FDA, HRSA, IHS, and SAMHSA.*

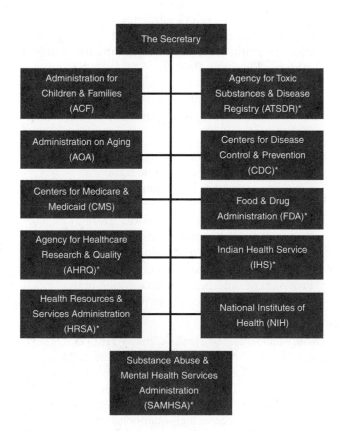

FIGURE 2-4: Organization of the U.S. Department of Health and Human Services

Delmar/Cengage Learning

Administration for Children and Families

Budget:	$46 Billion
Employees:	1,300+

ACF deals primarily with child abuse and neglect, foster care, adoptions, child support, Head Start, developmental disabilities, family assistance (welfare), Native American assistance, refugee resettlement, and legalized aliens (GovM, 2009). ACF also administers faith-based and community initiative programs.

Today, welfare programs are substantially controlled by federal legislation. Every five years, ACF conducts reviews of state programs to ensure they are in conformity with federal requirements; most states are not. At the same time, ACF is criticized for failing to adequately monitor state programs and its inability to sufficiently hold states accountable. Although states may be penalized for non-compliance or failure to comply with federal reporting requirements, a state would only lose a small portion of its federally allotted money for non-compliance. Congressional influence on ACF's oversight process results, without exception, in new promises of future compliance by the non-compliant states but no cut-backs in funding.

Transitions Out of Foster Care   For decades, ACF has met criticism for the nation's lack of oversight of state-administered foster programs. Recent concerns have been directed at how foster youth are generally unable to live independently once they reach eighteen years of age, with some youth resorting to sleeping in hospital emergency rooms (Sapp, 2008). A child welfare issue has evolved into a health care issue.

Sexually Transmitted Diseases in Young Americans   Over the past decade, Congress has allocated over $1 billion in funds into abstinence-until-marriage promotion. ACF also provides $50 million per year to fund responsible fatherhood programs focused on teens and young men. While not a program in and of themselves, virginity pledge programs are another government focus (GAO, 2006; Carbone, 2008).

ACF's Healthy Marriage Initiative has had a firm stance against use of condoms, a position that may be a factor in the increased levels of STDs among youth (GAO, 2004). Specifically, the Centers for Disease Control reports almost half of the nineteen million new STD infections are among young

Americans aged fifteen to twenty-four. One criticism is that the government presents abstinence as a way to prepare for a stable marriage, rather than as a method for reducing risky sexual behavior (Steib, 2008).

Administration on Aging

Budget:	$1.4 Billion
Employees:	100+

AOA helps Americans sixty-five and over to maintain independence in their homes through comprehensive community-based systems of care. This population of forty million comprised about 12 percent of the population in 2008 and is expected to represent 20 percent of the U.S. population by 2030. Three health care issues are of significant importance to the population served by AOA:

- Drug efficacy and the effect of the expanding number of drug withdrawals from the market
- Limited access to and increased non-affordability of basic health care
- Unreported elder abuse and neglect with lack of protective services

In partnership with the National Aging Network (which consists of over fifty state agencies on aging, almost nine hundred area agencies on aging, and twenty-nine thousand service providers), AOA seeks to promote the development of all-inclusive structures encompassing:

- Home health care
- Hospice services
- Long-term nursing care

Access to and Affordability of Basic Health Care   Americans sixty-five and over spend twice as much on health care compared to the rest of the population (AOA, 2005). While most older Americans have Medicare health insurance coverage, recipients must still contribute, and nearly half of all medical care costs come from non-Medicare sources. This places a heavy burden on this population, considering nearly six million Americans over the age of sixty-five are also poor or near poor and have limited access to medical care.

Drug Efficacy and Older Patients   Drugs produced by the pharmaceutical industry have helped to increase the life expectancy of Americans sixty-five and over to eighteen years longer than their predecessors (AOA, 2005). Therefore, as a

significant portion of the U.S. population grows older, the pharmaceutical industry will be placed under greater scrutiny to ensure its drugs are safe, as well as efficacious and affordable for older Americans.

Elder Abuse and Neglect   Between one and two million Americans sixty-five and older have been the victims of some form of abuse. AOA believes the reporting of abuse and neglect is as low as one in fourteen cases, despite mandatory reporting in all fifty states. Systems to address this public health issue do not exist in most communities (Wolfson, 2007).

Agency for Healthcare Research and Quality

Budget:	$325 Billion
Employees:	300+

Since 2005, AHRQ has issued two comprehensive annual reports that address statistical compliance on a range of issues and highlighting how the U.S. could improve the quality, safety, efficiency, and effectiveness of the nation's health care. Those reports are the National Healthcare Quality Report and the National Healthcare Disparity Report.

In addition, health services research to improve the quality of health care and promote evidence-based decision-making is supported by AHRQ, including research on:

- Access to quality health care by minorities and people of lower socioeconomic status
- Emerging standards in national health care information technology
- Patient injuries caused by medical errors
- Payments for the routine costs of clinical trials and treatment of trial-related complications
- Physician compliance with clinical guidelines
- Provision of emergency contraception in the nation's hospital emergency rooms

Quality and Access to Health Care   AHRQ Quality and Disparity Reports measure differences in the availability and use of health care services in various populations. Differences in quality and access to medical care do exist; people of lower socioeconomic status are less likely to receive high-quality health care.

Health Care Information Technology   Though AHRQ increasingly promotes the use of health care information technology, state efforts have driven most government progress. This dual-track regulatory strategy carries significant risks of interstate redundancy and incompatibility. A national policy of state experimentation would mitigate these risks by requiring interstate collaboration and adherence to emerging standards in return (Beaton, 2008).

Emergency Contraception   AHRQ research found the personal beliefs of physicians often supersede the proper care of sexual assault victims (AHRQ, 2003). Although the FDA approved over-the-counter access to emergency contraception for those over age eighteen in the pharmacy setting, few states have enacted explicit emergency contraception laws to require hospital emergency rooms to provide sexual assault victims with information regarding emergency contraception and then to furnish it in the hospital upon request. AHRQ has been clear in advising states that hospital emergency rooms must inform rape survivors of the availability of emergency contraception and provide information on how to access it, even though they may refer the patient to another facility to secure it (Boumil & Sussman, 2008).

Clinical Guidelines   AHRQ Quality and Disparity Reports on the terms of statistical compliance with clinical guidelines have demonstrated that even with clear-cut clinical guidelines, physicians ignore the guidelines more times than not. To improve physician compliance, AHRQ and the Institute of Medicine have recommended the need for a conceptual framework to analyze physician performance (McLean, 2007).

Medical Errors   Official AHRQ estimates of the rate of injuries caused by medical errors suggest American hospitals and health care providers bear some of the responsibility for as many as one hundred thousand deaths each year, a finding consistent with studies by the Institute of Medicine. AHRQ continuously monitors this phenomenon using outcomes research. For instance, AHRQ recently found that two-thirds of the serious injuries and deaths to newborn infants in the delivery room are the result of human error. Once AHRQ makes discoveries like this, national guidelines for common medical procedures are produced to address the problem.

Compliance with applicable guidelines is in turn monitored by the Joint Commission on Accreditation of Healthcare Organizations. Non-compliance could cause a health care provider to lose accreditation, which could provide grounds for insurers to deny payment for medical treatments

provided to patients (including public health programs like Medicare, Medicaid, and SCHIP).

Clinical Trials   Medicare, Medicaid, and SCHIP coverage of the routine costs of qualifying clinical trials, and medically reasonable and necessary services used to diagnose and treat clinical trial-related complications, is inconsistent. AHRQ, CMS, and the FDA are working with the health care industry and patients to resolve this payment issue (Dobbins & Scanlan, 2007).

Agency for Toxic Substances and Disease Registry

Budget:	$75 Billion
Employees:	300+

ATSDR is charged with the prevention of exposure to toxic substances and the prevention of the adverse health effects and diminished quality of life associated with exposure to hazardous substances from waste sites, or landfills, unplanned releases, and other sources of pollution present in the environment (GovM, 2009). Asbestos and lead contaminations are two of the more public areas the Agency works to improve.

Centers for Disease Control and Prevention

Budget:	$8.8 Billion
Employees:	6,900

The CDC is charged with protecting the public health of the nation by providing leadership and direction in the prevention and control of diseases and preventable conditions, and responding to public health emergencies (GovM, 2009). Within the CDC, there is the National Institute for Occupational Safety and Health, as well as six coordinating centers and offices:

- Environmental Health and Injury Prevention
- Global Health
- Health Information and Service
- Health Promotion
- Infectious Diseases
- Terrorism Preparedness and Emergency Response

Health law is a foundational public health tool for disease prevention and health promotion. For many traditional public health problems, both acute and chronic, the role of law has been crucial in attaining public health goals, both framing and complementing the roles of epidemiology and laboratory science. Recently, law has played a fundamental role in the control and prevention of emerging health problems such as the threat of pandemic influenza, food safety, and gun violence. The CDC's Public Health Law Program assists the six coordinating centers and offices to improve their understanding and use of law as a public health tool. CDC law initiatives have been developed in personal health records and retail-based health clinics.

Centers for Medicare and Medicaid Services

| Budget: | $704 Billion |
| Employees: | 4,200 |

Note: There are no reliable estimates of the number of CMS contractors. Estimates are contradictory within the same official publications, both within CMS and by oversight agencies. *See* CMS, 2009.

CMS administers Medicare, Medicaid, SCHIP, and related public health care programs. These programs served over ninety-two million beneficiaries in 2007, or one in three Americans, with 1.2 billion claims, making CMS the nation's largest purchasers of health care services.

Emergency Medicaid　While CMS funds Emergency Medicaid and promulgates policies the states must follow in administration of their own plans, defining emergency care has proven to be a problem (*see* Emergency Treatment Act of 1986, 42 U.S.C.A. § 1395dd (2003)). Several states are funding chemotherapy for immigrants regardless of status and are requesting reimbursement from CMS. This argument over whether chemotherapy should be covered under Emergency Medicaid highlights the government policy of only offering financial assistance for emergencies. Immigrants diagnosed with cancer suffer emergencies as the disease takes its course, but any emergency care given ultimately does little good because necessary follow-up treatment is unavailable.

For instance, CMS advised New York State it will no longer cover the cost of chemotherapy because it does not consider it to be emergency care under Emergency Medicaid. Whether CMS will attempt to recover prior-year funds for chemotherapy for undocumented immigrants by New York is debatable, but New York has pledged to continue funding chemotherapy (Shin, 2006).

Gainsharing Agreements　CMS has solicited hospitals to enter into gainsharing agreements with physicians in order to reduce costs while also improving patient care, authorized by Congress in the Deficit Reduction Act of 2005, 42 U.S.C.A. § 1396 (2009) and 20 U.S.C.A. §§ 1070a-1, 1092e (2009), and the Medicare Prescription Drug, Improvement, and Modernization Act of 2003, 42 U.S.C.A. §§ 299b-7, 1395, 1396 (2009) and 26 U.S.C.A. §§ 139A, 223, 4980G (2009). Under standard gainsharing agreements, hospitals pay physicians a share of any reduction in a hospital's costs attributable to the physicians' cost-saving efforts in providing medical services (Marcoux, 2008).

The merits of this approach are controversial. On one hand, properly structured arrangements could offer opportunities for hospitals to reduce costs without causing inappropriate reductions in medical services or rewarding patient referrals. On the other hand, gainsharing could reduce physician choice of medical devices and diagnostic tests and thus limit access to the most appropriate care (Marcoux, 2008). The medical device and diagnostic industries fear gainsharing might decrease incentives to invest in newer, more expensive technology and treatment procedures (Logarta, 2006). While the U.S. Department of Justice, which enforces health care fraud and abuse laws, will not prosecute gainsharing agreements authorized by CMS (Marcoux, 2008), this conditioned exception could vanish should gainsharing not produce positive results.

Food and Drug Administration

| Budget: | $1.7 Billion |
| Employees: | 10,000+ |

The FDA, the oldest federal regulatory agency in the nation, has garnered more than a century of scientific expertise. Federal concern for drugs started with the establishment of U.S. customs laboratories to administer the Import Drugs Act of 1848 (*see* 9 Stat. 237). The agency's roots date back to 1862, when the Division of Chemistry was created in the newly formed U.S. Department of Agriculture to analyze the food supply and provide advice on agricultural chemistry.

President Theodore Roosevelt signed the federal Pure Food and Drug Act in 1906, creating the FDA (*see* Pure Food and Drug Act of 1906, Pub. L. No. 59-384, § 3, 34 Stat. 768-769 (codified at 21 U.S.C.A. §§ 1-15 (1934) and repealed by 21 U.S.C.A. §392(a) (1938))). This legislation was followed thirty years later by the federal Food, Drug, and Cosmetic Act (FDCA), authorizing the FDA to regulate the manufacture and sale of therapeutic drugs, cosmetics, and food. The FDA was the first federal agency charged with consumer protection (*see* Federal Food, Drug, and Cosmetic Act of 1938, 21 U.S.C.A. §§ 301 *et seq.* (2009)). In the 1950s, the FDA moved away from Agriculture to the federal Security Agency and later to the U.S. Department of Health, Education and Welfare (now the U.S. Department of Health and Human Services), where it remains (*see* 21 U.S.C.A. § 141 (1927) notes).

Incremental Regulation   In the last seventy years, the FDCA has been amended several hundred times to narrow the broad mandates the FDA was originally given. This incremental approach to regulation has resulted in enormously complex ambiguities. Yet, Congress has not engaged in a comprehensive review of the FDCA since 1938, choosing instead to revise it word by word, provision by provision (O'Reilly, 2008). Today, the FDCA has slowly become inconsistent in both its terms and scope, specifically:

- Conflicting enforcement powers are provided for comparable violations
- Different words are used to mean the same thing in different parts of the FDCA
- Inconsistent types of authority are granted with respect to similar matters
- Relationships among all of the provisions in the FDCA are increasingly ambiguous

For instance, the FDA prohibits pharmaceutical companies from promoting the unapproved use of drugs, maintaining this information is detrimental to public health. At the same time, the FDA mandates that pharmaceutical companies provide open access to available data about unapproved uses so medical decision-making can be safer. One policy prohibits the same speech that another policy mandates. Despite these regulatory inconsistencies, the significance of the FDA's role in the U.S. economy continues to increase.

Regulation of a $1.5 Trillion Market   Growth in the medical products and food industries has resulted in the FDA regulating more than one-fourth of the U.S. economy, meaning about $1.5 trillion is regulated by this one agency (*see* GovM, 2009). The FDA is responsible for protecting the public health by ensuring the safety, efficacy, and security of the nation's food supply and seven categories of products:

- Biologicals
- Cosmetics
- Dietary supplements
- Human therapeutic drugs
- Medical devices
- Products that emit radiation
- Veterinary drugs

The FDA plays a significant role in addressing the nation's counterterrorism capabilities and ensuring the security of the food supply (GovM, 2009).

Drug Safety: Premarket Approval Process   Before a new medical product is introduced into the marketplace, the FDA must be provided reasonable assurances that the product is both safe and effective (Hutt, 2007). These assurances may be provided through the FDA's premarket approval (PMA) process. The PMA process permits the FDA to demand the submission of detailed information regarding the safety and effectiveness of the product under review (*see* 21 U.S.C.A. § 360e (2007) (describing the required contents of a premarket approval application)). The FDA then spends substantial time and resources reviewing these applications, with the average submission requiring 1,200 hours of review (over nine months of review time). Ordinarily, the FDA refers the product to an independent panel of experts, which prepares a report and recommendation on whether to approve marketing of the product. The FDA may also advise a company of any measures necessary to put its product in approvable form. Once the FDA determines the required reasonable assurances have been provided, an order is issued permitting product marketing, exactly as approved. Thereafter, changes affecting the safety or effectiveness of the product may not be made to the:

- Approved labeling
- Manufacturing process
- Product design

The FDA may withdraw its marketing approval if any such changes are made without prior approval. The U.S. Court of Appeals for the 11th Circuit provided a summary description of the premarket approval process in *Goodlin v. Medtronic, Inc.*, 167 F.3d 1367, 1369-70 (1999) that has since been cited by federal courts and the U.S. Supreme Court.

Post-Marketing Surveillance   Despite premarket review of medical products, active post-marketing surveillance for adverse effects is essential. Because all possible side effects of a product cannot be anticipated based on pre-approval studies involving only several hundred to several thousand patients, the FDA maintains a system of post-marketing surveillance to identify adverse events that did not appear during the approval process. The FDA monitors adverse events such as reactions and poisonings and uses this information to update labeling, and, on rare occasions, to re-evaluate or revoke product approvals or marketing decisions.

Product Safety and Adverse Event Reporting   The FDA's MedWatch program provides an avenue for health care professionals and the public to voluntarily report serious reactions and problems with medical products. It also ensures that new safety information is rapidly communicated to the health care community. All data contained on the MedWatch form is entered into the Adverse Events Reporting System, a computerized information database of safety reports that supports the FDA's post-marketing safety surveillance program for all approved medical products.

Industry Surveillance   After a product is approved and marketed, FDA field investigators and analysts conduct unannounced inspections of drug production and control facilities to assure:

- Companies adhere to the terms and conditions of approval described in the application
- The drug or product is manufactured in a consistent and controlled manner

Product Errors   Drug manufacturers are required by regulation to submit adverse event reports to the FDA. The MedWatch Web site provides information on mandatory reporting by manufacturers. In addition, manufacturers must submit either error and accident reports or drug quality reports when deviation from current good manufacturing practice regulations occurs.

The FDA receives error reports on marketed human drugs (including prescription drugs, generic drugs, and over-the-counter drugs) and non-vaccine biological products and devices. An error is defined as any preventable event that may cause or lead to inappropriate product use or patient harm. Such events may be related to professional practice or the medical products (including prescribing, product labeling, packaging, compounding, dispensing, distribution, administration, education, monitoring, and use).

Medical Product Shortages   It is the FDA's policy to attempt to prevent or alleviate shortages of medically necessary products. Medical product shortages may arise from varying causes, such as the unavailability of raw materials or packaging components, marketing decisions, and enforcement issues.

Drug Therapeutic Inequivalence Reporting   In the past ten years, the FDA has received an increase in reports of drug products that fail to work in patients

because the drug simply has no effect or is toxic. These problems are usually attributed to switching brands of drugs. As a result, the FDA created the Therapeutic Inequivalence Action Coordinating Committee to identify and evaluate reports of therapeutic failures and toxicity that could indicate that one drug product is not equivalent to another similar product.

Health Resources and Services Administration

Budget:	$6 Billion
Employees:	1,600+

The HRSA works to improve access to health care services through its primary care network of about 1,700 community health centers. The community health centers serve an estimated 16 percent of the nation's population, with more than twenty million people receiving services each year. Community health center services are targeted to those people who are:

- Isolated (people residing in inner cities, underserved, and rural communities)
- Medically vulnerable (pregnant women, people living with HIV/AIDS, people with brain injuries)
- Uninsured

In addition to the community health centers, the HRSA oversees the:

- Database on health care waste, fraud, and abuse
- Health care malpractice database
- National Health Services Corps
- National organ and tissue transplantation system
- Vaccine injury compensation programs

Shortage of Physicians   There is disequilibrium between the supply of physicians and the demand for their services (Iglehart, 2008). While Congress and private interests are again seriously exploring ways to provide health insurance to the uninsured, there is an inadequate number of health care providers to serve all Americans demanding health care. HRSA health centers have a shortage of more than 3,200 primary care providers, with larger shortages in rural and low-income areas, according to the National Association of Community Health Centers. Rural states (such as Nevada, Alabama, and Oklahoma) have the largest shortages. In addition, fifty-six million Americans do not have a regular source of health care because of physician shortages in their communities. This means that even if universal health care came into play tomorrow, not everyone would have access to health care providers without action to address physician shortages.

Diversity, Minority Health, and Health Disparities
The HRSA has a congressional mandate to seek to improve the diversity of the U.S. health care work-force and encourage the placement of health care professionals in communities where health care is scarce. There is also a separate National Center on Minority Health and Health Disparities within HHS with the mandate to develop NIH-wide policy issues related to research on health disparities (GovM, 2009).

While not all health disparities result from lack of diversity in the providers delivering health care, research on access to care would appear to demand a coordinated response to interrelated health care issues (Noah, 2008). Debate centers on whether a more effective response might be met by one government agency with the mandate to develop collaborative policies and one national program.

Indian Health Service

Budget:	$3.3 Billion
Employees:	19,800+

The Indian Health Service, a component of the U.S. Public Health Service, provides health services to American Indians and Alaskan Natives in almost six hundred registered tribal governments. It assists Native American tribes in developing their health programs and assists tribes in coordinating health planning and using available public health resources (GovM, 2009). The service also provides hospital and ambulatory medical care, rehabilitative services, and development of community sanitation facilities.

National Institutes of Health

Budget:	$28 Billion
Employees:	16,000+

NIH supports biomedical and behavioral research domestically and abroad, conducts research in its own laboratories and clinics, trains research scientists, and distributes public health information. Most of the NIH's funding is awarded through almost 50,000 competitive grants to more than 325,000 researchers at over 3,000 universities, medical schools, and other research institutions in every state and around the world. There are twenty-seven NIH institutes and centers, including eighteen National Institutes on:

- Aging
- Alcohol Abuse and Alcoholism
- Allergy and Infectious Diseases
- Arthritis and Musculoskeletal and Skin Diseases
- Biomedical Imaging and Bioengineering
- Child Health and Human Development
- Deafness and Other Communication Disorders
- Dental and Craniofacial Diseases
- Diabetes and Digestive and Kidney Diseases
- Drug Abuse
- Environmental Health Sciences
- Eye (Ophthalmological Diseases)
- General Medical Sciences
- Heart, Lung, and Blood Diseases
- Human Genome Research
- Mental Health
- Neurological Disorders and Strokes
- Nursing Research

Library of Medicine   The Library of Medicine serves as the nation's chief medical information source and provides medical library services and online bibliographic search capabilities, such as MEDLINE and TOXLINE (GovM, 2009).

Cancer Information Service   NIH coordinates the National Cancer Program, which conducts and supports research, training, and public education with respect to the cause, diagnosis, prevention, and treatment of cancer.

NIH Clinical Center   The NIH Clinical Center is the clinical research hospital for NIH. Through clinical research, physician-investigators translate laboratory discoveries into better treatments, therapies, and interventions. The Center conducts both clinical and laboratory research.

More than 350,000 patients have participated in clinical research studies since the Center opened in 1953. About 1,300 clinical research studies are currently in progress (GovM, 2009).

Center for Complementary and Alternative Medicine
This Center explores complementary and alternative healing practices in the context of rigorous

science, educating and training complementary and alternative medicine researchers, and disseminating authoritative information to the public and professionals. Through its programs, it seeks to facilitate the integration of safe and effective complementary and alternative practices into conventional medicine (GovM, 2009).

National Center for Research Resources   This Center provides laboratory scientists and clinical investigators with the resources, tools, and training necessary to understand, detect, treat, and prevent a wide range of diseases. With this support, scientists engage in basic laboratory research, translate these findings to animal-based studies, and apply them to patient-oriented research. Through its many collaborations, it supports all aspects of basic research, connecting researchers, patients, and communities across the nation.

Center for Scientific Review   The Center for Scientific Review (CSR) organizes the peer review groups that evaluate the majority of grant applications submitted to NIH. These groups include experienced researchers from across the country and abroad. Since 1946, CSR has ensured that NIH grant applications receive fair, independent, expert, and timely reviews free from inappropriate influences, so NIH can fund the most promising research. CSR also receives all incoming applications and assigns them to the NIH's institutes and centers that fund grants (GovM, 2009).

Substance Abuse and Mental Health Services Administration

Budget:	$3.2 Billion
Employees:	500+

SAMHSA funds and administers grant programs and contracts for a range of substance abuse treatment and mental health services, addressing such issues as suicide prevention and homelessness (GovM, 2009).

Internal Revenue Service within the U.S. Department of Treasury

Budget:	$11.7 Million
Employees:	100,000+

U.S. tax laws have a significant effect on the health care industry, affecting the payment for and delivery of health care. Established in 1862 as part of the U.S. Department of Treasury, the Internal Revenue Service

(IRS) has the authority to collect the proper amount of tax revenue (*see* 26 U.S.C.A. § 7802 (2000)).

The IRS administers and enforces the internal revenue laws and related laws with responsibility for:

- Determining, assessing, and collecting internal revenue taxes (individual income, social insurance, retirement, corporate income, excise, estate, and gift taxes)
- Operation of tax-exempt bonds (state and municipal governments and 501(c)(3) tax-exempt charitable organizations)
- Pension plan qualifications
- Status of tax-exempt organizations (health care system foundations and hospitals)

Many of the provisions in the internal revenue laws and related laws are direct government expenditures but are not included in the federal budget. For this reason, they are termed "tax expenditures." In recent years, tax expenditures have amounted to almost half the federal budget outlays. For instance, employer-paid health insurance benefits are non-taxable income. The federal government is forgoing taxes on health insurance premiums to promote a policy of encouraging employers to provide their workers with health insurance rather than higher salaries and wages. This policy was implemented after World War II in the 1950s when the economy shifted from workers being self-employed or working in family-run farms or businesses to industrial and urban wage-based jobs instead.

Limited Government

The architects of the U.S. Constitution took great care to form a limited government founded on personal responsibility and individual liberty. A fundamental policy issue facing the nation right now is whether the U.S. internal revenue laws promote or undermine these founding principles. When more than $2.5 trillion is collected in tax revenue each year, by over one-hundred thousand government employees, the meaning of "limited" arguably takes on an altogether different connotation.

Moral Dilemmas

1. Do Americans still have a limited government that exists to preserve freedom; for the most part, does this principle still apply to health care?

Social Policy Vehicle

An ongoing debate is whether the U.S. internal revenue laws are an appropriate vehicle for implementing sweeping social policies. If tax fairness is placed ahead of economic progress, will either be achieved? The perennial question is whether the wealthiest class of Americans and corporations should pay higher tax rates to help the poor and middle classes. Congress first received authority to levy taxes on the income of individuals and corporations in 1913, pursuant to the Sixteenth Amendment of the U.S. Constitution. Today, the percentage of tax filers paying no federal taxes has risen from about 18 percent in the 1980s to more than one-third in 2007 (CBO, 2007). The Tax Policy Center estimates that in 2008 nearly 40 percent of filers will have no federal income tax liability. There is serious debate about whether the removal of millions of taxpayers from the federal tax rolls is wise social policy.

Moral Dilemmas

1. Should American health care regulation authority be consolidated into one executive agency, or are there benefits to having multiple agencies involved?

Other Government Entities Affecting Health Care

There are fifty-nine independent federal regulatory agencies and government corporations. In addition, there are an additional fifty-two federal boards, commissions, committees, and councils established by congressional or presidential actions. There are at least four such agencies that significantly impact and regulate the health care industry:

- Consumer Product Safety Commission (CPSC)
- Federal Trade Commission (FTC)
- Pension Benefit Guaranty Corporation (PBGC)
- Medicare Payment Advisory Commission (MedPAC)

Debate about whether any of these government entities are truly independent is ever present. By placing limits on the President's power to appoint and remove heads of the government entities as well as mandating limits on the number of the President's own partisans that can be appointed, Congress has sought to limit presidential control (Devins & Lewis, 2008). Whether this is effective is debatable.

In addition to the preceding fifty-nine government entities, there are at least an additional fifty-two federal boards, commissions, committees, and councils established by congressional or presidential actions. Their functions are not strictly limited to the internal operations of their parent department or agency.

Consumer Product Safety Commission

Budget:	$80 Billion
Employees:	444+

The CPSC is an independent federal regulator with three commissioners on the agency's governing board appointed by the President, with the advice and consent of the Senate, who serve for terms of seven years. The Commission was established by the Consumer Product Safety Act of 1974, 15 U.S.C.A. §§ 2051-2055a, 2056-2058, 2060-2061, 2063-2089 (2009). With most consumer products imported, notably from China, and few products manufactured in the U.S., the CPSC helps protect the public against unreasonable risks of injury from such products by:

- Banning hazardous consumer products, such as lead-based paint
- Developing uniform safety standards for consumer products and minimizing conflicting state and local regulations
- Evaluating the comparative safety of consumer products
- Investigating product hazards, including product-related deaths, illnesses, and injuries

Through regulation, the CPSC tries to prevent harms before they occur; nevertheless, over twenty-eight thousand deaths and almost thirty-four million injuries are related to consumer products each year (Kelly & Fitzpatrick, 2008). In response to these unsafe conditions, the CPSC is responsible for implementing at least three federal consumer product safety laws passed by Congress regarding:

- Federal hazardous substances
- Flammable fabrics (Flammable Fabrics Act, 15 U.S.C.A. § 1191 (2008))
- Poison prevention packaging (Poison Prevention Packaging Act of 1970, 15 U.S.C.A. § 1471 (1976))

The Commission also monitors the prohibition on transportation of refrigerators without door safety devices under 15 U.S.C.A. § 1211 (1956). Manufacturers and importers are required to report defects in products that could create substantial hazards and take corrective action where appropriate if substantially hazardous consumer products are already in commerce. For instance, the CPSC was involved in managing the 2008 contamination of children's toys from China.

The CPSC also maintains a comprehensive Injury Information Clearinghouse. When harm does occur, frivolous litigation has often been reduced because of the CPSC's frequent resolution of consumer safety matters in which fines are imposed for product defects.

Nanotechnology   Nanotechnology offers the possibility of revolutionizing health care. Though a number of nanotechnology products are already on the market, the major developments are yet to come. Most discussion presents a polarized debate between those seeking rapid development unfettered by excessive regulation and those who advocate a stringent regulatory regime to protect against nanotechnology risks. For the second time in history, there is the opportunity for a federal governance system to develop simultaneously with an emerging technology, the FDA being the first time (Mandel, 2008). The governance model that is emerging for nanotechnology could provide important insights for reforming governance systems in general.[LN1]

> *Moral Dilemmas*
>
> 1. Should nanotechnology be allowed to develop unfettered or should it be strictly regulated?
>
> 2. How should the benefits of private development and public regulation be balanced?

Lead Poisonings   In 1978, the CPSC banned lead pigments in paints in a public health fight to eradicate lead poisoning. However, it was of limited effectiveness for a single, important reason: the CPSC only had the authority to ban future sales of lead pigment. The ban itself could do nothing to eliminate the harm posed from existing lead-based paint. Because of this limitation, today lead-based paint in older homes and lead-contaminated building dust and soil in urban areas are the most frequent sources of lead exposure for young children (Kelly & Fitzpatrick, 2008).

As a result, lead poisoning continues to cause harm nearly thirty years after banning the use of lead pigments. Because of the widespread nature of these harms, secondary prevention programs find poisoned children by screening their blood for lead. The CPSC then works with other government agencies to deal with environmental lead hazards.[LN2]

Federal Trade Commission

Budget:	$240 Billion
Employees:	1,044+

The FTC is the only federal agency with jurisdiction to enhance health care welfare and protect competition in broad sectors of the health care economy by:

- Enforcing laws that prohibit industry practices that are anticompetitive, deceptive, or unfair to health care entities

- Promoting informed choice and public understanding of the competitive process
- Seeking to accomplish its mission without impeding legitimate industry activity

The FTC's principal functions that affect the health care industry include the following:

- Barring interlocking directorates or officers' positions that may restrain competition
- Compelling hospitals and other health care providers to disclose in writing certain cost information, such as the annual percentage rate, before patients enter into credit transactions, as required by the Truth in Lending Act
- Prohibiting the dissemination of false or deceptive advertisements of health care products and services as well as other unfair or deceptive practices
- Promoting competition through the prevention of general trade restraints such as price-fixing agreements, boycotts, illegal combinations of competitors, and other unfair methods of competition
- Proscribing pricing discrimination, exclusive dealing, tying arrangements (where buyers desiring to purchase one product must purchase a second product that they may or may not want), and discrimination among competing health care providers and medical products companies
- Protecting patients with medical debt against circulation of inaccurate or obsolete credit reports and ensuring that credit bureaus, consumer reporting agencies, credit grantors, and bill collectors exercise their responsibilities in a fair and equitable manner
- Safeguarding the privacy of patients' personal information to prevent illegal or unwanted use of health data
- Stopping corporate mergers, acquisitions, or joint ventures that may substantially lessen competition or tend to create an illegal monopoly

(GovM, 2009)

The FTC was established by the Federal Trade Commission Act of 1914, 15 U.S.C.A. §§ 41-58 (2009). It is the only federal agency from which the American Medical Association (AMA) has sought special exemption from jurisdiction. The House passed a bill placing a moratorium on FTC investigations and lawsuits against physicians until Congress expressly approved such activity, but the bill was defeated in the Senate when the FTC challenged the AMA's rules banning physicians from engaging in contract medicine.

Competition in Health Care   One of the two major missions of the FTC is to encourage competition in the delivery of health care. The FTC seeks to prevent unfair practices that undermine competition and attempts to prevent mergers or acquisitions of health care systems if the results would inappropriately lessen competition.

The FTC challenges attempts by independent practice associations, hospital-contracting networks, physician-contracting networks, and preferred provider organizations to impede competition. It also prohibits physicians from discriminating among themselves in terms of price or other services provided and by:

- Denying reimbursement to physicians providing services to HMOs
- Jointly negotiating on behalf of their members with payers in a manner that constitutes unlawful horizontal price-fixing
- Penalizing physicians who accept salaries or payment on other than a fee-for-service basis

(*See generally* DOJ & FTC, 2004)

Health Care Advertising and Marketing   Health care consumer protection is the second of the two main missions of the FTC. The FTC works to:

- Ensure advertising is truthful and not false or misleading
- Prevent hospital and other health care providers from using unlawful practices when granting credit, maintaining credit information, collecting debts, and/or operating credit systems
- Reduce instances of fraudulent, deceptive, or unfair marketing and promotional practices

(DOJ & FTC, 2004)

The FTC initiates investigations in areas of concern to health care consumers, including health and nutrition claims in advertising. The rapid expansion of medical testing, especially the direct-to-consumer advertising of genetic testing, raises questions about the accuracy of such tests and their consequences for even the most educated of health care consumers (Gniady, 2008).

Medicare Advantage and Part D Prescription Drug Plan Compliance Activities   The deceptive sales tactics of private insurers running Medicare Advantage and Part D prescription drug plans (Channick, 2006) victimize Medicare beneficiaries. FTC audits of health-benefit options approved by Medicare, but sold and administered by private insurers, show widespread violations of patients' rights. Since 2006, when private Medicare coverage began, abuse of Medicare beneficiaries has grown as access to needed medications or coverage of medical treatments has been restricted under the private Medicare plans. This problem is not limited to a few rogue insurance agents; rather, insurers provide lucrative incentives to producers who sell the private plans and then fail to supervise their agents (Channick, 2006).

Unfortunately, weak CMS regulations pre-empt stronger state law protections (*see* 42 U.S.C.A. §§ 139w-26(b)(3)-112(g) (Supp. V 2007) (pre-empting all state laws and regulations related to private Medicare plans)). Through systematic review of the marketing of Medicare's private plans, the FTC is obtaining and maintaining compliance with its cease-and-desist orders. All private insurers against whom such orders have been issued are required to file reports with the FTC to substantiate their compliance. In the event compliance is not obtained, or if the order is subsequently violated, civil penalty proceedings may be instituted (Channick, 2006).

Agency Guidelines and Cooperative Procedures   Since the late 1960s, the FTC (like the FDA and CPSC) has relied increasingly on guidelines (Greene, 2006). A debate is ensuing in the health care industry about whether greater transparency is needed in the FTC's use of discretion. In carrying out its congressional directive to prevent unfair methods of competition or unfair or deceptive practices, the FTC makes extensive use of voluntary and cooperative procedures. Through these procedures, the health care industry obtains authoritative guidance and a substantial measure of certainty as to what it may do under the laws administered by the FTC. Guidelines provide the basis for voluntary abandonment of unlawful practices, while failure to comply with the guidelines may result in corrective action by the FTC.

Enforcement Powers   The FTC's law enforcement work falls into two general categories: actions to foster voluntary compliance with the law, and formal administrative or federal court litigation leading to mandatory orders against offenders. Compliance with the law may be obtained through voluntary and cooperative action in response to nonbinding staff advice, formal advisory opinions by the FTC, and/or guides and policy statements delineating legal requirements as to industry practices.

Formal litigation is instituted either by issuing an administrative complaint or by filing a federal district court complaint charging a health care provider or a medical products company with violating one or more of the statutes administered by the FTC. If the charges in an administrative matter are not contested, or if the charges are found to be true after an administrative hearing in a contested case, an order may be issued requiring discontinuance of the unlawful practices.

Investigations   Investigations by the FTC may originate through a complaint by a health care provider, competitor, Congress, or from federal, state, or local government agencies. Also, the FTC itself may initiate an investigation into possible violations of the laws it administers. No formality is required in submitting a complaint. It is the general policy of the FTC not to disclose the identity of the health care provider of any complainant, except as required by law or FTC rules. Upon receipt of a complaint, various criteria are applied in determining whether the particular matter should be investigated. An order issued after an administrative proceeding that requires the respondent to cease and desist or take other corrective action may be appealed. Appeals may go as far as the U.S. Supreme Court.

In addition to, or in lieu of, the administrative proceeding initiated by a formal complaint, the FTC may request a U.S. district court to issue a preliminary or permanent injunction to:

- Halt the use of unfair or deceptive practices
- Prevent an anticompetitive merger or unfair methods of competition
- Stop violations of any statute enforced by the FTC

Recently, the FTC initiated an investigation into children's advertising practices and the link between unhealthy food ads and childhood obesity. The consolidation of generic drug manufacturers is another area of ongoing FTC investigation as generics face a growing pressure to reduce costs. Lastly, the FTC is investigating the entire private equity industry, which may impact the pace of acquisition deals like the Hospital Corporation of America.

Pension Benefit Guaranty Corporation

Budget:	$1.4 Billion
Employees:	800+

Essentially, the PBGC is a federal insurance program to insure the employee defined-benefit pension plans of nearly forty-four million private-sector Americans in about thirty-one thousand plans (*see* Title IV of the Employee Retirement Income Security Act of 1974 (ERISA), 29 U.S.C.A. §§ 1301-1461 (2009); PBGC is subject to the Government Corporation Control Act, 31 U.S.C.A. §§ 9101-9109 (2009) and the Pension Protection Act of 2006, 26 U.S.C.A. §§ 430 *et seq.* (2009) and 29 U.S.C.A. §§ 1082-1085, 1202a (2006)). Defined-benefit plans provide a set benefit amount to retired employees based on such factors as length of service and compensation history. In 2008, PBGC generally limited annual benefits to $51,750 for sixty-five-year-

old retirees, exclusive of health and life insurance benefits. PBGC does not insure retirement plans that are not defined contribution pension plans, such as profit-sharing or 401(k) plans. Pension plans offered by professional service employers, such as physicians, with fewer than twenty-six employees, by church groups or by federal, state, or local governments usually are not insured. PBGC generally takes responsibility for paying retirement benefits to current and future retirees in the health care industry when:

- Health care provider liquidates with an underfunded pension plan
- PBGC ends a pension plan to protect participants and the insurance fund
- Pension plan of a sponsoring health care provider runs out of money
- Provider demonstrates it cannot continue funding a pension plan and stay in business

(PBGC, 2008)

For instance, the PBGC assumed the pension obligations for more than sixteen thousand retirees when the Allegheny Health Education and Research Foundation in Pennsylvania entered bankruptcy proceedings in the late 1990s. The Teamsters pension plans for about 1,600 retirees, who had worked for the Graduate Hospital Systems in Philadelphia, Pennsylvania, when its hospitals were acquired by Allegheny, are also being paid by the PBGC.

PBGC collects insurance premiums from employers that sponsor insured pension plans and receives funds from pension plans it takes over. While all insured pension plans pay premiums according to rates set by Congress, there is debate whether PBGC is in jeopardy of not being able to meet the needs of the growing current and future retirement population of pensioners (Steadman, 2008). Unless the PBGC becomes solvent, the U.S. Treasury, and ultimately taxpayers, will be responsible for a multibillion dollar bailout of this system, unless Congress reduces benefits to workers or raises premiums on employers.

Federal Deficit
PBGC is running a deficit in excess of $23 billion.
                    —2008 Annual Report on Social Security

Medicare Payment Advisory Commission

MedPAC is comprised of a seventeen-member governing board appointed by the U.S. Comptroller General. MedPAC works with the GAO to advise

Congress on payments to private health plans participating in Medicare and providers in Medicare's traditional fee-for-service program. MedPAC is tasked with analyzing access to care, quality of care, and other issues affecting Medicare.

USE OF GOVERNMENTAL POWERS

The American federal government is continually developing new health care programs and expanding its regulation of the health care industry.

However, this evolution has created overlap and excessive complexity in administrative responsibilities and regulatory powers. Further, there is confusion regarding how the federal government should construct health care spending plans that meet long-term objectives, while helping put the economy on a path to budget balance, and are at the same time expedited to the degree possible without causing waste and inefficiency. This will be particularly true should America venture into a national health care system.

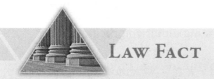

LAW FACT

COMPREHENSIVE HEALTH CARE REFORM

Should the U.S. health care system overhaul be passed through Congress's budget reconciliation process?

The Supremacy Clause of the U.S. Constitution is a powerful protection of the American principle of federalism because it allows federal action only if the precise procedures for lawmaking are followed (Clark, 2001). Budget reconciliation eliminates and lessens some of the major hurdles to enacting comprehensive federal legislation. Omnibus budget reconciliation acts, which typically include changes to revenue laws and entitlement programs, cannot be filibustered in the Senate (GAO, 2007); instead, a reconciliation bill is considered under rules that limit debate and allow passage by a simple majority (Wawro & Schickler, 2007). While budget reconciliation bills still must meet the constitutional requirements of bicameralism and presentment to the President for enactment, congressional passage is more likely because it eliminates internal impediments of the minority (Garrett, 2008).

—2 U.S.C.A. §§ 601-688, 900-907d (2009) (primary governing laws for the federal budget process).

CHAPTER SUMMARY

- American health care law has evolved out of the interpretation and application by the judicial, legislative, and executive branches of government of the fundamental principles contained in the country's founding documents: the Declaration of Independence, the U.S. Constitution, and the Bill of Rights.
- The separation of governmental powers is central to the U.S. Constitution.
- Americans have rights beyond those enumerated in the founding documents; this is based on the notions that it would be impossible to set forth every possible right and that some rights supersede the state.
- It is the province and duty of the judicial branch to interpret and apply the laws enacted by the legislative branch; the judiciary sometimes struggles to say what the law is, not what it should be.
- The U.S. Supreme Court is the highest American court, but it may only hear certain kinds of cases.
- "The People" are attempting to increase their influence upon American government, particularly through ballot initiatives.
- The legislative branch consists of Congress, which is comprised of the U.S. Senate and House of Representatives, who jointly draft and enact legislation.
- The Government Accountability and Congressional Budget Offices help to advise Congress and provide oversight and guidance.
- The executive branch is comprised of the President and various government agencies that administer and enforce legislation; two historic priorities have been to address health care fraud and drug safety issues.

- The U.S. Department of Health and Human Services has a pervasive influence on the American health care industry; its budget is greater than all of the other federal agencies combined.
- The nine Department of Health and Human Services agencies that significantly impact the American health care industry are the Administration for Children and Families, Administration on Aging, Agency for Healthcare Research and Quality, Centers for Medicare and Medicaid Services, Food and Drug Administration, Health Resources and Services Administration, National Institutes of Health, Public Health Service, and Substance Abuse and Mental Health Services Administration.
- The Food and Drug Administration regulates approximately one-fourth of the U.S. economy by ensuring the safety and efficacy of food, cosmetics, dietary supplements, therapeutic drugs, medical devices, radioactive products, and veterinary drugs.
- Beyond the Department of Health and Human Services, U.S. tax laws also influence how American health care is paid for and delivered.
- Nanotechnology provides the first opportunity since the formation of the Food and Drug Administration for governance to develop simultaneously with emerging technology.
- The Federal Trade Commission protects American health care by preventing unfair competition and deceptive business practices and protecting consumers.
- The Food and Drug Administration further protects Americans by requiring medical products manufacturers to prove that their products are safe and effective prior to marketing.

LAW NOTES

1. An example of the federal government's participation in emerging technology is the National Science and Technology Council, a federal council established by the Congressional Nanoscience, Engineering and Technology Subcommittees to regulate the industry. In addition, to CPSC's involvement, ten of the eleven cabinet departments and five independent regulatory agencies take part in regulating nanotechnology, in addition to the intelligence community:
   - U.S. Department of Agriculture
   - U.S. Department of Commerce:
     - Bureau of Industry and Security
     - Commerce and Technology Administration
     - National Institute of Standards and Technology
     - Patent and Trademark Office
   - U.S. Department of Defense
   - U.S. Department of Energy
   - HHS:
     - FDA
     - NIH
   - U.S. Department of Homeland Security
   - U.S. Department of Justice
   - U.S. Department of State
   - U.S. Department of the Treasury
   - U.S. Department of Transportation
   - Environmental Protection Agency
   - National Aeronautics and Space Administration
   - National Science Foundation
   - Nuclear Regulatory Commission
2. Other countries banned lead pigments for use in paints decades before the U.S. did. Outside the U.S., the dangers represented by lead pigments, in particular the application of white lead for interior painting along with the manufacturing, led many countries to enact bans on its use for interior paint: France, Belgium, and Austria in 1909; Tunisia and Greece in 1922; Czechoslovakia in 1924; Great Britain, Sweden, and Belgium in 1926; Poland in 1927; Spain and Yugoslavia in 1931; and Cuba in 1934 (Markowitz & Rosner, 2002).

CHAPTER BIBLIOGRAPHY

AHRQ (Agency for Healthcare Research & Quality). (2003). *Report to Congress: Medical examination and treatment for victims of sexual assault. Evidence-based clinical practice and provider training.* Rockville, MD: U.S. Department of Health & Human Services, AHRQ.

AMA (American Medical Association). (2007). *Health court principles.* Washington, DC: AMA.

AOA (Administration on the Aging). (2005). *Profile of older Americans.* Washington, DC: AOA.

Barnard, F. M. (2003). *Democratic legitimacy: Plural values and political power.* Montreal, Canada: McGill-Queen's University Press.

Beaton, B. J. (2008). Walking the federalist tightrope: A national policy of state experimentation for health information technology. *Columbia Law Review, 108,* 1670-1717.

Blackstone, W., & Cooley, T. M. (2003). *Blackstone's commentaries on the laws of England* (3rd rev. ed.). Clark, NJ: Lawbook Exchange.

Boumil, M. M., & Sussman, D. (2008). Emergency contraception: Law, policy and practice. *Connecticut Public Interest Law Journal, 7,* 157-188.

Carbone, J. (2008). Age matters: Class, family formation, and inequality. *Santa Clara Law Review, 48,* 901-958.

CBO (Congressional Budget Office). (2007). *The budget and economic outlook: An update.* Washington, DC: CBO.

Channick, S. A. (2006). The Medicare Prescription Drug, Improvement, and Modernization Act of 2003: Will it be good medicine for U.S. health policy? *Elder Law Journal, 14,* 241-245 (critiquing privatization).

Claremont Institute Center for Constitutional Jurisprudence. (2004). Brief of Amicus Curiae at 19, *Elk Grove Unified Sch. Dist. v. Newdow,* 542 U.S. 1 (U.S. Supreme Court 2004).

Clark, B. R. (2001). Separation of powers as a safeguard of federalism. *Texas Law Review, 79,* 1321-1459.

CMS (Centers for Medicare & Medicaid Services). (2009). *Justification of estimates for appropriations committees.* Washington, DC: U.S. Department of Health & Human Services, CMS.

___. (2007). *MMIS* (Medicaid Management Information System) *fiscal agent contract status report.* Washington, DC: U.S. Department of Health & Human Services, CMS.

Corrigan, J. M., et al. (2002). *Fostering rapid advances in health care: Learning from system demonstrations.* Washington, DC: Institute of Medicine.

Council of Economic Advisors. (2005). *Economic report of the President.* Washington, DC: Executive Office of the President.

Devins, N., & Lewis, D. E. (2008). Not-so independent agencies: Party polarization and the limits of institutional design. *Boston University Law Review, 88,* 459-498.

Dobbins, K., & Scanlan, K. (2007). Medicare's revised clinical trial policy and clinical trial-related provisions of FDAA (Food & Drug Administration Amendments of 2007): What is a sponsor to do? *Food & Drug Law Journal, 62,* 695-708.

DOJ & FTC (U.S. Department of Justice & Federal Trade Commission). (2004). *Improving health care: A dose of competition.* Washington, DC: DOJ & FTC.

GAO (General Accountability Office). (2007). *Health information technology: Early efforts initiated but comprehensive privacy approach needed for national strategy.* Washington, DC: GAO.

___. (2006). *Abstinence education: Efforts to assess the accuracy and effectiveness of federally-funded programs.* Washington, DC: GAO.

___. (2004). *Foster youth: HHS actions could improve coordination of services and monitoring of states' independent living programs.* Washington, DC: GAO.

Garrett, E. (2008). Symposium on separation of powers as a safeguard of federalism: Framework legislation and federalism. *Notre Dame Law Review, 83,* 1495-1539.

Gniady, J. A. (2008). Regulating direct-to-consumer genetic testing: Protecting the consumer without quashing a medical revolution. *Fordham Law Review, 76,* 2429-2475.

GovM (U.S. Government Manual). (2009). Washington, DC: Government Printing Office (official handbook of the federal government).

Greene, H. (2006). Guideline institutionalization: The role of merger guidelines in antitrust discourse. *William & Mary Law Review, 48* (3), 771-857.

Hazaray, N. F. (2007). Do the benefits outweigh the risks? The legal, business, and ethical ramifications of pulling a blockbuster drug off the market. *Indiana Health Law Review, 4,* 115-149.

Hilsenrath, J. (2008, December 13-14). The big numbers behind the bailouts. *Wall Street Journal,* p. A3.

Hutt, P. B. (2007). *FDA science and mission at risk: Report of the Subcommittee on Science & Technology.* Rockville, MD: FDA Science Board.

Iglehart, J. K. (2008). Grassroots activism and the pursuit of an expanded physician supply. *New England Journal of Medicine, 358,* 1742-1749.

Kaiser (Kaiser Family Foundation). (2008, November). *Kaiser Daily Health Policy Report: Medicaid paid nearly $198M for more than 100 unapproved drugs from 2004-2007.* Washington, DC: Kaiser.

___. (2008a, August). *Kaiser Daily Health Policy Report: Coverage and Access: U.S. faces serious shortage of primary care physicians, especially in low-income, rural communities, according to National Association of Community Health Centers.* Washington, DC: Kaiser.

Kelly, N. F. X., & Fitzpatrick, F. L. (2008). Access to justice: The use of contingent fee arrangements by public officials to vindicate public rights. *Cardozo Journal of Law & Gender, 13,* 759-781.

King, M. (2007). *Immigrants in the U.S. health care system, five myths that misinform the American public.* Washington, DC: Center for American Progress.

Locke, J. (2008). *The second treatise of civil government.* Scotts Valley, CA: CreateSpace.

Logarta, C. (2006). Provider response to cost containment: Fraud and abuse issues. *Annals of Health Law, 15,* 373-385.

Lowi, T. J. (1969). *The end of liberalism: Ideology, policy and the crisis of public authority.* New York, NY: W. W. Norton.

Mandel, G. (2008). Nanotechnology governance. *Alabama Law Review, 59,* 1323-1384.

Marcoux, V. M. (2008). Why healthcare fraud and abuse laws should allow appropriate hospital gainsharing. *Alabama Law Review, 59,* 539-559.

Markowitz, G., & Rosner, D. (2002). *Deceit and denial: The deadly politics of industrial pollution.* Berkeley, CA: University of California Press (recounting the manufacture, promotion, and sales along with the knowledge of the resulting childhood lead poisoning from lead pigments).

McLean, T. R. (2007). Telemedicine and the commoditization of medical services. *DePaul Journal of Health Care Law, 10,* 133-189.

Meyerson, M. I. (2008). *Liberty's blueprint: How Madison and Hamilton wrote the federalist papers, defined the Constitution, and made democracy safe for the world.* New York, NY: Basic Books.

Nation, G. A. (2008). Respondeat manufacturer: Imposing vicarious liability on manufacturers of criminal products. *Baylor Law Review, 60,* 155-228.

Noah, B. A. (2008). Prescription for racial equality in medicine. *Connecticut Law Review, 40,* 675-721.

O'Reilly, J. T. (2008). Losing deference in FDA's second century: Judicial review, politics, and a diminished legacy of expertise. *Cornell Law Review, 93,* 939-979 (describing the historical reputation of the FDA).

PBGC (Pension Benefit Guaranty Corporation). (2008). *Pension guarantees fact sheet.* Washington, DC: PBGC.

Perkins, R. E. (2007). A state guide to regulating ballot initiatives: Reevaluating constitutional analysis eight years after *Buckley v. American Constitutional Law Foundation. Michigan State Law Review, 2007,* 723-752.

Peters, P. G. (2008). Health courts? *Boston University Law Review, 88,* 227-287.

Rahdert, R. C. (2007). Comparative constitutional advocacy. *American University Law Review, 55,* 590, 553-665.

Rehfeld, A. (2008). *The concept of constituency: Political representation, democratic legitimacy, and institutional design.* New York, NY: Cambridge University Press.

Roberts, D. E. (2006). Legal constraints on the use of race in biomedical research: Toward a social justice framework. *Journal of Law, Medicine & Ethics, 34,* 526-533.

Sapp, J. (2008). Aging out of foster care: Enforcing the independent living program through contract liability. *Cardozo Law Review, 29,* 2861-2895.

Shin, H. J. (2006). All children are not created equal: PRWORA's (Personal Responsibility and Work Reconciliation Act) unconstitutional restriction on immigrant children's access to federal health care programs. *Family Court Review, 44 (3),* 484-497.

SSA (Social Security Administration). (2008). *Justification of estimates for appropriations committees.* Washington, DC: SSA.

Steadman, T. A. (2008). Fighting windfalls: The PBGC's battle for workers' pension benefits (and its own financial health). *Arkansas Law Review, 61,* 509-528.

Steib, D. (2008). Can "family values" lift Americans out of poverty? *Georgetown Journal of Gender & Law, 9,* 447-475.

Walker, D. M. (2005, February). Comptroller General of the U.S., GAO, at the Lecture: *Saving our future requires tough choices today,* at the Heritage Foundation, Washington, DC.

Wawro, G. J., & Schickler, E. (2007). *Filibuster: Obstruction and lawmaking in the U.S. Senate (Princeton studies in American politics).* Princeton, NJ: Princeton University Press.

Weinstein, J. B. (2007, November 28). U.S. District Judge, Eastern District of New York, at the 58th Annual Benjamin N. Cardozo Lecture: *The role of judges in a government of, for and by the people,* at New York City Bar Association, New York, NY.

Westmoreland, T. (2008). Health regulation and governance: Can we get there from here? Universal health insurance and the congressional budget process. *Georgetown Law Journal, 96,* 523-538.

Wolfson. S. A. (2007). AMA: National Advisory Council on Violence and Abuse: Screening for violence and abuse through the lens of medical ethics. *DePaul Journal of Health Care Law, 11,* 1-26.

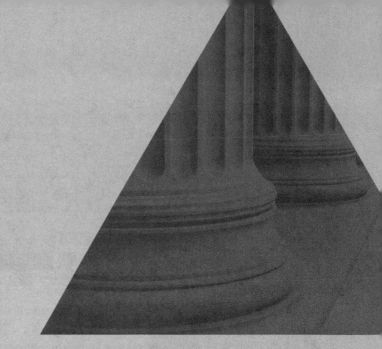

PART II

OVERVIEW OF SPECIFIC HEALTH LAWS

CHAPTER 3

HEALTH CARE COMPLIANCE PROGRAMS

> *"The greater the number of laws and enactments, the more thieves and robbers there will be."*
>
> —LAO-TZU (B.C.), CHINESE PHILOSOPHER

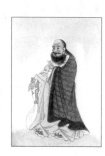

IN BRIEF

This chapter focuses on the prevention of health care fraud. Criminal and civil enforcement issues are reviewed within the framework of compliance and risk management in the health industry. A detailed overview of compliance regulations and safe harbors, designed to regulate health care costs through fraud prevention, is provided.

This is the only topic in this textbook where an appreciation of specific policy regulations is essential to understanding the political and ideological agendas dictating the direction and enforcement of health care activities. While expert legal advice is necessary to interpret conflicting compliance regulations, a simple awareness of the complexity of health care fraud in today's marketplace is the goal of this chapter. The regulations outlined in this chapter encompass reimbursement rules and standards of business conduct that each health industry segment is obliged to follow simply because it is the law for the health industry. Not all the compliance regulations necessarily address any inherently wrongful acts; most regulated activity considered fraudulent and abusive in health care is standard business practice and legal in other industries.

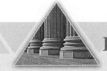

FACT OR FICTION

GOVERNMENT REIMBURSEMENT SYSTEMS

When does the use of regulatory loopholes constitute health care fraud?

Since nearly everyone agrees spending on health care is out of control, preventing obvious health care fraud should be rudimentary. Evidently not: Congress and state governors are resisting attempts to rein in a widely acknowledged abuse.

Medicaid and the State Children's Health Insurance Program (SCHIP), the open-ended government programs that provide health coverage for about fifty-nine million Americans, have expanded their enrollments annually. States determine eligibility and what services to cover; the federal government matches at least half the program costs. States exploit the ambiguities and loopholes in Medicaid and SCHIP reimbursement regulations to maximize their take of the federal coffers. By effectively controlling reimbursement arrangements, federal payouts are maximized and state health care costs are shifted onto taxpayers nationwide. Effective federal matching rates run as high as 83 percent for some states.

The government reimbursement systems often work as illustrated in Figure 3-1. States overpay providers, such as hospitals or nursing homes, for Medicaid and SCHIP benefits in excess of the conventional rates. Then the federal government reimburses the states for half of the inflated claims. Once the states receive the federal matching funds, providers are required to rebate the extra funds they received at the outset of these schemes. Cash thus makes a roundtrip from states to providers and back to the states, all to increase federal funding.

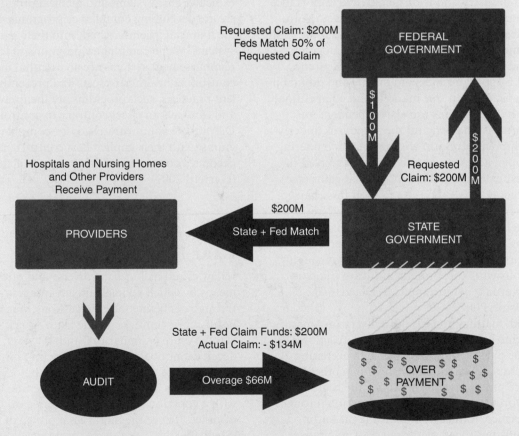

FIGURE 3-1: Government Reimbursement System

Delmar/Cengage Learning

(continues)

(continued)

The Government Accountability Office and other federal inspectors have abundantly documented these creative financing plans since the 1990s. For instance:

- Michigan and New York deposited their reconciliation proceeds in Medicaid accounts, recycling federal funds to decrease their overall state contributions
- Pennsylvania and Wisconsin expanded their state health care funding priorities to increase the amount of matching federal funds needed
- Oregon funded K-12 education using health care reimbursements during a state budget shortfall

A whole industry of lucrative contingent-fee consultants has arisen to assist states and the health industry to maximize their reimbursement systems and comply with government regulations. In this cat-and-mouse game, the federal government notices regulatory loopholes whenever they become too expensive and closes them. Other reimbursement cycles then start all over again.

—Zhang, 2008; Zhang, 2008a; Zhang, 2008b; GAO, 2006; GAO, 2005.
(See *Law Fact* at the end of this chapter for the answer.)

PRINCIPLES AND APPLICATIONS

The establishment of good governance is crucial for the health industry and is of heightened importance for hospitals and the medical products sectors. In the broadest sense, U.S. health care systems are built on the same foundation as American democracy: checks and balances, openness, and transparency. Sustained by good business judgments and profitability, and dependent on free markets and competition, U.S. health care systems are also dependent on medical professionalism and the standards underlying the Hippocratic Oath, with providers rendering fair and open access to health care, not swayed to the greatest extent possible by financial gains (*see* Harshbarger & Jois, 2007). As used in this chapter, whether an individual has perpetrated fraud within the health industry or the health care entities themselves are acting fraudulently, the term *provider* seems appropriate. Fraud by individuals is roughly synonymous with corporate health care fraud as defined internally within the U.S. Department of Justice (Ostas, 2007).

Indeed, malfunctions in the delivery of American medicine have usually involved a dereliction of duty on the part of those charged with exercising independent medical judgments. Among other things, compliance programs simply call for the health industry to perform its traditional role of reason through modern science. Rather than focusing on shifting strategies to stay ahead of the curve of reimbursement regulations, the health industry needs to center its attention on maintaining uncompromising commitment to scientific leadership and innovation in patient care and medical research.

Recognizing this new reality, increasing numbers of health care systems and medical products providers are developing compliance programs to regulate the financial incentives built into their reimbursement systems. While compliance programs to regulate reimbursement systems are an essential means of controlling health care costs and preventing fraudulent practices, such programs are themselves costly, and can have an effect contrary to controlling costs. Despite the administrative costs, compliance programs (with their implicit cost control agendas) could become a common health care trend of the future (Garrett, 2007).

DEFINITION OF HEALTH CARE FRAUD AND ABUSE

In law, fraud includes the diverse and often ingenious means by which people gain advantages over others through deliberate false suggestions, concealments, or misrepresentations of the truth (Black's Law, 2009). Abuse is similar to fraud; however, intent or deceit cannot be established (Black's Law, 2009). For simplicity, this chapter will refer only to fraud. In ethical terms, fraud combines deliberate deception with a conscious willingness to disregard the trust of others, hence the moral disapproval of such acts (Shell, 2006).

It is a mistake, however, to think of health care fraud only in terms perpetrators drawn to the trillion-dollar health industry to obtain easy cash. This category of fraud is indisputably the legitimate focus of government attention, but not the concern of this chapter on health care compliance programs. In reality, the boundaries between criminals and sophisticated criminal enterprises and those providers and complex health care ventures that respond improperly to the financial incentives built into legitimate reimbursement systems are sometimes far from clear. What actually constitutes health care fraud is unclear.

SCOPE OF HEALTH CARE FRAUD

The Centers for Medicare and Medicaid Services predict U.S. health care spending will reach $4.3 trillion by 2016 (CMS, 2008). Estimates are that at least 3 percent to roughly 10 percent of the total health care reimbursements are fraudulent (FBI, 2008; NHCAA, 2008). As illustrated in Figure 3-2, the National Health Care Anti-Fraud Association places a $13 billion annual price tag on health care fraud, while the Federal Bureau of Investigation, the Association of Certified Fraud Examiners, and the Blue Cross Blue Shield Association places the tag at about $43 to $57 billion.[LN1] The huge difference in cost estimates highlights the complexity of this health care issue.

The federal government, as the leading source of reimbursement for health care services, has focused on detecting health care fraud. The size of the Medicare program alone makes it vulnerable to health care fraud. Medicare spent approximately $400 billion in 2007 on more than forty-three million beneficiaries, and processed about 1.1 billion claims a year—on average, about twenty-five claims for every beneficiary in the U.S. (Zhang, 2008a; cf., Zhang, 2008 and 2008b).

FINANCIAL INCENTIVES

Providers certified to receive reimbursements under government programs (Medicare, Medicaid, and SCHIP) are the most likely targets for health care fraud investigations, including:

- Assisted living facilities
- Competitive medical plans (*CMPs* are insurance plans that pay providers on a fee-for-service basis for services)
- Durable medical equipment providers
- Health clinics
- Health maintenance organizations (*HMOs* are capitated managed care plans that pay providers a set amount per member per month for health care services)
- Hospitals
- Medical laboratories

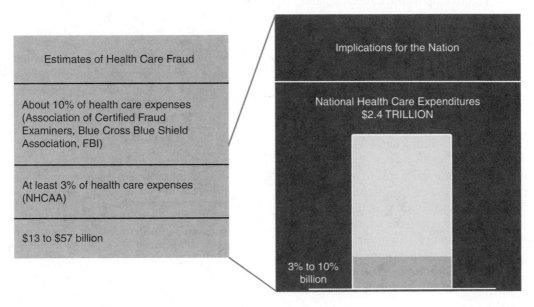

FIGURE 3-2: Fraud Risk Overview

Delmar/Cengage Learning

Data retreived from: Association of Certified Fraud Examiners (2009); Blue Cross Blue Shield Association (2009); Centers for Medicare and Medicaid Services, Office of the Actuary, National Health Statistics Group (2009); FBI (2008); NHCAA (2008)

- Nursing and rehabilitation centers
- Physicians and physician practice groups
- Prepaid health plans (*PHPs* are managed care plans that only cover specified health care services and medical products in return for prepaid premiums; similar to a capitated health maintenance organization)
- Providers of medical products

Moral Dilemmas

1. Should health care costs be regulated through anti-fraud enforcements?

Providers that deliver health care in a fraudulent or abusive manner can be subject to federal laws specifically targeting health care fraud:

- Anti-Kickback Prohibitions
- Health Insurance Portability and Accountability Act (HIPAA)
- False Claims Act (FCA)
- Self-Referral Limitations (Stark Amendments)

With this strong regulatory baseline, some would say the government is seeking to provide an ethical culture of financial incentives for the health industry. Up to now, U.S. health care markets, if left entirely to their own devices, often create precisely the wrong financial incentives in their economic relationships (Harshbarger & Jois, 2007), thus the need for government intervention to stop health care fraud and abusive practices.

Anti-Kickback Prohibitions

Criminal investigations often arise from kickback violations (*see* 42 U.S.C.A. § 1320a-7b(b) (2006)). Providers are prohibited from knowingly and willfully paying or receiving any payment in exchange for prescribing, purchasing, or recommending any health care services for which reimbursement will be made by any federally funded health care program. The anti-kickback prohibitions are broad in scope and apply to virtually all sectors of the health industry.

Not only are kickbacks prohibited, but also prohibited are an array of economic relationships significantly more complex than simple direct reimbursements for health care (Altshuler et al., 2008). As a result, anti-kickback prohibitions apply to many commonly accepted business practices, including:

- Business financial incentives
- Discount arrangements
- Gifts and business courtesies
- Payments for management and personal services
- Referrals from financially related parties

To convict for violations of the anti-kickback prohibitions, the government must prove three elements. It must show providers:

- Knowingly and willfully
- Solicited or received payment
- In return for, or to induce, patient referrals

The anti-kickback prohibitions do not define the meaning of "knowing and willful," and the definition of what constitutes "payment" is unclear. As such, it is not consistently required that agreements satisfy the mens rea, or criminal intent, condition before they are subject to investigation or sanctions. In some cases, providers must know their conduct is unlawful or must intend for it to be so; in other cases, a violation of the compliance standards alone is sufficient.

Any payment in return for patient referrals is prohibited. This includes rebates, as well as the transfer of anything of value. Courts apply the doctrine of fair market value in determining whether transactions fall within the safe harbor regulations (Altshuler et al., 2008). For instance, when Caremark paid dispensing fees to physicians who prescribed and administered an injectable synthetic growth hormone to patients, Caremark, as the exclusive non-hospital-based pharmacy distributor, had to pay nearly $200 million in fines to settle kickback charges.

Criminal and Civil Sanctions for Kickback Violations
Fines up to $25,000 per violation
Imprisonment up to five years
Automatic exclusion from federal health programs for no less than five years (includes exclusion from Medicare, Medicaid, and SCHIP)

Safe Harbor Regulations

While providers who pay or receive payments in order to attract business under federal health programs may be in violation of the anti-kickback law, this prohibition is interpreted so broadly it sometimes inhibits innocuous conduct. Even beneficial arrangements can be considered kickbacks. For instance, if a medical products provider seeks to persuade physicians to use the company's products, the company may violate the anti-kickback prohibitions when they give physicians too many free samples.

Because of this potential for liability, business practices, which might be considered kickbacks, have been safe harbored (*see* 42 C.F.R. § 1001.952 (2007) and 42 U.S.C.A. § 1320a-7b(b)(3) (2006) (codifying safe harbor regulations)). In this chapter, citations for the compliance standards are featured by section for each subject matter of the safe harbors in the Code of Federal Regulations. Multiple subdivision and part citations are not cited to avoid confusion. The standards are convoluted due to congressional incorporation of conflicting updates, interim standards and regulations, and advisory opinions.

In other words, payments paid in order to gain concessions are valid transactions if the government believes they are not kickbacks. Safe harbor regulations, fraud alerts, bulletins, and other forms of guidance are issued regularly to explain activities the government believes to be kickbacks. However, due to substantial uncertainty in the safe harbor provisions, advisory opinions often evaluate distinctive transactions on a case-by-case basis to determine whether the transactions constitute a kickback.

It should be noted that the criminal anti-kickback law and its civil counterpart, the Stark Amendments, are not consistent with one another. Thus, arrangements that comply with one may still violate the other. There are, however, two major differences between the anti-kickback and Stark provisions. First, the anti-kickback law is a criminal law; an improper intent is generally necessary to violate its provisions. This is not true of Stark, which is a civil law with no intent requirements for violation. Second, while activities must fall entirely within an exception to Stark to be legal, arrangements falling outside the anti-kickback safe harbor protections may not necessarily be unlawful. Compliance with the safe harbor regulations does not necessarily mean the transactions are also protected under Stark (Altshuler et al., 2008).

This is to say the anti-kickback and Stark provisions must be analyzed separately. While providers could comply with the anti-kickback law if they satisfy the requirements of the safe harbor regulations, it is often difficult to interpret and meet the safe harbor requirements because the kickback regulations incorporate other conflicting regulations.

Further, the burden of proving compliance rests with providers claiming safe harbor exemptions; the government does not need to prove conduct does not fit within a safe harbor. Moreover, failure to comply with safe harbor regulations does not necessarily mean the anti-kickback law has been violated, nor is it proof of unlawful activity (Altshuler et al., 2008). Compliance with the safe harbor regulations is required simply because it is the law (Ostas, 2007).

Investment Interests

The investment interest safe harbor was created because a literal interpretation of the anti-kickback provisions would prohibit providers from receiving payment from many investment activities (42 C.F.R. § 1001.952(a) (2007); 42 U.S.C.A. § 1320a-7b(b) (2006)). For instance, physicians could be prohibited from receiving dividends from a publicly traded pharmaceutical company if they prescribed too many of a the company's medical products for patients. This exception to the anti-kickback law protects physicians who hold health industry investments, provided they comply with the specific requirements enumerated in the anti-kickback laws. Investment interests include debentures, notes, bonds and shares, partnership units, or securities in health care entities.

The term *investor* defines anyone holding an investment interest. Holding an investment interest indirectly could include investing in another entity that holds an investment interest or having a family member hold the investment interest (McGuire & Scheider, 2007). Investors may be active, involved in the management of the entity, may be partners, or may be passive.

The safe harbor regulations distinguish between three categories of security investments in:

- Large entities with over $50 million in assets
- Small entities with less than $50 million in assets
- Entities located in medically underserved areas

While investments in each category must comply with different standards for returns-on-investments to qualify for safe harbor, there are some similarities between the three categories:

- Services cannot be marketed or provided to passive investors in a manner different than non-investors; investors with the power to generate patient referrals must be treated no differently than other investors
- Loans cannot be made or guaranteed that would allow anyone who has the ability to generate patient referrals to acquire an investment interest in the entity; although bank loans are not prohibited, loan guarantees and other similar arrangements made by an entity or its investors are prohibited
- Investment returns must be directly proportional to capital investments

In addition to the similarities shared by the three categories, a large entity must register its investment interests with the Securities and Exchange Commission. Investors in a position to generate patient referrals to the entity must obtain their investment interests on the same terms and at the same price available to the public.

Small entities and entities located in medically underserved areas must comply with five additional regulatory standards in addition to the three common standards:

- Investment interests offered cannot turn on investors' ability to generate referrals
- Investment interests offered to passive investors who can generate patient referrals cannot be different from the terms offered to all other passive investors
- No more than 40 percent of a small entity's gross revenue, or at least 75 percent of an entity located in a medically underserved area's gross revenue, comes from patient referrals generated by investors
- No more than 40 percent of the value of a small entity's investments, or 50 percent for an entity located in a medically underserved area, is held by investors with the ability to generate patient referrals
- Passive investors are not required to generate patient referrals to retain their investments

Independent physician associations may acquire investment interests in managed care organizations (MCOs) without meeting all the safe harbor requirements. Otherwise, MCOs that receive most of their patient referrals from physician-investors could not receive safe harbor protections. Such MCOs must make good faith marketing efforts to expand their patient bases.

Equipment Rental Contracts

Safe harbor regulations specify how contracts with providers must be written to ensure immunity from the anti-kickback law (Altshuler et al., 2008). The safe harbors created for equipment rental contracts, personal services, and management are similar (*see* 42 C.F.R. § 1001.952(c) (2007)). Payments under such contracts will not be the basis for kickback violations as long as:

- There is a written and signed contract
- Rental contracts are for at least one year
- Rental contracts cover all exchanges between the parties to the contracts, thereby preventing providers from entering multiple contracts with overlapping terms in an effort to circumvent the one-year restriction
- Equipment is appropriate for reasonable business purposes
- Rental payments are equal to fair market value and established in advance
- Schedules for use of the equipment are established upfront

The government is concerned termination provisions could be used to create sham equipment rental contracts. The contracts under this safe harbor may be terminated for cause as long as the conditions under which the contract could be terminated were specified and there is a prohibition on renegotiation

of the terms before the completion of the original one-year term (McGuire & Scheider, 2007).

Space Rental Contracts

Space rental contracts cannot be used to generate patient referrals, since rental fees are often disguised kickbacks to providers to make referrals (*see* 42 C.F.R. § 1001.952(b) (2007)). For instance, hospitals, clinical laboratories, and other providers are prohibited from leasing office space to physicians at below-market rates in anticipation of receiving patient referrals. Establishing the method of calculating rental charges, and not the specific rental amount, will not necessarily be a safe harbor (McGuire & Scheider, 2007).

Similarly, payments for rental space, traditionally provided free or for a nominal charge by hospitals, as an accommodation between hospitals and physicians for the benefit of patients, may be disguised kickbacks. In general, payments for rental of consignment closets in physician offices are also suspect (Altschuler et al., 2008). Rental of space in excess of needs, such as a medical product supplier's need for storage space or a clinical laboratory's need for space to test patients, creates a presumption that the rental charges are a pretext for giving kickbacks for patient referrals.

Personal Service and Management Contracts

Personal service and management contracts hold considerable potential for fraud. Such contracts are considered fraudulent when compensation for services is tied to the number of patient referrals or medical product sales (McGuire & Scheider, 2007). For instance, marketing contracts, where hospitals recommend durable medical equipment distributed by a particular distributor in exchange for a disproportionate share of the distributor's net profits, violates the anti-kickback provisions because compensation is directly tied to the number of sales generated (*see* 42 C.F.R. § 1001.952(d) (2007)).

Legitimate contracts are appropriate, but token arrangements should not be used to justify payments to providers. Characteristics of legitimate contracts include the retention of providers based on their expertise, rather than as an inducement for products or services, and retaining no more consultants than needed for specific programs. For instance, it would be inappropriate to retain ten thousand physicians for a clinical trial requiring no more than one thousand physicians, or to select them as a reward for high prescription rates.

Sale of Physician Practices

The safe harbor provision for the sale of physician practices is divided into two categories: sales to another provider and sales to a hospital or other entity (*see* 42 C.F.R. § 1001.952(e) (2007)). Each category of sale has different requirements, but sales to a hospital are generally not protected unless the physician practice is located in a medically underserved area (Altshuler et al., 2008).

It is common for physicians who sell their practice to another physician upon retirement to continue receiving consulting fees, an arrangement potentially in violation of the anti-kickback law. This safe harbor is designed to allow physicians to sell their practices to other physicians as long as the potential for fraud in such relationships is eliminated (McQuire & Scheider, 2007). To protect the sale proceeds by this safe harbor, physicians selling their practice to other physicians must complete the sale within one year, and after one year from the sale has passed, the selling physician must not be in a position to generate patient referrals for the purchasing physician's practice.

Hospital purchases of physician practices are not generally protected, because hospitals often purchase physicians' practices in order to ensure a steady stream of patient referrals into the hospital (Altshuler et al., 2008). The government believes such arrangements lead to increased health care costs and potential conflicts between the best interests of patients and physicians' business relationships. These are the very frauds the anti-kickback law is designed to prevent. The exception to this regulation is those practices with medical specialties in short supply in areas where the practices are located. If such a practice is sold to a hospital or other entity, it will be protected by this safe harbor if the:

- Physician has attempted to recruit another physician to take over the practice within one year of the sale under the standards established in the recruitment safe harbor
- Physician will not be in a position to generate patient referrals for the hospital once the sale has been completed
- Sale is completed within three years

(McGuire & Scheider, 2007)

Physician Referral Services

This safe harbor protects professional societies or consumer groups who operate fee-based referral services (see 42 C.F.R. § 1001.952(f) (2007)). The safe harbor is implicated where indirect payments are given for patient referrals. For instance, hospitals often operate free referral services for which physicians, in return, are expected to fulfill certain obligations such as sitting on hospital committees (McGuire & Scheider, 2007).

Referral services are prohibited from charging participating physicians fees based on the number of patients the physician accepts through referrals. To

qualify for safe harbor protection, referral contracts must meet the following standards:

- Fees paid by physicians to the referral service must be based on the cost of operating the service, not on the volume of patient referrals generated for physicians
- Physicians who meet the qualifications for participation cannot be excluded
- Referral services cannot establish requirements for the way physicians practice
- Service fees must be assessed equally against all participating physicians

In addition, physician referral services must keep records indicating:

- How patients are matched with participating physicians
- Patients seeking physician referrals were informed how physicians were selected for participation
- The nature of the relationship between the referral service and participating physicians
- What restrictions exclude physicians from participation in the referral service
- Whether physicians have paid fees to the referral service

Warranties Between Providers and Suppliers

Suppliers (sellers) of medical products often offer warranties to providers (buyers) that guarantee replacement of defective products. These warranties become fraudulent when providers receive product replacements or a reduced price because of a warranty, but then, for reimbursement purposes, report the purchases as new medical products (see 42 C.F.R. § 1001.952(g) (2007)). Another fraudulent warranty arrangement occurs when suppliers honor another manufacturer's warranties, but instead of repairing the medical products, replace them with their own brand, and then reimburse the provider for the replacement value. The anti-kickback law punishes such arrangements unless they fall within the protection of the warranty safe harbor. The safe harbor regulations impose requirements on both suppliers and providers (Altshuler et al., 2008).

Suppliers must:

- Accurately invoice price reductions
- Provide supplemental documentation explaining the warranty as needed
- Not pay for anything under the warranty other than the cost of the medical product itself
- Inform the buyer of its obligations under this provision

Providers must accurately report any price reductions on their cost reports. Upon request, providers must also present the government with invoices and warranty documentation.

Discounts Between Providers and Suppliers

The safe harbor for discounts, a common competitive practice, includes bundled sales arrangements where suppliers provide free medical products or services to induce the subsequent purchase of another service or product reimbursed in the same way (*see* 42 C.F.R. § 1001.952(h) (2007)). While discount arrangements are encouraged, situations where the government receives less than its proportional share of the discount are considered fraudulent.

While price reductions will not violate the anti-kickback law if the provisions of this safe harbor are met, payments in cash or cash equivalents, other than rebates, are not protected. If medical products or services are provided free or for a reduced price in order to induce the purchase of different services or medical products, the arrangement will not be protected unless they are reimbursed using the same methodology and the reduction is accurately reported (McQuire & Scheider, 2007). Price reductions that apply to one payer but not to government health programs, such as routine waivers of coinsurance or deductibles, warranties, and services provided through a personal or management services contract, are also not protected.

Separate standards are established for suppliers (sellers) and providers (buyers). The conditions that must be met to satisfy the requirements of this safe harbor depend on how providers are reimbursed.

Employment Contracts

This safe harbor is broad enough to cover most bona fide employment relationships (*see* 42 C.F.R. § 1001.952(i) (2007)). Employers are generally permitted to pay employees in whatever manner they choose. For instance, employment contracts that require physicians to refer patients to their employer-hospital are not considered inducements, nor are percentage compensation contracts that base compensation on personally performed services (McQuire & Scheider, 2007). These safe harbor regulations do not cover independent contractors, who may be protected under safe harbors for personal service and management contracts.

Group Purchasing Organizations

Payments to group purchasing organizations (GPO) by providers and medical product providers will fall within the GPO safe harbor if those payments meet two standards:

- GPOs must have a written contract with each medical products company from whom they purchase products and each provider to whom they sell products, specifying:
  - GPO fees will be no more than 3 percent of the purchase price
  - Maximum amount the GPO will be paid as a fixed sum or a fixed percentage of the value of the purchases
- GPOs must disclose to providers the medical products received from each supplier or medical products manufacturer annually, and the same disclosure must be made to the government upon request

(42 C.F.R. § 1001.952(j) (2007))

Advertisements and Promotions

Providers may generate business through advertising directly to patients or patient referral services. For these activities to avoid anti-kickback inquiry, they must fall within safe harbor requirements (*see* 42 C.F.R. § 1001.952(l) (2007)). Providers who attempt to attract patients by advertising a willingness to waive coinsurance or deductibles are potentially in violation of the anti-kickback law (Altshuler et al, 2008). While the government has proposed broadening the coinsurance and deductible safe harbor regulations, such waivers are presently only protected if patients for whom fees are waived qualify for Medicare, Medicaid, and SCHIP, or other government health programs and if the:

- Waived amount is not later claimed as bad debt
- Waivers are made irrespective of the reasons for admission, length of stay, or diagnosis
- Waivers are not part of a price reduction contract with third-party payers, unless the contract is part of a Medicare supplemental policy

(see Altshuler et al., 2008)

For instance, backup emergency ambulance services may waive coinsurance or deductibles because failure to collect fees would be unlikely to induce patient referrals, since use of the ambulance service is dependent on emergency needs and the inability of a primary ambulance service to respond (*see generally* GAO, 2005).

Reduced Fee Arrangements Between Providers and Health Insurers

Providers who contract with health insurers to provide health care for reduced fees may be protected by a safe harbor covering price reductions (*see* 42 C.F.R. § 1001.952(m) (2007)). Requirements vary depending on the health insurance plan and the reimbursement arrangements providers make with government health programs (Altshuler et al., 2008).

MCOs that have entered Medicare, Medicaid, or SCHIP at-risk contracts will be protected if they do not claim reimbursements from the government without prior approval. The burden of managed care contracts from health maintenance organizations, competitive medical plans, and prepaid health plans cannot be shifted onto the government.

Physician Recruitment in Medically Underserved Areas

Physician recruitment is frequently subject to fraud and is generally not protected from the anti-kickback law. Exceptions are made, however, for medically underserved areas (*see* 42 C.F.R. § 1001.952(n) (2007)). This safe harbor protects physician recruitment activities in areas having difficulty attracting physicians, enabling hospitals and clinics to offer financial incentives to potential physicians without being liable for kickback violations. Payments made to physicians to induce them to locate in medically underserved areas will be safe harbored if:

- There is a written, signed employment contract between physicians and their employer hospital or clinic
- At least 75 percent of the revenues of a physician leaving an established practice must come from patients the new physician has not previously seen
- At least 75 percent of the revenues of the new practice must come from medically underserved patients
- Employment contracts may not benefit anyone other than physicians with the power to generate patient referrals
- Financial incentives may not be tied to the amount of patient referrals physicians generate
- Financial incentives may only be provided for three years and employment contracts cannot be renegotiated during this term
- Physicians cannot be prevented from referring patients to or establishing staff privileges with other providers
- Physicians cannot be required to generate patient referrals, although physicians may be required to maintain hospital or clinic staff privileges
- Physicians must treat patients in a nondiscriminatory manner

(Altshuler et al., 2008; McGuire & Scheider, 2007)

The limitations of this regulation are that the safe harbor protection offered through compliance with these standards only lasts for three years and the protection is restricted to recruitment, not retention, contracts.

Obstetrical Malpractice Insurance Subsidies in Medically Underserved Areas

The safe harbor for obstetrical malpractice insurance allows hospitals or other providers to subsidize the costs of malpractice insurance for obstetricians practicing in underserved areas (urban or rural areas where there is a shortage of services) (*see* 42 C.F.R. § 1001.952(o) (2007)). Insurance can be fully subsidized for full-time obstetricians and nurse midwives; a portion of insurance can be subsidized for other providers.

Safe harbor protection requires that numerous standards be met:

- There must be a written and signed contract
- Malpractice insurance must be made for risk policies that share compensation for insured losses
- Providers must certify they believe at least 75 percent of their patients will be medically underserved during their first coverage year
- At least 75 percent of the provider's patients in the previous coverage period must be medically underserved during subsequent coverage periods
- Generation of new patient referrals cannot be a condition for receiving insurance subsidizes
- Providers cannot be prevented from referring patients to or establishing staff privileges at other hospitals
- Subsidies cannot be tied to the volume or value of patient referrals providers make to hospitals
- Obstetrical patients must be treated in a nondiscriminatory manner

(*see* McGuire & Scheider, 2007)

Cost-Based Managed Care

An additional safe harbor protects health insurers under contract with the government to increase health insurance coverage and reduce premiums or cost-sharing coinsurance and deductibles (*see* 42 C.F.R. § 1001.952(m) (2009)). If health maintenance organizations, competitive medical plans, and prepaid health plans cover services on a cost basis, the insurers must offer the same coverage increase (from reduced cost sharing to providers' waiver of coinsurance and deductibles) to all enrollees, unless the government approves otherwise. Such managed care insurers cannot claim the costs of the increased coverage as bad debt.

Physician to Physician Referrals

The referral safe harbor allows physicians to refer patients to one another (*see* 42 C.F.R. § 1001.952(s) (2007)). Physicians may refer patients to specialists, with the understanding patients will be referred back at a specified time or under certain conditions. Without the ability to create referral arrangements, physicians might hesitate to refer patients to specialists for fear they would lose their patients to the specialist; this fear could inhibit patient access to appropriate health care (Altshuler et al., 2008).

For instance, primary care physicians often refer patients to specialists with the understanding patients will be referred back when they have recovered.

Payments exchanged between the two physicians are protected from kickback charges if:

- Services for which referrals are made are not within the referring physician's specialty and are within the specialty of the physician to whom patients are referred
- Patients are sent back to the original referring physician at the medically appropriate time
- Payments or benefits exchanged between referring physicians and specialists are from patients or third-party payers
- Physicians do not receive payments from each other or split global fees from government health programs

(Altshuler et al., 2008; McGuire & Scheider, 2007)

Group Practices

Patient referrals between members of a group practice could create financial incentives for improper utilization because all members of the practice eventually share revenues. Investment in group practice is protected if:

- Interests in the practice are held by licensed medical professionals
- Interests are in the entire practice, not in particular subsets
- Practice is a unified business with unified decision-making, pooling of expenses and revenues, and a compensation system that is not based on satellite offices operating virtually independently
- Revenues from ancillary services only come from in-office services

(42 C.F.R. § 1001.952(p) (2007); Altshuler et al., 2008)

Cooperative Hospital Service Organizations

Cooperative Hospital Service Organizations (CHSO) are created by two or more tax-exempt hospitals to provide services such as purchasing and billing for their patron hospitals. Reimbursements exchanged between a CHSO and its patron hospitals may be protected under the CHSO safe harbor if the:

- CHSO is owned by at least two patron hospitals
- Reimbursements the patron hospitals make to the CHSO are for bona fide operating expenses
- Reimbursements made from the CHSO to the patron hospitals are a distribution of its net earnings

(42 C.F.R. § 1001.952(q) (2007); McGuire & Scheider, 2007)

Ambulatory Surgical Centers

Ambulatory surgical centers (ASCs), which exclusively conduct outpatient or same-day surgeries, operate as extensions of physicians' office practices. ASCs may be supported by physician-investors who refer patients to the center without violating the anti-kickback law.

Returns on physician investments in an ASC are protected if the:

- Ancillary services performed at the ASC are directly related to the surgeries performed at the ASC and are not billed separately
- ASC and its physician-investors are prohibited from making or guaranteeing loans for new investors to gain an investment interest in the ASC
- Center is a certified ASC
- Investment returns are proportional to capital invested
- Patients are not treated in a discriminatory manner
- Patients who are referred to the ASC by physician-investors are informed of the referring physician's investment interests
- Investment interests are not tied to the amount of patient referrals physician-investors generate for the ASC

(42 C.F.R. § 1001.952(r) (2007))

In addition, physician-investors in specialty ASCs must earn at least one-third of their medical practice income from surgeries at the ASC; the remaining two-thirds may come from surgeries and other services outside the ACS. While hospitals may also invest in ASCs, if at least one investor is a hospital, additional standards apply:

- ASCs are prohibited from using hospital space or equipment without a contract that conforms to the space or equipment rental safe harbor regulations
- Hospitals cannot generally claim reimbursement for any costs associated with the ASC on any cost reports or claims for reimbursement
- Hospitals cannot generate business for the ASC

(McGuire & Scheider, 2007)

Cost-Based Reimbursements

If providers receive reimbursement for patients on a cost or competitive at-risk basis, the following reduced fee standards must be fulfilled:

- Provider contracts with health insurers must remain in effect for at least one year
- Contracts must specify the services and medical products to be covered
- Price reductions must be completely and accurately reported on cost reports or claim forms for reimbursement
- Providers cannot submit claims to health insurers for reimbursement at reduced levels, without prior approval from the government

(42 C.F.R. § 1001.952(t) (2006))

When providers receive price reductions from health maintenance organizations, competitive medical plans, or PHIs with established Medicare, Medicaid, or SCHIP at-risk contracts, there is no need to report the discount. There is also no need for suppliers to report discounts to satisfy the requirements of this safe harbor.

Fee-for-Service Reimbursements from Health Insurers

If providers are not paid on an at-risk basis, these standards must be met:

- Provider contracts with health insurers must remain in effect for at least one year
- Contract must specify the services and medical products to be covered
- Fee schedules must be incorporated into the provider contracts
- Fee schedules must remain in effect for the entire contract term unless the government authorizes a reimbursement update
- Reimbursement claims cannot exceed the fee schedules
- Providers and health insurers must accurately report fee schedule amounts charged on cost reports
- Reimbursement amounts must be reported to the government upon request

(42 C.F.R. § 1001.952(t) (2007); McGuire & Scheider, 2007)

Reimbursements Between Managed Care Organizations and Contract Providers

Payments between MCOs and contractors, and those between contractors and subcontractors, are protected under the safe harbor for price reductions offered to MCOs if a signed, written one-year contract between the parties specifies what services will be covered (*see* 42 C.F.R. § 1001.952(u) (2007)). Neither party to such a contract may seek to give or receive reimbursement outside the scope of their contracts, if any government health care program is reimbursing the MCO on a fee-for-service or cost basis (Altshuler et al., 2008).

Generally, first-tier contractors cannot claim reimbursement from government health programs for services provided under their contracts with MCOs.[LN2] Special standards apply in these situations: first-tier contractors may claim reimbursement as long as the contract between the MCO and a health maintenance organization or competitive medical plans specifies first-tier contractors are responsible for making reimbursement claims (McGuire & Scheider, 2007). Reimbursements between first-tier contractors and subcontractors or between two subcontractors are only protected if the first-tier contractor is not an MCO. The financial burden of such contracts, however, may not be shifted to the government.

A separate safe harbor protects arrangements between MCOs and contractors and subcontractors

if the contracting entities bear some of the risk of patient care. Payments between MCOs and first-tier contractors are protected if a written, signed contract between the parties:

- Covers at least one year
- Specifies the services and medical products to be covered
- Requires participation in a quality assurance program
- Specifies how reimbursements will be determined and assessed:
  ○ Fixed charge per patient
  ○ Percentage of the premium
  ○ Diagnosis-related groups
- Details bonus and withhold arrangements, or the percentage of the capitation fees to be withheld for cost overruns

(McGuire & Scheider, 2007)

If the first-tier contractor has an investment interest in the health plan, the interest must fulfill the requirements of the investment interest safe harbor (Altshuler et al., 2008).

Reimbursements under Medicare, Medicaid, and SCHIP

Providers submitting cost reports to the government (hospitals and nursing homes) must fulfill four requirements:

- Discounts must be earned based on purchases made within one fiscal year
- Claims for discounts must be made within the fiscal year they were earned or the following year
- Discounts must be fully and accurately reported
- Documentation received about the discounts must be provided to the government

(42 C.F.R. § 1001.952(h) (2007))

The reimbursement standards are the same as those applicable to warranties between providers and suppliers.

Ambulance Replenishing

The regulations establish a safe harbor for ambulance restocking arrangements, or the practice of hospitals or other receiving facilities to restock ambulance providers with drugs and medical supplies used during the transportation of patients (*see* 42 C.F.R. § 1001.952(v) (2007)). Drugs or medical supplies transferred from hospitals to ambulance services will not violate the law when the following standards are satisfied:

- The ambulance and the hospital do not seek reimbursement for the same replenished drugs
- Records are maintained of the replenished drugs and restocked medical supplies

- The replenishing arrangement cannot be related to the volume or value of patient referrals generated on either side of the transaction
- Ambulances must serve the restocking hospital an average of three times per week
- Drug and medical supplies replenished were actually used by the ambulance during the transportation

(Altshuler et al., 2008; McGuire & Scheider, 2007)

Electronic Health Records

In an effort to promote the use of electronic health records, this safe harbor protects non-monetary services (hardware, software, health information technology, and training) for electronic prescription systems (*see* 42 C.F.R. § 1001.952(x), (y) (2007)). The intent is to promote such technology as a means of improving health care system efficiency and reducing medical errors; it is not intended to induce patient referrals.

> ### Moral Dilemmas
>
> 1. Has the health industry adequately addressed all the potential areas of high risk that have been identified by the government?
>
> 2. Besides the safe harbor provisions, are there any other potential areas of high risk?

The Health Insurance Portability and Accountability Act

HIPAA, the most comprehensive attempt to fight federal health care fraud thus far, extended the scope of the anti-kickback prohibitions to cover all health care programs and expanded the definition of a kickback (*see* 18 U.S.C.A. §§ 24 *et seq.* (2009)). The first federal law to regulate private health care, HIPAA significantly increased the enforcement power of the federal government by establishing programs to coordinate investigations of health care fraud at both the federal and state levels (*see* Altshuler et al., 2008).

HIPAA federalized health care fraud by making it illegal for anyone to knowingly and willfully:

- Defraud any health care program or obtain by means of false representations anything of value from a health care program (18 U.S.C.A. § 1347 (1996))
- Make false statements in any matter involving reimbursements for services or medical products (18 U.S.C.A. § 1035 (1996))
- Embezzle, convert, or steal any funds, property, or assets of a health care program (18 U.S.C.A. § 669 (1996))
- Obstruct, delay, prevent, or mislead the investigation of health care offenses (18 U.S.C.A. § 1518 (1996))

> **Sanctions for HIPAA Violations**
> Fines for individuals of $250,000 per violation
> Fines for organizations of $500,000 per violation
> Fines of twice the gain to the provider or loss to another because of the fraudulent conduct
> Source: 18 U.S.C.A. § 3571 (1987).

Self-Referral Limitations (Stark Amendments)

Self-referral limitations were enacted to enforce the FCA and counteract the rapidly increasing cost of health care resulting from physician self-referrals (McGuire & Scheider, 2007). Stark prohibits physicians from referring patients to providers in which the physician has a financial interest, absent a safe harbor provision, including:

- Clinical laboratory services
- Durable medical equipment and supplies
- Home health services
- Inpatient and outpatient hospital services
- Occupational therapy services
- Outpatient prescription drugs
- Parenteral and enteral nutrients
- Physical therapy services
- Prosthetics, orthotics, and prosthetic devices and supplies
- Radiation therapy services and supplies
- Radiology services, including magnetic resonance imaging, computerized axial tomography scans, and ultrasound devices

(see 42 U.S.C.A. § 1395nn (2008))

To establish a Stark violation and a conflict of interest, the government must show:

- Financial relationship between a health care entity and a physician
- Referral by the physician to the entity for designated health services
- Submission of a claim for services
- Absence of a safe harbor exception

(Altshuler et al., 2008)

A financial relationship includes an ownership or investment interest in an entity by physicians or the physicians' immediate family members, or a compensation arrangement between physicians or their immediate family members and the entity. Prohibited compensation arrangements can be any reimbursement, discount, forgiveness of debt, or other benefit. Because Stark does not have an intent requirement, strict liability is imposed for referrals if a financial relationship exists (Altshuler et al., 2008). An entity receiving a prohibited referral is forbidden from billing the government, any individual, third-party payer, or other entity.

The Stark Amendments contain several exceptions for certain financial arrangements where cross-referral arrangements are permissible. These exceptions fall into three categories:

- Exceptions applicable to both physician ownership or investment interests and compensation arrangements:
  - In-house ancillary services
  - Physician services
  - Prepaid plans
  - Other arrangements that do not pose a risk of program or patient fraud

(*see* Altshuler et al., 2008; McGuire & Scheider, 2007)

- Exceptions for hospital ownership and rural providers, or investment interests in publicly held securities
- Exceptions for compensation arrangements only:
  - Bona fide employment relationships
  - Group practice arrangements with hospitals
  - Isolated transactions
  - Personal service arrangements
  - Physician recruitment
  - Reimbursements by physicians
  - Rental of equipment
  - Rental of space
  - Payment unrelated to the provision of designated health services

A medical entity must also recognize that some transactions might comply with Stark while falling outside any of the anti-kickback safe harbors (Hubbell et al., 2005). For instance, a physician could make referrals to in-office ancillary services and, while this would likely comply with Stark, it might be a kickback violation since no safe harbor exists (McGuire & Scheider, 2007).

Sanctions for Violation of Self-Referral Limitations

Non-reimbursement for claims

Liability for claims already reimbursed

Fines up to $15,000 per claim violation

Fines up to $100,000 for prohibited cross-referral arrangements

Fines of $10,000 per day for failure to comply with reporting requirements

Mandatory exclusion of no less than three years from federal health programs

Source: 42 U.S.C.A. § 1395nn(g)(1-5) (2008).

False Claims Act

The FCA targets stealing (Smith, 2007). By creating liability for anyone who knowingly submits a false claim for reimbursement, the FCA has become one of the primary laws the government relies on to recover losses caused by health care fraud (*see* 31 U.S.C.A. §§ 3729-3731 (2009)).

To convict for violations of the FCA, the government must show that:

- A provider submitted a claim seeking reimbursement for services
- The claim was false
- The provider had both knowledge of the claim's falsity and an intent to submit that claim

To meet the statutory requirement, the false claim must have actually been submitted for reimbursement. While actions may be brought for incorrect submission of information on reimbursement claims, most FCA violations arise from misrepresentations including, but not limited to, submitting claims for medical products and services for:

- Patients never seen
- Services not personally rendered
- Medically unnecessary services
- Services not related to accidents
- Non-reimbursable costs (medically necessary services not covered by Medicare, Medicaid, or SCHIP)
- Unbundled diagnosis-related groups, or billing one bundled procedure as a group of smaller procedures
- Inflated costs
- Higher reimbursement levels than the codes for the services actually provided (upcoding)

A recent U.S. Supreme Court decision affecting all federal claims reimbursements involving Navy contracts and subcontracts clarified that the FCA requires intent to submit a false claim and knowledge of its falsity. The duty to know requires providers to understand the proper billing procedures and regulations. Knowledge and intent are often determining factors in whether prosecutions are pursued.

Allison affects Medicare, Medicaid, and SCHIP insurance reimbursements. All three public insurance programs rely on third-party contractors and subcontractors. Before this decision, only the potential to influence had to be demonstrated; actual reliance on the false statement was unnecessary. *Allison* makes it more difficult for the government to prove fraud based strictly on false claims reimbursed with government funds.

INTENT UNDER THE FALSE CLAIMS ACT

Allison Co. v. U.S. ex. rel. Sanders
[Federal Subcontractor v. Federal Government and Whistleblowers]
128 S.Ct. 2123 (U.S. Supreme Court 2008)

FACTS: This case surrounds a contract with the Navy and two shipyards to build guided missile destroyers. The shipyards subcontracted with Allison Engine Company to build generators. Allison in turn subcontracted with General Tool Company (GTC) to assemble the generators. The subcontracts required that each generator be manufactured according to Navy specifications. Former employees of GTC brought a qui tam action to recover damages under the FCA on the basis that the work had not been done in accordance with contract specifications.

The district court granted the government summary judgment. The Sixth Circuit U.S. Court of Appeals reversed in part and held that claims do not require proof of intent to cause a false claim to be paid by the government.

ISSUE: Is intent to defraud required for claims under the FCA?

HOLDING AND DECISION: Yes, intent to defraud the government is required for claims under the FCA.

ANALYSIS: First, the Supreme Court analyzed the plain language of the FCA and noted that intent to get a false claim paid by the government was required. The Court distinguished between getting a claim paid by a private entity and getting a false

or fraudulent claim paid with government funds. Under the FCA, Allison must have intended that the government itself pay the claim.

In addition, Allison must have intended for the government to rely on the false statements in paying the claim. Subcontractors violate the FCA if they submit false statements to the prime contractor, the shipyard in this instance, intending for their statements to be used by the prime contractor to get the government to pay a claim. The Court contrasted this with the situation where subcontractors make false statements to a private entity, but do not intend the government to rely on those false statements as a condition of payment. Subcontractors must intend that the false statements have a material effect on the government's decision to pay the false or fraudulent claim.

The Court reiterated its policy against transforming the FCA into an all-purpose anti-fraud statute. By requiring proof of intent to defraud the government, the Court sought to avoid drawing any causal links between false claims and the government's decision to pay a claim.

RULE OF LAW: Claims under the FCA must prove intent that the false statements were material to the government's decision to pay the false claim.

(See *generally* Blank, 2009; Morse & Wolff, 2009; Oretga, 2008; Reiss et al., 2008; Schindler, 2009.)

Now, the government must prove that there was "intent" that the false claim be reimbursed by the government, and that the false claim was "material" to the government's decision to pay the claim. Future cases will interpret how these heightened standards are applied to the health industry.

FCA liability does not extend to providers whose billing records are incorrect due to accounting errors, innocent mistakes, or good faith miscalculations. One lesson to take from this case is that it may be better to acknowledge an error, mistake, or miscalculation during a government investigation rather than attempting a cover-up.

Repeatedly, the cover-up is often worse than the actual original offense.

General Fraud Laws

In addition to using laws specifically targeting health care fraud, the government has brought charges for health care fraud under a panoply of about thirty-five different federal laws.[LN3] Two of the most common laws used by the government are the False Statements Act (FSA) and mail and wire fraud (including the Internet) (Altshuler et al., 2008). Because most health care occurs within legitimate business contracts, the mail and wire fraud laws provide additional options for the government.

CONVICTION OF PROVIDER UNDER THE FCA

U.S. v. Davis

[Federal Government v. Fraudulent Providers]

490 F.3d 541 (U.S. Court of Appeals for the 6th Circuit 2007)

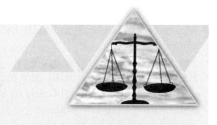

FACTS: A husband and wife team, the Davises, supplied oxygen to coal miners suffering from black lung disease. They founded the Kentucky Black Lung Association to help miners obtain black lung benefits, as well as access to disease-related medical products and services. The Association sent miners to a special clinic for pulmonary testing where Ms. Davis volunteered. From the clinic, miners were directed to a durable medical equipment company, owned by Mr. Davis, for their oxygen supplies, paid for by Medicare. Claims were submitted to Medicare for the miners' oxygen supplies with forged certificates of medical necessity; Ms. Davis signed the certificates of medical necessity, not the clinic physician as required by the anti-kickback regulation. While the Davises claimed their activities were a cost-efficient scheme to ensure miners received services to which they were entitled, the government maintained the couple failed to comply with the required safe harbor regulations. The Davises were initially charged with non-compliance of anti-kickback prohibitions; they were not accused of necessarily committing any wrongs or providing medical products and services to miners who were not entitled to black lung benefits. As the government investigation proceeded, the couple attempted to conceal their non-compliance with the law and misrepresented facts to the government investigators.

ISSUE: Can the required intent to commit health care fraud be inferred from circumstantial evidence?

HOLDING AND DECISION: Intent can be inferred from efforts to conceal the unlawful activity, from misrepresentations, from proof of knowledge, and from the providers' profits (*see* DHS, 2007).

ANALYSIS: Almost all the medical equipment company's business was from the one clinic where Ms. Davis handled the claims processing for miners referred to the clinic from her outreach association. Ms. Davis signed Certificate of Need forms requiring certification by an independent physician, as well as an independent supplier of medical equipment. The husband received a three-year prison sentence and the wife received a five-year sentence; together they were required to make restitution of $172,000.

RULE OF LAW: Because it is difficult to prove intent to defraud from direct evidence, circumstantial evidence of fraudulent intent may be considered and reasonable inferences may be made.

(*See generally* Altshuler et al., 2008; Blank, 2009).

Sanctions for False Claims

Fines range from $2,000 to $10,000 per claim

Treble damages and costs

Imprisonment ranges from five to twenty years per claim, up to life

Three- to five-year exclusion from federal health programs

Injunctive relief to freeze individual and corporate assets

Asset forfeitures

Adoption of government-supervised compliance programs

False Statements

FSA is a companion law to the FCA and broadly interprets false statements in the context of health care fraud (*see* 18 U.S.C.A. § 1001 (2006)). Providers who falsify reimbursement claims generally violate both the FSA and the FCA, which both prohibit false statements.

To violate the FSA, the government must prove the statement was:

- Submitted to a federal health care program or an intermediary of the government, such as a private insurance company
- False

- Material, but need not actually influence any government function
- Made knowingly and willfully
- Related to a federal health care program or private entities receiving federal funds or subject to federal regulation or supervision

To be material, the statement need only have a natural tendency or capacity to influence a government function; it need not actually do so. False statements made in any matter to a federal health program are within the scope of the FSA, including false statements to private entities receiving federal funds or subject to federal regulation or supervision.

Under the FSA providers must make false statements both knowingly and willfully, with the intent to defraud. Although the provision requires proof that the provider willfully made false statements, the government need not prove the provider knew its statements were unlawful; rather, the government need only prove the provider knew its statements were false (Altshuler et al., 2008). The government must show misrepresentations were not made innocently or inadvertently (McGuire & Scheider, 2007).

Sanctions for False Statements
Fines
Imprisonment up to five years per statement

Mail, Wire, or Internet Fraud

Providers who use the mail or any type of interstate electronic communications (including the wires or Internet) in their plans to defraud can also face charges of fraud (*see* 18 U.S.C.A. §§ 1341-1350 (2009) and 18 U.S.C.A. § 1343 (2008)). Mail fraud requires only the use of the mails, while wire and Internet fraud must involve the interstate use of communication for furtherance of the plan. *See* 18 U.S.C.A. § 1001 (2006). One can be convicted of mail, wire, or Internet communications fraud without being convicted of the primary charges of health care fraud (Altshuler et al., 2008).

For instance, the government must establish kickbacks occurred under the anti-kickback law, but only the plan to defraud and the use of the Internet are needed for Internet fraud. Charges can also be brought under special mail, wire, or Internet fraud provisions in HIPAA specific to health care fraud.

To prosecute for mail, wire, or Internet fraud, the government must prove providers:

- Intentionally participated in a plan to defraud
- Used the mails or any type of electronic communications to execute the plan

Several different variations of health care fraud can serve as the basis of the plan to defraud, including billing for services not rendered, false descriptions of services rendered, and false representations that services were medically necessary. Furthermore, a provider's plan to defraud patients of their right to honest services may also support a conviction. In contrast to the requirements of other fraud provisions, mere intent to defraud is, in itself, unlawful. In addition, the success of plans is not a necessary element for fraud convictions. Similarly, efforts to repay the funds obtained through a fraudulent plan do not necessarily indicate absence of fraudulent intent (Altshuler et al., 2008).

Unlike the high mens rea requirement of the first element, the second element of the mail, wire, or Internet fraud laws requires the government to meet only a minimal burden. Providers need not have personally used the mails or interstate electronic communications, nor must they have intended to use the mails or electronic communications. Rather, the link between the plan to defraud and the use of mails or electronic communications must only have been reasonably foreseeable (Altshuler et al., 2008).

Sanctions for Mail, Wire, or Internet Fraud
Fines
Imprisonment up to twenty years for each
   count of fraud
Mandatory exclusion from federal health
   programs of no less than three years for
   misdemeanor fraud, no less than five years
   for felony fraud (Medicaid Advisory
   Opinion 05-12)

GOVERNMENT ENFORCEMENT OF HEALTH CARE FRAUD LAWS

Few providers expect to become the subject of a government investigation, yet it happens every day. Government investigations cut across all sectors of the health industry. No provider is immune (Saul Ewing, 2006). Government agents often appear unannounced to execute search warrants and serve subpoenas. The key is planning for the unannounced government visit before it ever happens. Providers can position themselves best to respond to the unannounced visit by anticipating such an event and planning.

Triple Plays

Parallel criminal, civil, and administrative investigations for health care fraud generally occur. Indictments are usually filed first to investigate criminal activities, compelling providers to testify and submit documents to the government. Criminal charges are then filed, before or after arrests are made, to start the criminal justice process.

The government may seek to recover damages and assess civil penalties by bringing civil charges or by initiating administrative hearings (Altshuler et al., 2008). Health care fraud laws actually encourage the government to seek civil rather than criminal remedies, since financial recovery is usually much greater. In addition, once a criminal conviction has been obtained, civil recovery is often not available because the provider is no longer in business (McGuire & Scheider, 2007).

Finally, administrative procedures may determine whether providers must be excluded from participation in Medicare, Medicaid, and SCHIP (42 U.S.C.A. § 1320a-7 (2003)). The government often mandates the establishment of compliance programs during sentencing, pretrial diversion of criminal fraud charges, or settlements of civil fraud charges.

Qui Tam False Claims Actions

"Qui tam" is short for the Latin phrase "qui tam pro domino rege quam pro se ipso in hac parte sequitur," which means "he who brings an action for the king as well as for himself" (Black's Law, 2009). The government has shifted resources away from fraud investigations in the defense industry and toward qui tam health care cases, a growing method of health care fraud law enforcement (Rich, 2008). This shift in focus by the government has flooded the health industry with lawsuits. Almost five hundred U.S. hospitals were the subject of FCA investigations at the end of 2008; almost every major pharmaceutical and medical devices company faces qui tam claims (DOJ, 2007).

Private individuals, referred to as whistleblowers, can pursue enforcement of the FCA through qui tam actions (31 U.S.C.A. § 3730(b) (1994)). A whistleblower with knowledge of fraudulent practices first files a complaint under seal. The government then investigates the complaint and can intervene in the action and prosecute the claim if it chooses to do so. If the government intervenes and wins, the whistleblower receives 15 to 20 percent of the government's recovery (Altshuler et al., 2008).

When the government intervenes, whistleblowers can receive millions of dollars from successful qui tam actions:

Whistleblower Awards	
	(In millions)
AstraZeneca	$47.5
GlaxoSmithKline	$34.2
Schering Pharmaceutical	$31.6
Warner-Lambert	$24.6
Tenet Healthcare	$ 8.1
Source: U.S. Department of Justice.	

If the government does not intervene, whistleblowers can still sue on behalf of the government, and receive 25 to 30 percent of any recovery (from which legal fees must be deducted). Over the last twenty years, however, 94 percent of these lawsuits, totaling more than three thousand cases, were dismissed without recovering any funds (Rich, 2008). Today, with the government focus on health care fraud, whistleblower lawsuits in which the government does not find significant merit and attach any importance to, are exacting a heavy toll on the health industry and the American public. As whistleblower lawsuits, in which government does not intervene, progress through the judicial system, they are alienating providers and threatening public confidence in the legitimacy of the fight against health care fraud (Smith, 2007).

Deferred Prosecution Agreements

Providers suffer a peculiar vulnerability. While the standards of criminal liability allow the government to punish anyone falling within their jurisdiction, the health industry is facing the emergence of deferred prosecution agreements (DPAs) to force major changes in the governance of hospitals and providers of medical products (Wharton, 2005).

A DPA is a provisional settlement of a criminal lawsuit whereby the government agrees to suspend, but not dismiss, any prosecution in exchange for promises to reform in specified ways. Most settlements split the difference by having individuals pay half the maximum fines or serve half the sentence (Wharton, 2005).

DPAs take on an entirely different complexion in the health industry. The last thing a provider fears is the maximum fine from a successful criminal conviction. Rather, the deadly force of the DPA rests in a combination of two key factors: vicarious criminal liability and the collateral consequences of a criminal indictment prior to, and independent of, any eventual conviction (Epstein, 2006).

Vicarious Liability for Criminal Conduct

Vicarious liability, as first developed in civil tort law, allows innocent third parties to sue not only individual wrongdoers for damages, but also employers, so long as the wrongdoers' actions were within the scope of their employment. In the context of tort law, this ensures compensation for innocent victims, while giving employers the incentive to monitor employees (Wharton, 2005).

Beginning in 2003, the government imported this civil doctrine into the criminal arena. Today, the health industry faces criminal liability for the actions of employees, even if their wrongful actions were neither authorized nor condoned. The government uses vicarious liability to obtain favorable settlements to reform the health industry from the outside.

Providers receive a temporary reprieve from the government only if they remove individual wrongdoers and agree to DPAs with extensive federal monitoring and oversight (Wharton, 2005). Definitive numbers highlighting how extensively the government is involved in monitoring the health industry are difficult to come by, principally because the government does not have a policy of publicizing all DPAs (Garrett, 2007).

Collateral Consequences

In pursuing this DPA strategy, the government faces both a dilemma and an opportunity. The government's only credible threat against recalcitrant providers is a criminal indictment. Yet, simply filing an indictment triggers collateral repercussions sufficient to drive any provider out of business, since state and federal regulators are now duty-bound to suspend the licenses and permits under which providers do business.

Thus, while providers have strong protections against false convictions in the form of proof beyond a reasonable doubt of the elements of a crime and the ability to examine evidence or cross-examine witnesses, they are helpless to protect themselves prior to issuance of an indictment. At most, a conviction carries a fine, but an indictment, which lies wholly within the government's discretion, shuts down the provider's business. Faced with this pressure, the indictment is all that matters (Wharton, 2005).

Moral Dilemmas

1. Do DPAs serve the public interest?

Bristol Myers-Squibb

One notable DPA involved Bristol Myers-Squibb (BMS). BMS faced trouble because of a potential securities violation for inflating its quarterly earnings by a business practice known as channel stuffing.[LN4] BMS told its distributors they had to accept and inventory large amounts of BMS products immediately, with the understanding that, down the road, they could return the excess for a refund. Alleged securities violations arose from overstating quarterly earnings reports, without indicating any expected future write-offs (which could constitute common law accounting fraud by creating short-term gains at the expense of future sales). A settlement was reached with BMS before it could be determined whether the company engaged in legitimate earnings management or illegitimate channel stuffing. While channel stuffing by itself is generally legal, there is a fine line between having some reserves and raiding the "cookie jar" of all reserves and intentionally deceiving shareholders to believe that internal sales and earnings targets have been met. One action is legal, the other action is excessive use of reserves and is fraudulent under the FSA.[LN5]

What was decided was that BMS should not have aggressively managed its sales and earnings. The assumption was that the BMS DPA would prohibit the company from engaging in future channel stuffing. However, the government went beyond sanctioning this allegation alone (Epstein, 2006). For instance, the DPA required BMS to endow a business ethics chair at the alma mater of the U.S. Attorney prosecuting the case. Critics ask whether this was actually a kickback to the U.S. Attorney.

BMS agreed not only to abide by the law and to purge its ranks of the parties responsible for the channel-stuffing plan, but also to exhibit exemplary corporate citizenship (Wharton, 2005). To that end, oversight of all activities was required by an independent adviser, who had the power to attend all meetings and review all documents, and to report findings to the government. BMS was ordered to restructure its internal operations and appoint a new chief compliance officer to assist the government's adviser (Epstein, 2006). BMS also agreed to pay $839 million in restitution payments to shareholders and the Securities and Exchange Commission and to make contributions of $350 million to a fund for present and former shareholders arising from pending securities class action litigation to be used to restitute shareholders for the material risk to BMS's future sales and earnings (Christie & Hanna, 2006).

DPAs such as this erode the most elementary protections of the criminal law by turning the government into both judge and jury, thus undermining the principle of separation of powers (Epstein, 2006). In the case of a breached DPA, the government retains the right to file charges for the first time at any time. Statute of limitations concerns are addressed in the DPA itself, which typically waives all such rights (Spivack & Raman, 2008).

These powers were subsequently implemented when the government threatened to reinstate the indictment if BMS did not remove its chief executive for his role in an aborted contract with a generic company. This contract would have delayed the introduction of a generic competitor to one of BMS's best-selling drugs and led to a criminal antitrust investigation. While any connection between channel stuffing and price fixing was doubtful, BMS's sole remedy was to plead its case before the government in an environment devoid of the most rudimentary procedural protections (Wharton, 2005).

BMS is not the only instance of the government concluding corporate criminal investigations through DPAs. The government entered DPAs with the leading five artificial joint providers over kickbacks under which physicians accepted consulting fees in return for recommending their medical products. Biomet, DePuy Orthopaedics, Johnson & Johnson's Stryker, Smith & Nephew, and Zimmer paid a combined $311 million fine and agreed to implement compliance programs with federal monitoring (Spivack & Raman, 2008).

COMPLIANCE PROGRAMS

A first step in making tough choices about health care expenditures is the establishment of good compliance programs. Good compliance is based on the uncorruptible leadership of providers, characterized by independence and uncompromised medical judgments. When the medical judgments of providers become compromised by financial incentives and there is no true independence between the two, the outsider and the insider become one and the same, thus violating the cardinal rule that "no man is allowed to be a judge in his own cause" (Madison, 2005).

Uncompromised medical judgments include shared decision-making and shared responsibilities for compliance with the financial incentives appearing in the health care system's reimbursement systems. Today, rather than two independent entities sharing compliance in the nation's health care system, the medical judgments of providers have become commingled with the decision-making of reimbursement systems and the two have often become indistinguishable, thereby corrupting both in one too many instances.

Best Practices

Providers with effective compliance programs in place may receive reduced sentences after a conviction for health care fraud or the government may defer prosecution. Well-designed compliance programs elicit treatment that is more lenient if they incorporate some of the following best practices:

- Independent and empowered governing boards
- Transparent decision-making by executive management with open lines of communication
- Checks and balances with internal monitoring and audits of the reimbursement and expenditure processes
- Written policies and procedures documenting what practices may be illegal or potentially fraudulent
- Accountability, written codes of conduct, and ethics standards for providers, as well as the contractors, subcontractors, and suppliers
- Disciplinary guidance by compliance officers and compliance committees
- Aggressive clawback provisions to keep everyone accountable
- Compliance training and education that empowers providers to properly exercise independent judgment
- Regular independent compliance audits to ensure the adopted codes and standards are being followed

Provider Disclosures

Good governance standards are essential for providers. While the regulatory standards imposed are generally viewed as useful, there are downsides as well. On the affirmative side, there has been a tremendous amount of behavioral change in the wake of the anti-kickback laws. A culture of personal responsibility in the health industry has been driven in far more deeply by HIPAA, FCA, and Stark.

Many welcome the greater discipline forced on the reimbursement system by these laws, resulting in more consistency and greater transparency in patient reimbursement claims. Nevertheless, there is no substitute for honesty (Wharton, 2005). The focus on health care compliance may have come at a significant price. Some providers are devoting too much time to reputational risk and too little on medical innovation (Epstein, 2006).

While the government usurped the role of some providers in monitoring compliance programs, the pendulum is already swinging the other way (Useem, 2005). Responsibility is being shifted back to providers. To that end, many providers are redoubling their efforts to:

- Master the complexity of reimbursement systems
- Discover "creativity" in financial reporting
- Understand the tough compliance choices they must make

Not all health care fraud violations are the result of willful misconduct. When federal and state reimbursement laws conflict, providers must often select which high-risk regulations they will comply with and which lower-risk regulations they may ignore. Regulations are continually changing, as a result, compliance choices may become rapidly outdated or inadequate, depending upon how a provider is operating in a shifting marketplace. Despite such downsides, disclosure practices are helping spread consistent business practices throughout the health industry.

Governance Responsibilities

There are a number of practical steps for improving governance in any health care system. With intensifying demands on governing boards to take greater responsibility for tough decisions, boards face pressure to become more involved in day-to-day management decisions. There are at least two areas of concerted action for boards, and a host of steps for good compliance within each of the two:

- Setting reimbursement strategies
- Overseeing compliance and risk

(Useem, 2005)

Setting Reimbursement Strategies

While board directors cannot be expected to understand the overall strategy of the U.S. health care system of which their providers are only one part, they should be aware of the principles underlying their providers' business models. Directors are obligated to make a good faith effort to do their jobs and understand the financial interests they are charged with protecting. To build their understanding of reimbursement systems, directors might ask management the following questions:

- How does the provider make money?
- Where does its cash flow come from, and where is it going?
- How is the provider ranked compared to its competitors?
- Is the provider doing better or worse than its competitors are doing and why?
- How is the provider going to innovate, what is expected in terms of innovation, and can the provider afford to innovate at the projected pace it is envisioning?
- Is the provider living within its means?
- How well does bad news reach the governing board, and what can be done to improve its upward flow?

(Useem, 2005)

If board directors do not fully comprehend the chief executive's answers to their questions, the questions should all be asked again. Directors who allow others to make major decisions, without board supervision or oversight, may no longer defend themselves from personal liability for provider fraud based on their lack of knowledge (Wharton, 2005).

Overseeing Compliance and Risk

Holding board directors personally liable for failures to detect fraud has intensified the need for governing boards to be particularly vigilant in the areas of compliance and risk. For the moment, only small adjustments can be expected in implementation of the safe harbor provisions. Therefore, directors must learn to use the provisions in health care fraud laws to their advantage, especially laws that require providers to assess and guarantee their internal controls over reimbursement systems. By driving the health care fraud principles deeply into all aspects of the health industry, reimbursements that are more reliable might occur (see Useem, 2005).

The personal liability faced by directors is increasingly of concern and requires special attention. If individuals are preoccupied with minimizing personal risk and protecting their own assets against litigation, they may come to focus too much on private concerns and too little on health care innovations (Epstein, 2006).

Four steps are required for effective oversight of compliance and risk:

- Board directors should become more deeply engaged with strategic plans and executive decisions
- The audit committee of governing boards should accept full responsibility for overseeing audit issues so the remainder of the board can devote its time to other pressing reimbursement issues
- Governing boards should consider creating an operating exposure committee to focus on what could go wrong, thereby relieving the audit committee and the full board of this essential but difficult task
- Governing boards must insist on high ethical standards so everyone at all levels will recognize and eradicate conduct that cannot be legally justified, or conflicts with the law

(Wharton, 2005)

Moral Dilemmas

1. Does the health industry respond promptly enough to detected health care fraud?

2. Does the health industry voluntarily undertake effective corrective actions when problems are detected?

CONFUSION

The entire concept of why the government ever needs to threaten indictment of providers is confusing. Whether use of the doctrines of vicarious liability for criminal conduct in a corporate context gives government unwarranted and arbitrary power over the health industry is an issue vigorously debated.

Providers are just individuals tied together by an elaborate network of agreements and formal contracts (Epstein, 2006). While the government has a vital role in prevention of health care fraud, one might ask: why not go after individual wrongdoers the conventional, time-honored way, by careful investigations and skilled prosecution? One reason could be that DPAs allow the government to impose substantial reforms on the health industry without having to risk investigating and prosecuting individuals involved in health care fraud. Another reason is providers operating under DPAs usually bear the costs of any ongoing compliance programs and federal monitoring, thereby enabling the government to shift its resources toward investigating other providers.

Health Care Fraud on Trial

The high-profile DPAs negotiated by government prosecutors have focused attention on health care fraud and invited such questions as:

- What, if anything, has changed since fraud allegations started emerging against the health industry?
- Have the compliance programs the health industry has been forced to adopt served as a deterrent to individuals who might be tempted to disregard the standards of fair play?

(Wharton, 2005)

The government declared the DPAs negotiated with the five key providers in the orthopedic device industry created new compliance standards for the medical devices industry (U.S. Attorney's Office, 2007).

It may be too early to determine whether the most recent round of reform efforts addressing health care fraud (primarily the anti-kickback laws, HIPAA, FCA, and Stark Amendments) will have much impact on America's health care system. Moreover, there are limits to this compliance approach to ethics. Compliance is a hot topic, but there is perhaps inflated optimism about what good compliance programs can do (Wharton, 2005).

Simply rearranging the chairs does not prevent health care fraud. Fundamental reforms are required in the reimbursement systems of health care. Compliance systems are consistently unable to respond to a failed system of reimbursement. What is happening are *ad hoc* measures and regulations by the government and private insurers to try to deal with the emerging, growing, and increasingly severe problem of allocating limited financial resources in the health care sectors. Solutions to health care fraud must get at the heart of fraud—financial resources—and it really requires the emergence of a new set of actors with a new set of ideas. The wrangling over health care fraud involves a kind of closed group of actors that are part of the reimbursement problem; no new ideas are being brought forward. More regulations are continually being proposed to control reimbursement systems without changing the rules of the game first. The rules of the reimbursement game should be fundamentally changed in terms of health care system relationships before more regulations are injected into compliance programs. It is only with rule changes as a prerequisite that compliance programs will affect reimbursement systems. To the extent anyone believes compliance programs can completely prevent health care fraud, they may be disillusioned.

Moral Dilemmas

1. Are the primary sources of guidance from the health industry and government too mechanical or are they an effective means of defining health care compliance?

2. Are the fundamental elements of the health industry's compliance programs effective?

Cat-and-Mouse Compliance Games

A simple review of American history tells us fraud has always existed. In every fraud, several common factors are found, including risk-taking and competition. Yet risk-taking and competition are the very aspects of health care the government tries to regulate (Skeel, 2005). In the process, an elaborate reimbursement game of cat-and-mouse developed.

While government regulations are necessary, government is far removed from what is going on in detail inside the health industry. In all of the recent major scandals, the providers in question had elaborate corporate compliance programs in place. Future safe harbor regulations, fraud alerts, bulletins, and other guidance statements would likely just be more of the same. As rules pile up, providers tend to become increasingly bogged down with technicalities. Providers end up spending very little time focusing on the bigger picture of simply asking what is right and wrong (Wharton, 2005). Imagine what Hippocrates would say if there were only one reimbursement rule: "do no evil." Picture the government enforcing this rule.

For too long, a mythology has been fostered that codes of ethics and training about compliance would somehow prevent major frauds from ever occurring. There is abundant evidence that this simply does not work (Wharton, 2005).

From the legal perspective, there is a similar trap. As the push to prosecute health care cases in criminal, rather than civil, courts grows, providers will do whatever they can to avoid difficulty. While it may seem that the prospect of facing imprisonment and personal liability for fraudulent actions would keep providers on the straight and narrow, it can also encourage a kind of interpretation and implementation of the rules and regulations to remain just barely on the right side of the law. The line between civil and criminal law is quite fine, and often comes down to criminal intent, or willfulness (Wharton, 2005).

Icarus in the Health Care Industry

Fraud is not unique to the health industry, but something about the scientifically advanced U.S. medical institutions, with their elaborate systems of specialized knowledge and rules of behavior, allows fraud to happen more easily. There is a fascination with risk-taking. Greek mythology and the story of Icarus illustrate an important aspect of health care fraud. Icarus, while enjoying his newfound freedom, ignores his father's warnings and flies too close to the sun, finally melting his wings and dropping into the sea (Skeel, 2005).

It is a cautionary tale. The advanced technologies in American medicine are based on an individual's willingness to strap on wings and fly free, but people who are willing to take this kind of risk are also often the same people who refuse to heed warning signs of danger ahead. The U.S. rightly prides itself on the competitiveness of its health industry, but competition increases the odds of spectacular mistakes and failures (Wharton, 2005).

Perhaps it is simply too difficult to legislate a general sense of ethics and morality. Newly enacted health care reforms intended to control reimbursement systems, such as the anti-kickback laws, HIPAA, FCA, and Stark, are positive. Reimbursement systems do need to be carefully structured and monitored. For instance, financial incentives only for patient referrals or use of medical products are recipes for disaster. However, whether this structural reform should be a new goal for federal criminal law is not clear (Garrett, 2007).

Many in the health industry would like to see greater emphasis placed on certain aspects normally outside the scope of compliance. For example, a provider's culture is critically important. Some providers pride themselves on their integrity by focusing on the bigger picture, they simply ask, what is right and what is wrong?

Whether the purpose of fraud laws and regulations should be not to punish, but instead to change corporate cultures through compliance measures, is controversial (Henning, 2007). The truth is that there is only so much to gain from compliance programs. As the wise have always said, most people are honest, and they are even more honest when you watch them!

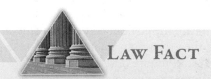 **LAW FACT**

GOVERNMENT REIMBURSEMENT SYSTEMS

When does the use of regulatory loopholes constitute fraud?

Federal audits of state Medicaid and SCHIP reimbursement systems resulted in twenty-nine states modifying their reconciliation practices since 2003. In 2007, attempts were made to make the reimbursement changes permanent through formal standards. The federal government would only pay for services and medical products actually received by Medicaid and SCHIP beneficiaries.

Most of the fifty state governors opposed this regulatory change, warning about cuts to the American social safety net, a net that costs U.S. taxpayers almost $156 billion a year. Congress prohibited enforcement of the federal regulations by slipping a regulatory moratorium into the Iraq-war-funding bill. Eventually a deal was reached to extend the regulatory moratorium in return for allocating an additional $25 million to combat health care fraud. Now, government anti-fraud forces watch and investigate after

(continues)

(continued)

state reimbursement systems have paid providers. The right word for this type of money laundering is fraud; a corporation caught in this kind of self-dealing, or inflating reimbursements to extract billions in federal funds and then laundering the money, would be indicted.

—Zhang, 2008; Zhang, 2008a; Zhang, 2008b; GAO, 2006; GAO, 2005.

CHAPTER SUMMARY

- Because the U.S. health industry is based broadly on many of the same principles of American democracy, it is important to uphold high ethical standards by prohibiting excessive influence from the prospect of financial gains.
- It is exceedingly difficult to define, measure, or regulate against health care fraud, as it exists in near-infinite forms.
- Government health programs are particularly subject to health care fraud due to their sheer size and generous funds.
- The horde of complex federal regulations prohibiting health care fraud make it difficult for many health care entities to comply due to lack of legal expertise and conflicts and ambiguities within the laws themselves.
- Criminal repercussions usually arise from violations in anti-kickback prohibition laws, which are extremely broad and encompass seemingly innocuous behavior at times.
- To convict for violations of the anti-kickback law, the government must show providers: (1) knowingly and willfully (2) solicited or received payment (including kickbacks, bribes, or rebates, as well as the transfer of anything of value) (3) in return for, or to induce, patient referrals; sanctions include fines, imprisonment, and/ or exclusion from federal health programs.
- There are over twenty-five exceptions, or safe harbors, to the anti-kickback law that prevent liability for nonfraudulent conduct; each exception has detailed requirements for qualification.
- HIPAA increases the federal government's power to investigate and punish health care fraud.
- Civil repercussions under the Stark Amendments exist for physicians whose conduct is meant to serve their own financial self-interests.
- To be successful under a Stark Amendment claim, the government must prove: (1) a financial relationship between the health care entity and the doctor, (2) the doctor referred the patient to the entity, (3) the entity submitted a claim for the patient's services, and (4) there is no applicable safe harbor exception.
- Unlike for anti-kickback prohibition violations, there is no intent requirement for a Stark Amendment violation; strict liability is imposed if the four criteria are met.
- Like the anti-kickback prohibition law, there are exceptions for some financial relationships and arrangements.
- Sanctions for Stark Amendment violations include non-reimbursement for claims, liability for claims that were already reimbursed, fines for each claim violation, each prohibited cross-referral arrangement, and for each day reporting requirements were not complied with, as well as exclusion from federal health care programs.
- It is possible to comply with the Stark Amendments while in violation of the anti-kickback law, and vice versa.
- The False Claims Act allows for criminal liability when the government can prove a provider knowingly and intentionally submitted a false claim for reimbursement for services or medical products.
- Sanctions for False Claims Act violations include fines, treble damages, imprisonment, exclusion from federal health care programs, injunctive relief freezing assets, asset forfeitures, and adoption of government-supervised compliance programs.
- The False Statements Act allows for criminal liability when the government can prove a provider knowingly and willfully submitted a false, material claim for reimbursement to a federal health care program or government intermediary related to an entity that receives federal funds or is subject to federal regulation or supervision; sanctions include fines and imprisonment.

- Use of the mail or interstate wire communication to perpetuate fraud subjects providers to fines, imprisonment, and exclusion from federal health care programs; the government need only meet a minimal burden to successfully prosecute under these provisions.
- Providers with well-designed compliance programs in place may receive lesser sanctions or deferred prosecution in return for the opportunity to address the problem and in order to prevent the imposition of sanctions.
- Despite the potential drawbacks of compliance programs (the complexity of complying with conflicting federal and state laws, the incentive to develop "creative" ways around the regulations, and the difficult choice providers face regarding which regulations to comply with because of the impossibility of complying with conflicting laws), such programs are spreading consistency and transparency in compliance practices throughout the health industry.
- Providers' boards of directors can improve compliance by setting reimbursement strategies, overseeing compliance and risk, and structuring the board properly.
- Government can act against health care fraud through criminal, civil, and administrative means; the newest tool in the government's arsenal is qui tam claims, or whistleblower claims, which unfortunately often tend to be non-meritorious.
- The current crop of anti-fraud laws aimed at health care is perhaps so complex and overwhelming that many are questioning whether it works to prevent fraud or actually works to encourage it by motivating providers to find ways of avoiding liability through questionable interpretation of the regulations.

LAW NOTES

1. The federal government won or negotiated approximately $2.2 billion in judgments and settlements in 2006 for fraud, while the Medicare Trust Fund received additional transfers of approximately $1.5 billion. Further:
   - U.S. Attorney Offices opened 836 new criminal health care fraud investigations involving 1,448 potential defendants
   - Federal prosecutors had 1,677 health care fraud criminal investigations pending, involving 2,713 potential defendants, and filed criminal charges in 355 cases involving 579 defendants
   - A total of 547 defendants were convicted for health care fraud-related crimes
   - The DOJ opened 915 new civil health care fraud investigations and had 2,016 civil health care fraud investigations pending

   (HHS & DOJ, 2008)
2. First-tier contractor refers to the first level of downstream income from an MCO; downstream income may run from the MCO through the first-tier contractor to subcontractors. First-tier contractors may also be referred to as primary contractors.
3. General criminal fraud laws include: Conspiracy to commit offense or to defraud the U.S., 18 U.S.C.A. § 371 (1994); Illegal remunerations (kickbacks), 42 U.S.C.A. § 1320a-7b(b) (2006); Laundering of monetary instruments, 18 U.S.C.A. § 1956 (2008); Racketeer Influenced and Corrupt Organizations Act (RICO), 18 U.S.C.A. §§ 1961-1968 (2009). The Travel Act, 18 U.S.C.A. § 1952 (2002) and the Public Contract Anti-Kickback Act (PCAKA), 41 U.S.C.A. § 53 (1986), have also been used.
4. Channel stuffing refers to the practice of inflating sales by inducing wholesalers to increase their purchases before they would in the normal course of purchasing medical products based on demand. If accounts receivables are accelerating much more quickly than revenues, channel stuffing is the likely reason. While this type of arbitrage is permissible, the gray area in accounting arose when BMS agreed to pay the wholesalers' carrying costs for the excess inventory and then guaranteed them a return on their investment until the medical products sold.
5. Drug wholesalers' pricing and inventory strategies are similar to what BMS did. Providers like McKesson, AmerisourceBergen, and Cardinal Health make a percentage of their revenue by arbitrage. They purchase more than they need before a manufacturer's price increase and then sell the same drugs at a markup after the manufacturer's price increase. When this practice becomes excessive and crosses the line is the issue; it is a gray area of aggressive accounting. The practice has the potential, however, to benefit end-consumers by giving wholesalers the flexibility to offer discounts to their retailers. Drug wholesalers traditionally charged retailers a percentage of the drugs shipped and bundled a host of services without additional charge (for packaging, distribution, inventory analysis and control). From the wholesaler's perspective, the rebate

for buying unneeded inventory was a cash flow unrelated to any particular sale. After BMS, fee-for-service pricing for the bundled services has generally replaced the rebate/discount/price hike model. Now, bundled services are often more profitable than the core distribution business itself. Since drug wholesalers still subtract rebates from the cost of inventory and recognize them as products sold without specifying the amounts, the end result remains unchanged.

CHAPTER BIBLIOGRAPHY

Allen, K. G., Director, Health Care, U.S. General Accounting Office. (2007, March 1). Children's health insurance: States' SCHIP enrollment and spending experiences and considerations for reauthorization. Hearing before the House Subcommittee on Health and the House Committee on Energy and Commerce, 109th Congress, Washington, DC.

Altshuler, M. et al. (2008). Health care fraud. *American Criminal Law Review, 45*, 607-664.

Black's Law Dictionary (9th ed.). (2009). Eagan, MN: Thomson Reuters West Publishing Co. (defining fraud as a knowing misrepresentation of the truth or the concealment of a material fact to induce others to act to their detriment).

Blank, S. M. et al. (2009). Health care fraud. *American Criminal Law Review, 46*, 701-759.

CMS (Centers for Medicare & Medicaid Services). (2008). *Growth in national health expenditures projected to remain steady through 2017: Health spending growth expected to continue to outpace economic growth and growth in general inflation.* Washington, DC: U.S. Department of Health & Human Services.

Christie, C. J., & Hanna, R. M. (2006). A push down the road of good corporate citizenship: The deferred prosecution agreement between the U.S. Attorney for the District of New Jersey and Bristol-Myers Squibb Co., *American Criminal Law Review, 43*, 1032-1061 (Christie and Hanna were the U.S. Attorneys prosecuting the BMS case).

DHS (U.S. Department of Homeland Security). (2007, October). *The federal law enforcement informer: Monthly legal resource and commentary for federal law enforcement officers and agents.* Washington, DC: DHS, Federal Law Enforcement Training Center.

DOJ (U.S. Department of Justice). (2007). *Fraud statistics, overview, October 1, 1986–September 30, 2007.* Washington, DC: DOJ Civil Division.

Edelman, T. (2006, September). *Issue brief: Oversight and enforcement of Medicare Part D plan requirements: Federal role and responsibilities.* Washington, DC: Kaiser Family Foundation Medicare Policy Project.

Epstein, R. A. (2006). *Overdose: How excessive government regulation stifles pharmaceutical innovation.* New Haven, CT: Yale University Press.

FBI (Federal Bureau of Investigation). (2008). *Financial crimes report to the public, fiscal year 2007.* Washington, DC: FBI (estimating the losses due to health care fraud as high as 10 percent of all health care expenditures, $226 billion year).

Fuhrmans, V. (2008, May 5). Medical specialties hit by a growing pay gap: Shortages develop in endocrinology, pediatric fields. *Wall Street Journal,* A1.

GAO (General Accounting Office). (2006). *Medicaid and SCHIP financial management: Steps taken to improve federal oversight but other actions needed to sustain efforts.* Washington, DC: GAO.

___. (2005). *Medicaid and SCHIP fraud and abuse: CMS's commitment to helping states safeguard program dollars is limited.* Washington, DC: GAO.

Garrett, B. L. (2007). Structural reform prosecution. *Virginia Law Review, 93*, 853-956.

Harshbarger, S., & Jois, G. U. (2007). Looking back and looking forward: Sarbanes-Oxley and the future of corporate governance. *Akron Law Review, 40*, 1-53.

Henning, P. J. (2007). The organizational guidelines: R.I.P.? *Yale Law Journal Pocket Part, 116*, 312-316.

HHS (U.S. Department of Health & Human Services) & DOJ (U.S. Department of Justice). (2008). *Health care fraud and abuse control program annual report for FY 2006.* Washington, DC: HHS & DOJ.

Hubbell, T. D. et al. (2005). Health care fraud. *American Criminal Law Review, 43*, 603-661.

Madison, J. (2005). *The Federalist Papers, No. 10.* New York, NY: Cosimo Classics (Original publication 1787).

Medicare vulnerabilities: Payments for claims tied to deceased doctors. (2008, July 17). Hearing before the Subcommittee on Investigations of the Senate Committee on Homeland Security and Governmental Affairs, 110th Congress, Washington, DC.

McGuire, D., & Scheider, M. (2007). Health care fraud. *American Criminal Law Review, 44*, 633-692.

Morse, M. A. & Wolff, P. S. (2009). Fraud Enforcement and Recovery Act of 2009, strengthens federal False Claims Act. *Lawyers Journal, 11*, 5-11.

NHCAA (National Health Care Anti-Fraud Association). (2008). *The problem of health care fraud: Consumer alert: The impact of health care fraud on you!* Washington, DC: NHCAA (estimating 3 percent of all health care spending, or $68 billion, is lost to health care fraud).

OIG (Office of Inspector General), U.S. Department of Health & Human Services. (2008). *Special Advisory Opinion OIG 08-07: Offering gifts and other inducements to beneficiaries.* Washington, DC: OIG.

___. (1998). *Advisory Opinion OIG 98-19.* Washington, DC: OIG.

Oretga, A. (2008). Recent development in health law: select recent court decisions. *American Journal of Law & Medicine, 34*, 585-587.

Ostas, D. T. (2007). When fraud pays: Executive self-dealing and the failure of self-restraint. *American Business Law Journal, 44*, 571-601.

Reiss, J. B. et al. (2008). Your business in court 2007-2008. *Food & Drug Law Journal, 63*, 753-798.

Rich, M. (2008). Prosecutorial indiscretion: Encouraging the Department of Justice to rein in out-of-control qui tam litigation under the civil False Claims Act. *University of Cincinnati Law Review, 76*, 1233-1277.

Saul Ewing. (2006). *Bulletin: The Justice Department revises guidelines for charging providers with crimes*. Philadelphia, PA: Saul Ewing.

Schindler, D.S. (2009). Pay for performance, quality of care and the revitalization of the False Claims Act. *Health Matrix, 19*, 387-422.

Shell, G. R. (2006). *Bargaining for advantage: Negotiation strategies for reasonable people* (2nd ed.). New Providence, NJ: Penguin.

Skeel, D. (2005). *Icarus in the boardroom: The fundamental flaws in corporate America and where they came from*. New York, NY: Oxford University Press U.S.

Smith, R. H. (2007). A key time for qui tam: The False Claims Act and Alabama. *Alabama Law Review, 58*, 1199-1214.

Spivack, P., & Raman, S. (2008). Regulating the "new regulators": Current trends in deferred prosecution agreements. *American Criminal Law Review, 45*, 159-190.

Useem, M. (2005). Global governance: The view from the 2005 World Economic Forum in Davos, Switzerland. *Leadership Newsletter, 2*.

U.S. Attorney's Office, District NJ. (2007, September 27). *Press release: Five providers in hip and knee replacement industry avoid prosecution by agreeing to compliance rules and monitoring* (stating compliance with the federal law by the medical devices industry going forward is the key element of these DPAs).

Wachino, V., & Rudowitz, R. (2006, July). *Key issues and opportunities: Implementing the new Medicaid and SCHIP integrity program*. Washington, DC: Kaiser Commission on Medicaid & the Uninsured.

Wharton (Wharton School at the University of Pennsylvania). (2005). Corporate fraud on trial: What have we learned? *Knowledge@Wharton*.

Zhang, J. (2008, August 26). Medicare ignored its claims policy, audit says. *Wall Street Journal*, p. A3.

___. (2008a, July 9). Medicare is hit by dead-physician billing scams; Senate report says false claims could top $100 million. *Wall Street Journal*, p. A4.

___. (2008b, May 19). Medicaid and SCHIP money laundering. *Wall Street Journal*, p. A14.

CHAPTER 4

ANTITRUST AND REGULATION OF HEALTH CARE PROVIDERS

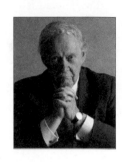

"If a firm has been 'attempting to exclude rivals on some basis other than efficiency,' it is fair to characterize its behavior as predatory."

—ROBERT H. BORK, HUDSON INSTITUTE AND HOOVER INSTITUTION,
FORMER U.S. SOLICITOR GENERAL AND FORMER CIRCUIT JUDGE OF THE
U.S. COURT OF APPEALS FOR THE DISTRICT OF COLUMBIA CIRCUIT

IN BRIEF

This chapter addresses how antitrust regulations influence hospitals and managed care. Often what makes good business sense conflicts with Americans' antitrust ideals. Antitrust rules and regulations can be difficult to understand and comply with, as the law only sanctions certain kinds of anticompetitive behavior and can be fairly nuanced as far as who is protected and who has standing to sue when wronged by monopolies and conspiracies in restraint of trade. Ideally, American antitrust laws should be based upon concrete wrongful conduct, and should not force the health care industry to adopt defensive, cumbersome business practices that actually impede their ability to compete.

FACT OR FICTION

PRICE FIXING BY PHARMACY BENEFIT MANAGERS

Are the purchases of pharmacy benefit managers (PBMs) a restraint of trade?

North Jackson, an independent community pharmacy, sued Caremark, a PBM, for violating antitrust laws in its efforts to negotiate reduced prices on behalf of its employers, health insurers, and other third-party payers of prescription drugs, as well as for price fixing with other PBMs. Independent pharmacies are forced into a choice between being included in PBM networks and accepting low reimbursement rates or leaving the PBM network and losing access to the large volume of business that such inclusion brings.

Caremark administers prescription drug benefit plans and helps control the cost of prescription drugs by creating a network of community pharmacies where subscribers can purchase discounted drugs. Caremark also lowers costs by processing claims, maintaining patient records, creating and managing formularies (lists of drugs preferred by a given plan), and negotiating discounts or rebates with drug manufacturers that want their drugs included on plan formularies. North Jackson entered into an agreement with Caremark to dispense prescription drugs to subscribers; in return for inclusion in Caremark's network, North Jackson must agree to dispense drugs to Caremark subscribers at a discount from prices charged to its cash-paying customers. Such discounted prices are usually determined using a formula based on a drug's average wholesale price plus a dispensing fee. North Jackson objects to Caremark's creation of community pharmacy networks and its negotiation of reimbursement rates. This lawsuit maintained Caremark's negotiation of low reimbursement rates was not a negotiation, but was instead a form of coercion that resulted from an illegal conspiracy to fix drug prices between and among Caremark and other PBMs and the third-party payers they represented.

—*North Jackson Pharmacy, Inc. v. Caremark Rx, Inc.,* 385 F.Supp.2d 740
(U.S. District Court for the Northern District of Illinois, Eastern Division 2005).
(See *Law Fact* at the end of this chapter for the answer.)

PRINCIPLES AND APPLICATIONS

The increasingly complex U.S. antitrust laws are commonly referred to as competition laws outside the U.S. (Bork, 1978, 2008). In theory, in a free enterprise system, the health care industry could direct its limited resources to the uses that would best satisfy patients with minimum intervention by the government. Of course, when the government pays for more than half of the health care provided in the U.S., with the remaining care regulated by government (McHugh, 2008), it is clear why the concept of free enterprise is totally theoretical in today's marketplace. Free enterprise in health care exists only in theory; it does not exist in reality.

When competition is stifled, the long arm of government antitrust enforcement should replace the invisible hand of the market as the regulator of dealings among health care providers and between providers and patients (Areeda & Hovenkamp, 2005). The court decisions described in this chapter contain some of the rules of the competitive game in which health care providers are the players, courts are the referees, and patients are the spectators.

In theory, in a competitive market comprised of integrated health care systems, the system that provided the best quality care for particular diseases would treat all the patients in a specific region diagnosed with certain diseases because no one else could obtain the treatment outcomes that this given health care system could. All the specialists in the region treating these diseases would be affiliated with this health care system because of its stellar patient care and reputation. Increased system specialization would drive efficiencies and medical costs downward. All the employers, health insurers, and other third-party payers would encourage patients in the region with certain diseases to utilize this health care system because of its treatment outcomes, innovative care, and prices for medical services (*see* Porter & Teisberg, 2006). None of this would violate any antitrust laws because no one else would be treating patients as well as this particular health care system.

After this health care system became the only provider in the region for treating specified diseases, antitrust law would prevent this system from artificially raising its prices for medical services once it monopolized treatment for particular disease states. In other words, an innocent health care monopoly obtained by merit, by providing the best quality patient care, is perfectly legal. Actions to create a coercive monopoly or dealings to artificially preserve the system's status as a monopoly would be illegal.

The purpose of antitrust law is to balance potential pro-competitive benefits against potential anti-competitive effects (Areeda & Hovenkamp, 2005). Antitrust law does not penalize health care providers who dominate their markets on their own merit, only those that intentionally dominate the market through wrongful conduct. Whenever antitrust violations are alleged to have arisen, except for per se violations, the government analyzes this competitive balancing on a case-by-case basis. Often it comes down to the government and the courts weighing what constitutes competition in today's health care markets and then deciding how best to maximize social welfare, in other words, answering the question of how high-quality, affordable health care can be made most accessible to all U.S. residents.

DEFENSIBLE THEORIES OF WRONGFUL CONDUCT

Antitrust cases brought against health care providers should be tightly tied to defensible theories of wrongful conduct (Epstein, 2007). Antitrust laws justifiably:

- Prohibit actions restricting competition, including unwinding the domination of multi-hospital health care systems in geographic regions of the country that have come to control health care in their markets and then have come to abuse their market powers by setting artificially high prices for medical care, accompanied by overly aggressive billing and collection procedures
- Ban wrongful conduct by health care systems dominating a geographic market, such as hospitals paying nurses below-market wages and benefits while artificially holding down staffing levels as the need for more nurses increases with the rising acuity level of hospital patients, as opposed to legitimate staffing levels based on patient needs with clinically accepted nurse-patient ratios
- Prevent anticompetitive practices that tend to lead to dominant positions in health care markets, including refusal to grant hospital privileges to physicians who refer patients to competing health care providers, as opposed to refusing hospital privileges to physicians who own interests in competing facilities, which is a legitimate competitive action by a competing hospital

- Observe the mergers and acquisitions of dominant health care systems, including joint ventures and strategic alliances that may threaten the competitive delivery of medical services and prohibit such actions altogether, or approve them subject to remedies such as an obligation to divest part of the merged health care delivery business

Antitrust remedies should not force the health care industry to adopt business practices and structural reorganizations that substantially impede the ability of providers to compete effectively (Epstein, 2007). For instance:

- Requiring brand pharmaceuticals to allow their generic competitors access to its patented molecules is not the same as regulating the drug industry
- Mandating 1,170 codes for angioplasty will not ensure the medical products industry is not overcharging hospitals for their advanced surgical stent products (Zhang, 2008)
- Prohibiting health insurers from practicing individual price discrimination in establishing premium prices (thereby encouraging preventable diseases and illnesses), while requiring community ratings, is not the same as regulating health insurance
- Requiring all health care providers to provide Medicare and Medicaid the lowest market price is not regulating the provision of health care

Moral Dilemmas

1. Is access to affordable health care a just outcome of antitrust regulations in the U.S.?

2. What is competitive health care, and is a competitive health care industry an end or the means to the higher end of ensuring every U.S. resident the right to health care?

3. Is the profitability of the health care industry hostile to or contributive to its social responsibilities?

4. Should the U.S. seek to minimize the necessity of resorting to government over-regulation and burdensome restrictions on the health care industry?

5. Is wealth creation a characteristic of wealth or does it tend to create more wealth, and what role should the government play in fostering wealth creation in the health care industry?

ANALYSIS OF COMPETITION[LN1]

Antitrust law directs itself only against conduct that unfairly tends to destroy competition (Stucke, 2006).

Defining Market Share

The first step in any analysis of competition involves defining the relevant market. This definition determines whether the business conduct actually harms competition and includes:

- Describing the medical services or products
- Locating appropriate geographic boundaries in which the competitive battle occurs
- Identifying other health care providers that supply the same medical services or products or that easily could do so

(*See generally* AEI, 2009)

The next step determines how much of all the business done by the providers in the relevant market is controlled by those allegedly involved in wrongful conduct. Only then can market share begin to be defined.

Analyzing Wrongful Conduct

The purpose of antitrust laws is not to protect health care providers from competition in relevant markets; it is to protect the public from the failure of providers being able to effectively compete (Hovenkamp, 2008). There are two basic types of anticompetitive conduct that are prohibited by antitrust laws.

Monopolization

While economists generally view monopoly power as an economic inequity, dominance of a market is not in itself illegal. In fact, the paradox of antitrust is that a merger of monopolists often makes consumers better off (Bork, 2008). Nowhere is this more evident than in the nation's leading vertically integrated academic medical centers. Antitrust laws do not prohibit strong, honest competition. It is only when unfair business tactics are used to attain or maintain monopoly status that conduct becomes illegal.

To prove an attempt to monopolize, there must be evidence of specific intent to destroy competition. Intent is determined by appraising competitive tactics within the context of a health care provider's general business behavior. Individual acts and practices, when viewed in isolation, may not be indicative of anything harmful. However, a pattern of actions, each one taken alone, may reflect intent to monopolize, such as seeking enforcement of fraudulent drug patent claims or price discrimination (AEI, 2009).

Arguments about predatory litigation are staples in antitrust law. For instance, this strategy is rampant in the pharmaceutical industry where generic manufacturers often pursue private advantage by seeking to mislead administrative agencies and the courts about the scope of the drug patents they invoke, arguing that branded drugs bar more competition than they do, or they may litigate to raise branded manufacturers' costs of doing business, not caring whether they prevail. *See generally* Bork, 1978; Posner, 1973; *In re Terazosin Hydrochloride Antitrust Litigation*, 335 F.Supp.2d 1336 (U. S. District Court for the Southern District of Florida 2004).

Conspiracies in Restraint of Trade

Conspiracies require a different antitrust approach. Because relationships among competitors in the health care industry can so easily evolve into conspiracies that threaten the competitive integrity of the medical marketplace, such relationships are subject to close scrutiny (AEI, 2009). Of course, most contacts among industry competitors elicit little antitrust concern:

- Purely social contacts
- Trade and professional association memberships
- Industry-wide lobbying for favorable legislation or regulation

(Shenefield & Stelzer, 2001)

However, any agreements among competing health care providers to control prices, or divide territory, customers, patients, or markets, are inherently illegal by themselves. The prohibition of contracts, combinations, and conspiracies in restraint of trade applies to agreements between manufacturers and distributors of medical products as well as agreements between health care providers. Of course, on numerous occasions the interests of manufacturers, distributors, and providers diverge. Manufacturers, for example, may wish to set minimum prices on a medical product, while distributors might wish to use the product as a traffic-generating loss leader. As a practical matter, manufacturers can certainly provide price lists or promotional materials that specify a desired price, as long as the distributor remains free to set their own price. Setting minimum or maximum resale prices may well trigger antitrust enforcement (AEI, 2009).

MEDICAL MERGERS AND ACQUISITIONS

Antitrust law is aimed at regulating competition.[LN2] The Federal Trade Commission (FTC) sees its antitrust effort as a potentially powerful force in reining in health care costs (FTC & DOJ, 2004). The American Hospital Association reports hospital costs in the U.S. exceed $648 billion a year in 2007 (AHA, 2008). Projections are that these costs will increase by

6 percent through 2012, driven primarily by increased utilization and population growth (PriceWaterhouseCoopers, 2008).

The federal government is targeting medical mergers and acquisitions that have resulted in higher hospital costs in recent years. While the consolidation of integrated health care systems should have made the industry more competitive and antitrust policy less important, instead it appears to be producing an increase in antitrust actions. It remains to be seen whether the government will seek to block or undo mergers in the hospital field to preserve independent hospital competitors after years of concentration in the industry.

The FTC shares responsibility with the U.S. Justice Department's Antitrust Division for enforcing antitrust laws in the health arena, with the Justice Department handling most insurance matters and the FTC handling hospital and medical products issues. Cases are heard and ruled on by an FTC administrative law judge. Any appeal of this ruling goes to the full five-member FTC for a vote. Further appeals go to a federal appeals court (Wysocki, 2005).

State attorneys general are increasingly bringing lawsuits under the federal antitrust laws, in addition to enforcing state antitrust laws. Private parties are also suing in federal courts for injunctions to prohibit violations of the antitrust laws and, importantly, for triple the damages they claim to have suffered (AEI, 2009).

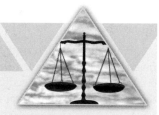

HOSPITAL MERGERS

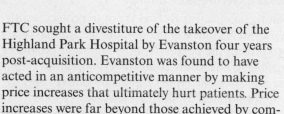

In the Matter of Evanston Northwestern Healthcare Corporation
Docket No. 9315 Opinion of the Federal Trade Commission
(2007, August 6)

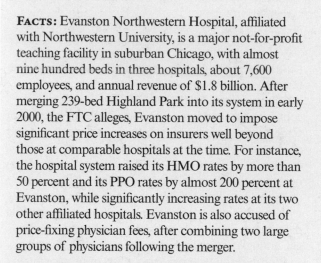

FACTS: Evanston Northwestern Hospital, affiliated with Northwestern University, is a major not-for-profit teaching facility in suburban Chicago, with almost nine hundred beds in three hospitals, about 7,600 employees, and annual revenue of $1.8 billion. After merging 239-bed Highland Park into its system in early 2000, the FTC alleges, Evanston moved to impose significant price increases on insurers well beyond those at comparable hospitals at the time. For instance, the hospital system raised its HMO rates by more than 50 percent and its PPO rates by almost 200 percent at Evanston, while significantly increasing rates at its two other affiliated hospitals. Evanston is also accused of price-fixing physician fees, after combining two large groups of physicians following the merger.

ISSUE: Did Evanston, which already operated two hospitals in suburban Chicago, use its post-merger market power with the acquisition of a third hospital to impose anticompetitive price increases on insurers and employers?

HOLDING AND DECISION: Yes, Evanston lessened hospital competition in suburban Chicago in its merger with Highland Park Hospital and therefore violated antitrust law.

ANALYSIS: Evanston acquired Highland Park in 2000; since that date, Evanston has operated the three hospitals as a single, integrated entity. The FTC sought a divestiture of the takeover of the Highland Park Hospital by Evanston four years post-acquisition. Evanston was found to have acted in an anticompetitive manner by making price increases that ultimately hurt patients. Price increases were far beyond those achieved by comparable hospitals during the same period of time.

An important factor to the FTC was the nonprofit status of Evanston, because in some previous mergers, courts pointed to hospitals' nonprofit status as a reason to let mergers go through. *See FTC v. Butterworth Health Corp.* 121 F.3d 708 (U.S. Court of Appeals for the 6th Circuit 1997) (FTC was not successful in blocking a Grand Rapids, Michigan, hospital merger based on an economic analysis that nonprofit mergers tended to reduce costs and prices; court also ruled nonprofit hospital boards, as community leaders, have an incentive to restrain prices). The FTC argued nonprofit hospitals have an incentive to maintain a surplus of revenue over expenses, and while they do not distribute these profits to shareholders, they should use them for salaries, equipment, or expansion.

The FTC had to prove its case by a process of elimination; it had to rule out other explanations, such as catch-up price increases, leaving market power as the only explanation. The FTC also found itself arguing over the proper definition of the market to determine how much concentration existed in the immediate Chicago region. Evanston

(continues)

(continued)

did not simply enable the Highland Park Hospital to compete more effectively with Evanston and Glenbrook Hospitals, by merging two financially healthy hospitals with a struggling hospital; rather, the merger lessened hospital competition in suburban Chicago. Patient alternatives for hospital care disappeared with the merger.

After a trial before an FTC administrative law judge, Evanston was ordered to divest the acquired assets of Highland Park. On appeal to the full Commission, the finding of anticompetitive actions by Evanston was affirmed, but the Commission reversed the divestiture order. Instead, the Commission found that a conduct remedy, rather than a structural remedy such as divestiture, was appropriate. The Commission ordered Evanston to establish two separate and independent teams for negotiating contracts with insurers and employers: one team for Evanston and Glenbrook Hospital, and another for Highland Park. The remedy was to be in effect for twenty years.

RULE OF LAW: The merger strategies of multiple-hospital systems that grow by acquiring neighboring hospitals will be judged and monitored for anticompetitive activities.

See In re Evanston Northwestern Healthcare, 2008 WL 2229488 (U.S. District Court for the Northern District of Illinois, Eastern Division 2008) (adjudicating five private causes of action against Evanston for its anticompetitive behavior). This case is ongoing and awaiting trial.

Pre-Merger Economics

This case against Evanston Northwestern Hospital was a high-stakes case and one of the FTC's major antitrust enforcement initiatives in health care over the last several years (Campbell, 2007). The twenty-year remedy sends a signal to large hospital systems that Evanston-type mergers are likely to face stiffer challenges and could even be blocked (Wysocki, 2005). A merger involving Inova Health System Foundation in Northern Virginia is being blocked by the FTC as it seeks to acquire a third hospital (Francis, 2008).

Since 2004, the number of hospitals involved in merger-and-acquisition deals has risen sharply with approximately two hundred hospitals being acquired or merged in the U.S. each year in transactions valued at more than $9 billion annually (Irving, 2008). In recent years, hospital and health systems have consolidated in Boston, Cleveland, Philadelphia, Salt Lake City, and Northern California, among other places (Wysocki, 2005).

For instance, Sacramento, California-based Sutter Health System, which has grown quickly by acquisition, has come under fire for its pricing policies. In 2007, the California Health Facilities Financing Authority required Sutter to contribute $8.5 million to clinics and rural hospitals before approving its $958 million bond application (BBW, 2007). The Authority was clear in stating that this bond restriction should send a message to Sutter and other nonprofit hospital borrowers that they have to take seriously their obligations to hold down the cost of patient care.

Post-Merger Hospital Pricing

The issue of post-merger hospital pricing is a controversial topic in the health care industry. The Evanston Northwestern Hospital case presented a rare opportunity to examine the actual effects of a merger on pricing in the hospital industry. Many analyses conclude hospital mergers either result in higher prices or have no effect on pricing (Posner, 2007). Before Evanston, most antitrust cases were brought pre-merger and therefore involved projections based upon economic theory.

When hospitals are nonprofit members of the community, one side of the debate views them as institutions with a strong humanitarian bent. The other side does not view the hospitals as existing on philanthropy; rather they are seen as existing based on their sales revenue and, therefore, they will exercise market power if they have the opportunity. This antitrust assault on nonprofit hospital systems occurs at a time when the hospital industry is under intensified scrutiny for misuse of its tax-exempt status. Hospitals are being criticized for charging uninsured patients the highest rates and aggressively pursuing patients for unpaid debts (Wysocki).

Moral Dilemmas

1. Is there a social mortgage on tax-exempt hospitals, in that the very existence of tax exemption is to ensure that the health care needs of every individual are met?

TERMINATION OF HOSPITAL PRIVILEGES BY PHYSICIAN-OWNERS OF SPECIALTY HOSPITAL

Arnett Physician Group, P.C. v. Greater Lafayette Health Services, Inc.
[Physicians Group v. General Hospital]
382 F.Supp.2d 1092 (U.S. District Court for the Northern District of Indiana 2005)

FACTS: The case involved contract disputes and negotiations between the Arnett Physician Group and its affiliated clinic, health plan, and HMO against the only existing general acute-care hospital in the Indiana community of Lafayette. The general hospital terminated Arnett's exclusive service contract and HMO agreement in response to the physicians' attempt to open their own specialty hospital. Twenty-one physicians subsequently left the Arnett Physician Group and became affiliated with the existing general hospital.

ISSUE: Did the general hospital unlawfully conspire with the physicians who left the Arnett Physician Group to join the hospital, and did the hospital violate antitrust law in denying the physicians who remained with Arnett access to the hospital's services?

HOLDING AND DECISION: No, staffing decisions at a single hospital cannot violate antitrust law.

ANALYSIS: The court held Arnett did not have antitrust standing resulting from a contract dispute with a single hospital. The hospital was found to have simply decided to substitute one exclusive radiology services provider for another. The hiring of physicians by the hospital did not amount to anticompetitive activity or confer antitrust standing. Further, there was no evidence connecting the hospital's termination of staff privileges by the Arnett Physician Group to their efforts to set up a competing acute-care hospital. A publicity campaign by the hospital against construction of a new hospital does not cause antitrust injury. Public expressions of opinion about competitors' plans cannot provide the basis for an antitrust claim and such conduct is clearly lawful.

RULE OF LAW: Antitrust laws protect competition, not competitors.

(*See generally* Miller).

SPECIALTY HOSPITALS

Texas and California are the states with the most specialty hospitals, followed by Louisiana and Oklahoma (GAO, 2005). While general hospitals are concerned that the number of specialty hospitals could grow rapidly, growth has been moderate and gradual.

Within their market niche, specialty hospitals are significant competitors to general acute-care hospitals. A controversial topic is the effect on general hospitals when specialty hospitals enter a market and target the most profitable patients, leaving less profitable patients to be served by general hospitals. To retaliate for loss of referrals, some general hospitals have terminated the privileges of physicians who have an ownership interest in specialty hospitals. Some physician-owners have consequently challenged such terminations in court. Stark and the anti-kickback laws generally prevent physicians from referring patients covered by government programs such as Medicare and Medicaid to hospitals in which the referring physicians have a financial relationship,

unless an exception or safe harbor applies. *See* 42 U.S.C.A. § 1395nn (2008).

Most cases like the Arnett Physician Group case have been won by the general hospitals on the basis that the markets at issue were competitive. The courts do not find it relevant whether or not physician-owners of specialty hospitals are excluded from privileges at particular general hospitals (Bartels, 2006). General hospitals are viewed as simply protecting their viability in the face of specialty hospital competition (GAO, 2005).

NURSING WAGES ANTITRUST LITIGATION

Fixing of wages may be prohibited if economic harm occurs and if it can be proved there was an agreement to fix wages. Registered nurses in five cities (Albany, Chicago, Detroit, Memphis, and San Antonio) have filed six almost identical antitrust class action lawsuits alleging that hospitals violated antitrust laws by fixing nursing wages and entering into information exchanges concerning nursing wages, resulting in lower nursing wages than would occur under market conditions (Miles, 2007).[LN3] The Service Employees International Union (SEIU) Nurse Alliance, representing more than 110,000 nurses as the nation's largest health care union, supports this antitrust litigation.

This litigation alleges that the hospitals acted as single entities paying nurses sub-competitive wages, but that they acquired the economic ability to do so as a group, despite a national nursing shortage. Specifically, the hospitals are accused of sharing non-public information about nurses' salaries and then agreeing to refrain from competing

with each other in setting nursing salaries. In addition, the litigation is examining how managed care has led hospitals to hold down nurse staffing levels, even as the average acuity level of patients has risen sharply (JCAHO, 2008).

PHYSICIAN PRIVILEGES AND CREDENTIALING

In the health care industry, private antitrust causes of action often involve physician privileges and credentialing.

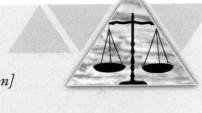

PHYSICIAN CREDENTIALING

Daniel v. American Board of Emergency Medicine
[Emergency Medicine Physicians v. Physician-Certification Organization]
428 F.3d 408 (U.S. Court of Appeals for the 2nd Circuit 2005)

FACTS: This is a class action comprised of approximately 14,000 uncertified, licensed physicians who practice emergency medicine throughout the U.S., but who did not complete formal residency training programs in emergency medicine. The non-certified physicians allege the American Board of Emergency Medicine (ABEM), the Council of Emergency Medicine Residency Directors (CORD), and the hospitals operating residency programs in emergency medicine and hiring ABEM-certified physicians colluded to restrain trade and competition in connection with the practice of emergency medicine in violation of antitrust laws. ABEM is a not-for-profit corporation that certifies physicians in emergency medicine who pass its examination. The Board is one of twenty-four medical certification boards who are members of the American Board of Medical Specialties.

ISSUE: Did ABEM and CORD manipulate the residency training requirement for emergency medicine certification to limit the number of physicians certified in order to guarantee super-competitive compensation for such physicians?

HOLDING AND DECISION: Issue never answered; non-certified emergency medicine physicians lacked standing to bring an antitrust action against physician-certification organizations.

ANALYSIS: When ABEM became a specialty board in the mid-1970s, only thirty emergency medicine residency programs existed in the U.S. In order to increase recognition of the specialty, ABEM proposed two eligibility tracks for physicians: the practice track, requiring seven thousand hours and five years of practicing or teaching emergency medicine; and the residency track, requiring completion of an approved residency training program. ABEM limited the practice track as an eligibility alternative for the first eight years. CORD is a national association that facilitates communication among the directors of emergency residency training programs.

Non-certified physicians, who would be eligible to take the ABEM exam if the practice track still existed, maintained that by closing the practice track and placing a premium on ABEM certification, ABEM and CORD unlawfully restrained trade and monopolized the market for certified physicians. Specifically, the non-certified physicians argued there was an attempt to limit the pool of eligible certification applicants, thus creating an artificial shortage of certified physicians, with the end goal of demanding super-competitive pay. While the American Academy of Emergency Medicine and the American Board of Osteopathic Medicine certify physicians in emergency medicine

(continues)

(continued)

and while ABEM certification is not required to practice emergency medicine in any state, the non-certified physicians asserted:

- ABEM certification is the most prestigious certification
- Leading hospitals only hire ABEM-certified physicians
- Most hospitals base compensation and promotion decisions on ABEM certification
- Non-ABEM certified physicians receive less salary than ABEM-certified physicians

Furthermore, non-certified physicians claimed they were denied positions solely by reason of not being certified and some were discharged, demoted, and assigned to undesirable work situations due to the lack of certification. Finally, it was asserted that CORD had an unfair interest in keeping the formal residency training as the only required path to ABEM certification.

In finding the non-certified physicians lacked standing, the court noted that even if private parties are injured by violations of antitrust laws, the party must still have standing to bring an antitrust claim. The court focused on two relevant factors for determining standing: the alleged antitrust injury and efficient enforcement of the antitrust claims.

First, the non-certified physicians alleged financial injury due to ABEM restricting the number of eligible physicians that take the certification exam, which in turn limits the number of such physicians and allows the certified physicians to charge higher costs. However, the non-physicians' injury was not that certified physicians commanded super-competitive salaries; their injury was their inability to do likewise. They never alleged they would have received the same pay but for ABEM's domination of the market. Rather, the non-certified physicians sued to restore the practice track as an alternative to residency training so they could qualify for the ABEM certification examination. The court ruled the non-certified physicians could not state an antitrust injury when their purpose was to join the cartel rather than disband it.

Second, the non-certified physicians were not the best enforcers for an antitrust violation; they had no interest in reducing the cost of emergency medical care. The relief they sought was to gain entry into an exclusive arrangement in order to share in the super-competitive salaries made possible by ABEM exclusivity.

RULE OF LAW: The inability of uncertified emergency medicine physicians, or would-be competitors, to command the same competitive salaries as certified physicians did not constitute an antitrust injury because, by requesting an injunction to temporarily restore the practice track so that they could qualify for certification, they sought to join the cartel.

(See generally Perry, 2007).

While the Second Circuit did not determine whether closing the practice track was an antitrust violation, the court noted that health insurers, and not physicians, would be best enforcers of any certification actions. The government and private health insurers, who compensate hospitals for most emergency care, have a direct and undivided economic interest in reducing the costs of emergency medical care.

EXCLUSIVE DEALING

Exclusive dealing, also known as tying or vertical integration, of contracting has received considerable attention in the health care industry with regard to competitive pricing of medical services and products. In its simplest form, an exclusive dealing arrangement is a contract restricting health care providers from acquiring medical products from any other manufacturer. The related practice of market share discounts, which reward health care systems for purchasing relatively more of a particular brand product, and bundled rebates also have the effect of impeding health care efficiency. While it is not illegal for manufacturers to agree to minimum prices, such agreements must be examined case by case for possible antitrust violations *(see generally* Lewis, 2006).

Moral Dilemmas

1. Is charging high super-competitive prices for medical products and services morally wrong?

EXCLUSIVE DEALING

United States v. Dentsply International, Inc.
[Government v. Manufacturer of Medical Products]
399 F.3d 181 (U.S. Court of Appeals for the 3rd Circuit 2005)

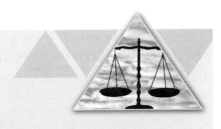

FACTS: Dentsply manufactured and sold artificial teeth for use in dentures and other restorative appliances to dental products dealers. The dealers, in turn, supplied the teeth and various other materials to dental laboratories, which fabricated dentures for sale to dentists. Dentsply excluded competitors from the artificial teeth market by prohibiting its authorized dealers from handling competitors' teeth, a policy designed to exclude its rivals from access to dealers. At the time of the antitrust action, the manufacturer controlled approximately 75 to 80 percent of the prefabricated teeth market in the U.S.

ISSUE: Can manufacturers of medical products prevent independent dealers from selling the products of other manufacturers?

HOLDING AND DECISION: No, manufacturers of medical products cannot lawfully maintain a monopoly over their products through exclusivity policies that prevent independent dealers from selling other manufacturers' products.

ANALYSIS: The Third Circuit found Dentsply had monopoly power in the relevant market of both sales to the laboratories and dental dealers. This market share was more than adequate to establish a prima facie case of market power. In addition, Dentsply's actions demonstrated its intent to exclude competitors and maintain monopolistic power by successfully prohibiting dealers from handling competitors' teeth. Another indication of Dentsply's market power was its control of prices, which it was able to set without consideration of its competitors' prices, something that a firm without monopoly power would not be able to do.

In addition, Dentsply used its market power to adversely affect competition in the market by preventing dealers from carrying competitors'

teeth. The ultimate users, the dental labs that buy the teeth at the point in the process where they are incorporated into other products, also could not purchase teeth of other manufacturers, and thus could not fulfill customer requests for alternative teeth lines. These requests were denied by dealers because of fear of being cut-off by Dentsply. Although not illegal in themselves, exclusive dealing arrangements can be an improper means of maintaining a monopoly and creating a barrier to entry to competitors in the market.

Dentsply also maintained resale prices by dental labs. Dental labs purchased artificial teeth through a network of authorized dealers. If a dealer did not have the requested teeth in stock, Dentsply would drop ship teeth directly to the labs, but billing and collection services were still handled by the dealers. Although Dentsply provided a suggested price list to dealers, which ordinarily is permissible, Dentsply went a step further by requiring any deviation from the suggested prices to be cleared with Dentsply; such deviations from the suggested price were permitted only when a lab was considering buying a competitor's teeth for reasons of price. In these instances, Dentsply, not the dealers, negotiated with the labs to determine a price at which the dealer would sell the teeth to the lab. Dentsply's control of the dealer network was the crucial point in the distribution chain where monopoly power over the market was established. This monopoly resulted in teeth being purchased at artificially high prices.

RULE OF LAW: A manufacturer of medical products has prima facie monopoly power to exclude competitors when it controls 75 to 80 percent of its product market for more than ten years.

(*See generally* BNA, 2005; Kovacic, 2007; Lambert & Wright, 2008; Miller, 2006; Novak, 2006; Rosch, 2008; Popofsky, 2008; Werden, 2006; Wildfang, 2006; Zain, 2008).

USING ANTITRUST LAWS TO THWART COMPETITION

Health insurers, including government health insurance programs, can grant, limit, and condition payments to providers. While these limitations are essentially turf wars for health care dollars, they are often challenged on antitrust grounds. The American Medical, Osteopathic, and Chiropractic Associations have each attempted to restrict competition by restricting medical services of the others.

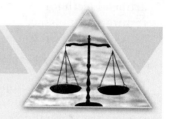

COMPETITIVE MANAGED CARE RESTRICTIONS

American Chiropractic Association, Inc. v. Leavitt
[Professional Association v. Secretary of the U.S. Department of Health & Human Services]
431 F.3d 812 (U.S. Court of Appeals for the District of Columbia 2005)

FACTS: The Medicare program subsidizes medical insurance for elderly and disabled persons. An enrollee selects a physician or obtains medical services through a managed care provider. Medicare then pays for covered care, such as a chiropractor's manual manipulation of the spine. The American Chiropractic Association (ACA), representing its chiropractic practitioners, maintained that Medicare only provides coverage when such services are performed by a chiropractor. The ACA also challenged the requirement that Medicare enrollees must obtain referrals from non-chiropractors for chiropractic corrections.

ISSUE: Does Medicare only provide coverage for spinal manipulation by chiropractors?

HOLDING AND DECISION: No, allopathic physicians and osteopathic physicians can receive Medicare reimbursement for performing spinal manipulation on Medicare beneficiaries.

ANALYSIS: The key question is whether the ACA could have its claims heard at the administrative level or if the claims could receive judicial review after channeling through the administrative system. Despite the fact that Medicare is federal legislation, claimants are prohibited from bringing claims grounded in the Medicare law directly in federal court with limited exceptions. This bar limits judicial review to claims already channeled through the administrative system; all administrative remedies must be exhausted before a claim can be brought in federal court. The only exceptions are when administrative regulations foreclose judicial review and when severe roadblocks cut off any avenue to federal courts as a practical matter.

The court determined the issue of non-chiropractor referrals could be brought at the administrative level. First, an enrollee must have the spinal manipulation performed by a chiropractor without a referral from a non-chiropractor. If health insurers then refuse to cover the service, enrollees could then file a grievance, claiming that the referral requirement was illegal under Medicare. This would then begin the administrative process, leading to judicial review. A second route could be for chiropractors to waive all rights to payment from enrollees and become their assignees, allowing chiropractors to bring the administrative challenge. The court said the minimum amount in controversy for judicial review was not a roadblock, since the amount could be met by aggregating claims. The court then analyzed standing as to whether chiropractors were the only practitioners under Medicare who could perform spinal manipulations. The court's analysis was the same as the question of the necessity of referrals from non-chiropractors.

RULE OF LAW: Federal courts are prohibited from interpreting the Medicare Act until all administrative options are exhausted.

(*See generally* Golding, 2009).

Following this case, forty-seven states now mandate health insurance coverage for spinal manipulation by chiropractors (Cogan et al., 2005). Most managed care plans, however, still require referrals from a non-chiropractor for chiropractic correction. While Medicare fee-for-service plans do not require referrals, most Medicare Advantage plans do under the guise of medical necessity.

LIFE-CYCLE MANAGEMENT OF DRUGS

Drug reformulation is one of the largest issues in antitrust and health care (Yoshitani & Cooper, 2007). It involves the use and misuse of intellectual property in the complex system of patents.

Branded drugs are generally reformulated by pharmaceutical companies to extend their patent protection. This reformulation requires a careful balance, as altering the drugs too much could result in new clinical trials through the FDA, while altering the drugs too little results in no additional patent protection. Between these two competing forces are the FDA and the U.S. Patent and Trademark Office, two federal agencies that do not often work together and whose regulations overlap and contradict one another.

Brand-name pharmaceuticals and generic manufacturers face the prisoners' dilemma: as long as any one of them can play the rigged patent game, they all have to play it. Usually there is a payment by brand-name pharmaceuticals to generics to stay off the market. That is a major antitrust concern and there are no explicit laws against this. Congress thought this would be an antitrust matter, and indeed, the FTC has recently accused a number of brand-name pharmaceuticals of paying off generic manufacturers to delay competition from generic medicines.

Certainly, both the branded and generic industries maintain this is not collusion at all, but a normal hedging of bets during litigation. While it is perfectly rational for parties in litigation to reach agreement on what the outer limits of liability would be, it raises flags. Anytime a patent holder is paying an alleged infringer, the money is flowing the wrong way and it raises flags. Of course, there are scenarios where all this is a sophisticated way of dealing with risk. Without more, this policy is not a *per se* antitrust violation, but it is disconcerting, and will likely continue to attract antitrust scrutiny (Wharton, 2002).

ANTITRUST COMPLIANCE

Almost everyone in the health care industry agrees on the need for antitrust compliance programs. Since imprisonment and multimillion-dollar fines can accompany slip-ups, it is best never to face antitrust investigations and litigation. Written policy statements, accompanied by recognized independent reference sources should be kept at employees' desks and work sites to give comprehensive compliance programs a permanence that compliance training alone cannot always claim, as well as continuous access to up-to-date online antitrust information.

There are no straightforward rules for the health care industry to follow when specific problems or questionable activities arise, since antitrust law is highly fact-specific and based on the detailed facts unique to each situation. Some basic antitrust guidelines, however, are standard:

- Join trade associations and participate in professional activities not affecting competition with fellow competitors, but never discuss business strategies, costs or service charges, or product pricing with competitors; this could result in charges of a price-fixing conspiracy (*see Drug Mart Pharmacy Corp. v. American Home Products. Corp.*, 472 F.Supp.2d 385 (U.S. District Court for the Eastern District of New York 2007))
- Never enter into agreements with competitors to stay out of each other's markets (*see* DPA, 2006)
- Never join forces with some competitors to the disadvantage and exclusion of other competitors; while some forms of cooperation, such as joint education and training activities are permissible if their main purpose is to improve competencies and industry effectiveness, other activities, especially those that deny excluded competitors access to essential information or facilities are problematic
- Aggressively and uncompromisingly compete for all business; antitrust laws do not penalize market success achieved by merit and lawful means
- Do not price services or products below some meaningful measure of cost with the intention of driving out the competition or discouraging new entrants, particularly if providers enjoy dominant market power and it is likely to seriously hurt the competition; consider the effect on competitors of any planned pricing actions and be sure that such harm is a consequence of supportable cost strategies with reliable business justifications

- Pay meaningful living wages with affordable health care benefits, particularly if providers enjoy significant market power in a high cost-of-living market or have sizeable profits with a considerable disparity between high-wage and low-wage workers, unless there is a credible business justification to do otherwise and the corresponding rationalization carries great weight with the public and government regulators (*see Unger v. Albany Med. Ctr.*, No. 06-CV-0765 (U.S. District Court for the Northern District of New York 2006))
- Suggest retail prices with distributors and dealers, but never coerce them to accept such prices on a take-it-or-leave-it basis; guide and persuade with aggressively bargained binding agreements, but do not refuse to negotiate, or intimidate or threaten (*see J.E. Pierce Apothecary, Inc. v. Harvard Pilgrim Health Care, Inc.*, 365 F.Supp.2d 119 (U.S. District Court for the District of Massachusetts 2005))
- Impose restrictions on distributors and dealers that contribute to competition with rivals; cancel non-performers, but keep credible records documenting their poor performance in case disputes arise about the circumstances
- Do not tie the sale of one product or service to another; such tying arrangements might be allowed in a few exceptional instances, but generally tying runs afoul of antitrust laws if they economically harm competitors in the tied market (*see Austrian, M.D. v. UnitedHealth Group, Inc.*, 43 Conn.L.Rptr. 852 (Superior Court of Connecticut 2007), citing *Jefferson Parish Hospital District No. 2 v. Hyde*, 466 U.S. 2 (U.S. Supreme Court 1984))
- Use exclusive dealing arrangements if business necessity justifies such deals, but the higher the market share and the longer the term of the agreement, the more imperative the need for a business justification
- Charge all patients and customers the same price, unless the cost of serving them varies, but freely cut prices to meet the lower prices of competitors

(*See generally* AEI, 2009; Bork, 1978, 2008; Epstein, 2007; Shenefield & Stelzer, 2001)

DIFFERENCES IN ANTITRUST PHILOSOPHY

Differences in antitrust philosophy[LN4] shape the different kinds of comprehensive settlements the government seeks and the courts grant when antitrust investigations arise (Epstein, 2007). These differences reflect the philosophical differences of two of the nation's founding fathers: Thomas Jefferson and Alexander Hamilton. Jefferson was a strict constructionist and believed in a very weak central government. Hamilton was a loose constructionist and believed in a strong central government. These opposing ideologies were a major factor in shaping American government and remain a major factor in shaping today's politics. The evolving democracy of the U.S. is based on reconciling the relationship between these two apparently different views of government. American politics has always been the art of making these apparent conflicting beliefs consistent. In the end, Americans have always championed Hamiltonian practicality to achieve Jeffersonian ideals. Success always centers on ideals and does not confuse methods of achievement with ideals.

One extreme wants strong federal antitrust enforcement and wants courts to loosely construct antitrust laws to best serve social welfare goals (health and general welfare of the public at large); the other extreme is strict constructionists of antitrust laws who oppose centralized control of competition. Rarely is either opposite played at its limits; most U.S. antitrust policies champion strong federal enforcement methods to achieve competitive ideals.

Today, rather aggressive enforcement strategies are being used to foster competition (Posner, 2007). Government power is fundamentally altering industry structures and the business practices of the health care industry, as found in the recent spate of consent decrees in the medical products industry. Health care companies are increasingly entering voluntary agreements to cease activities alleged by the government to be illegal in return for an end to charges of anticompetition.

Almost every major pharmaceutical company and all of the leading medical devices companies (including Biomet, Johnson & Johnson's DePuy Orthopaedics, Smith & Nephew, Stryker, and Zimmer) are operating under consent decrees with the federal government; more than five hundred hospitals are under investigation (Garrett). Government-imposed regulations and remedies that are not tightly tied to defensible theories of wrongful conduct often prove counterproductive; such measures typically force health care providers to adopt business practices and structural reorganizations that substantially impede their ability to compete effectively in the global medical marketplace (Epstein, 2007).

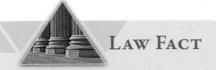

LAW FACT

PRICE FIXING BY PHARMACY BENEFIT MANAGERS

Are the purchases of pharmacy benefit managers (PBMs) a restraint of trade?

Caremark's purchases are not a restraint of trade; rather, they create pro-competitive efficiencies resulting in substantial benefits and cost savings to PBM patients.

—*North Jackson Pharmacy, Inc. v. Caremark RX, Inc.,* 385 F.Supp.2d 740
(U.S. District Court for the Northern District of Illinois, Eastern Division 2005).

CHAPTER SUMMARY

- Innocent monopolies obtained by meritorious competition are perfectly legal; actions to create a coercive monopoly or dealings to artificially preserve one's status as a monopoly are illegal.
- Antitrust law directs itself only against conduct that unfairly tends to destroy competition; it does not prohibit strong, honest competition.
- The purpose of antitrust laws is not to protect health care providers from competition in relevant markets; it is to protect the public from the failure of providers being able to effectively compete.
- Antitrust law does not penalize health care providers who dominate their market on their own merit, only those that intentionally dominate their market through wrongful conduct, or who use their market strength to promote abusive practices, such as paying sub-par wages or charging inflated prices.
- The two basic types of anticompetitive conduct that are prohibited are monopolization and conspiracies to restrain trade.
- To prove a prohibited attempt at monopolization, there must be evidence of intent to improperly destroy competition; this can be obtained by reviewing a pattern of individual acts and practices that alone are innocent, but when taken together are collusive.
- Conspiracies in restraint of trade are tricky to prove, as many contacts between competitors are not inherently unlawful; however, any agreement between competitors to control prices or to divide territory, customers, patients, or markets is inherently illegal.
- Medical mergers and acquisitions are generally intended to improve efficiency and lower costs; therefore, the FTC views mergers and/or acquisitions that result in higher costs with a suspicious eye, especially because the number of them has risen so sharply in recent years.
- Another recent area of concern for the FTC is the relationship between brand-name pharmaceuticals and generic manufacturers regarding artificial methods of protecting patents and keeping generics off the market.
- Antitrust cases and sanctions should be tightly tied to defensible theories of wrongful conduct in order to properly reflect what society thinks is wrong and clarify what is punishable conduct.
- Ideally, antitrust regulations would not force health care entities to adopt business practices that impede their ability to compete effectively, such as 1170 codes for angioplasty to ensure the medical products industry is not overcharging hospitals for their advanced surgical stent products.
- Health care entities can take steps to ensure that their conduct is not viewed an anticompetitive; some steps include refraining from making improper agreements with competitors, engaging in sustainable, justifiable forms of competition, keeping good records, and negotiating with rather than coercing competitors.

LAW NOTES

1. This section on antitrust analysis draws on the book by John H. Shenefield, a partner in the Washington, D.C. law firm of Morgan, Lewis, and Bockius, and former head of the Antitrust Division of the U.S. Department of Justice, and Irwin M. Stelzer, director of regulatory policy studies at the Hudson Institute.

2. There are three principal federal antitrust laws that impact the health care industry:
   - Sherman Act
   - Clayton Act
   - Federal Trade Commission Act (FTC Act)

   The oldest federal legislation, the Sherman Act, remains the core of antitrust law. Section I of the Act provides that "[e]very contract, combination in the form of trust or otherwise, or conspiracy, in restraint of trade or commerce among the several States... is declared to be illegal." The triggers are a contract, combination, or conspiracy. *See* Sherman Act of 1890, 15 U.S.C.A. §§ 1-7 (2009). In the absence of some cooperative conduct or joint action involving at least two distinct health care providers, the Sherman Act does not apply. It is also clear that the activity must have an effect on interstate commerce, which has been broadly interpreted by the courts to encompass almost any commercial activity (*see McElroy v. United States*, 455 U.S. 642 (U.S. Supreme Court 1982) (defining interstate commerce more broadly than merely as commerce crossing state lines)). Section II of the Act provides that "[e]very person who shall monopolize, or attempt to monopolize, or combine or conspire with any other person or persons, to monopolize any part of the trade or commerce among the several States... shall be deemed guilty of felony." Neither section of the Sherman Act specifies objectionable conduct or actions; thus it has been left to the courts to elaborate upon the general principles of this legislation on a case-by-case basis.

   Because there was minimal antitrust enforcement of the Sherman Act in the early twentieth century, Congress enacted the Clayton Act. This Act prohibits conduct whose effect "may be substantially to lessen competition or tend to create a monopoly in any line of commerce." *See* Clayton Act of 1914, 15 U.S.C.A. §§ 12-27 (2009); 29 U.S.C.A. §§ 52, 53 (1914). Congress subsequently enacted the FTC Act, which established the FTC as an independent regulatory agency with the power to prohibit unfair competitive practices, even though such conduct does not infringe either the Sherman or the Clayton antitrust laws. *See* Federal Trade Commission Act of 1947, 15 U.S.C.A. §§ 41-58 (2009).

3. *Unger v. Albany Med. Ctr.*, No. 06-CV-0765 (U.S. District Court for the Northern District of New York 2006); *Reed v. Advocate Health Care*, 2007 WL 967932 (U.S. District Court for the Northern District of Illinois, Eastern Division 2007); *Schultz v. Evanston Northwestern Healthcare*, No. 06-CV-03569 (U.S. District Court for the Northern District of Illinois 2006); *Clarke v. Baptist Memorial Healthcare Corp.*, No. 0602377 (U.S. District Court for the Western District of Tennessee, Western Division 2007); *Cason-Merenda v. Detroit Med. Ctr.*, 2008 WL 880286 (United States District Court for the Eastern District of Michigan, Southern Division 2008); *Maderazo v. Vanguard Health System*, 241 F.R.D. 597 (U.S. District Court for the Western District of Texas, San Antonio Division 2007).

4. The classical economic philosophies of the eighteenth and nineteenth centuries would restrain business to preserve liberty and competition (Smith, 1776; Mill, 1859). In the twentieth century there was a shift in economic theory with an emphasis on precise models of competition; this neoclassical model of free markets held that competitive free markets maximize social welfare (Samuelson, 2004). At the dawn of the twenty-first century, the Chicago school of economic philosophy, largely associated with the University of Chicago, is the theory most recently used by the U.S. Supreme Court (Bork, 2008; Posner, 1973, 2007). This school of thought allows vertical agreements (integrated health care systems) and price discrimination (managed care) if they do not harm society and prohibits only a few acts, namely:
   - Business alliances that fix prices and divide markets
   - Mergers that create monopolies
   - Dominant pricing that destroys other businesses for financial gain

CHAPTER BIBLIOGRAPHY

AEI (American Enterprise Institute) Event. (2009). *The antitrust burden: Can American companies still compete fairly abroad?* Washington, DC: AEI.

AHA (American Hospital Association). (2008). *Trendwatch: Beyond health care: The economic contribution of hospitals.* Chicago, IL: AHA.

Areeda, P. E., & Hovenkamp, H. (2005). *Antitrust law: An analysis of antitrust principles and their application.* New York, NY: Aspen Law & Business.

Bartels, J. (2006). The application of antitrust and fraud-and-abuse law to specialty hospitals. *Columbia Business Law Review*, 215-242.

BBW (Biotech Business Week). (2007, April 16). *Financing: California agency requires Sutter Health to pass through savings from tax-exempt bonds*, 312. Atlanta, GA: BBW.

BNA (Bureau of National Affairs). (2005). Dentsply's exclusivity policy illegally maintains its artificial tooth monopoly. *Antitrust & Trade Regulation Report, 88*, 207.

Bork, R. H. (2008). *A time to speak: Selected writings and arguments (American ideals & institutions)*. Wilmington, DE: Intercollegiate Studies Institute.

___. (1978). *The antitrust paradox: A policy at war with itself*. New York, NY: Basic Books (stating arguments about predatory litigation are staples in antitrust law).

Campbell, T. (2007). Defending hospital mergers after the FTC's unorthodox challenge to the Evanston Northwestern-Highland Park transaction. *Annals of Health Law, 16*, 213-237 (analysis written before the final FTC order was rendered).

Cogan, J. F. et al. (2005). Making markets work: Five steps to a better health care system. *Health Affairs*, 24 (6), 1447-1457.

DPA (Deferred Prosecution Agreement) between the U.S. Attorney for the District of New Jersey and Bristol Myers-Squibb (2006), Trenton, NJ.

Epstein, R. A. (2007). *Antitrust consent decrees in theory and practice: Why less is more*. Washington, DC: American Enterprise Institute (systematic study of the use of antitrust consent decrees and their effectiveness from both a historical and analytical perspective).

Francis, T. (2008, May 12). FTC will try to block Virginia hospital merger, *Wall Street Journal*, p. B2.

FTC (Federal Trade Commission) & DOJ (U.S. Department of Justice). (2004). *Improving health care: A dose of competition*. Washington, DC: FTC & DOJ.

GAO (General Accountability Office). (2005, May 19). *Specialty hospitals: Information on potential new facilities*. Washington, DC: GAO.

Garrett, B. L. (2007). Structural reform prosecution. *Virginia Law Review, 93*, 853-956.

Golding, E. (2009). Medicare Part D: Rights without remedies, bars to relief, and miles of red tape. *George Washington Law Review, 77*, 1044-1062.

Hovenkamp, H. (2008). *The antitrust enterprise: Principle and execution*. Cambridge, MA: Harvard University Press.

Irving (Irving Levin Associates). (2008). *The health care acquisition report*. (14th ed.). New Canaan, CT: Irving.

___. (2007). *Trendwatch chartbook*. New Canaan, CT: Irving.

JCAHO (Joint Commission on Accreditation of Healthcare Organizations). (2008). *Health care at the crossroads: Strategies for addressing the evolving nursing crisis*. Chicago, IL: JCAHO.

Kovacic, W. E. (2007). The intellectual DNA of modern U.S. competition law for dominant firm conduct: The Chicago/Harvard double helix. *Columbia Business Law Review, 2007*, 1-81.

Lambert, T. A. & Wright, J. D. (2008). The antitrust marathon: A roundtable discussion: Response to the antitrust marathon: Antitrust (over-?) confidence. *Loyola Consumer Law Review, 20*, 219-231.

Lewis, C. E. (2006). Appeals court rejects federal jurisdiction over chiropractors challenge to Medicare coverage. *American Journal of Law, Medicine & Ethics, 34* (2), 472-474.

McHugh, J. (2008, March). *Expanding access to health care: A free market perspective*. Midland, MI: Mackinac Center.

Miles, J. (2007). The nursing shortage, wage-information sharing among competing hospitals, and the antitrust laws: The nurse wages antitrust litigation. *Houston Journal of Health Law & Policy, 7*, 305-378.

Mill, J. S. (1859). *On liberty*. London, England: Longmans, Green, and Co. (advocating economic freedom of individuals from the state during the Victorian age in the nineteenth century).

Miller, I. (2006). Health care law: survey of recent developments in health law. *Indiana Law Review, 39*, 1051-1104.

Novak, J. J. (2007). United States v. Dentsply: The Third Circuit bites down on the 'alternative distribution channels' defense. *Iowa Journal of Corporate Law, 32*, 963-982.

Perry, A. B. (2007). Which cases are "such cases": Interpreting and applying section 12 of the Clayton Act. *Fordham Law Review, 76*, 1177-1224.

Popofsky, M. S. (2008). Section 2, safe harbors, and the rule of reason. *George Mason Law Review, 15*, 1265-1296.

Porter, M. E., & Teisberg, E. O. (2006). *Redefining health care: Creating value-based competition on results*. Boston, MA: Harvard Business School Press.

Posner, R. A. (2007). *Economic analysis of law* (7th ed.). New York, NY: Wolters Kluwer Law & Business (applying the Chicago-school economic philosophy to the law).

___. (1973). *Antitrust law: An economic perspective*. Chicago, IL: University of Chicago Press.

PriceWaterhouseCoopers. (2008). *Cost of caring: Key drivers of growth in spending on hospital care: Prepared for the American Hospital Association and the Federation of American Hospitals*. Washington, DC: PriceWaterhouseCoopers.

Rosch, J. T. (2008). The common law of section 2: Is it still alive and well? *George Mason Law Review, 15*, 1163-1173.

Samuelson, P. (2004). *Economics: An introductory analysis* (18th ed.). New York, NY: McGraw-Hill.

Shenefield, J. H., & Stelzer, I. M. (2001). *The antitrust laws: A primer*. Washington, DC: American Enterprise Institute.

Smith, A. (1776). *An inquiry into the nature and causes of the wealth of nations*. Hartford, CT: Cooke & Hale (advocating a free market economy at the dawn of the Industrial Revolution in the eighteenth century; Alexander Hamilton, David Ricardo, Thomas Malthus, and, later, Ludwig von Mises used this economics text as the starting point for their work).

Stucke, M. E. (2006). Morality and antitrust. *Columbia Business Law Review, 2006*, 443-547.

Werden, G. J. (2006). The "no economic sense" test for exclusionary conduct. *Iowa Journal of Corporate Law, 31*, 293-305.

Wharton (Wharton School of the University of Pennsylvania). (2002, June 19). Drug companies and the patent game: Fair play or foul. *Knowledge@Wharton*.

Wildfang, K. C. (2006). Predatory conduct under section 2 of the Sherman Act: Do recent cases illuminate the boundaries? *Iowa Journal of Corporate Law, 31*, 323-356.

Wysocki, B. (2005, January 15). FTC targets hospital merger in antitrust case: Agency expects vigilance on medical M&A to help rein in health-care costs. *Wall Street Journal*, p. A1 (discussing the FTC case against a hospital for price fixing and market power abuse).

Yoshitani, R. S., & Cooper, E. S. (2007). Pharmaceutical reformulation: The growth of life cycle management. *Houston Journal of Health Law & Policy, 7*, 379-409.

Zain, S. (2007). Sword or shield? An overview and competitive analysis of the marketing of "authorized generics". *Food & Drug Law Journal, 62*, 739-776.

Zhang. J. (2008, November 11). Why we need 1170 codes for angioplasty. *Wall Street Journal*, p. D1-2.

PART III

ACCESS TO HEALTH CARE

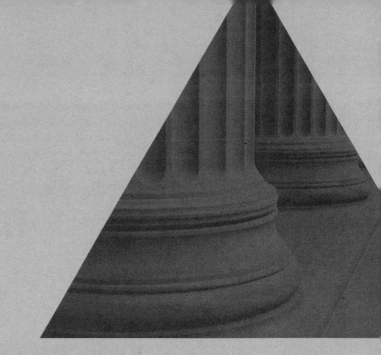

CHAPTER 5

ACCESS TO AND REIMBURSEMENT FOR MEDICALLY NECESSARY HEALTH CARE

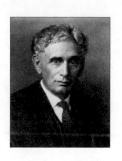

"It is one of the happy incidents of the federal system that a single courageous state may, if its citizens choose, serve as a laboratory, and try novel social and economic experiments without health risks to the rest of the country."

—JUSTICE LOUIS D. BRANDEIS (1856-1941), ASSOCIATE JUSTICE
OF THE U.S. SUPREME COURT

IN BRIEF

This chapter draws attention to the challenge of finding a way to provide access to medically necessary health care for all U.S. *residents,* including resident citizens and resident noncitizens, or more specifically, those in the U.S. without status and sometimes labeled undocumented, unauthorized, or illegal immigrants. Risk-pooling programs providing effective and affordable health coverage to millions of the uninsured and underinsured are examined. Also discussed are plans for the uninsured that cut through the ideological spectrum, from "pay or play" legislation that mandates universal health coverage and requires employers to either help "pay" for government-sponsored health care programs or "play" by providing their employees with adequate health insurance themselves, to tax credits that would offset much of the cost of buying health insurance policies from insurance companies.

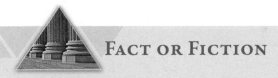

FACT OR FICTION

ACCESS TO BASIC HEALTH CARE

Is the federal government required to provide basic health care for residents at a veteran's retirement home?

The Armed Forces Retirement Home in Washington, D.C., provides full-time housing and health care for more than one thousand elderly veterans. Recently, the Home introduced a series of cost-saving measures that residents at the Home claim led to a severe decrease in the quality of health care. The deficiencies included the unavailability of physicians and dentists, medical neglect of residents, and delays in obtaining prescription drugs. The residents sued, requesting an injunction to force the Home to provide high-quality health care as required by law and asked the court to mandate that the Home maintain:

- Access to the medicines required for the treatment of residents
- Basic health care staffed by a physician
- Onsite x-ray, electrocardiogram, laboratory, and other primary care services
- Transportation for residents to nearby hospitals for necessary and urgent health care

The residents also requested that they be provided annual examinations to assess their overall physical and mental condition. The Home maintained the actual provision of basic health care was discretionary and that it was only required to maintain administrative procedures that provided for access to health care services for its residents.

—*Cody v. Cox*, 509 F.3d 606 (U.S. Court of Appeals for the District of Columbia Circuit, 2007).
(See *Law Fact* at the end of this chapter for the answer.)

PRINCIPLES AND APPLICATIONS

With health care access and reimbursement for health care at the forefront of public concern, various approaches are proposed to reform the U.S. health care system. The uninsured and underinsured are the nation's top health care challenges (Wharton, 2007).

ACCESS CHALLENGES

There is near unanimous agreement that the lack of access to health care services or health insurance coverage is one of the principal shortcomings of the U.S. health system, relative to health systems in other similar high-income, developed countries. Lack of universal access generally is believed to be the most significant contributor to the underperformance of the U.S. health care system in terms of broad population health measures, such as life expectancy (Schneider & Ohsfeldt, 2007).

About thirty-nine million working-age Americans reported cost as a barrier to receiving needed health care, a number that has been growing by an average of one million people annually over the past decade (DeNavas-Walt et al., 2008). As illustrated in Figure 5-1, the uninsured of limited means experienced the most consistent erosion in access, resulting

in a widening gap in access to care between the insured and uninsured (Hoffman & Schwartz, 2008).

COVERAGE FOR THE UNINSURED OR UNDERINSURED

It has been one of the most intractable problems facing public policy makers for years, which is how to provide health coverage to the millions of uninsured and underinsured in a way that is both effective and affordable. For more than forty years, there has been discussion about the fundamental question of how many households are uninsured and whether the uninsured are actually harmed due to lack of coverage (IOM, 2004). Today, there appears to be near universal agreement about:

- Who the uninsured are
- Why the uninsured are uninsured
- What happens to the uninsured of limited means when they need health care or the medical expense of the underinsured exceeds their coverage and ability to pay for care

About forty-two million Americans, or more than one in seven people in the United States,

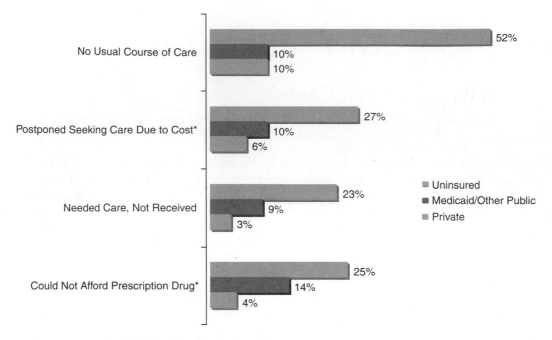

FIGURE 5-1: Barriers to Health Care by Insurance Status

* In the past twelve months.
Delmar/Cengage Learning
Data retrieved from: National Health Interview Survey (NHIS). (2009). Atlanta, GA: Centers for Disease Control & Prevention; *See also* Kaiser Commission on Medicaid & the Uninsured. (2008). Chartbook: Barriers to health care by insurance status. Washington, DC: Kaiser (analyzing 2007 NHIS data).

have no health insurance, and most of them have middleclass incomes (Tobert et al., 2008). The Congressional Budget Office notes that the uninsured population is not static; Americans fall into and out of coverage for various periods of time.

- Some thirty-seven million of the uninsured (almost nine out of ten uninsured) are working, however, either:
  ○ Their employers do not offer health insurance
  ○ They do not qualify for employer-sponsored insurance (ESI), or
  ○ They cannot afford their share of the health insurance premiums (Kaiser, 2007)
- The number of uninsured is expected to increase to forty-four million in 2010; an additional ten million will become uninsured by 2019 without major policy changes (CBO, 2008b)
- More than eight in ten of the uninsured are in low- or moderate-income families (Kaiser, 2008)
- Almost 20 percent of the individuals living with HIV/AIDS are uninsured (NASTAD, 2008)
- One in four of the nation's uninsured is eligible for either Medicaid or SCHIP (about twelve million uninsured) (Kaiser, 2008)
- A 1 percent rise in the nation's unemployment rate increases the number of uninsured by 1.1 million

and expands public spending on health care by $3.4 billion; an economic phenomena illustrated in Figure 5-2
- If all the uninsured were covered by insurance, overall health care costs would increase by $123 billion, or an additional 5 percent of national health spending (Hadley, 2008)
- Nearly seventy-seven million Americans went without health insurance for part or all of the year 2008, a number that has been increasing every year and is expected to increase in future years (Hadley, 2008)
- The uninsured spend about $30 billion dollars out-of-pocket and receive approximately $56 billion in uncompensated care while uninsured (Hadley, 2008)
- Government programs finance about 75 percent of the uninsured's uncompensated care (Hadley, 2008)

The effect of having millions of uninsured people is considerable. For one thing, the uninsured risk serious illness or death by delaying necessary health care. According to a report issued by the National Academy of Sciences' Institute of Medicine, lack of health insurance causes over eighteen thousand unnecessary deaths every year (IOM, 2004).

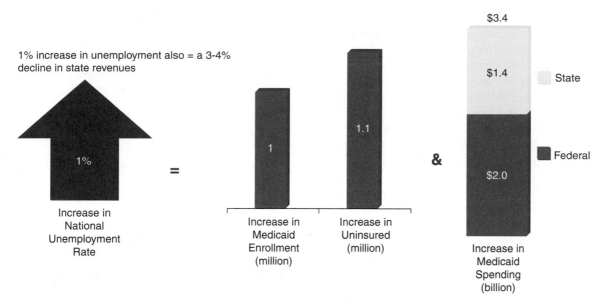

FIGURE 5-2: Impact of Unemployment Growth on Medicaid and the Number of Uninsured

Source: Kaiser Commission on Medicaid & the Uninsured.

ECONOMICS OF THE UNINSURED AND UNDERINSURED

The purpose of health insurance is to pool risks in order to provide access to affordable health care for all. The insured pay into the insurance risk pool, also known as guaranteed access programs, hoping they will never have to use it.

> **How does the issue of the uninsured affect the insured?**
> Everyone who pays into insurance risk pools is forced to pay higher health insurance premiums because it costs more to treat the uninsured when they become seriously ill as a result of a lack of routine, preventative care. Higher premiums lead to the insured being underinsured, who then do not have adequate coverage when a catastrophic injury or illness hits.

Societal costs in this situation, from the uninsured and the underinsured, may take non-economic forms such as a more unproductive workforce. Whether universal insurance mandates are effective in reducing societal costs is not always clear (Klick & Markowitz, 2003). What is clear is the long-term uninsured of sufficient means who can afford health insurance, but choose not to purchase coverage and instead spend their money on other things, are shifting their share of the insurance risk pools to everyone else.

Spillover Effect of the Non-Privately Insured

While the health care costs of the uninsured, in terms of uncompensated care, are driving up overall costs, the spillover effect of not being privately insured is more disturbing. According to the Agency for Healthcare Research and Quality, 1 percent of the U.S. population is responsible for about one-fourth of the nation's health care spending, and the top 5 percent accounted for half the spending (Zuvekas & Cohen, 2007). One widespread characteristic of this patient population is the seriousness and chronic nature of their illnesses. Moreover, their health conditions often arise from a general failure to receive preventive health care services and seek timely health care, two common attributes of being uninsured (Halpern et al., 2008). These hidden costs must be more visible and better controlled.

In addition, there is another spillover effect beyond the uninsured. In communities with large numbers of uninsured, even those who have insurance experience less availability of health care services and receive lower-quality health care than persons who live in communities with few uninsured persons. For instance, the burden on the charity care system is much higher because the uninsured often go to the emergency room for preventable illnesses (Pauly & Pagan, 2007).

Economic Cycle of Health Insurance

The best, most highly trained physicians are also often some of the most highly compensated citizens in the nation; the U.S. richly rewards its most skilled citizens who are at the top of the global knowledge pyramid.

The most highly regarded medical institutions in the U.S. are able to attract and retain the best physicians in the world with attractive compensation packages. These respected medical institutions, in turn, are part of comprehensive health care delivery systems with significant revenues; the top twenty-five hospital systems have revenues of more than $250 million a year (Carreyrou & Martinez, 2008). In turn, these health care delivery systems maintain their earnings from strategies pursued to increase revenues, including demanding upfront payments from patients (Martinez, 2008) and hiking list prices for health care to several times their actual cost. The uninsured are generally unable to afford this type of health care with its requirements for upfront cash payments and high prices (those with health insurance are required to pay their deductibles and co-pays before service is ever rendered). The economic cycle of health care follows the money: the highest-quality health care is near those patients who can afford the care, who are the insured.

By comparison, most of the hospitals under financial strain are in communities handling large numbers of uninsured. In turn, these hospitals are often unable to attract the best, most highly trained physicians with attractive compensation packages, nor are they able to invest in the latest medical technologies. Medical institutions with limited financial resources and average-skilled physicians, who are not the most highly trained, often provide lower-quality health care. It is the classic cycle of economic poverty; the least advantaged of society receive the least. In communities with large numbers of uninsured, even those who have insurance experience less availability of health care services than persons who live in communities with few uninsured persons (Pauly & Pagan, 2007).

Reframing Choices About Health Insurance

In seeking to address the challenge of insuring the uninsured, many different scenarios have been examined and tried

- Experimenting with employer mandates and taxes to provide health insurance
- Limiting medical malpractice liability and lawyers' fees
- Proposing targeted tax subsidies
- Creating state and local health care plans

No matter what solutions are adopted to deal with the uninsured, health risks continue to occupy center stage. Whether the U.S. decides to adopt the European style of maximizing health care outcomes or continue on its present course of allocating health risks is still undecided. There may, however, be better ways of defining the objectives of health care policy toward the uninsured and underinsured, or ways of framing the choices about health insurance.

DEFINING HEALTH RISKS

The allocation of health risks is a dominant force in the U.S. health care system (Hunter, 2008). The term *health risks* comes up frequently when medicine and health care are discussed. What are the health risks of:

- Going without health insurance if healthy?
- Dying from a complication of surgery or a medical procedure?
- Experiencing a life-threatening reaction to a drug or innovative treatment?
- Having a heart attack or being diagnosed with a serious illness such as cancer?

Most people do not necessarily use the term *health risks* in the same way health professionals and insurance experts do, which is a fact that can potentially lead to less than optimal political decisions about health care (Wharton, 2007). The language that describes access to health care, the uninsured and underinsured, and health spending sometimes gets in the way of clear thinking and sometimes implicitly reflects quite different ways of thinking (Pauly, 2007). There is no better example of this language confusion than use of the term *health risks*. Debates about health risks occur, often as if there were consensus on the meaning of the term, but in reality, everyone in the room uses the word in a variety of ways:

- Analyzing health risks in clinical decisions
- Pooling health risks through insurance
- Trading off between the health risks and benefits of medical interventions

Expected Utility Maximization

Flawed thinking about health risks can cause faulty decisions. One decision-making model that is increasingly followed in an attempt to make more rational decisions is known as expected utility maximization (Pauly, 2007). In the health care industry, utility is a measure of the relative satisfaction from consumption of health care. Used primarily by health economists, the expected utility model values risks as a weighted average of the possible outcomes with the:

- Weights being the probabilities of risks
- Values being the utility attached to changes in a person's well-being, in each situation

(Wharton, 2007)

For instance, at the individual level, when patients make decisions about what type of medical intervention to accept, each treatment outcome could be ranked. Suppose patients could:

- Do nothing
- Change their behavior and take medications
- Have surgery and take medications

If patients elect to change their behavior, then the patients strictly prefer changing their behavior to having surgery or are indifferent between them. If the consumption of health care by patients is ranked by the six generally preferred treatment outcomes,*

- Do nothing = 0
- Behavior change = 1
- Surgery = 3
- Behavior change and medications = 2
- Surgery and medications = 3
- Behavior change, surgery, and medications = 4

Then, as illustrated in Figure 5-3, patients prefer behavior change over surgery (with *one* being the most preferred choice), but prefer behavior change and taking medications over surgery and taking medications.

When deciding what can be done to address the challenges of health care access and reimbursement for health care, all the things that can be done at the systems level could be treated in the same manner. For instance, the patients are the U.S. health care system and the possible treatment outcomes are:

- Employer mandates and state or municipal fines on employers who refuse to provide health insurance for their employees
- Expansion of public health programs (Medicare, Medicaid, SCHIP, or other public programs)
- Targeted federal tax subsidies on employer-provided health insurance premiums that are subsidized by all taxpayers
- Regulatory reform of state insurance laws
- Consumer-directed health care plans
- Discounted drug programs

- Taxes on the excessive total compensation of individual executives in health industry sectors that are subsidized by public funds
- Corporate taxes on excessive profits in health industry sectors that are subsidized by public funds

If the maximization of utility is the criterion for organization of the U.S. health care system, one may speak meaningfully of increasing or decreasing utility and thereby explaining the behavior of patient in terms of attempts to increase their relative satisfaction with their health care.

Political Philosophy of Distributive Justice

The theory of distributive justice (Rawls, 2005a)[LN1] underlies the expected utility maximization model. As used in this text, distributive justice concerns what is just with respect to the allocation of health risks in the American health care system. Thus, if all U.S. residents were provided access to essential and affordable health care, the American health care system would be considered guided by the principles of distributive justice. Health care, however, is more than simply emergency care, it is health care that is *medically necessary;* primary and preventive care is a significant component of medically necessary health care.

For instance, in reform of the nation's health care system:

- What principles could Congress agree to if one side of the aisle cooperates with the other side of the aisle?
- What if each side of the aisle still prefers more of the benefits, and less of the burdens, associated with cooperation?
- What decisions about access to health care are both rational and reasonable, and according to whom?

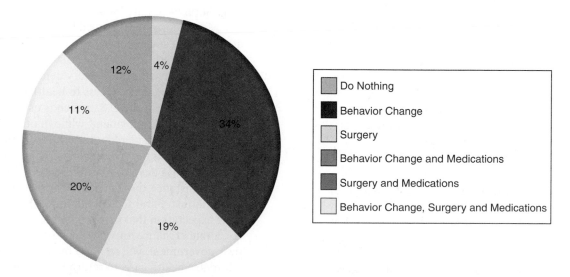

FIGURE 5-3: Expected Utility Maximization

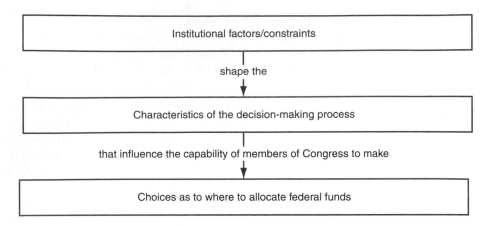

FIGURE 5-4: Determinants of Decision-Making by Congress

Delmar/Cengage Learning

Assuming members of Congress are rational, they have ends they want to achieve, but are also reasonable and open to compromise insofar as they would be glad to achieve these ends together if they could, in accord with principles that are mutually acceptable. Given how different the needs and aspirations are on each side of the aisle, how can Congress find principles that are acceptable to both sides? As illustrated in Figure 5-4, one decision-making model for this choice is expected utility maximization. The ideal health care reform would therefore be an overlapping consensus, because different and often conflicting needs and aspirations, will always overlap with each other (*see generally* Rawls, 2005, 2005a).

Fairness to the Least Advantaged
The theoretical approach to this decision-making model is based on the notion that inequalities should work to the benefit of the least advantaged in society.

A fair health care system provides *medically necessary health care* to the healthiest people at the top of the economic pyramid, as well as to people who are suffering the most from disease and illness and are at the bottom of the economic pyramid.

What is medically necessary is one of the million-dollar questions in the nation's debate about health care reform. The definition itself is a subject of frequent litigation that has been decided in conflicting ways by the courts. This policy approach is framed around two theories: the theory of social contracts and the theory of economic fairness.

Social Contracts   In a just society, there is an imaginary social contract between the governed and their

government. A social contract implies that a nation's citizens give up some rights to their government in order to receive and jointly preserve social order, the theoretical groundwork of democracy (*see generally* Locke, 2008; Rousseau, 2009). For John Locke, the purpose of government is to serve and benefit "the people"; government must be controlled by "the people" for which the government was made. For Jean-Jacques Rousseau, citizens of a nation place themselves and their authority under the supreme direction of the general will, and the group receives each individual as an indivisible part of the whole. As the Supreme Court has stated, a "fundamental principle of the social compact [is] that the whole people covenants with each citizen, and each citizen with the whole people, that all shall be governed by certain laws for the common good" *Jacobson v. Commonwealth of Massachusetts*, 197 U.S. 11, 27 (U.S. Supreme Court 1904).

Most people in the world believe their governments have a social contract to provide medically necessary health care, a belief that is shared by the majority of the citizens in every democracy in the world except the U.S. Access to health care is considered a privilege in the U.S., which is usually expressed as a benefit of employment, while in other democracies, access is considered a right of citizenship. This chapter is about the parameters of this social contract and how it has developed and is developing in the U.S.

For instance, a social contract exists between the health industry and society that gives the public a legitimate expectation that the companies, in return for their corporate existence provided by "the people" through their government, will respond by providing access to affordable health care. In return for the benefits of:

- Patent protection, the medical products industry will respond with drugs and medical devices that are reasonably accessible to the public

- Tax-exempt status, hospitals will make access to charitable health care available to patients in financial need
- Tax subsidies on employee health insurance plans, the insurance industry will provide a risk pool that offers affordable access to health insurance
- FDA market approval, the medical products industry is obligated to comply with the nation's anti-fraud laws

Economic Fairness   In making any decision, the essential question must always be: is this fair and does it make economic sense (Rawls, 2005)? There can be no fairness if something does not make economic sense. Wherever one ends up in society, everyone wants the transactions that affect their life to be reasonably just and understandable; the activities in life should be able to be transacted according to fair and socially acceptable rules that are in accordance with what is expected.

In addressing access to and reimbursement for health care, one framework for the decision process might be:

> **First Principle: Universal Health Care**
>
> - All U.S. residents have an equal claim to basic health care
> - The means to access this health care claim must be the same for everyone
> - Each person is free to select the health care system and providers for health care
> - Health care providers are guaranteed to receive fair value for the health care provided
>
> (*See generally* Rawls, 2005)
>
> **Second Principle: Maximization of Insurance Risk Pools**
>
> - Inequalities brought about by the inability to pay fair value for health care are permissible if the following two conditions are met:
>   - Health care must be accessible to all U.S. residents based on fairness; in other words, access to health care must be based on the medical condition of individuals and the health care provided must be of a minimum quality (the so-called equality of opportunity principle)
>   - The greatest assistance to access health care must be given to those at the bottom of the economic pyramid, or the least advantaged
>
> (*See generally* Rawls, 2005)

Equality of Opportunity

The equality of opportunity principle is not mandating that every U.S. resident have access to exactly the same health care; achieving this would offend American notions of individual autonomy and

responsibility. Nonetheless, access to health care would be assured *wherever* an individual is on the economic pyramid, but there would always be freedom to pursue additional health care based on the ability to pay fair value for that care (*see generally* Rawls, 2005).

Hierarchy of Principles

The first principle of universal health care has priority over the second principle of pooled health risks, and the first half of the second principle has priority over the latter half. The claim for universal health care would have priority over the claim for pooled health risks. The right to health care has a greater weight than the cost of the care. The ability to pay fair value for health care would have priority over the assistance provided to access the needed care (*see generally* Rawls, 2005).

Relationship Between Principles and Their Application

The principles and their application are two distinct, but related issues. The principles are not validated or invalidated by the ability or inability to apply them. For example, just because the U.S. health care system cannot have equal application of the principles does not mean the principles are not valid.

If these principles were applied perfectly and if the U.S. could find a way to pay for universal health care without any limitations, there would be no inequalities. If the U.S. had the ability to pay for every medical technology and every medicine needed by every U.S. resident, inequalities of access to health care would not exist. Essentially, if the U.S. had unlimited resources, there would be no inequalities. The point is that the U.S. does not have the financial resources to pay for everything. The scarcity of resources mandates that available financial resources be maximized. So, the nation must decide who gets what.

Application of the Principles

The expected utility maximization model could be used by employers to decide what type of health insurance coverage to purchase for their employees. Is it better to buy a health insurance policy with a high deductible but excellent catastrophic coverage, or a policy with a low deductible with more coverage for routine, lower-end expenses such as preventive care and routine provider visits? Alternatively, is it better yet to offer a cafeteria approach so individual employees can make the decision to meet their specific health care needs?

Health Risks

The key questions about health risks are:

- Which preferences should government use in designing medical interventions?
- Should the U.S. implement economically sensible solutions that may benefit only a fraction of the public?
- Or should the U.S. adopt less than optimal economic policies that are preferred by a wider constituency?

(Wharton, 2007)

By definition, health risks involve uncertainty. Uncertainty makes people uneasy. It is not just that people do not like bad outcomes; rather, they do not like not knowing what the outcome will be (Pauly, 2007). In the achievement of health and the use of health care, health risks seem to be everywhere at once:

- What will anyone's health be in the future?
- What accident or illness might occur?
- If sick, what:
  - Will be the outcome of treatments or medicines?
  - Adverse side effects could occur?
  - Future medical bills might arise?

While health economists use the expected utility model to explain how the public tends to make decisions in risky situations, in the real world people do not always make decisions this way (Wharton, 2007). There is still a lot of smoking in the U.S. and people who eat fast-food every day. Moreover, health consumers often misconstrue health risks when they are deciding among various medicines or treatments. Should they try an experimental drug versus a standard treatment? Or what type and level of coverage should they select when deciding whether to purchase health insurance?

Americans seem to value health insurance that reimburses them, so they get a return on their premium payments (Pauly, 2007). This perception is different than viewing health insurance as protection against the health risks of a catastrophic accident or illness, which probably will not happen but if it did, it could mean financial disaster. Most people reason that because they paid for insurance for so many years and hardly ever used it, that this purchase was a bad financial decision. The expected utility model says that was not a bad decision. If something

catastrophic had happened, they would benefit so much from the insurance that it would offset all the years of paying and getting nothing back.

Less Extensive Coverage for the Uninsured of Limited Means

Although most health insurance policies offer coverage for inpatient hospitalization, some insurers are attempting to attract the uninsured with low premiums that cover some outpatient services, which are more likely to be needed, while leaving less likely but far more expensive hospital costs uncovered or only partially covered. This could reduce treatments of minimal value, while enrollees would face higher costsharing or tighter control of their health care (CBO, 2008b).

While perhaps appealing, this approach is problematic from an economic standpoint (Wharton, 2007). Even though the uninsured are less likely to be hospitalized than require a physician's visit, everyone should be protected against hospital costs (Pauly, 2007). While individuals with less extensive coverage may be treated fairly from an economic perspective, they are not being treated fairly in terms of access to coverage.

Mutual Health Insurance Plans

Healthy people, in particular, fail to weigh health risks optimally, thinking they should not spend money on health insurance because their chances of falling seriously ill are small. In this case, one possible solution is designing health plans exclusively for healthy people who are unlikely to have preventable health conditions: for instance, nonsmokers who are not obese.[LN2]

The uninsured who are healthy could contribute insurance premiums into mutual health insurance plans, in return for the promise that if they are right and everyone is a low-user of health care services, premiums would be refunded. Mutual health insurance plans would pay dividends to policyholders if benefits payouts were low; these dividend payments would, in turn, be used to lower future premiums. Thus, healthy people would be in a risk pool with other healthy people like themselves and who have the same health risks as they do, whatever that health risk really is.

Mutual Fund for Young Adults

Health care economists at the Wharton School at the University of Pennsylvania have suggested a mutual fund for young healthy adults (ages nineteen to twenty-nine) since they account for such a large share of the uninsured (Pauly, 2007). In particular, more than four in ten uninsured young adults of limited means experience problems gaining access to needed health care, with adverse consequences for both their health and financial well-being (Kenney & Pelletier, 2008). This exposes young adults to the risks of high medical bills should they need care for a serious illness or injury.

Alternatives to Employer-Sponsored Insurance

On the issue of ESI, Americans are relying less and less on employers as the major source of their health insurance. More and more individuals are finding themselves in situations where they have to consider different options. Consequently, the challenge is to structure alternatives to ESI. This could possibly mean:

- Offering individuals access to tax-subsidized health insurance so they can use pretax dollars to pay for insurance, as they do now for ESI
- Allowing individuals to take advantage of group purchases and health insurance risk pooling

ESI coverage has been declining due both to the declining number of employees with access to employer insurance and decreasing rate of enrollment among employees (Kaiser, 2008). In addition, two of the fastest growing sectors of the economy, part-time entrepreneurial work and service sector jobs, traditionally do not supply ESI coverage (Pauly & Pagan, 2007). As a result, the uninsured rate for employees is increasing; it is also increasing for lower-income children with access to employer coverage. Employer coverage is likely to continue to decline as increasing premiums lead more employers to drop coverage. Employees will probably face greater challenges to obtaining coverage as they face increasing contribution amounts. In the absence of other affordable health coverage options, these trends can be expected to result in further growth in the number of uninsured employees (Cunningham et al., 2008).

Private Insurance Debate on Health Risks

The current controversy over ESI increases speculation that individual insurance will soon become a possibility for more Americans. Research on the relationship between premiums and expected medical expenses across the three major sources of private health insurance in the U.S. has exposed some common misconceptions about how these insurance markets work:

- Individual health insurance
- Large ESIs
- Small-group insurance

ESIs may not be performing as well, nor individual health insurance performing as poorly, as is generally believed (Pauly, 2003). Researchers at the Wharton School at the University of Pennsylvania examined three types of health insurance in terms of their extent of:

- Health insurance risk pooling, where all policyholders pay the same premium regardless of their level of expected expense
- Health risks segmentation, where premiums are proportional to the policyholder's estimated health risks

HEALTH INSURANCE RISK POOLING

The issue of health insurance risk pooling raises questions such as:

- Do health insurance premiums vary according to indicators of health risks? Should they?
- Should the young and the healthy subsidize the old and the not-so-healthy?
- Should public subsidies to health insurance vary according to economic status and health risks?

While the number of Americans covered by ESIs has been declining since 1997, the leading source of health insurance held by more than 158 million Americans is still employment-based (Hoffman & Schwartz, 2008). ESI receives a tax subsidy in excess of $300 billion a year (Kleinbard, 2008). Conventional wisdom gives high marks to ESI, asserting it manages to pool health risks across all customers. Individual health insurance, on the other hand, which is held by about 5 percent of Americans, gets the worst grade for supposedly seeking out low-risk customers while avoiding those considered high-risk (Claxton et al., 2008). While this information may be correct, the appearances that give rise to these judgments may be quite deceiving (Pauly, 2007).

Perceptions (or Misperceptions) About Health Risks

Perceptions (or misperceptions) about health risks affect the debate about how to best provide coverage for the uninsured and underinsured. In the U.S., it is hard to override public misperceptions, especially misperceptions about health risks (Pauly, 2007). There are at least four prevalent misperceptions about health risks:

- High-risk individuals with higher than average health risks pay higher health insurance premiums
- ESI pools health risks
- Individual health insurance policies carry higher premiums because of their high administrative costs
- Individual policies are not the best type of health insurance

High-Risk Individuals

First, do individual non-group insurers segment health risks? If so, does the health insurance industry rate people based on risks and do high-risk individuals pay more?

There is no relationship between individual health risks and the premiums people pay. While insurers attempt to segment health risks, the segmentation has never worked. Individuals holding individual insurance, whose anticipated medical expenses are twice the average, pay premiums only about 20 to 40 percent higher than other individual insurance customers (Wharton, 2007).

The result of these market forces in the individual non-group market is that the health insurance premiums paid by those with chronic conditions are not consistently greater than those paid by healthy people. What is more, there is no conclusive evidence that anyone seeking health insurance in the non-group market is deterred from obtaining coverage because they have higher than average health risks. Anecdotal reports exist, but on an aggregate scale, this misconception does not appear to be supported by the facts.

Insurance Risk Pools

Second, do ESIs pool health risks almost completely? The governance and distribution of risks are what drive the health care system. Interconnected policies and give-and-take practices are evident everywhere. All actors within the system (health insurers, health care providers, and health consumers) take on aspects of risk, and the system's viability is contingent on allocating these risks (Hunter, 2008).

In large employer groups, high-risk individuals pay somewhat more, either through higher premiums or lower wages because they exhibit some risk factors that influence their expected health expenses, such as age. Employees receive lower wages over their careers where they obtain health insurance than in organizations where they do not (Wharton, 2007). Thus, through lower wages, the more senior employees effectively pay more for their health insurance.

In addition, there is evidence location (for example, paying a higher insurance premium if based in New York where physicians and hospitals are more expensive, rather than in Iowa) and gender may also play a role in the premium rates employees pay (Pauly & Hoff, 2002). While wages of insured women are lower in states that mandate maternity benefits, there is no correlating research finding mandated contraceptive benefits lower insurance rates. It may simply be an issue of state mandates raising insurance rates.

Moreover, high-risk, low-wage employees in small groups are less likely to obtain health insurance than others. With ESI there is, of course, also a freedom of choice issue. There is currently a managed care backlash where employees are unhappy with what their employers are offering. Insurers stung by the cost in goodwill from this have developed product lines that shift elevated levels of risks to health consumers, through health savings accounts and higher co-payments and deductibles.

Maximizing Insurance Risk Pooling

To maximize risk spreading for all Americans, a federal level risk pool would have to be created using a single-payer system. Like Medicare, Social Security, and the Pension Benefit Guaranty Corporation, a social insurance system for health care would have to be funded by:

- Premiums paid by participants
- Taxes
- Additional general funds from the federal government (possibility on a match basis with the states)

In the existing third-party payer system in the U.S., insurance risk pooling will never be maximized (Pauly, 2007); private health insurers generally must be fully funded, whereas social insurance programs are often not fully funded, and some maintain full funding of social insurance programs is not economically desirable. Similarly, maximization will never be reached by private insurers regardless of how many mandated benefits are regulated (Monahan, 2007). Private insurers usually design health insurance programs with emphasis on fairness between individual purchasers of coverage, while social insurance programs usually place greater emphasis on the social adequacy of benefits for all participants.

Administrative Costs

Third, is individual health insurance not the best choice for universal coverage? Individual health insurance is too expensive, not because the insurance industry increases premiums for high risks, but because of the steep administrative costs. Individuals at all health risk levels are being charged premiums that are too high relative to the benefits they get back (Pauly, 2007). This high loading arises because this market, like all customized markets, such as automobile and homeowners insurances, is expensive to administer (Wharton, 2007). Unfortunately, faced with high prices and the absence of a tax subsidy for individual insurance, individuals with the greatest need of insurance assistance are the ones who are the most often discouraged from buying it.

Moral Dilemmas

1. Who should get included and excluded in any insurance risk-pooling process?

2. What type of systems of accountability and checks and balances should be sufficient to produce an insurance risk-pooling system that is equitable, as well as efficient and flexible?

Employer-Sponsored Insurance

Several issues are debated regarding ESI:

- Is ESI the best choice for universal coverage?
- Should employers be required to provide adequate ESI for their employees?

Not only does the tax subsidy to ESI lead to excessive levels of insurance coverage, but it is highly regressive and therefore inequitable (Wharton, 2007). This is because it favors those with higher incomes and those currently employed by businesses employing more than two hundred employees.

Challenges in the Individual Health Insurance Market

There is debate about directing the current ESI tax subsidy toward the individual health insurance market. Rather than focusing on risks segmentation, attention is now being directed toward the non-group market's problems: high loading costs and mistaken choices by policyholders.

ESI is no longer the norm for most Americans, especially for businesses employing less than two hundred employees. The Congressional Budget Office suggests the individual insurance market might be able to gain ground if the uninsured were given tax credits or subsidies (CBO, 2008b, 2008c). With the goal of getting more Americans insured, most likely there is going to be an increased reliance on the individual market. Understanding what is happening to those insured in the individual market is an important issue.

What Can Be Done?

The proposals to address this mass chaos cut across the ideological spectrum. Some plans call for a social insurance program, not subject to means-testing, that would give all U.S. residents a right to comprehensive health insurance coverage. Other plans rely more heavily on involvement by the private sector. Regardless, there is a great deal that can be done at the margins to address the challenge of the uninsured.

The Institute of Medicine recommends pursuing the goal of universal coverage by experimenting at the state level, so that the federal government can see on a lower level what might work on a national scale. Many would accept the proposition that encouraging local experimentation before implementation of national universal health care is a worthy idea.

The Kaiser Commission on Medicaid and the Uninsured suggests providing tax credits while expanding programs such as Medicaid and the State Children's Health Insurance Program (SCHIP). The SCHIP program, funded by the federal government and administered by the states, provides financial help for children whose families are not on Medicaid but cannot afford routine health care. SCHIP is a significant contributor in the effort to insure the uninsured that occurred in the late 1990s; by extending coverage and permitting states more latitude in administering SCHIP, an important group is being covered.

Moral Dilemmas

1. What standards should govern access to health care?

Employer Mandates or Taxes to Provide Health Insurance

Growing numbers of state and local governments are experimenting with universal health care plans. The basic similarity is most plans feature employer mandates or taxes aimed at changing employee benefit plans by requiring employers who are not providing adequate levels of health insurance for their employees to provide coverage.

"Pay or Play" Employer Mandates

In American legal scholarship, experiments in democracy are most closely associated with an approach to health law that emphasizes collaborative regulatory initiatives; principles of decentralization and stakeholder participation are used to develop new and less bureaucratic models of regulation and health care administration (Hunter, 2008). If Justice Louis Brandeis were to witness San Francisco's experiment with universal health care legislation, he might amend his characterization of the states as laboratories of democracy to include municipalities as well (Jacobs, 2008). San Francisco is seeking to provide access to affordable health care to the city's estimated 80,000 uninsured residents, roughly half of whom work.

"PAY OR PLAY" HEALTH REFORM MEASURES

Golden Gate Restaurant Association v. City and County of San Francisco
[Opponents of "Pay or Play" Reform v. Municipal Reformers]
546 F.3d 639 (U.S. Court of Appeals for the 9th Circuit 2008), rehearing denied, 2009
WL 605320 (U.S. Court of Appeals for the 9th Circuit 2009)

FACTS: In San Francisco, where 10 percent of the City residents have no health insurance and 15 percent of businesses provide no health coverage for their employees, the Board of Supervisors passed the San Francisco Health Care Security ordinance, which funds a network of primary care services for uninsured residents (S.F. Admin. Code § 14.2(d) (2007)). While the ordinance has met with general approval, its provision mandating contributions from local businesses that do not meet minimum health spending requirements was the subject of litigation.

The ordinance, adopted unanimously in 2006, creates a Health Access Program designed to make health care services available to the City's more than eighty thousand uninsured residents. Funding for the program, which provides primary care for the uninsured at both public and private facilities throughout the City, comes from:

- Mandatory contributions from businesses that do not meet designated health care contribution levels for their employees
- Municipal, state, and federal government grants
- Payments from individual enrollees

Employers can meet the required contribution levels in a variety of ways, by:

- Contributing to employee health savings accounts
- Donating to the City's new Health Access Program
- Paying a third party for health care delivery for their employees
- Reimbursing their employees directly for their health care expenditures

Such provisions are often called "pay or play" because employers must either help pay for government-sponsored health care programs or play by providing their employees with health insurance themselves.

Golden Gate Restaurant Association, representing the interests of over eight hundred San Francisco restaurants, brought an action challenging the ordinance. The Association claimed the 1974 Federal Employee Retirement Income Security Act (ERISA) pre-empted the ordinance's "pay or play" employer spending requirement. ERISA sets minimum standards for a wide array of employer-sponsored benefit plans, including most employer health plans. ERISA explicitly pre-empts state and local laws that relate to an employee benefit plan regulated by ERISA.

ISSUE: Does federal ERISA pre-empt the "pay or play" ordinance adopted by the City of San Francisco?

HOLDING AND DECISION: No, ERISA does not pre-empt San Francisco's "pay or play" ordinance.

ANALYSIS: A three-judge panel of the U.S. Court of Appeals for the Ninth Circuit unanimously agreed to stay the decision of the U.S. District Court pending a final ruling on the merits. The panel concluded that the public interest would be best served by allowing the ordinance to go forward in its entirety. The panel emphasized there was a presumption against ERISA pre-emption where laws fall within the state's traditional police power to regulate health and safety. It was unlikely, according to the panel, that the ordinance had an impermissible connection with an ERISA plan, because the ordinance did not require employers to:

- Adopt an ERISA plan
- Change the administrative practices of such plans
- Provide specific benefits through an existing ERISA plan

While employers would face an administrative burden in the form of required record maintenance, the panel noted this burden fell equally on employers who had ERISA plans and those who did not.

In addition, it was unlikely the ordinance would be pre-empted because of a reference to an

(continues)

(continued)

ERISA plan (since the ordinance may take ERISA health plan spending into account when calculating the required contribution of employers). The ordinance does not refer to ERISA plans specifically and could operate effectively, whether or not such plans existed.

Furthermore, the panel expressed confidence in the ordinance's political legitimacy, given that the San Francisco Board of Supervisors passed the ordinance unanimously, with the support of the Mayor. Citing the U.S. Supreme Court, the panel concluded federal courts of equity should exercise their discretionary power with proper regard for the rightful independence of local governments in carrying out their domestic policy.

RULE OF LAW: The spending requirements of San Francisco's "pay or play" ordinance do not establish an ERISA plan, nor do they have an impermissible connection with employers' ERISA plans, or make an impermissible reference to such plans.

(*See generally* Felstiner, 2008).

The San Francisco ordinance has forced retail and restaurant businesses with large populations of uninsured employees to adjust. Many businesses are passing the cost on to customers, with varying degrees of subtlety: a legal staffing agency bills clients a San Francisco health ordinance fee of $1.17 per hour, a cafe adds a 5 percent surcharge to bills and hands diners fliers describing the City's landmark solution to health care, a Mexican eatery notes a 3.5 percent charge for San Francisco affordable health care legislation (Dvorak, 2008). While some businesses raised prices and curtailed hiring, the ordinance shows early signs of doing what it was intended to do: push employers to defray medical costs for more of their employees (Dvorak, 2008). What is less clear is the extent to which mandated benefit laws affect the cost of coverage to employers (Monahan, 2007).

State Mandates for Universal Health Care Coverage

After a year-long struggle to provide universal health insurance to all state citizens, the California legislature defeated the measure. Like the San Francisco ordinance, the proposed California plan for universal health care coverage was explicit in requiring all employers to provide health insurance or pay a tax. The California law was to have applied to all employers with ten or more employees to provide adequate employee health care benefits or pay a 4 percent tax.

The Massachusetts plan is slightly different than the California plans; it does not feature a percentage tax. Massachusetts charges a $295-a-head fee to employers who do not provide employees with health insurance. Employers in Massachusetts are also liable for the catastrophic medical expenses of uninsured employees. Again, this may run afoul of ERISA because these penalties are aimed at changing employee benefit plans that are supposed to be voluntary according to federal law.

Attempts by Maryland and Suffolk County, New York, to require employers to provide adequate health insurance coverage for their employees were overturned by the federal courts following challenges by the retail industry (*see Retail Industry Leaders Association v. Fielder*, 475 F.3d 180 (U.S. Court of Appeals for the Fourth Circuit 2007); *Retail Industry Leaders Association v. Suffolk County*, 497 F.Supp.2d 403 (U.S. District Court for the Eastern District of New York 2007)). Maryland's legislation would have required employers with over ten thousand employees to spend at least 8 percent of their payroll on employee health care or remit such amount to the state. Maryland's percentage requirement was less than half what most employers in the U.S. pay to provide employee health insurance. The average employer in the U.S. spends at least 17 percent of its payroll providing health insurance coverage (Reich, 2008).

Suffolk County sought to require large retail stores selling groceries to pay a penalty for not providing health insurance that was equivalent to the cost to the public health care system of providing health care to one uninsured employee, or about $3.00 per employee. Both provisions would have largely affected Wal-Mart employees who were uninsured.

Such state mandates are clearly pre-empted by ERISA, the federal law that governs nearly all employee benefit plans. The incentive in the Massachusetts law, however, is not significant enough to force employers to make changes to their ERISA plans. Unlike the Maryland law, the rational action for employers to take in Massachusetts would be to pay the $295 per employee fee, a much less expensive option than making a fair and reasonable contribution to employee health coverage. Because the incentive under the Massachusetts law does not function as a mandate, the Massachusetts law is likely to survive any ERISA pre-emption challenge.

Can "Pay or Play" Survive ERISA Pre-emption?

The U.S. Supreme Court could take up the question of whether "pay or play" provisions can survive ERISA pre-emption (Jacobs, 2008). In doing so, several competing policy considerations would be at stake. When ERISA was enacted in the 1960s, there was widespread private employee benefit plan mismanagement. The goal of ERISA was twofold, to:

- Avoid conflicting health insurance requirements at the state and local levels
- Protect employees who were enrolled in private health insurance plans

Common Law Barriers to Health Care Reforms

ERISA opponents claim the law accomplishes its goal of regulatory uniformity at the expense of state and local governments' ability to provide innovative health care reforms. Although ERISA's legislative history makes it clear Congress intended to craft a broad pre-emption provision, it is unclear whether Congress ever anticipated the comprehensive influence the law has had on health care. There were sound reasons Congress decided to create a uniform national regulatory framework in 1974; employers were meant to be freed from the administrative burden of having to comply with a multitude of state and local requirements, leaving them with more money to spend on actual health care and other employee benefits.

The question is whether enough small businesses are providing adequate health care insurance to justify continued use of ERISA pre-emption. In 2008, the Kaiser Family Foundation annual survey of employers found:

- While almost all business with more than two hundred employees provided employee health insurance, less than six out of ten small businesses provided coverage
- Employees pay an average of $3,354 annually toward family coverage, which is more than double what they paid nine years ago
- The cost shift has been most dramatic for employers in small businesses, where more than one in three covered employees must pay at least $1,000 out of pocket before their plan generally will start to pay a share of their health care bills

(Kaiser, 2008a)

If the U.S. Supreme Court gives ERISA pre-emption the broader reading adopted by the Fourth Circuit when it invalidated the Maryland law, most, if not all, "pay or play" laws could be overturned. The resulting common law barrier to innovative solutions at the state and local levels would no doubt increase the already significant demands for a federal solution to the challenge of providing the uninsured with access to health care.

Limited ERISA Preemption

If the U.S. Supreme Court accepts the San Francisco experiment, and agrees with the Ninth Circuit, ERISA's pre-emptive reach will be limited to legislation with a direct impact on employee benefit plans. Alternatively, if the Court declines to hear the case and the Ninth Circuit decision stands, the nation is likely to spur the proliferation of provisions similar to the San Francisco ordinance. At least thirty states are considering legislation that requires employers either to provide minimum levels of health care to their employees or to pay the shortfall into public health care programs.

Federal "Pay or Play" Mandate

ERISA only pre-empts state and local law; therefore, a federal "pay or play" mandate could avoid this particular difficulty. The ultimate result of this ERISA litigation, therefore, may be to increase the demand for federal health care reform.

Health Care Ballot Initiatives

Health care initiatives in several states could resonate in national debate over the future of health care. Arizona's Proposition 101, Freedom of Choice in Health Care Act, was narrowly defeated in November 2008; the proposition would have blocked the state from enacting a universal health insurance plan. It would have amended the state's constitution to say that no law could impose any penalty or fine, of any type, for choosing to obtain or decline health care coverage or for participation in any particular health care system or plan.

So Arizona is free to adopt a state universal health insurance plan like Massachusetts, requiring everyone in the state to purchase health insurance or pay a fine. While opponents claimed the measure could have blocked regulations requiring insurers to maintain minimum solvency criteria and warned it could have increased Medicaid costs by forcing the state to pay for beneficiaries' out-of-network care, if it had passed, the measure could have been the basis of a legal challenge to the federal government creation of a national health insurance mandate.

Targeted Federal Tax Subsidies

Federal tax credits may be one way to provide coverage for the increasing number of uninsured. Problems in states with large-scale compulsory proposals for covering the uninsured have set the stage for the use of flexible, well-designed targeted subsidies, such as refundable tax credits to cover part of the premiums for private or public health insurance. A refundable tax credit is simply a credit that allows payments to taxpayers to exceed their tax obligations. Proposals that are now gaining acceptance are plans under which individuals or businesses could take advantage of tax credits for basic coverage that would vary inversely with income (Pauly & Hoff, 2002).

The Health Care Coalition for the Uninsured, an organization composed of sixteen of the nation's largest health care and community organizations, recently endorsed a program of tax credits that could be used to offset a large part of the cost of buying policies from insurance companies or from public insurance plans.[LN3] If tax credits or targeted subsidies permit the uninsured to buy mainstream insurance and use mainstream medical services, this will also improve quality for the insured by unleashing the power of the competitive market to provide more choices when it comes to securing affordable, quality insurance coverage (Pagan, 2007).

The insured may gain the most from helping the uninsured if the assistance is not targeted specifically at providing services to the uninsured only (Pauly & Pagan, 2007). While there is debate over the use of tax credits or vouchers to provide health insurance to low-income people versus expansion of Medicaid, proponents of this approach claim targeted tax subsidies would best address the issues of effectiveness and affordability.

Encourage the Purchase of Health Insurance for the Uninsured

While the U.S. uses the tax system to encourage the purchase of health insurance, the current system is upside-down. For instance, employer coverage premiums are excludable from income taxed at the federal and state levels. Therefore, for employees with high marginal tax rates (totaling over 50 percent for the highest wage earners), the tax incentive is high. With the current health insurance subsidy decreasing according to marginal tax rates, the lowest wage earners with lower marginal tax rates have little tax incentive to purchase health insurance.

The working poor generally receive no benefit from current tax subsidies. In other words, employees in the 50 percent tax category save half the cost of their premiums for health insurance compared to the 40 percent of Americans who do not pay any federal taxes and therefore save little when they purchase the same insurance. The Tax Policy Center estimates that for 2008, nearly 40 percent of filers will have no federal income tax liability. The current system provides the greatest tax benefits to persons who need it the least. Family households at the bottom of the income

pyramid get the smallest subsidy, but pay the highest share of their income for health insurance.

The Joint Tax Committee in Congress estimates current federal tax subsidies for the purchase of private health insurance coverage exceed $300 billion (Kleinbard, 2008). Tax credits to increase insurance coverage are a way to extend these tax benefits to lower-wage employees and to those currently outside the health insurance system.

The tax credit approach is essentially trying to fix the problem of the uninsured by relying on the private insurance market instead of direct government provisions. The tax credit acts as a targeted subsidy that effectively reduces the cost of private plans in the individual insurance market and encourages or mandates the uninsured to purchase insurance (Karakatsanis, 2007).

Initial Focus on the Uninsured of Limited Means

Under a comprehensive tax credit first proposed in 2002, uninsured lower-wage employees could be eligible for tax credits that would cover the full premium of a basic private insurance plan (Pauly & Hoff, 2002). Their eligibility for the tax credit would be on an income basis similar to many federal assistance programs.

For instance, individuals and family households with incomes ranging from 125 percent to about 450 percent of the poverty threshold could be eligible for tax credits, which is the same eligibility criteria for Head Start, Food Stamp Program, National School Lunch Program, Low Income Home Energy Assistance Program, and SCHIP. Poverty guidelines are updated periodically by the U.S. Department of Health and Human Services under the authority of 42 U.S.C.A. § 9902(2) (1998) and are currently $10,830 for an individual plus $3,740 for each additional person (Federal Register, 2009). For anyone unable to pay their insurance premiums out of pocket, vouchers could be issued to insurance companies or businesses, as long as family household incomes were less than $50,000 per year, which accounts for 45 percent of uninsured U.S. residents or about twenty-eight million uninsured (DeNavas-Walt et al., 2008), although the real median household income is $50,233 (DeNavas-Walt et al., 2008). Public Medicaid-like coverage could be provided for families below 125 percent of the poverty threshold who did not use the tax credits, which accounts for 17 percent of U.S. residents or about fifty-one million Americans (DeNavas-Walt et al., 2008; Pauly & Hoff, 2002).

Universal Expansion to All U.S. Residents

After using private markets to insure uninsured lower-wage employees, the tax credit program could be expanded to include other employees without insurance, but whose household incomes were greater than 450 percent of the poverty threshold, which is currently a household income greater than $46,800. Under most tax credit scenarios, the federal government would provide tax credits in the range of $2,500 per person, or $6,400 per family to purchase health insurance.

Participation in the tax credit program could be made mandatory for uninsured people, such as those with incomes greater than 450 percent of the poverty threshold. Most Americans in this income group have private insurance through their jobs, or they pay for insurance themselves out-of-pocket. Nevertheless, many Americans in this group do not have any coverage at all. They have some resources, but they are members of the middle class who need some assistance to cover the increased costs of their health care.

Under most proposals, tax credits would cover part of the premium for complete and comprehensive health insurance coverage. As a rule of thumb, the tax credit should be somewhere between one-half and two-thirds of the premium for a basic health insurance policy (Pauly & Hoff, 2002). The average annual premium for a health insurance policy is about $4,704 for

an individual; hence, a $2,500 credit would cover more than half of the premium cost, as shown in Figure 5-5. The average annual premium for a family is $12,680; thus, a $6,400 credit would cover more than half the cost (Kaiser, 2008a).

Tax Advantages

The availability of tax credits could help transform the private insurance markets in ways that could eventually change how the credits might be used. Tax credit plans are easy to administer and understand. Unlike bureaucracy-laden government programs, tax credit plans place no complex roadblocks in the way of people who need health insurance. Such ease of use is vital for universal health insurance coverage.

Tax credit plans rely as much as possible on private markets because they are seen as being the best positioned to satisfy customers' various needs. What is more, tax credits place minimal mandates on the kind of coverage people could buy; the only restriction that appears to be universally accepted is guaranteed renewability. While guaranteed renewability is required of all individual health insurance by the

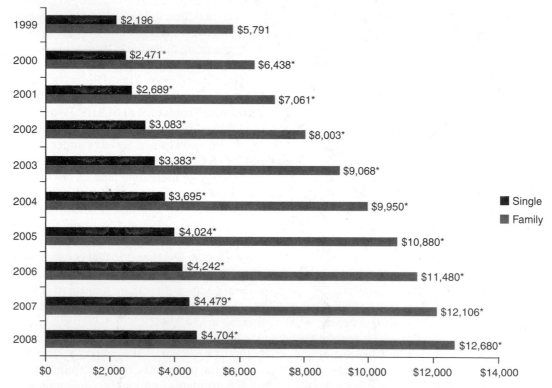

FIGURE 5-5: Average Annual Employee Contributions for Single and Family Coverage

* Estimate is statistically different from estimate for the previous year shown (p<.05).
Delmar/Cengage Learning
Data retrieved from: National Health Interview Survey (NHIS). (2009). Atlanta, GA: Centers for Disease Control & Prevention; *See also* Kaiser Commission on Medicaid & the Uninsured. (2008). Chartbook: Kaiser/HRET survey of employer-sponsored health benefits. Washington, DC: Kaiser (analyzing 1999-2007 NHIS data).

Health Insurance Portability and Accountability Act (HIPAA) of 1996, it is incomplete because the law fails to require that premiums be the same for all insured persons in a rating class (Pauly & Hoff, 2002). A tax credit is really a tax cut. It is simply a way for government to give taxpayers' money back to taxpayers.

Insurance Regulation

The U.S. spends a greater percentage of its gross domestic product (GDP) on health care than any other industrialized country (Angrisano et al., 2007); its system of insurance regulation is partly to blame for this. In the absence of comprehensive health care reform, the health share of GDP is expected to increase from 16.2 percent in 2007 to 20 percent by 2016 (CMS, 2009).

While the federal government regulates nearly all ESI coverage, states retain the power to regulate insurance contracts issued to their residents (*see* McCarran-Ferguson Act of 1945, 15 U.S.C.A. §§ 1011-1015 (2009)). As a result, employers who purchase insurance to cover their health plan benefits are subject to both federal and state regulation, while employers who self-insure plan benefits are exempt from all state insurance regulations and subject to only minimal federal regulations.

Employers who purchase insurance to cover their health plans are covered by federal insurance laws, such as the Newborns' and Mothers' Health Protection Act of 1996, 42 U.S.C.A. § 300gg-4 (1996) (requiring a minimum hospital stay of forty-eight hours following childbirth) and the Mental Health Parity Act of 1996, 29 U.S.C.A. § 1185a (2009) and 42 U.S.C.A. § 300gg-5 (2009) (requiring employers to provide the same health insurance coverage for health and mental health conditions). States, for instance, regulate the amount of financial reserves an insurance company must maintain. Employers subject to the state-based regulatory system have significantly higher compliance costs and have to comply with as many as fifty different sets of state laws. While insurance companies are likely to bear the brunt of the burden of technical compliance with individual state laws, having separate insurance contracts in different states does raise costs for multistate employers.

Regulatory Disparity

Employers who self-insure, as most employers with more than two hundred employees do, enjoy nearly complete freedom to structure their health plans, while those who purchase insurance, as most small firms and individual purchasers do, are often heavily regulated by their state (Monahan, 2007). This disparity in insurance regulation is difficult to justify. In both types of ESI plans, the insurance company typically processes all initial claims. However, employers have the ultimate authority to decide a claim on appeal from a self-insured plan, whereas the insurance company will decide all levels of an appealed claim in an insured plan pursuant to state law and regulations. While about one-third of Americans are covered by self-insured plans (Kaiser, 2008), most court cases challenging claim appeals appear to come from the more regulated health insurance plans rather than the self-insured plans.

The Congressional Budget Office found that health insurance would likely cost about 6 percent less if the insurance industry were allowed to get out from under some of the outmoded insurance regulations (CBO, 2008b). Insurance regulations provide employers who are most likely to provide health coverage with the lowest regulatory burden, while imposing a significant regulatory burden on smaller employers who are already least likely to provide health coverage to their employees (Monahan, 2007). President Clinton's Council of Economic Advisors suggested that as much as one-quarter of the uninsured lacked health insurance coverage due to the over-regulation of insurance.

Mandated Benefit Laws

Across the fifty states, the National Association of Insurance Commissioners finds that the average number of mandated benefit laws is thirty-two. One of the most expensive mandates is guaranteed issue, which defeats the actuarial logic of insurance by allowing individuals to wait until they are sick before they buy insurance without being penalized (Wharton, 2007). That leaves insurers little choice but to charge everyone else a little more to make up for the premiums the sick never contributed while they were healthy. Estimates are that by removing the average state's mandates, premiums could be reduced as much as 20 percent (Monahan, 2007).

If regulatory systems apply equally to all, there should be an incentive for the nation's largest employers to lobby for change. That is, if state-mandated benefit laws are adversely affecting coverage rates and leading to one in seven Americans being uninsured, Congress should be incentivized to take political action to lessen the regulatory burden. Under our current system, however, the most powerful players, which are large multistate employers, have no incentive to engage in the state-mandated benefit debate because they are exempt from the state mandates.[LN4]

Of course, right now there is great potential for inefficiency because there is no choice; mandated benefits prevent individuals from selecting an efficient level of insurance by failing to allow the individual to satisfy their preferences for coverage (Henderson, 2007). For example, not everyone needs maternity coverage, infertility services, erectile dysfunction drugs and services, or coverage for substance abuse treatment. For example, one cycle of in vitro fertilization costs between $10,000 and $15,000. The cost per live birth is significantly higher. One study at the University of Iowa found that the cost per live birth with the use of assisted reproductive technology was $44,000 to $212,000. Mandates reallocate limited resources within the common pool, but new or enhanced services are covered at the expense of other services or increased premiums, or both for everyone. In short, no one gets something for nothing.

Discounted Drug Programs

Into this mix, the U.S. health care system is faced with rising drug costs. Drug costs are increasing at a greater rate than any other part of the health care system. To address this concern, there are a variety of efforts that use the regulated drug supply to provide discounted drugs. For instance:

- Clearinghouse programs
- Comparison shopping sites
- Patient assistance programs

While critics contend the uninsured cannot afford access to physicians and other prescribers to obtain the prescriptions to participate in discounted drug programs, these programs are still steps in the right direction.

Clearinghouse programs appear to be the most effective in creating affordable prices for drugs for the uninsured with limited means and others with exceptional needs; the other methods are also effective in reducing the financial burden of medicines (Liang, 2008). In combination, these discount programs represent a foundation that could be consolidated and expanded to provide meaningful access to safe and affordable drugs for all who need them.

Clearinghouse Programs

By increasing access to prescription drugs, the health care system could see a drug dividend (improved health benefits in patients taking their prescribed medicines), resulting in better decreased health care expenditures as evidenced by:

- Decreased number of medical procedures
- Reductions in visits to hospitals

In addition to managing chronic diseases, many prescription drug treatments prevent hospitalizations and health complications. The U.S., however, will not realize the full benefits of a drug dividend of decreased health care expenditures until all people have access to the medicines they need. As illustrated in Figure 5-6, four out of ten Americans currently face problems accessing the prescribed drugs that they need.

The pharmaceutical industry itself has launched two national independent clearinghouse programs to assist in providing access to affordable drugs. State

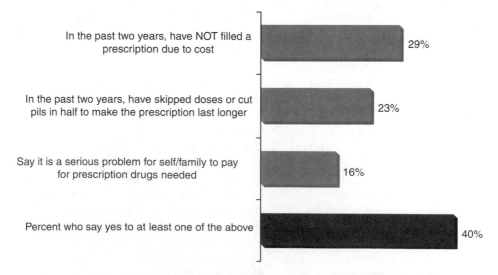

FIGURE 5-6: Serious Problems Paying, Not Filling Prescriptions, and Skipping Doses Because of Cost

Delmar/Cengage Learning

Data retrieved from: National Health Interview Survey (NHIS). (2009). Atlanta, GA: Centers for Disease Control & Prevention; *See also* USA Today, Kaiser Family Foundation & Harvard School of Public Health. (2008). The public on prescription drugs and pharmaceutical companies. McLean, VA: USA; Menlo Park, CA: Kaiser; Boston, MA: Harvard (analyzing a NHIS survey conducted on January 3-23, 2008).

programs[LN5] and other independent clearinghouse programs are also becoming available. These drug card programs alone, however, are not enough. While providing increased access to prescription drugs, millions are still without the protection of general health insurance.

Together Rx Access

Eleven pharmaceutical companies have joined together to voluntarily offer a health care card for the uninsured with limited means that provides significant savings on prescription drugs: Abbott, AstraZeneca, Bristol-Myers Squibb, GlaxoSmithKline, Johnson & Johnson, King Pharmaceuticals, Novartis, Pfizer, Sanofi-Aventis, Takeda, and TAP Pharmaceutical. Called *Together Rx Access,* this clearinghouse program affects up to 80 percent of the currently uninsured (Christenson, 2005). Savings are offered on almost three hundred brand-name prescription drugs used to treat the most common chronic health care conditions affecting Americans: allergies, arthritis, asthma, cancer, depression, diabetes, high cholesterol, and hypertension.

Eligible health consumers can save more than half on their prescription products directly from the manufacturers. Moreover, people applying for Together Rx Access are automatically notified if they are eligible for further savings (in some cases, free drugs) through each of the pharmaceutical companies' independently offered Patient Assistance Programs.

The Together Rx Access card is modeled after a similar program offered in 2003 to Medicare recipients. Of the pharmaceutical companies participating in this new program, seven participated in the parent program, Together Rx, which offered prescription drug savings for Medicare enrollees. To qualify for the Together Rx Access drug card, applicants must be:

- Legal U.S. residents under age sixty-five and otherwise not eligible for Medicare
- With incomes up to $30,000 for a single person or $60,000 for a family of four (adjusted for family size and location)
- Without public or private prescription drug coverage

Partnership for Prescription Assistance

The Partnership for Prescription Assistance brings together the pharmaceutical and biotechnology industries, physicians and other health care prescribers, patient advocacy organizations, and community groups to help health consumers who lack prescription coverage get the drugs they need. Many drugs are free, or nearly free, to the uninsured of limited means and others with exceptional needs

(Liang, 2008). The Partnership offers a single point of access to more than five hundred patient assistance programs, including more than two hundred programs offered by the pharmaceutical and biotechnology industries.

Comparison Shopping Sites

While greater price transparency might help curb rising drug costs, many overstate the likely magnitude of its contribution (Ginsberg, 2007). Nevertheless, comparison shopping sites using Internet price tools, as well as Web sites such as PillBot.com and DestinationRx.com can help reduce drug costs. PillBot.com offers a breakdown of the total prescription drug price, including price per unit information, referred to as the PPU in the pharmaceutical industry. For instance, the PPU for Ortho Neutrogena's Renova varied by as much as twenty dollars per PPU between the different online pharmacies (and was actually less at walk-in pharmacies), while the allergy medicine, Allegra cost $1.70 more per pill at one online chain pharmacy. Usually, the higher the dosage level, the higher the PPU, but this varies by pharmacy. CMS also has a prescription drug price comparison site for Medicare Part D enrollees and many states are developing sites for their residents.[LN6]

Patient Assistance Programs

For enrollees covered by Medicare Part D, pharmaceutical companies offer patient assistance programs that provide access to prescription drugs outside of the Part D benefit without any cost to the Medicare program (Federal Register, 2005). Most pharmaceutical companies have a data-sharing agreement with CMS to help coordinate drug utilization with plans providing Medicare prescription drug coverage. Medicare Part D benefit coverage has reduced the load on pharmaceutical assistance programs, enabling the pharmaceutical industry to expand such programs to lower-wage employees without health insurance, and others with exceptional needs.

CONSUMER-DIRECTED HEALTH CARE V. HIGH DEDUCTIBLE HEALTH PLANS

The rise in treatment prevalence, rather than rising treatment costs per case or population growth, accounts for most of the spending growth in health care (Thorpe, 2005, 2004).

Another approach is consumer-directed health care. At its heart, it means individuals pay more out of their own pockets. Although this approach is met with resistance, the only other proven way to restrain growth in costs is managed care, such as health maintenance organizations (Wharton, 2007). If health care spending is to be controlled, cost-sharing is the other alternative.

Under consumer-directed plans, the idea is to make the consumer more active in choosing their health care services and providers. Plan participants are given:

- Extensive information on prices for drugs, procedures, and other services
- Information to compare one health care provider with another
- Materials so they can assess what kind of health care they are likely to need

Humana, a health insurer in Louisville, Kentucky, was one of the first companies to offer its employees consumer-directed health care plans. The plans look more like auto insurance than health insurance. Employees choose which elements of coverage they want from a broad menu, based on their willingness to pay out-of-pocket expenses and their assessment of likely need. In such a plan, employees typically have the first $500 of annual health care expenses covered, as well as anything above $2,000 a year covered. Thus, employees can spend as much as $1,500 a year on their own; medical insurance covers anything over $2,000. Research has found that this approach does cut health care spending (Posner et al., 2005).

CHALLENGES OF ACCESS TO HEALTH CARE

Arguments presenting the uninsured and under-insured as being responsible for their own lack of health insurance are far easier to understand than arguments about market conditions that make coverage less available to residents at the bottom of the economic pyramid and those with serious or chronic illnesses. Employer mandates to provide coverage, federal tax credits, reform of state insurance laws, and drug discount programs are all important steps to incentivize greater health coverage and to make health insurance more affordable.

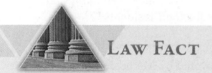

LAW FACT

ACCESS TO BASIC HEALTH CARE

Is the federal government required to provide basic health care for residents at a veteran's retirement home?

Yes, the federal government is required to provide high-quality and cost-effective health care consistent with the standards established by federal law.
          —*Cody v. Cox*, 509 F.3d 606 (U.S. Court of Appeals for the District of Columbia Circuit 2007).

CHAPTER SUMMARY

- The lack of access to health care by the uninsured and underinsured is one of the principal shortcomings of the U.S. health care system; it is a key reason the U.S. lags behind other similar nations in terms of health measures.
- About one-seventh of the American population has no health insurance, and most of them are earning middle-class incomes.
- The reasons some working Americans have no health insurance are because their employers do not offer insurance, they do not qualify for their employer's plans, or they cannot afford their employer's plan's premiums.
- Lack of health insurance causes over eighteen thousand deaths per year, and also results in higher health insurance premiums and underinsurance for those with insurance.

- Proposals for insuring the uninsured include employer mandates and taxes, limiting malpractice and legal fees, tax subsidies and credits, individual plans that take advantage of group pooling, and creating state and local health care plans.
- Regardless of how the term is used, resolution of the U.S. health care access problem involves allocating health risks in a way that makes fiscal and ethical sense and is just.
- Under the theoretical approach to addressing the nation's health care access problems, known as distributive justice, the right to basic health care has a greater weight than the cost of the care, and the ability to pay fair value for health care would have priority over the assistance provided to access the needed care.
- Proposals to reduce the cost of health care include providing less extensive coverage for the uninsured of limited means and mutual health insurance plans for people in good health.
- There is not yet a consensus on whether employer-sponsored plans or individual plans would provide the best method of reducing costs and allocating risks in terms of providing universal, comprehensive health care.
- One method for developing health care access solutions is to experiment at the state and local levels before pursuing a nationwide scheme; examples of this idea in operation are San Francisco's "pay or play" ordinance and Maryland's state mandate.
- The roadblock to experimenting on the state and local levels is ERISA, the federal law that governs nearly all employee benefit plans and pre-empts much health care legislation.
- Tax credits are a particularly enticing solution because they are easy to understand and administer, and they rely on the private markets to fulfill customers' needs by not limiting the kind of coverage people can buy, with the exception that coverage must be renewable.
- A major source of the cost of health insurance is the administrative costs necessary to comply with industry regulations, especially conflicts between federal and state regulations; the other major source of costs is the rise in treatment prevalence, rather than the rise in the cost of treatment itself.
- The drug industry has taken steps to address rising drug costs, such as clearinghouse programs, comparison shopping Web sites, and patient assistance programs.
- Other than managed care, consumer-directed health care plans are proven to control health care costs by giving consumers the opportunity to choose what kind of coverage they would like based on their willingness to pay expenses out-of-pocket.

LAW NOTES

1. John Rawls (1921-2002), Harvard University philosopher, is one of the leading twentieth-century figures in American law philosophy and is cited most frequently by the U.S. judiciary, especially the U.S. Supreme Court. Rawls received the National Humanities Medal from former President Bill Clinton in recognition of how his thought helped a whole generation of learned Americans revive their faith in democracy:
   - Rawls, J. (1999). *The law of peoples: With the idea of public reason revisited.*
   - ____. (1993). *Political liberalism: The John Dewey essays in philosophy.*
   - ____. (1971). *A theory of justice.*

   See John Nash, Princeton University mathematician, Nobel laureate, and subject of the book and film titled *A Beautiful Mind.* The Nash Equilibrium Theory was developed in four articles:
   - Nash, J. (1953). The bargaining problem. *Econometrica, 18,* 155-162.
   - ____. (1953). Two-person cooperative games. *Econometrica, 21,* 128-140 (discussing fairness in bargaining problems).
   - ____. (1951). Non-cooperative games. *Annals of Mathematics, 54,* 286-295.
   - ____. (1950). Equilibrium points in N-person games. *Proceedings of the National Academy of Sciences, 36,* 48-49.

   See also John Harsanyi, University of California-Berkeley mathematician, Nobel laureate with Nash.
   - Harsanyi, J. (1955). Cardinal welfare, individualistic ethics, and interpersonal comparisons of utility. *Journal of Political Economy, 63* (4), 302-321 (foreshadowing Rawls with a theory of distributive justice based on average expected utility maximization).

2. The University of Pennsylvania was an investor and one of the early backers of Collegiate Health Care Corp. (CHCC), the nation's first inter-university managed care organization. CHCC attempted to develop a mutual health insurance plan for college students in the late 1980s. More than one hundred schools participated in the nationwide effort before the concept was abandoned, primarily because of its complexity (like Hillary-Care). CHCC attempted to develop this insurance model at the same time as it tried to start an array of other innovative managed care services and products, and it could be said it failed because it did not focus on viable priorities in a competitive market. It tried to do it all as a start-up organization, from integrated delivery of campus health care services, to national conferences and Internet education, to sponsorship of population-specific medical research, to comprehensive inpatient and outpatient substance abuse and mental health services for the collegiate population.

3. Health Coverage Coalition for the Uninsured participating organizations include: AARP, America's Health Insurance Plans, American Academy of Family Physicians, American Hospital Association, American Medical Association, American Public Health Association, Blue Cross and Blue Shield Association, Catholic Health Association, Families USA, Federation of American Hospitals, Healthcare Leadership Council, Johnson & Johnson, Kaiser Permanente, Pfizer, United Health Foundation, and U.S. Chamber of Commerce.

4. Other clearinghouse models have been formed by states, consortiums of public and private providers, and corporate groups, to expand services beyond the discount drug programs offered by the pharmaceutical and biotechnology industries. The programs in California, Illinois, Indiana, Ohio, Rhode Island, Washington, West Virginia, and Washington, D.C. obtain demographic information and then match health consumers with eligible discount plans as well as assist in filling out enrollment forms for Medicaid assistance.

5. Arizona Rev. Stat. Ann. § 20-826.02 (Supp. 2006); Connecticut Gen. Stat. Ann. §§ 38a-493(f), 38a-520(f) (2008) (mandating that home health care may not be subjected to a deductible greater than $50 per person covered and may not have a coinsurance level less than 75 percent of the reasonable charges); Florida Stat. Ann. § 627.413 (2008); Kansas Stat. Ann. § 40-2,105 (2005) (requiring all health insurance policies to provide outpatient treatment of alcoholism, drug abuse, and nervous or mental conditions at levels not less than 100 percent of the first $100, 8 percent of the next $100, and 50 percent of the next $1,640 in any year and limited to not less than $7,500 in such person's lifetime); Maryland Code Ann., Ins. § 15-812(g)(2) (2008); New Jersey Stat. Ann. § 17:48E-35.27-28 (2008); New York Ins. Law §§ 3216, 4304, 4322 (2008) (prohibiting high-deductible health plans to be offered on the individual market; individual plans are required to include a maximum deductible of $1,000 per individual and $2,000 per family, a 20 percent coinsurance amount, no deductible for home health care services, and an out-of-pocket maximum of $3,000 per individual and $5,000 per family); North Dakota Cent. Code §§ 26.1-36-08(2)(d), 26.1-36-09(f)(4) (2007) (prohibiting requiring a deductible or co-payment for the first five substance abuse treatments in a calendar year; prohibiting a co-payment greater than 20 percent for remaining visits; prohibiting a deductible or co-payment for the first five hours of mental disorder treatment, or a co-payment of greater than 20 percent for remaining hours); Ohio Rev. Code Ann. § 1751.12 (2007); Oklahoma Stat. Ann. title 36, §§ 7002-7003 (2009); 72 Pennsylvania Stat. Ann. § 3402b.5 (2005) (eliminating the requirement that insurers provide coverage for at least one home health visit for new mothers who are discharged from the hospital less than forty-eight hours following a normal delivery or ninety-six hours after a Caesarean delivery; requiring coverage of medical foods for the treatment of several health conditions); Rhode Island Gen. Laws 27-69-3 (2006); Virginia Code Ann. § 38.2-5602.1 (Supp. 2008).

6. Some health experts express concern about the failure of online pharmacies to follow proper prescription procedures. Rogue online pharmacy sites are plagued with hoaxes and fake, tainted, contaminated, or unsafe medications that Customs and the U.S. Food and Drug Administration cannot provide even rudimentary controls over. There is also the inherent danger of patients obtaining medications from a variety of sources, thereby eliminating the potential for pharmacists to eliminate duplication and watch for interactions. Another concern is the online distribution of medications subject to licensing in the U.S. but not subject to licensing elsewhere in the world. Then there are sites such as ShopMedsNow.com where patients can order prescription medications without a required prescription. The one benefit of online pharmacies is their ability to provide emergency contraception for next-day delivery to women's homes, a need in states where access is restricted by state conscience laws that permit pharmacists to refuse dispensing of contraceptive prescriptions based on their religious convictions (*see generally* Liang, 2006; Rierson, 2008).

CHAPTER BIBLIOGRAPHY

Anderson, G. F. et al. (2006). Health care spending and use of information technology in OECD countries. *Health Affairs, 25* (3), 819-831 (analyzes the differences in uses of health information technology in the U.S. and the thirty member nations of the Organization for Economic Cooperation and Development, headquartered in Paris, France).

Angrisano, C. et al. (2007). A *framework to guide health care system reform*. San Francisco, CA: McKinsey Global Institute (analyzing why the costs of U.S. health care are so high).

Bieder, P. (2004). *Congressional Budget Office economic and budget issue brief: Limiting tort liability for medical malpractice.* Washington, DC: CBO (examines state activities related to reducing malpractice litigation and some possible causes for the rise in malpractice premiums; significant reductions in this rate of growth would only modestly affect overall health spending growth).

Bodenheimer, T. (2005). High and rising health care costs. Part 3: The role of health care providers. *Annals of Internal Medicine, 142* (12) 996-1002 (looks at how prices and quantities of health care services affect spending).

___. (2005a). High and rising health care costs. Part 2: Technologic innovation. *Annals of Internal Medicine, 142* (11) 932-937.

___. (2005b). High and rising health care costs. Part 1. *Annals of Internal Medicine, 142* (10), 847-854 (examines possible factors contributing to the rise in national health expenditures and cost-containment strategies that emphasize quality improvement as well as lowering spending).

Bodenheimer, T., & Fernandez, A. (2005). High and rising health care costs. Part 4: Can costs be controlled while preserving quality? *Annals of Internal Medicine, 143* (1) 26-31 (reviewing quality-enhancing strategies that might help slow the growth of health care costs).

Bodenheimer, T., & Grumbach, K. (2008). *Understanding health policy.* NY, NY: McGraw-Hill Medical.

Buntin, M. B. et al. (2006). Consumer-directed health care: Early evidence about effects on cost and quality. *Health Affairs, 25* (6) 516-530.

Carreyrou, J., & Martinez, B. (2008, April 4). Tax-exempt hospitals, once for the poor, strike it rich with tax-breaks, they outperform for-profit rivals. *Wall Street Journal,* p. A1.

Catlin, A. et al. (2008). National health spending in 2006: A year of change for prescription drugs. *Health Affairs, 27* (1), 14-29 (uses data collected by CMS to analyze the national trends of health spending in 2006 and the impact of Medicare Part D on prescription drug spending growth).

___. (2007). National health spending in 2005: The slowdown continues. *Health Affairs, 26* (1), 142-153 (in 2005, the health spending grew at a slower rate than the previous year).

CBO (Congressional Budget Office). (2008). *Geographic variation in health care spending.* Washington, DC: CBO (examining the amount of geographic variation in spending, the reasons for that variation, and its implications for evaluating the efficiency of the health care system).

___. (2008a). *Technological change and the growth of health care spending.* Washington, DC: CBO (describing the historical growth in spending on health care in the U.S.; examines the factors that determine health care spending and how they have contributed to spending growth over time).

___. (2008b). *Key issues in analyzing major health insurance proposals.* Washington, DC: CBO.

___. (2007). *Financing projected spending in the long run.* Washington, DC: CBO (analyzing the potential economic effects of increasing taxes to finance the expected increase in health spending over the next several decades).

___. (2003). *How many people lack health insurance and for how long?* Washington, DC: CBO.

Chernew, M. E. et al. (2004). Barriers to constraining health care cost growth. *Health Affairs, 23* (6), 122-128 (discussion of how to slow the growth of health care expenditures, looking specifically at managed care as a method of cost containment).

Christenson, V. (2005). Drug companies offer major discounts to uninsured. *Journal of Law, Medicine & Ethics, 33,* 399-402.

Claxton, G. et al. (2008). *Employer health benefits 2008 annual survey.* Menlo, CA: Kaiser Family Foundation & Health Research and Education Trust.

CMS (Centers for Medicare and Medicaid Services). (2009). *National health expenditure fact sheet.* Baltimore, MD: CMS.

Collins, S. R. et al. (2006). *Squeezed: Why rising exposure to health care costs threatens the health and financial well-being of American families.* NY, NY: Commonwealth Fund. (comparing adults with employer-based coverage and adults in the individual insurance market on a variety of factors including out-of-pocket payments, deductible rates, and percentage of income spent on health care).

Cunningham, P. J. et al. (2008). *The fraying link between work and health insurance: Trends in employer sponsored insurance for employees, 2000-2007.* Washington, DC: Center for Studying Health System Change (HSC) & Kaiser Commission on Medicaid & the Uninsured.

Cutler, D. M. et al. (2006). The value of medical spending in the U.S., 1960-2000. *New England Journal of Medicine, 355,* 920-927 (examining the value of increased medical spending by comparing gains in life expectancy with the increased costs of care).

Davis, K. et al. (2007). *Slowing the growth of U.S. health care expenditures: Where are the options?* NY, NY: Commonwealth Fund (reviewing factors that contribute to high spending on the health care system in the U.S, while analyzing strategies for accumulating savings, reducing spending growth, and improving health system performance).

DeNavas-Walt, C. et al. (2008). *Income, poverty and health insurance coverage in the U.S.* Washington, DC: U.S. Census Bureau.

Dvorak, P. (2008, May 5), Firms adjust to health-care law in San Francisco, businesses move to adapt to costs. *Wall Street Journal,* p. B4.

Farrell, D. et al. (2008). *Accounting for the cost of U.S. health care: A new look at why Americans spend more.* San Francisco, CA: McKinsey Global Institute.

Federal Register. (2009, January 23). 2009 poverty guidelines, 74 FR 4199-04

___. (2005, November 22). Bulletin on patient assistance programs for Medicare Part D enrollees, 70 FR 70623-03

Felstiner, A. (2008). *Golden Gate Restaurant Ass'n. v. City & County of San Francisco*: The Ninth Circuit limits ERISA preemption, expands pay-or-play options. *Berkeley Journal of Employment & Labor Law, 29,* 473-485.

Gabel, J. et al. (2005). Health benefits in 2005: Premium increases slow down, coverage continues to erode. *Health Affairs, 24* (5), 1273-1280 (accompanying the Employer Health Benefits Survey, published by Kaiser Family Foundation & Health Research and Educational Trust, discussing changes in the cost and scope of employer-based insurance since 2000).

Ginsburg, P. B. (2007). Shopping for price in medical care. *Health Affairs, 26* (2), 208-216 (analyzing the way in which individuals select health care services based on price and the influence that insurers and the government can have on price selection).

Hadley. J. (2008). Covering the uninsured in 2008: Current costs, sources of payment, and incremental costs. *Health Affairs, 27* (5), 399-415.

Halpern, M. T. et al. (2008). Association of insurance status and ethnicity with cancer stage at diagnosis for twelve cancer sites: A retrospective analysis. *Lancet Oncology, 9* (3), 222-231.

Hellander, I. (2008). The deepening crisis in U.S. health care: A review of data. *International Journal of Health Services, 38* (4), 607-623.

Henderson, D. R. (2007, January 10). Terminatorcare. *Wall Street Journal*, p. A17.

Hoffman, C., & Schwartz, K. (2008, October 15). *Trends in access to care among working-age adults, 1997-2006.* Washington, DC: Kaiser Commission on Medicaid & the Uninsured.

Hunter, N. D. (2008). Risks governance and deliberative democracy in health care. *Georgetown Law Journal, 97*, 1-59.

Hurley, R. E. (2005). A widening rift in access and quality: Growing evidence of economic disparities. *Health Affairs, 10*, 1377-1382.

IOM (Institute on Medicine) Committee on the Consequences of Uninsurance. (2004). *Insuring America's health: Principles and recommendations.* Washington, DC: IOM.

Jacobs, S. (2008). On the mend: The Ninth Circuit gives San Francisco's health care security ordinance the green light (for now). *Journal of Law, Medicine, & Ethics, 36*, 431-433.

Kaiser (Kaiser Commission on Medicaid & the Uninsured). (2008). *Issue brief: Five basic facts on the uninsured.* Washington, DC: Kaiser.

___. (2008a). *Employer health benefits 2008 annual survey.* Washington, DC: Kaiser.

___. (2007). *The uninsured: A primer.* Washington, DC: Kaiser.

Karakatsanis, A. G. (2007). Health insurance in America: Providing substance to America's values. *Journal of Medicine & Law, 11*, 337-375.

Keenan, P. S. (2004). *What is driving health care costs?* NY, NY: Commonwealth Fund.

Kenney, G., & Pelletier, J. (2008). *Spotlight on low-income uninsured young adults: Causes and consequences.* Washington, DC: Kaiser Commission on Medicaid & the Uninsured.

Kleinbard, E., chief economist for the Joint Tax Committee in Congress. (2008, July 31). *Tax expenditures for health care.* Testimony before the U.S. Senate Committee on Finance. Washington, DC.

Klick, J., & Markowitz, S. (2003). *Working paper: Are mental health insurance mandates effective?: Evidence from suicides.* Washington, DC: National Bureau of Economic Research.

Liang, B. A. (2008). A dose of reality: Promoting access to pharmaceuticals. *Wake Forest Intellectual Property Law Journal, 8*, 301-386.

___. (2006). Fade to black: Importation and counterfeit drugs. *American Journal of Law & Medicine, 32*, 279-323.

Locke, J. (2008). *Two treatises of government.* Birmingham, AL: Palladium Press (original work published 1689).

Martinez, B. (2008, April 28). Cash before chemo: Hospitals get tough, bad-debts prompt change in billing; $45,000 to come in. *Wall Street Journal*, p. A1.

Monahan, A. B. (2007). Federalism, federal regulation, or free market? An examination of mandated health benefit reform. *University of Illinois Law Review*, 1361-1416.

Mullins, C. D. et al (2005). Variability and growth in spending for outpatient specialty pharmaceuticals. *Health Affairs, 24* (4), 1117–1127 (documenting large expenditures on select specialty pharmaceutical categories and variation in spending across ten Blue Cross Blue Shield plans, age groups, and time).

NASTAD (National Alliance of State and Territorial AIDS Directors). (2008). *National ADAP monitoring project annual report.* Washington, DC: NASTAD & Menlo Park, CA: Kaiser Family Foundation.

Newhouse, J. (2004). Consumer-directed health plans and the RAND health insurance experiment. *Health Affairs, 23* (6), 107–113 (comparing consumer-directed health plans to the RAND Health Insurance Experiment of the 1970s and 1980s; suggests policy reforms to address the continual rise in health care costs, including a combination of managed care and cost sharing).

Owcharenko, N. (2005). *Backgrounder: Making association health plans a success.* Washington, DC: Heritage Foundation (outlining association health plans and their potential for lowering costs and expanding health care coverage).

Pagan, J. A., professor of economics at the University of Texas and senior fellow at the Leonard Davis Institute of Health Economics at the University of Pennsylvania. (2007, February 7). Beazley Symposium on *Access to health care: immigration from the Mayflower to border patrols: Who should have access to health care in the U.S.* at Loyola University Chicago School Law, Beazley Institute Health Law & Policy. Chicago.

Pauly, M. V., & Pagan, J. A. (2007). Spillovers and vulnerability: The case of community uninsurance. *Health Affairs, 26* (5), 1304-1314.

Pauly, M. V. (2007). Health risks and benefits in health care: The view from economics. *Health Affairs, 26*, 653-662.

Pauly, M. V. et al. (2005). Competition and new technology. *Health Affairs, 24* (6), 1523-1535 (discussing the effect of new technologies on health care prices and ways in which adopting different policies toward technology could increase competitiveness between insurers).

___. (2003). An adaptive credit plan for covering the uninsured. In Meyer J. A. et al., *Covering America: Real remedies for the uninsured* (Vol. 1). Washington, DC: Economic & Social Research Institute.

Pauly, M. V., & Hoff, J. S. (2002). *Responsible tax credits for health insurance.* Washington, DC: American Enterprise Institute for Public Policy Research (research on which most other tax credit proposals are based).

Posner, P. et al. (2005). *21st century challenges: Reexamining the base of the federal government.* Washington, DC: Government Accountability Office (report is intended to help

Congress in reviewing and reconsidering the basis of federal spending and tax programs, including a chapter that focuses on health care challenges).

Rawls, J. (2005). *A theory of justice*. Boston, MA: Belknap Press of Harvard University Press (original text).

___. (2005a). *Political liberalism*. NY: Columbia University Press.

Reich, R. (2008, January 29). America's middle classes are no longer coping. *Financial Times*, p. 8.

Remler, D. K., & Glied, S. A. (2006). How much more cost sharing will health savings accounts bring? *Health Affairs, 25* (4), 1070-1078.

Rierson, S. L. (2008). Pharmaceutical counterfeiting and the puzzle of remedies. *Wake Forest Intellectual Property Law Journal, 8*, 433-457.

Rousseau, J-J. (2009). *Discourse on political economy and the social contract*. (Oxford World's Classics). NY, NY: Oxford University Press (original work published 1762).

Schneider, J. E., & Ohsfeldt, R. L. (2007). The role of markets and competition in health care reform initiatives to improve efficiency and enhance access to care. *Cumberland Law Review, 37*, 479-511.

Thorpe, K. E. (2005). The rise in health care spending and what to do about it. *Health Affairs, 24* (6), 1436-1445 (examining causes for the growth of health spending, such as obesity and stress, over the past twenty years and suggests reform options).

Thorpe, K. E. et al. (2004). Which medical conditions account for the rise in health care spending? *Health Affairs*, w4, 437-445 (looking at the level and growth in health care spending attributable to the fifteen most expensive medical conditions and finding that a small number of conditions account for most of the growth in health care spending).

Tobert, J. et al. (2008). *Approaches to covering the uninsured: A guide*. Washington, DC: Kaiser Commission on Medicaid & the Uninsured.

Towers Perrin. (2005). *Managing health care costs in a new era: 10th Annual National Business Group on Health/Watson Wyatt Survey Report*. Stamford, CT: Towers Perrin (presenting a survey profile of trends in ESIs, including growing interest in consumer directed health plans, cost of private insurance, and employee cost-sharing).

Weinick, R. et al. (2005). Who can't pay for health care? *Journal of General Internal Medicine, 20* (6), 504-509 (using data from the Commonwealth Fund Health Care Quality Survey to examine barriers to health care).

Wharton (Wharton School at the University of Pennsylvania). (2007, September 5). A prescription for healthier medical care decisions: Begin by defining health risks. *Knowledge@ Wharton*.

White, C. (2007). Health care spending growth: How different is the U.S. from the rest of the OECD? *Health Affairs, 26* (1), 154-161 (comparing factors contributing to health care spending growth in the U.S. to that of other OECD countries).

Zuvekas, S. H., & Cohen, J. W. (2007). Prescription drugs and the changing concentration of health care expenditures. *Health Affairs, 26* (1), 249-257 (exploring the concentration of health care spending in various sectors and possible implications for cost containment).

CHAPTER 6

MEDICAID AND SCHIP ACCESS TO MEDICALLY NECESSARY HEALTH CARE

> *"In view of the Constitution, in the eye of the law, there is in this country no superior, dominant, ruling class of citizens. There is no caste here."*
>
> —Justice John Marshall Harlan (1833-1911), Associate Justice of the U.S. Supreme Court

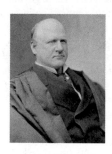

In Brief

Following chapter five, this chapter draws further attention to the challenge of finding a way to provide access to medically necessary health care for U.S. residents at the bottom of the economic pyramid. Attention is directed toward providing an overview of Medicaid financing, the *State Children's Health Insurance Program* (SCHIP). The Equal Access provisions of the federal Medicaid law are also examined. Finally, methods used to assess economic impact are explained. Medical assistance is generally referred to as *Medicaid insurance* in this chapter.

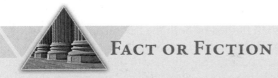

FACT OR FICTION

ACCESS TO MEDICALLY NECESSARY HEALTH CARE

Should the judiciary force a solution to shape the legislative dimensions of how to provide access to medically necessary health care for U.S. residents at the bottom of the economic pyramid, and in particular poor children?

Before 1965, health care in America was dual tracked: the insured received care from private physicians, while the uninsured, if they accessed health care at all, received treatment in ambulatory clinics and emergency rooms (Moncrieff, 2006). This was meant to change after Congress created the Medical Assistance program (Medicaid) in 1965 (*see* Medicaid Act, 42 U.S.C.A. §§ 1396-1396v (2009) (Congress created the Medicaid program by amending the Social Security Act, and as such, the program remains in the Social Security Act)). Since then, courts have examined whether the Medicaid-insured have an individually enforceable right to health care.[LN1] Courts are split on whether the federal Medicaid law creates a federally enforceable right of access to medically necessary health care, but generally agree U.S. residents eligible for Medicaid insurance have a federal right to financial assistance for:

- Early and periodic screening, diagnostic, and treatment services (EPSDT)
- Receipt of health care benefits with reasonable promptness
- Health services comparable in amount, duration, and scope to the insured in their geographic community

While courts generally hold there is a federally enforceable right to prompt and comparable payment for health services received by Medicaid-insured recipients, courts have failed to provide a uniform remedy when that right is violated (Sorkin, 2008).

The Oklahoma Chapter of the American Academy of Pediatrics, a professional organization of pediatricians and pediatric specialists, the Community Action Project of Tulsa County, and thirteen children and their parents representing a class of individuals filed a § 1983 federal civil rights lawsuit against the State of Oklahoma. The class maintained the State of Oklahoma and the Oklahoma Health Care Authority violated various provisions of the federal Medicaid law by failing to provide Medicaid-eligible children in the state with necessary health care.

The claim against the State of Oklahoma was twofold: the class contended state policies and procedures denied or deprived Medicaid-eligible children of the health and health care to which they were entitled under federal law, in particular EPSDT services with reasonable promptness. In addition, they claimed the state failed to have provider reimbursement rates set at a sufficient level to assure Medicaid-eligible children equal access to quality health care. The U.S. District Court found the state failed to ensure payments sufficient to enlist enough health care providers so that services were available to Medicaid-eligible children to the same extent such care and services were available to the general, non-Medicaid-insured population. Second, the state failed to furnish medical assistance with reasonable promptness to Medicaid-eligible children. The State of Oklahoma appealed the court's decision.

—*OKAAP v. Fogarty*, 472 F.3d 1208 (U.S. Court of Appeals for the 10th Circuit 2007), *U.S. Supreme Court certiorari denied*, 128 S.Ct. 68 (U.S. Supreme Court 2007), *on remand*, 522 F.Supp.2d 1353 (U.S. District Court for the Northern District of Oklahoma 2007). (See *Law Fact* at the end of this chapter for the answer.)

PRINCIPLES AND APPLICATIONS

Economic disparities, largely a function of different sources of insurance coverage, influence access to health care in the U.S. (Hurley, 2005). Many technological innovations and health care initiatives are focused on affluent communities and are accessible mainly to people with private health insurance. For the uninsured or people with Medicaid coverage at the bottom of the economic pyramid, access to routine medical procedures is often inadequate and not of the highest quality, if access exists at all.

Health care in the U.S. improves every year, since new drugs and new technologies appear constantly.

Health care in the U.S. also costs more every year and shows no signs of changing course. For those who have comprehensive health care insurance and the money to pay their deductibles, co-insurance, and out-of-network fees as needed, the U.S. health care system offers the best health care available anywhere in the world. For the one out of every four Americans who may be without health insurance for part or all of any given year, however, access to this quality health care is simply not affordable (MedPAC, 2008).

THE THREE W'S OF MEDICAID INSURANCE: WHO? WHAT? WHY?

Medicaid is the nation's public health insurance program for Americans of limited means and the severely disabled. It finances health care and long-term care services for more than sixty million people, many of whom face the highest burden of chronic disease of any population group in the U.S., owing to socioeconomic hardships (Kaiser, 2009).

Created by Title XIX of the Social Security Act, Medicaid insurance is a means-tested entitlement program funded by both the federal and state governments. Medicaid is the second largest line item in state budgets behind education, with over 21 percent of state funds being allocated to Medicaid on average (NASBO, 2009). Medicaid funds are the largest source of federal support for the states (Kaiser, 2009). Operated jointly by the federal government and the states, Medicaid insurance is projected to account for roughly 15 percent of the nation's health care spending in 2010, but more than half of all spending is for nursing home and other long-term care, as illustrated in Figure 6-1 (CMS, 2009).

Medicaid insurance is distinct from Medicare. The following chapter will address Medicare, the public health insurance programs for Americans sixty-five and older and for people with permanent disabilities who are under age sixty-five. Individuals contribute payroll taxes to Medicare throughout their working lives and become eligible for Medicare when they reach sixty-five, regardless of their income.

Federal Share of Medicaid Spending

The federal share of Medicaid spending, generally referred to as the Federal Medical Assistance

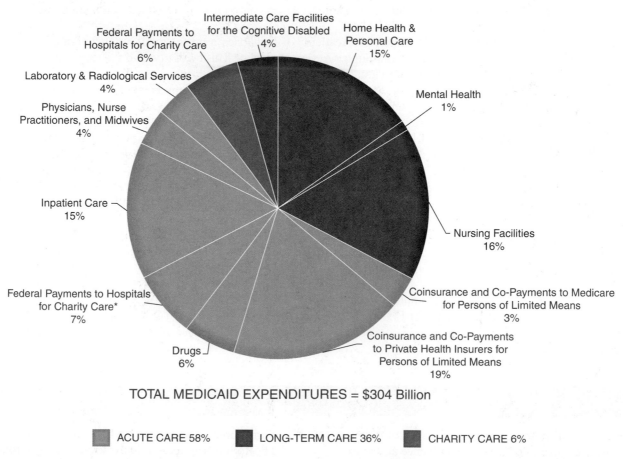

FIGURE 6-1: Total Medicaid Expenditures by Treatment Service (Exclusive of Administrative Costs)

Delmar/Cengage Learning

Data retrieved from: The Centers for Medicare & Medicaid Services. (2008). Medicaid at-a-glance. Baltimore, MD: CMS; see Urban Institute. (2009). Medicaid and SCHIP. Washington, DC: Urban Institute; see also Kaiser Commission on Medicaid & the Uninsured. (2007). Medicaid expenditures by service. Washington, DC: Kaiser.

Percentages (FMAP), is at least 50 percent in every state. FMAPs are what the Centers for Medicare and Medicaid Services (CMS) uses in determining the amount of federal matching funds for states. Federal contribution varies based on state per capita household income relative to the national income average. The highest federal contribution of 83 percent goes to Mississippi, the poorest state in the nation (*Federal Register,* 2008).

Overall, the federal government more than matches Medicaid spending by the states, paying an average of 57 percent of the nation's total Medicaid costs (Kaiser, 2008a). The federal government spent about $201 billion on Medicaid and the states spent an additional $158 billion in 2007, bringing the total Medicaid spending to over $359 billion for the year (NASBO, 2009), which only includes state funds used for federal matching purposes as defined by the Health Care Financing Administration, including state general funds and other funds and revenue used to match federal Medicaid contributions, such as local funds and provider taxes, fees, donations, and assessments. Amidst an economic recession, spending by the federal government for Medicaid benefits to the states reached $443 billion in 2008 (CMS, 2009).

Who Is Categorically Eligible for Medicaid Insurance?

Without Medicaid, most of the Medicaid-insured would be uninsured. To qualify for assistance, the Medicaid-insured must meet financial criteria and also belong to one of the categorically eligible groups. Medicaid is the principal safety net for:

- Low-wage working families with children
- Medicare-eligible beneficiaries with limited resources, who need assistance with filling gaps in their Medicare coverage
- Blind or severely disabled children and adults
- Uninsured pregnant women

Medicaid insurance does not, however, provide coverage for everyone at the bottom of the economic pyramid. Even under the broadest regulatory provisions, Medicaid insurance does not generally provide coverage for medically necessary health care, even for the very poorest persons in society, unless they are in one of the designated eligibility groups.

The regulations for counting income and resources vary from state to state and from categorically eligible group to group. There are also special regulations for those who live in nursing homes and for disabled children living at home. The regulatory obfuscations of the nation's public insurance system, for health care providers as well as individuals and families, are one of the most confusing areas of health law.

Low-Wage Earners with Children

Most of the Medicaid-insured are low-wage working parents with children (Kaiser, 2008a). Many of the Medicaid-insured adults are people from the middle class who are retired and now require care in a nursing home or other long-term care facility (MedPAC, 2008). Many of the severely disabled are blind or HIV/AIDS patients as illustrated in Figure 6-2; some 20 percent of the people living with AIDS are Medicaid-insured (NASTAD, 2008).

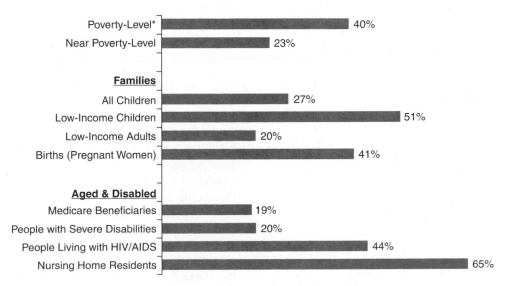

Percent with Medicaid Coverage:

Poverty-Level* — 40%
Near Poverty-Level — 23%

Families
All Children — 27%
Low-Income Children — 51%
Low-Income Adults — 20%
Births (Pregnant Women) — 41%

Aged & Disabled
Medicare Beneficiaries — 19%
People with Severe Disabilities — 20%
People Living with HIV/AIDS — 44%
Nursing Home Residents — 65%

FIGURE 6-2: Medicaid's Role for Selected Populations

*Families living at the federal poverty-level (FPL) have household incomes of $21,800 or less for a family of four; families near the poverty-level live at 133% of the FPL with household incomes less than $29,000.

Delmar/Cengage Learning

Data retrieved from: CMS, 2009; *Federal Register,* 2008; *See* Kaiser, 2008a.

Disabled Medicare Beneficiaries

One out of four people who are Medicaid-insured are disabled Medicare beneficiaries (MedPAC, 2008). This population group, however, accounts for more than 70 percent of the nation's Medicaid spending (Kaiser, 2008a).

Severely Disabled Children and Adults

Medicaid provides health insurance coverage for people with physical and mental disabilities and chronic illnesses, such as symptomatic HIV/AIDS patients. Often, these people cannot obtain coverage in the private insurance market, or the health insurance they have falls short of their medical needs.

One out of five people who are severely disabled are Medicaid-insured (Kaiser, 2008a). Almost half of the people living with HIV/AIDS in the U.S. are covered by Medicaid insurance (44 percent). This means nearly three out of every five Americans infected with HIV/AIDS are symptomatic and dying from a chronic illness that early care could have prevented before their symptoms manifest (Kaiser, 2009b).

Uninsured Pregnant Women

The birth mothers of four out of ten children born in the U.S. are covered by Medicaid insurance (Kaiser, 2009b). Medicaid provides access to prenatal care and neonatal intensive care for eligible women and their babies.

Most states offer expanded coverage of pregnant women beyond the federal income eligibility level of other Medicaid-eligible individuals. Twenty states covered pregnant women up to 185 percent of the federal poverty level (FPL) or $20,035 for a single mother in 2008; another twenty states provide eligibility criteria at higher income levels (Kaiser, 2009c). Poverty guidelines are updated periodically in the *Federal Register* by the U.S. Department of Health and Human Services under the authority of 42 U.S.C.A. § 9902(2) (1998), and were set at $10,830 for an individual plus $3,740 for each additional person in 2009 (*Federal Register,* 2009).

What Health Insurance Coverage Is Required for the Uninsured of Limited Means?

The following health services must be covered by Medicaid insurance:

- Dental services
- EPSDT services for children under twenty-one years of age
- Family planning and pregnancy services
- Home health services
- Hospital services, both inpatient and outpatient
- Laboratory and radiological services
- Licensed physician, nurse practitioner, and midwife services
- Nursing facility services for those over twenty-one years of age

Medicaid insurance payments are paid directly to hospitals and other health care providers, as illustrated in Figure 6-3.

Coverage Issues

Three-Month and Five-Year Rules

Medicaid insurance coverage may start three months prior to application for assistance with medical bills, if the individual would have been eligible during the retroactive period. Coverage generally stops at the end of the month in which a person's circumstances change. With many individuals facing unemployment as a result of serious injuries, illness, or disease, many people eligible for Medicaid assistance do not take advantage of this opportunity when faced with extraordinary medical bills. The primary reason for this failure to apply for Medicaid is that hospitals and other health care providers do not always advise patients of their possible eligibility for Medicaid until after the three-month eligibility period has lapsed. Whether this is simply an oversight or whether they prefer to bill the middle class at a higher rate than is available under the Medicaid fee structure is an issue of much debate (Doty et al., 2005). In addition, states administering the program have seldom developed active outreach programs to advise their residents of the benefits of Medicaid, nor have they actively sought to enroll state residents.

Most states have additional charity programs to provide medical assistance to residents who do not qualify for Medicaid, but face extraordinary circumstances requiring that society give them a helping hand. For instance, lawful permanent residents are not eligible for Medicaid insurance until they have been in the U.S. for five years. No federal funds are provided for these charity and patient assistance programs; they are strictly state-funded programs. The U.S. pharmaceutical industry has assumed a leadership position with their patient assistance programs. Since 2003, the industry has also provided discounted drug programs. Both programs are privately funded, without any government funding.

Definition of Medically Needy

Low income is only one test for Medicaid eligibility; assets and resources are also tested against established thresholds. Resources such as bank accounts, real property, or other items that can be sold for cash, generally must be used before individuals are eligible for Medicaid insurance. Medically needy persons, who would be categorically eligible for Medicaid insurance, except for income or assets, may become eligible for assistance, however, solely because of excessive medical expenses.

Medicaid insurance often becomes available to the American middle class facing nursing care or other long-term care costs or home care costs arising from chronic, non-terminal illnesses, such as

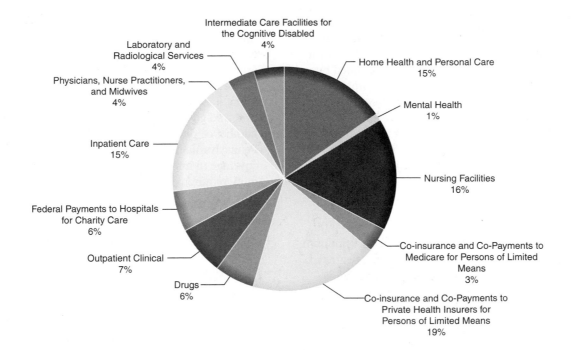

TOTAL MEDICAID EXPENDITURES EXCLUSIVE OF ADMINISTRATIVE COSTS: $339 Billion

FIGURE 6-3: Medicaid's Expenditures by Type of Service

Note: Percentage data excludes administrative costs, which are generally estimated to be an additional 4 to 6 percent of the total expenditures (CMS, 2009). In 2008, however, administrative costs exceeded $35 billion, almost twice the government estimates.
Delmar/Cengage Learning

Data retrieved from: The Centers for Medicare & Medicaid Services. (2008). Medicaid at-a-glance. Baltimore, MD: CMS; *see* Urban Institute. (2009). *Medicaid and SCHIP.* Washington, DC: Urban Institute; *see also* Kaiser Commission on Medicaid & the Uninsured. (2007). *Medicaid expenditures by service.* Washington, DC: Kaiser.

Parkinson's disease or dementia. The middle class is often covered by Medicaid insurance when their private insurance coverage is exhausted from medical situations, such as when:

- Expenses from a catastrophic injury or illness exceed the limits of their private insurance
- The medical treatments they elect to have are excluded from coverage by private insurers, who deem their care to be experimental
- They are treated out-of-network and their private insurance co-payment responsibilities were not capped

Moral Dilemmas

1. Should there be a limit on the total amount of coverage Medicaid will provide?

Emergency Health Services

One exception is generally for emergency services. However, emergency services must be life-threatening to be covered, and what constitutes a threat to life is determined by state agencies rather than by health care providers or injured or sick individuals.

Moral Dilemmas

1. What should be considered life-threatening?
2. Should coverage be revoked if it turns out an individual's experience was not life-threatening?

Delivery System Inequities

The federal government and the states jointly finance Medicaid. States increase Medicaid enrollments to qualify for more federal assistance, rather than being given incentives to increase efficiency and higher quality. This is theoretically easier said than practically achieved.

Coverage Incentives

One criticism of the current Medicaid delivery system is that coverage has become the end in itself (Hurley, 2005). States spread resources widely but thinly, without enough attention to:

- Accessibility
- Accurate and comparable payment rates
- Health outcomes, or whether coverage is actually improving health
- Quality of health care

States have no obligation to rigorously evaluate their programs in order to qualify for additional federal funds; funding is based on state demographics. For its part, the federal government has been restrained by coverage regulations when states have attempted to take steps to fix their own Medicaid programs, such as by devising outcome-based standards for evaluating performance, and de-emphasizing the goal of growing the number of covered people (Karakatsanis, 2007). Federal regulations also prohibit states from limiting Medicaid enrollments or establishing wait lists for entitlement programs.

State Waivers

States may expand Medicaid and the federal minimum standards, and they have done so to varying degrees. States cannot, however, use federal matching funds to provide insurance coverage to cover non-disabled adults without children, no matter how poor they are. States may use additional state funds, but no federal funds may be used for adults of working age who are not suffering from physical or mental disabilities.

A handful of states have received special permission, known as waivers, from federal regulators to take incremental steps to improve their Medicaid programs:

- Indiana is incorporating personal accounts to allow patients greater choice of health care providers and providing consumer incentives to patients who follow their treatment regimes

- Louisiana is providing tailored Medicaid services through managed care networks run by private, competing companies that are accountable for improving patient health outcomes
- North Carolina created a primary-care-based program that pays physicians to improve coordination of care, and gives patients more choice by expanding the number of physicians participating in the program
- Pennsylvania has sought to provide universal health coverage to uninsured families by expanding the eligibility requirements to qualify for Medicaid insurance

CMS, which regulates the program, recently gave states the flexibility to redesign their Medicaid benefits by modeling the programs after managed care plans already being offered in particular states (42 U.S.C.A. § 1315(f) (2000)). However, creating incentives for broader state accountability makes federal regulations far less significant, which probably means ending Medicaid's open-ended funding. Indeed, a series of waivers led to mandatory Medicaid managed care as a way to prevent unnecessary health care expenditures (Super, 2005).

Economics of the Medicaid-Insured

- Total Medicaid spending increased around 6 percent to over $329.4 billion in 2007 (Hartman et al., 2009)
- Medicare-insured and the disabled account for about 70 percent of Medicaid's expenditures

(Kaiser, 2008)

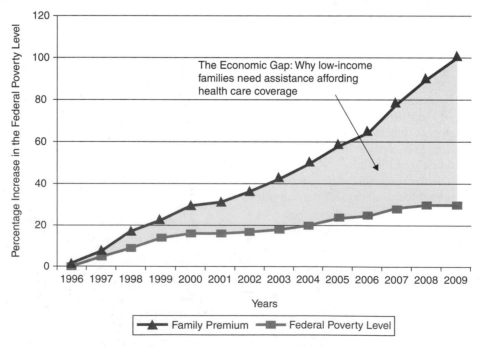

FIGURE 6-4: Cumulative Change in Family Health Insurance Premiums and Federal Poverty Level

Delmar/Cengage Learning

Data retrieved from: The Agency for Healthcare Research & Quality. (2009). *Medical expenditure panel survey: MEPS household component summary tables.* Rockville, MD: U.S. Department of Health & Human Services, AHRQ. *Federal Register,* 2009; *see* Holahan et al., 2009; *see also* Kaiser, 2008.

With health insurance premiums rising more rapidly than the federal poverty level, the protection offered to the sickest and poorest Americans by Medicaid, with eligibility tied to the poverty line, has not kept pace with rising health insurance costs over time (Kaiser, 2009). As illustrated in Figure 6-4, the federal poverty level has been increased 30 percent since 1996; during the same time period, private health insurance premiums have increased over 134 percent. Medicaid per capita spending has grown much more slowly than private health spending per capita.

Access to Medically Necessary Health Care

While Medicaid is an improvement over being uninsured, it often relegates the Medicaid-insured to inferior health care. In recognition of the disparity in health care available to the privately-insured and Medicare-insured, as compared to the Medicaid-insured, vigorous legislative and judicial debate is occurring about what constitutes access to health care in the U.S.

Eventually the nation will be forced to arrive at a political consensus. Whether the leadership to reach a compromise will arise from the executive branch, or the legislative branch will assume its leadership role, is not

EQUAL ACCESS TO HEALTH CARE

Equal Access for El Paso, Inc. v. Hawkins

[Medicaid-Insured Recipients v. Commissioner of the Texas State Medicaid Plan]

509 F.3d 697 (U.S. Court of Appeals for the 5th Circuit 2007),

U.S. Supreme Court certiorari denied, 129 S.Ct. 34 (U.S. Supreme Court 2008), on remand,

522 F.Supp.2d 1353 (U.S. District Court for the Northern District of Oklahoma 2007)

FACTS: Equal Access for El Paso is a nonprofit corporation designed to increase access to health care for individuals in El Paso County, Texas. Equal Access for El Paso and three health care providers (a physician, hospital, and health maintenance organization), all of whom sued on behalf of themselves, Medicaid-insured recipients, residents of El Paso County, and several individual Medicaid-insured recipients, brought suit against Hawkins, the Commissioner of the Texas Health and Human Services Commission and the administrator of the Texas Medicaid plan (Texas). Equal Access for El Paso claimed Texas set deficient Medicaid reimbursement and capitation rates, in violation of the Equal Access provision of the federal Medicaid law (*see* 42 U.S.C.A. § 1396a(a)(30)(A) (2009)). This deficient reimbursement resulted in inadequate access to health care for Medicaid-insured recipients living in the El Paso area. The inadequacy of the reimbursement and capitation rates, when combined with the disproportionately high percentage of Medicaid-insured recipients in El Paso, created a financial incentive for health care providers to practice outside the El Paso area and to seek out patients covered by private health insurance.

ISSUE: Do Medicaid-insured recipients and health care providers have the right to seek federal civil rights remedies for inadequate health care in their local communities under the Equal Access provision of the federal Medicaid law?

HOLDING AND DECISION: No, the Equal Access provision of the federal Medicaid law does not confer an individual private right of action that is enforceable under the federal civil rights law.

ANALYSIS: The Circuit Court began its analysis with examination of the federal civil rights law in which § 1983 imposes liability on any person who deprives a citizen of any rights secured by the U.S. Constitution and laws under color of state law or authority. Section 1983 provides in relevant part:

> Every person who, under color of any law, ordinance, regulation, custom, or usage, of any State or Territory or the District of Columbia, subjects, or causes to be subjected, any citizen of the U.S. or other person within the jurisdiction thereof to the deprivation of any rights, privileges, or immunities secured by the Constitution and laws, shall be liable to the party injured in an action at law, suit in equity, or other proper proceeding for redress.... 42 U.S.C.A. § 1983 (1996).

The U.S. Supreme Court restricted this civil right when it held that § 1983 provides a remedy only for the deprivation of rights secured by the

(continues)

(continued)

Constitution and laws of the U.S., not broader benefits or interests that may be enforced under the federal laws (*see Gonzaga University v. Doe*, 536 U.S. 273 (U.S. Supreme Court 2002)). Accordingly, the Circuit Court held there was no implied right of action in the federal Medicaid law without some rights-creating language showing Congress intended to create a right of access to health care. According to the U.S. Supreme Court, it is only violations of rights, not laws, that give rise to § 1983 actions.

The Circuit Court held the Equal Access provision of the federal Medicaid law did not show congressional intent to create individualized rights for Medicaid-insured recipients and health care providers. The Equal Access provision was interpreted as covering only institutional policy and practices in terms of the functions that must be performed by the states and the U.S. Department of Health and Human Services (HHS) in giving effect to the federal Medicaid law. The Circuit Court saw the federal Medicaid law as creating an affirmative duty on the part of states and HHS to enlist enough health care providers, so that health care was available to Medicaid-insured recipients to the same extent such care was available to the general non-Medicaid-insured population in the El Paso geographic area. The focus of the Equal Access

provision was interpreted as being aggregate, as opposed to individual, which is required to establish a private, individual right of action under § 1983.

As a result, the Equal Access provision of the federal Medicaid law does not create private, individual rights of action under § 1983. Rather the Equal Access provision simply provides that the states and HHS have a legal duty to ensure Medicaid-insured recipients as a group have access to health care on the same basis as the general non-Medicaid-insured population. The Equal Access provision is not concerned with whether Medicaid-insured recipients as a group have the right to access health care, or whether any particular Medicaid recipient has a right to access health care that is equal to the care provided to the privately insured in El Paso.

Rule of Law: The Equal Access provision of the federal Medicaid law confers no individual rights and thus cannot give rise to a presumption of enforceability under § 1983 of the federal civil rights law. Only laws that clearly confer private, individual rights of action may be enforced under § 1983.

(*See generally* Bobroff, 2008; Bobroff & Perkins, 2008; Jenkins & Ardalan, 2008; Lunsford, 2008).

yet clear. Whether the solution is a federalist approach or an approach arising from the states remains to be seen. What is certain is major reform of the U.S. health care system will require significant intergovernmental mandates for decades to come (*see generally* Lunsford, 2008).

The Fifth Circuit chose not to advance the rights of those historically denied access to health care and treatment. However, future litigants might seek relief in state courts. Today, it is the state judiciary that is expanding protection of individual liberties through interpretation of their own state constitutions (*see generally* Brennan, 1977, 1986).

Socioeconomic Inequities

For the people at the bottom of the economic pyramid in the U.S., health care is very different than it is for those at the top of the pyramid. Medicaid reimbursement rates are so low, and billing under the program is so complicated, that it is difficult for Medicaid-insured patients to access timely medical interventions or specialized care. Accumulating medical data shows the poor health outcomes of Medicaid-insured patients are not just a function of their underlying medical conditions, but a more direct consequence of the

shortcomings of Medicaid. For instance, Medicaid is replete with paperwork, regulations, and treatment rejections that make the program hard to navigate for health care providers, as well as the people it was established to serve, the Medicaid-insured patients.

Medicare/Medicaid-Insured

Data from the Medicare Payment Advisory Committee reveal the access problems faced by those who qualify for both Medicare and Medicaid insurance, generally referred to as being dual eligible. While the next chapter will explain the important protections provided by Medicare insurance, there are significant gaps in Medicare coverage, gaps that many meet with Medicaid and private health insurance. For instance, there are fairly high cost-sharing requirements for covered benefits and Medicare does not have a stop-loss benefit that limits out-of-pocket spending.

- Four out of ten physicians restrict access, because Medicaid reimbursement rates are so low and payments are often delayed
- About 30 percent of U.S. physicians refuse to accept new Medicare/Medicaid-insured patients,

while less than 3 percent refuse to accept new private-insured Medicare patients

• Access for the Medicare/Medicaid-insured is most limited in urban areas
• Most of the 6.2 million individuals who are dual-insured face restrictions on access to the latest medical technologies

(MedPAC, 2008)

Medicare beneficiaries who are Medicaid-insured are more likely to suffer from cognitive impairments and mental disorders, and have higher rates of diabetes, pulmonary disease, stroke, and Alzheimer's disease than peers in their age group who are privately insured. Nearly 40 percent are disabled. Relative to the Medicare-insured with private insurance, the Medicare/Medicaid-insured are:

• Spending a disproportionate share of Medicaid and Medicare funds
• Three times as likely to be in poor health
• Almost twenty times as likely to be institutionalized

(MedPAC, 2008)

For instance, the Medicare/Medicaid-insured account for 16 percent of the Medicare beneficiaries and 25 percent of Medicare spending. The costliest 20 percent account for more than 77 percent of Medicare spending (MedPAC, 2008).

Treatment of Serious Heart Conditions

The treatment of heart disease, which is among the most evaluated Medicaid services, discloses clinical disparities that can only be attributable to the influence of insurance status. While the clinical outcomes may have been a result of poorer long-term, follow-up care, most studies tried to control for the medical factors believed to influence patients' outcomes.[LN2]

• Medicaid-insured patients face significantly more angina, poorer quality of life, and higher risks of hospitalizations after myocardial infarctions (Rahimi, et al., 2007), with nearly twice the increased risk of complications and death (Sada et al., 1998)
• Patients with Medicaid coverage are almost 50 percent more likely to die after coronary artery bypass surgery than patients with private health insurance coverage (Zacharia et al., 2005)
• National Hospital Discharge Survey data, over a twenty-five-year period, reveal that more than 80 percent of the hospitalizations for heart failure are Medicare/Medicaid-insured patients, which is a rate of hospitalization reflecting the lack of timely interventions and medicines (Fang et al., 2004)

Diagnoses of Cancer

As illustrated in Figure 6-5, the probability of being diagnosed with late-stage cancers is two to almost three times greater for uninsured and Medicaid-insured patients than it is for people with private

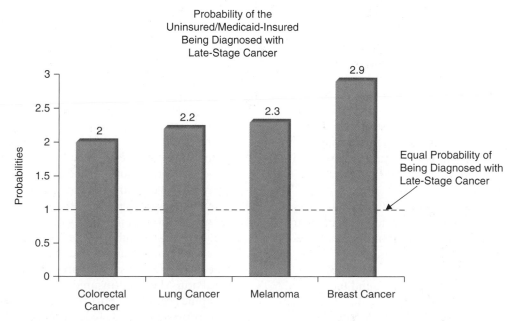

FIGURE 6-5: Diagnosis of Late-Stage Cancer, Uninsured/Medicaid-Insured v. Privately-Insured

Delmar/Cengage Learning

Data retrieved from: Halpern, 2008; *see* Weinick, R. et al. (2005). Who can't pay for health care? *Journal of General Internal Medicine, 20* (6), 504-509; *see also* Hoffman, C. (2009). *Health insurance and access to health care: The evidence.* Menlo Park, CA: Kaiser Foundation.

insurance coverage and access to health care, even after correcting for differences in the location of the tumor and its stage when diagnosed (Halpern, 2008).

People without private health insurance are unlikely to have access to comprehensive health care or participate in cancer-screening programs. Over the years, everyone in the health industry knew, and regional studies suggested, that uninsured and Medicaid-insured patients were more likely to present with advanced-stage cancer than privately insured patients (Halpern, 2007).

However, it was not until 2008 that these regional findings were assessed using national data. A national analysis revealed uninsured and Medicaid-insured patients had substantially increased risks of presenting with advanced-stage cancers at diagnosis (Halpern, 2008). Although many factors other than insurance status also affect the quality of care received, adequate insurance is a crucial factor for receiving appropriate cancer screening and timely access to health care. Individuals without medical insurance or with limited insurance are less likely than those

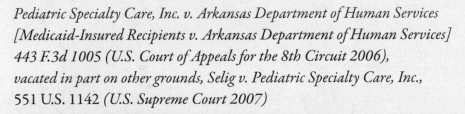

RIGHT OF ACCESS TO MEDICALLY NECESSARY HEALTH CARE

Pediatric Specialty Care, Inc. v. Arkansas Department of Human Services
[Medicaid-Insured Recipients v. Arkansas Department of Human Services]
443 F.3d 1005 (U.S. Court of Appeals for the 8th Circuit 2006),
vacated in part on other grounds, Selig v. Pediatric Specialty Care, Inc.,
551 U.S. 1142 (U.S. Supreme Court 2007)

FACTS: The directors of the State Arkansas Medicaid program implemented a policy of prior authorization that reduced the scope and duration of early intervention day treatment for disabled Medicaid-insured children. The primary motivation of the prior authorization policy action was to save money, even though federal Medicaid law requires states to act in the best interest of needy children who are disabled and require medically necessary rehabilitation and health care.

ISSUE: Do Medicaid-insured children and health care providers have the right to seek federal civil rights remedies for inadequate health care in their local communities under the Equal Access provision of the federal Medicaid law?

HOLDING AND DECISION: Yes, the Equal Access provision of the federal Medicaid law confers an individual private right of action that is enforceable under the federal civil rights law.

ANALYSIS: The Eighth Circuit found that the directors of the State Arkansas Medicaid program violated the providers' and the children's clearly established rights to provide and receive medically necessary health care. Medicaid-insured disabled

children are entitled to diagnostic, screening, preventive, and rehabilitative services. This includes any medical or remedial services provided in a facility, a home, or other setting, recommended by a physician. The services provided must seek to maximally reduce the physical or mental disability of children. In addition, the services must be continued until disabled children are restored to their best possible functional level. The court held the federal Medicaid law created an enforceable federal right to early intervention treatment when recommended by a physician that cannot be overridden by government policies or regulations.

The Equal Access provision of the federal Medicaid law requires state Medicaid plans to employ methods and procedures related to use of and payment for health care and services as necessary to ensure that the state's payments are consistent with efficiency, economy, and quality of care and are sufficient to enlist enough providers so that care and services are available under the plan at least to the extent such care and services are available to the general non-Medicaid-insured population in the geographic area. The court further held the Equal Access provisions of the federal Medicaid law created a clearly established federal right to access quality health care.

(continues)

(continued)

> **RULE OF LAW:** The rights to medically necessary health care conferred by the federal Medicaid law are clearly established federal rights, and those provisions of the federal Medicaid law are enforceable by both Medicaid-insured children and health care providers through federal civil rights causes of action.
> (*See generally* Bobroff, 2008 and Jenkins & Ardalan, 2008).

with broader insurance coverage to receive preventive services and to seek timely health care. The national analysis examined the association between insurance status and stage at diagnosis among women with breast cancer. These results are consistent with other reports that have documented less use of preventive services, including mammography, among uninsured women and the resulting delays in diagnosis and treatment.

The conflict between the two decisions in this chapter, the *Equal Access for El Paso* decision in the Fifth Circuit and the *Pediatric Specialty Care* decision in the Eighth Circuit, regarding the Equal Access provision of the federal Medicaid law, virtually ensures the U.S. Supreme Court will eventually step in to reconcile the differences. Judicial interpretations of the law regularly vary in the federal circuits and change over time, often going through conflicting stages of development before maturing into a coherent national policy. It is not uncommon for the federal circuits to go in different directions on the same issue. The role of Medicaid in providing access to basic health care is just one instance of this difference.

Treatment of HIV/AIDS

The uninsured and underinsured with inadequate prescription plans complain about being denied access to the antiretroviral drugs that can prevent their immune systems from being weakened to the point where they are disabled by full-blown Acquired Immune Deficiency Syndrome (AIDS) (Yamin, 2003). While infection with the Human Immunodeficiency Virus (HIV) has become a serious, but manageable, chronic condition for those with the resources to gain access to quality health care, lack of early access to care is the difference between life and death from AIDS (WHO, 2008).

While most young adults are relatively healthy, half of all new HIV infections occur among young people fifteen to twenty-four years of age. About twenty thousand young Americans are newly infected with the virus that causes AIDS annually; this is fifty-five new infections per day (WHO, 2008).

Twenty percent of the people living with HIV infections are uninsured (NASTAD, 2008). The cruel irony for them is that they do not qualify for Medicaid, and thus are not given access to the antiretroviral drugs that would have prevented their symptoms, until they manifest symptoms of the AIDS disease. This means treatment is withheld for most uninsured Americans of limited means until it is too late for preventative health care (Montaner, 2006). For the uninsured poor in the U.S., HIV/AIDS is a death sentence.

> *Moral Dilemmas*
>
> 1. Should states be able to place limitations upon enrollment in Medicaid, such as maintenance of a healthy weight, not smoking, and not abusing drugs?

SCHIP INSURANCE

The State Children's Health Insurance Program (SCHIP) was created in 1997 to address the growing challenge of uninsured children (*see* 42 U.S.C.A. §§ 1397aa-jj (2009) (subchapter XXI of the Social Security Act)). SCHIP is the single largest expansion of health insurance coverage since Medicaid was initiated in 1965. Five billion dollars was spent on SCHIP by the federal government in 2007, and another $7 billion in 2008 (CMS, 2009).

The Centers for Medicare and Medicaid Services is in charge of the SCHIP program, with joint financing by the federal and state governments. Administered by the states, within broad federal guidelines, each state determines:

- Administrative and operating procedures
- Benefit packages
- Design of its program
- Eligibility groups
- Payment levels for coverage

Who Is Targeted for SCHIP Insurance?

Covering roughly seven million children in 2009, SCHIP insurance plays an important role in reducing the number of uninsured children in America. The federal government provides a capped amount of matching funds to states for coverage of children, and some parents with household incomes too high to qualify for Medicaid insurance, but for whom private health insurance is unavailable or unaffordable. Although SCHIP is aimed mainly at covering children, a handful of states have obtained waivers from CMS to use SCHIP funds to cover adults, typically parents of Medicaid/SCHIP children.

SCHIP is designed to provide health insurance coverage to uninsured, low-income children who:

- Reside in a family with household income below 200 percent of the federal poverty level
- Whose family has an household income 50 percent higher than the state's Medicaid eligibility threshold

Certain children cannot be covered under SCHIP, including children who are:

- Insured under an employer-sponsored health insurance plan or have health insurance coverage through an association or individual plan
- Members of a family eligible for state or local government-sponsored health insurance based on employment with a public agency
- Residing in an institution for those suffering from mental illnesses
- Eligible for Medicaid insurance coverage

Expansion of Medicaid Insurance to Higher-Income Households

If a state elects to expand its Medicaid program using SCHIP insurance, the eligibility rules of Medicaid apply, including the inability to:

- Enforce residency requirements
- Enact lifetime caps
- Establish time limits for eligibility

For states that opt for a separate child health program, certain other federal restrictions affecting Medicaid eligibility are optional for SCHIP insurance. States may at their option:

- Choose to offer children one year of continuous eligibility
- Enforce enrollment caps for eligible children
- Have waiting lists for coverage of uninsured children

When screening and enrolling children for SCHIP insurance, however, all states must establish a system to determine if children are Medicaid eligible and provide a mechanism for enrollment into Medicaid. This is creating a dual system of public insurance eligibility for children. On the one hand, poor children may face more restrictive eligibility determinations and may not be continuously eligible, while children residing in higher-income households, who are not eligible for Medicaid insurance,

may face enrollment caps in some states, forcing them to remain uninsured, but waitlisted for SCHIP insurance coverage.

Limitation of SCHIP Coverage

For a period of time, the federal government required the states to restrict the availability of SCHIP insurance to children who were American citizens. Self-declarations of citizenship were abandoned in 2009; all children residing in the U.S. who meet need-based requirements for participation are now eligible for SCHIP insurance.

> *Moral Dilemmas*
> 1. Should SCHIP coverage be limited to American children?

Need-Based Cost-Sharing

States are permitted to impose different cost-sharing on SCHIP-insured enrollees on a need basis. More generous cost-sharing rules may apply, but are not required to apply, to children in the poorest households in the nation. While all courts acknowledge these federally imposed requirements, not all courts will offer families a remedy if state agencies or health care providers accepting SCHIP insurance refuse to follow the SCHIP regulations. In other words, some of the poorest insured families in America have unenforceable rights when their children are denied medical coverage.

Middle-Income Families

Costs may not be charged for preventive services or immunizations, nor may costs exceed 5 percent of a family's gross or net household income. States and health care providers may determine whether to base their cost-sharing on a gross or net basis and there is no mandate requiring uniformity.

Families must be advised of their maximum annual cost-sharing limit for each child. State plans must describe the:

- Consequences of not paying cost-sharing charges
- Disenrollment protections for families who cannot pay their cost-sharing obligations
- Methods used to determine cost-sharing amounts

States must permit families to pay their past due cost-sharing charges before being disenrolled; if household income declines, the failure to meet cost-sharing obligations may be waived, but waivers are not required. Again, some courts will not penalize states if they fail to follow their cost-sharing procedures.

Low-Wage Families

Where children reside in households at or below 150 percent of the federal poverty line, states may not impose more than:

- Nominal cost-sharing fees
- One cost-sharing charge for all services delivered during a single office visit
- One type of cost-sharing for a medical service

What Health Insurance Coverage Is Required for Uninsured Children?

For states that opt to expand Medicaid by participating in the SCHIP insurance program, the health services covered by SCHIP must mirror the health services covered by Medicaid insurance. States cannot simply restrict Medicaid coverage to focus on improving the health of their children; rather states are required to offer health services to all eligible individuals and families that meet specified financial criteria. This inability to target limited resources is a major weakness of the nation's public insurance system (Karakatsanis, 2007).

Why Is Public Health Insurance Economically Necessary?

Aside from the economic need to seek expected utility maximization, there are at least four additional reasons why public health insurance is economically necessary. In the health industry, utility is a measure of the relative satisfaction from consumption of health care. Maximization of utility is one of the key criteria for organization of the nation's health care system; by increasing utility, health care policies can seek to manage the behavior of patient-consumers in terms of increasing their relative satisfaction as consumers of health care with delivery of their care. The philosophical ideal of distributive justice underlies the expected utility maximization model with respect to the allocation of health risks in the nation's health care system, as well as the economic impact model in this chapter. In a democratic society like the U.S., there is an economic need for the federal government to:

- Support the nation's health care system and safety net
- Help generate economic activity in the states
- Maximize economic impacts on the nation's health care system
- Enhance state capacities for health insurance coverage

(*See generally* Kaiser, 2009a)

Nation's Health Care System and Safety Net

The guarantee of federal financing for Medicaid that matches state spending enables states to respond to:

- Aging population
- Chaotic economic downturns
- Emergencies and disasters
- Increases in health care costs
- Uninsured and underinsured populations

Generation of Economic Activity

As the largest source of federal support to the states, Medicaid is also a major economic engine in state economies. Medicaid supports millions of health care jobs across the nation and provides funding to thousands of health care providers who care for the Medicaid-insured, including:

- Community health centers
- Group homes
- Hospitals
- Managed care plans
- Nursing homes and other long-term care facilities

In turn, Medicaid funds generate economic activity, as follows:

- Economic impact of Medicaid funds is intensified because of the federal matching dollars
- State spending on behalf of the Medicaid-insured for health care pulls federal tax dollars into the state's local economies
- Medicaid funding to health care providers supports health care jobs and household income
- Health care jobs generate household income within the health care sector, and throughout other sectors of the local economy, due to the multiplier effect
- Additional tax revenues are derived from the health care jobs and household incomes generated

Economic Impact on the Health Care System

Government payments to health care providers, on behalf of U.S. residents eligible for Medicaid insurance, directly impact the providers by:

- Supporting health care jobs
- Creating household income
- Promoting consumer purchases associated with the provision of health care

Through the multiplier effect, new government spending creates larger impacts because of the influx of additional government funds. Other businesses and industries indirectly benefit from the multiplier effect through the economic chain. For instance, government funding of pharmaceutical drugs affects the downstream drug distributor's supply order, which affects the supply of drugs to the neighborhood retail pharmacy or pharmacy benefit manager, that are purchased by consumers, and so on. Upstream, the pharmaceutical industry's supply order for raw materials to produce and manufacture the drugs affects the intermediates who supply the compounds, which affects the global market for raw materials, and so on.

Finally, both the direct and indirect effects produce changes in household consumption. The taxes derived from household income being consumed are returned to the government, where the economic cycle repeats itself all over again, each time multiplying the economic impact on the overall economy.

State Capacity for Health Insurance Coverage

Apart from whichever model is used to assess the economic impact of Medicaid funds from the federal and state governments, consumer spending on health care has a positive impact on local economies.[LN3] The magnitude of the economic impact that can be contributed by the Medicaid-insured is dependent on at least three factors:

- Economic conditions of the state economy
- FMAP rates and federal funding to the states for Medicaid insurance
- Level of state funds available for Medicaid spending on health care

Reductions in Medicaid spending lead to declines in federal funding to the states, which decreases the flow of funds to health care providers, and consequently leads to declines in economic activity at the state and local levels. For instance, due to the federal match, a state with a 60 percent FMAP must cut overall Medicaid spending by $2.40 to save one dollar in state spending (Kaiser, 2009).

Moral Dilemmas
1. Is the argument for universal health care better supported by a financial or ethical basis?

UNAFFORDABILITY OF ADVANCED MEDICINE

The U.S. is the world leader in medical research and health care technology. Unfortunately, these advances provide little consolation as the prohibitive cost keeps them out of reach for people at the bottom of the economic pyramid, such as the:

- Medicaid insured
- Low-wage earners
- Uninsured
- Underinsured of limited means

This lack of access because health systems are inadequate and prices are unaffordable has been termed a health care crisis across America. Health care reform has become one of the leading concerns across the nation.

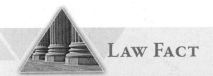 **LAW FACT**

ACCESS TO HEALTH CARE

Should the judiciary force a solution to shape the legislative dimensions of how to provide access to medically necessary health care for U.S. residents at the bottom of the economic pyramid, and in particular poor children?

Courts face real challenges when confronting questions with political implications without an accompanying political consensus on legislation, such as the federal Medicaid law. The role of the judiciary becomes more difficult when it faces making decisions regarding deeply contested health care values. In this class action, the Tenth Circuit held that the federal Medicaid law imposed no obligation whatsoever on the State of Oklahoma to deliver any health services. Rather, the Tenth Circuit concluded the state's obligation under the federal Medicaid law was merely to pay promptly for the health services of Medicaid-eligible children.

—*OKAAP v. Fogarty*, 472 F.3d 1208 (U.S. Court of Appeals for the 10th Circuit 2007),
U.S. Supreme Court certiorari denied, 128 S.Ct. 68 (U.S. Supreme Court 2007), *on remand*,
522 F.Supp.2d 1353 (U.S. District Court for the Northern District of Oklahoma 2007).

CHAPTER SUMMARY

- For those who have comprehensive health care insurance and/or money, the U.S. health care system offers the best health care in the world; for those at the bottom of the U.S. economic pyramid, access to basic medical care is inadequate, if it exists at all.
- Medicaid is the nation's public health insurance program for over sixty million Americans of limited means and/or who are severely disabled.
- Medicaid is funded and operated jointly by the federal and state governments; federal contributions to states vary based on state per capita income, and reached over $400 billion in 2008.
- People that qualify for Medicaid include low-wage working families with children, Medicare beneficiaries with limited resources, blind or severely disabled persons, and uninsured pregnant women.
- Medicaid covers services such as dental, preventative, screening, diagnostic, family planning and pregnancy, home health, hospital, laboratory and radiological, licensed professionals, and nursing facilities.
- Problems with obtaining Medicaid coverage include the timeline within which to apply for it, the requirement of being medically needy or suffering a medical emergency, and delivery system inequities.
- Whether access to quality health care in the U.S. will be developed by the executive branch, legislative branch, federal government, or states has yet to be seen.
- Even though some low-income people are able to secure coverage through Medicaid, they still suffer poor health outcomes due to Medicaid's shortcomings, including its paperwork, complexity, regulations, low reimbursement rates for providers, length of time required to obtain care, and lack of complete coverage.
- SCHIP is a program similar to Medicaid targeted toward covering children in low-income families.
- Public insurance makes good economic sense because it furthers the federal government's goals of supporting the nation's safety net, generating economic activity, maximizing the impact of dollars spent on health care, and enhancing the states' abilities to provide their own health insurance coverage.
- In resolving the American health care crisis, one of the fundamental questions is whether it remains more consistent with American notions of autonomy and responsibility for the government to simply encourage the desired result and ultimately leave the choice to the individual, or whether the time has come for government to mandate desired health outcomes.

LAW NOTES

1. *Oklahoma Chapter of the American Academy of Pediatrics v. Fogarty*, 472 F.3d 1208 (U.S. Court of Appeals for the 10th Circuit 2007) (assuming the EPSDT requirement creates a federally enforceable right); *Mandy R. v. Owens*, 464 F.3d 1139 (U.S. Court of Appeals for the 10th Circuit 2006) (agreeing with the Ninth and Third Circuits, which have held that the reasonable promptness and comparability requirements create a federally enforceable right); *Doe v. Chiles*, 136 F.3d 709 (U.S. Court of Appeals for the 11th Circuit 1998) (holding the reasonable promptness clause of the federal Medicaid law is enforceable under 42 U.S.C.A. § 1983 (1996)). *But see Sanders ex. rel. Rayl v. Kansas Department of Social and Rehabilitation Services*, 317 F.Supp.2d 1233 (U.S. District Court for the District of Kansas 2004) (holding that the reasonable promptness requirement does not create an enforceable right).

2. The prevalence and consequences of financial barriers to health care are well documented for patients with an acute myocardial infarction. One of the first research studies examined data from the National Registry of Myocardial Infarction to determine the influence of payer status on use of invasive cardiac procedures and patient outcome. Medicaid-insured patients were found to face a 100 percent increased risk of complications and death after myocardial infarction (Sada et al., 1998).

   Similar review of data from the Prospective Registry Evaluating Myocardial Infarction: Event and Recovery system showed financial barriers to health care were associated with worse recovery after symptoms manifested. PREMIER data, an observational, multicenter study of some 2,500 patients with acute myocardial infarction, shows Medicaid-insured patients who lack access to necessary health care have significantly more angina, poorer quality of life, and higher risk of rehospitalizations (Rahimi et al., 2007).

   A subsequent study looked at early or late coronary artery bypass surgeries and found Medicaid-insured patients have worse late surgery survival rates than privately-insured or Medicare patients. Medicaid-insured patients are almost 50 percent more likely to die after coronary artery bypass surgery than patients with private coverage or Medicare alone (Zacharia et al., 2005).

3. To assess economic impact, health economists generally use either the RIMS II (regional input-output modeling system) or IMPLAN (impact analysis for planning) input-output models. Input-output models account for economic relationships; the relationships between businesses and industries in an economy and the effects of changes in government expenditures can be estimated. Both models are based on a similar theory: a change in input (Medicaid expenditures) will produce direct impacts that will then ripple through other sectors of the economy, producing indirect and induced impacts (Kaiser, 2009a). The differences in the models are related to the types of multipliers each model uses and the approach used to compute the multipliers.

In Idaho, for every $1 million change in Medicaid spending:
- $2.4 million gained in federal dollars
- $5.2 million gained in business activity
- Sixty-nine jobs created
- $2.5 million total economic impact

(Pitz, 2006)

In North Carolina, for every $1 million change in Medicaid spending:
- $1.7 million gained in federal dollars
- $5.1 million gained in business activity
- 130 jobs created
- $6.0 million total economic impact

(Dumas et al., 2008)

In Oklahoma, for every $1 million change in Medicaid spending:
- $1.8 million gained in federal dollars
- $2.4 million gained in business activity
- Eighty-five jobs created
- $4.5 million total economic impact

(St. Clair & Doeksen, 2007)

CHAPTER BIBLIOGRAPHY

Bobroff, R. (2008). Section 1983 and preemption: Alternative means of court access for safety net statutes. *Loyola Journal of Public Interest Law, 10*, 27-85.

Bobroff, R., & Perkins, J. (2008). Recent developments in court access for Medicaid and Medicare cases. *Journal of Poverty Law & Policy, 42*, 246-250.

Bodenheimer, T., & Grumbach, K. (2008). *Understanding health policy.* New York, NY: McGraw-Hill Medical.

Brennan, Jr., W. J. (1986). The Bill of Rights and the states: The revival of state constitutions as guardians of individual rights. *New York University Law Review, 61*, 535-553 (classic text on state rights built on his influential article published ten years earlier).

____. (1977). State constitutions and the protection of individual rights. *Harvard Law Review, 90*, 489 (prominent text from a sitting U.S. Supreme Court Justice calling on state courts to take a more active role in protecting human rights and ensuring their residents' health, based on their state constitutions; cited thirteen times in U.S. Supreme Court decisions, over two hundred times in decisions by the highest appellate federal and state courts, and over eight hundred times by law review journals in the thirty some years since it was first published).

CMS (Centers for Medicare & Medicaid Services). (2009). *National health care expenditure data.* Washington, DC: U.S. Department of Health & Human Services, CMS, Office of the Actuary.

Cunningham, P. J. (2005). Medicaid cost containment and access to prescription drugs. *Health Affairs, 24* (3), 780-789 (examining the cost containment strategies applied to Medicaid and the impact of those strategies on enrollees).

DeNavas-Walt, C. et al. (2008). *Household income, poverty and health insurance coverage in the U.S.* Washington, DC: U.S. Census Bureau.

Doty, M. et al. (2005). *Seeing red: Americans driven into debt by medical bills.* New York, NY: Commonwealth Fund (analyzes data from the 2003 Commonwealth Fund Biennial Health Insurance Survey to examine trends in health care spending, medical debt, and the uninsured).

Dumas, C. et al. (2008). The economic impacts of Medicaid in North Carolina. *North Carolina Journal of Medicine, 69* (2), 78-87 (IMPLAN analysis).

Fang, J. et al. (2008). Heart failure-related hospitalization in the U.S., 1979 to 2004. *Journal of the American College of Cardiology, 52*, 427-434.

Fang, J., & Alderman, M. H. (2004). Does supplemental private insurance affect care of Medicare-insured hospitalized for myocardial infarction? *American Journal of Public Health, 94* (5), 777-782.

FR (Federal Register). (2009, January 23). 2009 poverty guidelines, 74 FR 4199-04.

____. (2008, November 26). Federal financial participation in state assistance expenditures; federal matching shares for Medicaid, the State Children's Health Insurance Program, and aid to needy aged, blind, or disabled persons for October 1, 2009 through September 30, 2010, *73* (229), 72051-72053.

Halpern, M. T. et al. (2008). Association of insurance status and ethnicity with cancer stage at diagnosis for twelve cancer sites: A retrospective analysis. *Lancet Oncology, 9* (3), 222-231.

___. (2007). Insurance status and stage of cancer at diagnosis among women with breast cancer. *Cancer, 110* (2), 403-411.

Hartman, M. et al. (2009). National health spending in 2007: Slower drug spending contributes to lowest rate of overall growth since 1998. *Health Affairs,* 28 (1), 246-261.

Holahan, J. et al. (2009). *Rising unemployment, Medicaid and the uninsured.* Washington, DC: Urban Institute & Kaiser Commission on Medicaid & the Uninsured.

___. (2007). *Characteristics of the uninsured: Who is eligible for public coverage and who needs help affording coverage?* Washington, DC: Kaiser Commission on Medicaid & and the Uninsured.

Hurley, R. E. (2005). A widening rift in access and quality: Growing evidence of economic disparities. *Health Affairs, 10,* 1377–1382.

Jenkins, A., & Ardalan, S. (2008). Positive health: The human right to health care under the New York State Constitution. *Fordham Urban Law Journal. 35,* 479-559.

Kaiser (Kaiser Commission on Medicaid & the Uninsured). (2009). *The role of Medicaid in state economies: A look at the research.* Washington, DC: Kaiser.

___. (2009a). *State fiscal conditions and Medicaid.* Washington, DC: Kaiser.

___. (2008). *Short term options for Medicaid in a recession.* Washington, DC: Kaiser.

___. (2008a). *Medicaid facts: The Medicaid program at a glance.* Washington, DC: Kaiser.

___. (2008b). *Health coverage of children: The role of Medicaid and SCHIP.* Washington, DC: Kaiser.

Karakatsanis, A. G. (2007). Health insurance in America: Providing substance to America's values. *Journal of Medicine & the Law, 11,* 337-375.

Kronick, R., & Rousseau, D. (2007). Is Medicaid sustainable? Spending projections for the program's second forty years. *Health Affairs,* 26 (2), 271-287 (examines the long-term fiscal sustainability of the Medicaid program).

Lunsford, J. (2008). Private rights of action under § 1983 to enforce the Equal Access Provision of the Medicaid Act: equal access for *El Paso v. Hawkins. American Journal of Law & Medicine, 34,* 85-87.

Marks, C. et al. (2009, January 9). *The role of Medicaid in state economies: A look at the research.* Washington, DC: Kaiser Commission on Medicaid & the Uninsured (synthesizing the results of twenty-nine studies in twenty-three states).

MedPAC (Medicare Payment Advisory Committee). (2008). *A data book: Healthcare spending and the Medicare program.* Washington, DC: MedPAC.

Moncrieff, A. R. (2006). Payments to Medicaid physicians: Interpreting the "equal access" provision. *University of Chicago Law Review, 73,* 673-704.

Montaner, J. S. et al. (2006). The case for expanding access to highly active antiretroviral therapy to curb the growth of the HIV pandemic. *Lancet 368,* 531-536 (citing studies that find a significant reduction in HIV transmission for patients on highly active ARV therapy).

NASBO (National Association of State Budget Officers). (2009). *NASBO fiscal year 2007 state expenditure report.* Washington, DC: NASBO.

NASTAD (National Alliance of State & Territorial AIDS Directors). (2008). *Report on findings from an assessment of health department efforts to implement HIV screening in health care settings.* Washington, DC: NASTAD.

Perry, M. et al (2008). *Turning to Medicaid and SCHIP in an economic recession: Conversations with recent applicants and enrollees.* Washington, DC: Kaiser Commission on Medicaid & the Uninsured.

Pitz, W. (2006). *Medicaid matters for Idaho's county economies.* Boise, ID: Northwest Federation Community Organizations and Idaho Community Action Network (IMPLAN analysis).

Rahimi, A. T. et al. (2007). Financial barriers to health care and outcomes after acute myocardial infarction. *Journal of the American Medical Association, 297* (10), 1063-1072.

Sada, M. J. et al. (1998). Influence of payer on use of invasive cardiac procedures and patient outcome after myocardial infarction in the U.S. *Journal of the American College of Cardiology, 31* (7), 1474-1480.

Sorkin, A. C. (2008). Financial assistance for Medicaid's continued existence: The need for the U.S. Supreme Court to adopt the Tenth Circuit's definition of medical assistance. *Denver University Law Review, 85,* 725-751.

Smith, V. (2009). *Medicaid in a crunch: A mid-FY 2009 update on state Medicaid issues in a recession.* Washington, DC: Kaiser Commission on Medicaid & the Uninsured (relaying the perspective of state Medicaid directors in describing the fiscal strain on Medicaid and other safety-net programs in 2008).

St. Clair, C. & Doeksen, G. (2007). *The economic impact of the Medicaid program on Oklahoma's economy.* Tulsa, OK: Oklahoma Health Care Authority (IMPLAN analysis).

Super, D. A. (2005). Are rights efficient? Challenging the managerial critique of individual rights. *California Law Review, 93,* 1051-1142.

Swartz. K. (2008). *Health coverage in a period of rising unemployment.* Washington, DC: Kaiser Commission on Medicaid & the Uninsured.

WHO (World Health Organization). (2008). *Progress report. Towards universal access: Scaling up priority HIV/AIDS interventions in the health sector.* London, England: WHO.

Yamin, A. E. (2003). Not just a tragedy: Access to medications as a right under international law, *Boston University International Law Journal, 21,* 325-371 (2003).

Zacharia, A. et al. (2005). Operative and late coronary artery bypass grafting outcomes in matched African-American versus Caucasian patients: Evidence of a late survival-Medicaid association. *Journal of the American College of Cardiology, 46,* 1526-1535.

CHAPTER 7
MEDICARE REFORMS

> *"Our current national health care system is simple: don't get sick."*
>
> —ANONYMOUS

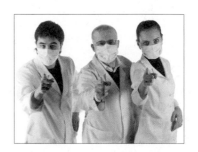

IN BRIEF

This chapter draws attention to the challenge of reforming Medicare, including Medicare's complex prescription drug plan. Debate about how much health care Medicare-eligible beneficiaries should finance versus how much should be financed by society is reviewed. How the federal government might pay for access to better quality health care and health services is discussed.

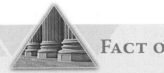

FACT OR FICTION

MEDICARE COVERAGE

Should employers be allowed to alter and decrease health insurance benefits for Medicare-eligible retirees to a level below that provided to non-Medicare-eligible retirees?

The Equal Employment Opportunity Commission proposed that employers be able to decrease their employer-provided health insurance benefits for retirees who reach the age of Medicare eligibility after many employers began dropping insurance benefits to avoid liability for age discrimination. Under the Age Discrimination in Employment Act, it is unlawful for employers to provide workers different benefits based on age, therefore making it difficult for employers to coordinate their retiree health insurance benefits with Medicare eligibility.

Although employers are not required to provide retiree health insurance benefits, about one-third of all Medicare beneficiaries rely on this private coverage to supplement Medicare and meet their health care needs, a drop from two-thirds in just two decades (Yamamoto et al., 2008). Medicare, on average, provides less generous benefits than employer-provided health insurance plans; Medicare has no out-of-pocket limits and greater cost-sharing, thereby imposing an additional burden on a population group that already assumes a greater share of health care costs. In addition, there is the coverage gap in the Medicare Part D prescription drug benefit and Medicare does not pay for long-term care, dental, or vision care.

—*AARP v. EEOC,* 489 F.3d 558 (U.S. Court of Appeals for the 3rd Circuit 2007),
U.S. Supreme Court certiorari denied, 128 S.Ct. 1733 (U.S. Supreme Court 2008).
(See *Law Fact* at the end of this chapter for the answer.)

PRINCIPLES AND APPLICATIONS

The Medicare program is the second largest social insurance program in the U.S., behind Social Security, offering guaranteed health insurance benefits to those eligible by virtue of their Social Security eligibility. Persons eligible for Medicare include individuals ages sixty-five and over, those with disabilities, and those with end-stage renal disease. *See* 42 U.S.C.A. § 1395c (1989). With over forty-five million beneficiaries and total expected expenditures of $477 billion in 2009 (Kaiser, 2008), plus an additional seventy-seven million baby boomers en route to Medicare (CMS, 2008), the challenge is one of growing needs versus limited federal resources.

Questions about funding and rapidly escalating costs suggest Medicare is not sustainable in its current form, which is growing without constraints because it is an entitlement program (Pauly, 2008). While Medicare beneficiaries make up less than 15 percent of the U.S. population, they account for most of the nation's health care cost; the rise in their treatment prevalence, rather than rising treatment costs per case or population growth, accounts for most of the spending growth in the nation's health care costs (Thorpe, 2005).

The sickest 25 percent of Medicare beneficiaries, or eleven million people, spend 90 percent of the U.S. health care dollars ($2 trillion) with an average of:

- Five diagnosed medical conditions
- One hospitalization yearly
- Ten prescriptions
- Twelve physicians
- $181,800 in health care expenditures yearly

They are the super-users of the U.S. health care system, and the key to cutting costs lies with the physicians who treat them (Crippen, 2007).

What can probably be said about this subgroup of Medicare beneficiaries is:

- Their care is not being coordinated by their multiple health care providers
- There is no medical evidence to support the drug cocktails they are ingesting
- At least two of their chronic medical conditions were preventable
- They are being over-treated and mistreated

According to the Medicare Payment Advisory Commission, the Medicare Trust Fund is projected to be depleted by 2019, with insufficient funds to pay benefits (MedPAC, 2008).

MEDICARE REFORM: FINANCING BY INDIVIDUALS OR SOCIETY?

Medicare, originally constructed in the 1960s to mimic the Blue Cross/Blue Shield mainstream approach to medicine, must be changed if it is to be sustained. Its benefits package still closely resembles the standard package available in the mid-1960s; 75 percent of Medicare enrollees have the traditional indemnity insurance at a time when less than 2 percent of the nation's health plan enrollees have conventional insurance that is not part of a managed care plan (Kaiser, 2008).

At the same time, Medicare payments are not intended to cover all the medical needs of enrollees, nor should society pay for all these expenses (Wharton, 2004). Only about one in ten individuals over sixty-five relies solely on Medicare; the rest have Medicaid, supplementary health insurance, or some other form of coverage in addition to Medicare. Although there is substantial variation in the ability of beneficiaries to supplement Medicare's basic benefits, basic care is available to all legal residents.

COMPLEXITY OF MEDICARE

The complexity of Medicare mirrors the nation's broader health care system with overlapping regions, services, and convoluted public/private

financing. To demonstrate the veracity of this statement, a brief overview of the types of Medicare plans is in order. As illustrated in Figure 7-1, Medicare itself is organized into four parts.

Part A: Medicare Hospital, Skilled Nursing, Home Health, and Hospice Care

Medicare Part A (Hospital Insurance) pays for over one-third of benefits spending. Most beneficiaries do not pay premiums for this benefit, because they have already paid for it through their payroll taxes. Part A does not cover custodial or long-term nursing care, and beneficiaries must meet certain eligibility criteria for home health and hospice care.

The home health care benefit is available to individuals certified by their physicians as being homebound. Eligibility is determined by the type of services needed (intermittent skilled nursing care, physical therapy, speech-language pathology services, and continued occupational therapy) (CMS, 2008). The Medicare hospice benefit is available only to individuals whose physicians have certified their expected mortality is less than six months (*Federal Register*, 2008).

Part B: Medicare Physician, Outpatient, Home Health Care, and Preventive Services

Medicare Part B (Physician Insurance) accounts for about 30 percent of benefits spending. Most people pay a monthly premium for this insurance; Medicaid may subsidize premiums based on income eligibility, which varies by state (*Federal Register*, 2005). Services are provided on a medically necessary basis.

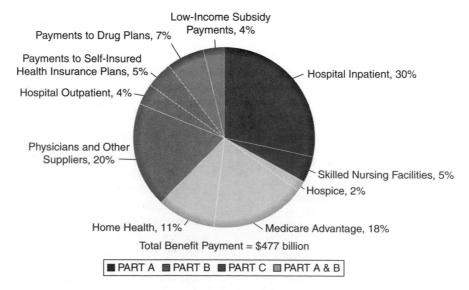

FIGURE 7-1: Medicare Benefit Payments by Type of Service

Delmar/Cengage Learning

Data retrieved from: The Congressional Budget Office. (2009). *Medicare anticipated annual payments.* Washington, DC: CBO.

Part C: Medicare Advantage Coverage

Part C refers to the private managed care plans, Medicare Advantage, in which beneficiaries can enroll, such as health maintenance organizations (HMOs), preferred provider organizations (PPOs), private fee-for-service plans (PFFSs), special needs plans (SNPs), and medical savings accounts (MSAs). There are twenty-six Medicare Advantage regions administering these programs, with most beneficiaries having a choice of six private plans (Kaiser, 2008).

The Medicare Advantage PFFS plans are not required to report quality measures, have Medicare review of services, or negotiate fees. Over 2.3 million beneficiaries are enrolled in PFFS plans.

The Medicare Advantage SNPs are restricted to dually eligible Medicare-Medicaid beneficiaries residing in long-term care facilities or are severely disabled. There are almost eight hundred SNPs serving about 1.2 million beneficiaries, coordinating SNP services in all 3,077 Medicaid offices in county boards of assistance with fifty state Medicaid agencies.

On top of this, the government allocated a $10 billion stabilization fund to develop regional PPOs from the local PPOs in each of the Medicaid Advantage regions. Utilization rates are not required to be reported by any of the Medicaid Advantage plans, so the federal government has no way to monitor access, use, or performance for over ten million Medicare beneficiaries enrolled in Part C. The result of this federal policy is shown in Figure 7-2, where the Medicare Payment Advisory Commission illustrates how costs are exceeding traditional fee-for-service Medicare.

Part D: Medicare Prescription Drug Coverage

Prescription drug plans generally have at least two economic objectives:

- Allow the health care system to improve the overall delivery of medical care
- Relieve the financial burden on those who have trouble affording their prescription drugs

While the Medicare Part D prescription drug program has value, it does not begin to address either of these economic objectives or the full extent of the Medicare crisis. It does, however, show how public perceptions, or misconceptions, can unduly influence decisions about health risks. The Medicare prescription drug plan is an example of health policy based not on a rational response to health risk, but rather on misperceptions of risks (Angrisano et al., 2007).

The drug plan, while providing coverage at the lower and upper ends of expenditures, allows for a coverage gap in the middle. As illustrated in Figure 7-3, the drug benefit is not catastrophic coverage above a deductible, but rather:

- Doughnut coverage with a modest deductible; then
- 75 percent coverage over a range of expenses; then
- 100 percent cost-sharing (the doughnut hole); and finally
- A return to complete coverage

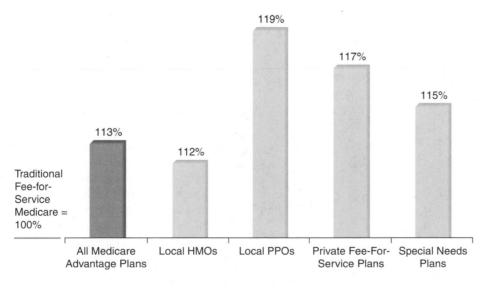

FIGURE 7-2: Average Payments to Medicare Advantage Plans Relative to Traditional Fee-for-Service Medicare

Delmar/Cengage Learning

Data retrieved from: MedPAC, 2008; Agency for Healthcare Research & Quality. (2009). *Medical expenditure panel survey: MEPS household component summary tables.* Rockville, MD: U.S. Department of Health & Human Services, AHRQ.

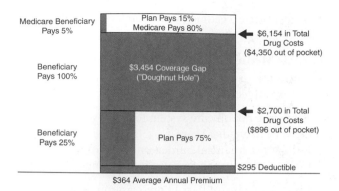

FIGURE 7-3: Standard Medicare Drug Prescription Benefit

Delmar/Cengage Learning
Data retrieved from: CMS, 2009.

Compared to traditional catastrophic coverage with a deductible, Part D reduced coverage for people with high expenses (where, in theory, people would have gotten the most economic utility value from coverage) to offer generous coverage for people with low expenses (where, in theory, coverage should be less valuable), to provide most beneficiaries with a return on their premium. While concentrating more of the Medicare prescription drug money on upper-end, catastrophic coverage makes more sense, the gap in the middle allows the federal government to provide the largest number of people with some benefit from this plan.

Supplemental Insurance Coverage

Medicare has high cost arrangements, no limit on out-of-pocket spending, and a coverage gap in the Part D prescription drug plan. Employer-sponsored health insurance, Medicaid, and Medigap (Medicare supplemental policies offered through private insurers) overlay each of the four types of Medicare and help with cost-sharing requirements and benefit gaps. Most Medicare beneficiaries have some form of supplemental health insurance.

> *Moral Dilemmas*
> 1. Should employers be required to fund retirees' health care costs?

STRUCTURAL REFORM OF MEDICARE

Little attention is being directed to the $65 trillion the U.S. needs to make Medicare whole (Wharton, 2004) or the over $1 billion private insurance takes in profits each year from Part C Medicare Advantage plans. In addition, little attention is directed to the $1 trillion in unfunded health care obligations for state and local government retirees (Kaiser, 2008). The nation is more focused on the revenue side of the equation than on addressing the rampant growth of benefit obligations that would require cuts for beneficiaries. Further, little attention is directed to insurance industry profits that were to be returned to Medicare beneficiaries in the form of reduced premiums or additional benefits (MedPAC, 2008a). Discussion generally centers on increasing payroll taxes or the premiums for Medicare insurance.[LN1]

Medicare is financed by a combination of sources of revenue, as illustrated in Figure 7-4:

- Payroll taxes (41 percent): 2.9 percent payroll tax on earnings
- General federal revenue (39 percent)
- Beneficiary premiums (12 percent): $96.40/month; individuals with incomes over $85,000, or $170,000 for couples, pay income-related premiums
- Payments from the states, taxation on Social Security benefits, and interest (8 percent)

Payroll taxes finance the majority of Part A, while general revenues fund three-quarters of Parts B and D.

There is not much talk about the real issue: how to control growth on Medicare spending. The Lahey Clinic Hospital case is one example of federal concern. government attempting to control costs (albeit, after-the-fact). From the Hospital's perspective, it maximized its revenue; unbundling its laboratory services made perfect economic sense. Medicare regulations did not preclude the practice at the time of the billings by the Hospital; the bundling and non-bundling practice was not foreseen and the re-testing was not defined as duplicative until later. Again, the complexity of Medicare presents itself. The Lahey case also demonstrates the problems that may arise under single-payor systems without competition; the physicians could compete for laboratory services and receive lower rates.

Obtaining more revenue for Medicare does not solve the problem until unnecessary spending like the Lahey case is controlled. While Social Security is still believed to be the most "untouchable" topic in politics, Medicare is a tougher problem politically because it does not involve a simple cash benefit; rather, Medicare puts a price tag on beneficiaries' health, perhaps even their lives.

RATIONING TREATMENT PREVALENCE

As mentioned, the rise in treatment prevalence, rather than rising treatment costs per case or population growth, accounts for most of the spending growth

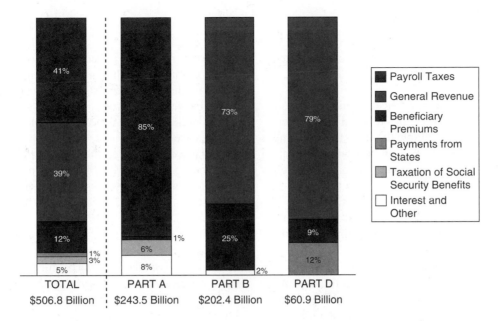

FIGURE 7-4: Estimated Sources of Medicare Revenue

COMMON LAW RECOVERY OF MEDICARE OVERPAYMENTS

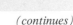

U.S. v. Lahey Clinic Hospital, Inc.

[U.S. v. Medicare Provider]

399 F.3d 1 (U.S. Court of Appeals for the 1st Circuit 2005),

U.S. Supreme Court certiorari denied, 546 U.S. 814 (U.S. Supreme Court 2005)

FACTS: A civil complaint was filed against the Lahey Clinic Hospital, claiming it billed Medicare and received payment for unnecessary tests and other diagnostic procedures for Medicare beneficiaries. The First Circuit was careful to acknowledge that Lahey, a renowned academic medical center, was not arguing that the U.S. may not recover overpayments, only that it has chosen the wrong approach in doing so; similarly, the U.S. has not alleged fraud on Lahey's part in this action. The U.S. sought restitution for over $311,000 in overpayments, under common law theories of unjust enrichment and payment under mistake of fact. Lahey maintained the Medicare Act and the administrative procedures promulgated by the Secretary of Health and Human Services (HHS) were the exclusive avenue for recovery of Medicare

overpayments and, as such, the federal courts had no subject matter jurisdiction (*see* 42 U.S.C.A. § 426 *et seq.* (2009)).

ISSUE: Can the federal government sue to recover alleged Medicare Part B overpayments using the common theories of unjust enrichment and payment under mistake of fact?

HOLDING AND DECISION: Yes, the federal government may use the common law to recover alleged Medicare overpayments.

ANALYSIS: The First Circuit summarized the background leading to this claim, namely how, beginning in the late 1980s, Medicare's escalating payments for laboratory services became a source

(continues)

(continued)

of increasing concern. Congress imposed payment caps on laboratory services, yet costs continued to escalate.

Medicare was paying twice as much as physicians for the same laboratory tests. Much of the added cost was attributable to laboratories billing Medicare separately and at the full rate for each individual tests in chemistry and urinalysis panels (known as unbundled billing). When physicians ordered the same panels, they were billed at a reduced rate to account for savings from performing the tests as a group (bundled billing). In addition, when physicians ordered certain hematology indices (which can be generated from the results of other tests), the laboratories repeated the test and billed Medicare for the duplicative test. Medicare overpaid laboratories in excess of $43.6 million for these two billing practices during a two-year period in the mid-1990s.

Laboratories might have saved an additional $15.6 million billed to Medicare by using available automated technology. Accordingly, the federal government sought to recover the overpayments from unbundled billing and duplicative tests that were medically unnecessary. A number of civil actions were instituted to recover some of these costs under various theories, and this is one of those cases.

The court rejected the argument that the U.S. could only recover overpayments through the administrative process established under the Medicare Act (*see* 42 U.S.C.A. § 405(g)-(h) (2008); *see also* 42 U.S.C.A. § 1395 (1965)). Nothing in the Medicare Act established that the administrative remedy mandated by Congress was the exclusive remedy for recovery of overpayments. The court also rejected the contention that the Medicare Act displaced underlying common law causes of action to recover overpayments.

RULE OF LAW: The federal government has broad power to recover overpayments wrongly paid from the U.S. Treasury, even absent any express statutory authorization to sue.

(Thorpe et al., 2004). Yet, rationing Medicare expenditures is rarely discussed. Politicians do not want to say "this person's life expectancy is only so many years, so this procedure is not worth the cost." Nevertheless, Americans are going to have this discussion soon. With educated baby-boomers aging and entering the Medicare system, access to health care will be a growing issue. Costs aside, demands simply for access, and for medical freedom, may yet breathe life into an ailing Medicare system (Thorpe, 2005).

Moral Dilemmas

1. Should some services be exempt from Medicare coverage?

OVERHAULING MEDICARE

Medicare is an inadequate health insurance plan in the sense that it does not protect individuals against long hospital stays or catastrophic expenses. Individuals pay the first $800 of hospital care and the first $100 of outpatient physician visits. Further, if they remain in the hospital for more than sixty or ninety days, they could end up paying another $250 per day for hospital care. This is not optimal health insurance. Insurance should protect people from financial ruin, but Medicare does not do that (Pauly, 2008). The least likely people to purchase supplemental Medicare coverage, which takes care of expenses not covered by Medicare, are low-income people. It is essential that Medicare protect people against catastrophic loss.

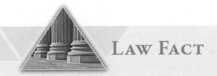

LAW FACT

MEDICARE COVERAGE

Should employers be allowed to alter and decrease health insurance benefits for Medicare-eligible retirees to a level below that provided to non-Medicare-eligible retirees?

The Equal Employment Opportunity Commission can provide an exemption to the Age Discrimination in Employment Act and allow employers to decrease or drop health benefits for retirees who reach the age of Medicare eligibility.

—*AARP v. EEOC,* 489 F.3d 558(U.S. Court of Appeals for the 3rd Circuit 2007), *U.S. Supreme Court certiorari denied,* 128 S.Ct. 1733 (U.S. Supreme Court 2008).

CHAPTER SUMMARY

- Medicare is one of the largest social insurance programs in the U.S., behind only Social Security.
- Soon, over one hundred million people will be eligible for Medicare, meaning the demand will likely exhaust the resources.
- Rise in treatment prevalence, rather than treatment cost or patient growth, accounts for most of the spending growth.
- About 90 percent of those receiving Medicare supplement benefits with other forms of coverage.
- Medicare is organized into four parts: A (Hospital Insurance), B (Physician Insurance), C (Medicare Advantage), and D (Prescription Drug).
- Medicare is financed by payroll taxes, general federal revenue, beneficiary premiums, and payments from states, taxation on Social Security benefits, and interest, but still suffers a serious budgetary shortfall.
- Medicare does not protect people from the kinds of medical expenses causing financial ruin, such as long hospital stays or catastrophic illnesses.

LAW NOTES

1. The government collects payroll taxes over time. These vary by individuals' wages and income, while providing a standard benefit to all enrollees. In this way, the program is able to ensure access to mainstream health care for beneficiaries at all levels of income. Medicare is a more progressive program than Social Security when both the contributions and benefits sides are considered; the benefits are the same, while contributions are higher from persons with high incomes (White, 2008).

CHAPTER BIBLIOGRAPHY

Angrisano, C. et al. (2007). A *framework to guide health care system reform.* San Francisco, CA: McKinsey Global Institute (analyzing why the costs of U.S. health care are so high).

Borer, E. C. (2008). Modernizing Medicare: Protecting America's most vulnerable patients from predatory health care marketing through accessible legal remedies. *Minnesota Law Review, 92,* 1165-1205.

Catlin, A. et al. (2008). National health spending in 2006: A year of change for prescription drugs. *Health Affairs, 27* (1), 14-29 (uses data collected by CMS to analyze the national trends of health spending in 2006 and the impact of Medicare Part D on prescription drug spending growth).

___. (2007). National health spending in 2005: The slowdown continues. *Health Affairs, 26* (1), 142-153.

CMS (Centers for Medicare & Medicaid Services). (2008). *Annual report of the Board of Trustees of the Hospital Insurance Supplementary Medical Insurance Trust Funds.* Washington, DC: CMS (on the past and estimated future financial operations of the Hospital Insurance, Supplementary Medicare Insurance Trust Funds, and prescription drug coverage).

Channick, S. A. (2006).The Medicare Prescription Drug, Improvement and Modernization Act of 2003: Will it be good medicine for U.S. health policy? *Elder Law Journal, 14,* 237-281 (critiquing privatization).

CBO (Congressional Budget Office). (2008). *Geographic variation in health care spending.* Washington, DC: CBO (examines the amount of geographic variation in spending, the reasons for that variation, and its implications for evaluating the efficiency of the nation's health care system).

___. (2008). *Technological change and the growth of health care spending* (describes the historical growth in spending on health care in the U.S., also examines the factors that determine health care spending and how they have contributed to spending growth over time).

Crippen, D., former director of the Congressional Budget Office at the Aspen Health. Aspen, CO (2007, October 5).

Cutler, D. M. et al. (2006). The value of medical spending in the U.S. *New England Journal of Medicine, 355,* 920-927 (examining the value of increased medical spending by comparing gains in life expectancy with the increased costs of health care).

Davis, K. et al. (2007). *Slowing the growth of U.S. health care expenditures: Where are the options?* New York, NY: Commonwealth Fund (reviews factors that contribute to high spending on the health care system in the U.S. and analyzes strategies for accumulating savings, reducing spending growth, and improving health system performance).

DeNavas-Walt, C. et al. (2008). *Income, poverty and health insurance coverage in the U.S.* Washington, DC: U.S. Census Bureau.

Farrell, D. et al. (2008). *Accounting for the cost of U.S. health care: A new look at why Americans spend more.* San Francisco, CA: McKinsey Global Institute.

Federal Register. (2008, June 5). Medicare and Medicaid programs: Hospice conditions of participation. 73 FR 32088-01

___. (2005). Office of Inspector General (OIG). Bulletin on patient assistance programs for Medicare Part D enrollees. 70 FR 70623-03

Ginsburg, P. B. (2007). Shopping for price in medical care. *Health Affairs, 26* (2), 208-216 (analyzes the way in which individuals select health care services based on price and the influence that insurers and the government can have on price selection).

Ginsburg, P. B., & Grossman, J. (2005). When the price is not right: How inadvertent payment incentives drive medical care. *Health Affairs* (examines inaccurate payment rates as a powerful driver of health cost trends by looking specifically at Medicare and how the program can address this issue).

Hartman, M. et al. (2006). Monitoring health spending increases: Incremental budget analyses reveal challenging tradeoffs. *Health Care Financing Review, 28* (1), 41-52 (examines the long term financial outlook of the Medicare program).

Kaiser (Kaiser Family Foundation). (2008). *Fact sheet: Medicare.* Menlo Park, CA: Kaiser.

Keenan, P. S. (2004). *What is driving health care costs?* New York, NY: Commonwealth Fund.

MedPAC (Medicare Payment Advisory Commission). (2008). *Report to the Congress: Reforming the delivery system.* Washington, DC: MedPAC.

___. (2008a). *Report to the Congress: Medicare payment policy.* Washington, DC: MedPAC.

___. (2007). *Report to the Congress: Promoting greater efficiency in Medicare.* Washington, DC: MedPAC.

Mullins, C. D. et al (2005). Variability and growth in spending for outpatient specialty pharmaceuticals. *Health Affairs,*

24 (4), 1117-1127 (study of ten Blue Cross Blue Shield plans documents large expenditures on select specialty pharmaceutical categories and much variation in spending across plans, age groups, and time).

Pauly, M. V. (2008). Studies on Medicare reform: *Markets without magic, how competition might save Medicare.* Washington, DC: American Enterprise Institute.

Poisal, J. A. et al. (2007). Health spending projections through 2016: Modest changes obscure Part D's impact. *Health Affairs, 26* (2), 242-253.

Posner, P. et al. (2005). *21st century challenges: Reexamining the base of the federal government.* Washington, DC: Government Accountability Office (report is intended to help Congress in reviewing and reconsidering the base of federal spending and tax programs, including a chapter that focuses on health care challenges).

Reinhardt, U. (2003). Does the aging of the population really drive the demand for health care? *Health Affairs, 22* (6), 27-39 (draws on the research literature and on data from the Medical Expenditure Panel Surveys to explore the impact that the aging of the U.S, population has on the annual growth in the demand for health care and in national health spending).

Riley, G. (2007). Long-term trends in the concentration of Medicare spending. *Health Affairs, 26* (3), 808-816 (analyzes the concentration of spending and cost containment efforts within the population of Medicare enrollees over the past thirty years).

Schlesinger, M., & Hacker, J. S. (2007). Secret weapon: The "new" Medicare as a route to health security. *Journal of Health Politics, Policy & the Law, 32* (2), 247-291 (arguing that Medicare's public/private hybrid gives the program flexibility).

Schneider, J. E., & Ohsfeldt, R. L. (2006/2007). The role of markets and competition in health care reform initiatives to improve efficiency and enhance access to care. *Cumberland Law Review, 37,* 479-511.

Thorpe, K. E. (2005). The rise in health care spending and what to do about it. *Health Affairs, 24* (6), 1436-1445 (examines causes for the growth of health spending, such as obesity and stress, over the past twenty years and suggests reform options).

Thorpe, K. E. et al. (2004). Which medical conditions account for the rise in health care spending? *Health Affairs, 4,* 437-445.

Weinick, R. et al. (2005). Who can't pay for health care? *Journal of General Internal Medicine, 20* (6), 504-509 (uses data from the Commonwealth Fund Health Care Quality Survey to examine barriers to health care).

Wharton (Wharton School at the University of Pennsylvania). (2004). Restructuring Medicare is a riskier operation than first thought. *Knowledge@Wharton.*

White, C. (2008). Why did Medicare spending growth slow down? *Health Affairs, 27* (3), 793-802.

Yamamoto, D. et al (2008). *How does the benefit value of Medicare compare to the benefit value of typical large employer plans?* Menlo Park, CA: Kaiser Family Foundation.

Zuvekas, S. H., & Cohen, J. W. (2007). Prescription drugs and the changing concentration of health care expenditures. *Health Affairs, 26* (1), 249-257 (explores the concentration of health care spending in various sectors and possible implications for cost containment).

PART IV

AFFORDABLE
HEALTH CARE

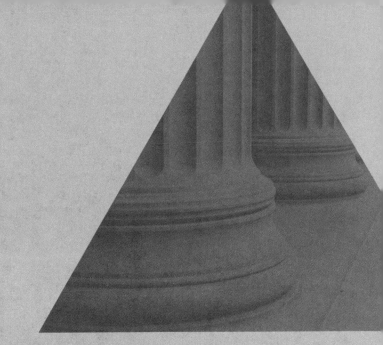

CHAPTER 8

MUTUALLY AFFORDABLE HEALTH CARE

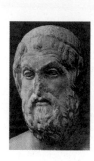

"Money: There's nothing in the world as demoralizing as money."

—SOPHOCLES (B.C.), GREEK PLAYWRIGHT, FROM *ANTIGONE*

IN BRIEF

This chapter examines whether nonprofit health care systems are required to provide fair and reasonable charges for medical services, or alternatively, mutually affordable health care, in return for substantial federal, state, and local tax exemptions. Amid growing concern about whether hospitals are doing enough to justify their tax exemptions, Congress and many state legislatures are calling on tax-exempt hospitals to make changes to their charitable care and financial assistance policies, as well as their billing and debt-collection practices.

It is important to note that while this chapter addresses the nation's two thousand tax-exempt hospitals, the pricing, billing, and collection principles, along with the corporate, tax, and consumer credit laws cited herein, are equally applicable to the nonprofit health care systems, of which tax-exempt hospitals are only one part.

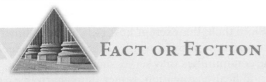

FACT OR FICTION

DISCRIMINATORY PRICING

Should the uninsured be charged the highest prices for health care?

Carlos Ferlini installed and repaired gutters for a living. Like millions of Americans, he made a decent living, but was not offered health insurance through his employer and could not afford to buy it on his own. In February 2006, Ferlini fell while working on a roof and badly injured himself, fracturing his skull and ribs and puncturing his lung. When he arrived at the hospital, Ferlini was close to death and the last thing on his mind was the cost. After spending eighteen days in Saint Joseph Medical Center, a tax-exempt hospital in Burbank, California, Carlos and his wife knew the resulting hospital bill was going to be a large amount. They fully intended to pay their bill, but they never expected it to be $246,000.

    K. B. Forbes is a community activist who has been pushing to protect uninsured patients' rights. When Ferlini asked him to look into his hospital bill, Forbes explained to him that what happened is very common. According to Forbes, hospitals charge uninsured patients four or five times more than what they would accept as payment in full from an insurance company. Forbes describes the hospital practice of charging the uninsured $20,000 for an appendectomy, a procedure that normally costs $5,000 for people with health insurance. Forbes investigated Ferlini's hospital bill and found that Saint Joseph Medical Center billed Ferlini $246,000, when slightly less than $50,000 would have been billed to an insurance company for the same exact treatment. At the same time, the Medical Center failed to advise Ferlini of his possible eligibility for Medicaid and Worker's Compensation, which covers the health care costs of employees injured on the job.

—Kuntze, 2008; Rosembaum, 2006.

(See *Law Fact* at the end of this chapter for the answer.)

PRINCIPLES AND APPLICATIONS

At issue in this chapter is how nonprofit health care systems carry out their charitable mission when attempting to allocate scarce health care resources in the most effective way possible. Most hospitals in the U.S. are recognized as charitable organizations exempt from federal taxes under Section 501(c)(3) of the U.S. Tax Code (*see* Exempt Organizations, 26 U.S.C.A. § 501 (2006) ("Exemption from tax.... (c) List of exempt organizations . . . (3) Corporations . . . organized and operated exclusively for . . . charitable, scientific.... no part of the net earnings of which inures to the benefit of any private shareholder or individual....")). In return for their tax exemptions, states and the Internal Revenue Service (IRS) previously required that tax-exempt hospitals provide a substantial amount of charitable care. Defining mutually affordable health care depends on health care financing, community federal poverty levels, existing state charitable care laws, and the charitable care policies of individual hospitals.

HISTORIC FOUNDATION OF TAX-EXEMPT HOSPITALS

Historically, relief of the poor has been viewed as a charitable purpose, at least since the Elizabethan Statute of Charitable Uses enacted by the English Parliament in 1601 (*see* An Act to Redress the Mis-Employment of Lands, Goods and Stock of Money Heretofore Given to Certain Charitable Uses, 1601, 43 Eliz. 1, c. 4 (Eng.), reprinted in 7 Stat. at Large 43 (Eng. 1763)). Providing charitable care has been an integral part of hospitals since the Middle Ages, when the first European hospitals were actually shelters for physically and mentally disabled individuals, homeless people, and a place to isolate portions of the population affected by epidemics. The early hospitals, however, actually provided more in the way of comfort care than health care.

    During this era, people who needed medical attention, and who could afford to pay for it, received health care at their homes by visiting physicians, surgeons, and nurses. However, with progressive technical advances in eighteenth-century Europe, in particular the discovery of anesthesia and antiseptics, the concept of the modern-day hospital, serving only medical needs, began to take hold.

The hospital movement began in England with the dual purpose of caring for the sick and removing the ailing from charity rolls, thereby reducing or removing the financial burden of their care from the community. In turn, the hospital patients served as clinical subjects for scientifically oriented physicians. For the same humanitarian, financial, and scientific reasons, the hospital movement spread to the American colonies (Morton & Woodbury, 1895).

The Social Contract for Hospital Care: 1751 to 1960s

The Pennsylvania Hospital in Philadelphia, the first hospital in the U.S., was chartered in 1751 from private subscriptions matched by funds from the Pennsylvania legislature. Founded by Benjamin Franklin and Dr. Thomas Bond, the hospital was established to care for the sick, poor, and insane. The story of the Good Samaritan was chosen by Franklin and Bond as the official seal, and the statement of mission was "Take Care of Him and I Will Repay Thee." This ushered in a new attitude of social responsibility in U.S. health care.

By the mid-nineteenth century, large public hospitals opened in all of the major cities in the U.S., along with academic research hospitals affiliated with medical schools. The first public hospitals in the U.S. were fully charitable and relied almost entirely on government support with no fee structures. The public hospitals provided health care to anyone who needed it, and expected no payment in return. While most private hospitals were tax-exempt due to their charitable purpose, they provided only a minimum of charitable care, in the form of free or discounted health care.

The Social Contract Evolves: 1969 to 2000s

After Medicare and Medicaid were created in the 1960s and the State Children's Health Insurance Program (SCHIP) was established in 1997, centuries of legal precedent of what constituted charitable purposes for hospitals changed. The hospital industry contended there would no longer be enough demand for charitable care to satisfy the IRS's tax-exemption standards because the government programs now reimbursed hospitals for health care previously provided free-of-charge (Becker, 2007). The industry maintained most Americans would be covered either by the new government programs or by private health insurance and pushed for a more flexible tax-exemption standard (Carreyrou & Martinez, 2008). This new standard, known as the "community benefit standard," was adopted by the IRS in 1969.

Since then, tax-exempt hospitals have qualified for tax exemption by providing other types of benefits to the communities they serve, such as emergency care and health education, rather than charitable care. For the first time since 1751, tax-exempt hospitals in the U.S. were no longer required to offer charitable care directly to the poor and financially distressed (Cohen, 2006). Prior to 1969, tax-exempt hospitals had to be involved in charitable care in order to be exempt. After 1969, the meaning of charitable care evolved from a connotation that tax-exempt hospitals had to provide charitable care to a community benefits standard with a commitment to the federal, state, and local governments to provide a benefit to the community that outweighed the benefit the governments would receive from tax revenue (Nie, 2007).

Private-Based, For-Profit Approach: 1997 to Present

By the twentieth century, the U.S hospital system was largely private-based with a for-profit approach to providing hospital care; few state-supported public hospitals remained. In the late twentieth century, chains of hospitals arose across the U.S., sponsored by nonprofit and for-profit corporations. Until recently, generous reimbursement rates from both private insurance and Medicare, Medicaid, and SCHIP permitted hospital chains to provide significant levels of charitable care for uninsured adults and the underinsured by cross-subsidizing that care from charges paid by insured patients.

Today, as the generosity of insurance reimbursements has tightened, most tax-exempt hospitals have become increasingly focused on financial performance and survival, and charitable care was the first casualty. The current debate is whether community benefits justify the tax dollars that the federal, state, and local governments forgo in granting exemptions to hospitals. As the demands for mutually affordable health care intensify, the tax dollars received by tax-exempt hospitals for the community's health are being scrutinized in litigation across the U.S. Estimates are that tax-exempt hospitals receive $12.6 billion in annual tax exemptions, on top of the $32 billion in government-assistance subsidies the hospital industry as a whole receives each year (CBO, 2006).

DUTY OF TAX-EXEMPT HOSPITALS TO PROVIDE MUTUALLY AFFORDABLE HEALTH CARE

"Mutually affordable" is undefined within the context of the current health care payment system. Does it mean everyone should be able to receive necessary and essential health care? If so, then what defines necessary and essential care? Once a consensus is reached on this definition, the next question is how can the U.S. develop a politically acceptable universal solution to the problem of paying costs for necessary health care for the uninsured and underinsured? Part of this solution is fair and mutually reasonable reimbursement to hospitals for the costs of health care.

The duty of tax-exempt hospitals to provide mutually affordable health care is at the center of the policy debate about how the U.S. might provide reasonably priced, comprehensive, and continuous health insurance to everyone. This debate tends to fall along two lines. One side endorses mandated health insurance for all Americans in order to guarantee that the nation's uninsured receive coverage. The other side also wants to improve access to affordable health care, but it places more emphasis on market-based solutions than government mandates. Both sides are debating universal coverage along with the issues of the uninsured and underinsured. At the core of this controversy is the responsibility of tax-exempt hospitals to provide charitable care (Aitsebaomo, 2004).

Congress is investigating tax-exempt hospitals, which represent almost half of the nonprofit sector's revenue, as part of a broader inquiry into possible abuses of tax exemptions by nonprofit organizations. Altogether the nonprofit sector accounts for over $1.4 trillion in revenue in the U.S. (Urban Institute, 2007). Many lawmakers are concerned about the plight of patients who are labeled as "self-pay," which includes the uninsured, in the wake of recent news reports that more and more people are being bankrupted by medical debts.[LN1]

The IRS is also checking to see if tax-exempt hospitals provide community benefits that set them apart from for-profit hospitals and justify their tax-exempt status (Becker, 2007). Moreover, some patients have sued tax-exempt hospitals, claiming the hospitals failed in their charitable mission by overcharging uninsured and underinsured patients for health care. Some of the lawsuits have been dismissed by federal courts; still more are pending in state courts.

Moral Dilemmas

1. When, under what medical circumstances, and why should tax-exempt hospitals be required to provide mutually affordable health care to patients?

Heightened Scrutiny of Charitable Care Practices

Tax-exempt hospitals have come under intense scrutiny over long-standing practices that often result in charging the highest prices to uninsured patients (Burns, 2004). Recently, several tax-exempt hospitals

across the country have been charged with billing their uninsured patients significantly more than their insured patients for the same health care, and then using overly aggressive collection practices to collect the resultant medical debt.

Legal proceedings and class-action lawsuits brought against nonprofit health care systems highlight the contradictory views underscoring concerns about the rising cost of health care and the increasing number of uninsured and underinsured patients (Moskowitz, 2005). Some hospitals are choosing to enter settlement agreements rather than litigate the myriad of unresolved issues as to what constitutes affordable health care. Regardless, this litigation has made hospital pricing, billing, and collection practices issues of public concern and serves as a signal to tax-exempt hospitals that they should expect closer inspection as the number of financially distressed patients continues to grow (Batchis, 2005).

Many nonprofit health care systems are under scrutiny and some tax-exempt hospitals have already been singled out for:

- Discriminatory pricing
- Overly aggressive collection practices
- Price gouging

Aggressive patient billing and collection practices by the entire hospital industry helped blur the distinction between for-profit and tax-exempt hospitals (Horwitz, 2007). Now, the various levels of government are examining this widespread discontent as they are squeezed by revenue shortfalls, and are eyeing the revenue bases of tax-exempt hospitals and challenging their tax-exempt status (Maples, 2007).

Evolving Health Care Delivery Systems

Propelling this conflicted situation is the changing business structure of tax-exempt hospitals. Their traditional foundation as compassionate caregivers is being transformed as they increasingly evolve into comprehensive health care delivery systems with significant revenues.

The size of tax-exempt hospitals' tax exemptions is increasingly criticized, in part because their revenues have risen so sharply in recent years, and because they represent such a big portion of America's health care spending. Thirty-one cents of every health care dollar is spent on hospitals (Carreyrou & Martinez, 2008). This figure includes health care at for-profit and tax-exempt hospitals.

Today, tax-exempt hospitals are being scrutinized for:

- Allowing for-profit entities to derive a profit from use of their tax-exempt facilities (e.g., food services, anesthesiology practices, physician practices, and parking)

- Charging uninsured patients the undiscounted cost for health care without regard to ability to pay, while discounting costs for insured patients and patients covered by government-assistance programs
- Charging patients more than the actual cost of health care rendered in order to cover the cost of unreimbursed care rendered
- Failing to use their assets and revenues to provide mutually affordable health care, while providing luxury facilities and excessive multimillion-dollar administrative salaries
- Refusing to provide emergency services without regard to the ability to pay

Moral Dilemmas

1. Should non-charitable, for-profit entities (physician group practices, pharmacies, cafeterias) be able to derive profits from the use of tax-exempt hospitals?

The Emergency Medical Treatment and Active Labor Act (EMTALA) creates an illusion about the availability of health care for the uninsured (*see* 42 U.S.C.A. § 1395dd (2003)). While EMTALA prohibits hospitals from refusing to screen, treat, and stabilize any person who seeks emergency treatment, the law does not require hospitals to cover the cost of treatment or any post-stabilization treatment.

Moral Dilemmas

1. What standards should govern the charges that tax-exempt hospitals can charge for medical services?

Public Benefit Corporations

Nonprofit health care systems are typically organized under a state's nonprofit corporation laws. Although nonprofit laws differ from state to state, the Revised Model Nonprofit Corporation Act has been adopted by most states to provide general uniformity of state laws nationally (Maples, 2007) (*see* Model Nonprofit Corporation Act § 2.02(a)(2)(i-iii) (1987)).

Since public benefit corporations are chartered by states to carry out benefits for the public, they receive tax-exempt status but are run almost identically to for-profits. According to the Internal Revenue Code (IRC), the definition of a "nonprofit" is any entity that serves the public interest. A nonprofit entity is one that does not declare a profit and uses all revenue available after meeting costs to serve the public

interest. In addition, most nonprofit entities are incorporated, which means they share many similarities with for-profits. Like other nonprofit organizations, tax-exempt hospitals do not have shareholders or owners to whom any profits can be distributed. Rather, any money they earn from their operations or from financial investments must be channeled back into the organization in some way.

Nonprofit entities have both paid and voluntary workers, but employment taxes and federal and state worker rules are no different than those applicable to for-profits. The perception that nonprofit entities are full of volunteers and low-paying jobs is a misconception. In fact, most nonprofit health care systems maintain salaries and benefits on par with their for-profit competitors. Chief executive officers of most tax-exempt hospitals have annual salaries in excess of $500,000 and some over $5 million (*see* Carreyrou & Martinez, 2008).

Today, about 60 percent of the 3,400 hospitals in the U.S. are nonprofit, tax-exempt entities. About 23 percent of hospitals are for-profit, and another 17 percent are run by the federal government, states, or counties (Charitable vs. nonprofit, 2008).

Profitability of Tax-Exempt Hospitals

The American Hospital Association (AHA), a trade association for the nation's hospitals, maintains that one-third of the nation's hospitals are losing money because government-assistance programs are often not enough to cover the hospitals' actual costs of treating patients. Most of the hospitals under financial strain are in communities handling large numbers of uninsured and underinsured patients, particularly those located in cities.

According to the American Hospital Directory, an information service company that compiles data hospitals report to the federal government, three out of four tax-exempt hospitals are solvent. This compares with about 60 percent of for-profit hospitals. This measure of solvency does not measure how solvent they are, whether they are just barely solvent or highly profitable. Thus, while it appears tax-exempt hospitals may have higher sustainability levels than their for-profit counterparts, no true financial comparison appears to be available.

It may be that this apparent disparity in solvency is the result of tax exemptions enjoyed while failing to return those tax benefits to the communities they serve. Tax-exempt hospitals are expected to channel the surpluses they generate back into their operations. Many tax-exempt hospitals, however, have used their growing surpluses to:

- Accumulate large cash reserves
- Build expensive new facilities

- Purchase the latest medical equipment and technologies
- Reward their executives with rich pay packages

(Carreyrou & Martinez, 2008)

As a result of the way tax-exempt hospitals have used their surpluses, some health care economists argue all hospitals should pay taxes (Reinhardt, 2006). They argue that tax-exempt hospitals differ little from for-profits in the provision of charitable care and, therefore, should either lose their tax-exempt status or adhere to new strict and specific requirements to provide care for the uninsured and underinsured (Horwitz, 2007).

Enjoying the pricing power that came from a decade of mergers, many tax-exempt hospitals saw earnings soar in recent years. The combined net revenue of the fifty largest tax-exempt hospitals jumped nearly eight-fold to over $4.0 billion according to the American Hospital Directory (Carreyrou & Martinez, 2008). One reason for hospitals' soaring profits is a gradual increase in Medicare reimbursements after federal budget cutbacks during the 1990s. By merging and gaining scale, many tax-exempt hospitals also gained leverage in price negotiations with health insurers. No fewer than twenty-five tax-exempt hospitals or hospital systems now have revenues of more than $250 million a year (Carreyrou & Martinez, 2008).

Much of the hospital industry's earnings growth comes from strategies it pursued to increase revenues. Among them:

- Demanding upfront payments from patients
- Focusing on expensive procedures
- Hiking list prices for procedures and services to several times their actual cost
- Issuing tax-exempt bonds, investing the proceeds in higher-yielding securities, and then keeping the untaxed investment gains
- Securitizing and then selling patients' debts to aggressive third-party debt collectors

(Martinez, 2008)

LACK OF AFFORDABLE HEALTH CARE

The number and proportion of Americans reporting no health care or a delay in obtaining needed health care have increased sharply in recent years, according to findings from the Robert Wood Johnson Foundation's Center for Studying Health Systems. One in five Americans, or fifty-nine million Americans, reported not getting or delaying necessary health care. This number is up from one in seven, or thirty-six million people, in 2003.

While access to affordable health care has deteriorated for both the insured and uninsured, insured people experienced a larger relative increase in access problems compared with the uninsured. In other words, health insurance no longer guarantees people will be able to access health care. Moreover, access declined more for people in fair or poor health than for healthier people. In addition, unmet medical needs increased for low-income children, reversing earlier trends and widening the access gap as compared to higher-income children (Cunningham & Felland, 2008). People reporting access problems increasingly cited:

- Cost as an obstacle to needed health care with rising deductibles and co-payments for both the insured and underinsured
- Health system barriers, such as health insurance restrictions and limitations, and the demands for upfront payments for health care before treatment services are rendered
- Rising rates of health insurance premiums, leaving little to cover the access fees required to obtain preventive, routine health care

THE UNINSURED AND UNDERINSURED: TWO GROWING PATIENT GROUPS

With the number of uninsured and underinsured Americans is climbing, the safety net tax-exempt hospitals provides for the uninsured and underinsured is stretched to the breaking point. The cost of caring for this population by major teaching hospitals is over $6 billion a year, a steady trend since 2004 (Kirch, 2008).

Health insurance is the most important determinant of access to affordable health care (Collins, 2007). People without adequate insurance coverage risk financial disaster if they find themselves in need of expensive health care.

Complete lack of health insurance is only one part of the problem today, as even the insured have serious gaps in coverage. A growing number of underinsured Americans also find themselves on shaky financial ground (Gerencher, 2007). Insurance coverage is the ticket into the health care system, but for too many Americans, that ticket does not buy financial security or genuinely affordable access to health care. People who have health insurance, but have coverage that does not adequately protect them from high medical costs, are generally considered underinsured if they have:

- Deductibles equal to or greater than 5 percent of their total household income
- Out-of-pocket medical, prescription, dental, and vision costs that amount to 10 percent or more of their total household income

- Out-of-pocket medical, prescription, dental, and vision costs that amount to 5 percent or more if they are a low-income individual with total household income below the federal poverty level of $10,400 (plus $3,600 for each additional family member)

(Davis, 2007)

Almost one-quarter of working-age adults face potential financial exposure from unaffordable health care. Much of this growth in the uninsured and underinsured comes from the middle class. While low-income people remain vulnerable, middle-income families have recently been hit the hardest. Although adults below the poverty level are at the highest risk of being uninsured or underinsured, insurance erosion has spread up the revenue distribution ladder well into the middle-class range. For those with annual incomes of $40,000 to $59,000, the underinsured percentage rate has reached double digits (Schoen et al., 2008).

Uninsured Patients

People who spend any time without health insurance report significantly higher rates of cost-related access problems, are significantly less likely to have a regular family physician, and are less likely to report that they always or often received the health care they need when they need it (Collins, 2007). Since 1998, the Kaiser Commission on Medicaid and the Uninsured has examined:

- How health insurance coverage is changing
- How many Americans lack health insurance coverage
- Who the uninsured are

The Kaiser Commission estimates there are about forty-seven million Americans without health insurance, which represents about 18 percent of the population under sixty-five years of age. Moreover, the number of uninsured is steadily growing. Most recently, the number of uninsured has increased by about 3.5 million between 2004 and 2006.

Most American families still obtain their health insurance through their employers, but that is not a guaranteed benefit for approximately 160 million employees and their dependents (Collins, 2007). In fact, 82 percent of the uninsured come from working families (Kaiser, 2008). The working poor comprise more than one-third of the uninsured; without employer-sponsored insurance, they cannot afford to pay the premiums themselves.

As the cost of health insurance continues to rise, fewer employers, particularly small firms, are able to provide affordable health insurance to their employees (Collins, 2007). In fact, employer-sponsored insurance decreased to 54 percent of the population in 2007. Government-assistance programs have filled some of the gap, but the assistance is mostly for children from financially distressed families, while many working-age Americans are left behind (Kaiser, 2008).

Underinsured Patients

More than twenty-five million working-age adults were underinsured last year according to the Commonwealth Fund, up 60 percent from the sixteen million who had inadequate coverage in 2003. The rate of underinsurance nearly tripled among middle- and high-income families, or those with at least $40,000 in family income.

The upward trend in the underinsured rate reflects how much rising health care costs have outpaced wage increases. The Kaiser Family Foundation found premiums for family coverage jumped 78 percent since 2001, while wages rose 19 percent and general inflation went up 17 percent during that time.

FEDERAL, STATE, AND LOCAL GOVERNMENTS AT ODDS

While the argument over hospital tax-exemption is ongoing at the federal level, the real battle is waged at the state and local levels. While tax-exemption is defined by the federal government, tax-exempt hospitals are also exempt from paying state and local taxes.

The state and local tax exemptions pre-date federal exemptions, originating when public hospitals functioned exclusively for the financially distressed members of the community. Tax-exempt hospitals relieved state and local governments from operating public hospitals and the burden of caring for those unable to afford health care, which offset the loss in state and local tax revenue.

Over time, tax-exempt hospitals evolved into huge business enterprises (Greaney & Boozang, 2005). The tax-exempt hospital changed its image dramatically, and is no longer looked at as a benevolent caregiver. Therefore, state and local governments have a vested interest when it comes to determining tax-exemption status for hospitals, and actively join in the debate as to what constitutes charitable care (Burns, 2004). In fact, the theories concerning charitable care are sharpened by states and localities and are used to attack or support the tax-exemption of hospitals.

It is clear that the federal approach to this debate differs from state and local approaches because of two opposing viewpoints. While the federal government has a strong incentive to support tax exemption to foster competition between for-profits and nonprofits, states and localities have noted the surpluses these tax-exempt hospitals accumulate and question whether community benefits from these hospitals really outweigh the benefit governments would receive from not only federal income tax revenues, but also state income and property tax revenues and tax-exempt bond financing. The most important benefit tax-exempt hospitals provide to governments is absorbing the unreimbursed costs from Medicare, Medicaid, and SCHIP (Bush, 2007).

FEDERAL CLASS-ACTION LAWSUITS

At the same time Congress is questioning the debt-collection policies of nonprofit hospitals, a coordinated effort is under way to file federal class-action lawsuits against nonprofit health care systems (Schwinn, 2006). Several national law firms with years of experience in mass tort litigation are participating in this litigation; several successfully led aggressive, coordinated actions against the tobacco industry in the 1990s (Moskowitz, 2005).

Since July 2004, class-action lawsuits alleging that hospitals have charged uninsured patients fees well in excess of those charged to insured patients have been initiated in federal courts. However, the consensus from the courts is that these cases do not present viable claims.[LN2] This consensus is consistent with the U.S. Supreme Court decision, *Eastern Kentucky Welfare Rights Organization. v. Simon*, 426 U.S. 26 (U.S. Supreme Court 1976), finding that uninsured patients had no standing to challenge IRS revenue rulings granting tax-exemptions under Section § 501(c)(3).

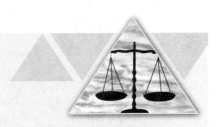

COORDINATED CLASS-ACTION LITIGATION

DiCarlo v. St. Mary Hospital

[Uninsured Patient v. Tax-Exempt Hospital]

530 F.3d 255 (U.S. Court of Appeals for the 3rd Circuit 2008)

FACTS: DiCarlo brought a class-action lawsuit against an acute-care medical/surgical hospital and its non-profit Catholic health care system operating the hospital, alleging breach of contract, breach of the duty of good faith and fair dealing, unjust enrichment, breach of fiduciary duty, and fraud. The hospital accepted discounted payments from various payers, including Medicare, Medicaid, and insurance or managed care plans that negotiated discounts with the hospital. The hospital also provided free or discounted care to patients eligible for charitable care.

DiCarlo was admitted to the hospital after experiencing an increased heart rate. At the time he was admitted, DiCarlo was uninsured and did not qualify for Medicare, Medicaid, or charitable care. Upon his arrival at the hospital, DiCarlo consented to whatever medical treatment was deemed necessary and guaranteed payment of all charges for services rendered. Following his treatment, the hospital charged DiCarlo $3,483 excluding separately billed physician fees.

ISSUE: Can tax-exempt hospitals charge uninsured patients greater amounts than those paid by privately insured patients, Medicare or Medicaid patients, or patients eligible for the charitable care?

HOLDING AND DECISION: Yes, tax-exempt hospitals may establish discriminatory pricing for its health care.

ANALYSIS: The court discussed the policy concerns about health care costs and found that the judiciary was ill-equipped to determine what fair and reasonable hospital costs were, or to make legislative determinations as to what constituted mutually affordable health care.

First, DiCarlo contended he only agreed to pay a reasonable price, which he defined as the Medicare, Medicaid, and charitable care rates: not the undiscounted rates charged the uninsured. This breach of contract claim goes directly to the heart of the federal class-action lawsuits: the charges to uninsured hospital patients for

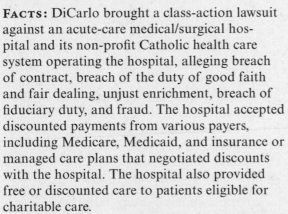

(continues)

(continued)

health care. All the same, the court dismissed this breach of contract claim, finding this contract claim did not reflect how hospital charges are actually set.

Hospitals have a uniform set of charges, known as the chargemaster, which applies to all patients. Discounted charges and computations apply in different situations (e.g., differing discounts are negotiated with managed care payors and insurance companies; another discount is accepted if patients are covered by a government-assistance program that legislatively imposes discounts; still other discounts are given to patients eligible for charitable care programs; while free care is available to patients that demonstrate financial need but are ineligible for any government programs).

Second, the court dismissed the breach of the duty of good faith and fair dealing claim built on the breach of contract claim. DiCarlo might have been entitled to relief under the covenant of good faith and fair dealing if his reasonable expectations of what he was obligated to pay were destroyed after he signed the consent form guaranteeing payment for medical services rendered, and if the hospital acted with ill motives and without any legitimate purpose. In signing the consent form,

however, DiCarlo promised to pay in full the definite price terms set by the hospital; his obligations were clear.

Third, in order to state a claim for unjust enrichment, the hospital must have received and retained a benefit from DiCarlo that would be unjust. However, DiCarlo did not give anything at all to the hospital. Therefore, the court dismissed this claim against the hospital.

Fourth, the court refused to expand the fiduciary duty of hospitals to their billing practices. Analogizing the practice to the debtor-creditor relationship, the breach of fiduciary duty claim was dismissed.

Finally, in dismissing the fraud claim, the court found the hospital's pricing and billing practices were not covered by state fraud laws. Hospital debt collectors are usually not covered by state consumer fraud statutes, so long as they are operating in their professional capacities.

RULE OF LAW: Tax-exempt hospitals are not required to provide free or reduced-rates for medical services to uninsured patients; moreover, it is not unreasonable to charge uninsured patients higher rates merely because various insurers have negotiated to pay lower rates.

How the duty of good faith and fair dealing applies, and appropriate remedies for breach of this duty, varies based on the circumstances. Health law issues such as the definition of standards of fair dealing in the hospital industry and the justified expectations of patients are being contested in ongoing litigation on mutually affordable health care. Many of the lawsuits are postured as class-actions against health care systems, of which tax-exempt hospitals are only one part. The AHA and other individual decision-makers (including officers, directors, and attorneys) are often listed as co-conspirators in the lawsuits for having drafted guidelines and provided advice that advanced discriminatory billing practices against the uninsured and underinsured. The complaints:

- Ask courts to impose constructive trusts on the hospitals' assets (Katz, 2005)
- Seek monetary damages
- Request injunctions prohibiting the hospitals from:
  ○ Billing uninsured patients the full, undiscounted cost of health care without utilizing a sliding scale payment scheme

○ Charging uninsured patients more than insured patients for the same treatment services
○ Prohibiting the use of aggressive and abusive collection practices by third-party collection agencies that have acquired securitized medical debt
○ Collecting unreasonable fees from uninsured and underinsured patients

The current lawsuits are likely part of the larger national debate on what charitable care means and whether nonprofits are deserving of their tax-exempt status. The first class-action lawsuits filed in federal court seeking monetary damages for uninsured patients have generally been dismissed or withdrawn.

Moral Dilemmas

1. Should disparate pricing for health care services be permissible?

DUTY TO PROVIDE MUTUALLY AFFORDABLE HEALTH CARE

Hutt v. Albert Einstein Medical Center
[Uninsured Patient v. Tax-Exempt Hospital]
2005 WL 2396313 (U.S. District Court for the Eastern District of Pennsylvania 2005)
and
Feliciano v. Thomas Jefferson University Hospital
[Uninsured Patient v. Tax-Exempt Hospital]
2005 WL 2397047 (U.S. District Court for the Eastern District of Pennsylvania 2005)

FACTS: Beginning in 2004, lawsuits were filed against hundreds of tax-exempt hospitals on behalf of uninsured patients in federal courts.

ISSUE: Do tax-exempt hospitals, as a result of their tax exemptions, have a contract with the federal government and the states to provide affordable health care to all patients and an obligation to abstain from overly aggressive debt-collection practices?

HOLDING AND DECISION: No, uninsured patients are not third-party beneficiaries to any government contract arising from tax exemption and tax-exempt hospitals never breached a public charitable trust to provide mutually affordable health care.

ANALYSIS: Under the third-party beneficiary claim, the uninsured patients argued the hospitals agreed to meet a number of specific obligations, including providing charitable care, in exchange for receiving tax exemptions. The uninsured patients claimed they were charged excessive medical fees and were subject to humiliating debt-collection tactics; therefore, they did not receive

the intended benefits of the hospitals' tax-exemption agreement with the government. However, the court dismissed the claim, finding the Internal Revenue Code (IRC) did not create a private cause of action. Furthermore, the court found that, even if such an action could be brought, the IRC did not create a contract between the government and the hospitals.

The uninsured patients also argued the hospitals created a public charitable trust to provide mutually affordable health care by accepting tax-exemption, and that their actions breached their trust obligations. The court again held the IRC did not create a private cause of action. Furthermore, under the Restatement (Second) of Trusts, the court held that a party must expressly intend to form a charitable trust. Here, the uninsured patients showed no intent on the part of the hospitals. Therefore, because there was no legal basis for the existence of a contract under 501(c)(3), and because there was no breach of a public charitable trust, the court dismissed the two lawsuits.

RULE OF LAW: There is no legal basis for a private cause of action arising from a hospital's tax-exemption status.

STATE CLASS-ACTION LAWSUITS

In addition to the federal class-action lawsuits, new pleadings are being filed in state courts (Olson, 2005). These complaints allege that tax-exempt hospitals are overcharging their uninsured patients. Specifically, these uninsured patients are charged more for the same health care than patients covered by private insurance or government-assistance plans. While the exact rate of discount that insured patients receive is unknown, many experts estimate

that the typical range of discounts nationally is between 45 and 50 percent (Anderson, 2007). One nationwide study cited in the complaints suggests that the uninsured pay 2.5 times the amount health insurance providers pay for the same treatment (Saar, 2008).The lawsuits also allege that hospitals are overly aggressive in their collection efforts toward the uninsured and underinsured, and that these unrelenting procedures together are followed more for private interests than for financial survival.

HEIGHTENED SCRUTINY OF CHARITABLE CARE AND COMMUNITY BENEFIT STANDARDS

There is heightened questioning on how much community benefit tax-exempt hospitals should provide to the communities they serve (Hanson, 2005). There is also debate on what means-based discounts tax-exempt hospitals should charge uninsured and underinsured patients.

Charitable Care Standard: IRC 56-185

IRC 56-185 described the traditional charitable care standard of tax-exemption. This rule considered the conventional role of public hospitals as health care facilities catering to the financially distressed.

The rule required tax-exempt hospitals to be organized as nonprofit entities whose main purpose was providing health care to the sick. Any surpluses over revenue incurred must never be used to benefit any private shareholder or individual. Under this rule, tax-exempt hospitals must provide health care to anyone, despite their ability to pay. The rule did not deny tax-exempt hospitals the right to charge uninsured and underinsured patients who had the ability to pay; rather, it provided an obligation to provide affordable health care to persons unable to pay. In addition, hospitals could charge patients a means-based rate and thereby render charitable care.

This ruling came under attack for several reasons, mostly because it was ambiguous. The ruling assumed hospitals could attain tax-exemption even if their primary function was providing health care to patients able to pay, as long as they provided free or reduced rates to those with no ability to pay. In addition, the ruling lacked clarity; it allowed hospitals tax exemptions based on behavior that might not represent sufficient activity to satisfy the "operated exclusively" requirement. Also, with the arrival of government-assistance programs, less free care was required. Ultimately, the IRS found it necessary to modify the ruling.

Community Benefit Standard: IRC 69-545

In return for not paying taxes, tax-exempt hospitals are expected to provide a community benefit, a loosely defined federal requirement whose most important component is charitable care. However, many tax-exempt hospitals include other costs in their community benefit accounting to the IRS, including unpaid patient bills. Often, such hospitals also include the difference between the list prices of health care they provide and what they are paid by government-assistance programs (see Carreyrou &

Martinez, 2008). Excluding those other costs, many tax-exempt hospitals spend less on charitable care than they receive in tax breaks (CBO, 2006).

In 1969, the IRS established the community benefit standard. In determining whether a nonprofit hospital qualifies for tax-exemption, the IRS applies the rules specified under the community benefit standard. Specifically, IRC 69-545 supports the underlying principle that tax-exemption is granted to tax-exempt hospitals that improve the overall health standard for the community, thus providing a benefit to the community. A key component is that the hospitals serve a public instead of a private interest. A tax-exempt hospital can demonstrate adherence to this standard by having a governing board of directors composed of individuals representing the community. They must also:

- Have an open admissions policy for patients who can pay by personal means or by third-party reimbursement
- Maintain an open medical staff policy whereby any qualified physician can have admitting privileges
- Operate an emergency room that is available to anyone needing health care regardless of ability to pay

Although several revisions have been made to the community benefit standard, the IRS never provided a detailed description of what the specific community benefits must be. Therefore, variations to the requirement proliferate as nonprofit health care systems individually interpret what *community benefits* means. For instance, the Catholic Health Association, comprised of over 1,200 Catholic hospitals, includes five activities when computing community benefits:

- Charges related to community development activities
- Development costs
- Education costs
- Research expenditures
- Unpaid patient bills

Many want to know how these activities directly benefit the community. Other tax-exempt hospitals have included the salaries of their employees as a community benefit, further obscuring the issue of affordable health care. At the same time, others maintain the impact of job production is a benefit that should be seen as promoting the community's well-being.

New IRS standards, due to take full effect in 2009, will require tax-exempt hospitals to explicitly state the specifics of their community benefit contributions (*Federal Register,* 2005). However, the new standards still will not require the hospitals to provide any minimum amount of charitable care.

NONPROFITS LOOK SIMILAR TO FOR-PROFITS

Nonprofits in the health industry are significant, revenue-seeking enterprises that compete vigorously, and for the most part, successfully, against their for-profit rivals (Greaney, 2005). Often, for-profits are accused of charging higher prices to patients; however, research shows that the only distinction between tax-exempt and for-profit hospitals in terms of affordable health care is market share. The higher the market share, the higher the prices to patients. While for-profit hospital pricing more strongly correlated with market concentration than nonprofit hospital pricing, price increases for both as the hospitals' market shares increase (Richman, 2006).

Many contend that the federal government is too far removed from the community to determine whether tax-exempt hospitals are really providing adequate benefits to outweigh the tax revenue benefits the governments give up. Since the federal government bears a large portion of the government subsidies to hospital care, it has a fiscal motive in wanting tax-exempt hospitals to operate at the same efficiency and performance levels as for-profit hospitals. Therefore, the federal government is not stepping in to disrupt the current state of affairs.

States and localities see things differently. They see the public hospital of the past being driven by advances in medicine, technology, and an abundance of money from insurance programs into efficient business enterprises that mimic for-profit hospitals. While tax-exempt hospitals continue to take advantage of their tax exemptions, states and localities argue they no longer provide meaningful charitable care. They argue such hospitals rarely care for the financially distressed as they used to and, in some cases, deny health care to the uninsured and underinsured altogether.

DISCRIMINATORY PRICING

The current hospital pricing system is based on a chargemaster, a list price for every infinitesimal procedure possibly delivered, along with a list price for every conceivable supply-item that might be used in the process of the treatment. In theory, this list price is updated annually by each hospital based on actual costs; in actuality, the reimbursement rates for federal programs such as Medicare, Medicaid, and SCHIP drive the list price. Chargemaster list prices can vary enormously across hospitals, depending on government payment methods, reportedly by a factor of up to seventeen even within a single community (Lagnado, 2004a).

While some may debate the shocking prices hospitals charge for individual treatments and medical supplies, this is really an unsuitable way to describe how hospital prices are determined, because it is based on an incomplete picture of the pricing system. Hospital pricing can be divided into two prices. First, there is the list price, similar to the salary advertised for jobs; it serves only as a beginning point for salary negotiations, for those who have the education and experience to negotiate. From these list prices, private insurers, Medicaid, Medicare, SCHIP, and other groups negotiate discounts with hospitals to arrive at so-called actual prices. Although list prices vary widely, the actual prices paid are relatively static (Reinhardt, 2006).

Given the list prices in the chargemaster, four general systems are used to actually pay hospitals:

- Commercial health insurers: discounted prices or per diems negotiated separately with each of the third-party insurers from which a hospital accepts reimbursement
- Medicaid/SCHIP: prices set by state governments based on per diem diagnosis-related groups
- Medicare: prices set by the federal government on a diagnosis-related group basis with outlier payments based on charges calculated with charge-to-cost ratios
- Self-paying and uninsured patients: full charges or means-tested discounts

Price discrimination, the practice of charging different prices to different patients for identical health care even when the actual costs are identical, is standard (Lagnado, 2004a). Hospital pricing becomes even more complex when it is noted that half of the revenue of most tax-exempt hospitals comes from government-assistance programs at levels that do not cover the actual costs incurred by hospitals. In fact, hospitals are paid about 38 percent of their list prices by patients or their insurers (Reinhardt, 2006). Given this pricing complexity, along with the additional out-of-pocket losses for bad debts and unreimbursed care, the rationale of hospitals behind seeking to maximize payments from the remaining segments of their private markets suddenly becomes much more understandable, if not logical.

Moral Dilemmas

1. Should self-paying patients be charged higher rates than insured patients for the same medical services, and if so, why?

Hospitals' Definition of Charitable Care

The way hospitals define charitable care and the implications of how unreimbursed care is released through bad debt write-offs is under examination. Tax-exempt hospitals have a certain degree of discretion regarding how they classify charitable care. In basic terms, six activities are classified together because of their common revenue character. All six definitions of charitable care can change just by changing how the care is defined.

Categories of Charitable Care

- Pure charitable care: hospitals can write off all or part of the costs of treatment services, determined prior to providing the services, and write off the remaining costs
- Uncompensated care (free care): bad debt combined with pure charitable care
- Bad debt: charges that cannot be collected from patients who are able to pay
- Care covered by government-assistance programs: care provided to individuals who are eligible for Medicaid, Medicare, SCHIP, or other state medical assistance programs
- Unreimbursed care: pure charitable care combined with the shortfall of contractual payments coming from government-assistance programs
- Total charitable care: pure charitable care combined with bad debt write-offs and unreimbursed care

Source: Siemens Medical Solutions, Credit and Collections Department.

Most tax-exempt hospitals offer free care to those demonstrating income up to 200 percent of the federal poverty level (individuals with a total household income below $21,660; $44,100 for a family of four in 2009) (*see e.g.*, New Jersey Charitable Care Program, N.J.A.C. § 10.52-11.8 (2008)). This represents about 65 percent of the uninsured (Kaiser, 2007). While this estimate represents over twenty-seven million people, free care is only provided to patients not eligible for government-assistance programs or state charity programs.

Bad Debt as a Contribution to Charitable Care

Given the complexity of the health care payment system, controversy ensues when tax-exempt hospitals write off bad debt and classify that write-off as a charitable care contribution to the community.

In many instances, what is reported as bad debt may be merely a book loss rather than an actual cash loss. This complexity appears as a theme in many of the class-action lawsuits on affordable health care, particularly the intersection of charitable care, uncompensated care, and bad debt, and how hospitals report these relative costs for the purpose of reimbursement.

Nearly all hospitals, whether nonprofit or for-profit, billing patients and collecting after health care is delivered will incur a certain amount of bad debt. Hospitals make allowances for bad debts and consider the financial implications in their fiscal budgets and forecasts. On average, tax-exempt hospitals charge patients 20 percent extra in order to make up for bad debt.

Moral Dilemmas

1. How should uncompensated care offered by tax-exempt hospitals be generally defined, and when should it become an implied obligation?

STATE GOVERNMENT MONITORING RESPONSIBILITIES

State governments monitor nonprofit health care systems to ensure their tax-exempt hospitals meet prescribed standards required to retain their tax-exemption. States ensure charitable care remains a determining factor in allowing tax exemption.

By taking a proactive role, states increase the amount of charitable care tax-exempt hospitals must provide. Most state laws are broad and flexible, but still require a minimum level of charitable care. States and localities are generally in the best position to understand what their various communities require in the form of health care for the uninsured and underinsured. They can also determine whether a tax-exempt hospital in a given community provides adequate charitable benefits to offset the tax revenue the governments could otherwise obtain from taxes.

Stricter State Requirements

Many states are debating whether to impose stricter requirements on tax-exempt hospitals (Schwinn, 2006). While it is too early to characterize this as a general trend (and so far, legislative efforts to enact new charitable care standards have not succeeded), what is clear is that a growing number of states are aggressively using tax exemptions as a means of extracting mutually affordable health care (Kane, 2007).

Illinois proposes requiring tax-exempt hospitals to spend at least 8 percent of their total operating costs on charitable care each year to retain their state tax exemptions, while a state debt collection law requires Illinois hospitals to:

- Publicize their free-care and financial aid programs
- Offer a reasonable payment plan to anyone (not just the financially disadvantaged) who cannot pay their hospital bills
- Adhere to serious procedural checks on when hospitals can go forward with bill collection proceedings (*see* Public Act 94-885, 2006-3A Illinois Comprehensive Statute Annotated Advance Legislative Service 252 (2006))

(Colombo, 2007)

Officials in Minnesota and Kansas have also expressed concern about the level of charitable care provided by tax-exempt hospitals and about their billing and debt-collection practices. Utah and Pennsylvania have used the federal government's community benefit standard, and then placed further requirements on their tax-exempt hospitals.

Charitable Care Accountability

At least one state requires greater accountability from tax-exempt hospitals than is required by the federal government. Hospitals in Texas are required to set aside 4 percent of their net patient revenues to provide charitable care to retain their tax exemption. While there is no evidence that hospitals cut off uninsured and underinsured patients once they have reached their 4 percent threshold the fact that it is legally possible should give people some pause about fairness in Texas (Colombo, 2007).

Charitable care is defined as the unreimbursed cost of providing health care for low-income patients, as distinguished from care covered by government-assistance programs. Charitable care is restricted to the unreimbursed cost of providing care to patients not covered by government-assistance programs.

To retain their tax-exemption, hospitals must provide charitable care at an acceptable level as defined by three criteria:

- Community needs assessment
- Resources at the hospitals' disposal
- Benefits the hospitals receive from their exemption

Charitable care must:

- Be provided in an amount equal to or greater than the hospital's monetary benefit from not having to pay state and local taxes
- Meet at least 4 percent of total patient revenue

Texas also requires tax-exempt hospitals to develop community benefit plans by including specific language in their corporate mission statements that clearly shows a commitment to serving the health care needs of the community. The statements must identify specific goals and objectives and provide a way to measure the effectiveness of the plans. The benefit plans are to be constructed after consulting and careful planning with local health departments, private businesses, consumers, and insurance companies. Finally the plans must provide a timeframe and specify budgets for carrying out the plans.

In addition, Texas provides a means to enforce the community benefit rules. Tax-exempt hospitals are audited every year and financial details are provided to the State Attorney General and to the State Comptroller who look for violations of the community benefit plans. Before strict charitable care requirements were imposed on its tax-exempt hospitals, Texas was one of three states with the highest percentages of uninsured people in the U.S. (along with Arizona and New Mexico) (Kaiser, 2007). The debate today is the provision of charitable care to illegal immigrants.

Moral Dilemmas

1. Should hospitals be required to serve illegal immigrants?

TAX-EXEMPT HOSPITALS

When the first federal class-action lawsuits were withdrawn or dismissed, there was an opportunity for hospital governing boards to prevent being drawn into the legal battles over what constitutes affordable health care. Tax-exempt hospitals now have the opportunity to increase oversight in many aspects of their pricing, billing, and collection activities. This includes, among other things:

- Examining how they handle billing for their uninsured and underinsured patients and determining whether the community is adequately informed about the hospital's charitable care and financial assistance activities
- Exploring in-house collection practices and agreements with third-party debt collectors to ensure that fair and appropriate collection practices are being followed
- Looking for obstacles that hinder the financially distressed when seeking health care and deciding whether the charge structure and the amounts of

charitable care and financial assistance the hospital can provide in light of its overall financial situation should be modified

- Reviewing patient intake procedures and policies to determine how charitable care and financial assistance practices are handled
- Performing a community assessment of service area demographics to see if hospital mission statements and community expectations are being appropriately applied to the hospital's patient population

(Duane Morris, 2004)

For instance, after the Yale–New Haven Hospital was named in a federal class-action lawsuit alleging improper charitable care practices, it:

- Closed accounts over five years outstanding
- Developed a sliding scale to provide means-tested discounts and free care to patients below certain incomes
- Removed property liens against former patients

This highly publicized case involved a husband who made regular payments to Yale–New Haven Hospital for twenty years after his wife died of cancer at the hospital. He eventually paid $16,000 on the $19,000 charge, but because of compounding interest accumulations, the principal of the debt grew to some $40,000 (Lagnado, 2004a). In instances like this, tax-exempt hospitals may need to rethink their overall role in the communities they serve (Davis, 2007). In fact, it is their approach to corporate social responsibility, and their disregard for community sentiment, that has raised questions about the billions of dollars in tax exemptions they receive (Carreyrou & Martinez, 2008).

Balancing Financial Viability and Mission

The lawsuits brought against the hospital community due to its billing and collection activities have resulted in some modification to the way tax-exempt hospitals are providing health care to their uninsured and underinsured patients. In fact, most hospitals have recently made changes and clarified their:

- Pricing
- Billing
- Collection policies
- Charitable care programs

Some hospitals are making changes quietly so as not to spur additional pressure against already stretched charitable care programs. However, with more than forty-seven million Americans uninsured or underinsured, tax-exempt hospitals are under tremendous pressure to correctly determine when patients are eligible for charitable care, or when patients can afford to pay.

While health care should ideally never be compromised due to the ability or inability to pay, tax-exempt hospitals have a responsibility to all of their patients to attempt to obtain payment from those who can afford to pay. These critical distinctions are a constant challenge to tax-exempt hospitals who strive to balance their charitable missions with running a fiscally responsible business.

As court cases show, aggressive pressure on uninsured and underinsured patients to pay more than their insured counterparts is not the way to obtain fiscal health. In fact, adapting aggressive collection policies usually requires added collection staff to contact patients for payment, and repeated attempts at cash collections likely turn into consulting sessions with patients on how to pay their medical bills. Overly aggressive collection activities often give way to assisting indebted, discharged patients with enrollment in government-assistance programs.

When debts cannot be collected, these non-cash collection situations should be seen as clear signals that there is something wrong with the way the business is being conducted, and in particular, something is fundamentally wrong with patient access to hospital care (Duane Morris, 2004). To find the proper balance between a hospital's charitable mission and financial viability, operational principles should be applied not just to cash collection processes, but to the entire hospital business.

Key "Should Be's"
- All debt-collection policies should be understandable and prominently available to everyone using the hospital; these policies should also be conveyed to prospective patients and local community service agencies
- Hospital financial and debt-collection policies should reflect the hospital's mission and value statements
- Financial aid policies should be consistent with hospital debt-collection policies
- Decisions regarding financial aid programs should become part of the admission procedures
- Financial aid determinations should be made in a timely manner
- Operational processes should be constantly explored for changes to improve cash-collection performance

Source: Siemens Medical Solutions, Credit and Collections Department.

Upfront Billing Practices

Many tax-exempt hospitals are adopting a new policy to improve their finances: making health care contingent on upfront payments. Typically, hospitals bill patients after they receive care. Now, pointing to their rising bad debt and charitable care costs, hospitals are asking patients for money before they receive treatment.

A recent survey found about 14 percent of tax-exempt hospitals required patients to make payments before receiving treatment (IRS). Hospitals say they have turned to the practice because of a spike in patients who do not pay their medical bills. Uncompensated care cost the hospital industry $31.2 billion in 2006; this figure was up 44 percent from $21.6 billion in 2000 according to the AHA. The bad debt is driven by a larger number of Americans who are uninsured or who do not have enough insurance to cover medical costs if catastrophe strikes. Even among those with adequate insurance, deductibles and co-payments are growing so large that insured patients also have trouble paying hospitals (*see generally* Martinez, 2008).

Tenet Healthcare and the Hospital Corporation of America, two of the largest for-profit hospital chains, also require patients to make upfront payments before they are admitted. While the practice has received little notice, some patient advocates find it harder to justify at tax-exempt hospitals with financial fortunes, given their supposedly benevolent mission.

Life-Threatening Medical Emergencies

While EMTALA requires hospitals to treat medical emergencies (*e.g.*, heart attacks or injuries from accidents), the law does not cover conditions that are not immediately life-threatening. EMTALA regulations address a hospital's ability to register and collect payment information from a patient seeking emergency services. These regulations allow a hospital to follow reasonable registration processes, including inquiries regarding a patient's insurance status and method of payment, as long as such processes do not result in a delay in screening or emergency treatment (*see* 42 C.F.R. § 489.24(d)(4) (2008)). Since determining credit capability can be done almost instantaneously by global credit information groups like Experian, Equifax, or TransUnion, hospitals can generally determine whether patients have the capability to guarantee payment of all charges, including collection costs, before medical treatment is rendered. The law actually allows hospitals to transfer a patient to another hospital for care as long as the patient is in stable condition.

Hospital registration processes, including all information obtained and forms signed by patients, should always be reasonable and not delay life-threatening treatment. EMTALA requires that Medicare-participating hospitals provide a medical screening examination to any person that comes to the emergency room; if a medical condition exists, hospitals are only required to provide stabilization services. Additional treatment can be conditioned on a determination of the ability to pay for such care and an agreement to sign contracts agreeing to pay incurred charges.

Adopting a Strategic Workflow Approach

The clichéd expression "cash is king" has significant insightful meaning to financial managers who understand how these three words depict much more than cash deposits on hand. The phrase is characteristically used in explaining the importance of cash flow as an indicator of the fiscal health of a hospital, although it goes well beyond just looking at cash flow as an indicator of operational well-being in responsibly managed hospitals.

As an example, if hospitals purposely or even inadvertently overcharge patients, they will find it difficult to collect the resulting receivable. In the same way, if hospitals charge a knowingly fiscally distressed patient, they should not hold much hope for the collections department to settle the debt.

When a hospital collects a receivable account, the cash receipt symbolizes the successful workings of the entire health care system, while uncollected accounts represent operational problems along the care-to-cash process. The success of any improvement in the care-to-cash process will ultimately be reflected in its effect on debts collected. For example, improvements in billing accuracy reduce reimbursement time and reduce billing remediation as well. Improvements to credit evaluation practices can determine charitable care candidates before they:

- Erode public confidence in hospital integrity
- Increase bad debt write-offs
- Reduce receivable performance ratios

Tax-exempt hospitals should constantly look for opportunities to leverage the human resource processes and the medical technologies that exist along the entire care-to-cash process. Many other operational spot solutions ultimately affect collections, including:

- Automatic cash applications
- Collection productivity
- Credit scoring and credit approval processes
- Deduction management
- Electronic funds transfers
- New patient processing procedures

Source: Siemens Medical Solutions, Credit and Collections Department

There are exponential gains available when hospitals tightly integrate front-end processes with back-end cash-collection performance. For instance, when an uninsured patient arrives at the hospital, they go through an admission process, are medically treated, released, billed, and referred to the collection department to follow-up for payment. Think of the various business processes within this care-to-cash route as a collage of business activities not independent from one another, but instead interacting and dependent on one another. Every step in this series of business events has potential to negatively or positively impact patient satisfaction and ultimately affects the way the hospital is perceived in the community.

From the abundance of overcharging and resulting aggressive collection activities, it appears many hospital collection departments operate as if they are within a vacuum where staff members are given the demanding task of collecting unsubstantiated medical charges from financially distressed patients. This "back-end" function exposes deficiencies in the "front-end" process, beginning with admissions procedures conducted regardless of the possibility of ever collecting payments for services. Ultimately, aggressive billing procedures must rely on overly aggressive collection actions to turn accounts receivable into cash, but instead ultimately turn into charge-offs or bad debts. This results in a skeptical public who sees the hospital community as abusing its mission statements.

Debt-collection policies should ideally accurately reflect the commitment the hospital makes to its community through its mission statement. Over time, these guiding principles become work procedures affecting the patient in the form of:

- Accurate billing practices
- Timely recognition of eligibility for charitable care
- Standardized charges

Source: Siemens Medical Solutions, Credit and Collections Department

Finally, collecting outstanding debts should be performed by professional credit and collection staffs that respect and uphold both creditor and debtor rights. Therefore, the succession of business events within a hospital can be scrutinized and improved in light of cash collections, beginning with admission policies that are fully transparent to all patients.

Improving Billing and Collection Transparency

The regulatory environment makes the billing and collection process for tax-exempt hospitals somewhat difficult. Additionally, nothing is standardized across the health industry as a whole when it comes to medical billing.

Regulatory Environment

There are several confusing laws intended to prevent discriminatory billing and overly aggressive collection actions. For instance, there are Medicare and Medicaid's bad debt rules and regulations requiring hospitals to make all reasonable attempts to collect reimbursement from a patient before discharging the uncollected debt as uncompensated care or bad debt (McGrath, 2007).

There was also the policy adopted by the AHA that since Medicare pricing policies required hospitals to bill all patients the same charge for each service, this meant the uninsured had to pay full price for their care. Hospitals nationwide chose to interpret this to mean they were precluded from offering discounts to the uninsured. Combine this with special fraud alerts and anti-kickback statutes specifying when hospitals can and cannot waive co-payments and deductibles, and the confusion about billing practices expands. The federal compliance program guidance for hospitals and advisory opinions from the Office of the Inspector General singularly and together make it difficult for hospitals to provide any type of means-tested discounts to uninsured or underinsured patients.

While these policies do not, and never have, prohibited hospitals from providing discounts to patients, they have often been misconstrued to require the uninsured to pay full price for their health care. These misconceptions that were never clarified by regulators also made it more difficult for hospitals to use discounts or other means of financial assistance for patients (OIG, 2004).

Moral Dilemmas

1. Should tax-exempt hospitals be forced to charge every patient the same price?

Standard Means-Tested Discounts

A critical first step that tax-exempt hospitals should take is a meticulous review of the policies and procedures that touch upon billing the uninsured and underinsured, and then ensuring that there is a standard means-tested discount for all eligible patients (Duane Morris, 2004). That would require a detailed evaluation of the state's billing regulations and comparison of them to the hospital's current billing practices. The AHA has published a statement of principles and guidelines governing hospital billing. Their principles are:

- Assist patients who cannot pay for part or all of the health care they receive

- Balance needed financial assistance for some patients with broader fiscal responsibilities in order to keep hospitals open and serving the needs of the community
- Serve the emergency health care needs of everyone, regardless of a patient's ability to pay
- Treat all patients equally

These principles are vague and leave plenty of room for interpretation for hospitals who may want to increase their profits through higher revenues and more effective collection tactics.

Moral Dilemmas

1. Should hospitals be required to explain their means-tested discount policies to all patients?

Provision of Price Information

One sound practice that leads to collection success is having documentation supporting outstanding medical bills. Patients should have an idea in advance of what the amount billed will be (in non-emergency situations), and be able to understand the bill when it arrives. The bill should detail what treatment, services, and materials it encompasses, and should set forth the expectation of prompt payment by a specified due date.

Consider a scenario in the commercial environment involving billing customers using the same practices as many hospitals use to bill their patients (*i.e.,* shipping a product to a customer without any discussion regarding the costs of the product and then invoicing the customer for the highest price the vendor can charge). This would be unheard of and likely wrought with problems. Instead of collecting the bill promptly, countless hours would be spent negotiating a fair price for what the customer bought. Besides the resulting slow turnover in the collection cycle, customers would be infuriated over this deceptive practice.

Likewise, hospitals should be obligated to notify perspective patients what the hospital plans to provide them in terms of health care and at the very least a reasonable estimate of the total price for the anticipated care. While handing patients detailed hospital charges for each and every conceivable service is unreasonable, patients should have an understanding of the nature of their financial obligations before any non-emergency treatment is accepted. Simply put, hospitals should provide patients with price information. One is hard-pressed to find reasons why hospitals should not model their business practices after those successful and accepted for cosmetic surgeries

and other elective medical surgeries that are self-pay (*e.g.,* most keratorefractive surgery and Lasik laser vision eye correction surgery).

Some hospital charges are certainly less precise than the price terms of ordinary contracts for goods or services. Hospitals cannot be expected specify an "exact" amount to be paid when emergency treatments are rendered or when unexpected medical conditions arise.

While general payment obligations of patients can be set forth for most hospital treatments, with emergency health care, usually nobody knows just what particular condition the patient has, or what treatments will be necessary to remedy the disease, sickness, or injury presented. It is incongruous to expect hospitals to fully perform their obligation to provide emergency health care to patients and then not send patients invoices for charges (including charges not covered by health insurance). This would be an absurd expectation.

Patients should know, before agreeing to non-emergency treatments, what is not covered by their health insurance. It bears repeating, price information should be provided before treatment is accepted.

Eligibility for Charitable Care and Other Forms of Financial Assistance

Providing clear and understandable price structures to potential patients for non-emergency health care is imperative to improving transparency, although hospitals may need to go further by taking the following factors into account in determining eligibility for charitable care and other forms of financial assistance:

- Amount owed to the hospital in relation to the patient's income
- Employment status
- Existing liabilities
- Level and type of assets

Source: Siemens Medical Solutions, Credit and Collections Department

Determining creditworthiness and granting credit terms is a common practice in a consumer-driven economy. For example, Experian's North American consumer database holds credit information on 215 million Americans. All of the credit bureaus heavily market their credit reporting service as well as regional credit statistics. They provide demographic information such as average credit scores by region and average household debt.

Improving the care-to-cash process should tightly link credit determinations that are made before, and not after, a hospital's admission process is set in motion for non-emergency health care. Once a patient is stabilized in an emergency medical situation, they and their families can then decide whether to accept additional medical treatment and whether they can afford to accept such treatment. Payment problems often arise when long term critical care is required for non-terminal conditions, as well as in many end-of-life situations when patients and families will not accept the process of dying. How to deal with these particular situations are inexorable problems without any political consensus at this time. Although these problems are societal, the business needs are incontrovertible.

Consumer Credit Laws

The federal consumer credit laws become very important when hospital accounts are securitized in the same manner as any other income-producing asset (Peterson, 2007). The hospital no longer retains any relationship with patients and servicing of the medical debt is done by a company specializing in collections activity. It is here, however, where the most credit abuse occurs. Some securitized medical debt is not subject to consumer credit laws and hospitals often deny any responsibility for medical debts that are packaged and sold to third parties. Whether tax-exempt hospitals have a responsibility to abide by consumer credit laws, when securitizing their medical debt, is another vigorously debated issue (Nix, 2007).

The Federal Trade Commission (FTC) regulates and enforces the laws that govern the right to get, use, and maintain credit. The FTC is the nation's consumer protection agency, working for the consumer to prevent abuses that occur in the market place, such as deception, fraud, and unfair business practices.

The FTC promotes consumer confidence by enforcing the federal laws enacted to protect the consumer. To promote consumer protection, this agency plans, develops, and implements national campaigns to alert consumers to their rights and to explain the business concepts regarding compliance to industries granting credit and collecting debts, including the health industry.

Regarding consumer credit, the FTC does not require creditors to extend credit, but does protect consumers when creditors do so. Hospitals are not required to extend credit to patients, but if they choose to do so, the FTC will monitor their billing and collection activities to make sure that they:

- Give patients an avenue to resolve disputes
- Make credit information available that is understandable and that fully explains the lending arrangements and all of the costs involved
- Protect the rights of patients by giving everyone a fair and equal opportunity to get credit

There are four federal consumer credit laws that influence a hospital's extension of credit to patients. Each law is contained in Title I of the Consumer Credit Protection Act:

- Equal Credit Opportunity Act (ECOA), 15 U.S.C.A. §§ 1691–1691f (2009)
- Fair Credit Billing Act (FCBA), 15 U.S.C.A. §§ 1666–1666i (2009)
- Fair Credit Reporting Act (FCRA), 15 U.S.C.A. §§ 1681–1681x (2009)
- Fair Debt Collection Practices Act (FDCPA), 15 U.S.C.A. §§ 1692–1692p (2009)

Equal Credit Opportunity Act

The federal ECOA regulates how hospitals may extend credit to patients based on credit-worthiness only, and not on factors that have nothing to do with their ability to repay their debts. For example, this Act makes it illegal for hospitals to take factors like race, sex, national origin, and marital status into consideration when extending credit. At the same time, hospitals must take into consideration all sources of regular revenue like alimony, child support, welfare payments, and veteran's benefits. While the Act prohibits hospitals from discrimination, the law also requires hospitals to inform patients if they were granted or denied credit within thirty days of receiving their application and if credit was denied, give the patient specific reasons why. Further, notification of any changes to a patient's account, such as interest rate changes or account closures, must be promptly given.

Moral Dilemmas

1. Would hospitals violate the ECOA if they made special provisions for religious communities to pay their medical bills?

Fair Credit Billing Act

The federal FCBA protects patients from unfair billing practices and gives patients an avenue to address a wide range of possible billing errors in a timely and fair manner. It addresses many billing errors, including incorrect amounts, charges for health care not received, and errors relating to missing payments.

The FCBA also helps patients know the exact credit terms of their agreements with a hospital and requires hospitals to divulge their exact credit terms to patients. For instance, full disclosure of monthly finance charges, annual interest rates, payment schedules, and late payment penalties promotes the informed use of credit.

Fair Credit Reporting Act

This federal law regulates the collection, dissemination, and use of credit information. Along with the FDCPA, it sets the hospitals' foundation for extension of credit to patients. The Act is specifically written to regulate the collection and distribution activities of the credit reporting agencies, which are the companies that hold the databases that generate credit reports. The FCRA is enforced by the FTC with the objectives to promote accuracy and protect the privacy of information that becomes part of a patient's credit profile.

Fair Debt Collection Practices Act

The federal FDCPA addresses abusive tactics used by third-party collectors retained by hospitals, such as collection agencies and collection attorneys. Its basic purpose is to eliminate abusive practices in the collection of patient debts. It also provides patients a way to dispute and obtain validation of their indebtedness. The Act creates guidelines governing the way debt-collection agencies can conduct their business, defines the rights of debtors, and spells out penalties for violations of the Act. This Act helps patients fight back against unfair, unethical, and illegal debt-collection activities on questionable debts:

- Debtor liens against liability insurance settlements to cover medical debts in excess of what a hospital would receive from the patient's medical insurance
- Overly aggressive tactics such as placing debtor liens on homes, garnishing wages, and placing attachments on bank accounts while refusing to negotiate deals that patients could afford
- Placing attachments on bodies, issuing arrest warrants for debtors who are absent for court proceedings

It contains explicit rules regarding how debt collectors can communicate with patients at home or at work in their attempt to collect legitimate debts.

Lawsuits have been filed in federal and state courts on behalf of patients against hundreds of hospitals, health care systems, and the AHA for overly aggressive collection tactics both for bills that were too high and for patients eligible for charity care, Medicaid or SCHIP insurance, or other state medical assistance at the time health care services were rendered or shortly afterwards (Batchis, 2005).

Moral Dilemmas

1. What constitutes reasonable and socially tolerable procedures for the collection of medical debt?

COLLECTING FROM THE UNINSURED AND UNDERINSURED WHO ARE ABLE TO PAY

The middle to lower middle class are the most vulnerable when it comes to access to affordable health care. By the time hospitals attempt to collect from many of these financially strapped individuals, they cannot be reached or refuse to volunteer information about their finances. Others qualify for government-assistance programs, but refuse to accept the assistance. One reason why a patient might refuse government-assistance is because liens will be placed on total assets over $100,000 or so for Medicaid and many charitable care programs. In these situations, hospitals have no recourse but to institute legal proceedings.

Generally, if a spouse or children live in the patient's primary residence, they do not have to sell the residence to be Medicaid eligible; they can keep about $100,000 of their total assets, an amount that varies from state to state. For instance, if a patient has $200,000 in equity in a primary residence, he or she will be required to re-title the property and have a lien placed on the residence for $100,000. Patients can also keep personal items, a car, and some life insurance. Savings and investments, real estate other than a primary residence, and excess life insurance must be used before patients are eligible for Medicaid.

More than half the working-age adults who are uninsured and 45 percent of the underinsured report problems paying medical bills or are paying off accrued medical debt (Schoen et al., 2008). In contrast, 26 percent of those who had adequate health insurance could not meet the costs of their medical bills and face financial stress. Medical debt forces families to make stark trade-offs. For example, 40 percent of insured adults with medical bill problems were unable to pay for basic necessities like food, heat, or rent and nearly 50 percent had used all of their savings to pay their medical bills (Collins, 2007). Many report they take on loans, a mortgage against their homes, or credit card debt to pay their medical bills. All this suggests that the current financial difficulties arising from unaffordable health care have the potential to linger into the future as long-term problems.

Transactional Transparency

Efforts to improve the care-to-cash turnover cycle will be compromised if the hospital collection department is not functioning at optimal levels of performance. In this regard, transactional transparency along the entire care-to-cash process is a key factor to collection efficiency.

Relevant patient data should be immediately available and accessible throughout the entire hospital process. Collection personnel should have ready access to patient account details, even if that requires open access to admissions and patient information, including background credit reviews and documented discussions regarding price and payment programs.

As discussed earlier, patients should know what to expect on their bills and be able to understand them. The admissions and billing departments must be accountable for the accuracy of the bills and should address any discrepancies the collection department finds. With today's computer programs, score-carding collection successes and failures can help pinpoint many of the upfront processes that need improvement until the collection success rate is optimal.

To increase cash collection success, hospitals might follow the collection practices of medical providers like Siemens Medical Solutions and contact patients within a week of discharge. Some may consider this an overly aggressive tactic, but this initial contact is more of a courtesy call, rather than a collection attempt. Almost immediately the collection department will know whether the proper party was billed, and that they acknowledge receipt of the bill. Questions regarding the charges may be discussed immediately and more difficult questions may be referred quickly to the billing department to address them directly with the patient. Subsequent calls might begin to take an increasingly stronger collection nature and ever firmer collection effort. This escalation approach could carry through to the point where the patient's account is outsourced to a third-party debt collector.

There are myriads of third-party debt collectors competing constantly for collection business, and some of their conduct can be alarming. However, many of the collection agencies and attorneys are very good at what they do, and they can be screened to verify they conform to the highest ethical standards. In addition, once they have been retained, their collection performance can be monitored. It is good business practice to utilize several agencies and attorneys at once. Using more than one agency or attorney helps monitor performance and allows comparisons of collection success rates and ethical standards.

Collection Agencies

The federal Health Insurance Portability and Accountability Act (HIPAA) allows hospitals to refer unpaid medical bills to outside third-party debt collectors and allows reporting of unpaid debts to credit reporting agencies (*see* 18 U.S.C.A. §§ 24 *et seq.* (2009)). From a business standpoint, debt collection agencies and attorneys are a valuable asset to a hospital collections department; when used appropriately, they help diminish bad debt write-offs.

HIPAA and FDCPA deal with two different rights: patient privacy and consumer protection. HIPAA protects patient confidentiality through its privacy provision; hospitals are required to protect the confidentiality of patients' medical records by not disclosing identifying information. The FDCPA protects patients through its validation requirements that oblige hospitals to substantiate claims for payment. The laws conflict, however, in the collection of medical debts through third-party debt collectors. The conflict results because the combination of the two laws may force patients to choose between divergent rights: if patients demand validation of their medical debts, they must allow third-party debt collectors to see their medical records in order to explain the source of charges (*see generally* Arnold, 2008). This, however, affects the patient's right to confidentiality when HIPAA defers to FDCPA for collection purposes. Even if the law allows minimum necessary disclosures of medical records, the conflict between these laws requires a solution that better protects Americans as both patients and consumers.

MEDICAL AND FINANCIAL VULNERABILITIES

While the U.S. has favored a market-based for-profit model, it has not been as successful as most might have liked. Perhaps it is time to revisit the pros and cons of this approach. Indeed, debate on mutually affordable health care suggests that continuing on the path where coverage decisions are based on clinical evidence alone, without consideration of costs, may no longer be feasible in the long run. The legal obligation to provide charitable care in lieu of taxes is uncertain. Determining who should be charged and how much to charge for health care is a complicated issue.

The next five years will likely bring major improvements in the nation's health care system. Everyone knows they are medically vulnerable because no one is going to live forever, but as more Americans realize they are also financially vulnerable, changes and solutions that work financially, medically, ethically, and politically will be in order (*see generally* Gerencher, 2007).

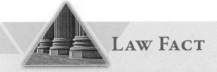

LAW FACT

DISCRIMINATORY PRICING

Should the uninsured be charged the highest prices for health care?

A few weeks after K. B. Forbes began probing Saint Joseph Medical Center for an explanation of the charges, the Ferlinis received an adjusted bill for $41,000, less than one-fifth the amount of the original medical bill of $246,000. While charges and computations are based on a uniform set of charges in each hospital's chargemaster, negotiated discount payments may apply in different situations.

—Kuntzc, 2008; Rosembaum, 2006.

CHAPTER SUMMARY

- In return for federal tax exemptions, tax-exempt hospitals are required to render a significant amount of community benefits, which do not necessarily consist of charitable care.
- Because community benefits can constitute almost anything, hospitals are not necessarily required to offer free or reduced-cost care to the uninsured or underinsured.
- While the 2,100 tax-exempt hospitals are heavily subsidized, with over $12.6 billion in tax exemptions and $32 billion in government-assistance subsidies each year, many fail to use their assets and revenues to provide mutually affordable health care to the uninsured and underinsured.
- Congress is investigating tax-exempt hospitals in light of the number of people bankrupted by medical debt and reports of hospitals abusing their tax exemption.
- The IRS is investigating whether tax-exempt hospitals provide enough community benefits to justify federal, state, and local governments forgoing the tax income they would otherwise receive.
- Patients have begun to sue tax-exempt hospitals, sometimes through class-action lawsuits, claiming the hospitals violate their charitable missions by overcharging uninsured and underinsured patients, price gouging, and employing overly aggressive debt-collection methods; this litigation has encouraged some hospitals to improve their pricing, billing, and collection methods before being sued.
- Uninsured and underinsured patients are often charged four to five times more for the exact same treatment as insured patients are charged.
- Today's tax-exempt hospitals compete effectively with for-profit hospitals, and in many cases are nearly indistinguishable, right down to state-of-the-art facilities and medical equipment.
- Government-assistance programs often do not reimburse tax-exempt hospitals enough to cover the actual cost of care rendered, forcing such hospitals to write off the remaining bad debt.
- One in four Americans are uninsured or underinsured, and nearly one in five Americans reported not seeking or delaying seeking necessary health care in 2007; only about half of the American population is able to obtain insurance coverage through employers.
- Many states are beginning to impose stricter regulation upon tax-exempt hospitals in order to ensure that the hospitals are justifying their tax exemption through meaningful benefits to their communities.
- One way tax-exempt hospitals might improve upon collecting their accounts receivable is to familiarize patients in advance of treatment with the costs and provide clear, detailed bills.
- Other ways tax-exempt hospitals can improve patient payments include better coordinating their overall business functions, charging patients based on a sliding scale or means-tested ability to pay, charging patients upfront for care, and modeling their business practices after other industries.
- The FTC along with four federal consumer credit laws all aim to help protect patients' credit rights, although hospitals are not required to extend credit to patients, and these consumer protection laws tend to conflict with patient privacy laws.

LAW NOTES

1. There are no accurate statistics as to how many personal bankruptcies are due to medical debt. Part of the problem with medical debt is its direct relationship to the consequences of lost income resulting from illness and hospitalizations. Additionally, unplanned spending may lead people to overstate the role of medical problems in their financial crises, as most of the research on bankruptcy filings is conducted by analyzing debtors' explanations. It is certainly more socially acceptable to admit to bankruptcy due to medical bills as opposed to acknowledging a history of undisciplined spending or failure to earn sufficient income to meet one's needs (or wants). The question of determining how many personal bankruptcies are due to medical debt is further complicated by the fact that hospitals routinely accept major credit cards as payment, while other people take out second mortgages to cover their medical bills; therefore, medical debt is often incorporated into regular personal debts. Thus, the precise number of people for whom medical debts are the primary cause of bankruptcy is unknown and difficult to estimate (Jacoby & Warren, 2006).

2. The Judicial Panel on Multidistrict Litigation rejected a motion to transfer and consolidate the actions pending around the country into one district. *See In re Not-For-Profit Hospitals/Uninsured Patients Litigation*, 341 F.Supp.2d 1354 (Judicial Panel on Multidistrict Litigation 2004). Plaintiffs voluntarily dismissed thirty cases prior to a court ruling on a motion to dismiss. In twenty-three additional actions, the district courts granted defendants' motions to dismiss. *See, e.g., Peterson v. Fairview Health Services*, 2005 WL 226168 (U.S. District Court for the District of Minnesota 2005); *Shriner v. ProMedica Health Sys., Inc.*, 2005 WL 139128 (U.S. District Court for the Northern District of Ohio, Western Division 2005); *Lorens v. Catholic Health Care Partners*, 356 F.Supp.2d 827 (U.S. District Court for the Northern District of Ohio, Eastern Division 2005); *Ferguson v. Centura Health Corp.*, 358 F.Supp.2d 1014 (U.S. District Court for the District of Colorado 2004); *Burton v. William Beaumont Hospital*, 347 F.Supp.2d 486 (U.S. District Court for the Eastern District of Michigan, Southern Division 2004); *Darr v. Sutter Health*, 2004 WL 2873068 (U.S. District Court for the Northern District of California 2004); *Amato v. UPMC*, 371 F.Supp.2d 752 (U.S. District Court for the Western District of Pennsylvania 2005); *Kizzire v. Baptist Health Systems, Inc.*, 343 F.Supp.2d 1074 (U.S. District Court for the Northern District of Alabama, Southern Division 2004). In an Illinois state case, the court granted defendants' motion to dismiss with respect to two claims and denied the motion with respect to the Illinois state law claims. *See Servedio v. Our Lady of the Resurrection Medical Center*, No. 04 L 3381 (Circuit Court of Cook County, Illinois 2006). No court has yet found for plaintiffs on the substantive legal issue.

CHAPTER BIBLIOGRAPHY

Aitsebaomo, G. O. (2004). The nonprofit hospital: A call for new national guidance requiring minimum annual charitable care to qualify for federal tax exemption. *Campbell Law Review, 26*, 1-25.

Anand, G. (2008, June 28). Opting out, "Old Order" Mennonites and Amish who shun insurance face rising bills. Should hospitals cut them a break? *Wall Street Journal*, p. A1.

Anderson, G. F. (2007). From "soak the rich" to "soak the poor": Recent trends in hospital pricing. *Health Affairs, 26* (3), 780-789.

Arnold, K. N. (2008). Getting payment for a clean bill of health: Reconciling the Health Insurance Portability and Accountability Act (HIPAA) with the Fair Debt Collection Practices Act (FDCPA) for health-care debt collection. *Iowa Law Review, 93*, 605-626.

Batchis, L. S. (2005). Can lawsuits help the uninsured access affordable hospital care? Potential theories for uninsured patient plaintiffs. *Temple Law Review, 78*, 493-541.

Becker, C. (2007). Community center of attention. IRS, finance poised to pounce on tax-exempt status. *Modern Healthcare, 37* (29), 8-9.

Burns, J. (2004). Are nonprofit health care systems really charitable? Taking the question to the state and local level. *Journal of Corporate Law, 29*, 665-683.

Bush, H. (2007, October). Regulations: Court ruling, IRS initiative highlight issues in debate over tax-exempt status. *Hospital Health Network, 81* (10), 24-25.

Carreyrou, J., & Martinez, B. (2008, April 4). Tax-exempt hospitals, once for the poor, strike it rich with tax-breaks, they outperform for-profit rivals. *Wall Street Journal*, p. A1.

Charitable vs. nonprofit: Hospitals exemption. (2008, April 4). *Wall Street Journal*, p. A10.

Cohen, B. (2006). The controversy over hospital charges to the uninsured. No villains, no heroes. *Villanova Law Review, 51*, 95-148.

Collins, S. R. (2007, November 4). *Widening gaps in health insurance coverage in the U.S: The need for universal coverage.* Invited testimony on Income Security and Family Support, Committee on Ways and Means, U.S. House of Representatives, Hearing on Impact of Gaps in Health Coverage on Income Security.

Colombo, J. D. (2007). Federal and state tax exemption policy, medical debt and healthcare for the poor. *Saint Louis University Law Journal, 25*, 433-457.

___. (2006). The role of tax exemption in a competitive health care market. *Journal of Health Politics, Policy & Law, 16*, 251-279.

___. (2005). Failure of community benefit. *Health Matrix 15*, 29-65.

CBO (Congressional Budget Office). (2006). *Tax-exempt hospitals and the provisions of community-benefits.* Washington, DC: CBO.

Cunningham P. J., & Felland, L. E. (2008). *Falling behind: Americans' access to medical care deteriorates. 2003-2007.* Princeton, NJ: Robert Wood Johnson Foundation: Center for Studying Health System Change.

Davis, K. (2007). Uninsured in America: Problems and possible solutions. *British Medical Journal, 334,* 346-348.

Duane Morris. (2004). *Non-profit hospitals: Reducing the risk of being accused of overcharging uninsured patients.* Philadelphia, PA: Duane Morris.

Federal Register. (2005, September 9). Standards for recognition of tax-exempt status if private benefit exists or if an applicable tax-exempt organization has engaged in excess benefit transactions. 70 FR 53,599 (to be codified at 26 C.F.R. pts. 1 and 53).

Gerencher, K. (2007, May 16). Groundswell builds in support of major health-care reform. San Francisco, CA: *Market Watch.*

Greaney, T. L. (2005). Oh, darling! 40 years later: The legacy of Darling v. Charleston Community Memorial Hospital and the evolution of hospital liability. New governance norms and quality of care in tax-exempt hospitals. *Annals of Health Law, 14,* 421-436.

Greaney, T. L., & Boozang, K. M. (2005). Mission, margin, and trust in the nonprofit health care enterprise. *Yale Journal of Health Policy, Law & Ethics, 5,* 1-87.

Hanson, J. (2005). Are we getting our money's worth? Charitable care, community-benefits, and tax exemption at tax-exempt hospitals. *Loyola Consumer Law Review, 17,* 395-418.

Horwitz, J. R. (2007). Does nonprofit ownership matter? *Yale Journal on Regulation, 24,* 139-204.

Interviews with Robert Mennor, Credit Manager, Siemens Medical Solutions, Credit and Collections Department (2007 to 2008) (generally recognized for its fair credit and non-discriminatory collection policies within the medical products community).

Jacoby, M. B., & Warren, E. (2006). Beyond hospital misbehavior: An alternative account of medical-related financial distress. *Northwestern University Law Review, 100,* 535-583 (summarizing news stories of, and the policy response to, hospital billing practices).

Kaiser (Kaiser Commission on Medicaid & the Uninsured). (2008). *Health insurance coverage in America.* Washington, DC: Kaiser.

___. (2007). *Distribution of the nonelderly uninsured by federal poverty level (FPL).* Washington, DC: Kaiser (based on the Census Bureau's 2006 and 2007 Current Population Survey: CPS Annual Social and Economic Supplements).

Kane, N. M. (2007). Tax-exempt hospitals: What is their charitable responsibility and how should it be defined and reported? *St. Louis University Law Journal, 54,* 451-473.

Katz, R. A. (2005). Let charitable directors direct: Why trust law should not curb board discretion over a charitable corporation's mission and unrestricted assets. *Chicago-Kent Law Review, 80,* 689-721.

Kirch, D. (2008). *Reform is no "either or": We must fix the payment system along with access.* New York, NY: Modern Access & Commonwealth Fund.

Kuntze, C. (2008). The fight for equal pricing in health care. *Journal of Legal Medicine, 29* (4), 537-552.

Lagnado, L. (2004, December 27). California hospitals open books, showing huge price differences. *Wall Street Journal,* p. A1.

___. (2004a, September 21). Anatomy of a hospital bill; Uninsured patients often face big markups on small items; "Rules are completely crazy." *Wall Street Journal,* p. B1.

Maples, A. M. (2007). State attorney general oversight of non-profit healthcare entities: Have we reached an ideological impasse? *Cumberland Law Review, 37,* 235-261.

Martinez, B. (2008, April 28). Cash before chemo: Hospitals get tough, bad-debts prompt change in billing; $45,000 to come in. *Wall Street Journal,* p. A1.

McGrath, J. (2007). Overcharging the uninsured in hospitals: Shifting a greater share of uncompensated medical care costs to the federal government. *Quinnipiac Law Review, 26,* 173-211.

Morton, T. G., & Woodbury, F. (1895). *The history of the Pennsylvania Hospital 1751-1895.* Philadelphia, PA: Times Printing House.

Moskowitz, E. (2005). Recent developments in health law: Class-action suits allege improper charitable care practices. *Journal of Law, Medicine & Ethics, 33,* 168-170.

Nie, D. L. (2007). Nonprofit hospital billing of uninsured patients: Consumer-based class actions move to state courts. *Indiana Health Law Review, 4,* 173-204.

Nix, J. B. (2005). The things people do when no one is looking: An argument for the expansion of standing in the charitable sector. *University of Miami Business Law Review, 14,* 147-192.

OIG (Office of Inspector General). (2004). *Hospital discounts offered to patients who cannot afford to pay their hospital bills.* Washington, DC: U.S. Department of Health & Human Services.

Olson, M. D. (2005). Defending the next round of nonprofit hospital class-action lawsuits. *Journal of Healthcare Finance, 31,* 75–89.

Peterson, C. L. (2007). Predatory structured finance. *Cardozo Law Review, 28,* 2185-2282.

Reinhardt, U. E. (2006). The pricing of U.S. hospital services: Chaos behind a veil of secrecy. *Health Affairs, 25,* 57–69 (discussing the variations in calculating hospital list prices).

Richman, B. D. (2006). The corrosive combination of non-profit monopolies and U.S.-style health insurance: Implications for antitrust and merger policy. *Law & Contemporary Problems, 69,* 139-158.

Rosembaum, M. (2006, March 5). *60 Minutes: Hospitals: Is the price right?* (CBS News television broadcast).

Saar, D. L. (2008). Blindsided (again): Iowa hospitals' abuse of the hospital lien statute and what has been done to correct it. *Drake Law Review, 56,* 463-501.

Schoen, C. et al. (2008). *How many are underinsured? Trends among U.S. adults.* New York, NY: Commonwealth Fund.

Schwinn, E. (2006, March 21). Senator [Charles E. Grassley, Chairman of the Senate Finance Committee] questions operating practices of tax-exempt hospitals, asks for changes. *Chronicle Philanthropy.*

Urban Institute. (2007). *Nonprofit almanac.* Washington, DC: National Center for Charitable Statistics.

Zarone, P., & Donaldson, I. (2006). Recent developments in Pennsylvania health law. *Duquesne Law Review, 44,* 459-470.

CHAPTER 9

PATIENT RIGHTS AND RESPONSIBILITIES

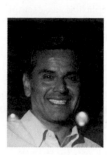

"Part of the American dream is the idea that health care is a right, not a privilege."

—ANTONIO VILLARAIGOSA, LOS ANGELES MAYOR

IN BRIEF

This chapter looks at patient rights and the responsibility to pay for health care. How do patients protect themselves when seeking available health care in today's managed care market? Who is the patients' agent in making health care decisions if it is no longer their physicians? This debate underscores the difficult job of trying to hold down health care costs while giving patients more say in the kind of medical treatment they can obtain. Based on this debate involving parties with incredibly divergent interests, this chapter examines the feasibility of providing a basic health insurance plan for every American citizen.

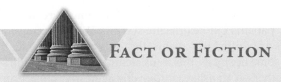

FACT OR FICTION

RIGHT TO EMERGENCY CARE

When is a patient entitled to emergency care?

Carolina Morales was diagnosed with a nonviable ectopic pregnancy. Two days later, while at work, she experienced severe abdominal pain accompanied by vomiting. Her employer called an ambulance. After placing Morales inside the ambulance, the ambulance crew set off for the hospital at which Morales's obstetrician regularly practiced. While in transit to the hospital, the paramedics called ahead to the emergency department to notify them of Morales's arrival and her need for emergency treatment. When the hospital received no assurance from the paramedics that Morales was insured, they abruptly terminated the call. The paramedics interpreted this as a refusal to treat Morales at the hospital emergency department. The hospital never claimed to be in diversionary status, that is, without adequate staff or facilities to accept additional emergency patients. Stymied by the actions of the hospital, the paramedics took Morales to a different facility where she was treated. In due course, Morales sued the first hospital and others for violating her legal right to emergency care. The hospital claimed that Morales was never entitled to emergency care since she had never physically come to its emergency department.

—*Morales v. Sociedad Espanola de Auxilio Mutuo y Beneficencia,* 524 F.3d 54
(U.S. Court of Appeals for the 1st Circuit 2008), *U.S. Supreme Court
certiorari denied,* 129 S.Ct. 898 (U.S. Supreme Court 2009).
(See *Law Fact* at the end of this chapter for the answer.)

PRINCIPLES AND APPLICATIONS

The patient rights debate underscores the difficult job of trying to minimize costs while giving American consumers greater freedom of choice in the kind of health care available. This debate largely affects the middle class rather than people who are covered by Medicare or low-income families who are often eligible to be covered by Medicaid, the State Children's Health Insurance Program (SCHIP), or other public health insurance programs (Dubay et al., 2007). While low-income uninsured families are eligible for charity care as needed, the middle-class insured lack a real safety net for catastrophic events when their deductibles and co-insurance exceeds their ability to pay for needed health care. The middle class is the only group in America that is unprotected, with nowhere to turn for assistance when their legitimate claims exceed their insurance caps or their health insurance is cancelled due to technicalities when they need it most.

The U.S. Census Bureau reports that one in three Americans without health insurance lives in a household with income greater than $50,000, but this is misleading. These higher-income uninsured people do not fit the profile of people who have the money but are unwilling to buy coverage. The higher-income uninsured have low individual incomes, but live with others, and only together are they considered higher-income. For the other higher-income uninsured, their higher income or lack of insurance is transient (Kuttner & Rutledge, 2007).

For the raison d'être of protecting middle-class America, many have come to favor a system of universal coverage: a reimbursement system that provides basic health insurance for every American citizen with the option of buying additional coverage. The fundamental issue in this patient rights debate concerns how patients protect themselves when confronted by illness or disease in today's health care marketplace. Physicians are no longer patients' agents (Wharton, 2008). The U.S. health care system is now comprised of parties with conflicting interests. The U.S. political system must take a comprehensive look at this pressing issue. For most, the answer seems to be a comprehensive system of reimbursement where everyone has health care coverage that is fairly broad and deep (Reinhardt, 2006).

The entire subject of health care is so complex that it does not lend itself to easy analysis or solutions. Nor does the current controversy over patient rights address the question of how policymakers and the private sector can find a way to provide affordable coverage to Americans who lack health insurance.

RIGHTS OR PRIVILEGES DEBATE

There is no need to agree on whether medically necessary health care is a right or a privilege before the U.S. begins to address the affordability question confronting the uninsured. Commonsense economics demands the U.S. address affordable health care coverage for one simple reason: it is cost-effective to do so. It is generally less costly to provide comprehensive health insurance that covers preventative and regularly administered health care than it is to provide delayed charity care on an as-needed basis (Kaiser Spotlight, 2004). It simply costs less to provide regular, basic preventative health care than it costs to provide delayed acute care, as every other developed economy in the world has long ago discovered.

Moral Dilemmas

1. Is health care a right and not a privilege?

2. Should health care be treated the same as every other service industry (such as restaurants, hotels, and dry cleaning); that is, those who can pay for it may have it?

PATIENT RIGHTS DEBATE

The debate over patient rights does not address the issue of how to find a way to provide affordable health care coverage to those uninsured Americans, nor does it address Medicare reform. While patient rights are attractive, this issue is really a red herring to avoid dealing with the more serious problems of the rapidly rising use of medical technologies, Medicare, and insuring the uninsured. The problem of patient rights is attractive to both sides of the political aisle, largely because it affects the middle class.

While a comprehensive Patients' Bill of Rights has not been debated in Congress for several years, state- and national-level legislative and judicial action on the issue of patient rights has recently occurred (Kaiser & Harvard, 2006). Proposals over the issue of patient rights are much like the information describing health insurance coverage. The proposals are complex, confusing, technical, legalistic, and generally unattractive. While it may be necessary to give patients a degree of additional leverage over managed care organizations (MCO), the benefits to be derived from giving patients the right to sue are uncertain (Wharton, 2001).

While patients are overlooked and sometimes even harmed by insurers, physicians, and many others in the current health care system, it is not necessarily knowingly. No one purposely wants to do harm to another. But in the course of events, patients do end up hurt

(Watson, 2007). For instance, cost-shifting hurts not only patients but health care systems. When excessive costs are shifted to patients, the costs may go unpaid. For some hospitals, this translates into a drop in funding; for others, it translates into overly aggressive collection actions against patients. For patients who can pay by credit cards, it may begin a cycle of debt that ends in personal bankruptcy. Therefore, the public backlash against managed care may sometimes be justified.

However, managed care is not as bad as spurious anecdotal stories of denied referrals and emergency-room treatment would indicate (Wharton, 2008). Current public debate is characterized less by careful analysis than by unfounded claims and harsh rhetoric (Kysar et al., 2006). For instance, the health care insurance tax credit, first proposed by health law economists, may well be one of the most misunderstood health care proposals (Pauly & Herring, 2007). Attacks on this idea are ruthless, but the tax credit is progressive and would provide an incentive for the uninsured to purchase health insurance, a feature that should endear opponents to the proposal.

Need for Fundamental Change

Research at the University of California at San Francisco looked at the issue of clinical quality and found that, on average, people in managed care get neither better nor worse health care than people with conventional fee-for-service insurance where there are no in-network and out-of-network benefits (Wharton, 2005). Other studies show there is great consumer dissatisfaction with managed care (*e.g.*, IOM, 2002). As illustrated in Figure 9-1, opinion polls support this research. In other words, managed care is not hurting patients; managed care is frustrating patients and physicians, and people are generally unhappy with the nation's health care system.

A Kaiser Family Foundation/Harvard School of Public Health poll recently found more than two-thirds of Americans believe the federal government spends too little on health care.

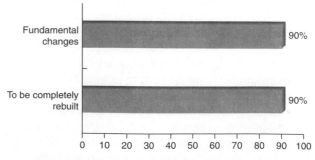

FIGURE 9-1: The U.S. Health Care System Needs

Delmar/Cengage Learning
Data retrieved from: CBS News Polls (2008, January 26).

COURT-APPROVED CLASS-ACTION SETTLEMENTS WITH TEN INSURERS

In re Managed Care Litigation

430 F.Supp.2d 1336 (U.S. District Court for the Southern District of Florida, Miami Division 2006), affirmed, 228 Fed.Appx. 927 (U.S. Court of Appeals for the 11th Circuit 2007)

FACTS: Medical providers in this class action alleged ten insurers (Anthem, Aetna, CIGNA, Coventry, Health Net, Humana, PacifiCare, Prudential, UnitedHealth, and Wellpoint) conspired to deny, delay, and reduce payments to them by:

- Bundling (only paying for some treatments provided during a single visit)
- Concealing the use of improper guidelines to delay or deny payments for medically covered services
- Downcoding (reclassifying treatments to categories with lower payments)
- Failing to disclose improper guidelines for compensation of medical providers operating under MCO capitation systems
- Misrepresenting or refusing to disclose fee schedules
- Refusing to promptly pay claims within contractually required time periods

The providers sought relief under the Racketeer Influenced and Corrupt Organizations Act (RICO), breach of contract claims, and various state laws violated over a thirteen-year time period.

Issues Being Settled: The court-approved settlements sought to simplify the reimbursement process and allow for greater physician involvement in determining what treatment procedures would be reimbursable in the future.

Court-Approved Settlements: In the court-approved settlements endorsed by the American Medical Association and nineteen state medical associations, less than 1 percent of the class members opted-out; the HMOs agreed to change their business and disclosure practices, establish medical foundations dedicated to the promotion of high-quality health care, and guarantee millions in payments to physicians. The settlement required the HMOs to, among other things:

- Increase the percentage of auto-adjudicated claims, or those processed electronically, to increase payment speed and efficiency
- Publically disclose their policies on bundling and downcoding
- Make their fee schedules transparent to participating physicians

- Restrict fee schedule changes to no more than once per year
- Apply a definition of "medically necessary" in accordance with generally accepted standards of medical practice
- Rely on scientific evidence published in peer-reviewed medical literature in determining clinical guidelines, taking into account physician society recommendations and other relevant factors
- Not include gag clauses in their contracts with physicians (restricting a physician's ability to discuss with patients treatment options not covered or treatment options covered by their health insurance plans but discouraged because of high cost)
- Implement an independent external billing dispute review process available for a claim or collection of similar claims with aggregate value above $500
- Allow physicians access to a medical-necessity-based external appeals process when authorized by the insured or when the service has already been provided
- Pay interest on all timely and properly submitted claims
- Form physician advisory committees

Future relief and system change have always been the primary focus of the class action, and these settlements could potentially help achieve several fundamental changes:

- Changes to the reimbursement system should generally simplify the billing and payment process, enabling physicians to better predict payments and reduce administrative costs
- Clinical recommendations by treating physicians should be considered when determining what is medically necessary
- Determination of the procedures as to what constitutes medically necessary should be more transparent
- Disclosure of reimbursement guidelines, if they exist, should make decision-making more apparent
- Medically necessary determinations should be based on scientific rather than financial concerns
- Review of medically necessary treatments should be considered in accordance with generally accepted medical practice

For instance, more than two-thirds of uninsured U.S. children are eligible for public coverage, yet there are hardly any community outreach efforts to reach families that are entitled to this government benefit (Sommers, 2007). Most Americans also believe Congress and the President can significantly improve health care if they would just choose to do so (Kaiser & Harvard, 2006).

While evidence of the quality gap between best practices and the current reality of everyday health care is widely documented and acknowledged, defects in quality are linked largely to system problems rather than individual errors or actions of medical providers. The federal Agency for Healthcare Research and Quality is helping to focus attention on the need to identify the characteristics that differentiate high-performing health care delivery systems from those that are not performing as well (*see* Gillies et al., 2006).

Patient Rights in Managed Care Plans

Patients covered by managed care plans have a number of rights, including access to:

- Emergency rooms, even if the hospitals are not affiliated with the patient's managed care plan
- Experimental medical treatments
- Legal proceedings, meaning they have a right to sue

Right to Emergency Care

President Franklin D. Roosevelt encouraged the U.S. to embrace the global recognition of a right to health in his State of the Union address in 1944, while advancing his idea of a second Bill of Rights, including the right to adequate health care and the opportunity to achieve and enjoy good health (Roosevelt, 1944). While the nation has not followed through with Roosevelt's overall vision, Americans do have a limited legal right to health care: the right to emergency care (Annas, 2008).

For instance, hospitals must provide for an appropriate medical screening examination within the capability of the hospital's emergency department to determine whether an emergency medical condition exists (*see* 42 U.S.C.A. § 1395dd(a) (2003)). Moreover, patients can obtain care at an emergency room even if the hospital is not affiliated with the MCO providing coverage for their health care. Many are demanding insurers implement policies whereby they will not deny payment for a visit to the emergency room, even when it is determined no medical emergency exists.

Right to Experimental Medical Treatments

Patients have the right to control their medical treatment. Terminally ill patients, especially those with cancer, are regularly treated with experimental medical treatments.

For instance, cancer drugs are ordinarily approved for very narrowly defined diseases. The federal Food and Drug Administration (FDA) generally approves such drugs for specific types of cancer and particular clinical indications. However, physicians frequently prescribe cancer drugs for unapproved or off-label uses outside of the narrowly defined indications. This right to off-label use of cancer drugs is based on the doctrine of informed consent, under which patients can choose experimental medical treatments if given sufficient information to understand the consequences, risks and benefits, and alternatives to such chosen treatments (NIH, 2007).

Since drugs are a type of medical treatment, off-label use of approved drugs raises the issue of whether the doctrine of informed consent should be extended to allow terminally ill patients to choose experimental drugs that have passed limited safety trials but have not been proven effective by the FDA. Is there a significant distinction between permitting patients to choose to end medical treatment, even if doing so would result in death, and permitting terminally ill patients to choose to have access to potentially life-saving drugs that have not been approved for efficacy by the FDA (Brady, 2006)? *See Cruzan v. Director, Missouri Department of Health*, 497 U.S. 261 (U.S. Supreme Court 1990).

The FDA can grant accelerated drug approval based on limited but promising clinical data. Proponents of access maintain the FDA should use fast-track regulations to give terminally ill patients the right to choose life-saving treatments while more lengthy definitive trials are undertaken (O'Reilly, 2008). The pharmaceutical industry, however, is concerned about accelerated deaths or harm to patients beyond the harm from their disease or illness, given the current uncertainties on the right to sue for deaths or injuries caused by experimental drugs. Currently, many lawsuits against the pharmaceutical industry are based on state consumer safety regulations that are stronger than federal FDA standards. Although the U.S. Supreme Court recently ruled in favor of preemption in a medical device case involving Medtronic, Congress may have other ideas to undo pre-emption and guarantee the right to sue in drug cases (Mundy & Wang, 2008). *See Riegel v. Medtronic, Inc.* 128 S.Ct. 999 (U.S. Supreme Court 2008).

Right to Sue Insurers

One of the most contentious issues in health care deals with when and where patients can take legal action if they feel an insurer wrongly denies them coverage and, as a result, causes them harm (Wharton, 2005; *see generally* Prieto-Gonzalez, 2004).

Moral Dilemmas

1. What is the distinction, if any, between requiring informed consent of patients who participate in clinical testing of experimental drugs for FDA approval and requiring informed consent for distribution of potentially life-saving drugs to terminally ill patients outside the clinical testing context?

One side of this debate maintains Congress should make certain insurers are held accountable when they deny treatments recommended by physicians. The other side argues increased liability on insurers will lead to increased costs, which will make health insurance even more costly, which is counter to congressional intent when ERISA was adopted in the first place.

STATE LAWSUITS AGAINST INSURERS ARE PRE-EMPTED BY ERISA

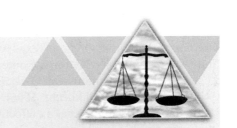

Aetna Health Inc. v. Juan Davila

[MCO v. Patients]

542 U.S. 200 (U.S. Supreme Court 2004)

FACTS: MCO patients from Texas claimed denial of proper health care by their insurers. Aetna denied payment to Juan Davila for the drug Vioxx prescribed by his physician for severe rheumatoid arthritis. While Vioxx was in Aetna's formulary (a list of medications Aetna decided it would cover), Aetna had a step-program requiring patients to try generic drugs before it would approve branded drugs. After three weeks on Aetna's step program, Davila developed severe internal bleeding and stomach ulcers from use of the generics, resulting in the inability to take any further oral pain medications. Ruby Calad developed complications after undergoing a complicated hysterectomy and being discharged from the hospital after one day, a limit set by Cigna. A Cigna discharge nurse decided, against the treating physician's judgment, that Calad's continued hospitalization did not meet the MCO's medical necessity criteria. As a result, Calad experienced severe complications and required readmittance to the hospital several days later. Both patients filed suit in state court.

ISSUE: Does ERISA pre-empt state claims for denial of proper health care so that insurers are not subject to medical malpractice rules if they make medical judgments affecting the quality of health care when determining health care coverage?

HOLDING AND DECISION: Yes, state claims are pre-empted by ERISA; as a result, if insurers negligently deny or delay a patient's treatment, the patient cannot sue the insurer for injuries. Rather, the patient can only recover severely limited ERISA remedies: the cost of the denied benefit or injunctive relief.

ANALYSIS: Most states require insurers to exercise ordinary care when making treatment decisions. Patients argued this protection extended to treatment decisions influenced by utilization review on the part of insurers. Utilization review is a review process designed to evaluate the appropriateness of health care services.

ERISA, a federal health benefits law passed to reconcile conflicting state laws regulating employer-sponsored health plans, provides wronged patients with the value of denied benefits from an MCO (*see* Employee Retirement Income Security Act of 1974 (ERISA), 26 U.S.C.A. §§ 219 *et seq.* (2009)). ERISA further provides that the federal law supersedes all state laws related to employer-sponsored health plans. This is known as the ERISA pre-emption doctrine. Because ERISA pre-empts state laws, the rights of patients exist only under ERISA, and patients can only sue to recover benefits due under the plan. There is no right to sue for state law claims under ERISA, such as for negligence, breach of contract, or any other state remedies. The Court further ruled denial of coverage for health care claims fell within the scope of ERISA, and were completely pre-empted by it.

RULE OF LAW: ERISA is the exclusive remedy for the denial of health benefits; since claims for denial of proper health care are not subject to state remedies, patients who receive their health care through employer-sponsored ERISA health plans cannot sue their insurers under state law for injuries resulting from their insurers' treatment decisions.

In *Davila*, the U.S. Supreme Court interpreted what constitutes a medical decision as opposed to a financial consideration. The Court reasoned that since utilization decisions are financial, ERISA pre-empts any state law claims against insurers. This means that a patient harmed as a direct result of an improper denial of treatment may recover only the value of that treatment, and nothing for the injuries that were a foreseeable consequence of such denial (Kim, J. W., 2005).

While the National Conference of State Legislatures reports this decision crushed patient bill of rights laws in twelve states (Arizona, California, Georgia, Louisiana, Maine, New Jersey, North Carolina, Oklahoma, Oregon, Texas, Washington, and West Virginia (*see* National Conference of State Legislatures, 2008)), many see *Davila* as having shifted political pressures (Schuknecht, 2006). The expectation and hope remains that an effective federal Patients' Bill of Rights will eventually render the *Davila* holding obsolete (Kim, J. W., 2005; *see generally* Miller, 2007).

Clearly, the federal courts have constructed substantial barriers to a state's ability to bring ERISA suits on behalf of its citizens. ERISA is viewed primarily as a federal concern outside the parameters of state interference. With a broad pre-emptive scope to occupy the entire field of regulation of employer-sponsored health plans, ERISA can exclude state laws and regulation.

Health Net establishes that the statutorily listed parties empowered to sue under ERISA should be viewed as having exclusive jurisdiction. The decision leaves unanswered questions as to whether patients of insurers are permitted to assign their rights for the purposes of a claim seeking ERISA enforcement. Nor did *Health Net* articulate what might constitute an injury and thus grant states standing to bring ERISA claims.

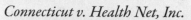

ERISA: STATUTORY STANDING OF STATES TO BRING CLAIMS ON BEHALF OF RESIDENTS

Connecticut v. Health Net, Inc.

[State v. Managed Care Organizations]

383 F.3d 1258 (U.S. Court of Appeals for the 11th Circuit 2004), U.S. Supreme Court certiorari denied, 543 U.S. 1149 (U.S. Supreme Court 2005)

FACTS: The State of Connecticut filed suit against eight insurers who had obstructed their patients' access to prescription drugs, failed to make timely payments to medical providers, failed to disclose health insurance plan information to patients, failed to respond to patients' letters and phone calls, and denied coverage based on arbitrary guidelines.

ISSUE: Do states have standing under ERISA to assert claims on behalf of their citizens?

HOLDING AND DECISION: No, states lack standing to assert ERISA claims on behalf of their citizens unless the state can show it suffered an injury.

ANALYSIS: The Judicial Panel on Multidistrict Litigation transferred this case to the U.S. District Court for the Southern District of Florida for coordinated pretrial management. Connecticut's claim was subsequently dismissed for lack of standing. Connecticut appealed to the Eleventh Circuit Court of Appeals. The Eleventh Circuit affirmed the District Court's dismissal of Connecticut's claim.

The Eleventh Circuit found Connecticut did not have a sufficient stake in the outcome of the ERISA claim to meet the constitutional minimum for standing in federal court. Connecticut was barred from bringing suit as an assignee on behalf of its citizens because Connecticut did not and would not suffer any type of injury as a result of the practices it claims violated ERISA. The Eleventh Circuit refused to consider whether Connecticut's parens patriae argument was constitutionally permitted and held Connecticut lacked statutory standing to sue in parens patriae to enforce the alleged ERISA violations because Connecticut failed to demonstrate Congress intended states to be able to bring actions. According to the Eleventh Circuit, the specific statutory language that only a participant, beneficiary, or fiduciary may bring suit implicitly indicates Congress never intended states to bring ERISA lawsuits on behalf of their citizens.

RULE OF LAW: States must suffer an actual or imminent injury to assert claims of ERISA violations on behalf of their citizens.

Private Rights of Action

Foundation Health v. Westside EKG Associates
[MCO v. Health Care Professionals]
944 So.2d 188 (Supreme Court of Florida 2006)

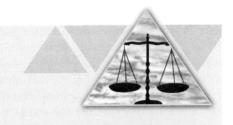

Facts: Westside, a group of physicians administering EKG interpretations, filed a breach of contract claim against seven insurers as a third-party beneficiary. Westside alleged its physicians provided MCO patients with health care under MCO policies; therefore, Westside was a third-party beneficiary to those patient contracts, and the insurers breached those contracts by repeatedly failing to promptly pay Westside. The insurers countered Westside lacked a private right of action to sue. At the time Westside brought its lawsuit, insurers were required by state law to promptly pay, contest, or deny claims, or pay interest; after a set time period, the MCO was required to pay the medical providers' claims.

Issue: Can medical providers sue for breach of a third-party beneficiary contract for an MCO's violations of a state law's prompt pay provisions?

Holding and Decision: Yes, medical providers are intended third-party beneficiaries of contracts between insurers and patients.

Analysis: The Supreme Court of Florida held that a medical provider may bring a cause of action as a third-party beneficiary to contracts between insurers and their patients based on allegations that the insurers failed to comply with the *prompt pay provisions* of state law. The elements of third-party beneficiary claims are:

- Existence of a contract
- The express intent of the contracting parties that the contract benefits the third party

- Breach of the contract by a contracting party
- Damages to the third party resulting from the breach

While the simple allegation that an MCO violated the prompt pay provisions of state law is not sufficient to establish a private right of action, when parties enter into a contract regarding matters that are the subject of statutory regulation, those regulatory provisions become a part of the contract. State law may be incorporated into MCO contracts for the purpose of establishing a breach of contract when the claims of medical providers are for a service state law requires insurers to provide. The court reasoned this was justified because the prompt pay provisions were integral to the rights of patients and the responsibilities of insurers established by state law.

Finally, the court considered whether, as a practical matter, non-participating providers were governed by these principles. The court answered in the affirmative, finding state law recognizes medical providers as third-party beneficiaries to MCO contracts. First, state law requires MCO contracts to compensate non-participating medical providers for emergency services and care. Second, state law prohibits insurers from waiving this benefit in their contracts; contractual provisions that contradict this law must be construed in accordance with state law.

Rule of Law: Medical providers may bring actions as third-party beneficiaries to contracts between insurers and their patients based on the MCO's failure to promptly pay the medical providers.

It is clear that states cannot bring ERISA claims as assignees for their citizens where alleged violations do not affect the state itself. *Health Net* does not prohibit patients, however, from combining their claims for a class-action suit alleging ERISA violations against insurers.

While future holdings may rely on *Westside* to incorporate state statutory requirements into other health insurance policies, thereby extending potential insurer liability (Miller, 2007), ERISA still precludes most patients from suing in federal courts to settle disputes over benefits, co-payments, and other non-medical judgments. This particular lawsuit issue has attracted the most attention with regards to patient rights, and the attention it has received is symptomatic of a breakdown in trust.

Patients have simply not found a constructive way to deal with tensions existing in the delivery of medical services by insurers. A mechanism is needed to allow for appropriate cost containment in health care decision-making and increased accountability of the people in charge of that cost containment. There is heated debate about the appropriate way to find a compromise (Wharton, 2008). However, almost everyone agrees (except trial lawyers) it is a shame anyone thinks lawsuits are the way to do it.

Alternative Dispute Systems

There is a strong government preference toward some type of alternative system to resolve health care disputes because of the belief it would be more efficient than litigation, less costly, and a better process for patients suffering some type of harm (*see* Federal Arbitration Act (FAA), 9 U.S.C.A. §§ 1-14 (2009)). The U.S. Supreme Court's expansive interpretation of arbitration has further fueled the widespread use of alternative dispute systems in medical settings and fostered the belief that tort law is not the best way to provide incentives for high-quality health care. *See Moses H. Cone Memorial Hospital v. Mercury Construction Corp.*, 460 U.S. 1, 24 (U.S. Supreme Court 1983) (upholding the enforceability of arbitration). Most Americans find it hard to believe there is not some method superior to litigation for resolving disputes between patients and medical providers (Galle, 2004).

Reasonableness of Arbitration Clauses   Critics of alternative dispute systems often say that when patients forgo their right to sue, the health industry strips them of a valuable right at a time when they might be at their most vulnerable (Moses, 2005). On this basis of unreasonableness, patients in health care contracts generally make one of five arguments when attacking arbitration clauses:

- Arbitration clauses are non-mutual because they are binding to medical providers but not to patients
- Arbitration clauses are unreasonable because they reduce patient rights
- Arbitration is too costly for patients to participate
- Lack of independent or neutral arbitrators
- Patients were coerced to sign arbitration agreements because there was no meaningful choice in obtaining needed medical services

(Galle, 2004)

Patients' rights to sue insurers often kicks in only after patients go through administrative review processes established by their insurers. The review processes are designed to provide a way to settle complaints in lieu of litigation. Patients who are able to demonstrate they were irreparably harmed by an insurer's refusal to pay for treatment must nonetheless often wait a period of time before filing a lawsuit.

During that time, a panel of independent experts often reviews the case, and the panel's findings are admissible in the court where the lawsuit is being heard (Wharton, 2005).

To better uphold patient agreements to use alternative dispute systems, health care providers should:

- Draft terms in the arbitration agreement clearly and unequivocally
- Educate patients about their right to sue insurers
- Encourage patients to ask questions regarding their right to sue
- Make arbitration agreements in insurance contracts optional, revocable, and mutual
- Prevent patients from bearing a large financial burden to arbitrate their claims

(Galle, 2004)

Potential Conflicts-of-Interest   Beyond the right to sue insurers is the issue of what constitutes a reasonable mechanism for ascertaining damages (Jost, 2008). The U.S. Supreme Court may address this issue when it examines how conflicts should be taken into account on judicial review of discretionary benefit determinations when administrators of insurers and self-insured health insurance plans both determine and pay patient claims. *See Metro. Life Ins. Co. v. Glenn,* 128 S.Ct. 2343 (U.S. Supreme Court 2008). Federal courts reviewing claim denials should take into account the conflicts-of-interest ERISA plan administrators face when they pay claims out of their own pockets while standing to profit by denying claims. The question is whether there is a conflict-of-interest when the same party administering a health insurance plan and paying claims out of its own pocket also stands to profit by denying patient claims.

Tort Reform

Legislative alterations to common law tort doctrines, otherwise known as tort reform, have been an intense political issue for at least thirty years. In particular, medical malpractice law has held a central place on many state legislative agendas with dozens of reforms enacted, struck down, and reenacted over the years. At the national level, no fewer than seventeen bills to federalize medical malpractice law, currently governed by state common law, have been recently debated in Congress (Avraham, 2006).

The Center for Public Integrity's *Lobby Watch* reports most interest groups agree lawsuits against insurers are acceptable, provided there are safeguards in place to prevent frivolous suits. While proponents of tort reform often exaggerate the dangers posed by such lawsuits, the judicial system already has the ability to throw out such cases before they go to trial. Tort reformers also often exaggerate the extent to which runaway juries award unwarranted damages that can financially harm insurers. The federal government finds evidence demonstrating that the rhetoric on tort reform is intentionally skewed by the American Medical Association (GAO, 2003). When jury awards are excessive, they can be, and commonly are, pared back by trial judges or appeals courts (Hyman et al., 2007).

Limitations on Damages   The Robert Wood Johnson Foundation finds limitations on damages are the only tort reform that continues to surface as effective (Mello, 2006). While limitations on noneconomic and punitive damages that could be awarded to patients may be acceptable, there is no simple prescription as to what those limitations should be (*see, e.g.,* Kenitz, 2006). Nor is there agreement on whether patient lawsuits should be allowed in state courts as well as federal courts. Should defense costs be recoverable when patient lawsuits are determined frivolous? How high a standard should be set for determining whether patient lawsuits are frivolous? Should there be limitations on joint and several liability? Should the collateral source rule be limited?

In federal courts, there are generally no limits on damage awards to patients for lost wages or pain and suffering, but punitive damages are often limited to around $5 million. In state courts, by contrast, patients are generally allowed to file suits if denied coverage based on a medical judgment. In state courts, there are no limits on awards for lost wages, pain and suffering, or punitive damages, unless state law imposes limits (Stanley, 2007). Both sides of the tort reform movement (Silver et al., 2006) debate the merit of paying damage awards in installments.

Federal Preemption of Tort Law   Today, with decisions in courtrooms being made by juries, class-action lawsuits, and contingency fees for trial lawyers, policy choices made about the legal system have ramifications in the U.S. health care system (Saiman, 2008). There is a national reform movement afoot for Congress to take a leadership position and begin addressing tort reform.

By concluding medical malpractice is a significant federal issue, perhaps because of its impact on interstate commerce, Congress could enact a jurisdictional statute shifting medical malpractice claims to federal courts (Allen, 2006). Once medical malpractice cases are in the federal system, the national reform effort could then take additional measures.

For instance, the federal system could shift medical malpractice cases within the federal system for consolidated handling by specialized medical courts under the Judicial Panel on Multidistrict Litigation (*see* 28 U.S.C.A. §1407 (1976)). Specialized courts may be more knowledgeable about medical treatments and monitoring of conditions, diseases, and disorders (Lang, 2004).

Most important, federal tort reform could serve the role of forcing state courts and legislatures to identify more clearly the substantive objectives of tort law (Rendleman, 2006). After all, since the federal government purchases a significant portion of the nation's medical services, it is in a position to make greater use of its spending power to leverage modifications in state tort laws that would otherwise be politically unfeasible to implement at the state level.

The cost of medical malpractice insurance, for instance, has driven OB/GYN specialists out of certain geographic areas (Kim, B., 2007) and medical devices are pricier in the U.S. than anywhere else, all a result of the current U.S. tort system. An issue of critical national importance is tort reform, not adequately addressed since the modern state tort reform movement began with California's 1975 Medical Injury Compensation Reform Act (Nelson, 2006).

Right to Sue Employers

Patients cannot sue their employers, unless the employer played a direct role in deciding whether a patient would receive health care. Generally, the courts favor allowing patients the right to sue employers involved in coverage decisions (Kim, J.W., 2005). If an employed physician played a significant role in making treatment decisions with regard to an employee, that employer will probably be sued, but employers are only sued if patients are actually harmed (*see Aetna Health Inc. v. Juan Davila,* 542 U.S. 200 (U.S. Supreme Court 2004)).

The most controversial part of tort reform is provisions expanding patients' right to sue employers (*see* Viscusi & Born, 2005). Businesses providing health insurance coverage to their employees are alarmed because they see a scenario in which they are sued, along with physicians and hospitals, when patients are harmed (Jost, 2008).

In general, patients have rights through disclosure rather than by regulation. If an employer tells its employees they cannot sue them, then employees can make a decision about whether they want to accept the employer's health insurance coverage. In *Davila,* the U.S. Supreme Court recently volleyed back to Congress the question of whether ERISA beneficiaries should have any remedy for damages caused by coverage decisions.

RATIONING AND COST-EFFECTIVENESS ANALYSIS

Some commentators distinguish between rationing, allocation of resources, and triage. In this chapter, however, rationing refers to the withholding of scarce resources from specific individuals so the resources will be available for others in the future.

The ability of patients to sue helps ensure a level playing field when rationing decisions are made. However, people who think lawsuits are a solution to U.S. health care problems are likely wrong. Lawsuits cannot possibly address the fundamental question at the heart of meaningful health care reform: how much is human life worth (Wharton, 2008)?

There is a near universal assumption that Americans' desire for health care exceeds their willingness to pay for it or to have others pay for their participation in public health insurance programs. But does it? There is a widespread but largely untested perception that Americans are unwilling to accept limits in health care (Gold et al., 2007).

Allocation of Scarce Health Care Resources

The paradox of the U.S. health care system is that total health care spending generates benefits far in excess of its total cost, while, at the same time, current expenditures are for services worth far less than they cost (Aaron, 2008). This contradictory statement obviously leads to questions about how to allocate scarce health care resources in the most effective way possible.

The entire issue of affordable health care, however, has become so complex it does not lend itself to easy analysis or cost-containment solutions. Health insurance plans and employers paying premiums for health care coverage are in a tough position. The public wants to cut costs, which inevitably involves rationing care, but then are outraged at the manner in which care is rationed. At the same time, most insurers have gone to excess in cost containment (Wharton, 2008, 2005).

To analogize, if a system contains excess fat, and if a scalpel is carefully used, the fat can be trimmed without harming the muscle or the nerves. But some insurers have used a meat cleaver to cut out the fat in health care and have harmed patients as a result. Although cost-containment strategies have been used in managing care, using health-based, cost-effectiveness analysis (CEA) to prioritize coverage decisions has not been among them (Gold et al., 2007). While CEA has the potential to consider a broad range of health care services, it has met with criticism because of the meat cleaver's potential to restrict access to health care by using criteria that discriminate against age and poor health status (Satz, 2008). This disapproval,

however, fails to understand that CEA is a benchmark strategy to carefully guide decision-making on health-related well-being. Moreover, critics often confuse this approach with health decisions on general well-being and the many other factors that are prioritized in this broader insurance analysis of whether to provide coverage.

Quality of Life Research

This section on quality of life research draws on articles by Chris P. Lee at The Wharton School of the University of Pennsylvania. Recent research from the University of Pennsylvania (Penn) and Stanford University offers guidance to engage in shaping some of the broadest resource allocation questions facing the U.S. health care system. Based on Medicare kidney dialysis data, CEA shows the average figure of $129,000 spent per year on each dialysis patient, resulting in one additional year of quality life for patients, is higher than prior studies have shown. This research used data from the U.S. Renal Data System on outcomes and costs from more than 500,000 patients initiating dialysis between 1996 and 2003, as well as from almost 160,000 patients who received a transplant during the same period. More importantly, this research puts a value on the cost-effectiveness of treatment across percentiles of the entire dialysis population in an attempt to develop a benchmark for health care coverage decisions.[LN1]

Quality-Adjusted Life-Year in End-Stage Renal Disease Patients

Dialysis for patients suffering end-stage renal disease (ESRD) is the one service Medicare provides for anyone, regardless of age. The program has been in effect since the 1970s and health care economists have long considered it a fair substitute for universal health care coverage and the value society places on a year of life, as measured by self-reported health and functioning (Wharton, 2008).

Before the Penn research, the number most commonly used to place a value on a year of quality life was $50,000 (Braithwaite et al., 2008). A Canadian study used an accounting ledger for more than two hundred ESRD patients during a time span of one year (Molzahn et al., 1996). The Penn research brings this older ESRD study up to date with costs and modern practices. While the gold standard was $50,000, this figure does not reflect the way dialysis is practiced today or the technology currently in use.

When it comes to health care, placing a value on life often leads to qualified coverage. Using rankings of the cost-effectiveness of medical interventions to make coverage decisions is clear and explicit. Without definite rankings, rationing is implicit because

Medicare has a finite budget. Medicare cannot provide coverage for everything. In the end, ESRD patients will not get everything they want. The mechanism for the rationing is performed in the name of what is medically necessary and reasonable. Medicare coverage is based on a clause stating patients must receive treatments that are necessary and reasonable (Wharton, 2008).

The $129,000 figure determined by Penn research compares to a range of $50,000 to $100,000 used in other countries running national health care systems, such as Australia and England, in guiding their coverage decisions. The World Health Organization has proposed $109,000 as the value of a disability-adjusted life-year, adding that, even though countries adopt spending thresholds in coverage decisions, they do not apply them without exceptions (WHO, 2006). Moreover, human health is just too unpredictable at the individual level for strict rationing of health care.

Indeed, continuing to base coverage decisions on clinical evidence alone, without consideration of costs, may not be feasible in the long run. Several researchers argue coverage decisions should be based on cost and effectiveness criteria. New technologies with cost-effectiveness ratios below $50,000 to $100,000 per incremental quality-adjusted life-year are deemed suitable for coverage, while others with higher ratios are too expensive (Wharton, 2005).

The Penn research concerns employers in several ways including employer and employee health benefit payments, insurance coverage, and malpractice cases. Health care costs are rising for employees, but employers are also paying more. Health insurance is expensive partly because of the degree of coverage. The fact is there are many medical procedures with high prices and minimal medical benefits. When is it justified for one person to subsidize the demands and wishes of someone else (Wharton, 2005)? The questions then are:

- How do universal health plans determine the right degree of coverage?
- At what point does coverage produce too little benefit for the costs demanded?
- How should preventable, detrimental behaviors and conditions affect all of these decisions?
- What line drawing problems exist?
- What is the acceptability of such limits for both physicians and patients?

One practical benchmark is based on ESRD. To the extent ESRD, given its unique historical status in the U.S., offers a reasonable point of reference for making coverage decisions, the Penn research can be used to guide those decisions. Although the $129,000 figure is substantially higher than the figure

of $50,000, using the former as the benchmark does not necessarily mean more funds will be spent. What it means is that resources could be allocated using ESRD as the reference point to define what is cost-effective treatment and what is not. In the same way, if applied to a case where malpractice cost a patient ten years of quality-adjusted life-years, a figure of $1.29 million could be used as a rough start for settlement negotiations.

Of course, cost-effectiveness is directly related to leading a responsible lifestyle. To the extent increased costs attributable to preventable behaviors and conditions are deducted from the $129,000 benchmark figure, increased costs would be borne by those who create the risk of the increased costs, rather than by those who do not pose the same economic risk. The Penn research does not address how the $129,000 figure would change if costs incumbent in the lifestyles choices of ESRD patients were factored into the benchmark, while at the same time relieving ESRD patients from bearing benefit costs not attributable to their own behavior. In short, the question is how the Penn research can help make people more accountable for their behavior with health insurance coverage consequences.

Moral Dilemmas

1. Should patient behavior be taken into account in determining whether a patient is eligible for health insurance? For instance, should a patient who took no steps to stop smoking, in spite of a physician's recommendations, be eligible for private or public health insurance funding of respiratory disease or lung cancer that is directly attributable to a smoking habit?

2. Similarly, should patients who fail to monitor their health with regular routine check-ups be compelled to pay higher insurance premiums for their health insurance plans?

Prospective Guidance for Allocation Decisions

If past trends continue, total health care spending will claim more than 30 percent of gross domestic product not long after 2030 (Kogan & Fiedler, 2007). As the spending on health care continues to rise unabated (right now it is growing at twice the rate of inflation and accounting for one out of every six dollars earned), the U.S. is coming to a point where compromises are inevitable (CMS, 2009). Either other forms of spending must be cut back to make room, or health care dollars must be spent more wisely (Keegan et al., 2008). There is just no other way (Aaron, 2008). Otherwise, spending on Medicare,

Medicaid, SCHIP, and other federal health care programs will rise to about 12 percent of gross domestic product over the same period, or nearly the current yield of income tax and payroll tax combined (OMB, 2007).

The Penn research provides guidance for making these decisions. These decisions are hard because they involve ethics and social values where there is no clear right or wrong. Given the opportunity to weigh in on ethical and normative issues that surround CEA, members of the public are appropriate parties to engage in shaping the broadest resource allocation questions (Gold et al., 2007). Public debate should continue on medical value and the difficulties involved.

DETERMINATIONS OF MEDICAL NECESSITY

The phrase *medical necessity* has been the benchmark by which coverage decisions are made affecting the medical treatment of patients. However, without incorporating the benefit derived from specific medical treatments, it is impossible to know what is medically necessary or reasonable. Moreover, this phrase is really subject to interpretation and, because of the subjectivity, decisions are not based on objective notions of medical benefit (Wharton, 2005).

Regulation intended to improve the flow of health information to patients is unequivocally desirable, based on either equity or efficiency grounds. Patients need to be able to compare their treatment options with the treatment of others when deciding which health providers achieve the best outcomes. Patients also need health information in determining what is reasonable for insurance coverage.[LN2]

Access to Health Information

Health care could be rationed if information measuring the relative quality of providers is collected (Aaron, 2008). If health care is to be rationed, insurance companies and medical providers need to produce meaningful information on outcomes, cost, and the performance and quality of physicians and hospitals. Currently, unbiased, easy-to-understand, comparative information evaluating health care services is lacking (Lansky, 2004). For instance, surgical success rates are almost impossible to find. Moreover, attempts to access the data to better understand how health care dollars are spent are met with stiff resistance from the medical establishment and its professional medical associations. One noteworthy exception is the New York State Department of Health Cardiac Surgery Reporting System, which collects and tracks clinical data on cardiac surgeries performed in New York hospitals.

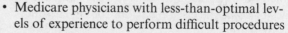

ACCESS TO THE MEDICARE DATABASE

Consumers' Checkbook v. U.S. HHS
[Consumer Group v. Federal Government]
554 F3d 1046 (U.S. Court of Appeals for the District of Columbia Circuit 2009)

FACTS: Consumers' Checkbook, a consumer group, requested Medicare claims information submitted by physicians for the purpose of identifying individual Medicare providers and determining each time a provider performed a particular service or procedure. No patient identifying information was requested.

The public interest at stake is the interest in obtaining information that would help the public make better-informed Medicare decisions and reveal how government funds are spent. Consumers' sought the Medicare records for purposes of quality studies on medical services provided by Medicare physicians. Specifically, Consumers' contended that analysis of the requested data would allow the public to examine, among other things, whether the government was allowing:

- Medicare physicians with less-than-optimal levels of experience to perform difficult procedures
- Medicare physicians with insufficient board certifications, histories of disciplinary actions, or poor scores on independent quality assessments, to perform high volumes of difficult procedures for which they might not be qualified
- Payments to Medicare physicians whose practice patterns did not conform with existing guidelines (e.g., whether physicians treating Medicare patients with specific diagnoses were providing annual exams and screenings recommended for those patients)

In order to perform these types of analyses, Consumers' maintained the Medicare claim information must include physician-identifying information linked to each Medicare service or procedure.

(continues)

(continued)

ISSUE: Should the government agree to disclosures of specific data about physicians from the Medicare claims database comprised of more than forty million Medicare patients and seven hundred thousand physicians?

HOLDING AND DECISION: No, the government is not authorized to exercise any supervision or control over the practice of medicine or the manner in which health care is provided, including the compensation of any health care professional.

ANALYSIS: The court agreed with the government that the requested information constituted an unwarranted invasion of the personal privacy of physicians.

According to the federal regulations, four factors are relevant to evaluating public interest. They are whether disclosure of the Medicare database:

- Advances the understanding of the general public as distinguished from a narrow segment of interested persons
- Pertains to the operations and activities of the federal government
- Reveals any meaningful information about Medicare not already part of public knowledge
- Significantly contributes to public understanding of Medicare

With regard to the third factor, the government maintained disclosure of the requested information would only advance the understanding of a small group of individuals, an argument rejected by the court.

With regard to the first factor, Consumers' stated the benefit to the public would be significant because the Medicare database would allow for analysis of Medicare services not presently available. For instance, studies show that, for some medical procedures, physicians performing a high volume of procedures produce superior quality outcomes for their patients. The Medicare data would allow analysis of this indicator of

quality for Medicare providers. The government contended the health information could not lead to quality analysis and the court agreed, stating there was no medical consensus on whether the number of procedures performed by a physician correlated to the quality of those procedures. The court added that any analysis would be incomplete because it would not reflect procedures performed on non-Medicare patients.

The court rejected Consumers' argument that the Medicare data would shed light on the government's compliance with its transparency initiatives. The court found that the government was already in the process of comparing the quality and price of health care, so consumers could make informed choices among physicians and hospitals. Once this data was compiled, regional health information alliances are to provide useful information for patients, exactly what is proposed by Consumers'.

Consumers' claimed the Medicare data would enable the public to determine if Medicare was paying physicians with insufficient certifications, disciplinary histories, or poor evaluations for a significant number of medical procedures. The court rejected this third factor, finding that the requested information was available through other publicly available sources.

Fourth, Consumers' claimed the Medicare data could be analyzed in conjunction with other treatment records to determine whether individual physicians were following standards of recommended care. However, the court stated Consumers' intended use of the data was irrelevant if it revealed little or nothing about the government's own conduct. The requested information must shed light on the government's performance of its duties versus providing information on private citizens.

RULE OF LAW: Access to the Medicare database would result in an unwarranted invasion of the personal privacy of participating physicians without a significant gain in public understanding of Medicare.

The availability of a Medicare database could be the beginning of an important patient choice movement that could help contribute to higher-quality health care and lower costs. Patients could benefit from a deeper understanding of the risks and benefits of a number of medical treatments provided by different providers. Patients could be further empowered

to make the best treatment choices, based on consideration of all the relevant factors, including which physicians have the best track records in treating their particular illness or disease.

Access to this health information could affect everything from elective procedures for non-serious conditions to complex medical treatments such as open-heart surgery and cancer therapy, since decisions would no longer be made just on the preconceptions of patients' physicians. Patients need information to compare national outcome and cost data in the context of their individual needs and health goals. An appeal of the *Consumers'* decision has not yet been filed.

Health Employer Data Information Set

In addition to the information in the Medicare database, health information is vital in the managed care marketplace for patients not enrolled in Medicare. In a managed care market, patients must estimate how frequently illness will strike and what their needs will be when they do get sick, in addition to estimating how much health care they will be permitted to access each time they need to use their managed care insurance plan.

Developing uniform sets of performance measures could provide benchmarks and promote the development of standards for quality. Development of the Health Employer Data Information Set by the nonprofit organization, National Committee for Quality Assurance, is an important step in this direction. This data provides a limited but important set of measures of differences in the rates at which patients use key medical services, such as pediatric immunization and blood-pressure screening.

Mandated Disclosure of Audited Outcome Data

Driven by patient choice, the federal government could establish an agency that requires the disclosure of audited outcome data from all insurance companies and medical providers nationwide (Herzlinger). With access to impartial data comparing health insurance plans and medical providers, patients could be empowered to make choices based on critical information that has been noticeably lacking in the health care marketplace. For instance, patients could review data on everything from surgeries to treatments for high cholesterol and diabetes, and then determine which physicians and hospitals have the most experience, best outcomes, least complications, and lowest costs (Falit, 2006). Without government mandated disclosure requirements, however, it is unclear how health information would ever be sufficiently uniform to produce meaningful results, let alone why insurance companies and providers would ever comply.

UNIVERSAL COVERAGE AND THE RIGHT TO HEALTH CARE DEBATE

Most Americans are now favoring a system of universal coverage that provides basic insurance for every citizen (Wharton, 2005). Just as there is a legal

right to emergency care, more energy and imagination is being directed to generalizing the right to health care (Annas, 2008). One challenge is to define exactly what constitutes this right. Much debate is centered on the issue of whether the U.S. should ensure everyone gets the basic care they need, while the rest is rationed.

Generally, a right to health care based on effective citizenship and fair equality of opportunity does not require that every member of society receive the most technologically advanced health care. It compels society to create a system of health care to aid its members in achieving the normal functioning required to enjoy equal opportunity. Thus, the right to health care imposes an obligation on society to provide health care to all, but does not create an unlimited right for individuals to access medical interventions without regard for effectiveness and resource limitations (Sandhu, 2007).

In addition to the moral appeal of universal coverage, strong economic arguments can be made for eliminating uninsured status (Falit, 2006). It usually costs less to provide preventative and regularly administered health care than it does to provide delayed charity care (Kaiser, 2004). This is especially true when the cost of lost productivity or unemployment as a result of medical problems is also taken into account. There is a quantifiable financial burden associated with the loss of income and quality of life that the uninsured experience because of poorer health and shorter life spans. According to the Institute of Medicine, the aggregate annual amount of lost health capital is between $65 billion and $130 billion (IOM, 2002).

State Plans Approaching Universal Coverage: Massachusetts and California

Massachusetts has adopted and California has proposed plans approaching universal health coverage (*see* Act Providing Access to Affordable, Quality, Accountable Health Care, M.G.L.A. 111M § 2 (2008); Bodaken, 2007; Chirba-Martin & Torres, 2008; Weeks, 2007). Central elements of both plans rely on individual mandates, purchasing pools, employer assessments, and shared responsibility. While health insurance plans are administered by private insurers, they are regulated, coordinated, and sold by the states.

Individual Mandates

Those with health insurance pay for the health care of the uninsured (Kaiser, 2004). This is one core problem of the U.S. health care system. In Massachusetts and California, everyone must participate equally. Under universal coverage, everyone pays through the state progressive tax systems. While the insured are still paying for the uninsured, universal coverage attempts to reduce the burden of people with a lower ability to pay health insurance premiums and shifts the incidence disproportionately to those with a higher ability to pay.

Individual mandates require all state residents to purchase health insurance for themselves and their children, or face a tax penalty. In Massachusetts:

- Minimum coverage plan costs: $3,000 to $6,600 annually
- Deductible: $2,000
- Limits on out-of-pocket expenses: $5,000
- Includes drug benefits
- Insurers are required to let parents add young adults up to age twenty-six

Massachusetts's individual mandate includes an affordability waiver that protects those who are ineligible for subsidies yet cannot afford private insurance. Rather than allowing more people to qualify for the subsidy in the first place (given the state's limited resources), the waiver is directed to assisting the working poor who are not eligible for Medicaid and individuals facing transient financial problems. In California:

- Minimum coverage plan costs: $1,200 annually
- Deductible: $5,000
- Limits on out-of-pocket expenses: $7,500

California lacks a safety valve like Massachusetts, which may affect universal coverage and premium rates (Gabel et al., 2007). With no waivers for individuals who cannot afford insurance, but who are ineligible for subsidies, more than half of the uninsured in California may still lack health coverage (Dubay et al., 2007). Both states provide subsidized insurance programs for low-income people while extending eligibility for Medicaid coverage (*see generally* Benson, 2007). The Current Population Survey is used to estimate what share of uninsured Americans are eligible for coverage through Medicaid or SCHIP, need financial assistance to purchase health insurance, and are likely able to afford insurance. This Surveys finds that 25 percent are eligible for public coverage, 56 percent need assistance, and 20 percent can afford coverage (Dubay et al., 2007).

Purchasing Pools

Non-group and small-group insurance markets merged into state-administered purchasing pools to provide a centralized location for individuals to purchase insurance. This consolidation created larger risk pools, thereby lowering premium costs.

Employer Assessments

In the context of universal coverage plans, a key issue is the role of employer-sponsored coverage. Such coverage has been slowly eroding and has been criticized for providing little meaningful plan choice (Ginsburg, 2008). Statewide universal coverage plans for individuals in Massachusetts and California could make employer-sponsored plans much less attractive down the road.

Employers with ten, eleven, or more full-time employees must enroll a percentage of their employees in employer-sponsored health insurance plans or pay a portion of the premiums for employee group insurance plans. Non-compliance results in annual assessments of employers, while tax penalties are imposed on uninsured adults without credible coverage. Employers must also offer Section 125 cafeteria plans, allowing employees to purchase insurance with pre-tax income, or risk the liability of state-sponsored care used by their employees if that usage exceeds a set limit. Finally, Massachusetts equalizes coverage for employees (Chirba-Martin & Torres, 2008); in contrast, California employers would be allowed to offer better plans and higher contributions to their higher paid employees. Neither state sets quality standards to prevent employers from offering plans that provide little real protection for workers (Benson, 2007).

Shared Responsibility

In California, where for-profit insurers dominate the market:

- Insurers are required to spend most of their premiums on patient care
- Responsibility for universal coverage is spread more broadly than Massachusetts
- Physicians and hospitals are required to pay a percentage of their revenues to help cover reforms
- Participating medical providers receive higher payments from Medicaid
- The use of nurse practitioners, physicians' assistants, and retail-based clinics is encouraged as a way to cut costs
- Quality of care is improved through the use of information technology

In Massachusetts, where not-for-profit insurers dominate, there is no mandate to spend most of their premiums on patient care. Both states require guaranteed issue and community rating, preventing insurers from denying coverage because of age or health status, or adjusting premiums based on health status. While the proposal requires insurers to promote healthy behaviors, other costly mandates are removed.

The Standards for Patient Rights and Responsibilities

Private and public health insurers, medical providers, and patients should work together to redesign health care processes in accordance with the following standards:

1. Care based on continuous care relationships. Patients should receive health care as needed and in many forms—not just face-to-face visits, but care provided over the Internet, by telephone, by remote monitoring, and by other technological means. This standard implies health care systems should be responsive at all times, twenty-four hours a day, seven days a week.

2. Customization based on patient needs and values. Health care systems should be designed to meet the most common types of medical needs, but have the capability to respond to individual patient choices and preferences.

3. Patients as the source of control. Patients should be given the necessary information and opportunity to exercise a chosen degree of control over health care decisions affecting them and their families. Health care systems should be able to accommodate differences in patient preferences and encourage shared decision-making.

4. Shared knowledge and the free flow of health information. Patients should have open access to their own medical data and to clinical knowledge. Medical providers and patients should communicate effectively and share information.

5. Evidence-based practice. Patients should receive health care based on the best available scientific knowledge. Medical treatments should not significantly vary from one provider to another or from one geographic location to another.

6. Safety. Patients should be safe from injury caused by health care systems. Reducing risk and ensuring safety requires greater attention to health care processes that help prevent and mitigate medical errors.

7. Transparency. Health care systems should make health information available to patients and their families to allow for making informed decisions when selecting health plans, hospitals, or physicians, or when choosing among alternative medical treatments. This should include information describing the performance of health care systems on safety, evidence-based practice, and patient satisfaction.

8. Preventive care. Health care systems should anticipate the medical needs of patients, rather than simply reacting to events.

9. Continuous decrease in waste. Health care systems should not waste resources or patient time.

10. Cooperation among providers. Medical providers should actively collaborate and communicate to ensure appropriate exchanges of health information and coordination of care.

Source: Institute of Medicine. (2003). *Hidden costs, value lost: Uninsurance in America*. Washington, DC: National Academies of Science, Academic Press.

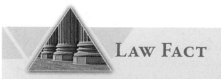 LAW FACT

RIGHT TO EMERGENCY CARE

When is a patient entitled to emergency care?

Patients have a legal right to emergency care without physically arriving on the hospital grounds as long as patients are en route to the hospital and the emergency department has been notified of their imminent arrival.

—*Morales v. Sociedad Espanola de Auxilio Mutuo y Beneficencia*, 524 F.3d 54 (U.S. Court of Appeals for the 1st Circuit 2008), *U.S. Supreme Court certiorari denied*, 129 S.Ct. 898 (U.S. Supreme Court 2009).

CHAPTER SUMMARY

- The main issue in the patient rights debate is how to balance costs with patients' choice of care.
- Many Americans support a system of universal coverage that would provide for basic health care needs, with the option of buying additional coverage.
- Patient harm seems to occur more due to problems with the health care system, rather than actual medical malpractice.
- Patients have a right to emergency care, experimental medical treatments in certain situations, and a limited right to sue.
- Under ERISA, a harmed patient can only recover the value of the treatment denied and nothing for any foreseeable injuries as a result of the denial, and states generally do not have standing to sue on behalf of their citizens; however, third parties may file a class-action suit alleging ERISA violations against insurers.
- Lawsuits, and even tort reform, are arguably not the best way to resolve problems in health care systems; arbitration and other alternative dispute mechanisms are gaining popularity, but still do not resolve the underlying problems with health care delivery, namely the questions of whether Americans' demand for health care outstrips available resources and how much a human life is worth.
- It is impossible to cut health care costs without rationing care, and it is impossible to ration care in a manner acceptable to all parties involved.
- One recently studied possible method of containing and managing health care costs involves cost-effectiveness analysis, but there is not yet a general consensus on how best to determine cost-effectiveness.
- Other methods of managing costs include redefining "medially necessary" and providing more public access to health care information.
- Uniform sets of performance measures and mandated disclosure of audited care outcome data would help patients make better health care decisions and perhaps lower costs.
- Massachusetts and California have come the closest to providing universal coverage for their citizens, but neither state has a perfect solution to the ethical and financial dilemmas involved in providing such a system.

LAW NOTES

1. Research from the University of Pennsylvania shows the incremental cost-effectiveness ratio of dialysis in current practice relative to the next least costly alternative is on average $62,000 per year, or about $129,000 for a quality-adjusted year of life (QALY). A quality-adjusted year of life is a measure that combines the length of time that life is extended and the quality of that life. However, the distribution of cost-effectiveness across the entire ESRD population is wide. For the lowest percentile, it costs only about $65,500 to provide an additional quality-adjusted life-year. For the top percentile, the figure is about $500,000. The higher costs per QALY were strongly associated with age and additional chronic illnesses in addition to ESRD. No health economist nor the strongest advocate for providing coverage would argue $500,000 for one year of life is reasonable. This would inflate health care spending by ten to fifteen times on top of current expenditures. The cost to preserve one QALY drops to $240,000 in the ninetieth percentile of expenditures. In effect, if this were to become the threshold, 90 percent of the dialysis patients could be treated for half what it would cost to treat the sickest for whom heavy expenditures do not effectively improve or extend quality or length of life (Lee et al., 2009, 2009a).

2. In reality, health insurers determine medical necessity and therefore reimbursement using guidelines published by actuarial firms such as Milliman in Seattle (Chu, 2004). In other words, medical necessity determinations are made on the basis of statistical calculations of financial benefit not medical benefit. Of course, the American Association of Health Plans and the actuarial firms deny their guidelines are based on financial objectives; instead, they claim they are designed to support quality health care. But, health insurance carriers often deny payment for health care because of actuarial guidelines, regardless of a patient's medical necessity. Critics of Milliman maintain health insurers seem to be using the actuarial guidelines 100 percent of the time and only consider the individual medical needs of patients on appeal of denied claims. Thus, claims for reimbursement other than routine claims are generally denied if they do not follow the so-called cookbook guidelines established by the actuarial firms. Milliman claims that health insurers who use their guidelines

as a basis for denying reimbursement for health care received are using them inappropriately; they are to be used to determine the risks and benefits of medical treatments (*see generally U.S. ex rel. Nudelman v. International Rehabilitation Associates*, 2006 U.S. Dist. LEXIS 17958 (U.S. District Court for the Eastern District of Pennsylvania 2006) (whistleblower case that settled for $3.2 million and included a three-year monitoring program of medical necessity determinations)).

CHAPTER BIBLIOGRAPHY

Aaron, H. J. (2008). Health care rationing: Inevitable, but impossible? *Georgetown Law Review, 96*, 539-558.

Allen, M. P. (2006). A survey and some commentary on federal tort reform. *Akron Law Review, 39*, 909-941.

Annas, G. J. (2008). Health care reform in America: Beyond ideology. *Indiana Health Law Review, 5*, 441-461.

Avraham, R. (2005). Putting a price on pain-and-suffering damages: A critique of the current approaches and a preliminary proposal for change. *Northwestern University Law Review, 100*, 87-119.

Benson, E. (2007). States lead the way on health insurance reform. *Journal of Law, Medicine & Ethics, 35*, 329-331.

Brady, T. (2009). Paternalism vs. patient autonomy: Is the FDA's "mothering" smothering grandma's and grandpa's choice of prescription drugs? *Elder Law Journal, 14*, 393-421.

Braithwaite, R. S. et al. (2008, April). What does the value of modern medicine say about the $50,000 per quality-adjusted life-year decision rule? *Medical Care, 46* (4), 349-356.

Bodaken, B., president and chief executive officer of Blue Shield of California. (2007, April 24). Fourth Annual World Health Care Congress: *State approaches to market reform and universal access: Massachusetts and California models*, at the Washington Convention Center in Washington, DC.

Chirba-Martin, M. A., & Torres, A. (2008). Special series on health care: Universal health care in Massachusetts: Setting the standard for national reform. *Fordham Urban Law Journal, 35*, 409-446.

Chu, M. (2004). Cigna settles with medical providers. *Journal of Law, Medicine & Ethics, 32*, 177-180.

CMS (Centers for Medicare and Medicaid Services). (2009). *National health expenditure data: Historical and projections. 1965-2017*. Washington, DC: CMS.

Dobson, A. et al. (2006). Mission vs. market: The cost-shift payment "hydraulic": Foundation, history, and implications. *Health Affairs, 25* (1), 22-33.

Dubay, L. et al. (2007). The uninsured and the affordability of health insurance coverage. *Health Affairs, 26* (1), 22-30.

Falit, B. P. (2006). The Bush administration's health care proposal: The proper establishment of a consumer-driven health care regime. *Journal of Law, Medicine & Ethics, 34*, 632-636.

Fuhrmans, V. (2003, September 4). Cigna settles suit by physicians over bills in $540 million pact. *Wall Street Journal*, p. D3.

Gabel, J. et al. (2007). Trends in the golden state: Small-group premiums rise sharply while actuarial values for individual coverage plummet. *Health Affairs, 26* (4), 488-499.

Galle, K. K. (2004). The appearance of impropriety: Making agreements to arbitrate in heath care contracts more palatable. *William Mitchell Law Review, 30*, 969-999.

GAO (General Accounting Office). (2003). *Medical malpractice: Implications of rising premiums on access to health care*. Washington, DC: GAO. (questioning the accuracy of studies by the American Medical Association).

Gillies, R. R. et al. (2006).The impact of health plan delivery system organization on clinical quality and patient satisfaction. *Health Services Research, 41* (4), 1181-1191.

Ginsburg, P. B. (2008). Formulas for compromise: Employment-based health benefits under universal coverage. *Health Affairs, 27* (3), 675-685.

Gold, M. R. et al. (2007). Medicare and cost-effectiveness analysis: Time to ask the taxpayers. *Health Affairs, 26* (5), 1399-1406.

Herzlinger, R. E. (2007). *Who killed health care? America's $2 trillion medical problem and the consumer-driven cure*. New York, NY: McGraw-Hill.

Herzlinger, R. E., & Parsa-Parsi, R. (2004). Consumer-driven health care: Lessons from Switzerland. *Journal of the American Medical Association, 292* (10), 1213-1220.

Hyman, D. A. et al. (2007). Do defendants pay what juries award? Post-verdict haircuts in Texas medical malpractice cases. *Journal of Empirical Legal Studies, 4*, 3-68.

IOM (Institute of Medicine). (2002). *Crossing the quality chasm: A new health system for the 21st century*. Washington, DC: IOM.

Iserson, K. V., & Moskop, J. C. (2007). Triage in medicine, part I: Concept, history, and types. *Annals of Emergency Medicine, 49* (3), 282-287.

Jost, T. S. (2008). "MetLife v. Glenn": The court addresses a conflict over conflicts in ERISA benefit administration. *Health Affairs*, 27 (5), 430-440.

Kaiser (Kaiser Commission on Medicaid and the Uninsured). (2004). *Issue update: The cost of care for the uninsured: what do we spend, who pays, and what would full coverage add to medical spending*. Washington, DC: Kaiser.

Kaiser & Harvard (Kaiser Family Foundation & Harvard School of Public Health). (2006). *The public's health care agenda for the new Congress and the presidential campaign*. Menlo, CA: Kaiser Family Foundation & Boston, MA: Harvard School of Public Health.

Kaiser Spotlight (Kaiser Public Opinion Spotlight). (2006). *The public, managed care and consumer protections*. Menlo, CA: Kaiser Family Foundation.

Keehan, S. et al. (2008). Trends: Health spending projections through 2017: The baby-boom generation is coming to Medicare. *Health Affairs, 27* (2), 145-155.

Kenitz, M. S. (2006). Wisconsin's caps on noneconomic damages in medical malpractice cases: Where Wisconsin stands (and should stand) on tort reform. *Marquette Law Review, 61*,

601-624 (criticizing the Wisconsin Supreme Court's disallowance of a cap on noneconomic damages in medical malpractice cases).

Kim, B. (2007). Current research on medical malpractice liability: The impact of malpractice risk on the use of obstetrics procedures. *Journal of Legal Studies, 36*, 79-116.

Kim, J. W. (2005). Managed care liability, ERISA preemption, and state "right to sue" legislation in *Aetna Health, Inc. v. Davila. Loyola University of Chicago Law Journal, 36*, 651-702.

Kniesner, T. J., & Viscusi, W. K. (2003). Why relative economic position does not matter: A cost-benefit analysis. *Yale Journal on Regulation, 20*, 1-24.

Kogan, R., & Fiedler, M. (2007). *CBPP (Center on Budget and Policy Priorities): The technical methodology underlying CBPP's long-term budget projections*. Washington, DC: CBPP.

Kuttner, H., & Rutledge, M. S. (2007). Data watch: Higher income and uninsured: Common or rare? *Health Affairs, 26* (6), 1745-1752.

Kysar, D. A. et al. (2006). The economics of civil justice: Medical malpractice myths and realities: Why an insurance crisis is not a lawsuit crisis. *Loyola of Los Angeles Law Review, 39*, 785-817.

Lang, A. R. (2004). A new approach to tort reform: An argument for the establishment of specialized medical courts. *Georgia Law Review, 39*, 293-320.

Lansky, D. (2004). Providing information to consumers. In R. E. Herzlinger (Ed.), *Consumer-driven health care: Implications for providers, payers and policymakers* (pp. 410-427). San Francisco, CA: Jossey-Bass.

Lavoie, D. (2008, February 26). Sex-change inmate says treatment stopped. *San Francisco Chronicle*.

Lee, C. P. et al. (2009). An empiric estimate of the value of life: Updating the renal dialysis cost-effectiveness standard. *Value in Health 12* (1), 80-87 (comparing cost, life expectancy, and quality-adjusted life expectancy of current dialysis practice for end-stage renal disease relative to three less costly alternatives and to no dialysis).

___. (2009a). Optimal initiation and management of dialysis therapy. *Operations Research, 55* (6).

___. (2008). Evaluating the potential effects of frequency and duration of hemodialysis on longevity, cost and cost-effectiveness. *Journal of the American Society of Nephrology, 19*, 1792-1797.

___ et al. (2006). A simulation model for estimating the cost and effectiveness of alternative dialysis initiation strategies. *Medical Decision Making, 26*, 638-643.

Mello, M. M. (2006). *The research synthesis project report 10: Medical malpractice: Impact of the crisis and effect of state tort reforms*. Princeton, NJ: Robert Wood Johnson Foundation.

Miller, W. (2007). Prompt payment: Florida Supreme Court allows private right of action based on MCO Act: Foundation Health v. Westside EKG Associates. *American Journal of Law & Medicine, 33*, 149-152.

Molzahn, A. E. et al. (1996). Quality of life of patients with end stage renal disease: A structural equation model. *Quality of Life Research, 5* (4), 1573-2649.

Moses, M. L. (2005). Privatized justice. *Loyola University Chicago Law Journal, 36*, 547, 535-550.

Mundy, A., & Wang, S. S. (2008, October 27). In drug case, justices weigh right to sue. *Wall Street Journal*, p. B1.

Murray, A. (2006, February 1). Health-care fixes should focus on quality. *Wall Street Journal*, p. A2.

Nelson, C. A. (2006). To truly reform we must be informed: Davis v. Parham, the separation of powers doctrine, and the constitutionality of tort reform in Arkansas. *Arkansas Law Review, 59*, 781-802.

NIH (National Institutes of Health). (2007). *Understanding clinical trials*. Bethesda, MD: NIH.

OMB (Office of Management & Budget). (2007). *Historical tables: Table 2-3: Budget of the U.S. government, fiscal year 2008*. Washington, DC: OMB.

O'Reilly, J. T. (2008). Losing deference in the FDA's second century: Judicial review, politics, and a diminished legacy of expertise. *Cornell Law Review, 93*, 939-979.

Pauly, M. V., & Herring, B. (2007). Health tracking: Risk pooling and regulation: Policy and reality in today's individual health insurance market. *Health Affairs, 26* (3), 770-779.

Power, III, J. D. (2004). The role of information: J. D. Power's paradigm lessons from the automotive industry. In R. E. Herzlinger (Ed.), *Consumer-driven health care: Implications for providers, payers and policymakers* (pp. 410-427). San Francisco, CA: Jossey-Bass.

Prieto-Gonzalez, M. (2004). Supreme Court rules HMO suits are preempted. *Journal of Law, Medicine & Ethics, 32*, 774-776.

Reinhardt, U. E. (2006). Pricing and payment: The pricing of U.S. hospital services: Chaos behind a veil of secrecy. *Health Affairs, 25* (1), 57-69.

Rendleman, D. (2006). A cap on the defendant's appeal bond?: Punitive damages tort reform. *Akron Law Review, 39*, 1089-1170.

Roosevelt, F. D. (1944, January 11). President's message to the 79th Congress on the State of the Union. *Published Papers, 12*, p. 41.

Saiman, C. (2008). Public law, private law, and legal science. *American Journal of Comparative Law*, 56, 691-702.

Sandhu, P. K. (2007). A legal right to health care: What can the U.S. learn from foreign models of health rights jurisprudence? *California Law Review, 95*, 1151-1192.

Satz, A. B. (2008). The limits of health care reform. *Alabama Law Review, 59*, 1451-1499.

Schuknecht, A. M. (2006). Aetna v. Davila: Absolution for managed health care organizations. *Loyola of Los Angeles Law Review, 39*, 947-977.

Silver, C. et al. (2006). *Georgetown Law and Economics Research Paper No. 981192: Physicians' insurance limits and malpractice payouts: Evidence from Texas closed claims*. Washington, DC: Georgetown University Law Center.

Sommers, B. D. (2007). Why millions of children eligible for Medicaid and SCHIP are uninsured: Poor retention versus poor take-up. *Health Affairs, 26* (5), 560-567.

Stanley, E. K. (2007). Parties' defenses to binding arbitration agreements in the health care field and the operation of the McCarran-Ferguson Act. *St. Mary's Law Journal, 38*, 591-640.

Tanner, M., & Cannon, M. (2007, April 5). Universal health care's dirty little secrets. *Los Angeles Times*, p. A23.

Viscusi, W. K., & Born. P. H. (2005). Damages caps, insurability, and the performance of medical malpractice insurance. *Journal of Risk & Insurance 72*, 23-43.

Watson, S. D. (2007, Winter). Consumer-directed Medicaid and cost-shifting to patients. *Saint Louis University Law Journal, 51*, 403-432.

Weeks, E. A. (2007). Failure to connect: The Massachusetts plan for individual health insurance. *Kansas Law Review, 55*, 1283-1312.

Wharton (Wharton School at the University of Pennsylvania). (2008). Cost-effective medical treatment: Putting an updated dollar value on human life. *Knowledge@Wharton*.

___. (2001). When taking two aspirin won't do: A primer on the Patients' Bill of Rights. *Knowledge@Wharton*.

WHO (World Health Organization). (2006). *Report of the Commission on Intellectual Property Rights, Innovation and Public Health*. Geneva, Switzerland: WHO.

CHAPTER 10

TORT REFORM AND REDUCING THE RISK OF MALPRACTICE

"Every man is a reformer until reform tramps on his toes."

—EDGAR WATSON HOWE (1853-1937), AMERICAN NOVELIST AND NEWSPAPER EDITOR

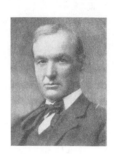

IN BRIEF

This chapter covers medical malpractice, as well as peer review processes, medical standards of care, and liability insurance. Also examined are selected proposals for tort reform, medical review boards, and no-fault policies that would eliminate provider liability for experimental or cutting-edge treatments that do not meet patient expectations.

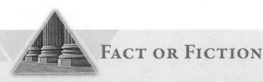

FACT OR FICTION

TORT REMEDIES FOR MEDICARE CLAIMANTS

Should a Medicare beneficiary be required to reimburse the federal government for medical expenses paid by Medicare after winning a settlement for a defectively designed product?

Bernice Loftin, a sixty-eight-year-old woman and Medicare beneficiary, underwent hip replacement surgery. One week after her surgery, Loftin dislocated her surgically repaired hip. X-rays subsequently revealed that the hip prosthesis was displaced and pressing against her sciatic nerve. Loftin underwent a second surgery, which led to a serious infection. Her physicians fought the infection with extensive medical procedures including radical debridement, the insertion of cement antibiotic beads, and prolonged physical therapy. At the time of these surgeries, Loftin's primary medical insurer was Medicare, which paid about $144,000 for Loftin's surgeries and subsequent medical care.

Loftin filed suit against the manufacturer of the hip prosthesis alleging defective design. As part of her claim for damages, Loftin cited the medical expenses paid by Medicare. Before trial, Loftin settled with the manufacturer, although it never admitted liability. The manufacturer paid the full settlement amount of $256,000 to Loftin's attorney, who, after deducting his contingency fee, distributed $153,600 to Loftin. The manufacturer paid all of the settlement; no part came from its liability insurance.

Within months of receiving her settlement, the federal government, through the Department of Health and Human Services (HHS), filed suit against Loftin, her attorney, and the manufacturer under the Medicare Secondary Payer Act (MSP). Under the MSP, the government is allowed to seek reimbursement from a primary insurer for payments made by Medicare to a Medicare beneficiary that the primary insurer should have paid or from any person that receives a payment from a primary insurer. Primary insurers are contractually committed to settling claims up to their applicable policy limits before any other insurer becomes liable for any part of the same claim, whereas secondary insurers are liable for settling any part of a claim not covered by primary insurers (*Black's Law Dictionary,* 2004). The government argued that, by making its own payment to Loftin, the manufacturer was self-insuring against any risk and was thus a primary insurer subject to the MSP law. As allowed under the MSP, the government sought reimbursement from Loftin and her attorney out of the payments received from the manufacturer. Under the MSP, HHS may seek double damages from a primary insurer; thus, HHS sought double damages from the manufacturer. If the government wins this lawsuit, Medicare will take almost all of Ms. Loftin's payment, leaving her less than $10,000 to compensate her for her pain and suffering.

—*Thompson v. Goetzmann,* 337 F.3d 489 (U.S. Court of Appeals for the 5th Circuit 2003).

(See *Law Fact* at the end of this chapter for the answer.)

PRINCIPLES AND APPLICATIONS

A tort is the legal term for a civil wrong for which a remedy may be obtained. Medical malpractice claims are torts that cause harm to patients for which patients may sue for damages. Actions in tort are derived from the common law. Common law is derived from court decisions, unlike the statutes developed by Congress and state legislatures. Congress and state legislatures, however, can change the common law that governs the tort system, and many states have enacted reform laws to reduce the risk of medical malpractice lawsuits.

Together, the U.S. legal and medical systems must make some difficult trade-offs and policy choices in

reforming the nation's tort system. The cost of medical malpractice, for instance, has driven obstetrician/gynecologist specialists out of certain geographic areas, making health care less accessible. Health care is also pricier in the U.S., in part due to the cost of malpractice insurance and lawsuits. But can it be said that the high cost of the nation's health care system is the result of a malfunctioning tort system?

Some maintain it is; most, however, maintain medical malpractice is a red herring—named for aromatic bait that apparently threw bloodhounds off the scent. Medical malpractice is of little consequence to the total cost of health care, but does serve to distract everyone from examining real reform of today's U.S. health care system. Any real reform must begin with a serious look at malpractice within the context of the largest provider of health care in the U.S., the publicly funded health care programs that provide care to over 103 million Americans.

PUBLICLY FUNDED HEALTH CARE PROGRAMS AFFECT TORT REFORM

Medicare was enacted in 1965 as part of the nation's federal social insurance program, along with need-based Medicaid, with the reluctant support of American physicians. The opening section of the legislation enacting Medicare and Medicaid reads:

> Nothing in this subchapter shall be construed to authorize any Federal officer or employee to exercise any supervision or control over the practice of medicine or the manner in which medical services are provided... or to exercise any supervision or control over the administration or operation of any such institution, agency, or person.

(Social Security Amendments of 1965, 26 U.S.C.A. § 6053 (1984); 42 U.S.C.A. §§ 424a *et seq.* (2009))

The three underlying premises of Medicare and Medicaid, inherent in this Social Security legislation, are:

- Health care providers will always be financially principled
- Patient care will be paramount at all times, rather than financial or corporate interests
- Providers will be clinically competent at all times

As it turns out, the three premises are clearly not always true. The theoretical foundation for publicly funded health care was arguably flawed from the start. Today, almost half a century after Medicare and Medicaid were first enacted, malpractice is more often than not blamed for the level of difficulty facing health care in the U.S. Some of the difficulties include:

- Quality of health care is comparably below other similarly developed, high-income countries around the world
- U.S. has the world's highest per capita expenditures on health care
- U.S. ranks twenty-eighth in life expectancy
- Preventable chronic disease affects more than four out of ten Americans
- Chronic diseases cost more than $500 billion annually
- Adherence to evidence-based clinical practice guidelines and best practices is distressingly low
- Avoidable medical errors are widespread

(Davis, 2008; Landro, 2004; Thorpe et al., 2007)

During the past half-century since the decision was made to provide health insurance for Americans sixty-five and over (the population group most likely to be living in poverty), some lessons have been learned from the nation's largest health coverage program covering low-income aged, blind, and disabled individuals, as well as parents and their dependent children on welfare:

- Health care delivery systems are important
- Institutional practices drive error rates more than individual failings of health care providers
- Coordination of care by physicians is essential to successful health outcomes
- Patient involvement is a factor in medical care quality
- Reliable information about the cost and value of medical services is needed
- Physician complaints seem to be a marker for clinically significant quality lapses in hospitals

(IOM, 2006; Kinney & Sage, 2008)

While few would defend the medical malpractice system as a cost-effective method of either compensation or quality improvement, it has become clear that preventable injuries are a more troubling problem for the U.S. health care system than frivolous lawsuits (Studdert et al., 2006). Choices made about the Medicare and Medicaid programs have ramifications in the legal and health care systems, and these choices must be addressed. Over fifty-nine million American adults have Medicaid coverage and over forty-four million have Medicare coverage (Kaiser, 2007). Tort reform cannot occur without reform of the public health insurance systems that reimburse more than one in three Americans.

DISRUPTIVE INNOVATION

The concept of "disruptive innovation" may be useful for the medical malpractice sector. The idea known in management circles for the past decade as "transformative innovation" is what Austrian economist Joseph Schumpeter had in mind when he borrowed the phrase "creative destruction" to describe his theories of how entrepreneurs sustain the capitalist system (Schumpeter, 2008). The development of new health insurance products of moderately higher risk-sharing and much lower cost may be useful for the medical malpractice sector.

New reimbursement methodologies for providing health insurance that is cheaper and more convenient must be developed if costs are to be lowered. Such insurance products are rarely offered and, when they are, as in the case of health maintenance organizations (HMOs), they are subject to intense criticism and resistance from those who have a vested interest in traditional reimbursement of health care providers. *See Aetna Health Inc. v. Davila*, 542 U.S. 200 (U.S. Supreme Court 2004) (class-action claiming injuries arising from HMO decisions not to provide coverage for treatment recommended by treating physicians and alleging HMOs failed to exercise ordinary care in the handling of coverage decisions).

Reframing State Regulations

The legal and health care systems have both been guilty of inhibiting discussion of tort reform alternatives as a way to reduce the risk of medical malpractice (Davies, 2007). While the applicability of the concept of disruptive innovation may be quite limited for regulators given today's political realities, theoretically, the possibility of reframing state insurance regulations could be the innovative change health care systems need. If there were sufficient changes in framing and regulating liability insurance by the states, it might be helpful if public health care programs also went through this process (Pauly & Herring, 2007).

Reform Market Exit Regulations

One regulatory change that could impact the cost of malpractice insurance is making it more difficult for national insurers to exit out of the professional liability insurance market in some states while continuing to operate in other states. Market exits of insurance carriers from a state leave that carrier's insured clients either uninsured or facing substantial premium increases for the same amount of coverage with new insurers (Pauly & Herring, 2007). Any hospital or health professional facing an open claim or having settled a significant malpractice claim will be uninsurable at comparable rates with a different carrier, regardless of fault.

In addition, switching to a new comparable insurer for the same liability coverage is always more expensive given the experience rating deductions that are based on claims-free policies. Policyholders obtain a deduction from their premiums for each year they remain free of filing any claims against their insurance carrier; the more years an insured remains claims-free, the higher the deduction, thus making it prohibitively expensive to switch carriers. When switches must be made, the malpractice premiums start from a higher base.

Reform Claims and Pricing Regulations

Concerns over liability insurance rate hikes appear to have cooled as the industry passes through another cycle. While premiums saw significant rate increases through the late 1990s, now the rate hikes have slowed down. Nevertheless, high premiums, at the top of a cycle, will at some point return as an issue (Pauly & Herring, 2007). Most state insurance agencies have

mediocre controls over claims and pricing to help smooth the behavior of insurers in cyclical markets. State regulators approve high-premium increases for one company and then tend to approve increases by other mimicking insurers, creating hot markets.

Compromise Reforms

Liability insurance costs have grown to unprecedented levels for physicians in states where tort reform has not occurred. After more than twenty years of debate, court battles, lobbying, and even ballot initiatives to amend state constitutions, several compromises are under consideration:

- Develop medical review panels where medical malpractice claimants present their claims before accessing the court system[LN3]
- Adopt non-economic damage ("pain and suffering") caps on malpractice awards
- Redefine malpractice
  - Limit the liability for innovative and experimental medical treatments that do not meet patient expectations
  - Extend enterprise liability to hospitals or managed care organizations (MCOs)
- Enhance the requirements for insurers to gain entry into state liability insurance markets (for instance, by mandating a greater capital base for entry)
- Develop compensation benchmarks for malpractice payouts
- Create specialized administrative health courts

(Cohen, 2005)

No one single compromise is the solution to reducing the risk of malpractice. However, some ideas have appeared to fall by the wayside:

- Restrictions of lawyers' contingency fees
- Legal limitations on medical malpractice claims (*see e.g., Kenyon v. Hammer*, 688 P.2d 961 (Supreme Court of Arizona 1984))
- Limits on punitive damages
- Abolishing the common law collateral source rule that allows damages to be recovered from third parties for losses already paid by first-party insurance (in other words, attempts to require damage awards to be reduced by the amounts received from collateral sources, such as health insurance, have not succeeded)
- Periodic payments of future damage awards (payment of awards periodically rather than in a lump sum)
- Limiting joint and several liability (requiring awards for injuries to be proportionately based on the health care provider's level of responsibility when more than one party may be liable for the injury)

States that have attempted to abolish the common law collateral-source rule have generally been struck down under equal protection concerns. *See e.g.*, *Coburn v. Agustin*, 627 F.Supp. 983 (U.S. District Court for the District of Kansas 1985); *Houk v. Furman*, 613 F.Supp. 1022 (U.S. District Court for the District of Maine 1985).

> *Moral Dilemmas*
> 1. Should there be a limit on the amount of damages permitted for non-economic pain and suffering, as distinguished from economic damages for costs, lost wages, etc.?

HOW MEDICAL MALPRACTICE OCCURS

Medical malpractice liability occurs when a health care provider engages in professional negligence or commits an intentional tort (Restatement, 1986). The core of a medical malpractice claim is that a health care provider failed to administer the care and skill ordinarily exercised by members of the medical profession practicing in the same or a similar location under similar circumstances.

The locality is a consideration because different locations have access to different resources; for instance, a hospital in a metropolitan area usually has access to better physicians and equipment than a hospital located in a remote or rural area. In other words, health care providers are expected to provide the best care possible based on the resources available to them.

While there are no national medical standards of care, the U.S. has moved away from the locality rule to a statewide level of reasonable skill and ability for practicing physicians. *See Gonzales v. Oregon*, 546 U.S. 243 (U.S. Supreme Court 2006) (holding that the federal government does not have the power to declare illegitimate medical standards for care specifically authorized under state laws).[LN1] Today, evidence-based clinical practice guidelines increasingly help define and establish medical standards of care. National guidelines published by the Agency for Healthcare Research and Quality (AHRQ), in partnership with the American Medical Association (AMA) and the American Association of Health Plans (AAHP), and available through the National Guideline Clearinghouse, help provide a shield against liability.

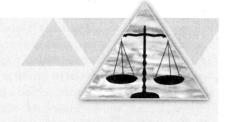

MEDICAL MALPRACTICE

Torres-Lazarini v. United States
[Patient v. Veterans Administration Hospital]
523 F.3d 69 (U.S. Court of Appeals for the 1st Circuit 2008)

FACTS: After Torres-Lazarini injured his shoulder in a fall, he went to the Veterans Health Administration (VA) hospital's emergency room in early September 2002 complaining of pain and limited range of motion and was treated by Dr. Rodriguez. Rodriguez examined his shoulder and ordered x-rays of the area. The x-rays revealed no damage from the fall, but did reveal a mild degenerative bone condition indicative of a precursor to osteoporosis. Torres-Lazarini was offered anti-inflammatory medication but refused it. Rodriguez suggested he apply ice to the shoulder and told him to return in two weeks if there was no improvement.

Torres-Lazarini returned to the VA with complaints of shoulder pain in mid-November 2002. Rodriguez examined the shoulder and concluded

that its condition had worsened. She offered to refer Torres-Lazarini to a physiatrist, a specialist who could determine if an MRI study was required and would recommend physical therapy, if appropriate. He turned down these suggestions. He returned to the VA again in December 2002 complaining of shoulder pain, but refused Rodriguez's offer to evaluate his shoulder.

In August 2004, he had another appointment with Rodriguez but refused further evaluation of his shoulder. Rodriguez recommended that he undergo an MRI, receive physical therapy, and schedule follow-up appointments. Torres-Lazarini underwent an MRI a few weeks later. The MRI revealed osteoarthritis and tearing of several tendons in the shoulder. The VA offered him surgery. Torres-Lazarini was told that although surgery

(continues)

(continued)

would not necessarily help restore his range of motion, it would ease his pain. He declined the surgery and sued the VA for malpractice.

At trial, an orthopedic surgeon who had never examined Torres-Lazarini testified that the VA breached its duty of care by failing to conduct an orthopedic evaluation shortly after the September 2002 fall and by waiting two years before conducting an MRI. He also testified that surgery soon after the accident would have restored his range of motion and alleviated his pain.

The VA presented the testimony of its expert, an orthopedic surgeon who physically examined Torres-Lazarini, asserting that severe osteoarthritis was causing the shoulder pain. He stated Rodriguez's recommendation of physical therapy was the proper treatment for loss of motion due to a dislocated shoulder. In addition, he testified that there was no breach of care because it was not standard practice to refer a patient with negative x-rays to an orthopedist. Rather, standard procedures were followed by immediately ordering x-rays, recommending a course of anti-inflammatory medication, and scheduling follow-up appointments. Finally, he stated that Rodriguez's recommendation that he receive evaluation from a physiatrist was proper.

ISSUE: Did the VA commit malpractice when it did not immediately order an MRI after x-rays came back negative?

HOLDING AND DECISION: No, Torres-Lazarini failed to prove that the VA committed malpractice; referral to a physiatrist to determine if an MRI was necessary was not a deviation from standard medical practice.

ANALYSIS: Professional negligence is defined as conduct "which falls below the standard established by law for the protection of others against unreasonable risk of harm" (Restatement, 1986). It generally arises from a failure to exercise the proper medical standard of care. The court found

the care Torres-Lazarini received for his shoulder was in full compliance with the standards of the medical profession for the type of soft tissue injury he suffered. While health care providers may still be found to have imposed an unreasonable risk on a patient even when they apply the standard diagnoses and carefully evaluate all possible medical treatments, the court also found that Torres-Lazarini refused the conservative treatment offered to him: he missed appointments, rejected physical therapy, and refused to cooperate with the VA in assessing and treating his shoulder injury.

Courts generally use the "but for" test to determine the existence of professional negligence. Courts use the substantial factor test when the "but for" test might allow each individual health care provider to escape responsibility because the conduct of one or more of the others would have been sufficient to produce the same result. Under the substantial factor test, a provider's conduct is a cause of the result if it is a substantial factor in bringing it about. In this case, Rodriguez was the only treating physician. Under the "but for" test, proximate cause is established when three elements are proven:

- Without the negligent action, the injury would not have occurred
- The injury is a natural and probable result of the negligence
- There is no other relevant intervening cause

While no negligence was found, the court noted the shoulder complications were caused by other intervening factors, such as age, multiple other falls, and degenerative joint illness, rather than by any negligent actions of the VA.

RULE OF LAW: When a medical malpractice claim alleges professional negligence against a health care professional with a duty to provide care, three elements must be demonstrated:

- Generally recognized medical standard of care
- Deviation from that standard
- The deviation was the cause of any injuries

MALPRACTICE MYTHS

The U.S. legal system's use of the tort system is often blamed for the lack of access to quality health care services due to the rising costs of liability insurance. The public is convinced there is a malpractice crisis due to excessive verdicts.

Myth: Medical Malpractice Costs Raise the Nation's Health Care Costs

The Congressional Budget Office found malpractice costs account for less than 2 percent of total health care spending. This may seem insignificant, until one realizes this is 2 percent of $2.8 trillion, the total spent on health care in 2008 (Keehan et al., 2008). The national cost of medical malpractice passed on to consumers now becomes approximately $50 billion (about $160 per capita).

In addition, the Congressional Budget Office estimated that a 25 to 30 percent reduction in malpractice costs would lower health care costs by less than half of 1 percent (about $12 billion). The likely effect on the nation's health care costs, however, would be comparably small (CBO, 2004). It seems that attention should be directed to areas where greater cost savings can be achieved. Malpractice costs are the red herring that diverts attention from the real issue of why many Americans lack access to quality health care. The health care delivery system has diverted its attention to the costs of medical malpractice, blaming the legal and insurance industries for the nation's rising health care costs, while failing to adequately address the costs associated with its own:

- Excessive administrative expenses
- Inappropriate care
- Inefficiencies
- Inflated prices
- Medical errors
- Poor management
- Waste and fraud

The total cost of medical malpractice is a valid cost to be examined, but this does not address the more important issue of how 98 percent of the "other" health care costs are being spent.

Myth: Malpractice Settlements Are Pervasive and Irrational

Research at the Harvard School of Public Health finds that more than 40 percent of all malpractice claims are not meritorious and most such claims are resolved without any payment of money (Studdert, 2006). Contrary to popular opinion, empirical research over the past two decades shows medical malpractice settlements are deliberate and rational. While the 1990 findings of the Harvard Medical Practice Study concluded that the merits of a malpractice claim have no bearing on the likelihood of a settlement, this finding is decidedly inconsistent with the growing body of empirical data accumulated by other researchers over the past two decades (Peters, 2007). Furthermore, no academic study has ever found a significant volume of frivolous malpractice claims (Hyman & Silver, 2005).

The amounts awarded to injured patients generally correlate to the merits of the underlying claims of professional negligence. Malpractice settlements are the product of an insurance-claims process that acts much like peer review in evaluating cases arising from

professional negligence or intentional torts. Insurance payments are:

- Most likely when the quality of medical care was inadequate
- Less likely when the quality of medical care was uncertain
- Least likely when the quality of medical care was high

In other words, settlement amounts are likely to be lowest when the quality of care was high, higher when care quality was too close to call, and highest when care quality was inadequate (Peters, 2007).

Moral Dilemmas

1. Should medical malpractice claims be permitted at all, or should physicians be permitted to make mistakes along with everyone else?

2. Should medical malpractice claims be permitted when the patient's initial need for medical care arose from the patient's own negligence or misconduct, such as an illegal drug overdose, an accident caused by driving under the influence, cancer due to smoking, etc.?

MEDICAL REVIEW PANELS

The idea of medical review panels is an example of disruptive regulation that first surfaced in the 1980s but did not survive judicial scrutiny. Different from peer review, these panels conduct preliminary hearings before a malpractice trial to determine the validity of the complaint. Recently, several regulatory proposals have taken on new life, the most notable being the proposal to establish a new complaint process for Medicare claimants.

Modifying Medicare's Complaint Process

Disruptive regulation could occur at key exchange points between the federal government and Medicare claimants to remove well-established but fundamentally misguided biases that diminish the effectiveness of Medicare (OIG, 2001). Faculty at Indiana University School of Law and the University of Texas at Austin have proposed a demonstration program for revamping Medicare's Quality Improvement Organizations (QIOs) entailing the use of medical review panels to:

- Hear and resolve real cases of medical injury
- Mediate discussions with patients

- Award reasonable compensation
- Provide feedback to participating health care providers regarding the safety and quality of their care

(*See* Peer Review Improvement Act of 1982, 42 U.S.C.A. §§ 1320c-1320c-12 (2009) (authorizing QIOs to handle beneficiary complaints; Kinney & Sage, 2008)

By modifying the complaint process for Medicare claimants, current peer review practices in both Medicare and conventional malpractice litigation could be constructively disrupted for a significant patient population. Restructuring the process between patient experience and system response would change the beneficiary complaint process from one that is relatively weak to one that could produce real results for meritorious Medicare claimants (IOM, 2006).

Financial Incentives Based on Quality and Efficiency

Opponents of Medicare's financial incentives posit several arguments: they maintain that not all patient complications (such as pressure ulcers, ventilator-associated pneumonia, and catheter-associated urinary tract infections) are necessarily reflective of medical errors or poor care, that complete avoidance of such conditions is impossible, and that complications generally occur with the sickest patients. The claim is providers will not want to care for the sickest patients, since they will be punished for the patient's poor health when complications arise. Providers can reduce the risk, but even with what is considered optimum care, bad things can happen.[LN2]

If Medicare aligned financial incentives with the dual goals of improving health care quality and efficiency (Davis & Guterman, 2007), this might enable collaborative quality improvement. For the first time since Medicare was established, health care providers might have the opportunity to promptly identify, resolve, and learn from medical errors as real malpractice cases are resolved through medical review panels (Hoffmann & Rowthorn, 2008).

NON-ECONOMIC DAMAGES CAPS

Non-economic damages caps appear to reduce premium growth (Danzon). States that have enacted caps on awards for non-economic damages have had significantly lower rates of malpractice premium increases than those without caps. For instance, in the late 1990s, general surgeons' medical malpractice premiums were increasing 75 percent each year in Dade County, Florida, but only 2 percent in Minnesota for a similar level of coverage (GAO, 2003). Determining non-economic damages is largely left to the discretion of the courts and juries, in particular. Such awards are often based on multiples of the economic damages (such as medical expenses, lost wages, rehabilitation costs); they are not discretionary, as claimed by many opponents of tort reform (Cohen, 2005).

Thirty-five states have placed limits on non-economic damages. Supporters maintain that caps balance the occasional need for lawsuits with the larger public need for affordable health care. According to the National Conference of State Legislatures, limits on malpractice awards have been adopted in all but fifteen states. Opponents are challenging non-economic damage caps (showing the principle that no tort reform is ever final), arguing that damage caps violate the separation of powers principle and the rights of juries. While these arguments have generally been unsuccessful, the challenges continue (Mello et al., 2008). Supporters counter by citing the rule of law that the legislative branch has always been able to alter common law remedies (whether in the form of changing laws by refusing to recognize punitive damages (Louisiana), shifting the burdens of proof, or limiting damage awards) (Nelson et al., 2008).

ENTRY AND EXIT RESTRICTIONS FOR THE LIABILITY INSURANCE INDUSTRY

Evidence on the role of aberrant pricing, in the severity of swings between hard liability insurance markets (when coverage is expensive and difficult to obtain) and soft markets (when coverage is plentiful and prices may become unrealistically low), supports the belief that insurers who undercharge, due to inexperience or excessive risk taking, contribute to excessive competition during soft markets. This has resulted in excessive price increases and insurer exits during a hard market. It is not the large insurance carriers with over one hundred years of experience selling policies and total assets in the hundreds of billions that start the atypical pricing cycles; rather it is the new players who simply have to show financial viability to enter today's insurance market (*see* Danzon et al., 2004).

It is only within the last decade of deregulation that insurance carriers were no longer required to provide performance guarantees and performance bonds to enter the industry. Appropriate regulatory policies must weigh the competitive benefits of easy entry and exit of new insurance businesses against the costs and disruption to the health industry of deviations from what is normal pricing of liability insurance. Some restrictions that are being returned to the books for the banking industry could also be applied to the insurance sector, such as:

- Activities restrictions and regulations
- Guidelines on capital maintenance and distributions of free cash flow
- Mandates requiring diversification of investments
- Regulation of management quality and investment policy

(Macey, 2006)

LIABILITY LIMITATIONS FOR INNOVATIVE AND EXPERIMENTAL MEDICAL TREATMENTS

The increasing pace of medical innovation and experimental treatments demands a better definition of malpractice. Physicians should not be liable, absent negligence, if cutting-edge treatments do not meet patient expectations (Fishman, 2004). Complicated medical procedures simply do not always work out due to their complexity.

The St. Paul Companies, the second largest U.S. commercial insurer, with business in forty states and covering one out of ten physicians in the nation, quit the medical malpractice business, citing millions in losses. St. Paul left the business after concluding it needed to raise its rates to break-even to a level where the premium increases would have accelerated the adverse selection for coverage. The environment was one in which the insurance mechanism had truly broken down (Fishman, 2004). The risk of a loss could no longer be equitably transferred from the insured to insurers, in exchange for a premium; guaranteed premiums could no longer prevent large, possibly devastating losses. For St. Paul and other insurers who either left the malpractice business or went bankrupt, it was an issue of solvency. They could simply no longer successfully manage the aberrant pricing and costs of medical malpractice. Unfortunately, St. Paul's departure decreased the incentive for others to keep malpractice rates competitive (Krella, 2007).

COMPENSATION BENCHMARKS FOR MALPRACTICE PAYOUTS

Recent research from the University of Pennsylvania and Stanford University on the value of a quality-adjusted life-year could be used in malpractice litigation, which has an impact on health care costs. For instance, the value of each life-year is about $129,000; therefore, in a case where negligence costs a patient ten years of life, a figure of $1.29 million could be used to begin settlement negotiations (Lee et al., 2009).[LN4]

Providing a benchmark is important, as it establishes a precedent for how compensation should be set. Increasing numbers of medical malpractice lawsuits have ended in higher payouts that have set new precedents. The costs of malpractice lawsuits, which are rising rapidly, have hurt the health care system in the sense that physicians and hospitals pay these costs and, ultimately, patients pay the bill (Lee et al., 2009). In addition, in order to avoid being hit with a malpractice lawsuit, physicians now:

- Practice defensive medicine, ordering excessive tests and treatments, which in turn drives up the overall cost of health care
- Curtail or halt their practice of medicine altogether
- Move their practice to more lucrative locations, leaving behind medically underserved areas
- Tailor their practice to a more lucrative specialty, resulting in a shortage of general practitioners

(AMA, 2005)

REDEFINING MALPRACTICE

While the benefits of enterprise liability far outweigh its disadvantages, there are differences on a number of issues, like the choice between hospitals and MCOs as the responsible enterprise. Regardless, it is agreed that there is a need for institutional, rather than individual, responsibility (Peters, 2007).

Boundaries of Liabilities

States must define the boundaries of vicarious liability. A Massachusetts case combined the duty to warn with the duty of care, which enlarges the field of physician liability (*see generally* Davis, 2008).

In practice, this decision raises the possibility that physicians may:

- Reconsider prescribing drugs they believe will be effective
- Over-warn patients about every conceivable side-effect of drugs, thereby deterring patients from taking their prescribed medications
- Be on notice of the consequences of prescribing drug cocktails that have never been clinically tested for their interactions together

Since physicians already owe a duty of care to patients, the decision does not impose a new duty, but perhaps unnecessarily expands a duty to non-patients

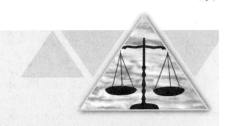

PHYSICIAN NEGLIGENCE

Coombes v. Florio

[Patient v. Accident Victim]

877 N.E.2d 567 (Supreme Court of Massachusetts 2007)

FACTS: Lyn-Ann Coombes brought this lawsuit on behalf of her ten-year-old son, Kevin Coombes, who was killed while standing on the sidewalk with a friend when David Sacca, a patient of Dr. Roland Florio, lost consciousness while driving and struck the boy when his car left the road. Coombes alleged the accident was a result of the side effects caused by the eight medications Florio prescribed to Sacca. By the date of the accident, Sacca was seventy-five years old and suffered from several serious medical conditions including asbestosis, chronic bronchitis, emphysema, high blood pressure, and metastatic lung cancer. While Florio had warned Sacca not to drive during his cancer treatments, he advised Sacca he could drive again when his treatments ended. Potential side effects of the combination of drugs Florio had prescribed to Sacca at the time of the accident included drowsiness, dizziness, lightheadedness, fainting, altered consciousness, and sedation.

Moreover, combining drugs often causes more severe side effects than the side effects resulting from individual use. The standard of care for a primary care physician includes warning elderly or chronically ill patients about the potential side effects of combination drugs, and their effect on a patient's ability to drive. Florio did not warn Sacca about any potential side effects of the various drugs prescribed or the possibility they could impair Sacca's ability to drive.

ISSUE: Does a physician's duty to warn patients of the side effects of drugs extend to foreseeable third-party non-patients?

HOLDING AND DECISION: Yes, the duty to warn extends to foreseeable third-party non-patients.

ANALYSIS: The court made clear this was an ordinary negligence claim and not a malpractice claim, which would require a direct physician-patient relationship. Florio was found negligent under ordinary common law negligence principles in prescribing drugs without warning Sacca of their potential side effects. The duty to warn extended

to Coombes because his injury was a foreseeable consequence of Florio's negligence.

To bring a negligence claim, Coombes had to show the existence of an act or omission that violated a duty owed to him by Florio. A precondition of the required duty is foreseeability, which is that the risk of the harm that occurred must have been foreseeable to Florio. Physicians have a duty of reasonable care, including the duty to warn their patients about side effects when prescribing drugs. When the side effects involved are likely to impair the patient's mental capacity, the foreseeable risk of injury in an automobile accident is not limited to the patient alone.

Turning to similar cases outside the medical context, the duty of reasonable care extends to all those involved when there is a foreseeable risk of an automobile accident. In addition, when the risk involved is large, it is irrelevant whether Florio did foresee, or should have foreseen, the particular circumstances even if Sacca was an intermediary actor.

The duty to warn patients about the effects of drugs has generally been limited to drugs taken in a physician's presence. This time, however, this distinction was not made. Instead, the court concluded the risk of potential side effects was foreseeable when the physician issued the prescription, regardless of where the drugs were taken. Finally, the court determined public policy favors imposing a duty on physicians under these circumstances, reasoning the duty will not impose a heavy burden on physicians because existing duties already require physicians to warn their patients of drug side effects. Additionally, the benefit of imposing the duty is significant because the duty protects the public from the foreseeable risk of known side effects impairing a patient's ability to drive.

In response to Florio's argument that fear of litigation arising from this duty would impose on a physician's decision about course of treatment, the court asserted the duty only involves warning a patient of side effects and does not imply negligence in choosing a course of medical treatment. Florio also argued increasing medical malpractice

(continues)

(continued)

rates are a strong reason against expanding a physician's duty to non-patients, but the court asserted that limiting physician liability to reduce medical malpractice rates is a decision best reserved for Congress and state legislatures.

When applying the foregoing analysis to the facts of this case, the court said the number and combination of drugs Sacca took increased the potential severity of any side effects and the likelihood that his driving ability would become impaired. The court further concluded that Florio owed a duty to all those foreseeably put at risk by his failure to warn, including Coombes. Ultimately, it will be a factual determination for a jury to decide whether Florio breached that duty, but the granting of summary judgment was inappropriately based on a

finding of no duty assigned to Coombes. Finally, the court clarified that Coombes did not assert Florio had any affirmative duty to control Sacca's actions and the claim asserted was limited to Florio's duty to warn Sacca of side effects. The court was clear that Florio was not the cause of Coombes's injury; Sacca was responsible for knowing how he was reacting to the medicines he was taking. The jury must decide what degree of responsibility, if any, was shared by Sacca's prescribing physician.

RULE OF LAW: The duty to warn patients of the side effects of drugs extends to non-patients foreseeably put at risk by a failure to warn.
(*See generally* Davis, 2008; Leonardo, 2008; Nicastro, 2008).

in ways that could become costly for the health care system (Davis, 2008). Physicians are not, in ordinary circumstances, legally responsible for the safety of others on the highway, or elsewhere, based on medical treatment afforded patients. The duty still resides with patients to know how drugs affect them; under this decision, however, some of that duty of care may be shifted to prescribing physicians. The decision enhances the duty-to-warn of the potential side effects of all drugs.

Enterprise Liability

Vicarious liability is an area of ever-expanding liability that arises under the common law doctrine of agency (*respondeat superior*). Any third person who has the right, ability, or duty to control the activities of a health care professional whose conduct resulted in an injury might be vicariously liable; all it takes is that the third party knew or should have known of the conduct and failed to take immediate and appropriate corrective action.

Enterprise liability could improve patient safety by changing existing laws to make hospitals or MCOs vicariously liable for the torts of individual physicians. While states will need to decide such issues as whether patient injuries occurring in outpatient facilities or those caused by medical errors during office visits following hospitalization should be covered by enterprise liability, these decisions are arguably relatively inconsequential. About 90 percent of the nation's malpractice claims arise out of medical care given inside hospitals (Peters, 2007).

In the rest of the health industry, the entity that delivers the medical products is vicariously liable for the errors of its workforce. Medical products manufacturers are liable for defective medical devices, not the individuals on the team who engineered the product. Liability is shifted entirely from individuals to the larger business enterprise. As a practical matter, the medical products industry operates under a system in which the enterprise bears all the costs of legal liability. By contrast, most malpractice claims are brought against physicians and other individual health care providers (Peters, 2007).

Corporate Practice Prohibitions

Private practice physicians have always been different. Unlike highly trained professionals in the pharmaceutical and medical device industry sectors, physicians have historically been treated as independent contractors, not employees, and have valued the independence associated with this status.

A century ago, when physicians feared that corporate employment of physicians would threaten the prevailing model of private practice, they successfully lobbied for enactment of corporate practice prohibitions. They have resisted corporate influence ever since, most recently in their alliance with patients to limit the power of HMOs (*see Davila*, 542 U.S. 200). However, physician independence has a cost.

Hospital-Based Physicians

Some states impose vicarious liability on hospitals for the conduct of physicians who are exclusively hospital-based, such as emergency medicine and anesthesiology physicians (*see generally* Lan, 2002).

VICARIOUS LIABILITY

Woodrum v. Johnson
[Patient v. Physician]
559 S.E.2d 908 (Supreme Court of West Virginia 2001)

FACTS: Timothy Woodrum brought a medical malpractice claim against Dr. Jerome Johnson for failing to properly diagnose and treat an infection-related empyema in his chest cavity. The lawsuit also named Monongalia General Hospital, since Johnson was an agent of the hospital and thus exposed the hospital to vicarious liability.

ISSUE: Do patients who settle with and release a physician from a lawsuit forsake their right to sue a hospital, whose only possible liability stems from the physician's actions?

HOLDING AND DECISION: No, patients who sue both a physician and a hospital, and then settle with the physician, do not release the hospital from possible vicarious liability.

ANALYSIS: Hospitals are barred from denying the agency status of physicians practicing in their emergency rooms. In settling with Johnson, Woodrum released the physician from his lawsuit against the hospital. The settlement agreement contained a specific provision reserving Woodrum's right to prosecute his cause of action against the hospital, including the claim that Johnson was the hospital's agent.

In response to the settlement between Woodrum and Johnson, the hospital filed a motion for summary judgment, arguing that because Johnson, an agent of the hospital, had been released from liability, the hospital could not be held liable. Specifically, the hospital argued the release of an agent should also release the principal, where the claim against the hospital is based solely upon agency.

While the court acknowledged technical differences between joint tortfeasors and those who are vicariously liable, there was no practical distinction between the two. Since Woodrum could originally have opted to sue only the hospital, the hospital is not prejudiced by a rule that permits Woodrum to proceed with the right to sue.

The second major argument made by the hospital was that allowing Woodrum to proceed against it would pave the way for a circular proceeding, since under the hospital's right to indemnity, any derivative action against it would ultimately be the responsibility of the physician. However, the fact that Johnson was released in a settlement has no bearing on the continued liability of the hospital unless the settlement was in full satisfaction of Woodrum's claims against both the physician and the hospital.

RULE OF LAW: A voluntary settlement with and release of a physician who is primarily liable for the patient's injury does not operate to release a hospital whose liability is vicarious.

While a 2001 state court decision, this was the first time West Virginia courts addressed this issue. This decision was subsequently followed in a non-medical case by the federal Fourth Circuit in 2005. A consensus, however, has not been reached in other trial-level jurisdictions.

Attending Physicians

Physicians who are not hospital-based are generally treated as independent contractors, rather than as agents or employees of the hospital. Hospitals therefore may escape vicarious liability for the errors of attending physicians.

Performance Improvement

Enterprise liability would more optimally use the resources hospitals or MCOs could bring to system quality activities. Only institutions can muster the resources to bring about systematic improvements in performance. Quality improvement theory, with its emphasis on systems design rather than individual fault, focuses on system strategies such as:

- Better monitoring of errors
- Thorough data analysis
- Examination of "hand-offs" and multi-person processes
- Accommodation of foreseeable human error

Hospitals and MCOs, of course, do not want any additional liability shifted to their organizations and often oppose enterprise liability. They are content with shifting liability onto individual providers, away from their institutions.

Anesthesiology Innovations

The power of enterprise liability is best illustrated by the reduction in anesthesia accidents in the late 1990s. It happened because Harvard was looking to lower the payouts made for anesthesia injuries in its nine teaching hospitals. Harvard's risk managers asked hospital anesthesiologists to investigate why their collective experience was so poor. As a result of their investigation, the anesthesiologists collectively devised new techniques and equipment to lower the risk of anesthesiology mishaps.

At the same time, the American Society of Anesthesiologists (ASA) conducted an intensive study of the causes of anesthesia-related injuries and developed better protocols (ASA, 2007). The improved standards of practice that resulted from these combined efforts have since become the medical standard of care. As a result, mortality rates from anesthesia accidents dropped from one in 10,000 to 20,000 to one in about 200,000 today, a ten- to twenty-fold improvement. Liability insurance premiums for the specialty of anesthesiology went from being among the highest in medicine to among the lowest.

These successful innovations in anesthesiology were prompted in part by the system of enterprise liability operating at Harvard. Like most medical schools, Harvard protected its anesthesiologists from the threat of liability by purchasing liability insurance on their behalf. Having done so, Harvard had a strong incentive to look for ways to bring down the cost of that insurance.

Risk Management

Today, the emphasis is on managing risks in health care systems, rather than focusing exclusively on the performance of individual health care providers. The greatest improvements in patient safety come from greater attention to the processes by which health care is delivered, since most medical errors are due to system breakdown not individual errors.

Greater attention to the system of delivery, rather than individual errors, enables risk managers to identify those stages of the process at which errors are most common and to redesign those stages to make errors both less common and more swiftly and effectively corrected. Accomplishing this objective requires both the capacity and the willingness to look at the entire health care delivery system. Hospital systems and MCOs are better situated to accomplish this than individual physicians.

Yet, the traditional system of individual physician liability greatly reduces the hospital's and MCO's incentive to take the necessary steps and then weather the possible backlash from physicians about interference with their discretion. Enterprise liability could produce that incentive.

Patient Safety

Many promising safety initiatives are led by hospitals and MCOs that already operate under a system of enterprise liability. For instance, the VA and Kaiser Permanente are leading an effort to improve diagnostic accuracy by using new tools, like computer decision-support systems, to:

- Help order correct tests
- Institute proper follow-up plans
- Obtain complete medical histories
- Perform adequate physical exams

The two hospitals at the forefront of patient safety voluntarily disclose errors: the VA hospital in Lexington, Kentucky, and the teaching hospital at the University of Michigan. Both hospitals also employ and insure their attending physicians (Landro, 2006).

Exclusive enterprise liability has two advantages regarding patient safety:

- The potential to increase physician participation in patient safety initiatives, along with physician willingness to disclose medical errors to patient safety committees. By eliminating individual liability, enterprise liability makes it easier for hospitals or MCOs to institute a blame-free culture that encourages open discussion of errors.
- Enterprise liability could permit physicians to discuss errors and near misses more freely. Enterprise liability is not risk-free; for instance, eliminating individual physician liability could theoretically dilute the effort physicians make to avoid patient injuries. Yet, that risk is already diluted by the availability of liability insurance that is not experience-rated and by the belief that physicians are not compensated for avoidance of patient injury.

(Peters, 2007)

Experience Rating

Hospitals or MCOs, unlike individual physicians, can be experience-rated. Insurance rates for hospitals or MCOs are based on actual claims rather than on the demographics of their geographic community (like individual physicians). Experience rating creates a powerful incentive to reduce medical errors. Health care causes far too many accidental injuries to avoid taking advantage of this potential to enhance patient safety.

While hospitals have an obvious financial reason to resist the transfer of legal responsibility entirely onto their shoulders, the issue is more complex for physicians. On the one hand, exclusive enterprise liability would take them out of the shadow of tort liability. On the other hand, physicians have traditionally opposed expanding hospital vicarious liability because they fear it will bring greater interference with their medical decision-making. Yet, this objection evokes a health care world that has long since passed. With rare exceptions, physicians already function as part of complex systems. Surely, physicians understand the importance of building those systems carefully. Furthermore, enterprise liability has existed in university hospitals and staff-model health maintenance organizations for many years.

Sooner or later, tort law must adapt. In hindsight, it is now obvious that the law's delay in doing so has been harmful for both physicians and patients, keeping individual physicians on the front line of malpractice litigation and depriving patients of the safety systems that enterprise liability will produce.

ADMINISTRATIVE HEALTH COURTS

There is increased momentum to take medical malpractice cases out of civil courts and assign them to administrative health courts modeled after the Social Security Administration hearings and appeals program (Peters, 2007). Congress has proposed legislation authorizing the creation of such specialized courts and legislation has also been proposed in about half a dozen states.[LN5] *See* Fair and Reliable Medical Justice Act, S. 1481, 110th Congress § 1 (2007); Fair and Reliable Medical Justice Act, H.R. 2497, 110th Congress § 1 (2007). Experiments with administrative health courts have also been recommended by the Institute of Medicine (IOM) and the American Medical Association (AMA, 2005).

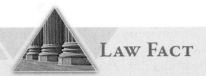

LAW FACT

TORT REMEDIES FOR MEDICARE CLAIMANTS

Should a Medicare beneficiary be required to reimburse the federal government for medical expenses paid by Medicare after winning a settlement for a defectively designed product?

No, while this case was the first federal appellate court to address this issue, it illustrates the government's refusal to accept the weight of jurisprudence comprising at least seven judicial rejections of its repeated attempts to have the MSP law construed beyond its plain terms.

—*Thompson v. Goetzmann*, 337 F.3d 489 (U.S. Circuit Court of Appeals for the 5th Circuit 2003).

CHAPTER SUMMARY

- Medical malpractice claims are civil wrongs caused by negligence or intentional conduct that cause harm to patients for which patients may sue for damages.
- Malpractice claims are blamed for some of the difficulties the U.S. health care system faces, such as quality of health care and relative health of patients being lower than that of similar countries, despite spending more per capita on health care.
- It is suggested that the focus be shifted to preventing injury or harm in the first place and away from the medical malpractice system in order to improve quality and cost-effectiveness.
- Liability insurance rates are highest in states where tort reform has not occurred.
- Some suggestions for reforming tort law include the implementation of medical review panels, pain and suffering damage caps, limited liability for experimental treatments, enterprise liability, and specialized administration health courts.
- To prove a medical malpractice claim, three elements must be demonstrated: (1) a generally recognized medical standard of care, (2) deviation from that standard, and (3) the deviation was the cause of any injuries.
- In reality, medical malpractice costs account for less than 2 percent of health care spending and a reduction in such costs would have little effect on premiums or quality of care.
- Contrary to popular belief, medical malpractice awards are generally rational and deliberate, and not usually obtained when the claim is frivolous or lacks merit.
- Despite the legal challenges that the idea of medical review panels has faced, the idea is still pursued by Medicare and states as a method of reducing medical malpractice litigation.

- Medical malpractice claims may be pressed by those other than the patient who were foreseeably harmed by the patient's medical treatment, or lack thereof.
- The greatest improvements in patient safety come from greater attention to risk management, since most medical errors are due to system failures rather than individual errors.
- Although enterprise liability may eliminate individual physician liability, it has the potential to greatly improve patient safety by increasing physician participation in patient safety initiatives and encouraging open disclosure and resolution of medical errors.

LAW NOTES

1. While health care providers, in fact, collectively set medical standards of care, at least three practical realities dispel the notion of national standards. First, there is the practical difficulty of proving exactly what the prevailing medical standard is, since the standard is generally custom-based for each patient. Second, to the extent the medical standard of care is ascertained, by continuing to give such medical care, providers are creating and perpetuating the very standard with which they may not want to comply. Third, medicine is regulated at the state level where physicians, nurse practitioners, and other health care professionals are licensed to practice within a certain locality.

2. The argument against Medicare's financial incentives is that it is too little, too late. Most non-Medicare markets already bear 100 percent of the financial costs of any medical errors.

   For instance, Medicare reimburses health care providers on a fee-for-service basis. This means that if a provider makes a mistake that injures a patient and the patient requires follow-up care, Medicare will pay for both the care that caused the injury and the follow-up care. Medicare thus rewards medical errors with extra payments. The Medicare Payment Advisory Commission acknowledges providers are paid more when quality is worse, such as when medical complications occur as the result of medical error. Medicare recently acknowledged this problem and no longer reimburses providers for hospital services attendant to hospital-acquired conditions (such as catheter-associated urinary tract infections) or hospital or physician services improperly delivered (such as performing the wrong test on a patient or a duplicate test).

   One alternative to fee-for-service Medicare is the adoption of Medicare prepaid group plans. Medicare would give health care providers a flat amount per Medicare recipient. When combined with an integrated delivery system, where the hospital and all the physicians work for the same entity, prepayment places the cost of avoidable medical errors squarely on providers. Following a medical error, the providers themselves have to pay the cost of any additional care. Under fee-for-service payment, providers lose money if they reduce medical errors; under prepayment, providers profit by reducing errors (Starr, 1984). This is how the Veterans Heath Administration operates.

3. At least twenty-three states have adopted medical review panels: Delaware Code Ann. tit. 18, §§ 6802, 6808, 6811 (1999) (restricted to medical negligence with authority to subpoena witnesses, administer oaths, and compel the production of documents; panel's outcome may shift the burden of proof at trial); Florida Stat. Ann. §§ 766.107, 766.209 (2005) (excludes admission of the arbitration result at trial and panel members may not be called to testify at trial; penalizes parties who reject their opponent's offer to arbitrate by limiting the amount or type of damages recoverable at trial); Hawaii Rev. Stat. §§ 671-12, 671-16 (2005) (excludes admission of the arbitration result at trial and panel members may not be called to testify at trial; no statement made in the course of the panel hearing shall be admissible in evidence either as an admission, to impeach the credibility of a witness, or for any other reason); Idaho Code Ann. § 6-1001 (2004) (informal and nonbinding arbitration, but nonetheless compulsory as a condition precedent to litigation); Indiana Code Ann. §§ 34-18-8-4, -6; 34-18-10-23 (1998) (requires panel review before filing any lawsuit involving more than $15,000; panel opinion is admissible at trial); Kansas Stat. Ann. §§ 65-4901, 65-4904 (2002) (panel must issue an opinion that is admissible at trial and either party may subpoena any member of the panel as a witness at trial); Louisana Rev. Stat. Ann. § 40:1299.47 (2007) (expert opinions are admissible at trial, but they are not conclusive and either party has the right to call any member of the panel as a witness at trial); Maine Rev. Stat. Ann. tit. 24, §§ 2851, 2852, 2857 (2000) (only unanimous panel findings are admissible at trial) and § 2853(5) (2006) (forbidding the panel to decide dispositive legal affirmative defenses and comparative negligence); Maryland Code Ann., Cts. & Jud. Proc. § 3-2A-06(d) (2006) (arbitration award is admissible at trial; the burden is on the party rejecting it to prove that it is not correct); Massachusetts Ann. Laws ch. 231, § 60B (2000) (panel opinion is admissible at trial and panel members may be called as witnesses at trial); Michigan Comp. Laws Ann. §§ 600.4915-4919 (2000) (compulsory mediation); Nebraska. Rev. Stat.

§§ 44-2840, 44-2841, 44-2844(2) (2004) (voluntary arbitration); Montana Code Ann. §§ 27-6-701, 27-6-704 (2005) (requiring panel review before filing any lawsuit and requiring nondisclosure of panel proceedings at trial); New Mexico Stat. Ann. §§ 41-5-15, 41-5-20 (1996) (requiring panel review before filing any lawsuit and requiring nondisclosure of panel proceedings at trial); Nebraska Rev. Stat. §§ 44-2840, 44-2841, 44-2844(2) (2004) (voluntary arbitration); Ohio Rev. Code Ann. § 2711.21 (2000) (nonbinding arbitration; requiring nondisclosure of panel proceedings at trial); Utah Code Ann.

§§ 78-14-12(1)(c), 78-14-15(1)-(2) (2002) (informal and nonbinding, but nonetheless compulsory as a condition precedent to litigation; requiring nondisclosure of panel proceedings at trial; panel members may not be called to testify at trial); Virginia. Code Ann. § 8.01-581.2 (2006) (allowing any party to convene a review panel) and § 8.01-581.8 (2000) (permitting admission of the panel opinion at trial and the right to call panel members as witnesses at trial); Vermont. Stat. Ann. tit. 12, § 7002 (2002) (voluntary arbitration); Wisconsin Stat. Ann. §§ 655.44(5), 655.465, 655.58 (2004) (requiring panel review before filing any lawsuit); Wyoming Stat. Ann. § 9-2-1518(a) (2005) (requiring panel review before filing any lawsuit and requiring nondisclosure of panel proceedings at trial).

4. The most commonly used benchmarks for the value of a quality-adjusted life-year are based on end-stage renal disease, the one disease for which Medicare has provided universal health care services since the 1970s. Recent cost-effectiveness analysis shows that, on average, $129,000 is spent per quality-adjusted life-year on each kidney dialysis patient suffering from this disease.

5. Maryland, New York, Oregon, Pennsylvania, and Virginia. *See* S. 508, 422d Gen. Assem., Reg. Sess. (Maryland, 2007) (establishing a medical liability division in circuit courts); H.B. 779, 422d Gen. Assem., Reg. Sess. (Maryland, 2007) (creating a task force to study the creation of a medical liability division within the Maryland circuit courts on the model of an existing, separate case management system for business and technology cases); H.B. 338, 422d Gen. Assem., Reg. Sess. (Maryland, 2007) (establishing a task force to study administrative compensation programs for birth-related neurological injury); H.B. 48, 422d Gen. Assem., Reg. Sess. (Maryland, 2007) (creating a medical malpractice review board of trained judges with the authority to hire neutral experts). *See also* S. 4149, 2007 Leg., 230th Sess. (New York, 2007) (authorizing health court pilot projects within the court system); S. 655, 74th Leg., Reg. Sess. (Oregon, 2007); S. 678, 2007 Gen. Assem., Reg. Sess. (Pennsylvania. 2007) (authorizing a demonstration program to examine an administrative medical liability system); S. J. Res. 90, 2006 Sess. (Virginia, 2006); H.R.J. Res. 183, 2006 Sess. (Virginia, 2006) (providing for continuance of the Joint Subcommittee to Study Risk Management Plans for Physicians and Hospitals, which is investigating the feasibility of establishing a pilot health court and subsequently a system of health courts).

CHAPTER BIBLIOGRAPHY

AMA (American Medical Association). (2005). *America's medical liability crisis*. Washington, DC: AMA.

ASA (American Society of Anesthesiologists). (2007). *ASA standards, guidelines and statements*. Park Ridge, IL: ASA.

Avraham. R. (2007). Current research on medical malpractice liability: An empirical study of the impact of tort reforms on medical malpractice settlement payments. *Journal of Legal Studies, 36*, 183-223 (first study to systematically explore the impact of tort reform on settlements).

___. (2006). *Law and economics research paper: Database of state tort law reforms* (DSTLR, 2nd ed.). Chicago, IL: Northwestern University School of Law.

___. (2006a). Putting a price on pain-and-suffering damages: A critique of the current approaches and preliminary proposal for change. *Northwestern University Law Review, 100*, 87-119.

Black's Law Dictionary (9th ed.). (2009) Eagan, MN: Thomson Reuters West Publishing Co.

Christensen, C. M. et al. (2009). *The innovator's prescription: A disruptive solution for health care*. New York, NY: McGraw-Hill.

Cohen, H. (2005). *CRS (Congressional Research Service) report for Congress: Medical malpractice liability reform: Legal issues and fifty-state survey of caps on punitive damages and noneconomic damages*. Washington, DC: CRS. (summarizing the law in all fifty states)

CBO (Congressional Budget Office). (2004). *Limiting tort liability for medical malpractice*. Washington, DC: CBO.

Currie, J., & MacLeod, W. B. (2006). *NBER working paper: First do no harm? Tort reform and birth outcomes*. Cambridge, MA: National Bureau of Economic Research.

Danzon, P. M. et al. (2004). *The "crisis" in malpractice insurance*. Research paper prepared for the Seventh Annual Brookings-Wharton Conference on Financial Services: Public Policy Issues Confronting the Insurance Industry at the Wharton School of the University of Pennsylvania, Philadelphia, PA.

Davies, J. (2007). Reforming the tort reform agenda. *Washington University Journal of Law & Policy, 25*, 119-159.

Davis, K., & Guterman, S. (2007). Rewarding excellence and efficiency in Medicare payments. *Milbank Quarterly, 95* (3), 449-468 (maintaining Medicare should align financial incentives with the dual goals of improving health care quality and efficiency).

Davis, M. (2008). Physician negligence: The Supreme Judicial Court of Massachusetts extends duty to warn patients of side effects of prescriptions to foreseeable third parties: *Coombes v. Florio. American Journal of Law & Medicine, 34,* 87-90.

Fishman, J. chairman and chief executive officer of St. Paul Companies, Inc. (2004, January 8). Seventh Annual Brookings-Wharton Conference on Financial Services: Public policy issues confronting the insurance industry at the Wharton School of the University of Pennsylvania, Philadelphia, PA.

GAO (General Accountability Office). (2003). *Malpractice insurance: Multiple factors have contributed to premium rate increases.* Washington, DC: GAO.

Harvard Medical Practice Study. (1990). *Patients, doctors, and lawyers: Medical injury, malpractice litigation, and patient compensation in New York: A report by the Harvard Medical Practice Study to the State of New York.* Albany, NY: New York State Department of Health (a study widely relied upon by tort critics).

Hoffmann, D. E., & Rowthorn, V. (2008). Achieving quality and responding to consumers: The Medicare beneficiary complaint process: Who should respond? *Indiana Health Law Review, 5,* 9-51.

Hyman, D. A., & Silver, C. (2005). The poor state of health care quality in the U.S, is malpractice liability part of the problem or part of the solution? *Cornell Law Review, 9,* 893-993.

IOM (Institute of Medicine). (2006). *Medicare's quality improvement organization program: Maximizing potential.* Washington, DC: IOM.

JCAHO (Joint Commission on Accreditation of Health Care Organizations). (2005). *Health care at the crossroads: Strategies for improving the medical liability system and preventing patient injury.* Chicago. IL: JCAHO.

Kaiser (Kaiser Commission on Medicaid & the Uninsured). (2007). *Enrolling uninsured low-income children in Mediaid and SCHIP.* Washington, DC: Kaiser.

Keehan, S. et al. (2008). Health spending projections through 2017. *Health Affairs, 27* (2) 146-155.

Kinney, E. D., & Sage, W. M. (2008). Dances with elephants: Administrative resolution of medical injury claims by Medicare claimants. *Indiana Health Law Review, 5,* 1-7.

Klick, J., & Stratmann, T. (2007). Does medical malpractice reform help states retain physicians and does it matter? *Journal of Legal Studies, 36* (S2), S121-S142.

Krella, J. C. (2007). Legislative malpractice: An analysis of Ohio's proposed mandatory medical malpractice arbitration program. *Dayton Law Review, 33,* 119-143.

Lan, I. (2002). Malpractice: Suit against hospital for vicarious liability allowed despite settlement with physician. *Journal of Law, Medicine & Ethics, 30,* 117-118.

Landro, L. (2006, November 29). The informed patient: Preventing the tragedy of misdiagnosis. *Wall Street Journal,* p. D1.

___. (2004, February 12). The informed patient: Preventive medicine gets more aggressive. *Wall Street Journal,* p. D1.

Lee, C. P. et al. (2009). An empiric estimate of the value of life: Updating the renal dialysis cost-effectiveness standard. *Value in Health, 12* (1), 80-87.

Leonardo, T. J. (2008). Tort law: Extending physician's duty of care to third parties for breach of duty owed to patient: *Coombes v. Florio,* 877 N.E.2d 567 (Mass. 2007). *Suffolk University Law Review, 42,* 277-284.

Letter from Dave Freudenthal, Governor of Wyoming, to the State of Wyoming Legislative Joint Judiciary Interim Committee & Joint Health, Labor, and Social Services Interim Committee (2004, June 21).

Macey, J. R. (2006). Commercial banking and democracy: The illusive quest for deregulation. *Yale Journal of Regulation, 23,* 1-27.

Mello, M. M. et al. (2008). Policy experimentation with administrative compensation for medical injury: Issues under state constitutional law. *Harvard Journal on Legislation, 45,* 59-105.

Nelson III, L. J. et al. (2008). Medical malpractice reform in three southern states. *Journal on Health & Biomedical Law, 4,* 9-151

Nicastro, D. P. (2008). Physician liability to non-patients: *Coombes v. Florio,* 450 Mass. 182 (2007). *Boston Bar Journal, 52,* 20-21.

OIG (Office of Inspector General). (2001). *The Medicare beneficiary complaint process: A rusty safety valve.* Washington, DC: U.S. Department of Health & Human Services, OIG.

Pauly, M. V., & Herring, B. (2007). Risk pooling and regulation: Policy and reality in today's individual health insurance market. *Health Affairs, 26* (3), 770-780.

Peters, P. G. (2007). What we know about malpractice settlements. *Iowa Law Review, 92,* 1783–1833 (comprehensively reviewing the empirical literature that tests the correlation between jury verdicts and evidence of negligence).

Restatement of the Law Second, Torts 2d. (1986). Washington, DC: American Law Institute.

Rabin, R. L. (2006). Pain and suffering and beyond: Some thoughts on recovery for intangible loss. *DePaul Law Review, 55,* 359-377.

Rubin, P., & Shepherd, J. (2005). *Emory law and economics research paper: Tort reform and accidental deaths.* Atlanta, GA: Emory University School of Law.

Schumpeter, J. A. (2008). *Capitalism, socialism, and democracy.* New York, NY: Harper Perennial Modern Classics (original 1942) (classic economics text that introduced the concept of *creative destruction*).

Sharkey, C. M. (2005). Unintended consequences of medical malpractice damages caps. *New York University Law Review, 80,* 391-512.

Silver, C. et al. (2006). *Georgetown law and economics research paper: Physicians' insurance limits and malpractice payouts: Evidence from Texas closed claims.* Washington, DC: Georgetown University Law Center.

Starr, P. (1984). *The social transformation of American medicine.* New York, NY: Basic Books (while more than twenty years old, this Pulitzer-prize winning text is a landmark in history).

Studdert, D. M. et al. (2007). Disclosure of medical injury to patients: An improbable risk management strategy. *Health Affairs, 26,* 215-226.

___ (2006). Claims, errors, and compensation payments in medical malpractice litigation. *New England Journal of Medicine, 35* (19), 2024-2033.

Swedloff, R. (2008). Can't settle, can't sue: How Congress stole tort remedies from Medicare claimants. *Akron Law Review, 41,* 558-607.

Thorpe, K. E. et al. (2007) Differences in disease prevalence as a source of the U.S.-European health care spending gap. *Health Affairs, 26* (6), 678-686.

Viscusi, W. K., & Born, P. H. (2005). Damages caps, insurability, and the performance of malpractice insurance. *Journal of Risk & Insurance, 72,* 23-43.

Wharton (Wharton School at the University of Pennsylvania). (2008). Cost-effective medical treatment: Putting an updated dollar value on human life. *Knowledge@Wharton.*

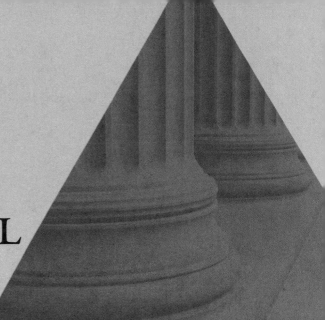

PART V

DEVELOPMENT OF HUMAN CAPITAL

CHAPTER 11

HUMAN RESOURCES DEPARTMENTS

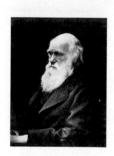

"It is not the strongest of the species that survives, nor the most intelligent; it is the one that is most adaptable to change."

—ATTRIBUTED TO CHARLES DARWIN (1809-1882), ENGLISH NATURALIST

IN BRIEF

Human resources (HR) departments are an essential partner in building many of the law topics in this text, from compliance and ethics programs to developing policies that ensure the health industry adheres to its social missions. This chapter addresses two fundamental ways of viewing HR: as a legal and technical department that works directly with senior management, providing crucial input into major business transactions, and focused on recruiting talent, promoting mobility and career development, and improving organizational effectiveness, versus the traditional role of administrators that involved many responsibilities that are now being outsourced. The need for the health industry to become more strategy-driven is emphasized in terms of the issues of pay and performance and management development.

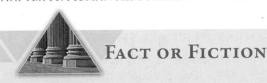

FACT OR FICTION

EXECUTIVE COMPENSATION

What should be the role of human resources when examining executive compensation?

Dr. William McGuire, the former chief executive officer (CEO) and chairman of the board of directors of UnitedHealth Group, departed from the company at the board's request after he illegally obtained executive compensation by backdating stock options worth over $1 billion. Backdating stock options brings an instant paper gain, which is equivalent to extra pay and thus is a cost to the company; failure to recognize this cost may mean the company has overstated its profits, possibly necessitating a restatement of past financial results (Forelle & Bandler, 2006). Backdating, in and of itself, is not illegal as long as it is authorized, fully disclosed and reported, and in keeping with tax rules (Narayanan et al., 2007). At his departure, Dr. McGuire was a named defendant in numerous class-action lawsuits: shareholder suits and federal securities class actions. In addition to the $1 billion, McGuire claimed United owed him millions in additional executive compensation.

The Securities and Exchange Commission filed its own lawsuit, which was settled when the board's Special Litigation Committee's report was released. McGuire agreed to settle the securities lawsuit against him by returning over $470 million to UnitedHealth and paying a $7 million civil fine, likely the largest securities fine ever assessed. In September of 2008, the shareholder lawsuits were settled when McGuire paid an additional $30 million in fines, returned over $3 million in unexercised stock options, and disgorged over $11 million in incentive-based cash bonuses received over the last two years of his employment; UnitedHealth paid over $895 million to shareholders.

—*In re UnitedHealth Group Inc. Shareholder Derivative Litigation,* 754 N.W.2d 544 (Supreme Court of Minnesota 2008); *In re UnitedHealth Group Incorporated PSLRA Litigation,* 2007 WL 1621456 (U.S. District Court for the District of Minnesota 2007); Forelle & Bandler, 2006; Wilmer Culter, 2006. (See *Law Fact* at the end of this chapter for the answer.)

PRINCIPLES AND APPLICATIONS

This chapter uses the term *human resources* rather than *work and employment relations* to better reflect the neutral perspective of this chapter and the need to fairly balance the needs of the employee and the employer. There are two different views of HR in the health industry. According to its critics, HR departments can be needlessly bureaucratic, obstructionist, stuck in the comfort zone of filling out forms and explaining organization benefits, too closely aligned with the interests of management, yet lacking the business knowledge to be effective strategic partners (Sirota et al., 2005). Dealing with this type of HR department is difficult. When employees are asked to rate the quality of different functions within their organization, this type of HR is repeatedly rated the lowest (Wharton, 2005).

The more positive view of HR is that it works directly with senior management, providing crucial input into major business transactions, such as mergers and acquisitions and restructurings. In this

scenario, HR departments have moved away from the traditional role of administrators, as many of those responsibilities are now outsourced, and toward a more creative focus on their primary role, including:

- Recruiting talent
- Promoting mobility and career development
- Improving organizational effectiveness

Unless HR reports to the CEO of the organization, the priorities of HR are likely set in the wrong direction and driven by inappropriate and ineffective motivators. For example, if HR reports to the chief financial officer, then HR and the organization are not in the best position to be successful in today's competitive health care market (Wharton, 2005). HR must be in a strategic position to affect and execute policy, not simply further down the organization's hierarchy and relegated to performing administrative functions and support services.

DEFINING THE ROLE OF HUMAN RESOURCES IN THE HEALTH INDUSTRY

Beginning in the 1920s, HR was a way to advocate for and protect employees, an orientation that became quite explicit in the 1950s and beyond as part of an effort by the health industry to prevent unionization. More recently, however, and especially over the past decade, the social contract between employees and employers, under which employers provided lifetime employment to their employees in return for loyalty and commitment to the employer, has ended.

Currently the health industry is pushing more and more work onto employees, and HR departments are becoming the mechanism for accomplishing this goal. As a result, the idea that HR represents employees, or at least deals objectively with their concerns, is obsolete. In addition, with the health industry continuing to cut back employee benefits, HR departments have increasingly found themselves serving as the bearers of bad news to employees.

Meanwhile, HR issues are very much a part of press coverage:

- The CEO of Ascension Health earned $2.4 million in salary compensation at the country's largest nonprofit hospital system, while Ascension closes money-losing hospitals in poor urban areas from Los Angeles to Chicago to Newark, New Jersey, where a large share of patients are uninsured
- The University of Pittsburgh Medical Center paid its chief executive more than $3.3 million, plus almost $37,000 from the hospital to cover a car allowance, spousal travel, and legal and financial counseling
- In Chicago, Northwestern Memorial Hospital's former CEO, Gary Mecklenburg, received a $16.4 million payout in 2006, while less than 2 percent of the hospital's revenues went to charity care
- The University of California San Francisco Medical Center provided its CEO and its chief operating officer low-interest mortgage loans of more than $1 million each
- The Cleveland Clinic continued to pay its former CEO, Floyd Loop, more than $1 million a year in deferred compensation, vacation pay, and consulting services, for two years after he retired

(Carreyrou & Martinez, 2008)

Moral Dilemmas

1. Why does the Conference Board survey of HR directors report job satisfaction in the U.S. health industry at its lowest level ever?

BUSINESS PARTNERSHIP

Looking at the history of HR in the health industry, changes usually require about a decade to take hold, such as:

- Outsourcing of administrative functions
- Establishing health care call centers and service centers
- Integrating work-life balance issues

For instance, most health care organizations are trying to more rapidly transform HR into a business partner, with less emphasis on those administrative functions that can be outsourced. To achieve this, it is vital to help key HR professionals accelerate their development of business skills. Many hospitals and medical products companies are doing this, but not very fast. There remains a tremendous attraction within HR to the comfort zone of more traditional and functional support-service relationships.

Strategic Mergers and Acquisitions

The number of mergers and acquisitions of health care services organizations rose rapidly throughout the 1990s, peaking at over 1,300. However, as merged entities confronted management difficulties, the number of mergers and acquisitions fell, dropping to its lowest level in 2003 at about four hundred, before returning to the typical range of five hundred per year (Levin, 2009). The classic area where HR departments can provide strategic input is anticipating these mergers and acquisitions. A very well-defined set of HR opportunities and experiences exists in these areas:

- Assistance in valuing mergers and acquisitions
- Developing integration plans
- Communicating with employees
- Matching talent

Some HR departments play a key role here. In others, they are still observers. For instance, mergers and acquisitions often involve crucial decisions about the future of the small health care organization.

One controversial area where HR departments play a critical communications role involves the mergers of Catholic and non-Catholic hospitals. Such mergers generally result in the elimination of most reproductive health services, including not only abortion, but sterilization, birth control drugs and devices, and in vitro fertilization. In California and the Midwest, where mergers between Catholic and non-Catholic hospitals have become increasingly prevalent, access to reproductive health services for isolated rural and economically disadvantaged areas has become a problem. Legislation has therefore been proposed in some states that, among other things, would expressly require all hospitals to provide a full range of reproductive health services as a condition of government funding and merger approval (Stabile, 2007). HR becomes entangled in issues of accommodating Catholic employees who do not want to be involved in the delivery of selected reproductive health services as a matter of conscience, as well as whether Catholic hospitals have to employ the employees from the non-Catholic hospital who practice or hold views contrary to Catholic teaching. Then, there is the separate issue of fostering tolerance of Catholic employees who hold differing religious views of health issues.

Operational Return on Investment

Over the last ten to fifteen years, HR has begun to have a serious impact on how the health industry operates. To put this in perspective, AstraZeneca had about $20.4 billion of non-interest expenses in 2007. Of that, more than $11 billion was related to personnel, including:

- Salaries
- Incentive plans
- Fringe benefits
- Talent retention programs
- Risk management strategies

If HR can effectively manage those dollars, with the goal of the highest possible return on human investment, the HR department will approach opportunities much differently.

Under this scenario, the HR department would have the operational mandate of:

- Growing revenue
- Increasing productivity
- Developing leadership

To effectively meet this mandate, the HR department should look very similar to any other high-level department in terms of employee skill-level. So, when HR participates in meetings with other departments, HR has the capability to talk about the business of delivery of health care services or medical products rather than focusing on HR alone.

Net Supplier of Management Talent

The HR department should be comprised of business managers and business partners, management professionals who can address the often unspoken critical facts regarding who is best qualified to be responsible for revenue production. HR managers should be included on replacement charts for other areas of the organization when management opportunities arise (when managers are replaced, the replacements should come from within HR departments versus the traditional approach of hiring new managers

from outside organizations). One of the goals of HR should be to serve as a net supplier of management talent; HR is where managers are trained, gain knowledge of the business, and become skilled at understanding how all parts of the organization contribute to the whole. HR professionals should have the ability to move into managing any part of the organization (Wharton, 2005).

Direct Tie-in with Strategic Development

Without the direct tie to strategy, there is no context for HR to work within. HR practice should be completely focused on aligning policies and procedures to the overall strategy of the health care organization. For instance, if a health care system converts from a nonprofit to a profit organization with private equity owners, a radical cultural shift occurs. HR must take the current set of HR practices and ensure they are consistent with organizational goals. At the simplest level, this means redesigning pay systems, not to increase employee pay, but to restructure the system to include smaller amounts of fixed compensation and to base pay largely on performance.

Cafeteria-Style Benefits

The health industry increasingly offers a cafeteria-style benefits approach. From flexible spending arrangements to health savings accounts to health reimbursement arrangements, cafeteria benefits are more suited to the type of consumer-driven organization most health care organizations strive to be (*Federal Register,* 2007). In this benefits approach, employees occupy the primary decision-making role regarding the type of benefits they receive.

Recruiting goals may have to shift and the way new employees are socialized may have to change. Nevertheless, HR can do much to align its mission from the employee point of view with the strategy of the health care organization. HR can help train employees to become more skilled at learning to take charge of their own lives, and to be more entrepreneurial and cost-conscious about the employee benefits they and their families need.

Leadership Development

Many CEOs see HR as the most critical function in any health care organization. Development of managers is the ultimate responsibility of every CEO and thus an integral part of HR. It is the responsibility of HR to allocate employees and dollars to opportunities. The CEO does not provide health care services or deliver medical products; the responsibility of the chief executive is placing employees in the right jobs, in partnership with HR.

To effectively meet this responsibility in partnership with the CEO, HR evaluation systems should be:

- Rigorous
- Non-bureaucratic
- Monitored as closely as financial reporting

While many HR professionals state their role is to serve as a strategic partner with senior management, critics question whether this is possible, given that HR departments often lack the business skills to understand strategy or their role in implementing it. Furthermore, some senior managers are not interested in having HR as a strategic partner; they simply want the department to hire the employees they (the managers) want. If top management does not see value in aligning strategically with HR, and if HR cannot think creatively in that role, then the partnership will likely never happen.

Of course, becoming a partner with senior management does not always happen immediately. The HR department must earn its way to the table. The key question should always be whether HR is successful at helping move the organization in the direction it wants to go. To do this, HR has a number of strategic imperatives, such as:

- Hiring the right employees in the right place at the right time
- Looking for breadth and depth of leadership talent within the organization
- Maintaining the right culture for the organization
- Risk mitigation
- Operational excellence

To meet these imperatives, HR should be out among the employees, patients, and the insurers, providing feedback on the pulse of the organization. Senior management must see HR as very valuable, especially in the areas of professional development and succession plans.

Branding
HR's influence should also extend beyond the HR department. Outside of the marketing function, HR has one of the biggest responsibilities related to branding (Wharton, 2005).

For example, every year the American health industry hires more than three hundred thousand employees externally, according to the U.S. Bureau of Labor Statistics Office of Occupational Statistics and Employment Projections. This is a branding opportunity to associate 1.5 to 3 million additional people with a health care service or medical product from a specific health care organization. As a rule of thumb, for every person hired, five to ten additional people hear detailed information and develop personal impressions about the employer (Wharton, 2005).

Each time HR interviews someone, it should look for talent that can be developed. The interviewee, in turn, has a chance to see the health industry from an insider's perspective. This is another branding opportunity. When HR interviews a potential candidate, even if that candidate is not hired, the experience should leave the interviewee with the desire to support the health care organization.

A TWO-TIERED HUMAN RESOURCES SYSTEM

Critics of HR development over the past decade suggest that HR has become a handmaiden of management, more concerned with carrying out directives from above than supporting the needs of employees (Kochan, 2005). While there might be some truth to this claim, it is largely because of the decentralization of HR functions.

The most common model today in the large health care systems and medical products companies is a smaller, highly expert central staff with HR support staff distributed throughout the organization. The reporting relationship may either be dual, to the head of the operating office and to the head of HR, or direct. Most often, the power dynamic seems to favor the relationship of HR to head executives. This distribution of the HR function has many advantages. However, one downside is a decrease in the view of HR as playing an ombudsperson role in the organization.

Pro-Management Perspective
The change toward the perception of HR as pro-management originated when the health industry began to outsource the administrative duties traditionally performed by HR. HR functions that were generally regarded by employees as positive employee relations (such as help with medical insurance, leave, and vacation issues) suddenly disappeared. Today, day-to-day contact between employees and HR departments is relegated to either voicemail or e-mail as opposed to conversations. At one time, employees could ask HR questions about benefits, compensation, and retirement. It was more transactional than strategic, but it was at least personal.

There is also the tendency of the HR department to treat employees as costs to be controlled rather than as human assets. It is often very difficult for the HR department not to feel the pressure to cut personnel costs. Given these two forces, it is no wonder employees view HR as an unnecessary evil.

Alternative Dispute Resolution System
HR systems are more effective when they are two-tiered. An alternative dispute resolution system

or some dispute resolution mechanism that gives employees a voice in the organization should be developed in every health care organization. Alternative dispute systems that mediate, arbitrate, or resolve workplace conflicts in other ways, in general, have certain advantages:

- Added flexibility
- Less formality
- Less focus on an adversarial nature
- More solution-oriented

Employee mediation and resolution of workplace conflicts is still part of the HR function. Employees need a means to exercise their right to challenge a performance appraisal, salary decision, or other personnel matter. Challenges are often handled in one of two ways:

- Appointment of an independent investigator, assigned by management, to look into the complaint
- A panel, comprised of randomly selected managers, hears and reviews the case and makes a decision

Where these alternative dispute resolution systems are in place, employees use them frequently and are generally satisfied with them (Sirota et al., 2005).

Social Contract

The social contract between the organization and its workforce no longer exists today; employees are on their own (Kochan, 2005). What HR must continually do is offer a compelling case to employees as to why they should want to work for their employer, rather than have employees feeling it is a privilege bestowed upon them to work. Things to be emphasized could include:

- Commitment to diversity
- Focus on performance differentiation
- Leadership development
- Leading-edge technology
- Skills training
- Workplace flexibility options

HR must show employees these opportunities exist with their employer. The most important issue for most health care professionals is the quality of culture and management the health industry supports:

- Fundamental respect for employees
- Long-term orientation toward them

(Sirota et al., 2005)

Many HR professionals are seeking policies to assist working families and lower-wage employees. Many in HR are also working to address the problems faced by temporary/contingent workers and the growing immigrant workforce. There is ongoing debate about how the health industry as a whole should achieve a more focused set of industry aims (Kochran, 2006).

SERVING EMPLOYEES AS THE CUSTOMERS

The health industry would do well to adopt one rule in the Nordstrom's employee handbook: use your good judgment in all situations (Sirota et al., 2005). Many HR departments are not interested in an open-minded approach when it comes to making exceptions to organization policies. Instead, they pursue standardization and uniformity in the face of a workforce that is heterogeneous and complex.

Bureaucrats everywhere abhor exceptions, not just because they may lead to charges of bias, but because they require more than rote solutions. Rather than sending the message that the organization values high-performing employees and is focused on rewarding and retaining them, HR bureaucrats often:

- Benchmark salaries, function by function and job by job, against industry standards
- Keep salaries (even those of star performers) within a narrow band determined by competitors

While HR often forfeits long-term value for short-term cost-efficiency, increasingly, general principles that value employees are being adopted for crafting workplace policies that serve employees as the customer. This means valuing employees as people. This is not being soft-hearted or naive, but rather is simply common sense. Valued employees far outproduce and outperform the average workforce: they step up to do the hard, even impossible tasks.[LN1]

For example, serving employees as the customer is about giving employees what they want most. What employees want most is best summarized in the so-called Three Factor Theory, and includes:

- Being treated fairly and equitably
- Feeling proud of their work and their employer
- Experiencing teamwork and camaraderie

(Sirota et al., 2005)

Sounds simple, but every HR professional and manager knows how challenging this can be.

Fair and Equitable Treatment

HR has a responsibility to ensure employees receive fair pay (which is defined as competitive pay), benefits, and job security. Health insurance is a significant issue. On the non-financial side, HR must ensure employees are treated respectfully. Unless these needs are met, not much else matters in any organization.

Sense of Achievement

HR also has the responsibility to ensure employees have a sense of achievement from their work; employees must feel proud of what they do and proud of the organization for which they are doing it. HR must ensure employees understand they are doing meaningful work, which is the primary reason so many employees are attracted to the health industry in the first place.

Team Camaraderie

Camaraderie involves supporting the organization's employees (not as a friend in the traditional sense of camaraderie, but as a valued customer). When an employee is sick, HR must be there. When there are occasions for grief or joy, HR must ensure the employee is treated as a valued customer. HR is ultimately responsible for managing this "customer" service. This means convincing other managers at the table that the workforce cannot be cut when there are economic uncertainties; trimming employees, without ensuring employees have comparable employment opportunities elsewhere within the health industry, destroys employees as customers and devastates any sense of camaraderie.

HUMAN RESOURCES' TRIPLE ROLES

HR has three roles in the health industry:

- Administrative functions
- Strategic partner
- Serving the employee as a customer

The most important part of this customer-centric approach for HR departments involves developing policies, practices, and philosophies geared toward creating a truly motivated and dedicated workforce. Generally speaking, this role is more notable by its absence (Sirota et al., 2005).

General Principles for Human Resource Policies, Practices, and Philosophies

U.S. employment regulations overlap with and in most cases agree with the core labor standards adopted by the International Labor Organization Declaration on Fundamental Principles and Rights at Work (2004, adopted in 1998). HR departments should assist health care organizations and medical products companies with complying with federal and state employment laws and regulations in order to:

- Ensure basic labor standards (hours of work, overtime compensation)[LN2]

- Ensure a safe and healthy work environment with minimal exposure to safety and health risks[LN3]
- Protect against workplace bias and discrimination in hiring, promotion, dismissal, and treatment of employees[LN4]
- Provide basic mechanisms for employee representation in the workplace[LN5]
- Protect against major downside risks associated with employment such as loss of pensions or health care benefits[LN6]
- Help cushion the impact of globalization and economic downturns[LN7]

(*See* Weil, 2007)

These existing labor regulations, however, do not completely and satisfactorily address many HR challenges involving new practices in the health industry, such as:

- Business process outsourcing
- Conversions of nonprofits to for-profits
- Employing independent contractors
- Reneging on long-term employment commitments
- Shifting production offshore
- Subcontracting
- Temporary workers
- Utilizing overseas suppliers

(Stone, 2007)

Moral Dilemmas

1. Should labor standards be legislated to address these new industry practices?

Employee Surveys

When HR professionals say they want to be business partners, what they often mean is they want to work for management. Most health care organizations say their employees are their greatest asset, but what they really mean is they are their biggest cost. HR should be proactive, actively involved in the organization, finding out the issues facing employees. The health industry regularly surveys patients and external customers; HR should survey its internal customers as well.

Employee Advocate

What is missing in the health industry, as well as in all other workplaces, is the view of HR as an employee advocate. HR should be able to handle hard conversations with employees about what must be done to improve and develop their individual talents on behalf of the organization. Employees must be allowed to question whether HR will actually provide skills training and leadership development, and whether HR will help employees move around the organization, or get positioned for a promotion, if employees do what is expected of them.

Administrative Functions

HR tends to push a number of functions onto managers that could be handled by HR staff, such as finding and downloading the forms needed when an employee retires. HR departments have delegated a number of jobs to others that they used to do themselves. Debate is ongoing about whether this is the direction to take.

Layoffs and Restructurings

One of the more difficult HR responsibilities is dealing with layoffs when there is a downsizing. The situation should be handled in a very humane way. Where major long-term issues are involved, such as restructurings and joint ventures, HR should actively be a part of those strategic discussions from the beginning, not just after the management decisions are made.

Flexible Work Environment

Flexible work in the health industry is a modern-day paradox. This is perhaps currently more so in the medical products sector, but may be upcoming industry-wide as the health care services sector transforms the delivery of medical treatments.

Current Paradox

Employers are introducing flexible policies needed by their workforces to help them maintain their dual work and family responsibilities. Today, as in the generation of the family farms, work and family are once again almost inseparable. In addition, technology has further blurred the lines between work and personal life. Work in the health industry must be better organized so employers can make full use of employee skills. Employees must be cross-utilized so HR departments can promote mobility and career development.

However, while flexible employment policies are required to increase or diminish the workforce and reassign and redeploy employees with ease, it is not always clear how this goal is to be accomplished. The health industry is debating how to adapt and yet preserve employee rights in the face of these challenges.

Employers want to motivate employees to contribute their knowledge. Yet the job security and job ladders of the past century, whereby employees had a stake in the well-being of their employers, have been dismantled in most organizations in the U.S. To address this paradox, HR departments are devising new organizational structures that embody flexibility while also promoting skill development and fostering employee engagement (Stone, 2007).

New Employment Relationship

This new employment relationship involves a change in the contract between employees and employers. Today's health care employees do not have a promise of lifetime employment security with a single employer. Instead, employers must promise "employability security" to employees, or the ability to acquire skills that will enhance employment opportunities in the health industry in general.

While today's employers can no longer promise employees orderly promotional opportunities, employers can promise employees opportunities to network and gain skills to prepare for jobs within the health industry itself. In this new relationship, HR should be helping employees to manage their own careers in the health industry, rather than expecting long-term employment from a single employer. Today, nowhere is this new employment relationship clearer than in the medical products sector; the health care information technology sector has been at the vanguard of this relationship change.

In-Sourcing

In-sourcing is another strategic imperative for HR departments. If someone within a health care organization wants to create a new business, HR should be there to negotiate about the employees and programs needed to get there.

Health care organizations are increasingly finding new businesses and needs they can provide and meet in-house (Friedman, 2007). A number of health care systems have established what used to be known as ancillary businesses that sell the expertise they have developed internally, including:

- Imaging and diagnostic centers
- Pharmacy benefit management companies
- For-profit pharmacies
- Physician practice management companies

The health industry may also start in-sourcing business process functions that were previously outsourced. For instance, recruiting has generally been outsourced because of the pricing, but the quality has been questionable in many organizations. HR must always look at trade-offs.

PERFORMANCE-BASED PAY

Given the controversies over excessive compensation packages, performance-based pay (merit pay and bonuses) continues to be an issue in the health industry. For instance, Congress adopted Internal Revenue Code section 162(m) in an effort to deter excessive executive pay packages by limiting the deductibility of non-performance-based compensation above $1 million. While tying compensation to results has been a relatively new focus in health care, performance-based pay represents the latest strategy to help everyone within a health care organization be more inclined to act in the best interest of the organization. Half of the corporations in the U.S., outside the health industry, have adopted performance-based pay (Gilson, 2006). Performance-based pay is viewed as one way to help improve the quality of health care services provided.

Simply stated, performance-based pay is an incentive program that measures several defined aspects of work and compensates employees according to the performance achieved by:

- Individuals
- Workplace teams
- Organization as a whole

The trend is to segment work across the organization as well as to segment the workforce in a way that allows differences to be defined and valued. The compensation system design in the health industry is an ever-evolving discipline tied closely to quantifiable metrics of value creation. This allows HR to move away from a system of treating everyone the same, to one where employees can be treated differently, and according to:

- Needs of the organization
- Individual preferences
- Employee performance

Individual performance is not the only measurement; it is also indispensable to have team and organization incentives (such as profit sharing or employee stock options). This threefold difference in total compensation is the underpinning of performance-based pay, whether it is pay, promotions, or the opportunity for incentive awards and recognition (Wharton, 2005).

Board Compensation Committees

Issues of pay and performance are now reaching boards of directors as well. One key factor in the evolution of HR departments has been Sarbanes-Oxley for the medical products sector and for-profit hospitals and health care providers in general, in particular, 15 U.S.C.A. § 7241(a)(5) (2002) (adopting requirement that chief executive officers and chief financial officers must discuss and review certain reports with the board's audit committee before filing). Committee members who rubber-stamp reports

face liability. For HR, this has radically changed the relationship with the board compensation committees.

The question arises as to where a board should obtain guidance on matters of pay and perks, from the HR department or consultants hired directly by the board. While board compensation committees now often hire consultants to advise them rather than rely solely on HR departments, the HR department still should be performing compensation analysis and bringing information and advice to the board.

Issues surrounding pay, including sensitivity to full disclosure of executive perks, are in the forefront for the health industry, as are issues of management development and succession. Sarbanes-Oxley, an area in which the HR function plays a key role, has had a profound effect on boards in the health industry.

Pay Issues and Equality

Pay issues are not always easy to resolve, especially at hospitals, where numerous constituencies believe they take precedence. It is often difficult to develop a clear strategy. One approach to setting compensation levels, a leftover from the culture of looking out for employees, is to have a model of equality: treat everyone roughly the same, especially on issues of compensation and benefits. Of course, organizations that do this get complaints from top managers claiming they lost employees because HR would not let them pay them enough. Top managers, who for the most part are high achievers, believe employees should be paid based on individual performance.

The problem is that perceived inequities drive employees to distraction. It is one thing to view an employee as a star performer and to want to pay some individuals more to prevent them from quitting. It is another to deal with what happens next. Employees who discover someone else is being paid more within an equal pay system object and charges of discrimination arise. So HR moves to a model where everyone is paid based on performance. However, this approach requires an objective assessment of performance that everyone should be willing to buy into; this is the hard part (Wharton, 2005).

Moral Dilemmas

1. Why does pay equity remain one of the most violated HR standards in the health industry?

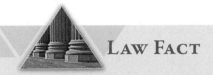

LAW FACT

EXECUTIVE COMPENSATION

What should be the role of human resources when examining executive compensation?

If HR is to be a strategic partner in the health industry, it can no longer be just with the CEO of an organization; it must be with the board and the board compensation committee.

—*In re UnitedHealth Group Inc. Shareholder Derivative Litigation*, 754 N.W.2d 544 (Supreme Court of Minnesota 2008); *In re UnitedHealth Group Incorporated PSLRA Litigation*, 2007 U.S. Dist. LEXIS 94616 (U.S. District Court for the District of Minnesota 2007); Forelle & Bandler, 2006; Wilmer Culter, 2006.

(See *Law Fact* at the end of this chapter for the answer.)

CHAPTER SUMMARY

- HR can be viewed as either an administrative function or a strategic function.
- While HR began as an employee advocate and protector, HR too often ended up treating employees as expendable, expensive liabilities.
- The media increasingly focuses upon HR issues as top executives are compensated seemingly without regard to performance, while top-performing lower-wage employees are often not paid living wages.
- One reason HR is slow to become an effective strategic business partner is because few HR employees have developed business skills necessary for this transition.
- Used effectively, HR departments could help health care entities grow revenue, increase productivity, and develop leadership.
- For HR to become an effective strategic business partner, senior managers must view it as more than just the department that hires and fires employees.
- An additional function HR could work to improve is that of a mediator between employees and employer; employees need a non-adversarial way to resolve grievances.
- The social contract between an organization and its workforce, as far as long-term employment and rewards in return for loyalty, has been broken; employees increasingly feel as if they are on their own and have lost their status as the employer's customer.
- Although HR is responsible for ensuring compliance with labor and employment laws, these laws do not satisfactorily address many challenges HR faces, or address them at all in some cases.
- Too many employees lack the motivation to contribute their knowledge to employers due to the lack of job stability, reward for performance, and flexibility in balancing personal and family obligations with work.
- Performance-based pay is difficult to administer because it is difficult to objectively determine; furthermore, it often subjects employers to distracted employees and charges of discrimination.

LAW NOTES

1. Valued employees create engaged external customers who foster organizational success by delivering positive financial outcomes (Dau-Schmidt & Haley, 2007). Research by David Sirota, Louis Mischkind, and Michael Irwin Meltzer found that companies where employees are valued outperform their competitors. Based on the results of 2.5 million employee surveys at twenty-eight companies employing 920,000 employees, the share price of fourteen companies where employees felt they were valued increased an average of 16 percent in 2004, compared to an industry average of 6 percent. Six companies where employees did not feel valued saw their share prices increase by 3 percent (Sirota et al., 2005).
2. Fair Labor Standards Act of 1938 (FLSA), 29 U.S.C.A. §§ 201-205, 206, 207, 209-219 (2009) (establishing national minimum wage, guaranteeing time-and-a-half for overtime in certain jobs, and generally prohibiting employment of minors); Davis-Bacon Act, 40 U.S.C.A. §§ 3141-3144, 3146, 3147 (2009); and Walsh-Healy Public Contracts Act, 41 U.S.C.A. §§ 35-45 (2009).
3. Occupational Safety and Health Act, Mine Safety and Health Act, 29 U.S.C.A. §§ 651-675, 677, 678, (2009) (establishing Black Lung disease program), and Drug Free Workplace Act, 41 U.S.C.A. §§ 701-707 (2009).

4. 29 U.S.C.A. § 206(d) (2007) (prohibiting wage differentials based on sex); Executive Order 11246 of 1965 (Equal Employment Opportunity) (prohibiting discrimination and requiring affirmative action to prevent discrimination); Age Discrimination Employment Act, 29 U.S.C.A. §§ 621-634 (2009); Americans with Disabilities Act of 1990, 42 U.S.C.A. §§ 12101-12103, 12111-12117, 12131-12134, 12141-12150, 12161-12165, 12181-12189, 12201-12205a, 12206-12213 (2009) and 47 U.S.C.A. § 225 (1996); Rehabilitation Act, 29 U.S.C.A. §§ 701-718, 720-728a, 730-732, 741, 751, 760-762a, 763-765, 771-776, 780-785, 790-794e, 795, 795a, 795g-795n, 796-796f-6, 798j-796l (2009); Surface Transportation Assistance Act of 1982 (STAA), 23 U.S.C.A. § 157 (1995) and 26 U.S.C.A. §§ 4051-4053, 9503 (2009); Anti-Retaliatory Provision-Surface Transportation Assistance Act, 49 U.S.C.A. § 31105 (2007); and Veterans' Reemployment Rights Act, 38 U.S.C.A. §§ 4301–4307 (2009).

5. National Labor Relations Act, 29 U.S.C.A. §§ 151-169 (2009); Labor Management Reporting Disclosure Act, 29 U.S.C.A. §§ 401, 402, 411-415, 431-441, 461-466, 481-483, 501-504, 521-531 (2009); and Railway Labor Act, 45 U.S.C.A. §§ 151-163, 181-185, 187, 188 (2009).

6. Employee Retirement Income Security Act (ERISA), 26 U.S.C.A. §§ 219, 408, 410-415, 4971, 4973-4975, 6047, 6057-6059, 6690, 6692, 6693, 7476 (2009) and 29 U.S.C.A. §§ 1001-1003, 1021-1031, 1051-1056, 1058-1061, 1081-1085, 1101-1114, 1131-1148, 1161-1169, 1181-1183, 1185, 1185a, 1185b, 1191, 1191a-1191c, 1201-1204, 1221, 1222, 1231, 1232, 1241, 1242, 1301-1303, 1305-1310, 1321, 1322, 1322a, 1322b, 1323, 1341, 1341a, 1342-1348, 1350, 1361-1371, 1381-1405, 1411-1415, 1421-1426, 1431, 1441, 1451-1453, 1461 (2009); Consolidated Omnibus Budget Reconciliation Act ("COBRA"), 7 U.S.C.A. §§ 1314g, 1314h, 1445-3 (2009), 10 U.S.C.A. § 1095 (2003), 15 U.S.C.A. §§ 687k, 687l, 697a, 697b, 1530 (2009), 19 U.S.C.A. § 58c (2007), 29 U.S.C.A. §§ 1001b, 1085a, 1143a, 1161 to 1168, 1369, 1370 (2009), 33 U.S.C.A. § 883j (1986), 38 U.S.C.A. § 1703 (2008), 42 U.S.C.A. §§ 238m, 300bb-1 - 300bb-8, 677, 1396r-3, 1395dd, 1395w-1, 1396v, 8287, 8287a to 8287c (2009), and 47 U.S.C.A. § 158 (1994).

7. Workers Adjustment & Retraining and Notification Act of (WARN), 29 U.S.C.A. §§ 2101-2109 (2009); Family Medical Leave Act, 5 U.S.C.A. §§ 6381-6387 and 29 U.S.C.A. §§ 2601, 2611-2619, 2631-2636, 2651-2654 (2009); and Trade Adjustment Assistance Act, 19 U.S.C.A. §§ 1431a, 1583, 2318, 2401, 2401a-2401g (2009), 26 U.S.C.A. §§ 35, 6050T, 7527 (2009), and 42 U.S.C.A. § 300gg-45 (2006).

CHAPTER BIBLIOGRAPHY

Carreyrou, J., & Martinez, B. (2008, April 4). Nonprofit hospitals, once for the poor, strike it rich with tax breaks, they outperform for-profit rivals. *Wall Street Journal,* p. A1.

Dau-Schmidt, K. G., & Haley, T. A. (2007). Governance of the workplace: The contemporary regime of individual contract. *Comparative Labor Law & Policy Journal, 28* (2), 313-349.

Federal Register. (2007, August 6). Cafeteria plans. 72 FR 43938-01.

Friedman, T. L. (2007). *The world is flat: A brief history of the twenty-first century.* New York, NY: Farrar, Straus & Giroux.

Forelle, C., & Bandler, J. (2006, March 18). The perfect payday. *Wall Street Journal,* p. A1.

Gilson, R. J. (2006). Controlling shareholders and corporate governance. *Harvard Law Review, 119,* 1641-1679.

Kochan, T. (2006). *Updating American labor law: Taking advantage of a window of opportunity.* Boston, MA: MIT School of Sloan Management, Institute for Work & Employment Resources.

____. (2005). *Restoring the American dream: A working families' agenda for America.* Boston, MA: MIT Press.

Levin (Levin Associates, Inc.) (2009) *Mergers and acquisitions database.* Norwalk, CT: Levin.

Narayanan, P. et al. (2007). The economic impact of backdating of executive stock options. *Michigan Law Review, 105,* 1597-1641.

Sirota, D. et al. (2005). *The enthusiastic employee: How organizations profit by giving workers what they want.* Philadelphia, PA: Wharton School Publishing.

Stabile, S. J. (2007). When conscience clashes with state law and policy: Catholic institutions. *Journal of Catholic Legal Studies, 467,* 137-159.

Stone, K. W. W. (2007). A new labor law for a new world of work: The case for a comparative-transnational approach. *Comparative Labor Law & Policy Journal, 28,* 565-581.

Taras, D. (2007, Winter). Reconciling differences differently: Employee voice in public policymaking and workplace governance. *Comparative Labor Law & Policy Journal, 28,* 167-191.

Weil, D. (2007). Crafting a progressive workplace regulatory policy: Why enforcement matters. *Comparative Labor Law & Policy Journal, 28,* 125-154.

Wharton (Wharton School of the University of Pennsylvania). (2005). Is your human resources department friend or foe? Depends on who's asking the question. *Knowledge@Wharton.*

Wilmer Cutler (Wilmer Cutler Pickering Hale & Dorr). (2006, March 18). *Report of Wilmer Cutler Pickering Hale & Dorr, LLC, to the Special Committee of the Board of Directors of UnitedHealth Group, Inc.* Washington, DC: Wilmer Cutler.

CHAPTER 12

EMPLOYERS' HEALTH CARE COSTS

"This is the greatest error of our day in the treatment of the human body, that physicians separate the soul from the body."

—PLATO (B.C.), GREEK PHILOSOPHER

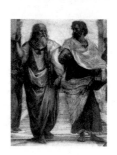

IN BRIEF

This chapter deals with the growing efforts to reduce and fairly allocate employers' health care costs. Particular attention is directed to smoking and the growing prevalence of obesity; that is to say, preventable behaviors and conditions that are both recognized as serious health issues that can no longer be ignored, as well as problems that can be addressed through environmental interventions. The challenges on this continuum of employer influence are twofold: first, to decide what type of medical interventions are legally permissible for preventable behaviors and conditions that are triggered by daily lifestyle choices, and second, whether the health industry should be working with employers to think about other preventive self-care issues, which effectively cost employers money and affect employee performance.

It is important to note that this chapter addresses only the actual medical diagnosis of obesity, and not simply employees who are "pleasantly plump." For adults, obesity ranges are determined by using weight and height to calculate a number called the body mass index (BMI), which correlates with their level of body obesity. According to the Centers for Disease Control (CDC), a person who is 5'9" and weighs between 125 pounds and 168 pounds is considered a healthy weight; the same person weighing between 169 pounds and 202 pounds is overweight; and the same person weighing more than 203 pounds is considered obese.

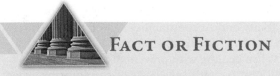

FACT OR FICTION

LIFESTYLE DISCRIMINATION

Can employees be fired for being obese?

Stephen Grindle weighed about 345 pounds when he was hired as a driver and dock worker with Watkins Motor Lines, where he loaded, unloaded, and arranged heavy freight. Following an on-the-job knee injury, he took a medical leave of absence for almost six months. When his medical leave was almost over, Grindle weighed 405 pounds, had a limited range of motion that prevented him from ducking and squatting, and became short-of-breath after a few steps.

After his medical leave expired, Watkins fired Grindle, claiming that he could not safely perform his job requirements as a dock worker, even though he had performed his job for five years when his weight ranged from 340 to 450 pounds. Grindle claimed that he was fired because of his obesity, in violation of the Americans with Disabilities Act (ADA), 42 U.S.C.A. §§ 12101 *et seq.* (2009); 47 U.S.C.A. § 225 (1996) (prohibits disability-based job discrimination).

—*EEOC v. Watkins Motor Lines, Inc.*, 463 F.3d 436
(U.S. Court of Appeals for the Sixth Circuit 2006).
(See *Law Fact* at the end of this chapter for the answer.)

PRINCIPLES AND APPLICATIONS

Preventable behaviors and conditions are often a topic of public conversation and debate, but preventive care has not been as successful as hoped for thus far. Health plans are reluctant to pay for preventive care, physicians are far more focused on treating disease, and employees are not motivated to maintain healthy lifestyles. As employers are trying to reduce the cost of their benefit programs, the epidemics of depression, diabetes, cardiovascular disease, and other chronic ailments[LN1] are bringing new urgency to the concept of preventive care (Landro, 2004). Consequently, employers are taking a much more aggressive look at preventable behaviors and conditions.

While preventable chronic diseases such as diabetes, arthritis, and circulatory disorders are responsible for the most direct medical costs among employees, the costliest medical condition overall is depression (Wharton School, 2005). Depression is more of a burden to the U.S. health care system than any other illness. Employees are often prescribed drugs before any other non-drug treatment options are explored, resulting in depression drugs being the leading cost among prescription drugs (Mark et al., 2008).

CURRENT QUALITY AND COSTS TRENDS

Two current trends in employer-provided benefits suggest that employers are inconsistent about how they want their health plans to work. One trend is investing

in improving the quality of employee medical care; the other trend is shifting the costs of this improvement to employees. This suggests that while employers want to improve the quality of employee health care, they do not want to foot the increased bill.

On one hand, many employers are investing in new programs to improve the quality of medical care, partly in response to recent concerns from the Institute of Medicine (IOM), the arm of the National Academy of Sciences that handles medical care issues, and others about the less-than-ideal state of the U.S. health care system (IOM, 2001). For example, a coalition of employers called the Leapfrog Group encourages hospitals to adopt computerized systems for entering medication orders as a way to prevent errors. General Electric has a program to identify the higher-quality physicians and hospitals used by its employees, thereby setting the stage for providing financial incentives for those employees who use better providers. In other words, many employers are willing to invest in quality improvements with the expectation that quality care will, in the long run, lower their health care costs. For example, employers are willing to pay for newer, higher-priced brand name drugs that have less adverse side effects today, so employees will be more compliant in taking their medications, thereby promoting better health conditions tomorrow.

At the same time, more employers are shifting the costs of their health plans to employees, partly because their costs have more than doubled during the past seven years. The highest-profile example of the cost-sharing trend has been the move to Health Savings Accounts (HSAs), championed as a way to combat health care inflation by giving consumers incentives to shop more astutely for care. HSAs, created early in 2004, allow pre-tax money to be put into accounts similar to 401(k) retirement accounts. Participants buy health plans with high deductibles, at least $1,000 a year for an individual and $2,000 for a family. High deductibles are meant to keep health plan premiums as low as possible. Money from the tax-free savings account is used to pay deductibles, and it could build up over the years. Proposals are circulating to make HSA benefit premiums tax deductible as well. HSAs also represent a way for employers to make employees more responsible for their own health care. High-profile HSAs aside, cost-sharing can also be something as simple as increasing employee co-pays.[LN2]

Taken together, the two trends illustrate that employers are struggling to accurately assess how decisions about health plans affect the bottom line. The cost-sharing trend, in particular, comes at a time when information is lacking about whether short-term savings will lead to long-term health problems and added costs. No one knows whether employees will avoid primary care for financial reasons, or whether employees will try to stay healthy to avoid paying more if they get sick.

Last, employers might just have to pay higher wages if health care benefits are reduced (CBO, 2006). This is not just an assumption of economic theory. Empirical evidence shows that the costs of health care benefits are fully shifted out of the wages employees receive (Gruber, 2000). What is missing in the debate about health care costs is a practical and accurate method to determine how much employers should invest in the health of their employees, and to identify the best benefit packages designed to encourage appropriate health care delivery and use. When measuring the true cost of employer-provided benefits, employers need to accurately measure and consider the payoffs that come from improving the health of their employees.

FORGET BIG BROTHER

Employees are always vulnerable to subtle forms of exploitation by their employers. This is one reason for federal privacy legislation known as the Health Insurance Portability and Accountability Act (HIPAA) that governs the collection of health care information about individual employees (see Health Insurance

Portability and Accountability Act of 1996 (HIPAA), 18 U.S.C.A. §§ 24 et seq. (2009)).

When dealing with preventable behaviors and conditions to control the costs of employer-provided benefits, it is important for employees not to conjure up images of their employer as "Big Brother" doing everything in their power to take advantage of them. Even though employers have access to broad-based information about the health conditions of their employees, most do not use it effectively and others do not always analyze it at all. The assumption is that larger self-insured employers with one thousand or more employees are very effective at understanding all of the different employer-benefit practices; they are not.

For example, despite the acknowledged benefits of wellness programs, employers continue to challenge their value. While most wellness programs require initial health screenings to develop a baseline for metrics (e.g, cholesterol levels, blood pressure, weight, and nicotine use), this baseline data is not always analyzed or evaluated. Employers are not always aware that initial screenings caught potentially serious health problems in their employees. In addition, aggregate data is seldom analyzed to detect systemic changes that could be made by employers.

PROSPECTIVE MEDICINE

The key to cutting employer-provided benefit costs is getting employees involved in their own health care when disease conditions can still be prevented.[LN3] What is really required is personalized prevention. For example, employers are increasingly making health risk assessments and personalized health plans available to their employees in hopes that they will become directly involved in avoiding preventable behaviors and conditions. In other words, the focus is shifting from treating preventable behaviors and conditions, toward tailoring treatments to individual needs so employees can develop healthy lifestyles and block preventable behaviors and conditions from arising. Although the U.S. is one of the world's most advanced countries, its population's overall health lags behind other similarly situated countries. This is perhaps because of the extreme lifestyle differences between the U.S. and other such countries, resulting in lower health care costs for those countries (Girion, 2007).

This new approach to health care is called prospective rather than preventive medicine. It uses individual medical histories to identify employees at the greatest risk of developing preventable behaviors and conditions, and takes steps to intervene early to prevent their onset (Landro, 2004). The issue for employers is how the value of preventive self-care can be raised so that employees will set priorities for their own health. This is the leading question surrounding the change in how employer-provided benefits will be managed in the future.

Traditional approaches put employees in disease-management programs once a health condition is diagnosed. However, employers are moving beyond disease management into focused, realistic ways to use early detection and early intervention to prevent conditions from ever developing into disease states (Landro, 2004). This change does not succeed with a cookie-cutter approach for all employees, but rather by tailoring programs for individual employees.

Clearly, employers are driving this prospective change. They provide health plans for 160 million employees (Kaiser, 2007). With the average cost of a family insurance plan having risen to $11,500 per year, according to the Kaiser Family Foundation, the need to trim employers' health care costs is undisputed.

Moral Dilemmas

1. What types of medical interventions are permissible for preventable behaviors and conditions triggered by voluntary lifestyle choices made on a day-to-day basis?

PREVENTABLE BEHAVIORS AND CONDITIONS

National business advocacy groups and associations now call smoking a *preventable behavior* and obesity a *preventable condition,* word choices that recognize these problems are avoidable and necessary to avoid. More than half of the adult U.S. population is overweight or obese. According to CDC standards, among developed countries, the U.S. has the most obese people. Americans are much heavier than they were ten years ago and much heavier than other people around the world. Life expectancy in the U.S., which is among the richest countries, only ranks forty-eighth in the world. Being overweight is comparable to having diabetes or high blood pressure. It is a true diagnosable disease that affects life expectancy (Power, 2003).

Recently, employers have declared war on smoking and obesity for one simple reason: smoking and obesity are now recognized as two real, and preventable, drains on employer-provided benefit costs. It is not the health behavior and condition of employees that is driving employers to take this seriously. The big driver is really the cost of health care, which

employers either have to bear or pass on to their employees. Employees with healthy lifestyles might ask why they are subsidizing the unhealthy choices of their counterparts on a day-to-day basis.

Smoking and obesity are two strong predictors of medical expenses. The business reason for doing something to diminish smoking and obesity is simply that expenses related to employer-provided benefits would be less. The general trend for most employers is that, sooner or later, the cost of health plans depends on how expensive employee health care needs are. Smoking and obesity in particular have come under attack because both conditions are directly related to rapidly rising health care costs, and both are seen as more easily avoidable than many other more preventable conditions that drive rising health care costs for employers.

Smoking Behaviors: Billion-Dollar Preventable Cost

In 1964, the Surgeon General first released a report stating that smoking is a health hazard and a primary contributor to lung disease (HEW, 1964). Since that report, substantial research has established that smoking dramatically increases the risk of death from a plethora of conditions. Despite widespread awareness and acceptance of the risks of smoking, one in five young Americans smokes (Smith, 2007; Warren, et al., 2006).

From the $1.9 trillion that the National Coalition on Health Care estimates employers spend on health care costs each year (Russell, 2007), the Centers for Disease Control (CDC) estimates that over 60 percent of the costs go toward treating tobacco-related illnesses. In addition to this direct cost, smokers cost the U.S. economy $98 billion a year in lost productivity (Wharton, 2006; *see also* HEW, 1964). Smokers miss work more often due to illness, take longer to recover from common illnesses, and take many more breaks throughout the average workday than their nonsmoking coworkers, all resulting in lost productivity.

Health care costs for smokers are estimated to be as much as 40 percent higher than those for nonsmokers (Chadwick, 2006). Many of the employment costs attributable to smokers, including increased health insurance costs, are ultimately shared by nonsmoking employees" (Chadwick, 2006). While employers pay an average of $1,429 per smoker per year in increased benefit costs when compared with the average cost of nonsmoking employees:

- Adverse health effects from smoking account for nearly one of every five deaths
- Smoking is responsible for 440,000 deaths annually

- 90 percent of the lung cancers, coronary heart disease, and chronic obstructive lung disease is attributable to smoking
- 8.6 million smokers suffer from serious illnesses attributable to smoking

(CDC, 2006; Valleau, 2007; Wharton, 2006)

Obesity Conditions: Billion-Dollar Preventable Cost

Obesity and weight-related conditions are significant contributors to health care costs, contributing as much as $93 billion to the nation's yearly medical bill. Of that $93 billion cost, the total cost of obesity to U.S. employers is estimated at more than $13 billion per year, a price tag that includes:

- $8 billion for added health insurance costs
- $2.4 billion for paid sick leave
- $1.8 billion for life insurance
- $1 billion for disability insurance

(DeFalco, 2006)

America does have a ray of hope; obesity levels seem to finally be leveling off (Stein, 2007). According to statistics compiled by the National Business Group, obesity is now considered a greater trigger for health problems and increased health spending than smoking (DeFalco, 2006).

The Rand Corporation found that individuals who are obese have 30 to 50 percent more chronic medical problems than those who smoke (Strum, 2002; Wharton, 2008). The CDC notes that being overweight increases the risk of many diseases and health conditions, including:

- Cancers (especially breast, colon, and endometrial)
- Dyslipidemia (high total cholesterol or high levels of triglycerides)
- Gallbladder disease
- Heart disease
- Hypertension (high blood pressure)
- Osteoarthritis
- Respiratory problems
- Sleep apnea
- Stroke
- Type 2 diabetes

The Rand study used a methodology to match obese nonsmokers with non-obese nonsmokers (and obese smokers with obese nonsmokers) in a fashion that could be described as an apples-to-apples approach that yielded sound results (Strum, 2002). When compared to a person of average weight, an obese person accounts for an additional $1,034.00 every year in doctor visits, medications, and medical procedures (Tsai & Wadden, 2005).

As obesity rises in the U.S., the medical conditions associated with obesity have helped trigger an increase in health care costs. The National Business Group notes that obesity accounts for approximately 9 percent of the health care costs each year, and that 8 percent of employers' medical claims are due to obesity. When analyzing increases in medical spending, the National Coalition on Health Care documented that obesity drove 27 percent of the increased costs of health care (Russell, 2007).

LIFESTYLE DISCRIMINATION AND CHOICES

There's no doubt that rising health care expenses increase the cost of medical care and health plans. The NCHC notes that employer health plan premiums are increasing at nearly three times the rate of inflation. In an effort to counter these statistics and to help employees adopt healthier lifestyles, employers are offering a variety of programs and benefits (Wharton, 2006).

Every state permits employers to penalize employees for smoking in the workplace or during working hours. Crucially, if a penalty is imposed on employees for smoking, reasonable alternatives must be available by law to employees who cannot quit smoking. For example, a smoker addicted to nicotine, a medical condition, could avoid being penalized by participating in a smoking-cessation program. Thus, employers with company policies on not smoking on company property may lawfully discipline or terminate employees who violate their smoking ban (Coil & Rice, 2004).

In many states, an increasing number of employers have enacted policies precluding the employment of smokers (Chadwick, 2006). The only protection from employment discrimination that smokers can rely on exists in the form of state laws prohibiting employment discrimination based on tobacco use, which exists in half the states, almost all of which are under challenge by public health organizations, such as the American Heart Association (Valleau, 2007). For instance, the World Health Organization's hiring policy rejects all applicants who smoke, as do an increasing number of employers from health care organizations to airlines. In contrast to this no-smoking approach by employers in states that tolerate lifestyle discrimination, other employers in those states have adopted a middle-of-the-road approach to employee smoking. Those employers, rather than proscribing employment of smokers, have passed on the additional costs attributable to smoking to employees who smoke.

Smoking opened the door for employers to also think about obesity-related issues, the leading preventable cost to the U.S. health care system. Obesity has not been examined critically in the same way as smoking has. Most employers see anti-obesity initiatives as beneficial. However, if employers start getting into other preventable behaviors and conditions that are not as costly, there might be push-back. For example, some employers already prevent their executives from participating in extreme sports (skydiving, motorcross and off-road racing, BMX racing and jumping, mountain and ice-climbing, street luge, and adventure racing) and offer cafeteria-style benefits that index employee costs according to the number of children receiving benefits (families with more than one child pay higher health plan premiums).

Moral Dilemmas

1. What ethical considerations should underlie lifestyle policies, such as the use of dynamic pricing in health benefit plans that charge smokers and obese employees higher premiums?

2. Having an unusually high number of children is also a lifestyle choice resulting in higher health care costs for employers; would charging such employee-parents just as much as smokers and obese employees without children be permissible?

Health Plan Ratings: Credible v. Demographic

There are two restraints on expansion of lifestyle discrimination beyond smoking and obesity: HIPAA and demographic benefit ratings for small employers. This is subject to HIPAA wellness rules that require all employees covered under the same employer-sponsored plan to pay the same premiums regardless of their health, with certain wellness programs being the exception. Under the July 2007 rules, employers can offer financial incentives of as much as 20 percent off the cost of covering an employee for participating in wellness programs. Two of the most popular incentives have become discounts to nonsmokers and those willing to submit to health risk assessments (including monitoring of weight, nicotine use, cholesterol, and blood pressure). This chapter focuses on this 20 percent incentive for employer-sponsored

plans. The first restraint is that HIPAA prevents employers from knowing which individual employees suffer from preventable diseases such as alcoholism, diabetes, emphysema, and heart disease. Employers have no proof of individual employees' preventable conditions.

Second, only larger employers have health plans with benefit costs credibly based on actual employee claims, and such employers are generally self-insured. They purchase re-insurance and only use health insurers as plan administrators. On the other hand, small employers with less than one thousand employees generally purchase health plans based on gender and age; their claims history has no relationship to the cost of their health plans. In other words, the costs of health plans for small employers are determined by demographics; when one or more members in their geographic community develops a costly medical condition, all the small employers in that community must pay higher premiums. Small employers cannot effectively manage their disease risk; their disease risks are based on the demographics of their geographic community, not on the actual claims of their employees.

In summary, health plan costs for large employers are based on actual claims; for small employers, costs are based on demographics in general. Large employers can effectively manage their employee claims; small employers cannot because they cannot control their risk pools.

Smoking Behaviors: A Lifestyle Choice

While employees have used the courts to challenge employment policies that consider off-duty behavior, such challenges have met with little success. Unless a state prohibits employers from participating in specific activities, such as smoking, employers have been successful in protecting their right to hire and fire employees as they please, meaning that employers can take an employee's health care costs into consideration in a decision to hire or fire that employee (Chadwick, 2006).

Ideally, employee policies should not be arbitrary and should be rationally connected to a legitimate goal. Challenges to policies often come about when a court compares the purpose and intent of a policy with its effect on the individual employee challenging it. The effect has to fit with the purpose. If challenged in a court of law, employers should be able to defend their employment policies and be able to demonstrate that they saw a rational connection between their policies and the specific interests served by the policies. If this connection is arbitrary or irrational, then the policy will fail. For example, policies prohibiting smoking should apply to all new hires or to current employees within a specific time period. Employers can also require job applicants to sign affidavits stating they have not used tobacco or tobacco products during a specified period preceding their job application if they can show that smoking would interfere with the employee's job performance or the operation of the business (Coil & Rice, 2004; Stewart, 1996).

To be sure, not all policies precluding the employment of smokers are permissible (Chadwick, 2006). The use of race or gender to somehow target smokers or other such discriminatory treatment is not permitted.

In addition, if employers use dynamic pricing to set the price of smokers' health plan premiums in such a way that it angers all employees, employers can spark a backlash against any prospective changes. However, dynamic pricing of health plan premiums is ever more common. This is subject to two federal regulatory restrictions: the HIPAA wellness rule and the 20 percent threshold rule. Under the wellness rule, group health plans cannot discriminate among individuals in eligibility, benefits, or premiums based on any health factor of an individual (health status, medical conditions, and genetic information are all

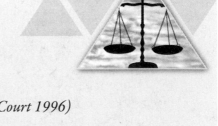

LIFESTYLE DISCRIMINATION: SMOKING

City of N. Miami v. Kurtz
[Employer v. Employee]
653 So.2d 1025 (Florida Supreme Court 1995),
U.S. Supreme Court certiorari denied, 516 U.S. 1043 (U.S. Supreme Court 1996)

FACTS: Arlene Kurtz attempted to apply for a clerk-typist position with the city of North Miami. At the time of her interview, she was informed that she was required to sign an affidavit stating that she had not used tobacco products for one year. Kurtz refused and brought suit.

ISSUE: Are employees entitled to protection against government intrusion into off-duty activities, namely smoking?

HOLDING AND DECISION: No. Smoking is not considered a private activity entitled to protection against government-employer consideration.

ANALYSIS: Initially, the trial court held that neither the Florida State Constitution nor the U.S. Constitution afforded Kurtz a right to privacy with respect to off-duty smoking and granted the City's motion for summary judgment. On appeal, the trial court decision was reversed, concluding that Kurtz did have a right to privacy with respect to smoking under Florida's state constitution, and that the City of North Miami's interests were insufficient to outweigh the intrusion into her privacy.

However, the Florida Supreme Court reversed and remanded with directions to reinstate the trial court's judgment. Florida, together with ten other states, incorporates privacy rights into its state constitution.

The Florida Supreme Court addressed whether the Florida constitution, with its right to privacy, protected Kurtz from governmental intrusion into non-work-related activities. In concluding that it did not, the court relied on the pervasive public nature of smoking. The court reasoned that smokers must frequently disclose whether they smoke in obtaining seating in restaurants, renting cars, and reserving motel rooms. Accordingly, the court held that smokers did not have an expectation of privacy within the meaning of the Florida constitution.

Turning to the U.S. Constitution, the court again concluded that Kurtz did not have a right of privacy with respect to smoking. First, the court examined whether the right to smoke constituted a recognized fundamental right entitled to protection absent a compelling state interest. The court concluded that smoking did not implicate fundamental rights. Notwithstanding this conclusion, the court concluded that even if the City's policy infringed upon a liberty interest, there was a sufficient rational basis for the rule given the cost savings realized by the City in refusing to hire employees who smoke.

RULE OF LAW: Smoking is not a fundamental right superseding governmental interests as it relates to employment.

(*See generally* Coil & Rice, 2004).

considered health factors). For example, employers cannot charge smokers higher health care premiums without offering those with a nicotine addiction access to supplemental wellness programs, such as smoking-cessation activities. Under the 20 percent threshold rule, employers cannot award employees more than a 20 percent reduction in their health plan premiums for being healthy (through lower co-pays, deductibles, or cash incentive payments). Increasingly, employees who smoke pay higher premiums to the same insurer than employees who have never smoked.[LN4]

Obesity Conditions: A Lifestyle Choice

While Santa Cruz and San Francisco, California, Michigan, and Washington, D.C., have passed laws barring employment discrimination because of weight (Capell, 2007), outside these areas, it remains very difficult for employees and job applicants to bring a successful case against employers for lifestyle discrimination based on obesity. For example, a 240-pound aerobics instructor in San Francisco successfully challenged Jazzercise Inc., which denied her a teaching position because she did not "look leaner than the public" (Ellin, 2006). Each case must

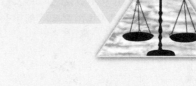

LIFESTYLE DISCRIMINATION: OBESITY

Cook v. Department of Mental Health, Retardation & Hospitals
[Interviewee v. Interviewer]
10 F.3d 17 (U.S. Court of Appeals for the First Circuit 1993)

FACTS: The State of Rhode Island refused to hire Arlene Cook, who weighed over 320 pounds, because of her obesity.

ISSUE: Can employers refuse to hire people who are obese?

HOLDING AND DECISION: Yes. Obesity need not be a physiological disorder to qualify for coverage under the Rehabilitation Act.

ANALYSIS: The trial court held that while obesity can be a disability under the Rehabilitation Act, it must be a physiological disorder and cannot be a transitory or self-imposed condition. The trial court found that the state discriminated against Cook because of a physiological disorder.

The state appealed the trial court's judgment. In response to the state's appeal, the Equal Employment Opportunity Commission (EEOC) filed an amicus brief with the First Circuit arguing that the issue of whether obesity is a disability must be determined on a case-by-case basis. Further, the EEOC argued that obesity may constitute a disability despite not being a physiological disorder; that is, obesity may be considered a physical impairment.

The EEOC further argued that whether obesity is substantially limiting should be analyzed by considering three factors: the nature and severity of the impairment, the duration or expected duration of the impairment, and the permanent

or long-term impact resulting from the impairment. Additionally, the EEOC argued that neither the Rehabilitation Act nor the ADA requires the consideration of how obese individuals become impaired. The EEOC maintained that voluntariness should not preclude the protection of obese individuals under either Act, and should only be relevant if someone could quickly change their weight by altering their behavior.

The First Circuit adopted the EEOC's reasoning that obesity need not be a physiological disorder to qualify for coverage under the Rehabilitation Act. Morbid obesity is a physiological disorder. The medical profession considers individuals morbidly obese if they weigh either more than twice their optimal weight or are more than one hundred pounds over their optimal weight. Morbid obesity involves a dysfunction of both the metabolic system and the neurological appetite-suppressing signal system, capable of causing adverse effects within the musculoskeletal, respiratory, and cardiovascular systems. Metabolic dysfunction, which leads to weight gain in the morbidly obese, lingers even after weight loss. Further, the court held that employers cannot deny employment on the grounds that obesity increases their benefit costs.

RULE OF LAW: As determined on a case-by-case basis, obesity is a disability protected against discrimination under the Rehabilitation Act.

(See generally Smith, 2007; Valleau, 2007).

be decided on a case-by-case basis with fact-specific and individualized inquiry.

The First Circuit Court of Appeals was the first federal appellate court to recognize that an employer violated the Rehabilitation Act by refusing to hire an obese job applicant. The Rehabilitation Act of 1973 provides protection from discrimination to handicapped employees; it preceded the ADA. Courts that have subsequently applied and discussed the decision, however, have generally found that obesity fails to meet the definition of a disability under the Rehabilitation Act or the ADA, the Rehabilitation Act's successor.[LN5]

Weight is a real dilemma for employers. They want employees to lose weight, but they do not want to fire them for being overweight. Practically, employers cannot refuse to hire overweight individuals, because two-thirds of Americans are overweight (Wharton, 2008).

> *Moral Dilemmas*
> 1. Should employers be permitted to penalize employees for smoking behavior and obesity conditions that increase employers' health care costs? If so, when? If not, why not?

HEALTH LAWS SUPPORTING LIFESTYLE CHOICES

Disability Legislation

Although some federal laws are specifically aimed at barring lifestyle discrimination, none reach so far as to regulate employer scrutiny of the smoking or weight status of employees. For example, the ADA prohibits employers from discriminating against disabled individuals on the basis of their disability in regard to job application procedures (hiring, advancement, or discharge), compensation, or job training. To be disabled within the meaning of the ADA, employees must establish that they have either a physical or mental impairment that substantially limits one or more of their major life activities, a record of an impairment, or that they are regarded by others as having such an impairment (whether or not the employee actually has an impairment). Major life activities include caring for oneself, performing manual tasks, walking, seeing, hearing, speaking, breathing, learning, and working. Other examples of major life activities include sitting, standing, lifting, and mental and emotional processes such as

thinking, concentrating, and interacting with others. The ADA prohibits employers from requiring medical examinations or making other disability-related inquiries to determine if an employee is disabled (or the extent of any such disability) unless the examination or inquiry is job-related and consistent with business necessity.

The ADA, with its focus on preventing discrimination against those with a significant physical or mental impairment, is inapplicable to claims brought by employees or job applicants who are not restricted in life activities. Although smoking and obesity may lead to eventual disability, neither, in and of itself, is a disability because neither limits major life activities as required under the ADA. Accordingly, while obese employees faced with lifestyle discrimination have recourse under the ADA, their legal protections are narrow and quite specific. Smokers have no such recourse.

Civil Rights Legislation

The federal Civil Rights Act prohibits discrimination in employment based on race, national origin, sex, and religion. Because discrimination against smokers and obese employees does not implicate race, national origin, sex, or religion, employees and job applicants subject to discrimination based on smoking or obesity have no recourse under the Civil Rights Act or similar state enactments.

In addition, as a result of the considerable body of evidence concerning the effect of secondhand smoke, there has been significant government regulation of smoking. For example, smoking is generally prohibited in the workplace and in public buildings. While policies aimed at protecting nonsmokers from secondhand smoke have not reached so far as to preclude smoking in private or to preclude employment consideration of private, off-duty smoking, absent state legislation, employers in most states are free to exercise their at-will right to exclude employees who smoke from the workforce. In Arkansas, California, Louisiana, Puerto Rico, and Bangor, Maine, citations can be issued to drivers or passengers smoking in a vehicle where a child under the age of eighteen is present (DeFao, 2007). Sixteen other states are considering similar legislation in homes and vehicles where children are present according to the National Conference of State Legislatures.

Invasion of Privacy

Employers' considerations of smoking and obesity do not usually violate privacy interests. Because there is no recognized state or federal constitutional right to be free from non-arbitrary employment considerations, absent lifestyle discrimination legislation,[LN6] employers can implement no-smoking and obesity policies.

Privacy claims, like the right to be free from intrusion upon seclusion, require that an employer's intrusion be unreasonable and intrusive upon private affairs. The mere fact that smoking may take place in private is insufficient to subject the activity to privacy protection. The same reasoning would apply to eating and/or not exercising.

Courts that have considered whether lifestyle smoking is a private affair that implicates a legitimate privacy interest have concluded that it is not. Today, smokers must reveal that they smoke in almost every aspect of life. No courts have considered whether eating and/or not exercising until obesity occurs is subject to privacy protection. However, claims for intrusion upon seclusion cannot be maintained where activities are habitually disclosed or undertaken in public.

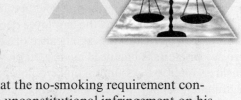

LIFESTYLE DISCRIMINATION: SMOKING

Grusendorf v. Oklahoma City

[Employee v. Employer]

816 F.2d 539 (U.S. Court of Appeals for the Tenth Circuit 1987)

FACTS: After a very stressful morning on his job as a firefighter trainee with the Oklahoma City Fire Department, Greg Grusendorf took several puffs from a cigarette during his lunch break. That afternoon, he was fired by his supervisor on the grounds that he had violated the terms of an agreement he signed as a precondition of employment that he would not smoke either on or off duty.

Grusendorf brought suit against the City of Oklahoma City and his supervisors at the Oklahoma City Fire Department, claiming his constitutional rights to liberty, privacy, property, and due process had been violated. Grusendorf claimed that he had a right to liberty and/or privacy while on his lunch break, or a right to be left alone, which included the right to smoke while off duty.

ISSUE: Can employees be fired for smoking in private?

HOLDING AND DECISION: Yes. An employer's no-smoking rules are enforceable if they are reasonable and balanced against an important interest that justifies the requirement. Such rules must be applied uniformly to all employees.

ANALYSIS: Grusendorf challenged the legality of a no-smoking-ever rule for firefighter trainees. He

claimed that the no-smoking requirement constituted an unconstitutional infringement on his rights to liberty, property, due process, and privacy. The federal district court dismissed his claims, finding no such infringement.

On appeal, the Tenth Circuit Court of Appeals addressed whether the regulation violated a federal constitutional right to privacy and concluded that it did not. As a threshold matter, the court addressed whether the right to smoke was a fundamental right subject to heightened constitutional protection. Nonetheless, the court concluded that there was a Fourteenth Amendment liberty interest involved in the right to smoke while off duty. Accordingly, to be constitutionally permissible, the no-smoking-ever regulation could not be arbitrary and must be rationally connected to public safety.

The Tenth Circuit found that there was a rational basis for the no-smoking rule because good health and physical conditioning are essential requirements for firefighters. In reaching its conclusion, however, the court invited constitutional attack on off-duty smoking regulations that may be arbitrary or irrational as applied.

RULE OF LAW: Smokers do not have a federal constitutional right to privacy.

(*See generally* Valleau, 2007).

DISCLOSURE REQUIREMENT OF LIFESTYLE CHOICES

Most employers who prohibit employee smoking or obesity require that employees agree to disclose their smoking or weight status. No intrusion into privacy occurs where employers have permission to commit the intrusive act or when the employee is on notice of the employment policy. Thus, where an employer has given notice of a no-smoking policy, the lifestyle smoker is caught between disclosing the smoking and being fired or refusing disclosure and being fired. Obesity is readily apparent, so it is difficult to claim a privacy intrusion.

Even if employees could establish that they had a reasonable expectation of privacy regarding their smoking or weight, employer scrutiny into employee smoking and obesity is reasonable. A balancing test is generally utilized in determining whether an employer's intrusion into an area the employee deems private is unreasonable. Thus, the significance of employee privacy interests is balanced against employer business interests. Assuming that employers have a legitimate business interest in reducing benefit costs, such as the increased health care costs incurred due to employees who smoke or are obese, employer policies requiring employee self-disclosure are not inherently unreasonable.

Tobacco-Free Policies

Weyco, an Okemos, Michigan, company specializing in employee benefit plans and benefit management, became famous as a result of its tobacco-free policy. As adopted, the Weyco policy required current employees to quit smoking or be fired, and employees who were identified as smokers on the target date were terminated. The Weyco policy provided that employees were to be subjected to random breath tests for carbon monoxide. A positive test result would be followed by a confirmatory urine test. After Weyco fully implemented its no-smoking policy, employees were required to maintain a tobacco-free status at all times (Schultz et al., 2005).

Regulation of Off-Duty Smoking

In response to Weyco's tobacco-free policy, some states enacted legislation prohibiting employers from basing employment decisions on off-duty smoking. Although many are broader, most of the state laws are aimed at preventing employers from firing, refusing to hire, or otherwise discriminating against employees who smoke. Not surprisingly, one of the biggest proponents of the right to smoke is the tobacco industry. Similarly, the American Civil Liberties Union has denounced lifestyle discrimination based on off-duty smoking as infringing on one's civil liberties or inherent right to privacy. Both argue that employers' consideration of lifestyle activities constitutes a slippery slope that will lead to discrimination based on other unhealthy or undesirable habits. The slippery slope argument centers on privacy issues and genetic testing. Already, concerns about discrimination against employees whose test results could become public have led most states to prohibit health insurers from using genetic information. In addition, federal agencies are prohibited from collecting genetic information from their employees or using such information to make hiring, promotion, or placement decisions (Executive Order, 2000).

Slippery Slope Arguments

A slippery slope has been defined as one that covers all situations where "A," which might be appealing, ends up materially increasing the probability that other situations will bring about "B," which is opposed. In the context of lifestyle discrimination on the basis of smoking and obesity, the argument is that where "A," the right to smoke in private and to be obese is not protected, then "B," employees will be subject to more offensive intrusions into their private lives.

Employees are always vulnerable to being taking advantage of by their employers. This is the reason for HIPAA privacy laws dealing with the collection of health care information about individual employees. What happens when a female employee gains weight during pregnancy and does not lose it right away? How would Weyco address the Pregnancy Discrimination Act of 1978?

Based on the slippery slope argument, if employers are allowed to discriminate against smokers and the obese, they might start targeting other groups as well. For example, women who choose to have children might have to pay for the health care costs associated with pregnancy and the costs associated with their children's health, people who break their legs while skiing might have to pay for the cost of the injuries they received as a consequence of their dangerous choice, even people who choose to take a busy highway home from work and then get in a serious car accident might have to pay for the cost of the injuries they received as a result of choosing to take that particular way home that day. On some level, practically all health care costs are a result of employees' own preventable choices. Based on this slippery slope argument, the only thing health care plans would have to pay for is preventive care itself.

One of the greatest problems with the slippery slope argument is that it is a convenient way of warning of the dire effects of lifestyle discrimination without actually having to address smoking or obesity. Thus, proponents argue that while self-identification at the outset of no-smoking or obesity policies may suffice, eventually employers will require universal medical testing of employees to enforce the policies.

Although most employers who discriminate based on smoking or obesity rely on voluntary disclosures, it is true that some employers, such as Weyco, have resorted to more intrusive measures to enforce their policies. However, when more intrusive means of policing off-duty behaviors are used, employers risk claims for invasion of privacy.

LIFESTYLE DISCRIMINATION IS GOOD BUSINESS

It is undisputed that employers incur costs as a result of hiring and retaining employees with unhealthy lifestyles. If employers do not impose a surcharge on such employees, then those additional costs are passed onto, or shared with, all employees.

There is no doubt that the greatest harm caused by smokers and obese employees is self-inflicted. Nonetheless, their lifestyle consequences have a ripple effect resulting in employer consequences. From the employer's perspective, given a choice between a nonsmoker and a smoker or between someone who is obese or non-obese, with all other things being equal, it would be an irrational business decision to choose the lifestyle smoker or obese employee. In dollars and cents, the employer who chooses to hire the lifestyle smoker or obese employee has opted to pay more for services that can be purchased for less. In other words, it is good business to hire nonsmokers and non-obese employees.

Nonetheless, employers who opt for lifestyle discrimination make a business decision to forego hiring from a segment of the available labor market. In certain industries, a ban on employment of employees with unhealthy lifestyles may be impracticable. For instance, because the highest incidence of smoking is among young unskilled employees, those businesses seeking a significant pool of unskilled laborers could ultimately limit their applicant pool to a point that any savings in benefit costs would be offset by the increased wages necessary to broaden the applicant pool.

At the same time, those in favor of lifestyle discrimination claim that no-smoking and obesity policies provide incentives for employees to adopt healthy lifestyles. In fact, there is some, albeit anecdotal, evidence supporting the proposition that no-smoking and healthy weight policies provide incentives for some employees to quit smoking or lose weight. When cast in these terms, employers' concerns for employees' health sounds virtuously noble; numerous news sources quote employees testifying that without incentives from employers, they would have never have quit smoking or lost weight. Moreover, evidence is beginning to emerge showing that incentivizing employees to lose weight may be effective (AP, 2007).

Paying for Lifestyle Choices

There are two sides to the lifestyle discrimination debate. On one hand, there is reluctance to allow employers to intrude into the health of employees with preventable behaviors and conditions. In reality, however, employers have a right to make hiring decisions based on the predicted efficiency of job applicants. Inevitably, employees with unhealthy lifestyles will cost more in employer-provided benefits and be less productive in general due to poor health.

Therefore, the question is whether there are alternatives to lifestyle discrimination. Many employers have opted to pass on health care costs attributable to preventable behaviors and conditions to those employees who smoke or are obese. Of course, this middle position is available only in those jurisdictions that have not enacted laws prohibiting discrimination and adhere to the premise that employment is at-will.

The middle approach of passing on employer costs attributable to preventable behaviors and conditions has two benefits. First, supplemental amounts paid by employees with preventable behaviors and conditions are intended to, and by all accounts do, offset at least some employer costs inherent in hiring these employees. Accordingly, to the extent that increased health care costs attributable to preventable behaviors and conditions are passed on to employees, the increased costs are borne by those who create the risk of the increased costs, rather than by those who do not pose the same economic risk to employers. Second, because it operates as a surcharge, it provides an incentive to employees to adopt healthier lifestyles, or stop smoking and lose weight.

Studies confirm that employers believe employees should be held accountable for their own health (Watson Wyatt, 2007). At the same time, employers believe employees are not held accountable.

One of the advantages of the benefits surcharge is that it forces employees to be responsible for the additional costs incumbent in their lifestyles, while at the same time relieving employees from bearing benefit costs not attributable to their own behavior. In short, it makes employees accountable for their behavior with employment consequences.

Balancing Costs: Preventable Behaviors and Conditions

Healthy lifestyles constitute a legitimate employment consideration. Employers need to know more about the nature of the risks they face, the likelihood of occurrence, and the health care costs that may result. Self-insured large employers and insurers that provide benefit plans to small employers are interested because they need to know how to set premiums for different types of risk within the context of their overall risk portfolio.

Although some states proscribe employment consideration of obesity and off-duty smoking, an increasing number of states continue the at-will tradition of employment, allowing employers to fire or refuse to hire employees at their option. In the middle are those employers who opt to hire smokers and obese employees, but only on the condition that those who smoke or are obese pay at least some of the benefit costs attributable to smoking or their weight. The prevailing view of employers is that policies covering preventable behaviors and conditions at the expense of all employees are not fair.

No one seriously disputes that smoking and obesity impact health and impose significant health and productivity costs on employers (PricewaterhouseCoopers & World Economic Forum, 2007). The World Economic Forum calls on business leaders to fight chronic diseases, many of which are related to smoking and obesity, in the workplace, not only to cut direct and indirect costs, but as a matter of social responsibility. There is considerable evidence that smoking and obesity are directly related to increased employer health care costs. An equitable approach to lifestyle discrimination should balance the concerns of employees with healthy lifestyles with those of employees who have preventable behaviors and conditions. Attempts should be made to balance individual employee privacy concerns with the cost burdens imposed on employers who are forced to hire employees with preventable behaviors and conditions. Under a balanced approach, employers could proscribe making hiring and firing decisions based on preventable behaviors and conditions. At the same time, legislation could also provide for employers to pass on the costs reasonably associated with the hiring and retention of employees with preventable behaviors and conditions to those specific employees. Under this scheme, it would be legitimate to charge a surcharge for employer-provided benefits to those employees who smoke or are obese.

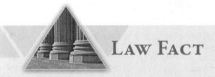

LAW FACT

LIFESTYLE DISCRIMINATION

Can employees be fired for being obese?

Obesity is not a disability unless it has a proven physiological cause.

—*EEOC v. Watkins Motor Lines, Inc.*, 463 F.3d 436
(U.S. Court of Appeals for the Sixth Circuit 2006).

CHAPTER SUMMARY

- HIPAA prevents employers from learning of individual employee health conditions.
- Large, self-insured employers usually have health plans with benefit costs credibly based on claims; smaller employers purchase demographic-based health plans.
- Employers may penalize employees for smoking behavior and obesity conditions unless there are state prohibitions against specific lifestyle discrimination activities.
- Lifestyle policies must not be arbitrary and must be rationally connected to a legitimate goal to survive being challenged in court.
- Neither gender nor race can be used to target smokers or obese employees for discriminatory treatment.
- Employers may use dynamic pricing in their health benefit plans and charge smokers and obese employees higher premiums.
- No federal legislation regulates employer scrutiny of the smoking or weight status of employees.

- The ADA prohibits employers from discriminating against the disabled in regard to job application procedures (hiring, advancement, or discharge), compensation, and training.
- To be disabled under the ADA, employees must have an impairment that substantially limits their major life activities, a record of impairment, or be regarded as having an impairment.
- The ADA prohibits employers from requiring medical examinations or inquiries to determine if an employee is disabled, unless the examination or inquiry is job-related and consistent with business necessity.
- The ADA, with its focus on preventing discrimination against those with significant impairments, is inapplicable to employees or job applicants who are not necessarily restricted in their life activities, such as smokers and obese individuals.
- Although smoking and obesity may lead to eventual disability, they are not, in and of themselves, a disability because they do not limit major life activities as required under the ADA.
- Because lifestyle discrimination against smoking and obesity does not implicate race, national origin, sex, or religion, employees and job applicants have no recourse under the Civil Rights Act or similar state enactments.
- Lifestyle discrimination against smoking and obesity does not violate privacy interests, since there is no constitutional right to be free from non-arbitrary employment considerations.
- Employers cannot unreasonably intrude upon the private affairs of employees; the fact that smoking may take place in private is insufficient to subject the behavior to privacy protection.
- Employers may require employees to agree to disclose their smoking or weight status; no intrusion into privacy occurs where employers have permission to commit the intrusive act or when the employee is on notice of the employment policy.
- Since employers have a legitimate business interest in reducing benefit costs, employer policies requiring employee self-disclosure are not unreasonable.
- Healthy lifestyles constitute a legitimate employment consideration.

LAW NOTES

1. Chronic diseases affect at least 125 million Americans and cost more than $500 billion annually (Landro, 2004). The federal Centers for Disease Control warned of an increased burden of heart disease and stroke on the health care system and calls for stronger prevention efforts. Also, the federally sponsored U.S. Preventive Services Task Force, which issues recommendations on screening tests, calls for physicians to screen their adult patients for preventable diseases and prescribes intensive behavior therapy to those who need it.

2. Humana, a health insurer in Louisville, Kentucky, asks its employees if they smoke. Those who said they do not smoke get a bonus in their paychecks each pay period. General Mills, Northwest Airlines, Continental Airlines, Sprint Nextel, Nissan, Gannett, and Scotts Miracle-Gro impose a surcharge on the employer-provided benefits of smokers. *See also* Forster, 2005; Higgins, 2005.

3. Prospective health programs with personalized planning are emerging. Landro (2004) describes how Duke University studied this idea in a randomized trial funded by the federal government's Center for Medicare and Medicaid Services before offering a prospective health program to its thirty-five thousand employees and their dependents. Emory University and other large academic medical centers and the Association of American Medical Colleges are also investigating the prospective health model for their own employees; medical schools that do research and provide health plans to their employees offer the perfect testing ground for this effort. Preventive care with more personalized planning is becoming more common in large nonprofit managed-care groups, such as Seattle's Group Health Cooperative, which covers 560,000 employees and their dependents in the Pacific Northwest.

   The lawn and gardening products company Scotts Miracle-Gro requires employees to take annual health assessments through a program affiliated with medical information Web site WebMD Health Corp., or pay extra benefit costs at a significant level. The health assessment starts with a form filled out online. Then, a health coach contacts the employee and arranges a treatment regimen to address any health issues. The employee must follow through with the recommendations or pay higher premiums. Whole Health Management Inc., a Cleveland company that also works with Continental Airlines, Sprint Nextel, and Nissan, among others, administers the program.

4. Vital Measures is one wellness program where credits are issued to employees under a supplemental health plan. Launched in July 2007 by UnitedHealthcare, the program is available to employers in Rhode Island, Pennsylvania, Colorado, and Ohio. Employees usually have a health plan with a $2,500 deductible and can then participate in a free, confidential health screening for body mass index, cholesterol, blood pressure, and

non-nicotine use. For each test that employees pass, they earn a $500 credit toward their deductible, issued under a supplemental plan administered by BeniComp Advantage. The earliest an employee failing a health test can earn the credit is the next year. However, there is an appeals process, and employees whose physicians say they cannot meet the standards for medical reasons are offered alternative ways of earning credits, such as participation in healthy lifestyle programs (smoking-cessation program or weight-loss program). Before the December 2007 regulatory guidelines were issued by the Employee Benefits Security Administration, Vital Measures was found to be in compliance with the HIPAA wellness rules, including the 20 percent threshold on rewards, by the U.S. Department of Labor.

5. Federal appeals courts considering whether obesity is a disability under the ADA or the Rehabilitation Act have held that it is not. *See McKibben v. Hamilton County*, 215 F.3d 1327 (U.S. Court of Appeals for the Sixth Circuit 2000) (weight was not a substantial limitation to job opportunities as a corrections officer); *Walton v. Mental Health Ass'n*, 168 F.3d 661 (U.S. Court of Appeals for the Third Circuit 1999) (perceived obesity is not a valid cause of action for discrimination); and *Francis v. City of Meriden*, 129 F.3d 281 (U.S. Court of Appeals for the Second Circuit 1997) (obesity is not a physical impairment within the meaning of the ADA unless it relates to a physiological disorder).

   Most federal trial courts have held that obesity fails to meet the definition of a disability. *See Dale v. Wynne*, 497 F.Supp.2d 1337 (U.S. District Court for the Middle District of Alabama, Northern Division 2007) (obesity must be based on a physiological disorder to be covered under the Rehabilitation Act); *Coleman v. Georgia Power Co.*, 81 F.Supp.2d 1365 (Northern District of Georgia, Atlanta Division 2000) (obesity must not only affect a bodily system but must also result from a physiological condition to qualify as an ADA impairment); *Furst v. Unified Court Systems*, 1999 WL 1021817 (U.S. District Court for the Eastern District of New York 1999) (weight was not a physical impairment that substantially limited a major life activity because there was no showing of obesity since there was no clinical diagnosis, no related medical problems, and no interference with any major life activity); *Hazeldine v. Beverage Media, Ltd.*, 954 F.Supp. 697 (U.S. District Court for the Southern District of New York 1997) (the threshold elements of an ADA claim were not met; there was no disability under the ADA due to obesity substantially limiting a major life activity or because of an employer's perception of an employee as disabled); *Fredregill v. Nationwide Agribusiness Insurance Co.*, 992 F.Supp. 1082 (U.S. District Court for the Southern District of Iowa, Central Division 1997) (claim that the employee was not promoted to senior management because of obesity failed to establish disability under the ADA); *Smaw v. Virginia Department of State Police*, 862 F.Supp. 1469 (U.S. District Court for the Eastern District of Virginia, Norfolk Division 1994) (employer did not violate the Rehabilitation Act or the ADA when it re-employed an employee as a dispatcher due to obesity and resulting inability to satisfy the maximum weight required for a trooper; obesity was regarded as an impairment for a particular position rather than an impairment from a class of jobs).

6. Twenty-one states have not enacted employee-privacy laws. Alabama, Alaska, Arkansas, California, Delaware, Florida, Georgia, Hawaii, Idaho, Kansas, Maryland, Massachusetts, Michigan, Mississippi, Nebraska, Ohio, Pennsylvania, Texas, Utah, Vermont, and Washington do not have employee-privacy laws. The states that have enacted employee-privacy laws include Arizona, Colorado, Connecticut, the District of Columbia, Illinois, Indiana, Kentucky, Louisiana, Maine, Minnesota, Missouri, Montana, Nevada, New Hampshire, New Jersey, New Mexico, New York, North Carolina, North Dakota, Oklahoma, Oregon, South Carolina, South Dakota, Virginia, West Virginia, Wisconsin, and Wyoming.

CHAPTER BIBLIOGRAPHY

AP (Associated Press). (2007, December 6). Drop cash; Workers may drop pounds. *Los Angeles Times*, p. C6 (employers cannot lose because they do not pay out until the employee actually loses the weight and keeps it off for a certain period of time).

Bosch, J. (2006). None of your business (interest): The argument for protecting all employee behavior with no business impact. *Southern California Law Review, 76*, 639-662.

Capell, P. (2007, October 2). Why weight-discrimination cases pose thorny legal tests. *Wall Street Journal*, p. B4 (proponents of weight-discrimination equate higher deductibles and higher co-pays to good-driver discounts and arguing that 70 percent of health care costs are lifestyle related; the logic is that higher out-of-pocket costs motivate employees to improve their health, which saves employers money and improves employee work performance).

CBO (Congressional Budget Office). (2006). *Potential effects on government revenues and outlays from an increase in the federal minimum wage.* Washington, DC: CBO.

CDC (Centers for Disease Control & Prevention). (2006) *State-specific prevalence of current cigarette smoking among adults and secondhand smoke rules and policies in homes and workplaces.* U.S. Morbidity & Mortality Weekly Report. Washington, DC: CDC.

Chadwick, K. L. (2006). Is leisure-time smoking a valid employment consideration? *Albany Law Review, 70,* 117-141 (examines the current approaches to employment discrimination against off-duty smoking).

Coil III, J. H., & Rice, C. M. (2004). When off-duty conduct becomes off limits: State laws expand to protect employees outside the workplace. *Employment Relations Today, 31* (3), 75-85.

Courtney, B. (2006). Is obesity really the next tobacco? Lessons learned from tobacco for obesity litigation. *Annals of Health Law, 15,* 61-105 (analyzes the parallels between obesity and smoking litigation; for example, both problems are attributed to intense marketing and advertising in their respective industries and both result in enormous medical costs and lost productivity).

DeFao, J. (2007, March 26). Proposed car-smoking ban angers foes of "nanny" laws: They don't want state dictating how kids are brought up. *San Francisco Chronicle,* p. A1.

___. (2006). *Wellness program management yearbook* (2nd ed.). Washington, DC: National Business Group on Health (nonprofit representing large employers).

Ellin, A. (2006, November 26). New breed of trainers are proving fat is fit. *New York Times,* p. G8.

Executive Order No. 13145, 65 *Federal Register* 286877. (2000) (to prohibit discrimination in federal employment based on genetic information).

Fletcher, M. (2004, November). Health risk appraisals address employees' individual problems. *Business Insurance, 38* (45), T3.

Forster, J. (2005, October 18). NWA smokers to pay more for insurance. *Detroit Free Press,* p.7 (Northwest Airlines charges its employees who smoke an additional fee for their health benefit plans).

Freudenheim, M. (2007, October 26). Seeking savings, employers help smokers quit. *New York Times,* p. A1 (". . . recent surveys indicate that one-third of companies with at least 200 workers now offer smoking cessation as part of their employee benefits package. Among the nation's biggest companies, the number may be nearly two-thirds of employers.... A survey by the nonprofit Kaiser Family Foundation found that smoking programs are offered by one in three companies with more than 200 workers. Among smaller firms, that was one in twelve.").

Girion, L. (2007, October 2). Europe healthier than U.S.: Older Americans have higher rates of serious diseases than aging Europeans, a study says. *Los Angeles Times,* p. C3.

Govan, R. C., & Mac, F. (2004). 33rd annual institute on employment law: Workplace privacy. *Practicing Law Institute, 712,* 245.

Gruber, J. (2000). Health insurance and the labor market. In J. Newhouse & A. Culyer (eds.), *The handbook of health economics* (pp. 645-706). Amsterdam, North Holland: Elsevier Science.

Hagan, R. P. (2005). Restaurants, bars and workplaces, lend me your air: Smoke-free laws as private property exactions: The undiscovered country for Nollan and Dolan. *Journal*

of Contemporary Health Law & Policy, 22, 144-145 ("397 municipalities and fourteen states have adopted smoke-free laws with respect to... restaurants, bars, or workplaces").

Heinen, L. (2004). *The big picture: U.S. employers combat weight-related health costs.* Washington, DC: National Business Group.

HEW (U.S. Department of Health, Education & Welfare). (1964). *Smoking and health: Report of the Advisory Committee to the Surgeon General of the Public Health Service.* Washington, DC: Public Health Service.

Higgins, M. (2005, October 19). Gannett smokers to pay. *Washington Times,* p. 1 (Gannett Company employees who admit to smoking are given the choice of enrolling in a company-funded cessation program or paying a $50 per month fee for their health benefit plans).

Hinton, K. (2005/2006). Employer by name, insurer by trade: Society's obesity epidemic and its effects on employers' healthcare costs. *Connecticut Insurance Law Journal, 12,* 137-171.

IOM (Institute of Medicine). (2001, March). *Crossing the quality chasm: A new health system for the 21st century* (Report from the Committee on the Quality of Health Care in America). Washington, DC: IOM.

Jurden, J. (2005). Spit and polish: A critique of military off-duty personal appearance standards. *Military Law Review, 184,* 1-65 (explaining the need for narrowly tailored rules that regulate off-duty behaviors).

Kaiser Daily Health Policy Report. (2008, January 22). *Administration news: Bush administration 2008 health care agenda will work to limit government role in health care system.* Menlo Park, CA: Kaiser Family Foundation.

Kaiser (Kaiser Family Foundation). (2007). *Health care costs: A primer.* Menlo Park, CA: Kaiser (examines the rapid growth in the nation's health care costs since 1970).

Landro, L. (2004, February 12). The informed patient: Preventive medicine gets more aggressive. *Wall Street Journal,* p. D1.

Lundborg, P. (2007). Smoking, information sources, and risk perceptions: New results on Swedish data. *Journal of Risk & Uncertainty, 34* (3), 217-240.

Mark et al. (2008). Mental health treatment expenditure trends, 1986-2003, *Psychiatric Services, 58,* 1041-1048.

Ott, C. H. (2005). Smoking-related health behaviors of employees and readiness to quit: Basis for health promotion interventions. *Journal of the American Association of Occupational Health Nurses, 53,* 249-256.

Power, C. (2003, August 11). Big trouble: Obesity is spreading to parts of the world that once worried about getting enough to eat. *Newsweek,* p. 42.

PricewaterhouseCoopers' Health Research Institute & World Economic Forum. (2007). *Working towards wellness: Accelerating the prevention of chronic disease.* New York, NY: PricewaterhouseCoopers (traditionally governments, not employers, have been responsible for the health of people; many business and policy leaders now believe that governments alone cannot prevent the spread of chronic disease... wellness must be inseparable from business objectives and long-term mission).

Raphael, J. (2007). The Calabasas smoking ban: A local ordinance points the way for the future of environmental tobacco smoke regulation. *Southern California Law Review, 80,* 393-423.

Russell, L. B. (2007). *Prevention's potential for slowing the growth of medical spending.* Washington, DC: National Coalition on Health Care (NCHC).

Rutkow, L. et al. (2007). Banning second-hand smoke in indoor public places under the Americans with Disabilities Act: A legal and public health imperative. *Connecticut Law Review, 40*, 409-458.

Schachte, V. (2005). Privacy in the workplace. *Annual Institute on Privacy Law: Data protection, the convergence of privacy and security, 6*, 153.

Schultz, M. et al. (2005, January 27). Workers fume as firms ban smoking at home, Michigan firms prohibit cigarette use, even off the job, angering privacy advocates. *Detroit News*, p. A1.

Silverman, P. (2005). Legal tools for cancer prevention and control. *Journal of Law, Medicine &Ethics (Special Supplement), 33*, 81-85 (smoking cessation programs cost approximately $7,000/quitter compared to a smoke-free workplace policy that leads to nearly nine times as many quitters and costs less than $800/quitter).

Smith, II, G. P. (2007). Cigarette smoking as a public health hazard: Crafting common law and legislative strategies for abatement. *Michigan State Journal of Medicine & Law, 11*, 251-302.

Stein, R. (2007, November 29). Obesity rates seen to level off: Plateau may answer question: How fat can Americans get? *Chicago Tribune*, p. 3.

Stewart, D. L. (1996). *City of North Miami v. Kurtz:* Is it curtains for privacy in Florida? *Nova Law Review, 30*, 1393-1414.

Sturm, R. (2002). The effects of obesity, smoking and drinking on medical programs and costs. *Health Affairs, 21* (2), 245-253 ("individuals who are obese have 30% to 50% more chronic medical problems than those who smoke or drink heavily").

Sugarman, S. (2003). Lifestyle discrimination in employment. *Berkeley Journal of Employment & Labor Law, 24*, 377-437 (examining the issue of how much employers should be able to intrude into the privacy of workers' off-duty lifestyle choices).

Tinetti, M., & Fried, T. (2004). The end of the disease era. *American Journal of Medicine, 116* (3) 179-185 (arguing that physicians must shift their focus from treating disease alone to tailoring treatments to individual patient needs).

Tolle, N. (2007, January). Non-physiologically caused obesity is not an impairment under ADA. *Employee Benefit Plan Review, 61* (7), 28.

Tsai, A. G., & Wadden, T. A. (2005). Systematic review: An evaluation of major commercial weight loss programs in the United States. *Annals of Internal Medicine, 142*, 56-66 (refining the financial costs associated with being overweight to include a per-person charge).

Valleau, C. (2007). If you're smoking you're fired: How tobacco could be dangerous to more than just your health. *DePaul Journal of Health Care Law, 10*, 457-492.

Volokh, E. (2003). The mechanisms of the slippery slope. *Harvard Law Review, 116*, 1026-1137 (evaluating the risk of slippery slope arguments).

Warren, C. W. et al. (2006). Patterns of global tobacco use in young people and implications for future chronic disease burden in adults. *Lancet. 367* (9512), 749-754.

Watson Wyatt. (2007, November 7). *Press release: More employers to offer workers financial incentives for healthy behavior*. Arlington, VA: Watson Wyatt (survey finds top employers integrate health management with business objectives).

Wharton (Wharton School of the University of Pennsylvania). (2008). From incentives to penalties: How far should employers go to reduce workplace obesity? *Knowledge@ Wharton* (noting that while an October 2007 Wall Street Journal Online/Harris Interactive survey found that two-thirds of 2,300 American adults polled said employers should not have the right to fire overweight employees or require enrollment in weight-loss programs, employers have gotten ahead of the culture on issues such as discrimination and sexual harassment in the past, and thus they may also be the logical leaders for behavior change with regard to obesity).

____. (2006). Efforts are growing to trim the fat from employees and employers' health care costs. *Knowledge@Wharton*.

____. (2005). Multiplier effect: The financial consequences of worker absences. *Knowledge@Wharton*.

Winokur, S. (2007). Seeing through the smoke: The need for national legislation banning smoking in bars and restaurants. *George Washington Law Review, 75*, 662-693.

CHAPTER 13

LABOR AND MANAGEMENT RELATIONS

> *"All that serves labor serves the nation. All that harms is treason. If a man tells you he trusts America, yet fears labor, he is a fool. There is no America without labor, and to fleece the one is to rob the other."*
>
> —ABRAHAM LINCOLN (1809-1865), SIXTEENTH PRESIDENT
> OF THE UNITED STATES OF AMERICA

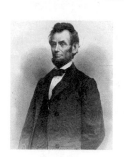

IN BRIEF

This chapter covers fundamental topics, such as employee free-choice reforms and unionization of physicians and nurses in an emerging stakeholder society. Nurse workload management and mandatory overtime are viewed in the context of their most severe consequences: adverse medical care and patient mortality. Health care staffing is placed alongside the recruitment and rights of foreign nurses and physicians who help the U.S. address staff shortages in the delivery of health care services in its health care systems.

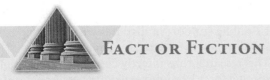

FACT OR FICTION

MANAGEMENT'S REFUSAL TO BARGAIN

What recourse do labor union employees have when management unilaterally makes decisions affecting employees and refuses to bargain over subjects contained in collective bargaining agreements?

The California Nurses Association (CNA) is the collective bargaining representative of the nurses at Enloe's facilities in Chico, California. The dispute in this case stems from management's unilateral adoption of a mandatory on-call policy that required nurses to work one four-hour on-call shift every four weeks, in addition to their regular shifts; nurses were permitted no more than thirty minutes to report when on call. Management indicated that if any nurse had a problem complying with the time requirement, that nurse should contact Enloe's clinical coordinator in order to make other arrangements.

When CNA learned of the on-call policy change, CNA told Enloe it could not unilaterally make the proposed change without first negotiating with the labor union. There is no disagreement between CNA and Enloe that the mandatory on-call policy was unilaterally adopted without consultation with Enloe's employees. The collective bargaining agreement included provisions spelling out Enloe's rights to manage the schedules of its employees, compensate nurses for on-call and call-back work, assign duties and hours to nurses, and establish standards related to patient care. It also contained a broad management rights clause.

There is a fundamental and long-running disagreement as to the appropriate approach to determine whether management has violated federal labor law when it refuses to bargain with its organized union employees over a subject contained in a collective bargaining agreement. Based on management's unilateral imposition of the new on-call policy, CNA filed a charge with the National Labor Relations Board (NLRB). The NLRB in turn issued a complaint against Enloe.

—*Enloe Medical Center v. National Labor Relations Board*, 433 F.3d 834
(U.S. Court of Appeals for the District of Columbia Circuit 2005).
(See *Law Fact* at the end of this chapter for the answer.)

PRINCIPLES AND APPLICATIONS

A new business model is needed for the delivery of health care in the twenty-first century in the U.S. A model that is less focused on treating diseases and more focused on public health needs and the prevention of disease may be required. The focus of health care must move away from just costs and bottom lines, and return to a place where science and innovation are once again the focal points of medicine. This would mean focusing on managing the health care of individuals rather than on just managing costs.

PUBLIC PERCEPTIONS OF LABOR AND MANAGEMENT

The recent global economic downturn has caused many to wonder whether traditional business models are broken. Most Americans believe the U.S. health care system is at a crossroads, facing both challenges to its funding and opportunities

for accelerating medical advancement. They believe significant reform of the system or even universal health care would be helpful in their struggle to access affordable, quality health care. At the same time, an image of ineffectiveness clouds the health care industry and its regulators. The only way to change this image of ineffectiveness is to change current reality (Maher, 2007).

Labor and management must appreciate that there are ways in which a partnership can catalyze change to add more value to the U.S. health care system, returning American medicine to its former place of global prominence. Both sides need to:

• Value markets and consumers of health care
• Understand their local, national, and global rivals that are competing to deliver the best medical care
• Appreciate where each partner can be most helpful: management with reforming the health care system and unions with increasing revenue from the public

and private sectors to bring about management's systemic reforms

- Level the playing field so medicine is about quality health care and efficiency and not about who can pay the least for staffing to provide the treatments and health care services

(*See generally* Maher, 2007)

MYTH: AMERICANS HATE LABOR UNIONS

Despite popular claims that labor unions are in decline, unions have maintained reasonably strong public support, as evidenced by:

- American National Election Study (Ohio State University)
- Current Population Survey (U.S. Bureau of Labor Statistics and U.S. Bureau of the Census)
- Gallup Surveys
- Hart Research National Opinion Surveys
- Roper Center for Public Opinion Research (University of Connecticut)

Although the data indicate that Americans remain skeptical about how much confidence they can place in labor unions and their leaders (the same can be said for management), the public recognizes the need for unions to protect the rights of employees (Panagopoulos & Francia, 2008). According to Harvard University research of both union and non-union private-sector employees, if employees were provided the union representation they desired in 2005, the unionization rate would be about 58 percent; almost eight times higher than the actual rate of 7 percent and considerably higher than the 44 percent found in Gallup and Hart Research polls from the mid-1990s (Freeman, 2007). As illustrated in Figure 13-1, the polls make clear that

labor's public support in disputes with business has remained steady over time (*see* Jones, 2008).

This research runs directly counter to what might be expected for a labor movement in decline. Moreover, as illustrated in Figure 13-2, most non-union employees now support labor unions.

RELEVANCE OF LABOR IN THE HEALTH CARE INDUSTRY

Almost everyone sees a window of opportunity for strategic trade-offs between the American labor movement and management. The most recent Q12 Gallup National Survey of 1.5 million employees in late 2008 found that almost three out of four employees were either underperforming or actively undermining their work (Thackray, 2008). This level of employee disengagement should be a wake-up call to management and opponents of organized labor who believe labor unions are a detriment to the nation. Organizations with high engagement scores exhibit lower turnover, higher growth, better productivity, better customer loyalty, and superior performance (Thackray, 2008).

Today, there is a unique opportunity for labor and management to come together, and find new ideas and new solutions to make working pay for everyone, not just the shareholders and the executives. While labor unions have the possibility of being more relevant today than at any time since labor first started in the U.S., there is a need for an attitude adjustment by both labor and management (Mahler, 2007).

While many American labor unions are losing members, the health care industry is becoming more unionized. Dominated by nurses and low-wage immigrant employees hoping for higher pay, health insurance, and retirement benefits, unions are successfully organizing nurses, maintenance staff, security

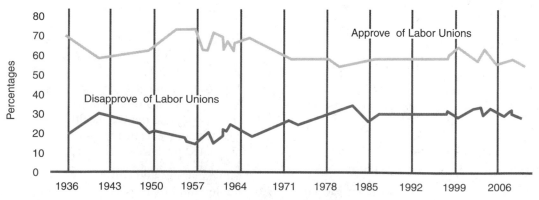

FIGURE 13-1: Current Fact: Americans Approve of Labor Unions by Two to One

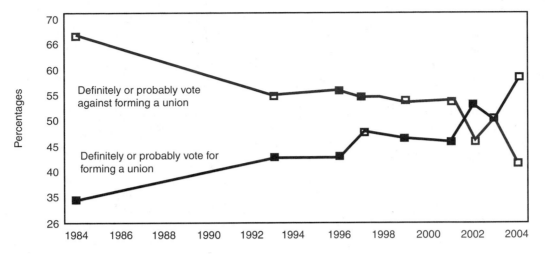

FIGURE 13-2: Current Fact: Most Non-Union Employees Support Unions

Delmar, Cengage Learning
Data retrieved from: Freeman, 2007.
Copyright Economic Policy Institute.

staff, and aides in hospitals, nursing homes, and other institutional health care facilities.

Labor union membership is high in the nursing profession (Kugielska & Linke, 2008). The Service Employees International Union (SEIU) claims that unions represent more than 3 million of the total 8.7 million registered nurses, practical and vocational nurses, paramedics, and aides (BLS, 2009). The Economic Policy Institute (EPI) estimates that if an additional five million health care employees joined a union:

- Five million employees would get a 22 percent raise on average, or an additional $7,000 per year
- $34 billion in total new wages would flow into the economy
- Nine hundred thousand jobs would be lifted above the poverty wage for a family of four ($10.22/hour)
- Between 1.8 million and 3 million dependent children would share in these benefits

(Vidal, 2009)

A valid question is the increased costs to the health care system from unionization. In answering the question, it might be more appropriate to focus attention on the top of the economic pyramid rather than the bottom. The nation might begin by addressing the merits of multimillion-dollar compensation packages. For instance, the average chief executive officer's pay has skyrocketed from 27 times more than the average employee's wages in 1973 to 344 times higher today (Vidal, 2009). While health care executives no doubt contribute to the economic development of the health care industry, there is growing debate about this income disparity when almost half of the three million aides are working for poverty wages, as are one in four support staff (BLS, 2009). Trickle-down

economics may not be working as once anticipated. Perhaps part of the nation health care reform should begin from this point and have the health care industry focus on reductions in its own employees' poverty and inequality.

Nevertheless, the cost from adding five million to the industry's unionized workforce would be $34 billion in new wages added to the nation's health care costs (Vidal, 2009). While this number would be offset by the economic benefits of poverty reduction when nine hundred thousand families would be brought above the poverty level, no definitive study exists to explain how wage increases would affect the nation's health care costs.

Moral Dilemmas

1. How should established health care providers and medical products companies think about labor and management, given the current economy?

Labor-Management Partnerships

In the health care industry, labor has generally shed its adversarial image and created labor-management partnerships. For instance, the SEIU has entered into a partnership with the American Association of Retired Persons and the Business Roundtable (an association of chief executive officers of U.S. companies with more than $5 trillion in annual revenues and nearly ten million employees; member companies comprise nearly a third of the total value of the U.S. stock markets and pay nearly half of all corporate income taxes paid to the federal government) to push Congress to act on health care reform (Maher, 2007).[LN1] At the same time, SEIU, with more than two million members, is feared by management in the health care industry because of its high success rate at waging aggressive organizing campaigns that usually include support from stakeholders (elected officials, clergy, community and patient activists), in addition to unremitting publicity.

The need for labor unions is far greater today than almost any time since the 1930s and 1940s (Maher, 2007). The compensation disparity between the average employee and the average chief executive officer (CEO) is wider than at any time in American history (Clemente, 2009). As illustrated in Figure 13-3, the average total compensation of CEOs in the health insurance sector was $9.4 million, while health aides are not covered by minimum wage laws.

In addition to concerns about the compensation of CEOs, health care employees want a voice in their jobs. With 7 percent of U.S. private-sector employees belonging to unions today, down from about 35 percent fifty years ago, the U.S. has one of the lowest percentages of private-sector employees covered by collective bargaining agreements as compared to other democracies around the world (Maher, 2007). The question is whether labor and management will become partners to respond to what is now a global service economy, or whether they will function as adversaries. Unions missed out on the growth of the new service economy, so the newest sectors of the medical products industry developed without unions, especially the biotechnology and health information technology sectors. Today, as regulatory changes, industry consolidation, and economic globalization are rapidly occurring, there is a unique opportunity for an engaged workforce through non-adversarial partnerships between management and labor (e.g., Freeman, 2007; Jones, 2008; Lafer, 2008; Panagopoulos & Francia, 2008; Thackray, 2008).

Debate is ongoing about whether management and labor want to address the differences in total compensation between employees and senior management executives. This difference in total compensation is the tip of the iceberg in seeking a balance between labor and management interests. For instance, on top of differences in total compensation between CEOs and senior management executives, many employees also bear associated medical costs, such as higher health insurance premiums and reduced wages due to co-payments/co-insurance fees that have a greater effect on them as compared to the burden placed on top executives.

Union organizing campaigns are very sophisticated today. There is now a wide range of consultants, lawyers, and strike breakers who have been battle-tested. Current labor law, however, has no remedial enforcement power without reforms (Maher, 2007; see Pattern

Makers' League v. NLRB, 473 U.S. 95 (U.S. Supreme Court 1985) (holding that union members who are strikebreakers have a protected right to resign from the union at any time); First National Maintenance Corp. v. NLRB, 452 U.S. 666 (U.S. Supreme Court 1981) (holding that plant closures are not a mandatory subject of bargaining even where employees lose jobs); H. K. Porter Co. v. NLRB, 397 U.S. 99 (U.S. Supreme Court 1970) (holding that the NLRB is not authorized to impose contract terms as a remedy)). Management and labor unions at the largest health care organizations have often violated labor laws and intimidated employees, sometimes without fear of repercussion. Toothless remedies fail to deter abuses by both management and labor (Specter & Nguyen, 2008).

Currently, federal court injunctions are required only for violations by unions; no such equitable remedy exists for unlawful acts committed by management. Furthermore, when management violates the law by refusing to bargain in good faith, the most common remedy issued by the National Labor Relations Board is for management to promise to act correctly in the future; no penalty is imposed on management (Lafer, 2008; see Republic Steel Corp. v. NLRB, 311 U.S. 7 (U.S. Supreme Court 1940) (limiting the NLRB to remedies designed to make employees harmed by unfair labor practices whole, not remedies designed to deter bad conduct)). It is statutorily impossible under current labor law to impose fines, imprisonment, or punitive damages on management.

Moral Dilemmas

1. What further innovative labor and management partnerships, if any, might emerge as alternatives to the traditional adversarial model?

2. Who will be the winners and losers under new labor and management partnerships, and how should winning and losing be defined given current budget constraints?

3. Which side do most Americans want to work for, management or labor, and why?

Employee Free Choice Reforms

One priority of labor is reform of the labor laws adopted in the 1930s and 1940s, a movement popularly known as Employee Free Choice (EFC) (see generally, Labor Management Relations Act of 1947 (Taft-Hartley Act), 29 U.S.C.A. §§ 141 et seq. (2009)). EFC reforms are built around three provisions that would:

- Force management to recognize unions seeking to represent employees on the basis of a showing of signed cards instead of a secret ballot election administered by the NLRB

- Increase penalties for management who hassle and seek to intimidate pro-union employees
- Provide for binding arbitration to resolve impasses in contract bargaining

Company	2000 Net Revenue ($ Millions)	2008 Net Revenue ($ Millions)	% Change 2008 vs 2000	Value of CEO's Total Direct Compensation ($ Millions)
Aetna	$ 127.1	$ 1,384.1	1,089.0%	$23.0
Amerigroup	$ 18.8	$ (50.7)	619.7%	$ 5.3
Centene	$ 7.2	$ 83.5	1,159.7%	$ 8.8
Cigna	$ 987.0	$ 292.0	(29.6%)	$12.2
Coventry Health Care	$ 61.3	$ 381.9	623.0%	$13.1
Health Net	$ 163.3	$ 95.0	(58.1%)	$ 3.7
Humana	$ 90.1	$ 647.2	718.3%	$ 4.8
UnitedHealth	$ 736.0	$ 2,977.0	404.5%	$13.2
United American	$ 22.9	$ 95.1	415.3%	$ 1.6
WellPoint	$ 226.0	$ 2,490.7	1,102.1%	$ 9.1
Total	$2,440.0	$84,414.3	3,460.0%	$94.3

	Value of Top Three Executives Total Direct Compensation ($ Millions)			Value of Total Direct Compensation to Top Four Executives ($ Millions)
Aetna	$5.1	$3.9	$2.5	$43.5
Amerigroup	$3.2	$2.4	$1.3	$12.2
Centene	$1.7	$1.5	$1.4	13.4
Cigns	$4.3	$4.2	N/A	$20.7
Coventry Health Care	$4.5	$2.7	50.8	$11.7
Health Net	$2.5	$1.6	$1.4	$9.2
Humana	$2.5	$1.8	$1.6	$10.7
UnitedHealth	$5.4	$5.3	$5.2	$29.1
United American	$1.1	$1.0	$0.8	$4.5
WellPoint	$8.8	$3.3	N/A	$21.2
Total				$176.2

FIGURE 13-3: Profits and Salaries of CEOs and Top Three Executives for Health Insurance Providers

Notes: Figures in parentheses are losses. Total direct compensation is the sum of salary, annual incentives, and long-term incentives. Amerigroup net income had a $234.2 million legal settlement expense that resulted in a $50.7 million charge to income. Cigna had a guaranteed minimum income benefits expense of $690 million from its guaranteed annuities; net income for 2007 was $1.1 million.

Delmar/Cengage Learning

Data retrieved from: 2000 and 2008 company filings with the U.S. Securities and Exchange Commission. Net revenue figures (profits) are from 2008 corporate annual income statements. Compensation data reflects year ended December 31, 2007.

In general, EFC might rebalance power between labor and management in the context of organizing and collective bargaining for an initial contract. Opponents of EFC claim the cost to individuals for this rebalance is too high since secret ballot elections are eliminated. This secret ballot claim, however, misreads EFC. Proponents, however, have not successfully explained the distinctions in current labor law and the proposed EFC law. Many large health care systems, such as Kaiser Permanente, the largest managed care organization in the U.S., currently allow employees to make their own choice in forming labor unions as proposed by the EFC.

Signed Cards v. Ballot Elections

Under current labor law, unions seeking to be certified as the bargaining representative for a group of employees must demonstrate that they have the support of the majority of employees in the group. Usually, unions will solicit employees to sign authorization cards showing their support for union representation; if a majority of employees signs cards, the union may present these cards to the employer and ask to be recognized. Management is not, however, obligated to recognize a union on the basis of signed cards. The only way to force management to recognize a union as its employees' representative is through a secret ballot election.

Currently, employers can insist on a secret ballot election if 30 percent of employees sign authorization cards. EFC reforms would change this; if more than 50 percent of the cards are signed, there is no election because union recognition is automatic. Under EFC, employees, rather than employers, can request a secret ballot vote when between 31 and 50 percent of the employees have signed authorization cards. Supporters of EFC maintain that the secret ballot election is still an option; opponents claim that the secret ballot is theoretical because unions will unduly pressure half of the employees to sign cards.

Under current labor law, management has an advantage over employees. The choice of whether to use an election process or majority sign-up to form the union is now exclusively controlled by management. From the time a union requests an election, and the actual date of the election, can last indefinitely under the EFC reforms, this extended pre-election period would vanish.

Financial Penalties

Management who fired or discriminated against pro-union employees would face more significant financial penalties than currently exist. *See* Employee Free Choice Act, H.R. 800, 110th Cong. (2007) (passed in the House of Representatives, sponsored

in the Senate by then-Senator Obama, but the Senate failed to act upon it; proposed legislation will have to be reintroduced and passed in a new congressional session in order for it to become law). Research shows that one-quarter of union-organizing drives lead to employee terminations, and that one out of every five employees who openly support a union is terminated. It can take years of hearings to have these employees reinstated, and the penalties management faces are minimal (Kochan & Shulman, 2007).

EFC laws would contain treble back pay. Treble back pay increases the amount management is required to pay to three times the amount of the employee's back pay when an employee is discharged or discriminated against during an organizing campaign or first contract drive. EFC also contains civil penalties, which provide for civil fines of up to $20,000 per violation for violating employees' rights during an organizing campaign or first contract drive.

Binding Arbitration

EFC also requires management to submit to binding arbitration to resolve negotiating impasses. In particular, if the two sides did not reach a first contract within ninety days of the commencement of bargaining, the matter would have to be submitted to an alternative dispute resolution process that could lead to binding arbitration upon the demand of either side. This represents a change from current labor law, which permits management to unilaterally put into place the terms of the last, best, and final offers upon reaching an impasse in negotiations. Under current labor rules, management must bargain in good faith with employees, but is not obligated to agree to any terms.

Prospects for Change

While management forces wield extraordinary clout in opposition of EFC, business's unity, or lack of it, will decide what happens. Majority sign-up is not a new procedure, as EFC opponents claim. Since the inception of the National Labor Relations Act in 1935, employees have been able to form a union when a majority signs authorization cards indicating their intent to be represented by a union. Currently, employers can demand a secret ballot election even if a majority of the employees have signed cards.

Comprehensive labor legislation is necessary to correct the fundamental problems facing management and labor. The most critical focus of this reform is protecting the right of employees to freely choose whether they wish to be represented (Specter & Nguyen, 2008).

General Bargaining Principles

General principles could serve as a reasonable starting point for crafting workplace policies that serve employees in today's economic environment. Much legislation already exists on these principles. For instance:

- Protect against major downside risks associated with employment to cushion the impact of globalization on individuals and local communities, loss of pensions or health care benefits, loss of job from major family emergencies:
  - Continuation of Health Benefits Coverage Act, 5 U.S.C.A. §§ 8901-8914 (2009)
  - Employee Retirement Income Security Act (ERISA), 26 U.S.C.A. §§ 219 *et seq.* (2009)
  - Family Medical Leave Act, 5 U.S.C.A. §§ 6381 *et seq.* (2009)
  - Trade Adjustment Assistance Act, 19 U.S.C.A. §§ 1431a *et seq.* (2009)
  - Unemployment Compensation, 5 U.S.C.A. §§ 8501-8525 (2009)
  - Workers Adjustment and Retraining Notification Act, 29 U.S.C.A. §§ 2101-2109 (2009)
- Assure basic labor standards: hours of work, overtime compensation:
  - Davis-Bacon Act, 40 U.S.C.A. §§ 3141-3144, 3146-3147 (2009)
  - Fair Labor Standards Act, 2 U.S.C.A. § 60k (1989); 29 U.S.C.A. §§ 210 *et seq.* (2009)
  - Minimum Wage Act, 29 U.S.C.A. § 206 (2007)
  - Service Contract Act, 41 U.S.C.A. §§ 351-358 (2009)
  - Walsh-Healy Act, 41 U.S.C.A. §§ 35-45 (2009)
- Ensure a safe and healthy work environment with low exposure to safety and health risks:
  - Drug Free Workplace Act, 41 U.S.C.A. §§ 701-707 (2009)
  - Occupational Safety and Health Act, 29 U.S.C.A. §§ 651 *et seq.* (2009); 42 U.S.C.A. § 3142-1 (2009)
- Protect against workplace discrimination in hiring, promotion, dismissal, and treatment of employees:
  - Civil Rights Acts, 2 U.S.C.A. §§ 60l *et seq.* (2009)
  - Age Discrimination Employment Act, 29 U.S.C.A. §§ 621-634 (2009)
  - Americans with Disabilities Act, 42 U.S.C.A. §§ 12101 *et seq.* (2009); 47 U.S.C.A. § 225 (1996)
  - President Lyndon B. Johnson, Exec. Order 11,246 (1965)
  - Immigration Reform and Control Act, 8 U.S.C.A. §§ 1160 *et seq.* (2009)
  - Pregnancy Discrimination Act, 42 U.S.C.A. § 2000e(k) (1991)
  - Rehabilitation Act, 29 U.S.C.A. §§ 701 *et seq.* (2009) (providing protection from discrimination to handicapped employees; it preceded the ADA); 42 U.S.C.A. § 2000d-7 (1986)
  - Equal Pay Act, 29 U.S.C.A. § 206(d) (2007)
  - Uniformed Services Employment and Reemployment Rights Act, 5 U.S.C.A. § 8432b (1999); 38 U.S.C.A. §§ 4301 *et seq.* (2009)
  - Veterans' Reemployment Rights Act, 38 U.S.C.A. §§ 4301-4307 (2009)
- Provide basic mechanisms for worker representation and voice at the workplace:
  - Labor Management Reporting and Disclosure Act, 29 U.S.C.A. §§ 401 *et seq.* (2009)
  - National Labor Relations Act, 29 U.S.C.A. §§ 151-169 (2009)

NURSE WORKLOAD MANAGEMENT

Nurses represent the largest single group of health care professionals in the nation (Hassmiller & Cozine, 2006). However, most hospitals struggle to maintain an adequate number of nurses on their staff. The reasons for this struggle are circular. One of the effects of managed care cost-cutting is understaffing, which leads to overworking existing staff. As hospitals run understaffed nurses are dissatisfied with the working conditions because they believe they cannot provide quality patient care. Thus, nurses leave hospitals for more satisfying positions and hospitals continue to run with understaffed nursing departments and overworked nurses. It is a perilous cycle.

In the midst of a current nursing shortage that is predicted to worsen over time, nurses claim that understaffing represents a danger to patient care. California was the first state to require mandatory nurse-to-patient ratios in all hospital units. This change ensured that staffing could no longer be ignored in the dialogue between hospital management and the nursing profession. Staffing concerns include:

- Fewer nurses on staff will significantly increase the risk of preventable hospital deaths and complications (Scott et al., 2006)
- There is a direct correlation between increased workload and lower nursing staff retention rates

Nursing shortages first manifested in the late 1990s in intensive care units and operating rooms, but spread to labor and delivery units, and general medical/surgical wards. Based upon current trends, the size of the nurse workforce will be nearly 30 percent below projected requirements within the decade unless change occurs.

Nurse Staffing Research

The nursing shortage, with the resulting increase in workloads, has also contributed to high rates of job dissatisfaction within the profession, with one in five trained nurses no longer working as nurses (BLS, 2009). Because of the unrealistic workloads:

- Nurses experience job dissatisfaction rates that are four times greater than the average for all other employees of any type in the U.S.
- Almost half of the nurses who reported high levels of burnout and job dissatisfaction intended to leave their jobs within the next year
- Higher professional skill mix, in other words more nurses versus nonprofessional caregivers, results in a lower incidence of adverse occurrences in inpatient care units (adverse occurrences in nursing literature include patient falls, medication administration errors, pressure ulcers, nosocomial infections, patient complaints, and mortality (*see generally* Kane))
- Fewer nurses on the night shift results in an increased risk for complications in intensive care units
- Decreased nurse staffing at night is related to postoperative complications and increased health care costs
- The higher the number of nurse-hours a patient receives, the better the patient care outcome
- A higher proportion of nurse care, plus more nurse-hours per day, results in shorter hospital stays and lower rates of upper gastrointestinal bleeding and urinary tract infections
- Higher proportion of nurse-hours relates to lower rates of failure to rescue:
  ○ The term *failure to rescue* is used by the federal Agency for Healthcare Research and Quality as a patient safety indicator and is defined as the death of a patient with one of six life-threatening complications, which can be largely influenced by early identification and medical intervention:
    - Acute renal failure
    - Deep vein thrombosis or pulmonary embolism (DVT/PE)
    - Pneumonia
    - Sepsis
    - Shock and/or cardiac arrest
    - Gastrointestinal (GI) hemorrhage and/or acute ulcer
- Registered nurse-hours affect patient outcome; there was no such connection between lower rates of adverse outcomes and increased numbers of licensed practical nurse-hours or aide-hours

(Aiken, 2002; Berney & Needleman, 2006; Carroll, 2006; Kane et al., 2007; IOM, 2004)

One of the most definitive research findings came out of the University of Pennsylvania, where low nurse staffing levels were linked to increased risks of mortality (Aiken, 2002):[LN2]

- In hospitals with high patient-to-nurse ratios, surgical patients experience higher risk-adjusted thirty-day mortality and failure-to-rescue rates, and nurses are more likely to experience burnout and job dissatisfaction
- Patient's chances of dying within thirty days after admission and the chances of experiencing failure to rescue each increased 7 percent for every additional patient per nurse
- When a nurse must care for six patients, instead of four, there is a 14 percent increase in mortality
- Mortality rises by one-third when the nurse workload increases to eight patients
- Applied nationally, some twenty thousand deaths could be prevented annually with adequate nurse-patient ratios

Recently, heart attack recovery rates were found to be higher in hospitals where nurses were unionized than in non-union hospitals where staffing levels were lower (Ash & Seago, 2004).

Various Approaches to Understaffing

Approximately five hundred thousand licensed nurses are not practicing nursing (IOM, 2004; *see also* Hassmiller & Cozine, 2006; Kugielska & Linke, 2008). There are three approaches to understaffing:

- Implement safe staffing plans in hospitals, with input from practicing nurses, to develop safe nurse-to-patient ratios based on evaluations of patient need
- Mandate specific nurse-to-patient ratios through legislation or administrative regulations
- Combination of both nurse-staffing plans and legislatively determined nurse-to-patient ratios

Mandatory Nurse-to-Patient Ratios

In the legislative preamble to the California nurse-to-patient ratio law, the state legislature declared that the quality of patient care was in jeopardy because of hospital staffing changes implemented in response to managed care. The legislature found that the quality of patient care was related to the number of nurses at the bedside, and wished to ensure a minimum number. The final set of nurse-to-patient ratios includes:

- 1:1 in trauma
- 1:2 in critical care units, intensive care newborn nursery, and post-anesthesia
- 1:4 in emergency, pediatrics, and telemetry units
- 1:5 in specialty care and step-down units
- 1:6 in medical surgical care units

22 CCR § 70217 (2009)

Regulations prohibit hospitals from assigning certain duties to unlicensed personnel, even if under the direct clinical supervision of nurses; criminal sanctions are authorized for willful or repeated violations.

Nurse Staffing Plans

Nurse staffing plans are based upon the premise, established by the American Nurses Association, that adequate nurse staffing is critical to the delivery of quality patient care (ANA, 2009; *see e.g.*, Aiken, 2002). These principles call for an individualized staffing model based upon a measure of unit intensity. The intent is for nurses to help develop these plans based upon a variety of factors, such as:

- Experience of the nursing staff
- Severity of patients' illnesses and medical conditions
- Available medical technology
- Support services available to the nurses

Nurse staffing plans are state law in California, Kentucky, Nevada, Texas, and Virginia. In addition, Florida, Hawaii, Illinois, Massachusetts, Rhode Island, and Washington have recently introduced legislation that would require nurse staffing plans at all health care facilities. The laws include a variety of components, such as:

- Civil penalties for enforcement purposes
- Daily posting of the numbers of nursing staff responsible for patient care
- Evaluation of the adequacy of the staffing plan through the collection of patient quality outcomes
- Requirement that American Nurses Association's principles for nurse staffing serve as a basis for development of staffing plans
- Requiring management to adopt and implement staffing plans with input from direct care nurses

Nurse staffing plans generally incorporate at least four of the following components:

- Appropriate mix of personnel that will allow nurses to practice according to their legal scope of practice
- Ongoing assessment done by nurses of the severity of the patient's disease, condition, and/or level of impairment or disability
- Professional standards of nursing practice
- Specific unit census to meet the needs of patients in a timely manner

(ANA, 2009)

Controversy: Merits of Nurse-to-Patient Ratios

Debate is ongoing about the merits of nurse-to-patient ratios. Supporters claim adequate nurse staffing is key to patient care and nurse retention:

- Understaffing endangers patients' lives
- Understaffing results in longer hospital stays (patients have a 3 to 6 percent shorter stay in hospitals with a high percentage of nurses)
- High turnover rates for nurses are expensive, and a direct result of the poor working conditions caused by understaffing
- Costs of implementing safe staffing ratios are offset by the improved quality of care and lives saved

(Rothberg, 2005)

Opponents maintain that minimum staffing ratios would only solve one aspect of nurses' job dissatisfaction, and that:

- Management would be stripped of its ability to make judgments about staffing levels
- Ratios do not provide the flexibility necessary to account for the changing needs of hospital patients
- Due to the massive nursing shortage, there are simply not enough nurses to meet mandated ratios, and thus units would be forced to close rather than operate in violation of the ratio mandates
- Costs of meeting the ratios are prohibitive and would decimate the already fragile health care systems in many parts of the nation

(*See* Bessette, 2006; Miles, 2007)

From an economic perspective, although staffing is a major concern, other aspects of the nursing profession are also important:

- Salaries
- Control of work schedules
- Input into hospital policy and management decisions
- Opportunities for advancement
- Support from hospital management
- Support staff to perform non-nursing tasks

(Carroll, 2006)

Opponents argue that hospitals would be compelled to cut spending for non-nursing staff to cover the increased costs for nurses. Another issue is the risk that hospitals could focus too narrowly on staffing issues, rather than using resources for other factors that are also critical to quality patient care. Critics maintain that hospitals with the best patient outcomes have organizational cultures that give nurses an important role in decision-making, the implication being that other factors can play just as important a role as staffing ratios (Albro, 2008).

Mandatory Minimum Nurse-to-Patient Ratios

Despite the various arguments put forth by hospitals in favor of shifting staffing plans, there appears to be a need for definitive minimums in order to provide safe, effective patient care. Studies demonstrate the clear threat to patient health when nurses are given too many patients in an effort reduce costs. Ironically, cutting costs has led to increased damage awards to some hospitals and increased mortality for their patients (Carroll, 2006).

Furthermore, the perceived short-term costs that hospitals will avoid absent mandatory ratios may be counterproductive when understaffing results in poor patient care. Low staffing levels are a dangerous choice when scientific studies quantitatively identify the increased risks to hospital patients. Cost reductions should not take precedence over adequate patient care.

OTHER CRUCIAL ISSUES IN HEALTH CARE STAFFING

Mandatory Overtime

Problems are associated with mandatory overtime, the most severe consequence being adverse medical care (Kugielska & Linke, 2008). Nurses average about eight and a half weeks of overtime per year (Hassmiller & Cozine, 2006). Yet, only three states have mandatory overtime laws: Illinois, Maine, and Washington include protection from retaliatory behavior.

The role of unions in negotiating contract provisions limiting mandatory overtime is especially important in states that do not currently have laws banning mandatory overtime. For instance, some contracts limit mandated overtime to four hours in one shift. Other contracts specify overtime can only be mandated after an unforeseen emergency and limit the shift of any nurse, even those normally working twelve hours, to thirteen hours. Other negotiated contracts simply ban mandatory overtime and are aimed at retaining currently employed nurses and attracting new nurses (*see generally* Kugielska & Linke, 2008).

The Department of Labor (DOL) has issued numerous opinion letters in an attempt to clarify the Fair Labor Standards Act (FLSA) overtime regulations issued in 2004. Several regulations involve hospitals and health care systems.

Joint Employees

The DOL issued an opinion letter in response to a question from a health care system about its obligation to pay overtime under the FLSA. The health care system had a nurse who held positions at two different companies within the system. Based on a review of the facts provided, the DOL determined that the health care system had to pay overtime to the nurse if the nurse's combined hours at the two companies exceeded forty hours in a workweek.

The DOL's determination was based on its interpretation of joint employer regulations, which state that an employee who performs work that simultaneously benefits two or more hospitals at different times during the workweek generally will be jointly employed, where the hospitals are not completely disassociated with respect to the employment of the particular employee. If the hospitals have common control, especially in personnel matters, they will be treated as the same employer for employment purposes. Separating personnel functions may not be enough to avoid being considered joint management. Each hospital within the health care system had its own:

- Federal identification number
- Human resources department
- Payroll system
- Retirement plan

While there was no regular interchange of employees between the hospitals, the DOL found they were joint employers. The DOL looked at the facts and found the two hospitals:

- Shared a common president and board of directors
- Shared a system for posting job openings
- Non-union employees had common health care plans
- One human resources department occasionally provided administrative support to the other
- Personnel policies were the same, although in different handbooks
- Senior executives and managers had responsibility for more than one entity within the system

Because of these multiple associations, the DOL found that both hospitals were responsible for combining the hours an employee worked at both hospitals for purposes of calculating overtime. The joint employer analysis is fact-sensitive; several factors need to be considered and each relationship has to be reviewed separately. To avoid being a joint employer, hospitals need to remain as separate as possible, and stay away from multiple associations.

Exempt Status

Issues often arise with regard to exempt and salaried employees. Exempt employees are salaried employees who are not subject to overtime compensation under the Fair Labor Standards Act as hourly workers. Whether exempt employees perform the same duties as others within the same job classification who are paid on an hourly basis does not affect the status of the other employees, assuming those who are considered exempt truly meet the duty and salary basis requirements necessary for the exemption.

At issue is whether paying otherwise exempt employees a shift differential for working evenings and weekends affects their salary basis, and therefore invalidates the professional exemption (*see* 29 C.F.R.

§ 541.300 (2009)). The DOL's opinion is that the predetermined amount of salary necessary to support an exemption need not include all of the compensation that the employee will be paid. Exemptions are not based on job title or classification, but rather upon the salary and duties of the individual employee (*see* 29 C.F.R. § 541.2 (2009)). Further, the exemption is not lost if an employee who is paid the proper salary also receives additional compensation based on hours worked for work beyond the normal workweek. The DOL relied on 29 C.F.R. § 541.602, which states that an employee is compensated on a salaried basis if the employee regularly receives each pay period, on a weekly or less frequent basis, a predetermined amount constituting all or part of the employee's compensation, which amount is not subject to reduction because of variations in the quality or quantity of the work performed (*see* 29 C.F.R. § 541.602 (2009)). Such additional amounts of compensation may be paid on any basis:

- Bonus
- Flat amount
- Paid time off
- Straight-time hourly amount
- Time and one-half of a calculated hourly amount

Exempt employees may be paid overtime premiums or shift differentials without invalidating their exempt status (*see* 29 C.F.R. § 541.604(a) (2009)).

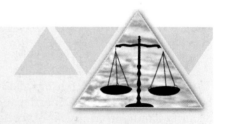

Moral Dilemmas

1. What key policy changes are most likely between labor and management?

Worker's Compensation

Another area of controversy in the workplace is worker's compensation.

EXCLUSIVE REMEDY OF WORKER'S COMPENSATION

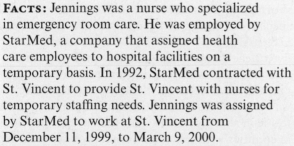

Jennings v. St. Vincent Hospital and Health Care Center
[Nurse v. Hospital]
832 N.E.2d 1044 (Court Appeals of Indiana 2005)

FACTS: Jennings was a nurse who specialized in emergency room care. He was employed by StarMed, a company that assigned health care employees to hospital facilities on a temporary basis. In 1992, StarMed contracted with St. Vincent to provide St. Vincent with nurses for temporary staffing needs. Jennings was assigned by StarMed to work at St. Vincent from December 11, 1999, to March 9, 2000.

Jennings allegedly contracted Hepatitis C after being stuck by an angiocatheter while performing nursing duties in the emergency room at St. Vincent Hospital. Jennings filed a claim for worker's compensation benefits against StarMed. He also filed a civil suit against St. Vincent claiming negligence. St. Vincent responded with a motion to dismiss based on lack of subject matter jurisdiction, claiming that Jennings was a co-employee of St. Vincent and StarMed, thus invoking the protection of the exclusive remedy provision of the

Worker's Compensation Act. Under this provision, an injured employee is entitled to worker's compensation benefits only, and may not sue the employer for damages. The trial court granted St. Vincent's motion, and Jennings appealed that determination.

ISSUE: Are employees working for health care facilities through a staffing agency in a joint employment situation?

HOLDING AND DECISION: Yes, employees working for health care facilities through a staffing agency are employees of both entities and are subject to the exclusive remedy provision in the Worker's Compensation Act.

ANALYSIS: The court held that Jennings was a co-employee of St. Vincent and StarMed. The Worker's Compensation Act explicitly recognizes that a worker may have more than one employer at

(continues)

(continued)

a given moment. To determine whether a worker was engaged in a joint employment situation, seven factors must be evaluated and weighed as a balancing test. The factors include:

- The right to discharge
- Mode of payment
- Supplying tools or equipment
- Belief of the parties in the existence of an employer-employee relationship
- Control over the means used in the results reached
- Length of employment
- Establishment of the work boundaries

After analyzing each factor, the court determined that St. Vincent's right to discharge Jennings, the tools and equipment that St. Vincent supplied Jennings, and, most important, its control over

Jennings's performance of his duties led to the conclusion that Jennings was a co-employee of St. Vincent and StarMed. Weighing against this determination was the belief of the parties in the existence of an employer-employee relationship and the length of employment factors. The court found that the mode of payment factor was not determinative. Because the more significant factors weighed in favor of an employer-employee relationship, the court concluded that both StarMed and St. Vincent were management entities protected by the exclusive remedy provision.

RULE OF LAW: An injured employee is entitled to worker's compensation benefits only, and may not otherwise sue the employer for damages.

(*See generally* Miller, 2006, 2007; Romaniuk, 2007).

RECRUITMENT AND RIGHTS OF FOREIGN NURSES AND PHYSICIANS

The U.S. Bureau of Citizenship and Immigration Services within the U.S. Department of Homeland Security handles recruitment of foreign nurses and physicians.

J-1 Waivers for Foreign Medical Graduates: Conrad Program

Foreign medical graduates (FMGs) usually enter the U.S. on temporary J-1 exchange visitor visas to complete their graduate medical education and training. Upon completion of such programs (often medical residency and fellowship training), the FMG must return home to satisfy a two-year home residency requirement before becoming eligible for any other U.S. visa category or lawful permanent residence (*see* Inadmissible Aliens, 8 U.S.C.A. § 1182(e) (1999)).

Many FMGs, however, seek a waiver of their home residency requirement to pursue employment opportunities in the U.S. Any federal agency or state health department may request a waiver on behalf of an FMG (*see* The Immigration and Nationality Technical Corrections Act of 1994, 8 U.S.C.A. § 1184 (2009)). One waiver option is the Conrad 30 program, which allows each state health department to grant thirty such waivers to FMGs. In exchange, the FMG must agree to practice

medicine for three years in a designated health care shortage area. Once the two-year home residency requirement of the J-1 visa status is waived, the physician is able to pursue other immigration options, including sponsorship for H-1B visa status and eventually lawful permanent residence (*see* 8 U.S.C.A. § 1182(e) (1999)).

Foreign-born physicians are permitted to practice in either primary care or specialty medicine. Specialists may qualify if there is a demonstrated shortage of physicians able to provide the medical specialty in designated geographical areas (*see* 8 U.S.C.A. §§ 1182 and 1184 (2009)). Additionally, five of each state's thirty waivers may be granted to a physician who practices in areas not designated as underserved if the physician receiving the waiver practices in facilities that serve patients who reside in shortage areas. This may permit providers in counties with less than a whole county Health Professional Shortage Area (HPSA) or Medically Underserved Area (MUA) designation to qualify as a waiver sponsor. Finally, physicians sponsored for a waiver by either a federal or state agency are exempt from the H-1B cap (*see* 8 U.S.C.A. § 1184 (2009)).

H-1B Annual Quota

Although not exclusively affecting the health industry, the current annual quota of sixty-five thousand on the number of H-1B visas has caused considerable difficulty for many management teams (*see* 8 U.S.C.A. § 1184(g)(1)(A) (2009)). Management in the health industry regularly utilizes the H-1B visa category to sponsor foreign physicians and other health care employees (8 U.S.C.A. § 1184(i) (1)(B) (2009)). The H-1B visa category is only available to individuals working in specialty occupations, which is generally interpreted to mean the position must require a minimum of baccalaureate-level education in a particular discipline. As such, most nursing positions do not qualify for H-1B classification.

H-1B caps are reached weeks prior to the start of the federal fiscal year on October 1. Enacted December 3, 2004, the H-1B Visa Reform Act of 2004 did not directly raise the annual cap; however, additional foreign nationals are now exempt from the sixty-five thousand annual limitations (*see* 8 U.S.C.A. § 1184 (2009)). The visa fee is now $2,000. For instance, twenty thousand visas are set aside for foreign nationals with a Master's or higher degree from a U.S. institution of higher education. Foreign nationals with offers to work at institutions of higher education or related or affiliated nonprofit entities and those who already have been counted against the cap continue to be exempt from the numerical cap (*see* 8 U.S.C.A. § 1184(g) (2009)). Nonprofit health care entities with formal affiliations with institutions of higher education may qualify for an exemption from the cap. The current quota still has not been sufficient to meet the demand for H-1B professionals, and new legislation to further increase and extend the quota will be the subject of continuing debate.

Lawful Permanent Residence

The health industry sponsors valued foreign national employees for lawful permanent residence or green card status (*see Federal Register,* 2004; 20 C.F.R. pts. 655 and 656). This labor certification process is often the initial requirement for permanent residence based on an offer of employment. This avenue of entry to the U.S. is only available where qualified U.S. employees are not available for the work offered to foreign nationals. For instance, nursing and physical therapy have long been recognized as job shortage areas.

CONTINGENT EMPLOYEES

Part-time and temporary employees, and independent contractors or employees of a subcontracting employer, are reaching new heights and changing the employment relationship, especially in the medical products sector. Contingent employees face continued downward pressure on their wages with generally no health insurance or pension benefits and no expectation of long-term employment. With jobs that are not well defined, few contingent employees are offered training or educational benefits. Moreover, most contingent employees spend their careers with multiple employers with none of the employment advantages of traditional workers in years past.

One of the most critical impacts on the health care industry is that contingent employees in the American economy often face periods of unemployment between jobs and are a key part of the nation's uninsured problem. Employers with high numbers of contingent employees are often more concerned with ensuring low prices than with maintaining a stable workforce; in effect shifting their workforce costs to the American taxpayer in the name of flexibility. When Manpower, Inc. is the nation's largest employer with almost four million contingent employees worldwide, there is a need for comprehensive reform of U.S. labor law (Dau-Schmidt, 2007). The common misconception is that the federal government or Wal-Mart are the nation's largest employers; the Bureau of Labor Statistics reports, however, that Wal-Mart employs 1.2 million employees and that one in ten of the 1.8 million federal employees are contingent employees (often through Manpower).

NEED FOR COMPREHENSIVE LEGISLATIVE REFORM

Existing labor law no longer improves the plight of American workers or betters the American economy. The nation's failure to adopt comprehensive health care legislation has placed unionized employers at a competitive disadvantage with companies abroad, and sometimes with non-union domestic employers. Corporations outside the U.S. do not make the substantial contributions to health care and pension payments to workers covered by collective bargaining agreements, as is the case with unionized American employers in the U.S. Such assistance is mainly provided by the government with all corporations unionized and non-unionized, bearing the tax burden equally. It is difficult to see how labor law reform alone can make a significant contribution to improving the American workplace under these circumstances, when organized American companies are at such a competitive disadvantage (Gould, 2007).

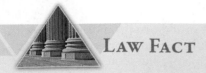

LAW FACT

MANAGEMENT'S REFUSAL TO BARGAIN

What recourse do labor union employees have when management unilaterally makes decisions affecting employees and refuses to bargain over subjects contained in collective bargaining agreements?

If, as the court concluded, the collective bargaining agreement gave the employer the right to adopt and implement its new policy without bargaining with the union, Enloe would have the authority to ameliorate or make individual exceptions to the policy without discussing those ancillary matters with the union.

—*Enloe Medical Center v. National Labor Relations Board*, 433 F.3d 834
(U.S. Court of Appeals for the District of Columbia Circuit 2005).

CHAPTER SUMMARY

- Nurses are the largest single group of health care providers in the country; the most severe consequence of nurse shortages is increased patient mortality.
- Labor and management in the health industry have the opportunity to work together to improve efficiency and value in the delivery of health care.
- Although many unions are losing members, the health industry is becoming increasingly unionized.
- Labor law has not undergone much reform since it was first enacted in the earlier part of the twentieth century; many are calling for reforms that would allow employees to unionize more easily, be prevented from employer backlash, and allow for problem resolution through arbitration.
- The general legal principles that already exist could also serve the health industry in crafting workplace policies.
- Nurse shortages are a severe problem; unless something changes, the nurse workforce will be nearly 30 percent below projected requirements within the decade.
- Because of the workload increase due to shortages, nurses have a very high rate of job dissatisfaction; however, simply involving nurses in the workplace discussion tends to reduce dissatisfaction despite the workload.
- California has enacted mandatory minimum nurse-to-patient ratios.
- Although mandatory overtime helps address the nurse shortage issue, it contributes to reduced quality of care for patients.
- One possibility to address the shortage of nurses and other health care workers is to attract foreign workers, but employers face legal and regulatory hurdles in doing so.

LAW NOTES

1. Seven labor unions recently organized themselves in a new Change to Win Coalition comprised of almost seven million employees to address affordable health care:
    1. International Brotherhood of Teamsters (1.4 million members)
    2. Laborers' International Union of North America (500,000 members)
    3. Service Employees International Union (2.0 million members)
    4. United Brotherhood of Carpenters and Joiners of America (520,000 members)
    5. United Farm Workers of America (50,000 members)
    6. United Food and Commercial Workers International Union (1.3 million members)
    7. UNITE HERE (840,000)
2. The landmark Aiken study was a cross-sectional analysis of data from over ten thousand nurses surveyed and over one-quarter million general, orthopedic, and vascular surgery patients discharged from 168 general hospitals in Pennsylvania (Aiken, 2002). The Aiken research was subsequently confirmed by international research. *See* Rafferty (2007) (nurse staffing levels in hospitals in England have the same impact on patient

outcomes and factors influencing nurse retention as found in the U.S. by Aiken), *but see* Halm et al. (2005) (finding staffing was not a significant predictor of mortality or failure to rescue, nor did clinical specialty predict emotional exhaustion or job dissatisfaction in analysis of data from 149 nurses and over 2,700 general, orthopedic, and vascular surgery patients discharged from one Midwestern hospital).

CHAPTER BIBLIOGRAPHY

AFL-CIO (American Federation of Labor and Congress of Industrial Organizations). (2005). *The costs and benefits of safe staffing ratios*. Washington, DC: AFL-CIO Department of Professional Employees.

Aiken, L. (2002). Hospital nurse staffing and patient mortality, nurse burnout, and job dissatisfaction. *Journal of the American Medical Association, 288* (16), 1987-1993 (landmark research on nurse staffing).

Albro, A. (2008). Rubbing salt in the wound: As nurses battle with a nationwide staffing shortage, an NLRB decision threatens to limit the ability of nurses to unionize. *Northwestern Journal of Law & Social Policy, 3*, 103-130.

ANA (American Nurse's Association). (2009). *Principles on safe staffing*. Silver Spring, MD: ANA.

___. (2009). *Utilization guide to the principles on safe staffing*. Silver Spring, MD: ANA.

Ash, M., & Seago, J. A. (2004). The effect of registered nurses' unions on heart-attack mortality. *Industrial & Labor Relations Review, 57* (3), 422-442.

Berney, B., & Needleman, J. (2006). Impact of nursing overtime on nurse-sensitive patient outcomes in New York hospitals. *Policy, Politics, & Nursing Practice, 7* (2), 87-100.

Bessette, J. M. (2006). An analysis in support of minimum nurse-to-patient ratios in Massachusetts. *Quinnipiac Health Law Journal, 9*, 173-218.

BLS (Bureau of Labor Statistics). (2009). *Occupational outlook handbook: Registered nurses*. Washington, DC: U.S. Department of Labor, BLS.

Carroll, A. N. (2006). Mandatory nurse-to-patient ratios: Can ratios bring better health care to Kentucky? *Brandeis Law Journal, 44*, 673-693.

Clemente, F. (2009). *A public health insurance plan; Reducing costs and improving quality*. Washington, DC: Institute for America's Future.

Dau-Schmidt, K. G. (2007). The changing face of collective representation: The future of collective bargaining. *Chicago-Kent Law Review, 82*, 903-930.

DOL (U.S. Department of Labor). (2005, April 11). Overtime for joint employees of health care system. *FLSA Opinion Letter 2005-15*. Washington, DC: DOL, Employment Standards Administration.

___. (2005, August 19). Exempt status of nurse practitioners. *FLSA Opinion Letter 2005-20*. Washington, DC: DOL, Employment Standards Administration.

Federal Register. (2004, December 27). Labor certification for the permanent employment of aliens in the United States; implementation of new system. 69 FR 77326-01 (codified at 20 C.F.R. pts. 655 and 656 (2009)).

Freeman, R. B. (2007). Briefing paper: Do workers still want unions? More than ever. Washington, DC: *Economic Policy Institute*.

Gould, W. B. (2007). Independent adjudication, political process, and the state of labor-management relations: The role of the National Labor Relations Board. *Indiana Law Journal, 82*, 461-496.

Halm, M. et al. (2005). Hospital nurse staffing and patient mortality, emotional exhaustion, and job dissatisfaction. *Clinical Nurse Specialist, 19* (5), 241-251.

Hassmiller, S. B., & Cozine, M. (2006). Addressing the nurse shortage to improve the quality of patient care. *Health Affairs, 25* (1), 268-274.

IOM (Institute of Medicine), Committee on the Work Environment for Nurses and Patient Safety. (2004). *Keeping patients safe: Transforming the work environment of nurses*. Washington, DC: IOM.

Jones, J. M. (2008, December 1). *The Gallup poll briefing: Americans remain broadly supportive of labor unions*. Washington, DC: Gallup.

Kane, R. L. et al. (2007). *Nurse staffing and quality of patient care. Evidence report/technology assessment. 151*, 1–115. Rockville, MD Agency for Health Care Policy & Research (AHRQ) (meta-analysis tested the consistency of the association between nurse staffing and patient outcomes).

Kochan, T., & Shulman, B. (2007, February 22). *Briefing paper: A new social contract: Restoring dignity and balance to the economy*. Washington, DC: Economic Policy Institute.

Kugielska, L., & Linke, M. (2008). Balancing the Red Cross: An examination of hospital malpractice and the nursing shortage. *Hofstra Labor & Employment Law Journal, 25*, 563-599.

Lafler, G., professor at the University of Oregon's Labor Education and Research Center. (2008, April 2). Before the U.S. Senate Committee on Appropriations, Subcommittee on Labor, Health & Human Services, Education & Agencies. Hearing on NLRB representation elections and initial collective bargaining agreements: Safeguarding workers' rights?

___. (2007, July). *Neither free nor fair: The subversion of democracy under NLRB elections*. Washington, DC: American Rights at Work.

Lee, C. J. (2006). Federal regulation of hospital resident work hours: Enforcement with real teeth. *Journal of Health Care Law & Policy, 9*, 162-206 (discussing the controversial nature of the adoption of federal regulations governing the eighty-hour medical residents' workweek).

Maher, K. (2007, January 22). Are unions relevant? *Wall Street Journal*, p. R5.

Mantese, T. et al. (2006). Nurse staffing, legislative alternatives and health care policy. *DePaul Journal of Health Care Law, 9*, 1171-1193 (noting that while some states have focused on improving nurse-to-patient ratios to ensure higher-quality patient care, other states limit the amount of mandatory overtime a nurse can be forced to work).

Miller, I. (2007). Survey of recent developments in health law. *Indiana Law Review, 40*, 931-962.

___. (2006). Survey of recent developments in health law. *Indiana Law Review, 39*, 1051-1104.

Miles, J. (2007). Antitrust and health care symposium: The nursing shortage, wage-information sharing among competing hospitals, and the antitrust laws: The nurse wages antitrust litigation. *Houston Journal of Health Law & Policy, 7*, 305-378.

Panagopoulos, C., & Francia, P. L. (2008). The polls: Trends: Labor unions in the U.S. *Public Opinion Quarterly, 72* (1), 134-159.

Rafferty, A. M. (2007). Outcomes of variation in hospital nurse staffing in English hospitals: Cross-sectional analysis of survey data and discharge records. *International Journal of Nursing Studies, 44* (2), 175-182 (confirming the Aiken research internationally).

Romaniuk, M. J. (2007). Year in review: A survey of significant 2006 developments in the area of labor and employment law and the impact upon Indiana employers. *Indiana Law Review, 40*, 821-862.

Rothberg, M. B. (2005). Improving patient-to-nurse ratios is a cost-effective safety intervention. *Medical Care, 43* (8), 785-791 (confirming the link between nurse staffing and patient outcomes).

Scott, L. D. et al. (2006). Effects of critical care nurses' work hours on vigilance and patients' safety. *American Journal of Critical Care, 15*, 30-37.

Specter, A., & Nguyen, E. S. (2008). Representation without intimidation: Securing workers' right to choose under the National Labor Relations Act. *Harvard Journal on Legislation, 45*, 311-334.

Stampalia, H. J. (2006). Inadequate staffing kills. *Quinnipiac Law Review, 25*, 173-209.

Thackray, J. (2008). *Gallup Management Journal: Feedback for real.* Washington, DC: Gallup.

Vidal, N. (2009). *Organizing prosperity: Union effects on job quality, community betterment, and industry standards.* Washington, DC: Economic Policy Institute.

PART VI

STRATEGIC HEALTH CARE RESTRUCTURINGS

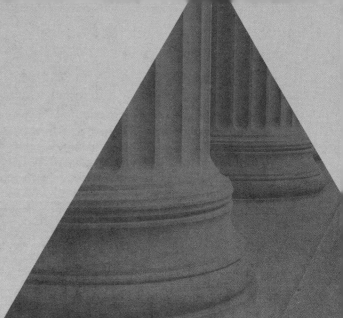

CHAPTER 14

TRENDS IN HEALTH CARE RESTRUCTURINGS

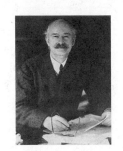

"[Professionals] may, as in the case of a successful doctor, grow rich; but the meaning of their profession, both for themselves and for the public, is not that they make money but that they make health, or safety, or knowledge, or good government or good law.... [Professions uphold] as the criterion of success the end for which the profession, whatever it may be, is carried on, and [subordinate] the inclination, appetites and ambition of individuals to the rules of an organization which has as its object to promote the performance of function."

—R. H. TAWNEY (1880-1962), ECONOMIST, HISTORIAN, AND SOCIAL CRITIC, FROM
THE ACQUISITIVE SOCIETY (1921)

IN BRIEF

This chapter examines the movement of the U.S. health care system into integrated delivery systems that are multi-tiered. Within these integrated health systems are numerous restructured programs, such as the emergence of medical homes, retail clinics, and medical tourism.

FACT OR FICTION

COMPARATIVE-EFFECTIVENESS RESEARCH

Should medicines and medical treatments that are found to be less clinically effective and more expensive not be prescribed?

The 2009 economic-stimulus bill allocates $1.1 billion for comparative-effectiveness research to determine which drugs are best for certain illnesses and medical conditions. Some see this research as a way to help the government and the insurance industry curtail the use of expensive medicines and medical treatments that do poorly in the comparative studies, though the official purpose is not cost reduction. The issue is: how should this comparative-effectiveness research be carried out in the U.S.?

The federal government hopes to expand health care coverage while limiting use of medicines and medical treatments that do not work well. Part of the political debate is whether the:

- Medical products industry should re-engineer the way its products are developed?
- U.S. Agency for Health Care Research and Quality should restructure and enhance its post-approval system for identifying and interpreting pharmacovigilance indicators (this oversight system is termed *pharmacovigilance* by the World Health Organization, which defines it as "the science and activities relating to the detection, assessment, understanding and prevention of adverse effects or other drug-related problems" (WHO, 2008))?
- U.S. Food and Drug Administration should be restructured to ratchet up the approval criteria for new medical products?

These options are not as easy as they seem. Research out of Dartmouth Medical School shows health care spending varies wildly between regions, often with little or no correlation to health outcomes. IMS Health reports there are about 4 billion prescriptions written every year in the U.S., and close to one-half million adverse events reported to the Food and Drug Administration. More than half of the insured population in the U.S. is taking prescription medicines, often more than one and more than 20 percent of the time the use is off-label, according to the Drug Information Association. Errors in prescribing or administering medicines by prescribing health care professionals, self-medication with supplements and over-the-counter products and alternative treatments by patients, further confound detection of effectiveness.

—*See* Orszag, 2009; Elmendorf, 2009.

(See *Law Fact* at the end of this chapter for the answer.)

PRINCIPLES AND APPLICATIONS

The legend of Alexander the Great arriving in the Kingdom of Phrygia in what is now central Turkey is like health care in the U.S., where anywhere from 25 to 50 percent of what is spent each year is unnecessary (Morreim, 2006; Schneider & Haw, 2009; *see also* Asch et al., 2006; McGlynn et al., 2003). Like Alexander, the U.S. faces a unique challenge. In Phrygia, the gods had assisted Gordius, the King, with tying his oxcart to a pole with an intricate knot. The man who could undo the Gordian knot would rule all Asia. When Alexander could not untie the knot, he unsheathed his sword and sliced it with one stroke, producing the Alexandrian solution.

Clearly, the U.S. health care system needs an Alexandrian solution if it hopes to develop effective,

integrated delivery systems. The U.S. reimbursement system is like the Gordian knot: it has become a complex, impossible-to-resolve system of interrelated rules and regulations that no one can rationally understand or direct.

TRENDS IN HEALTH CARE

With health care reform, the prediction is that three important trends will emerge in the U.S.

Multi-Tiered Delivery of Health Care

The movement of the U.S. toward a multi-tiered health care system was first recognized in the mid-1990s (Reinhardt, 1995). While critics maintain this policy direction

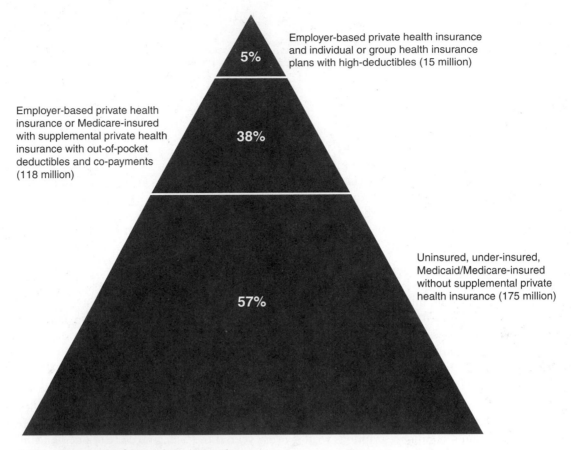

FIGURE 14-1: Pyramid of Health Care Delivery

Delmar/Cengage Learning
Data retrieved from: Jost, 2007; Reinhardt, 1995 (Princeton University economist who first predicted the three-tiered health care system).

is contrary to the intent of the Medicaid and Medicare legislation, which envisioned integrated uniform health care based on need, this is where the U.S. health care system is moving, as illustrated in Figure 14-1 (*see* Reid et al., 2005). For those who are able to pay, there will be a level of service that goes beyond what is now provided by the health industry (Wharton, 2002).

- The top tier of the pyramid, the high-income wage earners, pays handsomely for access to tomorrow's medical technology; some higher-income insured individuals may have high deductible policies through individual/non-group health insurance plans or receive employment-based coverage
- In the next tier down are the employed with employer-sponsored health insurance and the Medicare-insured with supplemental private health insurance; they spend more out-of-pocket to receive care from tightly managed health care organizations
- Those at the bottom tier of the pyramid are eligible to receive health care wherever they can find it,

but more often than not they go without basic and preventive care; low Medicaid payment rates generally restrict the choice of health care provider, but if they can find providers who participate in Medicaid, the services and products of those providers will be covered in full

Moral Dilemmas

1. If *essential health care* (also referred to as medically necessary health care in this text) is provided to every U.S. resident, should access to the latest medical technologies be based on need or the ability to pay?

Provider Segmentation

Because not everyone receives the same health care, other parts of the health industry will be required to segment themselves into tiers that make more intelligent use of patient information. Some of this will be aimed at more effective use of treatments and drugs (Wharton, 2002). If, for example, a hospital system has a regional primary care network of thirty physician practices, the system might expand to a national network of three hundred specialists and begin accepting referrals from a national network of physician practices. Several levels of fine cost segmentation could then occur, and treatment costs could be spread among this larger network of providers.

Cost-Based Reimbursement

The more accurately treatment services are priced, the better it will be for patients with little or no insurance coverage at the lower tier. If patients who cost $700 a month to treat pay a health care provider $300, and patients who cost $50 a month to treat also pay a provider $300, what the provider is reimbursed can be adjusted to better reflect each patient's risk status. In other words, what is the cost difference for treating these two patients with different health conditions? Once this question is answered, the differences in patient costs can be converted into cost differences in what the providers will be reimbursed.

For instance, instead of reimbursing a health care provider a set amount each time a patient is treated for a given medical condition, the provider could be reimbursed for a full treatment cycle. This creates an incentive for providers to provide the most effective, innovative care available rather than cheaper treatments. As a result, providers would be forced to compete in the prevention, diagnosis, and treatment of individual health conditions, disease by disease and patient by patient. It is here where enormous differences in costs can occur. When this occurs, providers face the choice of becoming limited-volume, high-price, high-cost specialists, or high-volume, low-cost providers of standard health care. Providers can treat both segments with great benefits in lowering the average costs. To do this, however, it must be possible to provide treatments at different prices at the level of the health condition of each patient. Costs must match value in each disease and patient segment. Different disease and patient values require different prices to cover different medical costs. Over time, providers will be forced to choose one segment or the other. The alternative is what we have today with the absence of price differentials: providers are reimbursed below cost in one segment and are non-competitive in another because reimbursement is based on average costs that hide more than they disclose. With cost-based reimbursement the number of uninsured and underinsured Americans might decrease and basic preventive care might become more affordable (Wharton, 2006a).

RESTRUCTURING HEALTH CARE SYSTEMS

When the managed care movement began in the 1970s, the problems it was supposed to solve were clear: the financial incentives associated with the traditional third-party payment system were inflationary, and the delivery of care across the board was poorly coordinated (Wharton, 2000). Today, it is difficult to determine where the U.S. health care system should go, after four decades of reform with managed care. One thing is certain: given the amount of frustration expressed by the American public, the U.S. does not have it right yet. The integrated health maintenance organization and all the different managed care organizations that have been developed have not worked as expected.

In addressing the future of U.S. health care, it is critical to realize that for many people, the term *managed care* has become synonymous with a number of significant breakdowns in the health care system. Managed care cuts prices without integrating service delivery, which means there is continued overall lack of coordination and integration in patient treatment. Three strategic restructurings are emerging to address the coordination and integration of patient health care:

- Access to research comparing medicines and medical treatments
- Access to quality health care
- Development of incentives for preventive care

(Asch et al., 2006; Falit & Sclar, 2006; Sage, 2004)

Comparative-Effectiveness Research

In an era of more and more high-powered and expensive therapeutics, the dissatisfaction with health care is only going to get worse without fundamental change on who has access to research comparing medicines and medical treatments (Sage, 2004). Although *comparative efficacy* would be a more precise term, this chapter uses the term *comparative-effectiveness* because it is what is more familiar, even though the two nouns are not synonyms.[LN1] Under Health Maintenance Organization (HMO) insurance plans, physicians and hospitals have to undergo prior utilization review in an attempt to reduce unnecessary medicines and medical treatments. However, the public's dissatisfaction with HMOs forced this managed care sector to dilute or end most of its cost-control strategies that were implemented starting in the 1980s. Today, it is acknowledged by many that managed care may work only if government is the one doing the managing. That is, cost can be controlled only with a new government entitlement of essential health care to all U.S. residents. As the nation seeks to expand health care coverage, medicines and medical treatments that do not work have to be limited, but there is no consensus as how this limitation is to take place. One proposal is that medicines and medical treatments found to be less effective but more expensive should not be prescribed. Yet any effort to reduce health care coverage based on costs alone still seems to be untenable to most Americans.

No matter what, there is a push to determine which medicines and medical treatments work best at the lowest cost in particular patients.[LN2] The Institute of Medicine and the Commonwealth Fund have recommended establishing a National Center to integrate information about the relative clinical and cost-effectiveness of alternative treatment options into health care purchasing and coverage decisions (IOM, 2006; Schoen et al., 2007). One goal of a National Center would be to make effectiveness determinations on the best unbiased science possible in cooperation with the National Institutes of Health and other national research institutes. This research into comparative-effectiveness would help the nation's health care system direct its dollars to medicines and medical treatments that are worth the money. While there is concern that useful medicines and medical treatments may not become available just because they cost too much or some medicines and medical treatment options for patients may be limited, the greatest concern is about conflicts of interest among those asked to generate the research. Despite these concerns, there is widespread agreement on the attributes that need to be associated with comparative-effectiveness research:

- Objectivity in the selection of what is studied
- Independence from political pressures generated either by government or by private-sector stakeholders
- Credibility in the findings

(Wilensky, 2006)

To date, the medical products industry has controlled this clinical trial data and research, how it is reviewed and evaluated, and whether the public and the government finds out about it and uses it.[LN3] The goal of comparative-effectiveness research has to be how to obtain more value from the nation's health care spending, not how to avoid expensive medicines and medical treatments, a critical distinction that has not always been adequately addressed. Transparency of health costs, effectiveness, quality, and the ability to use such information are critical prerequisites for coordinated health care and the development of policies that encourage such care (Davis et al., 2008).

Medical Homes

Physicians cannot understand all the health care being provided to their patients because no single physician is responsible for a patient's overall care (*see* AAFP, 2007). This indicator is important because having a *medical home* or regular provider of care is crucial to efforts to ensure access to timely quality care (Asch et al., 2006).

Under this model of care, every individual and family would have a primary care professional, such as a physician, physician's assistant, or nurse practitioner, to:

- Facilitate their timely and coordinated health care
- Coordinate referrals for testing and specialty services
- Monitor management of chronic conditions

(Goldman, 2008)

From a patient's perspective, this represents an industry best practice. Patients benefit from a single point of entry into the health care system, as well as the continuity of a relationship with a primary care professional to direct their plan of care (Goldman, 2008). From a systems perspective, emphasizing primary care and preventive services is widely recognized as producing:

- Fewer hospitalizations
- Improved health outcomes
- Lower health care costs

(Kruse, 2007)

Numerous groups advocate this model to expand and enhance the role of primary care physicians in coordinating care and medical homes, including the:

- American Academy of Family Physicians
- American Academy of Pediatrics
- American College of Physicians
- American Osteopathic Association

In recent years, working conditions for primary care physicians have deteriorated, with salaries among the lowest and work-hours among the longest of all physicians (Woo, 2006). This combination has resulted in a significant decrease in the number of U.S. medical graduates selecting careers in family medicine and general internal medicine (Mullan, 2008). While international medical graduates, as well as nurse practitioners and physician assistants, have filled some of the gaps in the primary care base, this new and important concept of the medical home gives promise to a re-conceptualization of primary care (AAFP, 2007).

Nonetheless, a quality health care system that is affordable will not exist without a robust primary care base that is trained for the job and competitively compensated for the work (Mullan, 2008). Payment reforms are required to strengthen primary care to provide better coordination and more accessible and patient-centered care through enhanced medical home approaches that help integrate care (Davis et al., 2008). Some preferred provider organization (PPO) medical home networks are being developed, but thus far, primarily for Medicaid populations.

Quality Incentives for Improvements in Patient Health

For health care providers, health care restructurings are a mixed bag. Sometimes it changes the incentives for doing more by doing less, but not often. The current health care system does not provide incentives to providers for preventative care; rather it rewards providers for providing medicines and medical treatments. For instance, when hospitals develop preventive programs that significantly reduce hospitalizations, they are penalized when their patients stay healthy rather than rewarded. When Duke University's hospital system saved $8,000 per patient by creating an integrated program for treating congestive heart failure, the episode-centered payment system penalized Duke by reducing the compensation its hospitals received; as the number of reimbursable episodes fell, so did the hospitals' revenue (Falit & Sclar, 2006).

Such perverse incentives also affect physicians. Insurers typically dictate the reimbursement for every discrete episode of care. Since patients with chronic conditions cost physicians more because they require more time, but often do not result in additional revenue per treatment, physicians have an incentive to establish a practice that selects the healthiest patients. Additionally, payer's reimbursement prevents providers from creating bundles of related services that patients with chronic conditions typically require (Falit & Sclar, 2006). Financial incentives need to be realigned to enhance value and achieve savings when physicians provide quality health care that reduces costs.

In addition, medicines and medical treatments found to be less effective and in some cases more expensive should no longer be prescribed. The nation's health care system has to direct its dollars to treatments that are worth the money. While the financial pressure on physicians and hospitals has been significant, there are few financial incentives for providing coordinated, quality health care. The disease management movement of the 1990s that was developed by employers slowly became intertwined with the performance-for-pay movement developed by the insurance industry; cost savings came to the forefront under the guise of coordinated quality care, which may in fact cost more.

PROBLEMS WITHOUT SOLUTIONS

According to prominent studies, adults in the U.S. receive the generally accepted standard of preventive, acute, and chronic care only about half the time (Asch et al., 2006; McGlynn et al., 2003). What is more, and contrary to popular misconceptions, there is only moderate variation in quality-of-care scores among socioeconomic groups (McGlynn et al., 2003). In other words, the U.S. health care system is uniformly failing to serve everyone half the time (Asch et al., 2006).

While most Americans understand the need for a better system of health insurance and increased access to health care, an inevitable stalemate exists. Problems have been identified, but there is no political consensus on what the solutions should be.

Americans seem resolved to wanting the best health care, but are not always willing to pay for it. What the U.S. has with managed care is not managed health care, but managed costs. What the nation must consider is how to deliver a quality health care system, where health care problems are avoided and where people obtain care before it is too late. Health care has to move its focus away from solely on costs and toward encompassing quality as well, where:

- Medical problems are avoided
- People obtain care before it is too late

Health care has to unequivocally move its focus away from solely on costs and toward quality. Tiered health insurance plans would not necessarily charge more for higher-quality services. In fact, plans should charge more for low-quality services that are high cost, as a means of encouraging patients to choose more efficient care (Madison, 2007).

Cost-Shifting

Health care systems can no longer continue to just shift costs. Cost-shifting in health care has been going on for a long time. Most health care systems were fine while Medicare reimbursed them all of the costs they incurred in treating individuals with Medicare insurance. Medicare stopped overpaying in 1983 when it implemented the prospective payment system (PPS) for inpatient hospital care. Health care costs had mushroomed partly because health care systems tried to bill Medicare for as many services for each patient as they could. Under PPS, Medicare pays hospitals a predetermined amount for each Medicare patient discharged, based on the patient's diagnoses or procedures. Today, Medicare pays the costs that should be incurred by an efficient health care provider when it provides necessary and appropriate health care.

But it is important to remember that Medicare payments are made not simply to reimburse hospitals for treatment of patients covered by Medicare insurance, but for maintaining a certain level and quality of care, both for the hospital and the community the hospital serves. In practice, however, what the actual rates of reimbursement are for Medicare is determined as much by political calculations as by hospital costs; there is no rational analysis driving Medicare payments. The issue is: what can the political market bear and how does this translate to all the individual payments?

Understanding the Pyramid of Health Care

No one can resolve the U.S. health care crisis without understanding the nation's pyramid of health care.[LN4] People at the bottom of the pyramid behave the same way with small amounts of dollars for health care as people higher up the pyramid; they save their dollars for something important to them. In the U.S. health care system, too many public policies do not understand that people at different levels of the pyramid just have different amounts of money to spend on health care, some more and some less. Despite differences health concerns are indeed paramount for most Americans. For instance, it is estimated that 40 percent of the hits on the Internet are for health care information; most people are going to their physicians and then checking the Internet to find out more, or vice versa.

Light at the End of the Tunnel

As amazing as emerging medical technologies are, they will not improve the health care delivery system by themselves. Anyone who sees a light at the end of this tunnel probably is not being realistic. The U.S. health care system cannot survive in its present form, if all the nation does is cut costs. The nation must move to a system that recognizes the importance of bringing new biosciences into the service of health, as well as a management philosophy based on distributive justice (Executive Order 13497, 2009). The medical products sector is an integral part of the nation's health care system, yet its value is not understood by the rank-and-file health care professionals and the consumers of health care. New pharmaceuticals, biopharmaceuticals, medical devices, and health information technology hold

significant promise for patients facing illnesses and diseases, or medical conditions that are often life threatening. All parts of the system will have to pay their fair share for medicines and medical treatments, but it will never work until there is more concern about quality than finances. Squeezing one part of the nation's health care system has unintended impacts on another.

While debate is occurring about the role of the government, the uninsured, and rising health care costs, it may be worthwhile to take another look at integrated health systems. Integrated health systems emerged in the 1980s, amid promises that they could achieve more cost-effective delivery along with value-added services for patients, and improved provider satisfaction (Burns et al., 2005). Today, however, very few integrated health systems have delivered on that promise: Kaiser Permanente, the University of Pennsylvania Health Care System, and the Veterans Health Administration are three systems that did deliver for the most part. One might ask, what happened to the rest?

INTEGRATED HEALTH SYSTEMS

It could be said that answers were not sought from the right places; in pursuit of the perfect integrated health system, attention went to the various structural vehicles, such as physician hospital organizations that have been developed to enable physicians and hospitals to jointly contract with integrated health systems (Burns & Pauly, 2002). Rather than concentrating on the *structures* of integration, focus should have been directed to the *processes* of integration, such as:

- Developing collective groups of physicians and other health care professionals
- Partnering with physicians and other health care providers, such as home health agencies and long-term care facilities
- Representing all health care professionals in governance

Integration Processes

Integrated health systems are built by bringing multiple hospitals, physicians, and other health care professionals together under one system to establish, at least in theory, a single cohesive market force. Because the hospitals, physicians, and other health care professionals often span across various markets, however, tensions and conflicts often arise from the clash of different cultures and philosophies existing within the different medical groups (Burns & Pauly, 2002). In fact, these tensions and conflicts are inherent to the structure of integrated health systems and exist at various different levels, such as:

- Hospital-to-hospital
- Physician-to-physician
- Physician-to-other health care professionals
- Physician-to-integrated health system

Progress has been stymied in large part because integrated health systems did not adequately attend to these tensions and conflicts. Until these tensions and conflcits are acknowledged and managed, the future success of integrated health care may be limited. Research has identified numerous tensions and conflicts that exist in any integrated health system (Burns et al., 2005). Generally, tensions and conflicts arise because integrated health systems encompass multiple entities with competing interests. For instance:

- While integrated health systems seek interdependence and centralization, physicians and other health care professionals seek decentralization and autonomy
- Hospitals, physicians, and other health care professionals often want to maintain control of provision of care to their patients and are threatened by integrated health systems that seek to centralize activities
- Hospitals, physicians, and other health care professionals are often reluctant to embrace integrated health-system-led objectives because they require cooperation with other hospitals and physicians, many of whom were once considered rivals
- Tensions often arise because physicians and health≈care professionals are neither informed nor consulted on issues of integration, despite the fact that integrated health systems need their buy-in

Not surprisingly, the challenge is addressing and managing these inherent tensions and conflicts. The issues that integrated health systems face are not unique to the delivery of health care, however. In fact, much can be learned from the medical products industry, such as Johnson & Johnson, a $61 billion global pharmaceutical company that employs some 120,000 employees in 250 operating companies in 57 different countries. For Johnson & Johnson, it is critical to achieve global product standardization while still maintaining market responsiveness and flexibility at the local level. Successful global pharmaceutical companies balance the simultaneous needs to be both:

- Large and small
- Centralized and decentralized
- Global and local

One might ask how Johnson & Johnson does this. Johnson & Johnson does it by using centralized integrative structures, which appear to be more financially successful than less centralized structures (Burns et al., 2005). Like Johnson & Johnson, successful integrated health systems centralize their administrative power within an executive office responsible for policy planning, with executive authority residing in the individual hospitals, physicians, and professional groups.

In integrated health systems, problems often arise when the executive office meddles in the affairs of individual hospitals, physicians, and professional groups, such as drawing up plans over trivial issues. Autonomous hospitals, physicians, and professional groups end up acting as extensions of the executive office, merely executing plans already decided by the executive office. Recognizing that it cannot resolve all the tensions and conflicts it faces, Johnson & Johnson developed processes that allow the company to balance these tensions and conflicts and pursue them simultaneously. For instance, the presidents of Johnson & Johnson's operating companies report to both a global head, who has responsibility for a product line, as well as regional country coordinators who have responsibility for a geographical line. In this way, Johnson & Johnson enures that neither interest, global or local, is ignored. Integrated health systems face similar challenges when the executive office enters reimbursement contracts with the health insurance industry and the individual hospitals, physicians, and professional groups encounter utilization barriers as they attempt to provide medically necessary health care to their insured patients. Likewise, they must learn to navigate the narrow channel between conflicting objectives.

Collective Groups of Physicians and Other Health Care Professionals

In integrated health systems, a key issue for physicians and other professional groups is how to maintain professional autonomy without sacrificing economic security. One way many physicians and other health care professionals have attempted to reconcile these seemingly incompatible interests is through a process called collectivization. They organize themselves into medical groups with collective control (by function, such as anesthesiology and physical therapy, or by medical specialty, such as cardiology or orthopedics). Essentially, physicians and other health care professionals organize themselves into collectives, such as:

- Economic contracting vehicles
- Large physician and professional groups
- Specialty clinics

Although collectivization requires some sacrifice of autonomy at the individual level, the payoff is collective autonomy and increased economic security. The size of the medical group provides increased visibility and leverage for physicians and other health care professionals within integrated health systems. These medical groups also enjoy enhanced representation in governance and other integrated health system benefits, such as strategic planning and financial assistance. Integrated health systems benefit from this process because unorganized physicians and other health care professionals are pressured to form their own collective medical groups.

No Formula for Successful Integration

During the mid-1990s, many hospitals pursued several integration efforts:

- Development of managed care plans (vertical integration into health insurance products)
- Loose alliances with and acquisitions of physician practices (vertical integration into primary care services)
- Mergers and affiliations with other hospitals (horizontal integration of health care products and services)

Hospitals pursued these efforts both individually and jointly (Burns et al., 2005). While numerous approaches have been used by integrated health systems to resolve tensions and conflicts, there is no formula for successful integration. The structures, or contractual vehicles, however, are never the answer. Processes must be developed to manage the tensions and conflicts within integrated health systems in a way that creates meaning for all of the participants, including:

- Patients
- Hospitals
- Physicians and other health care professionals
- Integrated health systems
- Wider service community of health care consumers

Diversification Strategies

Conceptually, these integrated health system arrangements represent a variety of diversification strategies. Diversification is said to exist when a system operates in two or more markets. Thus, for instance, the hospital diversifies when it begins to produce services in upstream primary care markets, or downstream in long-term care markets. Such diversification is typically unrelated to the hospital's core inpatient and outpatient, mostly specialty care.

Diversification can also exist when an integrated health system moves into new geographic markets or related lines of business. In the hospital industry, such diversification can take the form of multi-hospital systems that cross metropolitan and state lines, with different levels of market risk, as well as hospital systems that combine academic medical centers with outlying community hospitals. In all of these instances, diversification requires changes in administrative mechanisms, which are multi-divisional structures, to enable management of the increased number of services and geographic markets in which the integrated health system operates (Burns et al., 2005).

Conflict Management

Recognition that conflicts exist and are interdependent and not mutually exclusive is key. One medical group's position cannot be supported at the expense of another. Conflict management calls for a careful balancing of rival perspectives that, most of the time, requires that multiple directions be simultaneously pursued. The goal should be to create strategic alliances that accomplish the objectives of the integrated health system while balancing the often divergent needs of the individual hospitals, physicians, and professional groups.

RESTRUCTURED HEALTH CARE PROGRAMS

Two emerging areas of interest are retail clinics and medical tourism. Two major players are: RediClinic, a health care start-up created by America Online founder Steve Case (*see generally* Sage, 2004), and Apollo Hospitals, the largest health care system in India (*see generally* Cortez, 2008).

Retail Clinics

A new strategic innovation is walk-in medical clinics at retail stores and malls, operated by firms such as RediClinic. Wal-Mart has over fifty retail clinics, and while they may not be profit centers themselves (at least not yet), the clinics boost pharmacy sales and draw shoppers into Wal-Mart. Currently, of those visiting the clinics at Wal-Mart:

- 30 to 40 percent are uninsured
- 20 to 40 percent would have sought emergency room care
- 10 to 20 percent would have gone without medical treatment

(Wharton, 2002)

While retail clinics are getting leverage from Wal-Mart, they pose new issues of supply chain management specific to health care, as opposed to product inventory, where Wal-Mart is viewed as the master. It makes sense for Wal-Mart to provide the retail clinics; they compliment Wal-Mart's optical and pharmacy services. The challenge for Wal-Mart is managing consistent, quality health care. Health care is consumed as it is produced, unlike a shelf product that sits around until customers want it. Quality health care often rests on the dependability of the health care professionals delivering the care. Consistent, quality health care requires retail clinics to maintain excess capacity for times when they are not busy in order to meet patient needs when they arise. It is still an exercise in balancing supply and demand, but the factors at play are different.

Retail clinics also fit into Wal-Mart's push to present itself as a kinder company, particularly after unions generated reports showing that Wal-Mart employees generally lacked health insurance coverage and that the company's employees were the top users of Medicaid.

Medical Tourism

Medical tourism, the phenomenon in which health care providers in emerging markets offer a vacation and surgery together at low prices to patients from developing economies, is gaining in popularity. In 2007, over half a million U.S. citizens sought health care outside the U.S. (Cortez, 2008). While India lags behind countries like Thailand, as a result of airport infrastructure, health care providers such as Apollo Hospitals are expanding their medical tourism from the U.S. and Europe at 10 percent a year (Wharton, 2008).

There is high value in terms of clinical outcomes and high-quality care at one-fifth the cost of care in the U.S. (Milstein, 2006). Hospitals that are medical tourism sites have Joint Commission International (JCI) accreditation, which puts them on par with hospitals in the rest of the world. JCI was formed in 1994 by the Joint Commission on Accreditation of Healthcare Organizations (JCAHO), and the nonprofit arm of JCAHO, Quality Healthcare Resources, Inc. In 1998, JCAHO formed a subsidiary, Joint Commission Resources, Inc. (JCR). JCI is now a division of JCR.

JCI launched its international accreditation program in 1999 in response to growing interest in worldwide accreditation and quality improvement. For instance, JCI ranks three Apollo hospitals (Chennai, Hyderabad (only accredited for acute stroke care), and Indraprastha) shoulder to shoulder with the Mayo Clinic and the Cleveland Clinic.

The case mix of most of the work that goes to India is tertiary care and acute care. It is not the plastic surgeries found in Bangkok. It is high-end orthopedic work, cardiology, and some oncology. Apollo Hospitals is developing packages to assist patients to use Indian facilities and is in conversation with private medical insurers for coverage (Wharton, 2008, 2006). Apollo accepts U.S. health insurance. United Group Programs, a Florida-based insurer, with offices in Pennsylvania and Georgia, sells self-insurance policies to small businesses that offer a plan that sends patients to Bumrungrad Hospital in Bangkok. Dunkin Donuts and Manpower are two United Group clients. Blue Shield of California and Health Net of California offer policies allowing patients to seek treatment in Mexico.

The single hurdle facing U.S. patients going to emerging countries for health care is legal liability and the fact that they cannot address their concerns through a legal forum in the U.S. They can, of course, use the legal system where they receive their health care, but generally patients want a legal system they are familiar with to back them up in case there is a problem (Cortez, 2008). Currently, the incidence of problems is not even 1 percent at Apollo Hospitals in India; its success rates and clinical outcomes are also very good (Wharton, 2008). While patients have the same rights in India as they would in the U.S., it is a hurdle for India to address the legal forum issue.

Apollo Hospitals combines elements of both Western care and Eastern medicine. Allopathic medicine is used for actual treatment in terms of surgery and diagnosis, but where rehab and well-being are concerned, the systems of *ayurveda* (traditional Indian medicine) and yoga are integrated into patient care. The key here is that many patients find value from integrating *ayurveda* and yoga with allopathic care and are willing to travel to India to obtain this integration (Wharton, 2008).

Moral Dilemmas

1. How should governments retain their jurisdiction to respond to important legal and ethical questions in medical tourism?

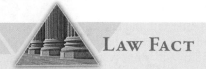

LAW FACT

COMPARATIVE-EFFECTIVENESS RESEARCH

Should medicines and medical treatments that are found to be less clinically effective and more expensive not be prescribed?

Three federal agencies will be coordinating the $1.1 billion in federal funds for comparative-effectiveness research: the National Institutes of Health, U.S. Agency for Health Care Research and Quality, and the U.S. Department of Health and Human Services. For purposes of effectiveness comparisons in determining which medicines and medical treatments are safe and which ones work, there are two research categories:

- Post-marketing surveillance
- Post-approval research

Post-marketing surveillance focuses on signal detection. Information is collected on outcomes from health care professionals, patients, and the medical products industry. Information is collected through two types of health information systems:

- Passive retrieval systems (adverse event reporting)
- Active systems (data-mining of health records from third-party payers and registries)

Post-approval research consists of surveys, studies, or trials to further ascertain whether signals actually represent a health effect related to a specific medicine or medical treatment (as opposed to confounding due to background prevalence of symptoms in the patient population or some other cause). Research conducted post-approval also elicits data that will help to clarify the magnitude and frequency of adverse events as well as mitigating factors:

- Co-morbidity (multiple cofounding medical conditions)
- Polypharmacy (use of multiple prescription drugs and self-medications)
- Patient demographics

—*See* Orszag, 2009; Elmendorf, 2009.

CHAPTER SUMMARY

- Managed care was meant to control health care costs and coordinate health care delivery, but four decades after its inception, it has accomplished neither goal.
- Health care providers lack the financial incentives to provide quality care.
- Policymakers should understand that people at the bottom of the economic pyramid behave the same as those at the top; they save their health care dollars to put toward what is important to them.
- Integrated health systems are meant to combine hospitals and health care providers together into one system.
- Integrated health systems are difficult to accomplish because of the difference in practice, culture, and philosophy between different medical groups.
- The unresolved polarities and tensions between different medical groups hinder the progress of integrated health systems; there is no formula for successful integration.
- As with other industries, global health care companies must balance the need to be simultaneously large and small, centralized and decentralized, and global and local.
- Physicians in particular desire to retain autonomy within integrated health systems, and so they organize into collectives in order to maintain their influence.
- A diversification strategy is needed within an integration strategy because once an integrated system comes into existence, it is usually operating within more than one market.

LAW NOTES

1. Congress defined *effective* in the Federal Food, Drug, and Cosmetic Act, declaring that the federal government must prohibit the sale of any drug if "there is a lack of substantial evidence that the drug will have the effect it purports or is represented to have under the conditions of use prescribed, recommended, or suggested in the proposed labeling thereof...." 21 U.S.C.A. § 355(d) (2008). This meaning of *effective* distinguishes effectiveness from efficacy. Efficacy refers to the propensity of a drug to achieve intended, observable clinical improvement. An anti-hypertensive drug is efficacious if it lowers blood pressure. Effectiveness, by contrast, refers to the fit between what happens to patients and what the drug manufacturer promises on drug labels. An example of a drug that achieves efficacy but not effectiveness might be an anti-hypertensive drug that functions to lower blood pressure but not by as many millimeters as its manufacturer claims it will (*see* Bernstein, 2007).

2. The Care Focused Purchasing project involves a group of large private employers working with health plans to assemble claims data for millions of individuals in order to assess provider effectiveness (Rowe et al., 2006). Twenty Blue Cross plans have also joined to create Blue Health Intelligence, a program under which they will pool data from about 80 million subscribers. They will share the information initially with employers and eventually with consumers (Madison, 2007).

3. No research studies are considered as critical or useful in determining clinical effectiveness as those using human participants, also known as clinical trials. It is only in the past few decades that the clinical trial has emerged as the preferred method in the evaluation of medical interventions (Cahoy, 2007). More specifically, randomized controlled clinical trials are considered the gold standard of medical research for evaluation of therapeutic efficacy (*see* Weed, 2008). In medical products review, any conclusion regarding a medical product's safety or efficacy depends on what is found in controlled clinical trials on humans. Of course, a number of pieces of information are relevant to the effectiveness analysis. For example, an explanation of the chemical structure, studies on stability, and descriptions of the physiochemical characteristics can tell scientists much about how a drug will be likely to act in a human physiological setting (Cahoy, 2007). *See* FDA, 2001 (explaining the rationale for the non-clinical pharmacology studies in drug approval applications).

4. For instance, one health care policy came about by chance. Medicare beneficiaries would not get flu vaccinations until they were completely free, which was not a big budgetary issue, but this understanding came about in a peculiar way. The federal government's fiscal year starts October 1, which is when the Medicare deductible recycles. October is also the start of the flu vaccination season, but many Medicare participants did not want to use their deductible right away, preferring to save it for something more important. Once the flu vaccinations were free, flu vaccination participation doubled and tripled. This is just one example of how decisions on how to manage health care are complicated in many ways. (*See* Wilensky, 2006).

CHAPTER BIBLIOGRAPHY

AAFP (American Academy of Family Physicians), American Academy of Pediatrics, American College of Physicians, and American Osteopathic Association. (2007). *Joint principles of the patient-centered medical home.* Leawood, KS: AAFP.

Asch, S. M. et al. (2006). Who is at greatest risk for receiving poor-quality health care? *New England Journal of Medicine, 354*, 1147-2619.

Bernstein, A. (2007). Regulating pharmaceuticals and scientific issues regarding asbestos: Enhancing drug effectiveness and efficacy through personal injury litigation. *Journal of Law & Policy, 15*, 1051-1101.

Burns, L. R. et al. (2005). The financial performance of integrated health organizations: Practitioner application. *Journal of Healthcare Management, 50* (3), 181-191 (examines thirty-six large integrated health systems and the impact integration strategies have on the financial performance of hospitals, physicians, and health plans over time).

Burns, L. R., & Pauly, M. V. (2002). Integrated delivery networks: A detour on the road to integrated health care? *Health Affairs, 21* (4), 128-143.

Cahoy, D. T. (2007). Medical product information incentives and the transparency paradox. Indiana Law Journal, *82*, 623-671.

Cortez, N. (2008). Patients without borders: The emerging global market for patients and the evolution of modern health care. *Indiana Law Journal, 83*, 71-132.

Davis, K. et al. (2008). Setting the context for health reform: Aiming high for the U.S. health system: A context for health reform. *Journal of Law, Medicine & Ethics, 36*, 629-642.

Elmendorf, D. W., Director, Congressional Budget Office. (2009, February 10). Key issues and budget options for health reform. *Congressional Budget Office*. Senate Budget Committee.

Executive Order 13497. (2009, January 30). Regulatory planning and review. Washington, DC: The White House (calling for a regulatory review that will "address the role of distributional considerations, fairness, and concern for the interests of future generations").

Falit, B. P., & Sclar, D. (2006). The Bush administration's health care proposal: The proper establishment of a consumer-driven health care regime. *Journal of Law, Medicine & Ethics, 34*, 632-636.

FDA (Food & Drug Administration). (2001). *Guidance for industry: Safety pharmacology studies for human pharmaceuticals*. Rockville, MD: FDA.

Goldman, B. P. (2008). City & County of San Francisco: The San Francisco Health Care Security Ordinance: Universal health care beyond ERISA's reach? *Stanford Law & Policy Review, 19*, 361-376.

IOM (Institute of Medicine). (2006). *Performance measurement: Accelerating improvement*. Washington, DC: IOM (proposing creation of a National Quality Coordination Board).

Jost, T. S. (2007). The Massachusetts health plan: Public insurance for the poor, private insurance for the wealthy, self-insurance for the rest? *University of Kansas Law Review, 55*, 1091-1102.

Kruse, J. (2007). Improving care with the patient-centered medical home. *American Family Physician, 76* (6), 744-756.

Madison, K. (2007). Regulating health care quality in an information age. *University of California–Davis Law Review, 40*, 1577-1652.

McGlynn, E. A. et al. (2003, June 26). The quality of health care delivered to adults in the U.S. *New England Journal of Medicine, 348* (26), 2635-2645.

Milstein, A., chief physician, Mercer Health and Benefits and medical director, Pacific Business Group on Health. (2006, June 27). The globalization of health care: Can medical tourism reduce health care costs? *Hearing before the Special Senate Committee on Aging*.

Morreim, E. H. (2006). High-deductible health plans: New twists on old challenges from tort and contract. *Vanderbilt Law Review, 59*, 1207-1261.

Mullan, F. (2008). Beyond coverage: Building capacity to promote and protect the public's health: Aging, primary care, and self-sufficiency: Health care workforce challenges ahead. *Journal of Law, Medicine & Ethics, 36*, 703-708.

Obama, B. (2009, January 30). *Memorandum for the heads of executive departments and agencies: White House Task Force on Middle-Class Working Families*. Washington, DC: The White House.

Orszag, P. R. (2009, March 10). *The President's fiscal year 2010 budget proposal*. Washington, DC: Office of Management and Budget.

Reid, P. R. et al. (2005). *Building a better delivery system: A new engineering/health care partnership*. Washington, DC: Institute of Medicine & National Academy of Engineering (making the assumption that because systems-engineering tools have been effective in other industries, these tools will be effective in the health care field).

Reinhardt, U. E. (1995). Turning our gaze from bread and circus games. *Health Affairs, 14* (1), 33-35.

Rowe, J. W. et al. (2006). The emerging context for advances in comparative-effectiveness assessment. *Health Affairs, 26* (5), w593-w595.

Rowland, D., & Schwartz, A. (2008). America's uninsured: The statistics and back story. *American Society of Law, Medicine & Ethics, 36*, 618-660.

Sage, W. M. (2007). Implementing universal coverage: Might the fact that 90% of Americans live within 15 miles of a Wal-Mart help achieve universal health care? *University of Kansas Law Review, 55*, 1233-1245.

___. (2004). Managed care's Crimea: Medical necessity, therapeutic benefit, and the goals of administrative process in health insurance. *Duke Law Journal, 53*, 593-666.

Schneider, C. E., & Haw, M. A. (2009). The patient life: Can consumers direct health care? *Journal of Law and Medicine, 35*, 7-65 (stating that 25 percent of American health care is unnecessary).

Schoen, C. et al. (2007). *Bending the curve: Options for achieving savings and improving value in U.S. health spending*. New York, NY: Commonwealth Fund.

Weed, D. L. (2008). Truth, Epidemiology, and general causation. *Brooklyn Law Review, 73*, 943-957.

Wharton (Wharton School at the University of Pennsylvania). (2008). Apollo Hospitals' Suneeta Reddy: Medical tourism is a huge market. *India Knowledge@Wharton* (one of the three regional editions, including *Universia Knowledge@Wharton* and *China Knowledge@Wharton*).

___. (2006). A brave new world beckons Indian innovators and entrepreneurs. *India Knowledge@Wharton*.

___. (2006a). Wal-Mart: Is there a downside to going upscale? *Knowledge@Wharton*.

___. (2002). Business processes are moving from the West to other parts of the world. *Knowledge@Wharton*.

___. (2000). Drug prices: Let the competition begin. *Knowledge@Wharton*.

WHO (World Health Organization). (2008). *Policy perspectives on medicines: Pharmacovigilance: Ensuring the safe use of medicines*. Geneva, Switzerland: WHO.

Wilensky, G. R. (2006). Developing a center for comparative-effectiveness information. *Health Affairs, 25*, w572-w585 (suggesting creation of a federal agency responsible for comparative-effectiveness information).

Woo, B. (2006). Primary care: The best job in medicine. *New England Journal of Medicine, 355* (9), 864-866.

CHAPTER 15

INTEGRATION DEALS IN THE HEALTH CARE SECTOR

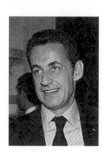

"A new form of capitalism is needed, based on values which put finances at the service of business and citizens, not vice versa."

—NICOLAS SARKOZY, PRESIDENT OF FRANCE

IN BRIEF

This chapter looks at the two sides of the restructuring coin: mergers and acquisitions and bankruptcies. On one side, nonprofit to for-profit conversions and private equity acquisition activities in the health care sector have experienced the greatest expansion of any industry group in recent years, with transactions and dollar amounts doubling across the globe. On the other side, the largest nonprofit health care failure in the U.S., the bankruptcy of the Allegheny Health, Education, and Research Foundation (AHERF), is discussed. A popular integration strategy among academic medical centers, namely that of acquiring physicians, researchers, and medical facilities in order to corner patient markets, is examined. While AHERF did not survive its bankruptcy, the ever-evolving understanding and lessons to be taken from AHERF's fall are as relevant today as when it filed for bankruptcy in 1998 (Cobb & Hotchkiss, 2004). It could be said that the demise of AHERF foreshadowed the for-profit corporate scandals that began with Enron, up to the current financial environment that is impacting the health industry today.

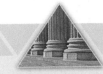

FACT OR FICTION

VOLUNTARY CLOSURE OF INSOLVENT HOSPITALS IN MEDICALLY UNDERSERVED COMMUNITIES

Should states consider the needs of individual patients before approving the closure of insolvent hospitals in medically underserved communities?

St. Vincent's Catholic Medical Centers (St. Vincent's) was one of New York City's most comprehensive health care systems and the largest provider of emergency health care in the city. Before filing for bankruptcy, St. Vincent's had seven hospitals with 2,500 affiliated physicians and employed 12,500 full- or part-time employees. Over the course of its bankruptcy, St. Vincent's divested itself of all its acute care hospitals, except its flagship hospital in Greenwich Village.

St. Vincent's filed a Debtor's Motion for (A) an Order Approving (i) Bidding Procedures with Respect to the Sale of Mary Immaculate Hospital and St. John's Queens Hospital, and Related Assets, (ii) the Time, Date, Place, and Form of Notice for Each of the Auction and Sale Hearings, and (iii) a Break-Up Fee and Expense Reimbursement and (B) an Order Approving (i) the Sale of the Hospitals and Related Assets Free and Clear of Liens, Claims, Encumbrances, and Other Interests, and (ii) the Assumption and Assignment of Executory Contracts and Unexpired Leases. *See In re St. Vincent's Catholic Medical Centers of New York et al.*, No. 05 B 14945 (ASH) (U.S. Bankruptcy Court for the Southern District of New York 2007).

Two communities, Central Brooklyn and Southeast Queens (Jamaica) were especially impacted by St. Vincent's divestment activities. Both communities suffer from some of the worst health care outcomes in the nation. Both Central Brooklyn and Jamaica have an infant mortality rate that is more than quadruple the rate in Greenwich Village. Additionally, the percentage of adults with diabetes in both Central Brooklyn and Jamaica is more than double the percentage in Greenwich Village.

New York City designated the Central Brooklyn neighborhoods of Crown Heights, Bedford-Stuyvesant, and East New York/Brownsville as neighborhoods with the most severe health-related problems in the city. Compared to New York City overall, adults have a 20 percent higher rate of heart disease hospitalizations, more than twice the rate of HIV-related deaths, a 35 percent higher rate of mental illness hospitalizations, a more than 70 percent higher rate of alcohol-related hospitalizations, a 60 percent higher rate of drug-related deaths, a 25 percent higher rate of deaths from cancer, and a 66 percent higher rate of asthma-related hospitalizations. While similar to Central Brooklyn, Jamaica—which has toxic sites from aluminum, glass, metal, plastics, steel, and textiles manufacturing activities for the aerospace, apparel, automotive, building, computer, electronics, and telecommunications industries—has the second highest asthma hospitalization rate for children, and the highest rate of asthma prevalence for adults in the city. Jamaica also houses the city's transitional housing program for homeless men and women living with AIDS, who in turn relied on a St. Vincent's hospital for their treatment needs.

This was the backdrop behind St. Vincent's divestment plans. Residents in Central Brooklyn and Jamaica claimed the hospital closures in their communities would amount to a health care catastrophe and urged the state to consider their needs in determining the future of the hospitals. Specifically, the residents asked the state to determine whether patients would have alternative sites for health care, and requested that the public be allowed to participate in the decision-making process before closing hospitals affecting local health care.

As part of the bankruptcy reorganization, St. Vincent's directed $800 million in funds derived from the divestment of its six hospitals in Central Brooklyn and Jamaica to reconstruction of its Greenwich Village hospital. St. Vincent's reasons for closing or selling its hospitals were never based on the health needs of the communities, but rather on the need to cover its costs.

—*Verified Petition PP 8-9, McCloud v. Novello*, Index No. 22406/05 (New York Superior Court Kings County July 22, 2005) and *Stipulation and Order Dismissing Adversary Proceeding, St. Vincent's Catholic Medical Centers of New York v. McCloud* (*In re St. Vincent's Catholic Medical Centers of New York*), Case No. 05-2351A (U.S. Bankruptcy Court for the Southern District of New York January 19, 2006); *see also* Lee, 2008.

(See *Law Fact* at the end of this chapter for the answer.)

PRINCIPLES AND APPLICATIONS

The health industry is at risk in the current economic environment, with weaker and slower members of the group facing a greater chance of restructuring or even bankruptcy (Alvarez, 2008). Hospitals, in particular, are likely to see a significant rise in restructurings. The intersection of the managed care system and the issues of strategic health care restructurings is substantial and important and explained with broad strokes rather than overly technical details. The way in which hospital organizations choose to change the way in which they provide health care will determine the direction of the next movement in the upcoming decade or so.

When the managed care movement began in earnest in the 1970s, the problems it was supposed to solve were clear:

- Financial incentives associated with the traditional third-party payment system were inflationary
- Delivery of care was poorly coordinated

(Wharton, 2000)

What is infinitely harder to solve is where the health industry will go from the present. There are really only two sure things: first, the U.S. has not yet achieved success in the health care arena, and second, integration deals and other strategic restructurings, particularly hospital bankruptcies, will be part of the next attempt to give Americans the highest standard of care, with continued innovation and broader access to new technologies at a lower and more affordable cost.

COMPETITION IN HEALTH CARE

Several factors contribute to the changing landscape of the health industry and the increasing need of nonprofit providers to compete with for-profits. With governmental regulation of the industry blurring and market forces becoming more dominant, medicine has taken on a primarily business rather than service orientation, and the line between the standards governing for-profit and nonprofit enterprises has blurred.

Nonprofit to For-Profit Conversions

While the current conversion phenomenon has been hyperbolically characterized as the largest redeployment of charitable assets in the Anglo-American world since Henry VIII closed the monasteries in 1536-1540 (Fishman & Schwartz, 2006), there is no denying the last decade has seen the proliferation of billion-dollar deals in health care. While it is nearly impossible to accurately estimate the number of nonprofit to for-profit conversions in the health industry, they have generally occurred as changes in corporate form for the hospital and HMO sectors rather than as straightforward mergers and acquisitions (Greaney & Boozang, 2005).

Hospital Conversions

For-profit hospitals unquestionably generate a healthier profit margin than other hospitals. Private for-profit hospitals hover around a 9 percent profit margin, while the margins for private nonprofits come in at around 4 percent. Public hospitals (owned by local governments, states, and the federal government) fall slightly behind the nonprofits (Greaney & Boozang, 2005). Private nonprofit hospitals are generally affiliated with research universities or religious orders of the Roman Catholic Church.

Many of the converted nonprofit hospitals were the victims of insolvencies and bankruptcies. For instance, Tenet Healthcare (Tenet) of Santa Barbara, California, owner of between fifty and sixty for-profit hospitals in twelve states in 2008, obtained ownership of several significant hospital systems affiliated with academic medical centers during bankruptcy proceedings. Tenet is the nation's second-largest hospital chain behind Hospital Corporation of America (HCA), with $8.7 billion in net operating revenue in 2007; the for-profit chain has about 14,600 acute care beds and employs over 62,000 employees. Tenet acquired eight hospitals in eastern Pennsylvania out of the bankruptcy of AHERF and retained two as acute care facilities; the other six hospitals were sold and subsequently converted to other uses, such as rehabilitation, skilled nursing, or outpatient-care centers, or closed.[LN1]

Health Plan Conversions

Most of the converted health maintenance organizations (HMOs) have merged with one another or with historically for-profit insurers. Six firms now dominate the national HMO market: Aetna, CIGNA, Kaiser Permanente, Humana, UnitedHealthcare, and Wellpoint.

Significantly, the regional Blue Cross (covering hospitals) and Blue Shield plans, which were established during the Depression to provide expansive hospital and physician coverage and were historically nonprofit in their orientation, recently changed their corporate status by eliminating the requirement that their licensees be organized as nonprofit corporations (Greaney & Boozang, 2005). When the largest, and often dominant, nonprofit institution in health care finance and delivery moves toward a for-profit model, the extent of the conversion phenomenon becomes clearer (Hall & Conover, 2003).

For instance, research by the Milbank Fund indicates that the time has passed when nonprofit Blue Cross plans were much more lenient underwriters in assessing the eligibility of individuals to receive health insurance coverage than other for-profit commercial insurers. Underwriting practices and policies at Blue Cross plans are now broadly consistent with those of for-profit insurers. Underwriters place similar lifetime caps on how much coverage individuals should receive for their health care and establish comparable ranges of deductibles and co-payments that are available for any given premium. Underwriting decisions on whether even to accept the risk and insure certain individuals with certain diseases and illnesses are the same; certain individuals are simply uninsurable. While the underwriting practices of the converted Blue Cross plans are generally similar in comparison to for-profit insurers, if not more lenient, conversions adversely impacted the risk selection in some states. For-profit insurers are not as willing to accept the risk of losing money as their nonprofit counterparts when examining the health status of the insured.

The Milbank research further established that nonprofit to for-profit conversions of the Blue Cross plans increased profit incentives. Therefore, such conversions should result in:

- Higher health insurance rates in market segments where Blue Cross plans hold considerable market power and as a result are subject to less aggressive rate regulation
- Lower medical loss ratios, which can be achieved by tougher negotiations with health care providers and more refined underwriting and risk selection practices
- Improved operational efficiency and customer service
- Unlocked wealth that can be devoted explicitly to health-related charitable purposes

(Hall & Conover, 2003)

For health care providers, however, for-profit conversions of Blue Cross and HMO plans remain a jumbled hodgepodge of unrelated profit incentives. Sometimes the conversion changes the incentives, but not often. Also, while the financial pressures on the health industry are significant, there are still few rewards for providing quality preventive health care.

Private Equity Buyouts of For-Profits

For-profit hospitals have made attractive buyout targets because many have strong cash flows and large capital expenditure budgets with endowments that can be used to reduce the debt from going private. However, hospitals can also be risky buys, thanks to industry head winds over the last several years. Some for-profit hospitals are opting to go private because expansion through joint ventures and strategic alliances takes time to pay off, which is time they do not have as publically traded entities.

The largest publicly traded hospital chain, HCA of Nashville, Tennessee, was the first for-profit to go private in 2006. A trio of buyout firms, Bain Capital, Kohlberg Kravis Roberts (KKR), and Merrill Lynch Global Private Equity, paid almost $21 billion plus the assumption of about $12 billion in debt. For-profit organizations may be publicly owned or privately owned, just as nonprofits in most states; only nonprofits may be tax-exempt, however. With almost $28 billion in revenue, HCA owns 166 hospitals in twenty states and England, plus another 120 outpatient centers.

Within months, the nation's third largest hospital chain, Triad Hospitals (Triad) of Plano, Texas, agreed to convert from a public to private company. In 2007, Triad had a buyout agreement with private equity investors, CCMP Capital Advisors, and the private equity arm of Goldman Sachs for $4.7 billion, plus the assumption of about $1.7 billion in debt (Francis, 2007). Before the conversion occurred, Triad changed its mind and merged with Community Health Systems of Franklin, Tennessee. The combined company has a market capitalization value of about $7.2 billion.

With number-two-ranked Tenet perhaps too heavily leveraged to be attractive, the most likely remaining buyout candidate is LifePoint Hospitals of Brentwood, Tennessee, with a market capitalization value of about $2 billion. A hindrance to future buyouts, however, may be the growing belief among private equity investors that the reimbursement problems facing the hospital industry will not be solved anytime soon.

BANKRUPTCY RESTRUCTURINGS

More than half of U.S. hospitals are not seeing enough patients to provide sufficient revenue to fund operations and are on the brink of insolvency or already are insolvent. Restructuring firm Alvarez & Marsal recently found:

- More than 2,000 of the nearly 4,900 acute-care hospitals do not make a profit treating patients
- Nearly 750 hospitals that do turn a profit earn less than what they need to fund day-to-day operations
- One-fifth of the nation's acute-care hospitals do not have enough funds for their most basic capital expenditures, such as making facility repairs or meeting essential maintenance needs
- While many hospitals continue to operate despite insolvency, an increasing number are filing for bankruptcy

(Palank, 2008)

Moreover, capital expenses are underfunded in the range of $10 billion to $20 billion because hospitals are using capital funds to support their day-to-day operations. While hospital insolvencies and hospital bankruptcies are rampant, the U.S. Trustee Program, the government agency charged with ensuring the integrity of the bankruptcy system, projects there will be continued insolvencies and more bankruptcies moving forward.

A top tier of about five hundred to one thousand hospitals:

- Are consistently profitable
- Have excellent credit ratings
- Claim a substantial share of the market

The problem facing some four thousand hospitals is widespread overcapacity: too many beds and too few patients (Bertrand, et al., 2005). Hospitals are also competing with same-day surgery centers and outpatient clinics and all sorts of innovative ways to deliver health care.

While hospital occupancy levels move downward:

- Costs continue to increase
- Reimbursement rates continue to decline
- There is an increasing number of uninsured patients

Nor are hospitals immune to the nation's credit crunch; they are forced to take on costly loans, if they can get financing at all. Lenders willing to finance a hospital at an amount that was five or six times its cash flow in mid-2008 are now making loans only in amounts that are double or triple the hospital's cash flow. What was a relatively secure financial environment in health care has now become rather tense.

Hospitals then turn to other, often unsteady, sources of revenue:

- Cash from auxiliary operations (*e.g.*, thrift shops, gift shops, parking lots)
- Local and state government assistance
- Philanthropy

Band-aid fixes, however, cannot cover gaping wounds that continue to get bigger. Some see the whole hospital industry sliding slowly into insolvency. Before the hospital industry can bottom out, which may not be until 2010 or later, more hospitals will have to seek mergers or bankruptcy filings to cure their balance sheets. Most hospitals can get by even if they are insolvent, but they do not have much of a future unless their capital structures are fixed (Palank, 2008).

> ### Moral Dilemmas
> 1. Is it time for hospitals to challenge under-reimbursement by the Medicare, Medicaid, and SCHIP entitlement programs?

The Nation's Largest Nonprofit Health Care Bankruptcy

Before filing for bankruptcy, AHERF and its fifty-five corporate affiliates:

- Reported $2.05 billion in revenues
- Were comprised of fifteen hospitals in the Philadelphia and Pittsburgh markets with more than five hundred physicians in their management practice
- Employed almost thirty thousand employees
- Enrolled about 3,300 students a year at the nation's largest medical school, the Philadelphia-based Allegheny University of Health Sciences (formerly the Medical College of Pennsylvania and Hahnemann University; now the merged medical schools are known as MCP Hahnemann University of the Health Sciences, managed by Drexel University)

(Burns et al., 2000; Greaney & Boozang, 2005)

When AHERF finally entered bankruptcy in 1998, it had been losing more than $1.0 million every day for over a year; it left behind $1.5 billion in debt and 65,000 creditors. *See In re Allegheny Health, Education & Research Foundation*, 292 B.R. 68 (U.S. Bankruptcy Court for the Western District of Pennsylvania 2003). When bankruptcy proceedings were finally concluded, unsecured creditors received about 12 cents on the dollar from the bankrupt estate (Cobb & Hotchkiss, 2004). According to the American Bankruptcy Institute, the AHERF bankruptcy meant the dismantling of the nation's largest nonprofit health care provider (DeMarco & Valentine, 2005). It led to thousands of layoffs and the sale of six Philadelphia hospitals to Tenet, an investor-owned corporation. Further, it called into question a strategy popular among academic medical centers in the mid-1990s of acquiring, at almost any cost, physicians, researchers, and medical facilities in order to corner health care markets (Wharton, 2000).

Breakdown in Accountability

No one single factor led to the bankruptcy of AHERF. Instead, there was a breakdown in accountability at almost every level. Indeed, much of the intrigue of this bankruptcy stems from the fact that so many actors, both inside and outside AHERF, played a part in its demise (Burns et al., 2000). Among those who failed both AHERF and the communities it served were:

- Senior management
- Board of Directors
- Accountants
- Auditors
- Bond-rating agencies

(Wharton, 2000)

Even with this cast of hundreds, however, Sherif Abdelhak, the former AHERF chief executive officer, and David McConnell, former chief financial officer, are particularly deserving of criticism (Burns et al., 2000). While they were never found to have used AHERF for their own personal gain (Fisher, 2002), their flawed assumptions, fiscal irresponsibility, and questionable ethical decisions remained the topic of litigation for more than a decade after their downfall (Burns et al., 2000). McConnell paid a $40,000 Securities and Exchange Commission (SEC) fine and entered an accelerated rehabilitative disposition program that permits non-violent, first-time offenders a chance to wipe their records clean upon completion of program requirements (Cobb & Hotchkiss, 2004); Abdelhak faced nearly 1,500 criminal charges and pled no contest to a single misdemeanor count of misusing charitable funds and was sentenced to eleven to twenty-three months of prison with work-release; he was paroled in three months (Cobb & Hotchkiss, 2004). Following the bankruptcy, the two executives, along with several members of AHERF's management team and board, were the subject of over sixty unsecured creditors' lawsuits (Greaney & Boozang, 2005). Investigations by the SEC, the Pennsylvania Attorney General, and the federal Pension Benefit Guaranty Corp. are still not finalized. Additional lawsuits were also filed against AHERF's auditor, Coopers and Lybrand, now part of PricewaterhouseCoopers (Burns et al., 2000). Three auditors were sanctioned by the SEC; one paid a fine of $40,000 (Cobb & Hotchkiss, 2004).

Flawed Corporate Strategy

AHERF had a mandate from its board to develop a premier medical education and research system. The strategy was to:

- Develop the nation's first statewide integrated delivery system grounded in academic medicine
- Build regional market share to leverage managed care payers
- Negotiate contracts from HMOs that covered all the costs of enrollees' health care
- Achieve synergies among the assets acquired
- Use community/suburban hospitals to refer private-pay patients to AHERF's teaching hospitals

For various reasons, all five elements of AHERF's strategy were problematic:

- Pennsylvania had few statewide payers that could contract with a statewide integrated delivery system
- Few of its delivery systems had enough market share to leverage managed care payers, especially in markets such as Philadelphia with an excess of hospital beds and physicians
- Hospitals' enthusiasm for assuming risk, and the willingness of HMOs to pass it on, meant huge hospital losses
- Synergies and economies of scale through mergers are difficult to realize, especially with rapid expansion
- Academic medical centers had trouble persuading suburbanites to use older teaching hospitals in the cities, even as suburban hospitals were developing revenue-generating services that attracted urban patients

(Burns et al., 2000)

While these five assumptions were serious miscalculations, it is important to remember they were commonsense wisdom at the time:

- Everyone believed them
- Consultants were propounding them
- Trade literature was repeating them

After a while, if enough people repeat something, it becomes believable. A lot of other academic medical centers, including the University of Pennsylvania Health Care System, went the same route.

The expansion of AHERF into Philadelphia was conducted at a breakneck pace over a ten-year period (mid-1980s to the mid-1990s), with major acquisitions every two years:

- Medical College of Pennsylvania and its two affiliated hospitals
- United Hospitals' four hospitals and Suburban Medical Associates
- Hahnemann Medical College and hospital
- Graduate Health System and its six hospitals

None of the acquisitions were strong financial performers; most were financial underperformers and highly leveraged. The purchase of the Graduate Health System was the straw that broke the back of AHERF. It was a huge debt load and the Graduate hospitals were marginal performers financially. There was simply no way to manage it all (Wharton, 2000).

Lessons Learned

1. Hospital mergers do not generally result in economies of scale and lower prices unless the hospitals are small and the markets are competitive (Burns et al., 2000).
2. There is no firm evidence that large health care systems enjoy economies of scale in their operations, and some evidence shows they take years to learn how to operate (Wharton, 2000).
3. Acquisitions based on the arguments of expansion, greater size, and greater market presence still require prudence and due diligence; there is no substitute for precise financial analysis and close scrutiny.
4. Disciplined growth strategies need to be supported by rigorous financial planning and feasibility analysis (Goldstein, 2008).

Overloaded Debt

Debt was a major problem for AHERF. During the 1980s, when the newly established AHERF consisted of Pittsburgh-based Allegheny General Hospital, the hospital had just $67 million in debt. With a teaching affiliation with the University of Pittsburgh Medical Center, Allegheny was one of only a few hospitals nationwide with an "Aa" bond rating (Burns et al., 2000). By 1998, a hugely expanded AHERF, which by then had been using Allegheny General Hospital and other facilities in the western part of the state to subsidize its eastern operations, had a debt of $1.3 billion (*In re Allegheny Health, Education and Research Foundation*, Case No. 98-25773 (U.S. Bankruptcy Court for the Western District of Pennsylvania 1998)). Its margins during the mid-1990s fell to between 0 and 3 percent, compared to 6 to 12 percent at competing hospitals.

Lessons Learned

1. Drops in debt service are a red flag; they generally reflect a lower ability of borrowers to pay their debt principle and interest payments (Burns et al., 2000).

Faulty Integration of Primary Care Practices

As part of its vertical integration strategy, AHERF purchased physician practices in the mistaken belief this would help secure inpatient referrals to the system's hospitals. Unfortunately, its competitors were following the same strategy and the bidding wars that resulted meant physicians were frequently overpaid for their practices. Purchase agreements filed in the Philadelphia Court of Common Pleas showed that physician practices acquired by AHERF generally received:

- $70,000 to $150,000 for their assets irrespective of actual value (which was considerably less in almost all instances)
- Average annual salary of $220,000 to $250,000 for five years
- 60 percent of their revenues above $470,000 to $570,000

In addition, the contracts included no means to monitor practice productivity (Burns et al., 2000). Along with aggressively acquiring physician practices, AHERF was also recruiting clinical and research faculty, which it hoped would:

- Attract federal funding
- Enhance its research reputation
- Result in more patients and thus new revenue sources

Again, high payments were the norm. Before its bankruptcy, AHERF was recruiting three orthopedists a year and guaranteeing salaries of about $3.9 million a year. At the time, the average salary for a surgical orthopedist in Philadelphia was $67,000, which was lower than the national norm because of the regional oversupply of orthopedists.

Lessons Learned

1. Physician integration is critical to grow market share, but needs to be methodical and measured (Goldstein, 2008).
2. Know your market when hiring; the vertical integration into primary care through acquisition of physician practices generally resulted in losses of $75,000 to $100,000 per physician per year for AHERF (Burns et al., 2000).
3. Commission-based acquisitions in the health industry provide too strong an incentive to cut deals rapidly; the chief operating officer of AHERF's physician network received a $15,000 commission for each physician practice acquired, which resulted in overpaying for most practices (Burns et al., 2000).

Dominant Bargaining Power of Payers

While AHERF engaged in full-risk, fully capitated contracting with local health insurers, that is, accepting a fixed payment per year for each enrollee for agreed-upon health care its precarious financial condition was significantly aggravated by Philadelphia's competitive health care environment. AHERF lost over $100 million each year as it attempted to become a player in the HMO market (Weinstein, 2000).

Pittsburgh, in western Pennsylvania, had only five health plans and 15 percent HMO penetration. By contrast, Philadelphia, in eastern Pennsylvania, had eleven health plans and a 30 percent HMO penetration. Moreover, two plans dominated the HMO market, which meant they had enormous power over providers in Philadelphia (Burns et al., 2000). With five major academic medical centers (University of Pennsylvania Health Care System, Jefferson Health System, Temple University Health System, Philadelphia College of Osteopathic Medicine, and the combined MCP-Hahnemann Health System) and more than eighty teaching and community hospitals vying for market share and research funding.

> **Lessons Learned**
>
> 1. Over-bedded, over-doctored, over-staffed, and over-used health care markets only increase the bargaining power of the health insurance industry (*see* Wharton, 2000).

This was all at a time when neither the Federal Trade Commission nor the U.S. Department of Justice pursued antitrust actions against insurers for their activities to control health care markets. Thus, AHERF was receiving HMO premium payments that were increasing at a decreasing rate while the cost of providing health care for its expanded health care system was escalating (Weinstein, 2000). AHERF's expansion occurred just as the state's entire Medicaid population was switched to mandated managed care. At the same time, federal efforts were reducing hospital reimbursements for Medicare patients. On top of all this, private health insurers were all lowering their reimbursement rates (Burns et al., 2000).

The combined decline in revenues relentlessly hit an already overextended AHERF. In the end, AHERF spent a lot on building an integrated health care system but achieved little leverage over the payers (Weinstein, 2000).

Faulty Financing Mechanisms

Months before the bankruptcy, senior management was praising AHERF's:

- Growing market share
- Organizational growth
- Physician networks
- Productivity improvements

What was not disclosed were the financing mechanisms used to fuel the decade of growth, including:

- Enormous debt from all the acquisitions
- Hidden internal cash transfers between the fifty-five affiliated corporations
- Internal subsidies not justified by business activities
- Raids on restricted assets and hospital endowments
- Misuse of research and scientific grants
- Misappropriation of funded depreciation and reserve cash accounts for operating expenses
- Invasion of restricted funds from employee pension funds
- Failing to account for bad debt reserves from uncollectible accounts receivables

(Burns et al., 2000)

> **Lessons Learned**
>
> 1. Disclosure of the financial performance of all of a health system's operations creates greater transparency and builds credibility (Goldsteinm 2008).

Complex Tax-Exempt Hospital Bonds

Economic thinkers have said for at least two centuries that the more important a given kind of thing becomes to society, the more likely there will be hard-edged rules to manage it. Ever sharper lines are drawn around entitlements so everyone knows who has what (Freyermuth, 2006).

Unfortunately, the rules surrounding hospital debt and bond-rating mechanisms are complex and little understood. The need for clarity is lacking and it is safe to assume many actors, both inside and outside AHERF, failed to understand that the credit ratings given to AHERF's debt referred to the rating of its insurer, not the rating of the health care system. This lack of clarity produced a greater level of misunderstanding for AHERF to resolve, as its hospitals were largely stuck in a zero-sum game posture with payers. AHERF was trying to maximize its position with payers, just as funds to reimburse hospitals became scarce, making bond funds more highly valued. Confusion like this, all along the debt line, helped conceal AHERF's true financial condition.

One instance outlined by faculty at The Wharton School at the University of Pennsylvania illustrates the complexity involved in debt financing of large integrated health care systems like AHERF (Wharton, 2000). Moody's Investor Service (Moody's) covered debt issued by five sets of AHERF hospitals, some of which found their debt publicly downgraded as AHERF's financial problems grew (Burns et al., 2000).

The hospital debt of one health care system was junk bond status with a "Ba2" rating at the time its hospitals were acquired by AHERF. However, another AHERF had hospital bonds separately rated as "Aaa" insured, "Baa" (barely above investment grade), and "Ba" (below investment grade). AHERF:

• Called five sets of outstanding bonds on thirteen hospitals in eastern Pennsylvania
• Refinanced their debt
• Reissued new bonds under DVOG
• Insured the DVOG bonds using MBIA Insurance

(Burns et al., 2000)

MBIA, the nation's largest health care bond insurer, was the underwriter of the newly issued bonds. By insuring the debt, AHERF garnered an "Aaa" rating for DVOG's debt (the highest quality rating possible). Yet in reality this rating had nothing to do with any improvement in the underlying financial health of the system issuing the bonds. Rather, the rating reflected the underlying health of the insurance company (MBIA's rating by Moody's) to insure that debt. The financial troubles at AHERF thus remained hidden from the public (Weinstein, 2000).

Meanwhile, although Moody's internal assessment noted weak operations at AHERF, underlying bond ratings are not published unless requested by the issuers. AHERF never requested that its ratings be made public until it was forced to do so. When Moody's finally released its underlying rating of DVOG, debt that had been rated "Aaa" suddenly had a publicized underlying rating of "B3" (not much assurance that bond interest and principal payments will ever be paid). Within days, the DVOG ratings fell to "Caa1" (poor-quality rating, such issues are dangerous and may be in default) and AHERF was forced to declare bankruptcy (Burns et al., 2000). During the hospital debt financings, no one apparently examined how DVOG's bond ratings matched up with standard financial fundamentals:

• Debt-to-cash flows
• Debt-to-equity ratios
• Falling or rising revenue streams

Lessons Learned

1. The credit-rating agencies (Standard & Poor's, Moody's, and Fitch Ratings) are constrained in providing ratings to risky health system bonds.
2. Bond insurance masks the underlying credit quality of bonds (Burns et al., 2000).

Hidden Cash Transfers

AHERF's use of hidden cash transfers to cope with the system's growing financial problems was another factor leading to the bankruptcy filing. This situation came about because AHERF's corporate bylaws allowed management of the parent company to move cash from one operating affiliate to another, without the consent of the affiliate or the knowledge of the board.

Financial management of AHERF was in boxes, so each person or entity within AHERF could see only one piece of the overall financial position. Moreover, the operating revenues and endowment funds from the scattered operations of AHERF were commingled in a structure that permitted funds to be transferred between fifty-five operating affiliates as needed and financial results to be manipulated to make affiliate operations look as favorable as possible (Burns et al., 2000).

Lessons Learned

1. For health care systems with multiple subsidiaries and operating affiliates, intra-system financial arrangements should be treated as loans from the parent to the affiliates, as appropriate. This enhances the ability of the parent to be treated as a legitimate creditor of the affiliates in the event of any affiliate's bankruptcy or other similar condition (Kaplan & Peregrine, 2002).

AHERF's external auditors, Coopers and Lybrand, gave AHERF a clean bill of health in its last audit before its bankruptcy. Included in this audit was a large, improperly recorded loan and financial statements that were later retracted, precipitating an investigation by the SEC (Burns et al., 2000). AHERF was the first nonprofit health care system the SEC ever pursued (Weinstein, 2000).

Inadequate Governance Structure

Following AHERF's bankruptcy, hospital governing boards were held to a higher standard of corporate governance (Harper & Schreiber, 2007). The weak governance structure of AHERF included a parent board of between twenty-five and thirty-five directors, rather than the standard thirteen to seventeen, and a network of 132 directors on ten different boards responsible for AHERF's various operations (Burns et al., 2000). There was little overlap in membership.

Another area of debate among hospitals is the composition of their boards of directors. Should physicians serve on hospital boards? One factor used by the Internal Revenue Service for determining tax-exempt status is board composition. Tax-exempt hospitals operate to serve public rather than private interests. *See* Revenue Ruling 69-545 (1969).

AHERF also suffered from weak board composition and several inherent conflicts of interest. Two months before the bankruptcy of AHERF, a $89 million loan was repaid to a bank consortium including Mellon Bank without board discussion or approval. Five board members were current or former directors or executives with Mellon, including its former chairman, who was AHERF's chairman in 2000 (Burns et al., 2000).

Lessons Learned

1. Strong governance and oversight of management are needed to ensure accountability (Goldstein, 2008).
2. When in the zone of insolvency, boards should pay particular attention to the financial impact of proposed corporate transactions; financial advisors should be retained to advise on the fairness of any such transactions (Katz, 2000).

Wealth Destruction

The eight hospitals owned by AHERF in the Philadelphia region were valued between $500 million and $550 million before the bankruptcy filing, based on various bids received from Vanguard, a potential buyer. The final acquisition of the eight Philadelphia hospitals to Tenet for $345 million suggests a loss of $200 million. In actuality, eight nonprofit hospitals were converted to for-profit entities and then all but two were subsequently sold or closed. In addition, the eight Philadelphia hospitals had more than $206 million in endowments and other restricted accounts that disappeared. AHERF's bankruptcy also spelled the demise of its western hospitals in Pittsburgh, including its one-time star performer and flagship, Allegheny General Hospital (Burns et al., 2000).

Unfunded Pension Funds

The sale of the Philadelphia hospitals owned by AHERF required termination of its pension plans. *See* e.g., *Burstein v. Retirement Account Plan for Employees of Allegheny Health Education and Research Foundation*, 334 F.3d 365 (U.S. Court of Appeals for the 3rd Circuit 2003). However, AHERF was $40 million short in funds needed to terminate plans in its Philadelphia operations, a shortfall that became the responsibility of the federal Pension Benefit Guaranty Corp. (PBGC).[LN2]

Lessons Learned

1. Clear and precise financial reports and related disclosures should be made to the governing board to better enable its directors to identify when financially distressed subsidiaries and affiliates may enter the zone of insolvency.
2. Corporate governance policies and executive employment agreements should confirm the obligation of management to advise the governing board regularly on financial conditions (Katz, 2000).

Excess System Capacity

The state of Pennsylvania and local officials in Philadelphia and Pittsburgh stepped in to make sure the AHERF hospitals did not close. In terms of saving jobs, this was a good strategy, but in terms of maintaining excess bed capacity, capacity that was expensive and not needed, it was a dangerous public policy. The poor performance of AHERF's integration strategies was cloaked by inaccurate, misleading financial results and certain institutional structures that limited the scrutiny and efficient response of the health care markets (Burns et al., 2000). Nevertheless, actions were taken for political, not economic, reasons. For instance, what was the academic justification for a fifth medical school in a metropolitan market with four nationally renowned schools of medicine?

Lessons Learned

1. If the troubles of a health care system are the product of managerial decisions that initially succeed but then fail in the face of new market forces, bankruptcy is not necessarily an undesirable outcome (Wharton, 2000).
2. Bankruptcy may not, however, be the best course of action if the troubles are more the product of:
   - Management's unethical and lax behavior
   - Lack of due diligence by the governing board
   - Presence of inflexible and rigid organizational forces
   (Burns et al., 2000)

The Message to Other Integrated Health Care Systems

While few other health care systems operate in exactly the same way AHERF did, there is a significant segment of the hospital industry that is facing multimillion-dollar losses and financial trouble due to:

- Increasing costs of keeping up with medical technology
- High costs of hiring top physicians
- Continued pressure on reimbursement payments
- Eroded hospital endowments and investments from stock-market turbulence
- Paucity of gifts and pledges that most depended on over the past decade
- Mounting debt collection problems and defaults by patients unable to pay their medical bills
- Growing competition from specialty care centers, such as diagnostic imaging boutiques

(Francis, 2007; Goldstein, 2008; Lundstrom, 2004)

It should be kept in mind that what happened at AHERF occurred years before the corporate scandals of the so-called "Enron era" were brought to light. Health care entities are well advised to stay grounded and do honest business even in times of relentless frustration and financial stress (Wharton School, 2000).

HOSPITAL BANKRUPTCIES

Given the nation's economic turmoil, there may be a number of other health care system bankruptcies down the road.[LN3] State budget deficits could mean further cuts in Medicare, Medicaid, and SCHIP entitlement payments, hurting the bottom lines of health care providers and pushing more hospitals into bankruptcy before growth and a full-blown recovery returns. Growth and recovery both depend on the political aftermath.

In the meantime, most hospitals are cutting costs and raising short-term revenues in whatever ways they can. Moreover, the thousands who have lost and will lose their jobs in an economic recession will be without coverage when their health insurance benefits run out, further straining health care systems already overburdened by the uninsured and underinsured (Lagnado, 2008).

BASIS OF EXPECTATIONS

English legal and social reformer Jeremy Bentham said long ago, property is "nothing but a basis of expectation" of wealth creation (Bentham, 1789).

Moral Dilemmas

1. Although the government has a legitimate interest in keeping the costs of health care as low as possible, are hospitals being unfairly coerced to accept society's financial burdens when they take a loss on each entitlement case admitted?

2. Should bankruptcy courts consider the health needs of medically underserved communities in bankruptcy reorganizations?

3. Should bankruptcy courts ever approve the reorganization of a health care system that chooses to divest all of its hospitals in medically underserved communities while it reallocates the funds from their closures and sales to a flagship hospital in a higher-income community?

4. Should the legal privilege of bankruptcy be available to health care systems that abuse the tax-exempt hospital bond system and/or other standard financial controls, or should such systems be forced to go out of business and simply close their doors?

The merger and acquisition rules in this chapter are the very substance of property. The rules are the beliefs that:

- Nonprofit to for-profit conversions improve profit margins
- Private equity buyouts permit businesses that are generating revenue but are not yet profitable enough to realize their economic potential with the opportunity to grow their capital bases by expanding into new markets or financing acquisitions
- Tax-exempt hospital bond financings provide needed capital for growth
- Bankruptcy reconstructions repair capital structures

Their great advantage, or so it is commonly thought, is that the rules signal, in a clear and distinct language, precisely what the financial obligations are for health care businesses and how health care systems may take care of their interests (Freyermuth, 2006). The American health industry is in for an era of innovative medicine if it puts finances at the service of scientific advances and not vice versa (Wharton, 2000).

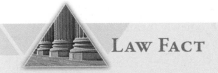

LAW FACT

VOLUNTARY CLOSURE OF INSOLVENT HOSPITALS IN MEDICALLY UNDERSERVED COMMUNITIES

Should states consider the needs of individual patients before approving the closure of insolvent hospitals in medically underserved communities?

No, public needs analysis or community input is not required before states approve the voluntary closure of insolvent hospitals, as opposed to involuntary, state-mandated closures. Hospitals need only provide information to patients regarding their ability to obtain future health care and establish a plan for the storage and safekeeping of patient medical records. *See* 11 U.S.C.A. § 351 (2005) (portion of Bankruptcy Abuse Prevention and Consumer Protection Act of 2005 (BAPCPA) describing procedure to dispose of patient records in health care bankruptcy).

— *Verified Petition PP 8-9, McCloud v. Novello,* Index No. 22406/05 (New York Superior Court Kings County July 22, 2005) and *Stipulation and Order Dismissing Adversary Proceeding, St. Vincent's Catholic Medical Centers of New York v. McCloud (In re St. Vincent's Catholic Medical Centers of New York),* Case No. 05-2351A (U.S. Bankruptcy Court for the Southern District of New York January 19, 2006); *see also* Lee, 2008.

CHAPTER SUMMARY

- Because of the current turbulent economy, hospitals are increasingly facing restructurings and/or bankruptcy.
- The managed care framework failed to solve high costs and poor-quality-of-care problems; restructuring is the next step being taken in hopes of improving the delivery of American health care.
- One popular method of restructuring involves nonprofit hospitals converting into for-profit hospitals.
- Other methods involve private equity buyouts of for-profit hospitals and bankruptcy restructurings.
- Very few hospitals are consistently profitable, have excellent credit ratings, and claim a substantial share of their market.
- Beyond patients' failure to pay medical bills and lack of full reimbursement from third-party payers, hospitals are also faced with over-capacity and competition from other forms of health care delivery, all contributing to hospitals' financial viability problems.
- One of the most shocking health care bankruptcies was that of the Allegheny Health, Education, and Research Foundation (AHERF), the nation's largest nonprofit health care provider, which had been rapidly expanding just prior to filing for bankruptcy.
- Among the problems that contributed to AHERF's financial failure were a breakdown in accountability, flawed corporate strategy, overloaded debt, faulty integration of primary care practices, lack of bargaining power as compared to third-party payers, faulty financing mechanisms, improperly rated bonds, hidden cash transfers, inadequate corporate governance, and excess system capacity.
- Results of AHERF's bankruptcy included wealth destruction and unfunded pension funds.
- Despite AHERF's failure, other academic medical centers continue to engage in and suffer from some of the same behaviors that led to AHERF's downfall.
- Hospital bankruptcies are likely to continue because, although health care is viewed slightly differently than other service industries, it is subject to the same financial constraints as all service industries in a tumultuous economy.

LAW NOTES

1. Of the eight hospitals with close to 2,500 licensed beds acquired by Tenet during the AHERF bankruptcy, only two facilities remain as acute-care hospitals:
   - Hahnemann University Hospital, 618 beds
   - St. Christopher's Hospital for Children, 183 beds

- Medical College of Pennsylvania Hospital, 465 beds (closed and sold to newly formed for-profit Solis Healthcare and now in bankruptcy)
- Graduate Hospital, 330 beds (sold to the University of Pennsylvania Health Care System and converted to a rehabilitation center)
- City Avenue Osteopathic Hospital, 228 beds (closed)
- Parkview Hospital, 200 beds (closed and then sold to Cancer Treatment Centers of America and converted into a skilled nursing home)
- Elkins Park Hospital, 280 beds (sold to the Albert Einstein Medical Network and converted to a rehabilitation center)
- Warminster Hospital, 180 beds (sold to Solis and then resold to current owners, nonprofit Abington Memorial Hospital and since converted into an outpatient-care center)

2. PBGC currently guarantees payment of basic pension benefits earned by American workers and retirees participating in private-sector defined benefit pension plans. The percentage of defined benefit plans, however, has dropped dramatically in the last ten years (today, most employers have switched their plans to cash balance plans or defined contribution plans, such as 401(k) plans, which employees are responsible for funding, often matched by employer contributions but with no guaranteed retirement benefits and subject to market risks).

   PBGC receives no funds from general tax revenues but is facing future retiree shortfalls, as is Social Security. Operations are financed by insurance premiums set by Congress and paid by sponsors of defined benefit plans, investment income, assets from pension plans trusteed by PBGC, and recoveries from the companies formerly responsible for the pension plans. In 2008, the maximum monthly guarantee for a straight-life annuity at age sixty-five was generally $51,750 per year (with no survivor benefits); financial problems arise for retirees of bankrupt companies when they expected to receive significantly higher annual retirement incomes. But, most retirement plans are not covered by PBGC; for instance, retirement plans offered by professional service employers (such as physicians and lawyers), employers with fewer than twenty-six employees, by church groups, or by federal, state, or local governments usually are not insured. In addition, profit-sharing and 401(k) pension plans are not covered by PBGC.

3. The outlook for Philadelphia-area hospitals in particular has not been helped by the bankruptcy of AHERF. Both new issue and secondary market hospital bonds in this region became unpopular. As a result, even before the 2007 economic downturn, it was more difficult and expensive for hospitals to upgrade their existing plant and capacity as they competed.

CHAPTER BIBLIOGRAPHY

Alvarez II, T. (2008, September). Managing director of the Manhattan restructuring firm Alvarez & Marsal at the Reuters Restructuring Summit in New York, NY.

Becker, C. (2003). Early release: Abdelhak wins parole after serving three months. *Modern Healthcare, 33* (5), 18-19.

Bentham, J. (1789). *Introduction to principles of morals and legislation.* London, England: W. Pickering.

Bertrand, M. et al. (2005). Does managed care change the management of nonprofit hospitals? Evidence from the executive labor market. *Industrial & Labor Relations Review, 58,* 494-513.

Burns, R. et al. (2000). The fall of the house of AHERF: The Allegheny bankruptcy. *Health Affairs, 19,* 7-41 (analysis by University of Pennsylvania faculty of the developments behind the dramatic rise and equally dramatic fall of AHERF).

Cobb, A. L., & Hotchkiss, H. G. (2004). AHERF: It may have started with a bang, but did it end in a whimper? *American Bankruptcy Institute, 23* (8), 30-31.

DeMarco, D. A., & Valentine, N. A. (2005). Health care hazards and eleemosynary elocutions: Bankruptcy Abuse Prevention and Consumer Protection Act changes the sale of nonprofit health care assets. *American Bankruptcy Institute, 24* (8), 16-58.

Fisher, M. (2002). *Press release: Pennsylvania Office of Attorney General Michael Fisher: Former AHERF official pleads to raiding endowments; CEO sentenced to 11 to 23 months.*

Fishman, J. J., & Schwartz, S. (2006). *Nonprofit organizations: Cases and materials* (University Casebook Series). Eagan, MN: Thomson West Foundation Press.

Francis, T. (2007, February 6). Hospitals look healthy for now: After Triad deal, buyout players may find few gems. *Wall Street Journal,* p. C3.

Freyermuth, R. W. (2006). Interdisciplinary perspectives on bankruptcy reform: Crystals, mud, BAPCPA, and the structure of bankruptcy decision-making. *Missouri Law Review, 71,* 1069-1078.

Goldstein, L. (2008, August). The failure of AHERF: Five important lessons. *Healthcare Financial Management, 62* (8), 52-57.

Greaney, T. L., & Boozang, K. M. (2005). Mission, margin, and trust in the nonprofit health care enterprise. *Yale Journal of Health Policy, Law & Ethics, 5,* 1-86.

Hall, M. A., & Conover, C. J. (2003). The impact of Blue Cross conversions on accessibility, affordability, and the public interest. *Milbank Quarterly, 81,* 509-542 (summarizing studies and concluding that although the evidence is mixed, it suggests that members of nonprofit HMOs are more satisfied and receive better service and a somewhat higher quality of care).

Harper, R. T., & Schreiber, S. W. (2007). Health law developments: Hospital boards of directors—the challenges of being a hospital director—fiduciary duties, governance issues and board composition. *Pennsylvania Bar Association Quarterly, 78*, 130-133.

Jacoby, M. B. (2007). Individual health insurance mandates and financial distress: A few notes from the debtor-creditor research and debates. *University of Kansas Law Review, 55*, 1247-1257 (maintaining the long-term income effects of health care problems are more financially devastating than the medical bills themselves).

___. (2007). The debtor-patient revisited. *Saint Louis University Law Journal, 51*, 307-324.

___. (2007) Bankruptcy reform and the costs of sickness: Exploring the intersections. *Missouri Law Review, 71*, 903-918.

Jacoby, M. B., & Warren, E. (2006). Beyond hospital misbehavior: An alternative account of medical-related financial distress. *Northwestern University Law Review, 100*, 535-584 (discussing the economic impact of health care).

Kaplan, H. L., & Peregrine, M. W. (2002). Health care enters the zone of insolvency. *American Bankruptcy Institute, 21* (8), 32-33.

Katz, Judge G. (2000, June 30). Administrative proceeding File No. 3-10245. Order instituting cease-and-desist proceedings, making findings, and imposing cease-and-desist order. Washington, DC: U.S. Securities & Exchange Commission.

Lagnado, L. (2008, September 22). The financial crisis: Hospital boards feel Street's pain. *Wall Street Journal*, p. A6.

Lee, J. H. (2008). A civic Republican view of hospital closures and community health planning. *Fordham Urban Law Journal, 35*, 561-600.

Lundstrom, T. (2004). Under-reimbursement of Medicaid and Medicare hospitalizations as an unconstitutional taking of hospital services. *Wayne Law Review, 50*, 1243-1256.

NAAG (National Association of Attorney Generals). (1998). *Model legislation on conversion of nonprofit entities to for-profit status*. Washington, DC: NAAG.

Nelson, L. J. (2006/2007). A tale of three systems: A comparative overview of health care reform in England, Canada, and the United States. *Cumberland Law Review, 37*, 513-542.

Palank, J. (2008, May 1). Many hospitals on brink of insolvency, study finds. *Wall Street Journal*, p. B7.

Weinstein, S. (2000, August 1). Attorney, Office of Municipal Securities, U.S. Securities & Exchange Commission before the AICPA (American Institute of Certified Public Accountants) National Healthcare Industry Conference. Speech: Understanding AHERF:Observations on the recent settlements Involving Allegheny Health, Education and Research Foundation. Washington, DC.

Wharton (Wharton School at the University of Pennsylvania). (2000). The patient died: A post-mortem on America's largest nonprofit health care failure. *Knowledge@Wharton*.

Zywicki, T. J. (2005). An economic analysis of the consumer bankruptcy crisis. *Northwestern University Law Review, 99*, 1463-1541.

CHAPTER 16

BUSINESS PROCESS OUTSOURCING

> *"I cannot say whether things will get better if we change; what I can say is they must change if they are to get better."*
>
> —GEORG CHRISTOPH LICHTENBERG (1742-1799), GERMAN SCIENTIST

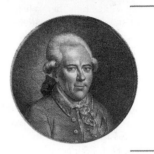

IN BRIEF

This chapter addresses the rapidly expanding integration and outsourcing industry surrounding the health care market. Outsourcing of business processes in health care, from general administrative services to clinical data analysis, is proliferating. Outsourcing of knowledge processes, from telemedicine to cyber-surgery to drug development, continues to increase with innovations in health information technologies. This chapter provides an overview of outsourcing principles applicable to a variety of health care settings.

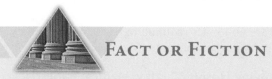

FACT OR FICTION

GLOBAL DRUG OUTSOURCING

Are imported drug ingredients inspected by the U.S. Food and Drug Administration?

Baxter International, of Deerfield, Illinois, procures the active pharmaceutical ingredient for the anti-clotting, generic drug heparin from Scientific Protein Laboratories of Waunakee, Wisconsin. Scientific Protein is owned by a buyout and financing firm called American Capital Strategies, based in Bethesda, Maryland. American Capital Strategies receives the active ingredient, which mainly originates from the mucus of pig intestines and other animal tissues, from a majority-owned U.S. joint venture called Changzhou SPL, located in Changzhou, China. The generic heparin active pharmaceutical ingredient, which is used primarily for kidney dialysis, heart surgery, and a procedure called apheresis in immune disorder patients, has been tied to nineteen deaths and several hundred extreme allergic reactions resulting in vomiting, diarrhea, low blood pressure, speeding heartbeats, and fainting.

—Burton et al., 2008.

(See *Law Fact* at the end of this chapter for the answer.)

PRINCIPLES AND APPLICATIONS

Business process outsourcing (BPO), the use of outside vendors for the performance of general administrative services (finance, accounting, human resources, claims processing, customer relationship management, and procurement) is a critical issue for health care providers as the demand to reduce overall costs continues to multiply. The effective use of outsourcing is commonsensical given that at least one-third of U.S. health care costs are attributed to overhead and management expenses (Relman, 2005).

The value of the integration and outsourcing market for the health industry worldwide is estimated at about $31 billion (Wharton, 2006). Clearly, outsourcing remains a legitimate strategic option for health care systems currently operating at margins of 2 to 3 percent (BCG, 2006). While discretionary patient spending expands due to the growth of consumer-directed health care, the demands for cost-effective care will only increase.

As acceptance of BPO accelerates, the health industry is continually seeking to outsource non-strategic services that can be accomplished more cost-efficiently by BPO providers (Jain, 2007). Outsourcing transfers responsibility for ongoing management tasks and execution of business activities, processes, or functional areas to BPO providers in order to improve efficiency and performance (Singh, 2003). BPO arrangements are often exceedingly complex and complicated because they involve the transfer of one or more complete business processes or entire business functions to an external contractor who will perform them.

BPO is generally recognized to stand for *business process outsourcing*. In this text, for purpose of simplicity, BPO also stands for *business process offshoring*, the practice of running the business functions of health care organizations by their own foreign captive units or by BPO providers in offshore locations.

OFFSHORING OF HEALTH CARE OUTSOURCING

The use of offshore BPO providers has increased dramatically in recent years due to the increased flexibility in services offered by new health information technologies (AMA, 1996). The leading BPO providers serving the U.S. health industry are in India. The largest BPO is Tata Consultancy Services (TCS), with annual revenues of more than $3 billion, followed by Wipro with earnings in excess of $2.4 billion, and Infosys with revenue of over $2.2 billion (BCG, 2006). Such services as technical information support, transcription, collation, billing, insurance claims processing, and X-ray analysis are sent offshore with growing frequency, as hospitals and health plans come under heightened pressure to cut costs (Rashbaum, 2004). For example, as the cost of telecommunications time falls, the volume of medicine practiced in cyberspace is expected to steadily increase (Merrell, 2005).

It has been estimated that the $20 billion industry that transcribes physicians' dictated notes into written form outsources as much as half of its work offshore (Lazarus, 2004). Similarly, almost half of the claims processing for Medicare is outsourced offshore (GAO, 2005).

FLATTENING OF THE U.S. HEALTH CARE SYSTEM

The boundaries of health care providers are being flattened at the same time that they are being expanded (Friedman, 2007). With this connectivity, globalization and technology have made it possible to do business, or almost anything, instantaneously worldwide. For instance, when a health care provider tells a BPO contractor to handle certain medical services in exchange for a fee, what was once handled inside a hospital or physician's office now becomes a market transaction handled outside the hospital or physician's office. As a result, the boundaries of the health care provider are flattened or connected to the BPO contractor; the playing field becomes level as the provider and contractor are linked together in a logical and intelligible way (Fund et al., 2007). Meanwhile, a different game is starting. An extended organization is developing in which health care providers relinquish control in return for monitoring knowledge. Since the purpose of outsourcing is to delegate one or more functions to an external contractor, the decision to outsource the function allows health care providers to focus their resources on their strategic services, clinical care, medical education, and research (Yeun, 2008).

Outsourcing also allows a greater focus on core competencies, from epidemiology to genetics. Core competencies consist of the fundamental parts of a provider's value package, or the medical functions that constitute the provider's competitive advantage (Yeun, 2008). For instance, most teaching hospitals do not engage in business functions unrelated to their core functions (such as maintenance, food services, security staffing, patient billing, and insurance claim processing); they focus instead on clinical care, medical education, and research.

With this flattening, the BPO industry has now achieved critical mass in its quest for providing knowledge process outsourcing services, where skills, judgment, and discretion are the tools (BCG & Wharton, 2007). The outsourcing of American medical jobs will only surge with technological innovations in the fields of telemedicine and cyber-surgery (Anvari, 2005; Klaus, 2006). As used in this text, *telemedicine* is the diagnostic practice of medicine over distance using telecommunications and interactive video technologies (AMA, 1996). Telemedicine is distinguished from e-health, which is broader in scope, as it includes not only health care delivery but also health information technologies. Digitalization of medical data in virtually every medical discipline, coupled with recent advancements in telecommunications, means that physicians and their clinical support

staff are no longer required to reside on the same continent as their patients (McLean, 2006).

Supplying Hospital Staff v. Medical Expertise

When examining outsourcing, there is a difference between the supply of staff and the supply of medical expertise (Wharton, 2002). Health information technology enables the establishment of deep, information-based linkages between a health care provider and its BPO contractor. For example, with radiology services, each sees the same patient X-rays; the provider takes the X-rays (records the medical data) and the BPO contractor interprets the X-rays (explains the meaning of the medical data). At one level, a hospital and the BPO contractor engage in a market transaction, but at another level, the BPO contractor is an extension of the hospital.

Today, most U.S. hospitals are part of vast, complex networks.[LN1] The issue for many hospitals is how multifaceted they need to be; how many different functions does a hospital need to perform itself, as opposed to having a BPO contractor perform them for the hospital? U.S. auto manufacturers realized in the early part of the nineteenth century that there was no reason for them to own rubber plantations in the Amazon so that they could make their own tires; another entity could make the tires while they could focus on assembling automobiles. In the same way, hospitals are beginning to recognize that they do not need to do everything to support their organizations (Wharton, 2002). Some levels of better-quality medical expertise and clinical support functions, as well as business functions, can be acquired far less expensively from outside their organizations by BPO providers (Weiss & Azaran, 2007). There are BPO specialists for almost every business process who are better at providing the service for many health care providers than any one provider on their own (TES, 2007), from health care standards for health care system integration, bioinformatics, regulatory compliance, to telemedicine.

- In health care systems integration, BPO contractors can integrate data standards for use in electronic medical records (EMRs), computerized provider order entry systems (CPOEs), and genetic databases, within technical frameworks to clean and integrate quality health care data
- In nomenclature integration, BPO contractors can integrate Systematized Nomenclature of Medicine (SNOMED), developed by the College of American Pathologists and used in EMRs, CPOEs, and genetic databases
- In bioinformatics, BPO contractors can provide high-performance computing technology to

enhance the storage and analysis of molecular information in areas ranging from protein structure production to machine learning techniques for target identification to molecular modeling to lead identification and optimization

- In regulatory compliance, BPO contractors can provide comprehensive solutions to resolve compliance issues, rather than isolated applications, for managing GxPs, Sarbanes-Oxley, and privacy regulations, while improving validation processes across teams and aligning compliance strategies with broader business goals; GxP refers to quality guidelines used in the health industry (*see* 21 C.F.R. §§ 1271.1–1271.85 (2009))
- In telemedicine, health care providers face high patient volume in remote locations, BPO contractors can provide leading-edge technology and strategies for the transfer of medical information online and in real-time for use in diagnosis, treatment, and education across distances

There is a need for access to complete and accurate medical data; however, most health care providers have multiple, patchwork applications running on disparate platforms that cannot provide rapid and integrated patient information at the point of service. In addition, different health care providers and health care networks use different clinical terms that mean the same thing. For instance, the terms *myocardial infarction*, *heart attack*, and *MI* may mean the same thing to a cardiologist, but, to a computer, they are different. There is a need for access to consistent medical data between different health care providers, and because patient information is recorded differently from place to place, a comprehensive medical terminology system is needed as part of any information infrastructure.

Teleradiology

As discussed, the traditional system of providing health care is in the process of being flattened (Terry, 2007). Statistics show radiological outsourcing growing by 7 percent per year, with 12 percent of hospitals currently engaging in such a practice (Hwang, 2004). Reliable estimates as to the size of the offshore market do not exist, however, since teleradiology is currently provided primarily by a number of private companies that are not obligated to file public reports (Levy & Yu, 2006).

Teleradiology is the largest component of international telemedicine today in terms of complexity, and hence cost; it is roughly midway between teleconsultations and cyber-surgery (Alexander, 2007). For instance, when X-ray analysis is moved from a U.S. hospital to an offshore BPO contractor, the hospital

stops exercising control over medical personnel analyzing patient X-rays. Now, the hospital looks at the number of errors per number of X-rays processed and controls the level of quality. In addition, the hospital randomly samples X-rays to monitor the quality of the analysis. The hospital no longer tells the physicians and technicians how to analyze patient X-rays; now the hospital and BPO contractor agree on the outcomes of the analysis and the hospital pays the BPO contractor depending on the number of X-rays analyzed (BCG & Wharton, 2007). Thus, the extended health care organization is one in which the hospital relinquishes local control. The BPO contractor actually hires the physicians and technicians who analyze patient X-rays, while the hospital monitors their analyses and attempts to control overall quality.

Telecardiology, Teledermatology, Teleophthalmology, and Telepathology

The points raised concerning the practice of radiology apply equally to any branch of medicine that is primarily concerned with the evaluation of images or medical data that can be reduced to an image format. Most branches of medicine are ripe for business process outsourcing offshore, including cardiology (Liu et al., 2006), dermatology (Bowns et al., 2006; Wooton et al., 2000), ophthalmology (Johnson et al., 2007; Barclay, 2002), and pathology (Horbinski et al., 2007). Some endoscopy procedures are already being replaced by innovative radiology techniques that render endoscopy obsolete (Pickhardt et al., 2003).

BPO Centers-of-Excellence

In a world of telemedicine, it is possible to concentrate expertise in BPO centers-of-excellence (CoEs)[LN2] that would receive health data from multiple health care systems. For example, it is not hard to imagine BPO CoEs where radiologists would work around the clock, in full eight-hour shifts, to perform all of the data interpretations for images generated in several states in the U.S. (Nyberg & Lanzieri, 2007). With health data concentrated into BPO CoEs, wherever the best skill set exists, the economies-of-scale would cause the net unit cost for radiographic interpretation to fall below the costs currently generated by radiologists interpreting films under exclusive contracts in community hospitals.

Other BPO CoEs could be staffed by cardiologists and still others by pathologists. Additionally, nothing would prevent such BPO CoEs from competing to provide services on the third shifts in hospitals in countries eight time zones ahead or behind. Such BPO CoEs could be located in U.S.

health care facilities where patient care is offered at an exemplary level on a wide range of measures or in emerging economies in health care facilities with exemplary patient care in Eastern Europe, India, China, or South Africa; BPO CoEs would have the manpower to compete with radiologists, cardiologists, or pathologists on a global basis.

Medical Products Outsourcing

In the majority of areas of medical products outsourcing, most of the concerns boil down to audit of standardized procedures, including:

- Clinical trials
- Cost and price analyses
- Early-stage drug development
- Environmental health and safety
- Manufacturing
- Production planning
- Quality assurance and quality oversight

(Cekola, 2007)

FDA regulations that standardize procedures and verification work make it easy for the non-core functions of clinical research and development and commercialization to be outsourced. *See* Regulations Relating to Good Clinical Practices (GCPs) and Clinical Trials, 21 C.F.R. §§ 11, 50, 54, 56, 312, 314, 601, 812, 814 (2009). Producers of medical products must document what their systems do and prove that the systems function consistently within a certain margin of error, and these producers must also perform audits whenever called upon to do so by the FDA (*see* Bellman & Koppel, 2005). For instance, global pharmaceuticals have between five hundred and eight hundred environmental health and safety workers, from regulation statisticians to analysts and other back-office function workers.

FDA guidelines also provide a system of business processes to ensure that the medical products produced by manufacturers have the identity, strength, composition, quality, and purity that they are represented to possess. GMPs address operating procedures and documentation requirements for:

- Distribution
- In-house testing
- Production and process controls
- Qualifications of manufacturing personnel
- Raw materials quality assurance
- Record-keeping of substances throughout the manufacturing process
- Standards for cleanliness and safety
- Warehousing

From this perspective, it is advantageous for producers of medical products to use BPO providers for outsourced work. If the procedures are in writing and are auditable, the producers of medical products and the BPO providers will each be familiar with them and know how to evaluate them.

Risk Management of BPO Relationships

Understanding and defining acceptable risk levels is one of the first hurdles for outsourcing. Companies involved in outsourcing offshore are incorporating detailed clauses into their BPO contracts. They are setting up integrated metrics within the outsourcing relationship with clear deadlines, standards for accuracy, and database locks that prevent reopening the data after it is finalized (COM, 2007). There are hundreds of line items that are agreed upon in industry-wide, standardized master agreements and statements of work (Baird, 2006).

The key point is that information transferred offshore is only protected insofar as the terms of the BPO contract provide and as the destination country permits. Thus, a U.S. health care provider's ability to safeguard the personal medical data it transfers to BPO providers in countries with weaker data protection laws is largely limited to the ability to enforce any data protection clauses in its BPO contract (Yeun, 2008). Providers also have to weigh operational risks such as natural disasters and technology failures, and performance risks such as pricing traps and

Good Automated Manufacturing Practices (GaMPs)

- A Risk-Based Approach to Compliant Electronic Records and Signatures
- Calibration Management
- Electronic Data Archiving
- Global Information Systems Control and Compliance
- IT Infrastructure Control and Compliance
- Validation of Laboratory Computerized Systems
- Validation of Process Control Systems

non-delivery on service-level agreements. All of these risks can be managed by the right:

- Acceptable service-level agreements
- BPO delivery model
- Clear-cut price negotiations
- Proper contractor selection

Providers should also check the geo-political stability and infrastructure capabilities, among the other factors, in the BPO contractor's country. Above all, health care providers should consider a risk-mitigation approach by hedging their operational risks in multiple locations (BCG & Wharton, 2007).

> *Moral Dilemmas*
>
> 1. Does the FDA have a moral responsibility to protect the U.S. population by becoming more accountable for inspecting and monitoring overseas BPO providers?
>
> 2. Is the U.S. relinquishing too much control to developing countries by outsourcing processes overseas?

Protection of Tacit Knowledge

The health industry is often concerned about the misuse of residual knowledge about strategy when considering outsourcing (Hodges & Block, 2005). Such concerns, however, can be mitigated by requiring BPO providers to be quarantined after sensitive projects, which means they cannot work with competitors for a limited period of time (Bellman & Koppel, 2005).

This loss of tacit knowledge, of how things are done, is constantly a concern with BPO providers. Nonetheless, outsourcing is so cost-effective that health care providers and producers of medical products are often tempted to outsource, without worrying about tacit knowledge. This unstated oversight, however, could lead to real problems with execution.

There is no easy way to pass along tacit knowledge to BPO providers, unless companies are very good at formalizing their business processes and documenting everything that is done (Bellman & Koppel, 2005). Corporate epistemology must be documented before outsourcing can be successful (Polanyi, 2007). Epistemology is the branch of philosophy that explains how experts gain and verify knowledge. The intuitive process of how knowledge is acquired without any explicit direction must be converted into detailed requirements that can be given to BPO providers for proper implementation.

Alternatives to thorough documentation of tacit knowledge could include running captive centers or

adopting other business relationships that are at an arm's length with respect to outsourcing, rather than using BPO providers. The less tangible the work, though, the more closely strategic activities should be held and not outsourced (BCG & Wharton, 2007).

> *Moral Dilemmas*
>
> 1. Should labor, human rights, and environmental standards be considered in BPO contracts and costs?
>
> 2. Does offshore contracting of BPO services decrease U.S. employment opportunities, and in turn hurt the U.S. economy?

GLOBAL DRUG MANUFACTURING IN CHINA

China occupies center stage for outsourcing of raw materials for the drug industry. The manufacturers, in turn, are responsible for sourcing raw materials and appropriately processing the material (Fairclough & Burton, 2008). The quality of exported chemicals from China is the responsibility of importers and importing countries (Mathews & Burton, 2008). The Chinese State Food and Drug Administration (Chinese State FDA) works with its foreign regulatory counterparts to monitor drug-ingredient production to ensure that raw materials are consistent, clean, and traceable (Fairclough, 2008). Based on international practice, however, safeguarding the legality, quality, and safety of active pharmaceutical ingredients is the ultimate responsibility of the global drug manufacturers and the importing countries, not the exporting countries (FDA, 2008). While approximately 80 percent of the active pharmaceutical ingredients in U.S. drugs originate from foreign manufacturers, the FDA currently only inspects about 10 percent of foreign drug producers due to insufficient field-force funding (Wechsler, 2008).

The generic heparin case that started this chapter highlights regulatory gaps that have opened as drug manufacturers globalize their purchase of ingredients. Most drug suppliers in China that export to the U.S. are not licensed, nor are they inspected by the Chinese State FDA or the U.S. FDA. Due to federal cost constraints, the U.S. FDA conducted, at most, twenty-one inspections of Chinese drug-making facilities annually in fiscal years 2002 through 2007, according to the U.S. Government Accountability Office (GAO). This represents a small fraction of the more than seven hundred Chinese facilities that, as of the end of fiscal year 2007, the GAO reports were involved in making drugs or drug ingredients for the

U.S. market (Fairclough & Burton, 2008). In China, few raw material suppliers are certified by Chinese drug regulators as drug producers; most are registered as chemical makers or agricultural byproducts companies and are not checked by state drug authorities (Burton & Dooren, 2008).

EARLY-STAGE MEDICAL PRODUCTS RESEARCH IN INDIA

Instead of routine data work, outsourcing is moving toward information extraction, which involves interpretation and inference (Rashbaum, 2004). More and more of this trend is occurring with medical products research. Instead of data entry, BPO contractors are now offering high-end research services. The most popular service for outsourcing is performing clinical trials.[LN3] As medical products pass through the clinical trial process, data regarding their safety and efficacy must be gathered to support an application to the FDA, because it is only through FDA approval that a company can capitalize on its products. BPO providers supply the necessary staff to appropriately collect, store, question, report, and analyze that data to provide justification for FDA approval to market a medical product.

Producers of medical products have become much more efficient by outsourcing to BPO providers (Agarwal et al., 2005). Earlier concerns about protection of intellectual property in India diminished significantly after the Indian government introduced patent legislation allowing medical product companies to obtain patent protection on almost every aspect of product development, from molecules and microorganisms to processes (Hason & Shimotake, 2006; Helm, 2006).

There is a growing desire among producers of medical products to conduct their clinical research in India due to the relatively easy access to participants in clinical trials (McGee, 2006). Research indicates that conducting clinical trials in India can lower early-stage drug discovery costs by $35 to $50 million per new drug due to rapid enrollment of participants in trials and shortened enrollment timelines for clinical trials (Hazelwood et al., 2005). While the cost of creating a new drug can be as high as $900 million, it takes $350 to $500 million to take a new chemical entity through all the stages of clinical trials and reach the market.

More important than the cost-efficiencies, producers of medical products can avoid fiduciary status and some liability claims by designing protocols to comply with FDA regulations and outsourcing their clinical research (Geis, 2007). The leading federal court decision on fiduciary duty of BPO contractors has led to discussion of federal legislation to address the liabilities of offshore BPOs, but there is no groundswell of public demand for any legislative change (Wharton, 2007).

It is India that currently occupies center stage for outsourcing in health care because of the country's large educated labor force, especially its reservoir of research and engineering graduates. The sheer numbers of India's talent force make a compelling case for outsourcing to India. India has some 22 million university graduates, including:

- 6 million science graduates
- 1.2 million with engineering degrees
- 600,000 physicians

India's educated population is growing rapidly, with nearly 2.5 million graduates added in 2004 alone, including 25,000 physicians and nearly 600,000 science and engineering graduates (NASSCOM & McKinsey, 2005). Wage arbitrage is another reason. Health care providers must pay a 40 to 80 percent cost premium in direct wages alone to obtain the quality of labor they can obtain more cheaply from BPOs in India (Click & Deuning, 2005). It is estimated that the cost of conducting clinical drug trials in India is only one-seventh of that in the U.S. or Europe (Clendenin, 2006). Even with all these advantages, India is still facing intense competition from BPO providers in other emerging markets in China, South Africa, and Eastern Europe.

Cost-Effectiveness of Captives and Business Process Organizations

A study by consultants McKinsey & Co. and the National Association of Software and Service Companies–India (NASSCOM & McKinsey, 2005), the Indian technology and outsourcing industry trade group, found that on average, back-offices (or captives, as they are referred to in the information technology and outsourcing industries) are less efficient than BPO providers that specialize in integration and outsourcing. NASSCOM represents information technology companies and BPO providers, which are also known as IT-enabled services (ITES) providers. For some types of back-office work, captives' costs were 30 percent higher (Range, 2008). At the same time, higher captive costs did not lead to lower staff turnover or better-quality work (Click & Deuning, 2005).

Outsourcing of health care service functions began with setting up domestic captive service centers. These centers began by executing enterprise-wide operations that involved the conversion of medical records from patient charts to electronic medical records (Wharton, 2002). Today, these domestic captive centers are starting to move their information extraction and reporting tasks offshore. Two factors are making this possible: the convergence in health care computing platforms and the rapid advances in communications technology. As enterprise-wide platforms, such as relational databases and networking standards, become standardized and software tools become available that facilitate porting large medical data sets between dispersed information technology systems, the flow of medical data and personal health information within health care systems should become more practical and cost less.

As the flow of medical data between computers swells, so will the extent of human intervention and the degree of expertise required to transform data into information. As a result, the costs of providing accurate and timely personal health information to support clinical decision-making will begin mounting by orders of magnitude (McLean, 2005). As this happens, the U.S. health industry will be faced with a two-pronged cost escalation: providers will need to hire more staff and at the same time increase the expertise levels of existing staff (Wharton, 2002). The move to centralize non-strategic functions in lower-cost labor regimes is an obvious response to the cost frontier faced by the U.S. health industry (O'Rourke, 2003). Initial reports suggest that some health care providers benefit through up to 60 percent in cost savings in lower-wage markets (Wharton, 2005a).

Hybrid "Program Offices"

Indian BPO firms have developed businesses for the delivery of higher-end health care services that are a hybrid between captive organizations doing business in-house and traditional work outsourced by contractors (WHO, 2004). The BPO captive work model, executed by traditional managerial authority, has been merged with the outside work model, facilitated by price and contract, to create what are known as program offices, also known as program management offices, project offices, project management offices, and project control centers. Program offices are actually centralized centers that monitor, influence, and control projects to make them more efficient. What makes program offices unique is that they have no responsibility for the activities of projects; they are uninvolved in project management. With the development of health information technology, Indian program offices can work very closely with U.S. health care providers, to the point where the BPO's employees become almost like the U.S. provider's employees.

BPO PRIVACY CONCERNS

Isolated data security and privacy violations have become high-visibility issues disproportionate to the ground realities of BPO providers (Bertram, 2006). Nonetheless, most Americans remember headlines about the disgruntled medical transcripter in Pakistan who threatened to disclose the University of California–San Francisco Medical Center's patient records if she was not given her back-pay (Lazarus, 2003). At the same time, it is often forgotten that most privacy violations of personal health information occur in the U.S. and are the result of individuals not protecting their own medical data (Brantley, 2004); many voluntarily relinquish their privacy online in chat rooms and through participation in Internet surveys.

Even so, with outsourcing, there has been a rise in the privacy concerns of patients with regard to improper disclosures of personal medical data, and fraud, such as medical identity theft (Davis, 2004). As the health industry moves toward greater use of health information technology, particularly in the transition to electronic medical record systems, this concern will need to be addressed (Moshell, 2005). With the movement toward electronic health records, the health industry will face many of the same privacy concerns and risks that have confronted financial institutions. (HHS, 2002) Thus, the recommendations of the Federal Deposit Insurance Corporation (FDIC) with regard to consumer privacy risks can serve as a model for health care entities. The FDIC recommends that three general areas be considered when outsourcing offshore:

- Privacy risks in the offshore BPO contractor's country
- Ongoing oversight of all third-party contractors, their activities, and the status of data protection in the contractor's country, including the use of independent audit reports
- Contract provisions that protect the privacy of patients and their medical data, including:
  - Choice of law
  - Local legal review of the BPO contractor's contract to determine enforceability of all aspects of the contract
  - Prohibition on use or disclosure of offshore data except to carry out the contracted services

(FDIC, 2004)

WHAT LIES AHEAD FOR BPOS?

At present, most outsourcing of medical services in the U.S. is done to provide medical coverage at community hospitals on the third shift (11:00 PM to 7:00 AM), when it is hard to find physicians. Yet because BPOs' contractors allow hospitals to tap into low-wage labor pools in developing nations, the U.S. health care system could potentially lower costs by outsourcing more medical services (IDC, 2008). Independent of the potential for system-wide efficiencies, increased use of BPO providers could:

- Improve access to care
- Create economies-of-scale
- Reduce medical errors
- Improve competition amongst providers

(IBM, 2006)

If such efficiencies can be documented, it is likely that more services will be outsourced on the first and second shifts, not necessarily because physicians cannot be found, but rather because it will cut costs and/or improve efficiency.

As the U.S. health industry struggles with restructuring the delivery of existing medical services, new opportunities will emerge to improve efficiencies and medical treatments that do not yet exist. This

will lead to the next wave of integration and outsourcing. For instance, over the years, many health care providers have collected mountains of personal medical data on their patients. BPO providers could offer to interpret that data. If analyzed, that medical data could provide valuable insights into new ways to effectively restructure the strategic functions of health care providers. While waiting for that to unfold, no BPO industry observers have placed bets on what other unprecedented services await discovery (BCG & Wharton, 2007).

Moral Dilemmas

1. Do the cost-efficiencies of utilizing BPO providers outweigh the risks of contaminated supply chains?

2. Should consumers have a more active say in whether U.S. medical product companies outsource processes to developing countries?

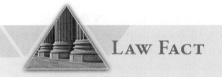

LAW FACT

GLOBAL DRUG OUTSOURCING

Are imported drug ingredients inspected by the U.S. Food and Drug Administration?

The legal requirement for drug manufacturers to get inspected every two years applies only to domestic plants, not offshore facilities.

—Burton et al., 2008.

CHAPTER SUMMARY

- It is estimated that at least one-third of U.S. health care costs are a result of overhead and management expenses, non-strategic services that can be accomplished more cost-efficiently by BPO providers.
- Technical information support, transcription, collation, billing, insurance claims processing, and X-ray analysis are sent offshore with increasing frequency, as health care systems come under greater pressure to reduce costs.
- When examining health industry outsourcing, there is a difference between the supply of staff and the supply of expertise.
- Any branch of medicine that is primarily concerned with the evaluation of images or the evaluation of medical data that can be reduced to an image format is suitable for BPO contracting.
- The U.S. FDA's regulations that standardize manufacturing, clinical trials, drug development procedures, and verification work make it easy to outsource the non-core functions of research and development and commercialization.

- India's patent legislation allows medical product companies to obtain patent protection on almost every aspect of product development, from materials to processes.
- There is a growing desire among producers of medical products to conduct their clinical research in India due to the relatively easy access to clinical trial participants, which can lower early-stage drug discovery costs by $35 to $50 million per new drug.
- As important as the cost-efficiencies are for BPO providers, producers of medical products can avoid fiduciary status and some liability claims by designing protocols to comply with FDA regulations and then outsourcing their clinical research.
- When outsourcing offshore, detailed clauses should be incorporated into BPO contracts that define the integrated metrics that will be used to monitor the outsourcing relationship with clear deadlines for performance, as well as the standards to be used for informational accuracy and database locks.
- Information transferred offshore is only protected insofar as the terms of the BPO contract provide and as the destination country permits, in terms of enforcement and recognition of a right to legal action.
- India possesses the largest advantage for outsourcing health care because of the wage arbitrage of its large educated labor force, which has the potential to save about 80 percent in direct wages alone.
- Captive organizations are significantly less efficient than BPO providers that specialize in integration and outsourcing.
- The misuse of implicit knowledge about strategy and best practices can be mitigated by restricting BPO providers from working with competitors for a limited period of time.
- The less tangible the work, the more closely health care providers and producers of medical products should hold strategic activities inside their organizations rather than outsource.
- As the U.S. health industry struggles to restructure the delivery of existing medical services, new opportunities to improve efficiencies and medical treatments that do not yet exist will be revealed. This will likely result in another round of integration and outsourcing.

LAW NOTES

1. For example, the Children's Hospital of Philadelphia (CHOP) is a 430-bed hospital receiving over 1 million outpatient and inpatient visits per year. Founded in 1855, CHOP is now the largest integrated pediatric health care network in the U.S., with nine outpatient specialty centers, four primary care centers, inpatient and intensive care (neonatal intensive care unit (NICU) and pediatric intensive care unit (PICU)) units at five community hospitals, a poison control center, and twenty-eight primary care (Kids First) practices throughout Pennsylvania, New Jersey, and Delaware. It is the pediatric teaching site for the University of Pennsylvania School of Medicine, although it operates autonomously medically, administratively, and financially.

2. National CoEs for comprehensive health care were first established in the U.S. in 1996 by the U.S. Department of Health and Human Services to improve the health status of women. Located in academic medical centers, they bring together the work of their schools and departments to address women's health care. CoEs on Women's Health unite:
   - State-of-the-art health care services addressing all of a woman's needs
   - Gender-based research
   - Education and training
   - Community linkages
   - Leadership positions for women in academic medicine

3. The largest global BPO providers for clinical trials, or contract research organizations (CROs), are Quintiles, Covance, and Parexel. Quintiles, headquartered near Research Triangle Park, North Carolina, has more than $2.0 billion in annual revenues, global operations in more than fifty-two countries, and more than 19,000 employees. Covance, headquartered in Princeton, New Jersey, is the second largest, with annual revenues greater than $1.4 billion and more than 8,700 employees. Parexel, headquartered near Boston, Massachusetts, has more than 7,300 employees and annual revenues of about $1.3 billion.

CHAPTER BIBLIOGRAPHY

Agarwal, S. et al. (2005). Destination India: Offshore outsourcing and its implications. *Computer & Telecommunications Law Review, 11* (8), 246-262.

Alexander III, A. A. (2007). American diagnostic radiology moves offshore: Is this field riding the "Internet wave" into a regulatory abyss? *Journal of Law & Health, 20,* 199-251.

AMA (American Medical Association). (1996). *Joint report of Council on Medical Education and Council on Medical Services, the promotion of quality telemedicine.* Washington, DC: AMA.

Anvari, M. (2005). Remote telepresence surgery. *Laparoscopy Today, 4,* 5-7 (experience with non-physician astronauts suggests that telemedicine supervision of physician extenders may allow the latter to perform surgical procedures, thereby eliminating the need for local physicians).

Baird, D. G. (2006). "Boilerplate": Foundations of market contracts symposium. *Michigan Law Review, 104,* 821-826 (discussion of the benefits and concerns presented by contractual boilerplate language).

Barclay, L. (2002). Telemedicine may improve screening for diabetic retinopathy, diabetes care. *Medscape 25,* 1384-1389, 1477-1478.

Barth, A. S. (2006). Recent developments in health law: Select recent court decisions. *American Journal of Law & Medicine, 32,* 405-408.

BCG (Boston Consulting Group) & Knowledge@Wharton. (2007). *What's next for India: Beyond the back office.* Boston, MA: BCG & Philadelphia, PA: Wharton School of the University of Pennsylvania.

BCG. (2006). *Performance outcomes of onshore and offshore business process outsourcing (BPO).* Boston, MA: BCG.

Bellman, E., & Koppel, N. (2005, September 28). More U.S. legal work moves to India's low-cost lawyers. *Wall Street Journal,* p. B1.

Bertram, B. (2006). Building fortress India: Should a federal law be created to address privacy concerns in the U.S. and Indian business process outsourcing relationship? *International & Comparative Law Review, 29,* 245-268.

Bhattacharya, A. et al. (2004). *Capturing global advantage: How leading industrial companies are transforming their industries by sourcing and selling in China, India and other low-cost countries.* Boston, MA: Boston Consulting Group.

Bowns, I. R. et al. (2006). Telemedicine in dermatology: A randomized controlled trial. *Health Technology Assessment, 10* (43), iii-iv, ix-xi, 1-39.

Brantley, D. et al. (2004). *Innovation, demand and investment in telehealth.* Washington, DC: U.S. Department of Commerce, Office of Technology Policy.

Burton, T. M., & Dooren, J. C. (2008, March 15). FDA orders heparin shipments to be tested at the U.S. border. *Wall Street Journal,* p. B9.

Burton, T. M. et al. (2008, February 15). Heparin probe finds U.S. tie to Chinese plant. *Wall Street Journal,* p. B1.

Cekola, J. (2007). Outsourcing drug investigations to India: A comment on U.S., Indian, and international regulation of clinical trials in cross-border pharmaceutical research. *Northwestern Journal of International Law & Business, 28,* 125-145.

Clendenin, G. S. (2006). Allaying the outsourcing tempest: A candid look at outsourcing vis-a-vis the future of American jobs. *University of Miami Business Law Review, 14,* 295-312.

Click, R. L., & Deuning, T. N. (2005). *Business process outsourcing: The competitive advantage.* Farmington, MI:

Thomson Gale (discusses the how and why of BPO with a straightforward how-to approach).

COM (Commission of the European Communities). (2007). *Communication on the follow-up of the work programme for better implementation of the data protection directive.* Brussels, Belgium: COM.

Davis, B. (2004, May 10). As jobs move offshore, so does privacy. *Wall Street Journal,* p. A2.

Fairclough, G. (2008, February 28). China puts drug-safety onus on buyers. *Wall Street Journal,* p. D6.

Fairclough, G., & Burton, T. M. (2008, February 21). The heparin trail: China's role in supply of drug is under fire. *Wall Street Journal,* p. A1.

FDA (Food & Drug Administration) Import operations and actions. (2008). In *FDA regulatory procedures manual.* (Chapter 9). Silver Spring, MD FDA, Division of Import Operations & Policies.

FDIC (Federal Deposit Insurance Corporation). (2004). *Offshore outsourcing of data services by insured institutions and associated privacy risks.* Washington, DC: FDIC.

Friedman, T. L. (2007). *The world is flat: A brief history of the twenty-first century: Further updated and expanded.* New York, NY: Picador (introducing "flat" metaphors to describe the affects of globalization and international competition that have been sparked by technological change, particularly from developing countries such as India and China).

Fund, V. K. et al. (2007). *Competing in a flat world: Building enterprises for a borderless world.* Upper Saddle River, NJ: Wharton School Publishing.

GAO (General Accounting Office). (2005). Privacy: Domestic and offshore outsourcing of personal information in Medicare, Medicaid, and Tricare. Washington, DC: GAO.

Geis, G. S. (2007). Business outsourcing and the agency cost problem. *Notre Dame Law Review, 82,* 955-1003.

Hason, A. K., & Shimotake, J. E. (2006). Global interdependence and international commercial law: Recent developments in patent rights for pharmaceuticals in China and India. *Pace International Law Review, 18,* 303-315.

Hazelwood, S. E. et al. (2005). Possibilities and pitfalls of outsourcing. *Healthcare Financial Management, 44,* 45-46.

Helm, K. A. (2006). Outsourcing the fire of genius: The effects of patent infringement jurisprudence on pharmaceutical drug development. *Fordham Intellectual Property, Media & Entertainment Law Journal, 17,* 153-206.

HHS (U.S. Department of Health & Human Service). (2002). *HIPAA privacy technical guidance.* Washington, DC: HHS, Office of Civil Rights.

Hodges, M., & Block, D. (2005). *Business process outsourcing: Current trends and best practices.* New York, NY: National Contract Management Association.

Horbinski, C. et al. (2007). Telepathology for intraoperative neuropathologic consultations at an academic medical center: A five-year report. *Journal of Neuropathology & Experimental Neurology, 66* (8), 750-759.

Hwang, N. H. (2004). The concerns of electronically outsourcing radiological services overseas. *Journal of Legal Medicine, 25* (471), 469-484.

IBM. (2006). *The business impact of outsourcing: A fact-based analysis.* White Plains, NY: IBM (companies engaged in IT outsourcing experienced significant gains, compared to their competition: 12 percent higher growth in earnings, 10 percent lower expenses, and 9 percent higher return on assets).

IDC (Interactive Data Corp.) (2008, January). *Health industry insights.* U.S. life science top ten predictions. Framington, MA: IDC.

Jain, A. (2007). *Examining the evolving offshore business process outsourcing model.* Plano, TX: Perot Systems.

Johnson, K. S. et al. (2007). Semi-automated analysis of retinal vessel diameter in retinopathy of prematurity patients with and without plus disease. *American Journal of Ophthalmology, 143* (4), 723-725 (finding that semi-automated analysis of retinal vessel diameters may be useful in telemedicine screening strategies).

Klaus, M. (2006). Outsourcing vital operations: What if U.S. health care costs drive patients overseas for surgery? *Quinnipiac Health Law Journal, 9,* 219-247.

Lazarus, D. (2004, March 28). Outsourced UCSF notes highlight privacy risk. *San Francisco Chronicle,* p. A1.

___. (2003, October 22). A tough lesson on medical privacy: Pakistani transcriber threatens UCSF over back pay. *San Francisco Chronicle,* p. A1.

Levy, F., & Yu, K. H. (2006). *Offshoring radiology services to India* (Working Paper No. IPC-06-005). Boston, MA: Massachusetts Institute of Technology Industrial Performance Center.

Liu, F. et al. (2006). Aortic valve calcification as an incidental finding at CT of the elderly: Severity and location as predictors of aortic stenosis. *American Journal of Roentgenology, 186* (2), 342-349 (finding telemedicine case management improved glycemic control, blood pressure levels, and total and LDL cholesterol levels).

Mathews, A. W., & Burton, T. M. (2008, March 6). Contaminant is found in heparin batches. *Wall Street Journal,* p. A3.

McGee, P. (2006). Clinical trials on the move: Dropping enrollment for clinical trials in the U.S. and Western Europe has companies looking to countries like India and China as a solution. *Drug Discovery & Development, 9* (6), 16-22.

McLean, T. R. (2007). Shaping a new direction for law and medicine: An international debate on culture, disaster, biotechnology and public health: Telemedicine and the commoditization of medical services. *DePaul Journal of Health Care Law, 10,* 131-175.

McLean, T. R., & Richards, E. P. (2006). Teleradiology: A case study on the economic and legal considerations in international trade in telemedicine. *Health Affairs, 25,* 1378-1385.

McLean, T. R. (2006a). The future of telemedicine and its Faustian reliance on regulatory trade barriers for protection. *Journal of Law & Medicine, 16,* 443-509.

___. (2006b). International law, telemedicine & health insurance: China as a case study. *American Journal of Law & Medicine, 32,* 7-51.

___. (2005). The off-shoring of American medicine: Scope, economic issues and legal liabilities. *Annals of Health Law, 14,* 205-264 (discussing in detail the rationale for the potential outsourcing of virtually all professional medical positions).

Merrell, R. C. (2005). Telemedicine and telesurgery in the operating room. *American College of Surgeons Bulletin, 90* (8), 9-13.

Moshell, R. (2005). And then there was one: The outlook for a self-regulatory U.S. amidst a global trend toward comprehensive data protection. *Texas Technical Law Review, 37* (357), 356-443 (international momentum has swung decidedly toward comprehensive data protection frameworks modeled on the EU's breakthrough effort).

Mueller, J. M. (2007). The tiger awakens: The tumultuous transformation of India's patent system and the rise of Indian pharmaceutical innovation. *University of Pittsburgh Law Review, 68,* 491-641.

NASSCOM (National Association of Software & Service Companies–India) & McKinsey. (2005). *Extending India's leadership in the global IT and BPO industries.* New Delhi, India: NASSCOM & New York, NY: McKinsey (estimating that offshore services will grow to $60 billion by 2010).

NSB (National Science Board). (2008). *Science and engineering indicators* (volume 1, NSB 08-01; volume 2, NSB 08-01A). Arlington, VA: National Science Foundation.

Nyberg, E. M., & Lanzieri, C. F. (2007). American diagnostic radiology moves offshore: Surfing the "Internet wave" to worldwide access and quality. *Journal of Law & Health, 20,* 253-264.

O'Rourke, D. (2003). Outsourcing regulation: Analyzing non-governmental systems of labor standards and monitoring. *Policy Studies Journal, 31,* 1-29.

Pickhardt, P. J. et al. (2003). Computed tomographic virtual colonoscopy to screen for colorectal neoplasia in asymptomatic adults. *New England Journal of Medicine, 349,* 2191-2200 (discussing how some radiologic imaging techniques are equivalent to endoscopic examinations).

Polanyi, M. (2007). *Personal knowledge towards a post-critical philosophy.* London, England: Taylor & Francis (a classic first published in 1958 by a twentieth-century epistemologist who studied how humans acquire and authenticate tacit knowledge).

Range, J. (2008, February 11). Rethinking the India back office, some Western firms weigh selling their units as costs rise, dollar weakens. *Wall Street Journal,* p. A6.

Rashbaum, K. N. (2004). Offshore outsourcing of health data services. *Health Lawyer, 16,* 24-70.

Reid, P. R. et al. (2005). *Building a better delivery system: A new engineering / health care partnership.* Washington, DC: Institute of Medicine & National Academy of Engineering (making the assumption that because systems-engineering tools have been effective in other industries, these tools will be effective in the health care field).

Relman, A. S. (2005). Reforming the U.S. health care system: What the legal and medical professions need to know. *Journal of Law & Medicine, 15* (428), 423-431.

Saver, R. S. (2009). Regulation and reimbursement: At the end of the clinical trial: Does access to investigational technology end as well? *Western New England Law Review, 31,* 411-451.

Singh, K. D. (2003). *Understanding the business of business process outsourcing, in business process outsourcing: Trends and insights,* 56-57. New Delhi, India: Associated Chambers of Commerce & Industry of India.

Sinha, K. (2005, October 23). India to follow US, UK lead on trials. *Times of India.*

Skarda-McCann, J. (2006). Overseas outsourcing of private information & individual remedies for breach of privacy. *Rutgers Computer & Technology Law Journal, 32,* 325-347.

Solomon, J. S. (2004, April 26). Traveling cure: India's new coup in outsourcing: Inpatient care. *Wall Street Journal,* p. A1.

Terry, N. P. (2007). The politics of health law: Under-regulated health care phenomena in a flat world: Medical tourism and outsourcing. *Western New England Law Review, 29,* 421-472.

TES (T-Systems Enterprise Services). (2007). *White paper: Business process outsourcing.* New York, NY: TES (a division of Deutsche Telekom).

Wechsler, J. (2008). Supply chains without borders: International outsourcing carries risks for marketers and regulatory challenges for FDA. *Pharmaceutical Executive,* 28-30.

Weiss, R. M., & Azaran, A. (2007). Outward bound: Considering the business and legal implications of international outsourcing. *Georgetown Journal of International Law, 38* (738), 735-767 (expertise of foreign contractors compares favorably with domestic expertise).

Wharton (Wharton School of the University of Pennsylvania). (2007). Indian BPO firms step out of the back office, toward knowledge process outsourcing and beyond. *Knowledge@Wharton.*

___. (2006). *A brave new world beckons Indian innovators and entrepreneurs.* Knowledge@Wharton.

___. (2005). *Human capital: Can India bridge the knowledge gaps needed for research?* Knowledge@Wharton.

___. (2005a). *How some BPOs seek to build and protect their turf.* Knowledge@Wharton.

___. (2002). *Business processes are moving from the west to other parts of the world.* Knowledge@Wharton.

WHO (World Health Organization). (2004). *Report to India, country report for mode 1: BPO border trade for health services,* 63-65. Washington, DC: WHO.

Winter, J. D. (2008). Is it time to abandon FDA'S no release from liability regulation for clinical studies? *Food & Drug Law Journal, 63,* 525-536.

Wooton, R. et al. (2000). Multicenter randomised control trial comparing real time teledermatology with conventional outpatient dermatological care. *British Medical Journal, 320,* 1252-1256.

Yeun, S. (2008). Exporting trust with data: Audited self-regulation as a solution to cross-border data transfer protection concerns in the offshore outsourcing industry. *Columbia Science & Technology Law Review, 9,* 41-86.

PART VII

PRODUCERS OF MEDICAL PRODUCTS

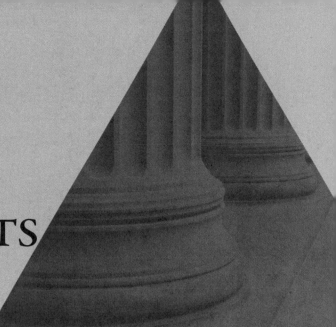

CHAPTER 17

PHARMACEUTICALS

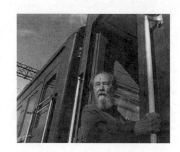

> "It is impossible to stand with only the support of a legalistic structure. A society without any objective legal scale is a terrible one indeed. But a society with no other scale but the legal one is not quite worthy of man either. A society which is based on the letter of the law and never reaches any higher is taking very scarce advantage of the high level of human possibilities."
>
> —ALEXANDER ISAYEVICH SOLZHENITSYN (1918-2008), NOBEL PRIZE IN LITERATURE RECIPIENT

IN BRIEF

While the pharmaceutical industry is frequently criticized by patients, consumer groups, and others for charging high prices, a realistic view of the industry involves the interplay of high risk and long timelines for product development. This chapter focuses on drug pricing and the impact of managed care on regulating drug prices. Particular attention is directed to off-label drug uses, the latent effects of drugs, and the effect of generic competition on the brand-name pharmaceutical industry. No pharmaceutical overview would be complete without looking at the vaccine industry as it garners new interest in response to flu-shot shortages, concerns about global pandemics, and the development of potential vaccines targeted at new ailments, including cancer. Vaccines are an important part of our normal health care system; the rationale as to why vaccines should be covered by insurance and how they effectively reduce costs is explained.

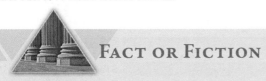

FACT OR FICTION

STATE PRE-EMPTION OF DRUG LABELING

When do drug labeling judgments of the FDA pre-empt state law product liability claims?

Vermont guitarist Diana Levine lost an arm to gangrene after Wyeth's anti-nausea drug Phenergan was inadvertently injected into one of her arteries during an IV-push injection. Levine had gone to a clinic for treatment of a migraine headache.

Levine argued Phenergan's labeling was defective because although it was approved by the FDA, it did not provide proper warnings of the risk of administering the drug through an IV-push injection instead of using an IV-drip. A Vermont jury awarded Levine $6.7 million in damages. The Vermont Supreme Court upheld the award; FDA drug regulations do not prevent a company from being sued under state law over drug labeling.

Wyeth maintained Levine's failure-to-warn claim, which was based on Vermont law, should be pre-empted by federal drug labeling regulations. Wyeth claimed it fully complied with federal labeling law. The FDA knew of the drug's risks and benefits and instructed the company to use labeling that encompassed both. Wyeth maintained federal law prohibited the company from revising the warnings on its product label as the Vermont court required.

—Wyeth v. Levine, 129 S.Ct. 1187 (U.S. Supreme Court 2009).
(See *Law Fact* at the end of this chapter for the answer.)

PRINCIPLES AND APPLICATIONS

The U.S. pharmaceutical industry is maturing and moving away from the growth strategy perfected in the 1990s, a strategy based on blockbuster drugs that generated over a $1 billion in revenue per drug each year. The pace of drug discovery has since slowed amid tougher regulatory scrutiny. At the same time, revenue has declined as blockbuster patents have expired and generic competition has expanded. Together these forces have resulted in an increased urgency to add new lines of business to offset the weak core drug business (*see e.g.*, Rockoff, 2009).

Today, the pharmaceutical industry is rapidly consolidating into more diversified companies, as illustrated in Figure 17-1, becoming less reliant on traditional pharmaceutical research and the attendant unpredictability of drug development. The historical divide between the pharmaceutical and biotechnology sectors is quickly closing. For instance, Pfizer's acquisition of Wyeth added biotechnology drugs, vaccines, and consumer health products to its lineup (Rockoff, 2009). Merck's takeover of Schering-Plough brought biotechnology, consumer health, and animal health care to its ledger. These two multibillion-dollar mergers, along with Roche's purchase of Genentech, a biotechnology stand-alone, are uniting pharmaceuticals with biotechnology.

While the growing convergence of pharmaceutical and biotechnology companies was expected, how the intersection of small-molecule (pharmaceutical) and large-molecule (biotechnology) businesses will play out is still debated within the health care industry (Chang, 2009). In the trade, pharmaceutical drugs are generally referred to as small-molecules and drugs from the biotechnology industry as large-molecules. Drug molecule proteins manufactured in living cells are much larger and more complex than small-molecule drugs produced by synthesizing chemicals. Pharmaceutical companies are looking outside their own laboratories for new drugs and there is significant outsourcing to smaller life science companies to develop medical products. Global pharmaceutical companies are competing intensely for new ideas as a new global paradigm slowly emerges.

Health care investors are pulling back from early-stage investments to focus on compounds that have been proven safe in the short term and are in Phase II studies to determine whether they actually work against targeted diseases. While there is a higher chance of giving up a blockbuster drug, there is greater certainty of the drug being approved and actually making it to market (Wharton, 2006).

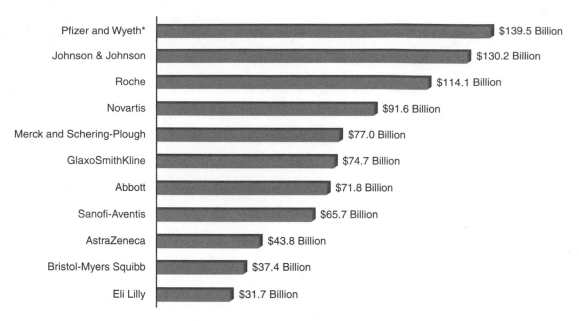

FIGURE 17-1: U.S. Pharmaceutical Industry

Delmar/Cengage Learning
Data retrieved from: 2008 company filings with the U.S. Securities and Exchange Commission; revenue figures are from 2008 corporate annual income statements ended December 31, 2008. *See* Rackoff, J. (2009, March 10). Merck to buy rival for $41 billon: Schering-Plough deal is latest bid to diversify: Roche nears Genentech takeover. *Wall Street Journal*, p. A1.

Government and Pharmaceutical Industry Funding	Pharmaceutical Industry Funding				Government & Insurance Industry Funding				
Academic Research	Basic Research & Drug Discovery	Drug Development	Clinical Trials	Manufacturing, Quality Assurance, & Quality Control	Sales, Marketing, & Distribution	Screening & Diagnostics	Medicines & Medical Treatment	Point of Care Administration	Reimbursement for Medicines & Medical Treatment

FIGURE 17-2: View of the Pharmaceutical Market

Delmar/Cengage Learning

OVERVIEW OF THE PHARMACEUTICAL MARKET

The pharmaceutical industry has traditionally been research driven. According to the Congressional Budget Office, the pharmaceutical industry is one of the most research-intensive industries in the U.S., investing five times as much in research and development relative to sales than the average U.S. manufacturing firm (CBO, 2006). Domestic research and development spending by both pharmaceutical and biotechnology companies equaled roughly $65,000 per direct employee in 2006, or about eight times the published estimates of research and development spending per employee in all manufacturing industries (Burns, 2009).

The key segments in the pharmaceutical industry's landscape are often misunderstood: from the basic academic research that builds understanding of human biological processes to treat diseases and illnesses through drug discovery, development, clinical trials, manufacturing, sales and marketing, and distribution. Figure 17-2 provides an overview of this pharmaceutical market.

Academic and Basic Research (Three to Six Years)

Drug discovery is the result of laboratory collaboration between the global pharmaceutical industry, small drug companies, the nations' academic research groups, and the National Institutes of Health (PhRMA, 2007). Scientists work to understand the disease to be treated and the underlying cause of the condition. They try to understand how the genes are altered, how alterations affect the proteins they encode, how those proteins interact with each other in the cells, how those affected cells affect the specific tissue they are in, and finally how the affected tissue affects individual patients (PhRMA, 2007). NIH and the pharmaceutical industry are the major sources of funding for this basic research.

Drug Discovery and Development (Ten to Fifteen Years)

For the first time in history, scientists are beginning to understand the inner workings of human disease at the molecular level. Recent advances in genomics, proteomics, and computational power present new ways to understand illness. The task of discovering and developing safe, effective drugs is even more promising as knowledge of disease increases (PhRMA, 2007).

As illustrated in Figure 17-3, it can take fifteen years to develop one new drug from the time of the initial drug discovery to the point of care where it is administered to patients. Hundreds of people are engaged in this process; depending on the complexity of the drug, as many as two thousand can be involved. Many of the new drugs coming to market in 2009 were in the early stages of discovery in 1994. In 1994, President Bill Clinton delivered his first State of the Union address calling for health care reform, the first summit was held to discuss the Internet, George W. Bush was

elected governor of Texas, and the first version of the Netscape web browser was released. The average cost to discover and develop each successful new drug is now between $800 million and $1 billion. This number includes the costs of thousands of failures. For every five thousand to ten thousand compounds entering the drug discovery pipeline, one new drug product receives FDA approval (PhRMA, 2007).

Clinical Trials (Six to Seven Years)

The drug candidate then goes into clinical trials in humans, where the drug must be proven to be safe and effective before the FDA will approve it. This process involves a series of trials, each with its own clinical goals and regulatory requirements. Physicians carry out each trial with patients in hospitals, offices, and clinics, in coordination with the sponsoring pharmaceutical company.

Before any clinical trials can begin, an Investigational New Drug (IND) Application must be filed with the FDA. The IND includes the results of the pre-clinical work, the drug candidate's chemical structure, how it is thought to work in the body, a listing of any anticipated side effects, and how it is to be manufactured. The IND also provides a detailed clinical trial plan outlining how, where, and by whom the clinical trial will be performed. The approved IND grants authority for the medication's sponsor to ship this unapproved medicine in interstate commerce for clinical testing.

In addition to the IND, all clinical trials must be reviewed by the Institutional Review Board (IRB) at each institution where the trials are to take place. Throughout the clinical trial process, the sponsoring pharmaceutical company must provide information to the FDA and the IRBs about how the trials are progressing.

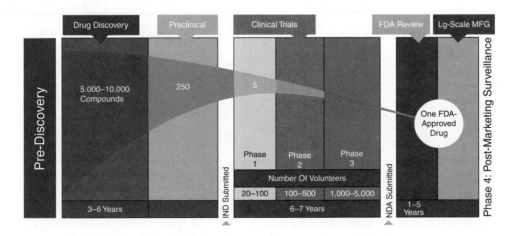

FIGURE 17-3: Drug Discovery and Development

Delmar/Cengage Learning

Data retrieved from: Pharmaceutical Research and Manufacturers of America. (2007). *Drug discovery and development: Understanding the R&D process*. Washington, DC: PhRMA.

New Drug Application and Approval (One-half to Two Years)

Once the clinical trials are complete, the sponsoring pharmaceutical company reviews all the data. If the company decides the drug candidate is both safe and effective, it prepares and files a new drug application (NDA) requesting FDA approval to market the drug. The NDA describes the decade of testing and generally runs one hundred thousand pages or more. The NDA is reviewed by the FDA and independent advisory committees of experts appointed by the FDA, who then decide under what market conditions the drug should be approved. The FDA is not required to accept the recommendations of the advisory committee, but it generally does.

Drug Manufacturing

Going from small-scale manufacturing of supplies for clinical testing to large-scale manufacturing for the public market is a major undertaking. In many cases, a new manufacturing site must be constructed because the manufacturing process is different from drug to drug. Moreover, each manufacturing facility must meet strict Current Good Manufacturing Practices (CGMP) standards. Drug manufacturing is not only one of the most highly skilled forms of manufacturing, but it is also one of the most regulated (PhRMA, 2007).

Ongoing Research and Monitoring

Even after a drug is approved for marketing, ongoing research and monitoring of the drug continues.

Pharmaceutical companies must continuously monitor the usage of their drugs and report adverse events to the FDA. In addition, the FDA may require the company to conduct Phase IV studies to determine long-term safety or how the drug affects specific subpopulations. The dramatic increase in research and development expenditures by the pharmaceutical and biotechnology industry is illustrated in Figure 17-4.

GLOBAL PRICING OF DRUGS

Global drug pricing is a complex process lacking a clear, simple explanation (Reinhardt, 2004). In most discussions about the cost of drugs, three parts of the cost equation are left out of the equation:

- Cost of disease and illness
- Economic benefits of improved health
- Global complexity of drug pricing

Cost of Disease and Illness

The cost of disease and illness includes the cost of drugs, hospitalizations, physician visits, physical therapies, and surgeries (PhRMA, 2007). When a drug can significantly reduce or eliminate these other costs, that reduction is a factor in determining the price of the drug, especially when the drug can permanently cure or alleviate previously fatal or debilitating conditions. As illustrated in Figure 17-5, if patients adhered to their recommended drug regimes, the savings to the health care system could

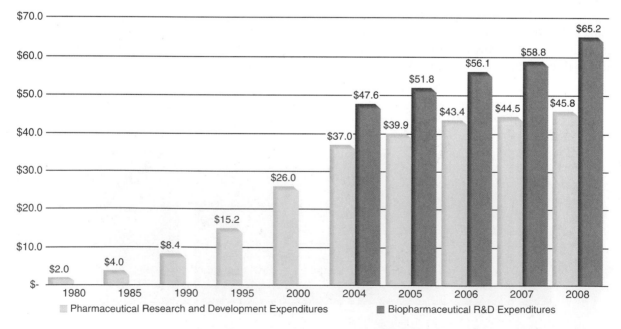

FIGURE 17-4: Pharmaceutical Expenditures on Research and Development (in Billions $)

Delmar/Cengage Learning

Data retrieved from: Burrill & Company. (2008). Analysis for Pharmaceutical Research & Manufacturers of America. Washington, DC: PhRMA; Pharmaceutical Research & Manufacturers of America. (2008). *PhRMA annual member survey.* Washington, DC: PhRMA.

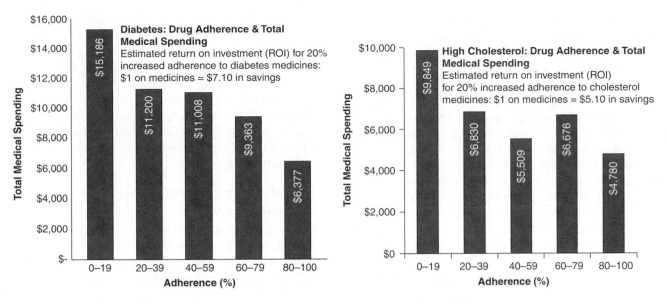

FIGURE 17-5: Greater Adherence to Drug Regimes Decreases Total Health Care Costs

Delmar/Cengage Learning

Data retrieved from: Sokol, M. C. et al. (2005). Impact of medication adherence on hospitalization risk and healthcare costs. *Medical Care, 43* (6), 523–530.

be dramatic. For instance, for every dollar spent on diabetes drugs, $7.10 is saved on health care costs; for cholesterol drugs, there is $5.10 in savings (Sokol et al., 2005). It is noteworthy that the cost of ingredients on production can be a very minor contribution to total product cost (akin to women's high-fashion shoes).

Economic Benefits of Improved Health

Drugs are increasingly priced to reflect economic benefits to individual patients. This includes making economic calculations as to how much money a drug saves when it prevents a patient from having surgery, or the economic benefit of allowing a patient to continue working when, without the drug, employment would not have been possible.

The key measure used to assess the marginal value of a drug for different patient groups is generally the additional cost per quality-adjusted life-year (QALY) gained (Wharton, 2006). If appropriate data on quality of life is unavailable, cost-effectiveness is estimated using alternatives such as cost per life-year gained (*see generally* Henry et al., 2005; Rawlins et al., 2005). At the same time, the industry considers:

• The degree of uncertainty surrounding these price estimates
• Particular features of the medical condition
• Innovative nature of the drug
• Where appropriate, the wider societal costs and benefits

(Rawlins & Culyer, 2004; Reinhardt, 2004)

Global Complexity of Drug Pricing

Nearly everyone wants lowered drug prices, but no one (including the health care industry) knows how

to deliver them while maintaining resources for future innovative research and development. This quandary is due to the multitude of factors influencing global pricing decisions:

• Competing stakeholders' interests between developed and developing nations
• Complex regulatory policies that differ by country and have contradictory pricing goals
• Costs of global research and development
• Economic objectives behind drug pricing in negotiation and management of price decisions by insurers and governments worldwide
• Desire to donate drugs for the uninsured and patients in the lower economic pyramid, both in the U.S. and globally
• Social welfare differences between higher-income and lower-income patient communities

Facing a situation where costs to market drugs to physicians and the public are increasing enormously while company laboratories are having trouble developing new blockbuster drugs to drive revenue, something will have to give. Almost everyone within the industry agrees the blockbuster model of drug development has to go, as its costs have become astronomical (*see* Epstein, 2008). While some companies operate as if they were in a growth industry, delivering 10 or 12 percent growth per year, pharmaceuticals is now a mature global industry focused on product quality and innovative product improvement (Vagelos & Galambos, 2004).

Correlation Between Global Drug Prices and International Per Capita Incomes

In general, global drug price differences correlate with per capita income differences between countries. This is a critical fact to consider when high drug prices in the U.S. are criticized. Pricing occurs on a global basis and the gross domestic product (GDP) purchasing power parity per capita of the U.S. in relationship to the rest of the world is five times higher. As illustrated in Figure 17-6, GDP purchasing power parities standardize cost-of-living differences worldwide.

While the ability to pay higher drug prices is about five times greater for Americans compared to other citizens in the world, drug prices in the U.S. are generally 6 to 33 percent higher than in other countries. In terms of global fairness and equity, it could be argued Americans should be paying higher prices for their drugs, given their comparable wealth. For instance, the average income for Americans is $48,000 according to the International Monetary Fund, compared to $10,500 for most non-Americans. Therefore, by way of illustration, a $10.00 tablet in the U.S. should cost $2.00 in the rest of the world, or five times less.

At the same time, the use of generic drugs is higher in the U.S., and prices for these are lower (Danzon, 2005). Further, the differences in drug pricing are not as significant when exchange rates and gross domestic product rates are being considered. Even if per capita income is used as the basis for comparison, price differences as they relate to income are relatively proportionate globally (Danzon, 2005). In summary, drug pricing is complex, in part because of the need to balance the interests of industry innovation with public need and entitlement.

Two Policy Proposals: Drug Pricing

Differential Pricing System

One possible solution to high drug prices in the U.S. is to adopt the European differential pricing system. Under this system, developed countries help underwrite the cost of drug research and development, and developing countries help pay for the costs associated with manufacturing the drugs.

This system also supports global patent protection so brand-name drugs can receive premium pricing in order to help fund innovative drug development. Lastly, this system aims to control global spillover, which occurs when low-priced drugs gain entry back into high-priced markets, thereby reducing

Country	Rank	IMF	Rank	WB	Rank	CIA
Brunei	6	$54,100	N/A	N/A	5	$50,596
Canada	15	$40,200	12	$35,729	13	$39,339
Kuwait	4	$60,800	N/A	N/A	9	$40,943
Liechtenstein	1	$118,000	N/A	N/A	N/A	N/A
Luxembourg	3	$851,000	1	$78,985	2	$81,730
Mexico	64	$14,400	50	$12,780	57	$14,582
Norway	5	$55,750	2	$53,334	3	$55,199
Qatar	2	$101,000	N/A	N/A	1	$86,670
Singapore	7	$52,900	3	$50,299	4	$51,649
United States	8	$48,000	4	$45,790	6	$47,025
World		**$10,500**		**$9,900**		**$10,539**

FIGURE 17-6: Countries' Gross Domestic Purchasing Power Parity per Capita

Note: GDP at purchasing power parity ("PPP") per capita is the value of all final goods and services produced within a country in 2008 divided by the average population for 2008. The CIA (Central Intelligence Agency) and the two international organizations that oversees the global financial system, the IMF (International Monetary Fund) and the Word Bank, calculate gross domestic purchasing power parity differently.
Delmar/Cengage Learning
Data retrieved from: IMF. (2008). *World economic outlook database*. Washington, DC: IMF; Word Bank. (2007). *World development indicators database*. Washington, DC: World Bank per CIA (2008). *The world fact book*. Washington, DC: CIA.

demand and prices in those markets. Advantages of a differential pricing system include:

- Efficient use of existing drugs by market forces
- No harm to consumers of health care in developed, high-income markets
- Allows drug consumption at marginal cost

Further, this system opens markets; developing countries are better off while developed countries are no worse off. This is not a cost-shifting scheme, as the cost of research and development would be a joint cost, not attributable to a single country. If developing countries pay any portion of the manufacturing costs, then it is possible that drug prices will be lower in the U.S.

One-Price Policy for Drugs

The other policy proposal is for the pharmaceutical industry to adopt a one-price policy when selling drugs in different countries, a strategy that would neutralize the debate over drug imports and also would spread out the costs of research more evenly across consumers in different countries (Vagelos & Galambos, 2004). Achieving a one-price policy would be difficult (Wilson, 2004). With companies bringing similar drugs to market, the pharmaceutical industry would have to compete on price, something it has not done traditionally; as a result, prices would decrease.

Re-importation and Secure Global Supply Chains

In an effort to work with the pharmaceutical industry in systematically improving global production and distribution efficiencies, the FDA recently initiated a voluntary pilot program to promote the safety of drugs and active pharmaceutical ingredients produced outside the U.S. To qualify, companies need to maintain control over their drug products from the time of manufacture through entry into the U.S.

The goal is to develop secure global supply chains. Such a program would assist the agency in its efforts to prevent the importation of drugs not in compliance with applicable FDA requirements; this would allow the agency to focus its resources on foreign-produced drugs that may not be compliant. A secure global supply chain will also help mitigate risks such as contamination and counterfeiting (FDA, 2009).

MARKET CHANGES: COST MANAGEMENT

Managed care (or more accurately, cost management) has affected the pharmaceutical industry in several ways; some but not all of which improve the quality of health care. Moreover, these market changes exacerbate three issues relating to FDA regulation of the industry:

- Managed care forces that focus on reducing costs while seeking improvements in the effectiveness of drugs
- Managed care has come to function as the intermediary between physicians who actually prescribe drugs and the pharmaceutical industry by screening drugs for placement on drug formularies
- Impact of increasing cost pressures on a maturing industry

(Epstein, 2008)

It has been argued that cost management has induced the pharmaceutical industry to curtail its research and development of new drugs. Regardless of the merits of this contention, managed care has considerable leverage to negotiate drug prices, and indeed, pharmaceutical companies now directly market their drug products to managed care organizations (MCOs).

Some of the two areas most affected by managed care are the use of:

- Cost-effectiveness data
- Off-label use promotion

"New" Targets of Promotional Information

Unlike physicians who seek information in order to prescribe specific drugs, MCOs and the government seek information in order to make cost-benefit trade-offs between different drugs. The pharmaceutical industry caters to this need for information, creating at least two issues for the FDA:

- Pharmacoeconomics as a tool to manage drug costs
- Information provided to the MCOs about off-label uses

Pharmacoeconomics

Pharmacoeconomics is the study of the relative cost-effectiveness of treatments. MCOs use such studies to create their drug formularies. The primary benefit is economic; pharmacoeconomics helps lower health care costs by helping to select the least expensive, but still effective, drugs for placement on formularies.

The pharmaceutical industry may provide pharmacoeconomic information about drug products to formulary committees, MCOs, and similar large-scale buyers of health care products. The law, however, does not permit the dissemination of pharmacoeconomic information that could affect prescribing choices to individual prescribers.

While the law is intended to provide MCOs with dependable facts about the economic consequences of their procurement decisions, the pharmaceutical industry uses pharmacoeconomic studies as marketing devices to promote specific drugs. Because the FDA has the power to regulate advertising and marketing, it needs to determine whether it is wise to review these cost-effectiveness claims with the same rigorous validation procedures it uses for claims of safety and effectiveness in drug marketing, labeling, and advertising (*see* 21 U.S.C.A. § 331(a), (d), and (k) (2007)).

Off-Label Drug Use

The FDA has taken the position that if off-label use must occur, then it should be limited to the confines of individualized treatments requested by a physician. MCOs have an interest in off-label uses in order to create formularies and guidelines that constrain costs and limit physicians' treatment decisions (Garrett & Garis, 2007). However, an MCO's formulary decisions are usually made in advance, creating a problem when a potential use is unapproved and the MCO cannot gain access to information to evaluate that use. MCOs request information months ahead of actual availability about a then-unapproved drug in order to create formularies for the next one to two years.

The learned intermediary doctrine imposes an obligation on pharmaceutical companies to warn physicians of foreseeable risks associated with the use of its drugs (Restatement § 6(d)(1), 1998). The justification for this doctrine is that physicians are in a better position to supply patients with information about the drugs, and to warn them of the risks appropriate for the patient's individual circumstances so the patient is in the best position to make an informed decision regarding treatment. In prescription drug cases involving the learned intermediary doctrine, when a warning specifically mentions the circumstances complained of, the warning is generally considered adequate as a matter of law (Cook, 2007).

While any advertising of off-label uses directed to patients is prohibited, peer-reviewed journal articles about an off-label use of drugs may be disseminated, provided the company commits itself to file, within a specified time frame, a supplemental FDA application based on appropriate research to establish the safety and effectiveness of the unapproved use. The primary assumption is MCOs and physicians can view such information critically, but this does not hold true for patients. How the FDA should protect health care consumers in off-label use of drugs is an issue of continued debate.

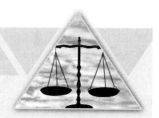

PRODUCTS LIABILITY FOR OFF-LABEL DRUG USE

McNeil v. Wyeth

[Patient v. Pharmaceutical Company]

462 F.3d 364 (U.S. Court of Appeals for the 5th Circuit 2006)

FACTS: Sue McNeil claimed Wyeth did not adequately warn physicians of the increased risk of tardive dyskinesia (TD), a severe neurological disorder, associated with long-term use of Reglan, a drug manufactured by Wyeth to treat gastroesophageal reflux disease (GERD). Dr. Eduardo Wilkinson, McNeil's primary physician, prescribed Reglan to treat symptoms related to McNeil's GERD. Reglan's labeling warned the drug could produce TD.[LN1]

Dr. Wilkinson gave McNeil a six-month prescription of Reglan, even though the FDA only approved Reglan's use for three months. Two additional physicians subsequently renewed McNeil's prescription for a total of eight additional months. After taking Reglan for fourteen months, McNeil went to an emergency room complaining of shortness of breath and an involuntary chewing motion of her mouth. The emergency room physician diagnosed her with extrapyramidal symptoms (EPS), which he believed was likely caused by her long-term exposure to Reglan. Dr. Wilkinson confirmed the EPS diagnosis, and discontinued her use of Reglan. When her EPS symptoms failed to improve, she consulted a neurologist and two physicians specializing in movement disorders. All three specialists diagnosed McNeil with Reglan-induced TD and Reglan-induced EPS, confirming Reglan was the cause of her condition.

McNeil sued Wyeth in state court, claiming Wyeth failed to provide adequate warnings to physicians and consumers of the increased risk of TD associated with the long-term use of Reglan.

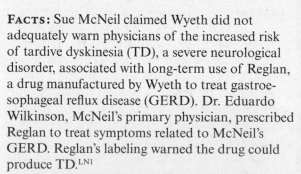
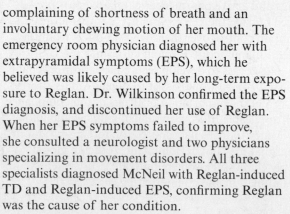

(continues)

(continued)

Wyeth maintained Reglan's labeling sufficiently warned of the dangers of Reglan.

ISSUE: Does understating the risk of side effects render drug labels misleading and ineffective?

HOLDING AND DECISION: Yes, when there is a warning of a much lower risk than the actual risk, the warning label is misleading and ineffective; drug labels should explain the higher risks of developing side effects from long-term use of a drug.

ANALYSIS: The Fifth Circuit distinguished the case from other cases based on the learned intermediary doctrine; McNeil did not claim the warning was inadequate because her condition was not mentioned, but rather that the warning was misleading as to the level of risk associated with developing the condition. The court found that warning a learned intermediary, such as Dr. Wilkinson, of a much lower risk than the actual risk of developing a condition renders a warning both misleading and ineffective.

Wyeth maintained it did not have a duty to warn about risks related to using Reglan beyond a period of three months because Reglan's labeling stated it was not intended for use over longer periods. The court, however, disagreed with Wyeth's argument, finding Reglan was routinely prescribed for long-term use. Wyeth's own marketing data indicated most patients were using Reglan for periods beyond the recommended three months. In addition, medical journals drew attention to the common use of Reglan as a long-term treatment. Because of the widespread use of Reglan for more than three months, a jury could infer the warning was ineffective and inadequate.

While Wyeth claimed it was not required to update its label because studies indicating the risk of developing TD due to long-term use of Reglan merely demonstrated an association between the two, without actually showing causation, FDA regulations require drug labels to be revised to include a warning as soon as there is reasonable evidence of an association of a serious hazard with a drug; a causal relationship need not be proved. Furthermore, Wyeth was not relieved of this duty to warn solely because no clinical trials proved actual causation. The pharmaceutical industry frequently warns physicians certain drug use is not recommended even if clinical trials do not confirm risk or causation.

The court further found it was a question of fact for the jury to determine whether Wyeth should have warned physicians of the risks of the long-term use of Reglan. The side effects of EPS and TD are highly predictable for drugs, such as Reglan, that block dopamine receptors. Thus, the court found there was a genuine issue of fact concerning whether Reglan's labeling was adequate. Wyeth failed to warn that the risk of developing TD increased significantly with long-term use.

Finally, the court found there was a genuine issue of material fact as to whether the label's inadequate information caused Dr. Wilkinson to prescribe the drug to McNeil. If an adequately informed learned intermediary would have adequately informed a patient of the risks of a disease had a label been sufficient, but failed to do so because of the lack of information provided on the label, and if the patient would have rejected the drug if informed, then an inadequate label could be considered to have produced the injury. The rationale for this rule is that the ineffective label essentially defeats the purpose behind the learned intermediary doctrine. Thus, because Dr. Wilkinson gave conflicting testimony concerning whether he would have prescribed the drug had he known of the significant risks, the court concluded that this was an issue of fact for the jury to decide.

On the issue of whether the label was clearly misleading, the Fifth Circuit held there were enough arguments on either side that the issue should be decided by a trial court. Furthermore, there was a genuine issue concerning whether, had the warning label accurately conveyed the level of risk involved, McNeil's physician would have nevertheless prescribed the drug.

RULE OF LAW: Drug labels may be misleading, even without evidence proving a causal relationship connecting long-term use with the serious side effect; all that needs to be shown is some association between long-term use and increased risk for the alleged side effect.

(See generally Cook, 2007; Reiss et al., 2007).

The *Wyeth* case suggests the pharmaceutical industry may be held liable for warnings of a much lower risk than the actual risk of developing side effects from their drugs if:

- Use beyond the package insert is widespread
- Pharmaceutical company knows, or should know, of the common off-label use of its drugs

In light of this decision, the pharmaceutical industry may need to update its warnings to address these risks, even if the risks are only merely associated with the drug and causation has not been definitively proven (Cook, 2007).

Pharmaceutical Benefit Managers

Pharmaceutical benefit managers (PBMs) also directly affect the provision of health care. PBMs administer and process drug benefits claims, and are often electronically linked to the community pharmacies participating in their programs. PBMs also seek to lower managed care costs by restricting patient choices of drugs to cheaper generics or to preferred brands; often these substitutions rely on formularies chosen by the MCO to reduce drug costs (Garrett & Garis, 2007).

More often than not, PBMs seek to actively encourage physicians to alter prescription patterns within the same therapeutic class. Furthermore, many MCOs use PBMs to educate individual professionals and patients about drugs. Thus, in some instances, a PBM may offer services that fall within a traditional definition of health care provision rather than just cost management. Disease management programs deepen these concerns because they provide information on dosage and choices available to patients. Although such substitutions based on price may seem health-neutral, consider the effect pharmacoeconomic data could have: instead of merely trading price, if the PBM trades price for quality, then more than just the cost of health care is being affected (*see generally* Garrett & Garis, 2007).

EXPOSURE GAME

For years, the traditional requirements needed to prove consumers were injured by drugs created insurmountable obstacles to recovery from the pharmaceutical industry. Generally, four elements must be proven in any tort (civil wrong) lawsuit:

- Duty: consumers must show the companies owed them a duty
- Breach of duty: the companies breached that duty
- Causation: the breach of duty caused personal injury to consumers

- Damages: proven with a reasonable degree of certainty

As between injured health care consumers and the pharmaceutical industry, the task of tort law is to determine who should bear the loss. Tort law protects individual autonomy by compensating victims for intrusions of their bodily integrity (Weeks, 2007). The law also enforces standards of conduct. When pharmaceutical companies market drugs that unreasonably endanger the safety of consumers, they must pay for the harms they inflict. However, the goal of tort law extends beyond compensation; optimal drug safety does not mean perfect drug safety, but instead seeks to balance the risks and benefits of drugs against the individual consumer's interest in being effectively treated for a medical condition (*see* Weeks, 2007).

Causation Requirement

The burden of proof required to show causation is fourfold:

- Consumers were exposed to the drug
- General causation: drug was capable of causing the injury complained of
- Specific causation: drug actually caused the injury
- The particular pharmaceutical company was responsible for manufacturing the drug that caused the injury

(Restatement § 15, 1998)

Proving general causation involves introducing statistical evidence comparing the incidence of an injury in the general population and the incidence of the injury in the patient population exposed to the drug. Proving specific causation involves testimony that the drug in question was produced by the pharmaceutical company and probably caused the injury. Both of these proof requirements involve scientific and statistical evidence, the admissibility of which can be controversial (Cohen, 2005).

The standard for admitting scientific evidence in courts is a two-part test, known as the Daubert principle:

- Whether testimony conveys scientific knowledge grounded in the methods and procedures of science and is more than subjective belief or unsupported speculation
- Whether it is relevant

Daubert v. Merrell Dow Pharmaceuticals, Inc., 509 U.S. 579 (U.S. Supreme Court 1993)[LN2]

The legal standard for admissibility remains high because of the standards the scientific community imposes on itself. In science, a hypothesis is never proven. It is either rejected or not rejected with a certain degree of certainty. The degree of certainty is generally 95 percent, a difficult standard to meet because of scientific uncertainty and because of the limited data available. Where statistical analysis is performed and a mean and standard deviation are calculated, the 95 percent confidence interval is a range from the mean minus the standard deviation to the mean plus the standard deviation. This means there is 95 percent confidence that a value will be in that range. Because the burden of proof is on the injured consumer, these difficulties work in favor, in theory at least, of the pharmaceutical industry (Cohen, 2005).

Vioxx was part a new class of anti-arthritis drugs called COX-2 blockers. Unlike traditional anti-arthritis drugs (non-steroidal anti-inflammatory drugs), COX-2 blockers selectively targeted the COX-2 enzyme (bad enzyme) without affecting the function of the COX-1 enzyme (good enzyme). As a result, COX-2 blockers reduced symptoms o0f arthritis with minimal side effects. In the first Vioxx jury trial in Texas, however, the lack of scientific evidence of causation was not an obstacle to a multimillion-dollar damage award. The case turned on juror impressions of Merck's corporate behavior. Jurors reportedly believed Merck had marketed a drug it knew to be dangerous, and this belief overcame the causation requirement. This jury decision was, nevertheless, subsequently overturned in the following decision.

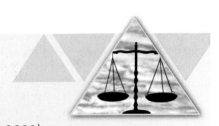

EVIDENCE OF CAUSATION

Ernst v. Merck & Co., Inc.

[Widow v. Pharmaceutical Company]

2009 WL 1677857 (Court of Appeals of Texas, 14th District, Houston 2009)

FACTS: Robert Ernst, a marathon runner, fitness trainer, and manager for a Texas Wal-Mart, died of a cardiac arrhythmia and atherosclerosis after taking Vioxx for seven months. In her lawsuit against Merck, his wife, Carol Ernst, alleged negligent failure to warn of the dangers associated with the drug and civil conspiracy to conceal the danger. By the time the case went to trial, it was one of about 4,200 Vioxx lawsuits nationwide.

Right before the Ernst trial was scheduled to begin, Texas filed widely publicized charges against Merck for falsely advertising the safety of Vioxx and defrauding the state Medicaid program. *See Texas v. Merck & Co., Inc.*, 385 F.Supp.2d 604 (U.S. District Court for the Western District of Texas, Austin Division 2005). Although Merck filed for a continuance, claiming the publicity prejudiced any possible jury member and prevented a fair trial, the Ernst trial proceeded in an untraditional way.

The jurors awarded Ernst $253.4 million, $229 million of which was punitive damages. Ernst had asked for $40 million. This appeal followed, in which Merck claimed the causation requirement was not met.

ISSUE: Was Ernst's death caused by a blood clot triggered by Vioxx?

HOLDING AND DECISION: No, there was no competent and legally sufficient evidence on the issue of causation and the existence of a blood clot, therefore, Ernst could not collect any damages.

ANALYSIS: The Ernst trial was not a causation case about heart attacks and strokes being increased by the use of Vioxx; it evolved around corporate accountability. While Ernst had to establish to a reasonable degree of medical certainty that Vioxx probably (not possibly) caused her husband's fatal cardiac arrhythmia, causation was not an issue for this Texas jury.

Following this overturned trial verdict, Merck attempted to refute evidence it knew Vioxx to be dangerous. In doing so, Merck acknowledged the battleground was the morality of Merck's actions, not the legal validity of the injury claims. The issue shifted toward whether Merck knowingly

(continues)

(continued)

marketed a dangerous drug and away from the evidence of causation. No reliable scientific evidence demonstrated Vioxx caused cardiac arrhythmias and no epidemiological study with a placebo demonstrated a statistically significant effect from Vioxx taken for less than eighteen months.

RULE OF LAW: Legally sufficient evidence of causation must be presented in order for damages to be awarded in a personal injury and wrongful death lawsuit against a drug manufacturer; testifying experts may not simply speculate as to whether a drug caused an injury.

(*See* Cohen, 2005).

Doctrine of *Res Ipsa Loquitor*

In most pharmaceutical cases, the central issue is proof of causation, because the standard for admissibility of scientific evidence can be very high and such evidence is expensive and often unavailable (Restatement § 6, 1998). In some lawsuits against the pharmaceutical industry, however, the requirements of causation can be relaxed, such as when an injury is of a type that does not occur except as a result of negligence, using the doctrine of *res ipsa loquitor*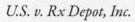

(Restatement § 328D comment (a), 1965). In these situations, the occurrence of an injury is enough to infer both negligence and causation.

Latent Effects from Approved Drugs

The number of successful lawsuits over latent effects from FDA-approved medicines might indicate the research required by regulation is often not enough to assess all of the harmful effects of a drug (Cohen, 2005).

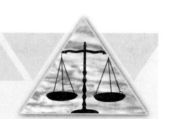

RESTITUTION UNDER THE FOOD, DRUG AND COSMETIC ACT

U.S. v. Rx Depot, Inc.

[Federal Government v. Re-Importer]

438 F.3d 1052 (U.S. Court of Appeals for the 10th Circuit 2006),

U.S. Supreme Court certiorari denied, 549 U.S. 817 (U.S. Supreme Court 2006)

FACTS: Rx Depot helped U.S. patients obtain reduced-priced prescription drugs from Canada by acting as the middleman in a re-importation scheme. Customers gave Rx Depot information about their prescriptions from American physicians. Rx Depot then transmitted information to cooperating Canadian physicians and pharmacies. Once Canadian physicians rewrote the American prescriptions, Canadian pharmacies dispensed these prescriptions and sent them directly to patients in the U.S.

The federal government filed a lawsuit against Rx Depot claiming the company violated the federal Food, Drug and Cosmetic Act (FDCA) by re-importing prescription drugs originally manufactured in the U.S. and

introducing new drugs into interstate commerce without approval. *See* 21 U.S.C.A. §§ 301 *et seq.* (2009). The parties subsequently agreed to a consent decree, which confirmed Rx Depot violated the FDCA and prevented the company from resuming business operations. The consent decree, however, left it to the courts to determine what equitable relief to award the federal government.

ISSUE: Does the FDCA permit courts to order restitution for violations?

HOLDING AND DECISION: Yes, courts may order violators of the FDCA to pay restitution to the federal government.

(continues)

(continued)

ANALYSIS: The Tenth Circuit analyzed whether courts may order restitution when a federal law invokes equity jurisdiction, and determined that courts may use all equitable powers available to exercise jurisdiction unless the law restricts the form of equitable relief by clear and valid legislative command or necessary and inescapable inference.

Because restitution is a traditional equitable remedy, courts are permitted to grant restitution unless the:

- FDCA contains clear legislative language preventing courts from ordering restitution
- Purposes of the FDCA are inconsistent with granting restitution

Additionally, cases involving the public interest provide courts with broader and more flexible equitable powers. Since the U.S. brought this case to protect public health and safety, the court has broader and more flexible equitable powers.

Rx Depot maintained language within the FDCA implies only forward-looking remedies are available (21 U.S.C.A. § 332(a) (1993)). The U.S. Supreme Court has, however, declined to determine whether laws similar to the FDCA's language permit courts to order restitution. The court therefore found the FDCA's language does not prohibit courts from ordering restitution.

Rx Depot also asserted that since the FDCA expressly authorizes certain remedies, a court should be reluctant to infer additional remedies. Congress, however, authorized courts to provide all traditional equitable remedies when it granted courts general equity jurisdiction under the FDCA. Additionally, express remedies do not limit courts to providing only these remedies listed in the FDCA. The FDCA's express authorization of certain remedies does not prohibit courts from ordering equitable remedies not listed in the FDCA.

Additionally, Rx Depot claimed that since the FDCA specifically authorizes restitution for certain medical devices, Congress did not intend to allow restitution under other FDCA provisions. Restitution refers to the return of unlawful gains, in this case whatever profits Rx Depot obtained as a result of its re-importation activities, also referred to as disgorgement (Garner, 2009). The restitution the FDCA specifies refers to powers the FDA has to order restitution payments, powers that are not limited to the equitable powers the FDCA grants to courts.

Finally, Rx Depot argued the FDCA's legislative history prohibits courts from ordering restitution because Congress intended for seizure to be the harshest remedy available. This argument fails, however, because seizures can be harsher than restitution. For instance, the FDCA permits seizures based on the FDA's request to a court upon a showing of reasonable belief that a party is in violation of the FDCA, without hearing from the party, while a court can only order restitution after a party is found to be in violation of the FDCA. In addition, seizures under the FDCA deprive a company of its capital investment and potential profit, while restitution only deprives a company of its profits. Therefore, the court held the FDCA permits restitution when it furthers the purposes of the FDCA, because the FDCA does not contain a clear legislative command or compel a necessary and inescapable inference precluding restitution.

RULE OF LAW: Courts can order restitution because the FDCA invokes general equity jurisdiction and does not contain a clear legislative command prohibiting restitution.

(See generally Barth, 2006; Hall & Berlin, 2006; Hall & Sobotka, 2007; Noah, 2008; Pyle, 2006).

FDA PREEMPTION

Pain Management

Controlled substances can be used for legitimate medical purposes to relieve pain and suffering and allow management of medical and surgical conditions, whether acute or chronic in duration. However, because opiate analgesics to treat chronic pains are attractive, addicting drugs, diversion from physicians and pharmacists can lead to serious health problems (Miller, 2006). Consequently, the public has a vested interest in protecting the medical uses of pain management drugs, while reducing the morbidity and mortality from their misuse (Miller, 2006).

Of concern is the level of increased federal and state criminal investigations and prosecutions of physicians for their prescribing practices. There has been substantial regulatory policy development to address this issue, with medical boards adopting regulations, guidelines, and policy statements to provide guidance to licensees about using opioids to treat pain (Gilson, 2007).

STATE PREEMPTION: MEDICAL MARIJUANA

Gonzales v. Raich

[Federal Government v. Patient]

545 U.S. 1 (U.S. Supreme Court 2005),

affirmed on remand, 500 F.3d 850 (U.S. Court of Appeals for the 9th Circuit 2007)

FACTS: Angel Raich has been using marijuana every two hours, every day for more than eight years to control the symptoms of a number of painful conditions, including an inoperable brain tumor, endometriosis, scoliosis, uterine fibroid tumors, and life-threatening weight loss. Raich had tried thirty-five other medications to control her symptoms without success before turning to marijuana. Diane Monson used marijuana to alleviate severe back pain and spasms resulting from a degenerative disease of the spine. Their marijuana use is legal under California's Compassionate Use Act; patients with serious medical conditions and their primary caregivers may cultivate and possess marijuana on the recommendation of a physician without being subject to criminal prosecution or sanction (Cal. Health & Safety Code § 11362.5 (1996)). Federal authorities, however, seized six marijuana plants from Monson on the grounds she was violating federal laws, which make possession of marijuana for any purpose illegal. In order to secure access to what they believe is their last-resort treatment, Raich and Monson filed a lawsuit in federal court to enjoin enforcement of the Controlled Substances Act (CSA) against them. *See* 21 U.S.C.A. §§ 801 *et seq.* (2009).

The Ninth Circuit, ruling for Raich and Monson, declared the federal CSA is unconstitutional as applied to use of marijuana for medical purposes. Specifically, the court held intrastate, non-commercial cultivation, possession, and use of marijuana for personal medical purposes on the advice of a physician is not commerce and therefore is beyond the reach of federal legislation. The federal government appealed the Ninth Circuit's ruling to the U.S. Supreme Court, which refused to directly find California's Compassionate Use Act unconstitutional and remanded the case back to the Ninth Circuit to clarify whether there was a fundamental right to medical marijuana.

ISSUE: Is the right to medical marijuana claimed by Raich a fundamental right?

HOLDING AND DECISION: No, the right to use medical marijuana has not gained the traction on a national scale to be deemed a fundamental right.

ANALYSIS: While the U.S. Supreme Court found the CSA preempts contrary state medical marijuana laws, the Supreme Court did not clarify whether the right claimed by Raich was a fundamental right, and remanded the case to the Ninth Circuit on this issue. Although Raich claimed the CSA was unconstitutional because it infringed her fundamental rights protected by the Fifth and Ninth Amendments, the Ninth Circuit ruled against her on this claim, but it left open the possibility she had a defense of necessity. The U.S. Supreme Court vacated the Ninth Circuit's opinion and held that Congress's Commerce Clause authority includes the power to prohibit purely intrastate cultivation and use of marijuana.

RULE OF LAW: Raich might qualify for the common law defense of necessity if she were ever to be criminally prosecuted by the federal government for violation of the CSA.

(*See generally* Barnett, 2007; Carhart, 2006; Ingram, 2008; Kmeic, 2005; Lindsay, et al., 2006; Pedersen, 2008; Somin, 2006 for review of the U.S. Supreme Court decision; *see generally* Carcieri, 2007; Dorn, 2008; Pedersen, 2008 for discussion of the Ninth Circuit decision).

State and Local Medical Marijuana Laws

Earlier, in an unpublished opinion, the Ninth Circuit indicated that this activity is strictly limited. The Ninth Circuit distinguished and upheld the conviction of a dealer in medicinal marijuana, noting that while small amounts of marijuana for personal use would be within acceptable limits, the dealer admitted to possessing thirty-seven pounds of marijuana for distribution. *See U.S. v. Real Property Located at 5300 Lights Creek Lane*, 116 Fed.Appx. 117 (U.S. Court of Appeals for the 9th Circuit 2004).

Moral Dilemmas

1. Should health care professionals, including pharmacists, have First Amendment constitutional protections that allow them to discuss marijuana use with patients?

2. How far should state health laws be constrained when they conflict with federal power?

REGULATION BY LITIGATION

Federal regulators, state attorneys general, and attorneys for health care consumers increasingly rely upon litigation to impose regulatory constraints on the pharmaceutical industry. Through such regulation by litigation, government officials and private attorneys bypass traditional processes and reorient regulatory priorities (Morriss et al., 2009). Some claim regulation by litigation is attractive to regulators and activists because it provides an inappropriate and undemocratic shortcut to imposing regulatory burdens on private pharmaceutical companies and needs to be curbed. Others argue regulation by litigation is an important regulatory tool that can help control corporate abuses and encourage the adoption of needed consumer protections. The real issue to be addressed is why regulation by litigation is on the rise (Shell, 2004).

Moral Dilemmas

1. Is regulation of the pharmaceutical industry by litigation a problem, and, if so, how should it be controlled?

NO-COMPETE AGREEMENTS WITH GENERIC MANUFACTURERS

There is a controversial debate concerning the validity of no-compete agreements between the brand-name pharmaceutical industry and generic manufacturers. More broadly, the issue is defining the appropriate balance between the seemingly competing interests of patent and antitrust laws (Liu, 2008). Today, two out of three drug prescriptions in the U.S. are dispensed using generics, much higher than other developed nations in the world (Danzon & Furukawa, 2008).

Federal antitrust law finds contracts that restrain trade are illegal. *See* Sherman Antitrust Act, 15 U.S.C.A. §§ 1-7 (2009). The ban on contracts that restrain trade has been interpreted to include only unreasonable restraints on trade, that is, those that impair competition. A per se violation of the Sherman Act occurs when an agreement is obviously anticompetitive and the court can predict with confidence the rule of reason will condemn it. *See In re Cardizem CD Antitrust Litigation*, 332 F.3d 896 (U.S. Court of Appeals for the 6th Circuit 2003).

The U.S. Supreme Court has articulated an antitrust immunity, referred to as the Noerr-Pennington doctrine, under which the First Amendment protects companies actively seeking to protect their economic and business interests from infringing competitors. *See Eastern R.R. Presidents Conference v. Noerr Motor Freight, Inc.*, 365 U.S. 127 (U.S. Supreme Court 1961). However, this protection does not extend to lawsuits without a sufficient basis or that are simply seeking to harm competitors, rather than actually achieve favorable action from regulatory agencies and the courts.

Approval for new medicines to enter the U.S. market must be granted by the FDA. In 1984, Congress passed the Drug Price Competition and Patent Term Restoration Act (Hatch-Waxman) to accelerate the development and introduction of generic drugs in the U.S. market. Hatch-Waxman, intended to encourage generics to challenge invalid or unenforceable branded drug patents:

- Gives the first mover a 180-day exclusivity period to market a generic drug
- Allows generic manufacturers to rely on the safety and efficacy tests of the original branded-name drug, which results in an expedited process of filing an abbreviated new drug application (ANDA), rather than the previously required NDA

When a generic manufacturer files an ANDA, it must show the patent for the branded drug:

- Was never filed with the FDA
- Has expired or will expire
- Is invalid or will not be impinged by the generic drug (a paragraph IV certification)

21 U.S.C.A. § 355(b)(2)(A) (2008)

If the generic manufacturer attempts to demonstrate the last of these three options and challenge the patent itself, then the filer of the ANDA must inform the holder of the patent that a claim is being made that its drug is not a unique or non-obvious development (meaning a claim that the drug itself is not patentable). The patent holder (RGWB) has forty-five days to sue for patent infringement.

A lawsuit results in a thirty-month moratorium preventing the filer of the ANDA from bringing the product to market. The *Valley Drug* case illustrates the competitive nature of the pharmaceutical industry and how the low barriers to generic entry under Hatch-Waxman make patent protection crucial to the survival of the nation's pharmaceutical industry (Liu, 2008).

NO-COMPETE AGREEMENTS

Valley Drug Co. v. Geneva Pharmaceuticals, Inc.
[Drug Wholesaler v. Generic Manufacturer]
350 F.3d 1181 (U.S. Court of Appeals for the 11th Circuit 2003).
Rehearing en banc denied by Valley Drug Co. v. Abbott Labs., 92 Fed.Appx. 783
(U.S. Court of Appeals for the 11th Circuit 2004), class certification granted in part and denied in part by In re Terazosin Hydrochloride Antitrust (U.S. District Court for the Southern District of Florida)

FACTS: In this ongoing litigation, a consolidated group of health insurance companies, pharmacy benefit managers, and pharmacy chains claimed they were injured by the antitrust activities of branded drug company Abbott Laboratories and generic pharmaceutical companies Geneva Pharmaceuticals and Zenith Goldline Pharmaceuticals when they entered into agreements not to compete.

Abbott registered its patent for branded drug Hytrin (terazosin hydrochloride) to treat hypertension and enlarged prostate in 1987. Geneva subsequently filed four ANDAs in pursuit of FDA approval for its generic version of Hytrin, claiming its generic did not infringe any valid patent by Abbott. Zenith also filed an ANDA for a generic. Abbott sued each company within the forty-five-day window set by the FDA, thereby delaying FDA approval for the generic drugs for at least thirty months.

Although the litigation remained unresolved, the thirty-month stays were nearing expiration in 1998 when Abbott struck agreements with Geneva and Zenith to prevent introduction of their generics. The generic drugs cost sixty cents less per tablet than Abbott's name-brand drug. Abbott paid Zenith $3 million up front and promised an additional $6 million per quarter if Zenith did not produce its generic. Geneva received $4.5 million per month in exchange for not marketing its generic until a final, unappealable judgment that Abbott's patent was invalid was handed down. At the time the Abbott-Geneva and Abbott-Zenith agreements were struck, the FDA had

a successful defense requirement for generic manufacturers that required them to successfully defend their applications before they could begin exclusively marketing their generics. In 2000, this class action was filed against Abbott and the two generic manufacturers. The U.S. District Court granted summary judgment against the three companies;[LN3] the companies appealed to the Eleventh Circuit.

ISSUE: Are agreements in which pharmaceutical companies pay generic manufacturers not to compete valid?

HOLDING AND DECISION: Agreements in which brand-name pharmaceutical companies pay generic manufacturers not to compete are valid if they merely confirm the exclusivity of a patented drug.

ANALYSIS: The Eleventh Circuit focused on the existence of a patent. If Abbott had made payments to Geneva and Zenith in return for their exiting and refraining from entering the market, this would have violated antitrust laws. However, this is not what Abbott did, because it owned a patent with the lawful right to exclude the generics from the market. This exclusionary right is granted to allow patentees to exploit whatever degree of market power they might gain as an incentive to induce investment in drug innovations and the public disclosure of such innovations.

(continues)

(continued)

The anticompetitive and exclusionary nature of patents does not necessarily lead to antitrust violations. If the Abbott agreements only provided for payments before the patent expired or were declared invalid, then they did not prolong the exclusionary effect of the patent.

The Eleventh Circuit further addressed the invalidity of one of Abbott's patents and the impropriety of paying potentially infringing competitors. First, Abbott's patent rights were declared nonexistent after the agreements were entered into; therefore, their subsequent invalidity is irrelevant. Only patents procured by fraud are relevant to antitrust claims. Second, payments alone from Abbott to the generic manufacturers do not demonstrate the exclusionary effect was beyond that allowed by the patent.

RULE OF LAW: Agreements between pharmaceutical and generic companies not to compete are not *per se* unlawful if these agreements do not expand the existing exclusionary right of patents.

(*See generally* Chamblee, 2004; Greene, 2005 for discussion of the Eleventh Circuit's 2003 decision).

With the influx of cases at the federal appellate level and congressional discussion of further amendments to the federal Hatch-Waxman Act, the debate about no-compete agreements is warming up as the judicial and legislative branches attempt to balance the incentives for innovation with the incentives to lower drug costs.[LN4] A number of debates, however, fail to put the multimillion-dollar payments by pharmaceutical patent owners into appropriate perspective. The issue is really about how the regulatory system can assist the pharmaceutical industry to make its drugs affordable while balancing the industry's need to recoup its research and development investments (*e.g.*, Liu, 2008,).

In this particular case, Abbott invested $1.3 billion to develop Hytrin over a ten-year period by the time its patent was filed in 1987. Abbott was entitled to exclusive marketing of its patented brand drug until 2008. However, the Hytrin patent was challenged by two generic manufacturers when Abbott had thirteen years remaining on its patent. The issue is how Abbott should best protect its billion-dollar investment when faced with a generic challenge halfway through its market exclusivity period. At the time of the generic challenge, Hytrin brought in $540 million a year in revenues and was 20 percent of Abbott's sales. It may make economic sense to pay Zenith and Geneva $78 million a year to protect $540 million in annual revenue. The issue is whether the entire regulatory system has broken down when pharmaceutical companies are forced to pay generic manufacturers simply to confirm the exclusivity of their patented drugs.

Pharmaceutical companies are often forced to defend their patents in order to recoup their investments. Patent challenges are occurring as early as four years after a product launch (*see e.g.*, Gongola, 2003). For instance:

- Bayer obtained the patent covering the antibiotic Cipro (ciprofloxacin hydrochloride) in 1987 and obtained FDA approval of the drug three months later; within four years, Barr, a generic manufacturer, filed an ANDA for a generic version of Cipro, although Cipro had ten years remaining on its patent (*In re Ciprofloxacin Hydrochloride Antitrust Litigation*, 166 F.Supp.2d 740 (U.S. District Court for the Eastern District of New York 2001), *affirmed,* 735 N.W.2d 448 (Supreme Court of Wisconsin 2007); *In re Ciprofloxacin Hydrochloride Antitrust Litigation*, 261 F.Supp.2d 188 (U.S. District Court, for the Eastern District of New York 2003))
- Sanofi-Synthelabo and its U.S. partner Bristol-Myers Squibb obtained FDA approval of their blood-thinning drug Plavix in 1997; within four years, Apotex, a generic manufacturer, filed an ANDA for a generic version of Plavix, although Plavix had ten years remaining on its patent (*Sanofi-Synthelabo v. Apotex Inc.*, 488 F.Supp.2d 317 (U.S. District Court for the Southern District of New York 2006), *U.S. Supreme Court certiorari denied,* 2009 WL 2251300 (U.S. Supreme Court 2009)).

Generic manufacturers can obtain windfalls when they prevail in patent lawsuits, while if they lose, they incur insignificant economic risks. The high profitability potential, coupled with low litigation risks, makes generic manufacturers willing to invest millions of dollars in these patent challenges (Liu, 2008). At the same time, the pharmaceutical industry is struggling to fill the financial holes resulting from patent expirations or early generic entry in the U.S. market. Faced with patent challenges from generic manufacturers at increasingly early stages of their patent terms, the pharmaceutical industry has been trying to protect the exclusive rights for their patented drugs, while being forced to compromise in negotiating patent settlement terms with generic manufacturers. The no-compete agreements are just one form of these compromises (Liu, 2008).

For several years, Congress has proposed legislation to penalize generics for entering into agreements with pharmaceutical companies that pay the generics not to compete. Both the House and Senate passed Medicare bills with provisions stating that if a generic signs an agreement not to market its generic drug in exchange for a payment from a pharmaceutical company, it forfeits its right to the 180-day exclusivity period under the Hatch-Waxman Act. In addition to this provision, the bills provide for only one, rather than multiple, thirty-month stays when a pharmaceutical company sues for patent infringement (the FDA amended its rules governing patent submissions to include this provision), and they allow generic manufacturers to file counterclaims when sued for patent infringement. These efforts are targeted to eliminate loopholes that allow the pharmaceutical industry to repeatedly extend patents and keep generics off the market. The federal government estimates that by making it more difficult for the pharmaceutical industry to stop generics from entering the market, Medicare and consumer costs could be reduced by $3.5 billion per year.

However, some argue these provisions give too much benefit to generics, a result that will provide a disincentive to pharmaceutical innovation. Proponents of this view point out the average effective patent life of approved drugs is far below that of other non-drug patented products. Reducing the patent life further could result in the pharmaceutical industry being less willing to incur the costs of research and development to stimulate innovation. In short, the current regulatory scheme appears to favor generic manufacturers while increasing litigation costs. The intensified patent challenges and early entry of generics have adversely affected the financial stability of the pharmaceutical industry, and thus its ability to fund new research and development.

VACCINES

Many pharmaceutical companies are increasing their stake in the vaccine market:

- GlaxoSmithKline acquired both the Pennsylvania vaccine plant where Wyeth once made flu vaccine and the Canadian flu-vaccine producer ID Biomedical

- Novartis has taken a controlling stake in Chiron, a California vaccine maker
- Pfizer-Wyeth, on the strength of its childhood vaccine Prevnar, opened a research and manufacturing plant in Ireland
- Sanofi-Adventis, the world's largest vaccine maker, has secured $200 million in U.S. government contracts to boost flu-vaccine production and test new technology to produce vaccines more efficiently

This new interest in vaccines represents a significant uptick for the industry. For years, vaccines were on pharmaceutical firms' backburners as manufacturers pulled out of what had come to be viewed as a high-risk commodity business. In the late 1960s, there were twenty-six vaccine manufacturers in the U.S. market; today, four firms produce almost all routine childhood vaccines (GlaxoSmithKline, Novartis, Pfizer-Wyeth, and Sanofi-Aventis) and many of the recommended pediatric vaccines have a single supplier (*see* Wharton, 2005). Now, after decades of decline, vaccines are gaining new interest from:

- Concerns about public emergencies from bioterrorist attacks
- Development of potential vaccines targeted at new therapeutic markets (including diabetes, cancer, and smoking cessation)
- Fears about pandemics from the avian and swine influenzas
- Pharmaceutical industry and the federal government in response to flu-shot shortages

Despite this growing interest and the emergence of new vaccine technologies, vaccines remain a small piece of the overall health industry market. With sales of over $16 billion, vaccines comprise less than 5 percent of the global pharmaceutical industry (IMS, 2008). While vaccines do not face significant generic competition due to their high entry and manufacturing costs, vaccine companies continue to face lengthy and expensive research and development costs and low return on investment rates.

Anti-Vaccine Movement

The strength of this sector of the pharmaceutical industry is that vaccines work: they effectively create induced immunity for many infectious diseases. With the historic success of vaccines in virtually eliminating many life-threatening and debilitating diseases, their obvious benefit is preventing disease before it occurs. As of the beginning of 2009, vaccines prevent twenty-two diseases and illnesses, as listed below.

Vaccine-Preventable Diseases and Illnesses
- Cervical Cancer/Human Papillomavirus (HPV)
- Chickenpox and Shingles
- Cholera
- Diphtheria
- Haemophilus Influenzae Type b (Hib) Diseases
- Hepatitis A and Hepatitis B
- Influenza
- Japanese Encephalitis
- Measles
- Meningococcal Diseases
- Mumps
- Pertussis
- Polio
- Rotavirus Diseases
- Rubella
- Streptococcus Pneumoniae Infections
- Tetanus
- Tick-Borne Encephalitis
- Tuberculosis
- Typhoid
- Yellow Fever

Source: Kalorama, 2008.

Despite this success, the vaccine industry faces an active anti-vaccine movement, which includes:

- Campaigns against cervical cancer vaccines (Gardasil)
- Controversy surrounding mercury-containing vaccines
- Misinformation about the side effects of vaccines

(Kalorama, 2008)

Vaccinations for Children

The U.S. has a patchwork system of paying for childhood immunizations. One anomaly of this system is that for children whose health insurance does not cover newly recommended vaccines, it is better to have no insurance at all, since free vaccines are available to children who are uninsured or qualify for public insurance (Lee et al., 2007). Many states do not help children with inadequate private insurance (Landro, 2008). One estimate is that current policy puts more than a million children at risk for diseases such as chickenpox, pneumonia, and hepatitis A (Landro, 2008; Lee et al., 2007).

Figure 17-7 illustrates the eleven recommended vaccines for children from birth to six years of age. Unfortunately, health insurance plans are not keeping up with new vaccines for children; the private-sector cost for all recommended childhood immunizations averages $300 per child every year for the first six years of each child's life (CDC, 2009). The average annual per-child cost was $26 in 1995 (Landro, 2008), meaning there has been a thirteen-fold increase over a decade for recommended vaccines.

Childhood vaccines have become a $1-billion-a-year endeavor since the discovery of polio vaccine in the 1950s. In 2007, the number of U.S. births set a record of over 4.3 million. With about 40 percent of the births to unwed mothers, much of the responsibility for immunizations is falling to the government.

About fifty-five million employees and their dependents get coverage through self-insured plans that are exempt from state immunization mandates; these children are the most likely to be underinsured for vaccines (Lee et al., 2007). While other employer-provided plans provide vaccine coverage, co-payments and deductibles apply.

The CDC opposes prioritizing vaccines and instead favors better coverage by insurers and more government funding (Landro, 2008). With costs rising, a debate is emerging concerning whether it may be time to decide at a national level which vaccines are most important:

- Sixteen states require health insurers to cover all recommended vaccines, but this policy does not cover employees covered by self-insured health insurance plans
- Seventeen states did not give meningitis vaccines to children with inadequate private insurance
- Eight states do not give pneumococcal shots to underinsured infants and toddlers
- A handful of states do not provide shots for chickenpox and hepatitis A to the underinsured
- Two states do not provide TDaP, the combined booster shot for tetanus, diphtheria, and pertussis (whooping cough), for eleven- to twelve-year-olds.
- More than 1 million insured children are unable to get the meningococcal vaccine, leaving them vulnerable to potentially deadly infections

(Lee et al., 2007)

No information was available for two vaccines newly recommended in 2008: an oral vaccine for infants against rotavirus, a common cause of childhood diarrhea and vomiting, and a vaccine for girls against human papillomavirus, which can cause cervical cancer.

Vaccine	Age	Birth	1 month	2 months	4 months	6 months	12 months	15 months	18 months	19–23 months	2–3 years	4–6 years
Hepatitis B		HEP B	HEP B				HEP B					
Rotavirus				RV	RV	RV						
Diphtheria, Tetanus, Pertussis				DTaP	DTaP	DTaP		DTaP				DTaP
Haemophilas Influenza Type b				Hib	Hib	Hib	Hib					
Pneumococcal				PCV	PCV	PCV	PCV				PPSV (revaccination)	
Inactivated Poliovirus				IPV	IPV		IPV					IPV
Influenza					Annual seasonal flu vaccine at 6 months and up							
Measles, Mumps, Rubella							MMR					MMR
Varicella							Varicella					Varicella
Hepatitis A							HepA (2 doses)					HepA Series
Meningococcal												MCV

☐ Range of recommended ages.   ■ Certain high-risk groups.

FIGURE 17-7: Recommended Immunization Schedule for Children

Delmar/Cengage Learning

Data retrieved from: Advisory Committee on Immunization Practices. (2009, February 18). Recommended immunization schedules for persons aged 0 through 18 years–United States, 2009. *Journal of the American Medical Association, 301* (7), 715. The recommended immunization schedules for children have been approved by the Advisory Committee on Immunization Practices, the American Academy of Pediatrics, and the American Academy of Family Physicians.

Vaccine	Cost	Age and dosage
TDaP	$65	19 to 64 years old, one dose.
Tetanus booster	$45	All adults over 19, every 10 years.
MMR	$50-$65	19 to 49, one or two doses if not previously vaccinated or infected. Over 50, one dose if risk of disease is present.
Shingles	$220	Over 50, one dose.
Pneumonia	$45	19 to 64, one or two doses when risk of disease is present. One dose after age 65.
Influenza	$20-$30	19 to 49, one dose seasonally when risk of disease is present. Over 50, one dose seasonally.

FIGURE 17-8: Common Vaccines to Prevent Diseases in Adults

Delmar/Cengage Learning
Data retrieved from: CDC, 2009; Landro, 2008; Temte, 2009.

Adult Vaccinations

Figure 17-8 illustrates the six vaccines that are recommended for adults. Although immunization rates for children are high, and young people rarely die from diseases vaccines can prevent, that is not the case for adults. For instance, pediatric hospitalizations associated with laboratory-confirmed influenza infections are monitored by two population-based surveillance networks: Emerging Infections Program (EIP) and the New Vaccine

Surveillance Network (NVSN). As many as seventy thousand adult Americans die each year from vaccine-preventable diseases like influenza, pneumonia, and complications of hepatitis, according to the CDC; such diseases also sicken hundreds of thousands of adults, at a cost of treatment exceeding $10 billion annually.

One problem is a lack of any national system to promote and monitor adult vaccinations (Landro, 2008). The Kaiser Foundation reports only about

60 percent of adults aged sixty-five and over have ever had a pneumonia vaccine.

While the federal Vaccines for Children Program provides vaccines at no cost to children who cannot afford them, and carefully monitors supply and demand, the infrastructure to ensure the adult vaccination pipeline is inadequate (Temte, 2009). There is currently little coordination between federal public health agencies, private medical providers, and the private companies that make adult vaccines (Landro, 2008).

Targeted Medicines with Hybrid Pricing

The traditional view of vaccines as a bulk-order commodity is changing. In fact, it is almost a misnomer to call some of the new products vaccines. They are patented, targeted treatments and can command hybrid pricing (Wharton, 2005). For instance, Wyeth's childhood MMR vaccine Prevnar, has proven itself as such a superior product that it commands $84 per dose from insurers, compared to competitors' $47 per dose (CDC, 2009).

Insurers are increasingly willing to support new, high-priced vaccines that are proven to keep immunity long term and are a very efficient way to prevent illness. Prevention of disease has significant economic advantages (Wharton, 2005). The pharmaceutical industry is at a point in the market where developing vaccines is attractive, which has not been true in the recent past. The role the government and the insurance industry increasingly plays in determining what is valuable in the pharmaceutical market cannot be underestimated.

GlaxoSmithKline has more than twenty new vaccines under development, including products to combat strep, meningitis, and rotavirus. In the past, attention was directed to childhood vaccines, but more and more research and development is focusing on vaccines for adolescents and young adults, and adult vaccines for diseases such as cancer (Danzon & Furukawa, 2008). The U.S. health care system approach to vaccines really has to adapt to accommodate these new products by focusing on disease prevention through vaccines versus treatment of disease (Wharton, 2005). Prevention is much more cost-effective than treatment of diseases.

Gardasil: Cervical Cancer Vaccine

Gardasil, a new vaccine by Merck to prevent cervical cancer, is an example of a new generation of vaccines for expanded markets that is able to fetch a premium price from government and private insurers. Texas was the first state to attempt to require school-aged girls to be vaccinated against the sexually transmitted disease, human papillomavirus, or HPV, that causes cervical cancer. By issuing an executive order, the governor tried to sidestep legislative opposition but was stopped by the state legislature. Virginia and the District of Columbia are the only two jurisdictions to mandate Gardasil vaccinations (Javitt et al., 2008).

Merck is bankrolling efforts to pass state laws across the country mandating Gardasil for girls as young as age eleven. It has funneled money through Women in Government, an advocacy group made up of female state legislators around the country. The federal government recommends all girls get the shots at age eleven, before they are likely to be sexually active. Merck could generate billions in sales if Gardasil, at $360 for the three-shot regimen, is made mandatory across the country. Gardasil was also recently approved for boys.

Opponents to mandatory Gardasil vaccinations maintain:

- HPV does not pose imminent and significant risk of harm to others and therefore should not be subject to mandates
- Mandates will financially burden existing government health programs and private physicians
- Mandating HPV vaccination for minor females is premature since long-term safety and effectiveness of the vaccine has not been established
- Sex-specific mandates raise constitutional concerns
- The vaccine can never completely eradicate HPV as long as it is only administered to females under schemes with a multitude of exemptions

(Dowling, 2008; Javitt et al., 2008)

Vaccine Shortages

The U.S. vaccine market is prone to shortages. This is an industry with a relatively small market where prices are set, so it tends to gravitate to the best producer in a sole-supplier situation (Danzon, 2005). When a supplier experiences a problem or cuts back production, shortages arise. For instance, a severe influenza vaccine shortage occurred during the mid-2000 influenza season because of the loss of all vaccines made by Chiron for U.S. distribution when the company faced contamination issues at its manufacturing site (McQuillan et al., 2009).

The U.S. must find a better way to finance vaccines and expand insurance coverage, while facing single or few suppliers. National mechanisms to stockpile vaccines are needed, as well as a backup system to bring vaccines back into the system quickly when they are needed (Danzon, 2005). Some of the vaccine shortages in recent years have come as a result of stepped-up FDA review of vaccine manufacturing. The more serious the FDA became about manufacturing site inspections, the more shortages arose. For instance, Wyeth produced an influenza vaccine for the U.S. market for more than twenty years, but after the company was fined $30 million for manufacturing violations and an additional $15,000 for every day it remained out of compliance, Wyeth announced it would exit the flu market in 2002, leaving only two companies to manufacture an influenza vaccine (Wharton, 2005).

Over-Regulated Market

The role of government in the vaccine market cannot be overlooked. Assertions that a market-driven system for vaccines has failed are wrong. While the pharmaceutical industry provides vaccines, this market sector has never had a chance to be a free market (Pauly, 2005). Vaccine production is among the most heavily regulated sectors in the health care products industry since they are derived from living organisms (Wharton, 2005).

The Institute of Medicine found that the federal government often mandates vaccine protection, but does not provide enough money to encourage vaccine manufacturers to develop new products or maintain production (IOM, 2008). Some argue that if government is going to require vaccination protection, it should pay for it. Essentially these vaccines are thought of as a public good, and thus they are an obligation for the government to finance (Pauly, 2005).

Vaccines should be thought of as an important part of our normal health care system and should be covered by insurance because they are so effective in reducing health care costs (Danzon, 2006). The IOM report on vaccines has been met with stunning silence. The insurance industry is disinterested in receiving government subsidies for mandated programs because such companies fear they might ultimately be left with the mandate, but not the subsidy (Pauly, 2005).

At the moment there is a total lack of trust between these three parties: government, insurers, and the vaccine industry. The government generates additional mistrust when it threatens to step in and cut pharmaceutical prices when demand is high, as it did with the antibiotic Cipro during the anthrax attacks on U.S. postal facilities in 2001. There is talk about better planning, but no movement yet (Pauly, 2005).

One proposal is a system that provides some government pricing guarantees to encourage vaccine manufacturers, especially for flu vaccines, to remain in business. The flu market is particularly complicated because vaccines are formulated each year based on strains expected to be most prevalent. They cannot be stockpiled if they go unused. Governments could:

- Set a trigger price at which vaccine manufacturers could not raise prices if shortages develop

- Make concessions to compensate for the price cap, such as extended patent life, to avoid temporary spikes

(*See generally* Wharton, 2005)

Commodification of Mandatory Vaccines

Increasing the relative prices paid for new vaccines to levels more closely reflective of their social value compared to other new drugs is essential to achieving appropriate incentives for allocation of research and development (Danzon & Pereira, 2005). The biggest obstacle vaccine manufacturers face is little payback for their risk because many of their products are purchased in bulk by governments and other public health authorities, including humanitarian agencies. These large buyers are able to negotiate low prices. In the U.S., the government is paying for over half of all vaccines for children, and the vaccine industry is more or less forced to take low prices (Wharton, 2005). It is difficult to pursue innovative vaccine research and development with negotiated low prices.

National Vaccine Injury Compensation Program

The National Vaccine Injury Compensation Program (VICP) is one example where there has been some meeting of the minds when it comes to differing perceptions of health risk (Pauly, 2005). In 1986, Congress created VICP, which established a no-fault system for compensating those who may have been injured by routine childhood vaccines (Wharton, 2005).

This program arose in part because different groups had very different views on the health risks posed by pediatric vaccines. Some people believed there was a high health risk of side effects; others believed it was low. The strategy was to levy an excise tax on vaccine sales, use the proceeds to set up a trust fund, and pay claims for actual damages on a no-fault basis. After an initial flurry of payments for previous injuries, the level of payments fell dramatically, and the trust fund balance grew. Those who thought adverse effects would be common turned out to be wrong. The point is those who thought side effects were unlikely expected to get money back, and those who thought they were likely felt they were protected; both groups could agree with the VICP proposal. Nevertheless, while VICP was designed to streamline and limit vaccine manufacturers' liability, lawsuits continue to be brought against vaccine manufacturers by using opt-out provisions in the VICP legislation (Wharton, 2005).

Demand Side of the Vaccine Market

The demand side of the vaccine market is crucial to keeping the vaccine industry vibrant. Even with successful development of safe vaccines:

- People need to know about vaccines and believe they are beneficial
- People must be willing to pay for vaccines
- Health care professionals must be willing to administer vaccines

(Wharton, 2005)

Vaccine Litigation

Lawsuits filed against the vaccine industry alleging its products have harmed patients are another reason the pharmaceutical industry has become wary of vaccine production. Because vaccines have the potential to reach millions of patients, a bad outcome has the potential to bankrupt a manufacturer. In the case of widely distributed vaccines, a company is engaging in a bet-the-firm risk if things go badly (Pauly, 2005). This discourages research and development on certain types of vaccines and discourages production and marketing (Wharton, 2005).

FUTURE CHALLENGES FACING THE PHARMACEUTICAL INDUSTRY

Few areas of pharmaceuticals have seen the fast-moving developments in the marketplace the vaccine market has recently had (Sahoo, 2008). The new interest in vaccines comes at a time when the pharmaceutical industry is struggling with few new products coming to market. While there are challenges on the revenue side of the business, the process of developing vaccines is more predictable, cheaper, and faster than it is for other drugs (Wharton, 2005). Today, the pharmaceutical industry is primarily focused on currently non-vaccine-preventable diseases, as listed below.

Non-Vaccine-Preventable Diseases
- Cancer
- Dengue Fever
- Epstein-Barr Virus (EBV)
- Helicobacter Pylori Infections
- Hepatitis C and Hepatitis E
- HIV/AIDS
- Malaria
- Nosocomial Infections
- Respiratory Infections
- Roundworm and Hookworm Infection
- Sexually Transmitted Diseases (STDs)
- Tobacco
- West Nile Virus Infections

Source: Kalorama, 2008.

If insurers increase interest, vaccine manufacturers will invest in manufacturing plants in the U.S. (Danzon, 2006). Today, there is a tremendous amount of research activity in vaccines by both the pharmaceutical and biotechnology industries. With adequate reimbursement, the problem of innovation will take care of itself (Wharton, 2005).

Financing Basic Pharmaceutical Research

The most important issue in the debate over vaccines is how to finance new vaccine research and development. Right now, the best route to development of novel vaccines is continued investment in basic pharmaceutical research that might lead to wide-ranging discoveries that could be applied to vaccine development. The real need is a way to fund basic research. Only a few global firms can take upon themselves the risk of developing and testing vaccine products (Wharton, 2005).

Value of Pharmaceutical Innovation

The pharmaceutical industry has made significant advances in helping health care consumers live longer and better lives. Today, drugs treat health care conditions once thought to be untreatable. Both mortality and disability rates have fallen consistently over the years as a result of new drugs being brought to market. Drugs prevent the need for hospital, emergency, and long-term care for heart attacks, strokes, HIV/AIDS, and many cancers that at one time debilitated individuals. Today, even without full cures, drugs greatly delay the onset and severity of major diseases and illnesses, and reduce expensive and unproductive time spent in hospitals, nursing homes, and under the care of family members (Sokol et al., 2005). All too often, however, discussions center on the increase in spending on health care rather than the benefits of improved health care the spending brought (PhRMA, 2007). The pressure to control drug prices is targeted well beyond their actual contribution to overall health care cost increases.

A focus on drug prices alone often overlooks the value health care consumers and society derives from improved health. While high drug prices must be part of any debate on health care, the cost of drugs should be considered in the context of the total benefits received from increased longevity without disabilities, as well as total savings achieved from not having to use hospitals and nursing homes. The basic question is whether Americans find the increase in health care spending for new life-saving drugs and disease-eradicating vaccines is worth it. Perhaps pandemic fears will answer this question sooner than anticipated.

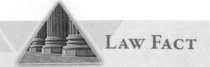 LAW FACT

STATE PRE-EMPTION OF DRUG LABELING

When do drug labeling judgments of the FDA pre-empt state law product liability claims?

When the risk of gangrene from IV-push injection of the drug became apparent, Wyeth had a duty to provide a warning adequately describing that risk. While the warnings on the drug's label were deemed sufficient by the FDA, Wyeth failed to demonstrate it was impossible for it to comply with both federal and state requirements. FDA regulations permitted Wyeth to unilaterally strengthen its warning, and the mere fact the FDA approved the drug's label did not establish it would have prohibited such a change.

—*Wyeth v. Levine*, 129 S.Ct. 1187 (U.S. Supreme Court 2009).

CHAPTER SUMMARY

- Global pharmaceutical companies are moving away from a growth strategy based on blockbuster drugs and toward a growth strategy based on acquiring and merging with biotechnology companies in order to have a more diverse product base.
- High prices for drugs without significant health care value are increasingly unjustified, so pharmaceutical companies are moving toward pricing drugs based on the economic value they provide to patients.
- The pharmaceutical industry is one of the most research-intensive industries in the U.S., investing five times as much in research and development relative to sales than the average U.S. manufacturing firm; the stages of research and development include academic and basic research, drug discovery and development, clinical trials, NDA and approval, drug manufacturing, and ongoing research and monitoring.
- Global drug pricing is incredibly complex and does not have one methodology that can please everyone.
- The FDA struggles to efficiently and effectively regulate drugs imported into the U.S.
- MCOs exercise great power over the pharmaceutical industry in terms of determining drug prices and perhaps hindering the development of new drugs in the process.
- The learned intermediary doctrine imposes an obligation on pharmaceutical companies to warn physicians of foreseeable risks associated with the use of their drugs, including potential off-label uses.
- Of the four elements consumers must prove to win a products liability lawsuit against a drug manufacturer (duty, breach, causation, and damages), causation is the hardest element to prove because of the high standard of scientific evidence required.
- The number of successful lawsuits over latent effects from regulated and approved pharmaceuticals is an indication the research required by regulation is often not enough to assess all of the harmful effects of a drug; however, there is little regulatory incentive for companies to do more comprehensive research.
- There is an ongoing battle between federal and state law over whether consumers may use marijuana for medicinal purposes.
- Because federal drug regulations are incomplete, litigation is increasingly used to force drug companies to better protect consumers.
- Balancing the competing interests of patent and antitrust laws in the pharmaceutical and generic industries is difficult; because it is easier for generics to gain FDA approval, branded drug companies often seek to discourage generic competition through no-compete agreements under which they pay the generic manufacturers not to compete.
- After decades of declining interest in the vaccine market, pharmaceutical companies are increasing their interest in this market due to its potential value and the decline in the profitability of the blockbuster drug model of business; focus is increasing on vaccines for adults and on how to surge vaccine production, if necessary.
- Vaccine laws and funding for them vary immensely between the states; a higher emphasis is placed on vaccinating children than adults, and much more funding is available for childhood immunizations.
- The American government highly regulates and monitors vaccines, and has set up a fund to reimburse those who were likely injured by routine childhood vaccines.
- The attention given to vaccinations as opposed to other health care concerns is due in part to the fact that vaccinations makes good economic sense in terms of the costs they save by preventing illness in the first place.

LAW NOTES

1. Reglan aids in controlling GERD by blocking dopamine receptors in the brain and throughout the body, enhancing movement or contractions of the esophagus, stomach, and intestines. By blocking these receptors, Reglan can cause EPS, which is an adverse drug reaction involving the extrapyramidal nervous system. TD is a particularly severe form of EPS causing grotesque involuntary movements of the mouth, tongue, lips, and extremities, involuntary chewing movements, and a general sense of agitation.

2. *Daubert v. Merrell Dow Pharmaceuticals, Inc.*, 509 U.S. 579 (U.S. Supreme Court 1993) involved children with serious birth defects, in which scientific experts testified *in vitro* and *in vivo* testing (test tube and animal studies) showed the drug Bendectin, used during pregnancy for anti-nausea, could cause limb-reduction birth defects. The lower court ruled testimony was inadmissible because it was not generally accepted by the scientific community, and Merrell was granted summary judgment. The U.S. Supreme Court vacated the judgment and remanded so the expert testimony could be reevaluated in keeping with the new standard for admission of scientific evidence; heretofore, scientific evidence had to be generally accepted by the scientific community. On remand, the Ninth Circuit applied the two-part Daubert standard and found that none of the children's experts based their testimony on preexisting or independent research, published their work in scientific journals, or adequately explained their methodology. The court concluded the proffered scientific testimony was not derived by scientific method. *See Daubert v. Merrell Dow Pharmaceuticals, Inc.*, 43 F.3d 1311 (U.S. Court of Appeals for the 9th Circuit 1995), *U.S. Supreme Court certiorari denied,* 516 U.S. 869 (U.S. Supreme Court 1995).

3. In *In re Terazosin Hydrochloride Antitrust Litigation,* 164 F.Supp.2d 1340 (U.S. District Court for the Southern District of Florida 2000), the U.S. District Court for the Southern District of Florida held the agreements Abbott had with Geneva and Zenith violated § 1 of the Sherman Antitrust Act because they represented horizontal collusion that impaired domestic competition and restrained the trade of terazosin hydrochloride products. Abbott and both generic manufacturers would otherwise be competing in the same market, which would increase competition and decrease prices.

    It found Abbott was solidifying its monopoly through monetary payments: Geneva and Zenith forswore competing with Abbott in the U.S. market for terazosin hydrochloride drugs and promised to take steps to forestall others from entering that market for the life of their respective agreements in exchange for millions of dollars. The court rejected the companies' claims that the agreements were pro-competition because they prevented costly patent litigation and removed barriers to entry for the generic manufacturers. Moreover, the court found the Abbott-Geneva agreement did not resolve the patent litigation since Geneva could begin marketing its product if Abbott chose to stop payments. The court further held it was unreasonable to suggest Abbott paid Geneva to spur competition in its own lucrative domestic market for terazosin hydrochloride products. The Abbott-Zenith agreement, with its provisions to forestall market entry, was also found to curtail competition. While the companies maintained they were immune from prosecution under the Noerr-Pennington doctrine because their agreements arose out of ongoing litigation, the court ruled immunity does not apply to restraints adopted by private entities; it extends only when restraint of trade is the intended consequence of public action. These agreements served to harm competition, not to encourage favorable governmental action.

    The District Court held that the agreements were a *per se* violation of the Sherman Act. The appellate court held that the agreements were not a *per se* violation to the extent they had no broader exclusionary effect than that provided by the disputed patents, and remanded the case for further proceedings. *See In re Terazosin Hydrochloride Antitrust Litigation*, 344 F.3d 1294 (U.S. Court of Appeals for the 11th Circuit 2003).

4. An issue not addressed in this chapter is pharmaceutical patents held by research universities and public-sector research institutes in developed nations. Universities Allied for Essential Medicines, an international student group with over forty campus chapters (with the slogan "Our Labs, Our Drugs, Our Responsibility"), is advocating segmented market pricing where universities and public research institutes in developed nations open access to their patented drugs to people at the bottom of the world's economic pyramid (Hickey, 2007; Kesselheim, 2008; Wasan, 2009).

CHAPTER BIBLIOGRAPHY

Aggarwal, S. (2005). Clearing the air: What the latest Supreme Court decision regarding medical marijuana really means. *American Journal of Hospice & Palliative Care, 22* (5), 327-329.

Barnett, R. E. (2006). Access to justice: The social responsibility of lawyers: The presumption of liberty and the public interest: Medical marijuana and fundamental rights. *Journal of Law & Politics, 22,* 29-45.

Barth, A. S. (2006). Recent developments in health law: Select recent court decisions. *American Journal of Law & Medicine, 32,* 405-408.

Bouchard, R. A. (2007). Balancing public and private interests in the commercialization of publicly funded medical research: Is there a role for compulsory government royalty fees? *Boston University Journal of Science & Technology Law, 13,* 120-191.

Burns, L. R. (2009). *The biopharmaceutical sector's impact on the U.S. economy: Analysis at the national, state, and local levels.* Stamford, CT: Archstone Consulting.

Carcieri, M. D. (2007). *Gonzales v. Raich:* Congressional tyranny and irrelevance in the war on drugs. *University of Pennsylvania Journal of Costitutional Law, 9,* 131-1165.

Carhart, C. L. (2006). Will the ever-swinging pendulum of Commerce Clause interpretation ever stop? A casenote on *Gonzales v. Raich. Whittier Law Review, 27,* 833-865.

CBO (Congressional Budget Office). (2006). *Research and development in the pharmaceutical industry.* Washington, DC: CBO.

CDC (Centers for Disease Control). (2009). *CDC vaccine price list.* Atlanta, GA: CDC.

Chamblee, L. E. (2004). Between "merit inquiry" and "rigorous analysis": Using Daubert to navigate the gray areas of federal class action certification. *Florida State University Law Review, 31,* 1041-1090.

Chang, N., chairman and managing director, Asia Orbimed. (2009, February 20). Pharmaceutical-biotechnology panel: The blurring line between pharmaceutical and biotechnology at the 14th Annual Wharton Health Care Business Conference on catalyzing change: Accelerating health care advancement. Philadelphia, PA.

Cohen, J. G. (2005). Merck and the Vioxx decision: Playing by the changing rules of the chemical exposure game. *Journal of Law, Medicine & Ethics, 33,* 866-869.

Cook, L. (2007). Products liability: Genuine issue of material fact over whether understating risk of side effects renders pharmaceutical drug labels misleading and ineffective: *McNeil v. Wyeth. American Journal of Law & Medicine, 33,* 141-145.

Danzon, P. M. (2005). Vaccine supply: A cross-national perspective. How do the economics of vaccines differ in the U.S. from other countries, both industrialized and developing? *Health Affairs, 24* (3), 706-717.

Danzon, P. M., & Furukawa, M. F. (2008). International prices and availability of pharmaceuticals. *Health Affairs, 27* (1), 221-233.

___. (2006). Prices and availability of biopharmaceuticals: An international comparison. *Health Affairs, 25* (5), 1353-1362.

Danzon, P. M., & Pereira, N. S. (2005). Why sole-supplier vaccine markets may be here to stay: Vaccine markets tend to evolve toward a single dominant supplier, which has advantages as well as disadvantages. *Health Affairs, 24* (3), 694-696.

Das, R. (2005). Regulation of medical marijuana. *Journal of the American Medical Association, 294* (24), 3091.

Dorn, A. (2008). The untimely death of the Commerce Clause: *Gonzales v. Raich's* threat to federalism, the democratic process, and individual rights and liberties. *Temple Political & Civil Rights Law Review, 18,* 213-252.

Dowling, T. S. (2008). Mandating a human papillomavirus vaccine: An investigation into whether such legislation is constitutional and prudent. *American Journal of Law & Medicine, 34,* 65-84.

Epstein, R. A. (2008). *Overdose: How excessive government regulation stifles pharmaceutical innovation.* New Haven, CT: Yale University Press.

FDA (Food & Drug Administration). (2009, January 14). *Press release: FDA launches pilot program to improve the safety of drugs and active drug ingredients produced outside the U.S.* Bethesda, MD: FDA.

Garner, B. A. (2004). *Black's law dictionary* (8th ed.). Eagan, MN: Thomson Reuters West Publishing.

Garrett, A. D., & Garis, R. (2007). Leveling the playing field in the pharmacy benefit management industry. *Valparaiso University Law Review, 42,* 33-79.

Gilson, A. M. (2007). State medical board members' beliefs about pain, addiction, and diversion and abuse: A changing regulatory environment. *Journal on Pain, 8* (9), 682-691.

Gongola, J. A. (2003). Prescriptions for change: The Hatch-Waxman Act and new legislation to increase the availability of generic drugs to consumers, *Indiana Law Review, 36,* 787-825.

Gostin, L. O. (2005). Medical marijuana, American federalism, and the Supreme Court. *Journal of the American Medical Association, 294* (7), 842-844.

Greene, S. (2005). A prescription for change: How the Medicare Act revises Hatch-Waxman to speed market entry of generic drugs. *Iowa Journal of Corporation Law, 30,* 309-355.

Hall, R. F., & Berlin, R. J. (2006). When you have a hammer everything looks like a nail: Misapplication of the False Claims Act to off-label promotion. *Food & Drug Law Journal, 61,* 653-677.

Hall, R. F., & Sobotka. E. S. (2007). Inconsistent government policies: Why FDA off-label regulation cannot survive First Amendment review under Greater New Orleans. *Food & Drug Law Journal, 62,* 1-48.

Harper, R. M. (2008). A matter of life and death: Affording terminally-ill patients access to post-phase I investigational new drugs. *Journal of Medicine & Law, 12,* 265-295.

Henry, D. A. et al. (2005). Drug prices and value for money: The Australian pharmaceutical benefits scheme. *Journal of the American Medical Association, 294,* 2630-2633.

Hickey, B. (2007). The public research in the Public Interest Act. *Journal of Law, Medicine & Ethics, 35,* 332-334.

IMS Health. (2008). *Global pharmaceutical market and therapy forecast.* Plymouth Meeting, PA: IMS.

Ingram, J. D. (2008). Medical use of marijuana, *Oklahoma City University Law Review, 33,* 589-602.

IOM (Institute of Medicine) Committee on Review of Priorities in the National Vaccine Plan. (2008). *Initial guidance for an update of the national vaccine plan: A letter report to the National Vaccine Program Office.* Washington, DC: IOM.

JAMA (Journal of the American Medical Association). (2009). Recommended immunization schedules for persons aged 0 through 18 years. See U.S., 2009. *Journal of the American Medical Association, 301* (7), 715.

Javitt, G. et al. (2008). Assessing mandatory HPV vaccination: Who should call the shots? *Journal of Law, Medicine & Ethics, 36,* 384-394.

Kalorama (Kalorama International). (2008). *Vaccines: World market analysis, key players, and critical trends in a fast-changing industry*. Rockville, MD: Kalmorama.

Kesselheim, A. S. (2008). Think globally, prescribe locally: How rational pharmaceutical policy in the U.S. can improve global access to essential medicines. *American Journal of Law & Medicine, 34*, 125-139.

Kmeic, D. W. (2005). Enumerated powers and unenumerated rights: *Gonzales v. Raich* and *Wickard v. Filburn* displaced. *Cato Supreme Court Review, 2004/2005*, 71-100.

Landro, L. (2008, July 9). The informed patient: Get your shots: Adults need vaccines, too; Public-health experts push for national inoculation plan; A rise in whooping cough. *Wall Street Journal*, p. D1.

Lee, G. et al. (2007). Gaps in vaccine financing for underinsured children in the U.S. *Journal of the American Medical Association, 298* (6), 638-643.

Lindsay, L. A. et al. (2006). Access to justice: The social responsibility of lawyers: Hastened death and the regulation of the practice of medicine. *Journal of Law & Politics, 22*, 1-28.

Liu, W. J. (2008). Balancing accessibility and sustainability: How to achieve the dual objectives of the Hatch-Waxman Act while resolving antitrust issues in pharmaceutical patent settlement cases. *Albany Law Journal of Science & Technology, 18*, 441-492.

McKee, G. (2006). Keeping drugs out of the toilet: The need for federal action to allow consumer drug donation. *Quinnipiac Health Law Journal, 10*, 45-76.

McQuillan, L. et al. (2009). Impact of the 2004-2005 influenza vaccine shortage on pediatric practice: A national survey. *Pediatrics, 123* (2), E186.

Miller, N. S. (2006). Failure of enforcement controlled substance laws in health policy for prescribing opiate medications: A painful assessment of morbidity and mortality. *American Journal of Therapeutics, 13* (6), 527-533.

___. (2004). Prescription opiate medications: Medical uses and consequences, uses and control. *Clinical Psychiatry, 27*, 689-708.

Morriss, A. et al. (2009). *Regulation by litigation*. New Haven, CT: Yale University Press.

Muldrew, B. L. (2004). Drug enforcement: Controlled Substances Act inapplicable to medicinal marijuana. *Journal of Law, Medicine & Ethics 32* (2), 371-372.

Noah, L. (2008). The little agency that could (act with indifference to constitutional and statutory strictures). *Cornell Law Review, 93*, 901-925.

Pauly. M. V. (2005). Improving vaccine supply and development: Who needs what? *Health Affairs, 24* (3) 680-690.

Pedersen, S. L. (2008). When Congress practices medicine: How Congressional legislation of medical judgment may infringe a fundamental right. *Touro Law Review, 24*, 791-848.

PhRMA (Pharmaceutical Research and Manufacturers Association). (2007). *Drug discovery and development*. Washington, DC: PhRMA.

Pyle, K. R. (2006). *FDA v. Ephedra*: Is it time to lift the ban? *Food & Drug Law Journal, 61*, 701-751.

Rawlins, M. D. et al. (2005). Quality, innovation, and value for money: NICE and the British National Health Service. *Journal of the American Medical Association, 294*, 2618-2622.

Rawlins, M. D., & Culyer, A. J. (2004). National Institute for Clinical Excellence and its value judgments. *British Medical Journal, 329*, 224-229.

Reinhardt, U. E. (2004). An information infrastructure for the pharmaceutical market. *Health Affairs, 23* (1), 107-112.

Reiss, J. B. et al. (2007). Your business in court. *Food & Drug Law Journal, 62*, 305-341.

Restatement (second) of torts. (1965). Philadelphia, PA: American Law Institute (national compilation and interpretation of trends in tort decisions and policy).

Restatement (third) of torts: products liability. (1998). Philadelphia, PA: American Law Institute.

Rockoff, J. (2009, March 10). Merck to buy rival for $41 billion: Schering-Plough deal is latest bid to diversify; Roche nears Genentech takeover. *Wall Street Journal*, p. A1.

Sahoo, A. (2008). *Vaccines: World market analysis, key players, and critical trends in a fast-changing industry*. New York, NY: Kalorama Information (covers current world revenues and forecasts through 2013 for pediatric and adult vaccines, and provides pipeline analysis and company profiles).

Sampat, B. N. (2009). Ensuring policy and laws are both effective and just: Academic patents and access to medicines in developing countries. *American Journal on Public Health, 99* (1), 9-18.

Schwartz, V. E. et al. (2009). Marketing pharmaceutical products in the twenty-first century: An analysis of the continued viability of traditional principles of law in the age of direct-to-consumer advertising. *Harvard Journal on Law & Public Policy, 32* (1), 333-388.

Seamon, M. J. (2006). The legal status of medical marijuana. *Annals of Pharmacotherapy, 40* (12), 2211-2215.

Seamon, M. J. et al. (2007). Medical marijuana and the developing role of the pharmacist. *American Journal on Health-System Pharmacy, 64* (10), 1037-1044.

Shell, G. R. (2004). *Make the rules or your rivals will*. New York, NY: Crown Business, Random House.

Smith, J. C. et al. (2009). Immunization policy development in the U.S.: The role of the Advisory Committee on Immunization Practices. *Annals of Internal Medicine, 150* (1), 45.

Sokol, M. C. et al. (2005). Impact of medication adherence on hospitalization risk and healthcare costs. *Medical Care, 43* (6), 523-530.

Somin, I. (2006). *Gonzales v. Raich*: Federalism as a casualty of the war on drugs. *Cornell Journal of Law & Public Policy, 15* (3), 507-550.

Temte, J. L. (2009). ACIP releases adult immunization schedule. *American Family Physician, 79* (2), 152-156.

Vagelos, R., & Galambos, L. (2004). *Medicine, science, and Merck*. New York, NY: Cambridge University Press.

Wasan, K. M. (2009). The global access initiative at the University of British Columbia (UBC): Availability of UBC discoveries and technologies to the developing world. *Journal of Pharmaceutical Science, 98* (3), 791-794.

Weeks, E. A. (2007). Beyond compensation: Using torts to promote public health. *Journal of Health Care Law & Policy, 10*, 27-59.

Wharton (Wharton School at the University of Pennsylvania). (2007). A prescription for healthier medical care decisions: Begin by defining health risk. *Knowledge@Wharton*.

___. (2006). Will it pay off, or become a write off? Managing risk in venture capital investing. *Knowledge@Wharton*.

___. (2005). After decades of malaise, the vaccine industry is getting an injection. *Knowledge@Wharton*.

Wilson, J. F. (2004). Cheaper drugs in foreign markets increase the focus on domestic drug prices. *Annals of Internal Medicine, 140* (8), 677-681.

CHAPTER 18
BIOTECHNOLOGY AND BIOPHARMACEUTICALS

> *"Since the 1980s, biotechnology has moved us, literally or figuratively, from the classroom to the boardroom and from the New England Journal of Medicine to the Wall Street Journal."*
>
> —LEON ROSENBERG, FORMER DEAN OF YALE UNIVERSITY SCHOOL OF MEDICINE

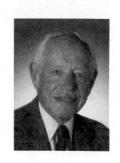

IN BRIEF

This chapter explains the laws affecting gene and protein therapy and other biotechnology fields, such as genomics, bioinformatics, and proteomics, which hold the potential to transform health care delivery. Already, there are almost two hundred marketed biopharmaceuticals worldwide, many of which have substantially impacted patients' lives. The U.S. health care industry, however, will only be able to capitalize on these opportunities if it understands this research and the legal restraints affecting these producers of medical products. The two U.S. Supreme Court decisions presented in this chapter's Fact or Fiction represent two sides of the same biotechnology patent coin. One side of the coin involves patent disputes pursuant to licensing agreements; the other side of the coin involves patent disputes where there are no licensing agreements.

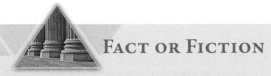

FACT OR FICTION

BIOSCIENCE RESEARCH

How should the interests of patent holders, users of patented inventions, and the general public, all involved in a bioscience patent dispute, be balanced by the courts?

The patented invention in this case was a tri-peptide. Integra Lifesciences used the tri-peptide to test its tumor-suppressing function without obtaining the patent holder's approval or first entering into a license agreement with Merck, the patent holder. Merck sued Integra Lifesciences for patent infringement.
—*Merck KGaA v. Integra Lifesciences I, Ltd.*, 545 U.S. 193 (U.S. Supreme Court 2005).

The patented invention in another case was an experimental process called coexpression technology, a research tool used to produce immunoglobulin chains in a recombinant host cell. MedImmune was assigned the right to use the coexpression technology to manufacture a drug under a license agreement with Genentech, the patent holder. MedImmune paid the demanded royalties under protest, but sought declaratory relief claiming that the patent at issue was invalid and unenforceable.
—*MedImmune, Inc. v. Genentech, Inc.*, 549 U.S. 118 (U.S. Supreme Court 2007).
(See *Law Fact* at the end of this chapter for the answer.)

PRINCIPLES AND APPLICATIONS

Over the past thirty years, biotechnology has come to represent an American success story. With 1,500 public and private companies employing tens of thousands of people, the U.S. is universally considered to be the global biotechnology leader. U.S. biotechnology companies capture about 75 percent of the global revenue in biotechnology sales (Mullen, 2007). While several global European pharmaceutical companies outsource bioscience research and development operations to the U.S., it should be noted that although the revenue may be captured in the U.S., a lot of the work associated with bringing biopharmaceuticals to market (research and development, manufacturing, fill finish, packaging, and labeling) is done outside the U.S. to take advantage of specific tax strategies.

The availability of venture capital, combined with the willingness of investors to support the development of the nation's biotechnology companies with initial public offerings, has put the U.S. as much as five to ten years ahead of Europe and Japan in developing a biotechnology industry.

The most important metric, however, is the biotechnology industry's impact on combating diseases and illnesses, including cancer, multiple sclerosis, rheumatoid arthritis, and rare genetic disorders, as illustrated in Figure 18-1. With over six hundred drugs under development for over one hundred diseases (PhRMA, 2008), the biotechnology sector has been at the forefront of scientific medical innovations. Biotechnology companies have also assumed

leadership roles in developing vaccines for pandemic influenzas.

Biotechnology will be one of the major wealth creators in the next two decades, and, even more importantly, a new science that will significantly improve the lives of health care consumers (Burns, 2005). Admittedly, there is considerable social and political debate about how to best use this emerging technology. However, health care providers cannot be on the sidelines of biotechnology; the stakes are much too high (Wharton, 2006).

CHALLENGES FACING THE BIOTECHNOLOGY INDUSTRY

Many of the same challenges facing the pharmaceutical industry in bringing new medical products and services to the market are also faced by the biotechnology sector. The challenges of getting to the market are simply magnified in the biotechnology sector, where the:

- Roles of government agencies in regulation of biotechnology products are unclear
- Need for providers of health insurance to be involved in biopharmaceuticals pricing to treat rare orphan diseases (defined as those diseases that affect fewer than two hundred thousand people) is just being worked out

Regardless of the market challenges, the potential for scientific breakthroughs is enormous, and the

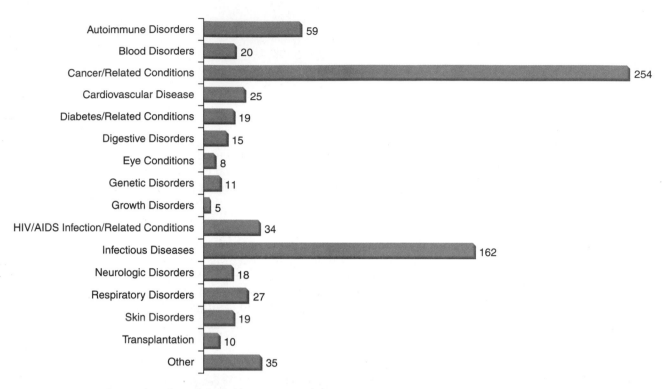

FIGURE 18-1: Biotechnology Medicines in Development

Note: Some medicines are listed in more than one category.
Delmar/Cengage Learning
Data retrieved from: PhRMA, 2008.

marketplace is responding with a willingness to continue investing in new opportunities. While the complex patterns of regulatory and scientific change in biotechnology leads to more surprises[LN1] than in traditional pharmaceutical companies, investors in the biotechnology industry must recognize that biotechnology companies are partners with the market in developing new biosciences.

Unclear Regulatory Structure

While the FDA has the mandate to regulate the biotechnology industry, federal regulations have not kept pace with the rapidly developing biosciences. Some newly emerging areas of the biotechnology industry have largely escaped regulation, such as reprogenics and synthetic biology, while other areas face regulations that appear contradictory on their faces. For instance, chemically synthesized gene therapy products meet the current drug definition but not the biologic product definition for regulation by the U.S. Food and Drug Administration (21 C.F.R. pts. 20, 312, and 601 (1993)); but RNA interference therapy does not meet the definition of human gene therapy (McKnight, 2004). Given the rate of change in the biotechnology industry, the issue is whether the current regulatory definitions should be brought up to date; certainly a more accurate definition of biologics can be provided today than was the case in 1993.

Defining and Understanding Biopharmaceuticals

The dynamic nature and complexity of biotechnology makes it difficult to understand, much less differentiate between biopharmaceutical and pharmaceutical drugs. This confusion is a potential danger that can lead to less than optimal policy and political decisions about issues involving the biotechnology industry (Pauly et al., 2005). There are no better examples of this confusion than references to:

- Global pricing of pharmaceutical and biopharmaceutical drugs
- Pharmacoeconomics and the cost-effectiveness of drug therapies
- Biopharmaceutical therapies compared to non-treatment of orphan diseases
- Similarities and clinical differences between brand-name innovator biopharmaceuticals and biosimilars

There is no consensus on these issues and, in reality, debate participants often fail to appreciate that they are using words in a variety of conflicting and imprecise ways. For instance, rare orphan drug status can be given to older drugs, if they are being used in new ways, a policy allowing biotechnology companies that did not pay development costs to receive protection from competition (Anand, 2005a).[LN2]

Definition of Pharmaceutical Drugs

Traditional pharmaceutical companies make small-molecule drugs, usually in the form of tablets and capsules. Most drugs are produced by synthesizing chemicals in a series of well-defined steps through the processes of chemistry with a predictable outcome. The chemicals have well-defined molecular structures that result from, or take part in, chemical reactions during manufacturing; the chemical reactions change the properties of the small-molecule as drugs are manufactured into pills.

Biopharmaceuticals Defined

While biopharmaceuticals are also known as bioengineered drugs, biotechnology drugs, and specialty pharmaceuticals (the term health insurance providers use), this chapter consistently uses the term *biopharmaceutical* to refer to drug molecule proteins manufactured in living cells, as distinguished from the term *pharmaceuticals*, which refers to small-molecule drugs produced by synthesizing chemicals. In other words, biopharmaceuticals are engineered from living cells instead of from chemical molecules like most pharmaceuticals (*see* Walsh, 2003).

Biopharmaceuticals are a new class of drugs derived from proteins manufactured in living cells. Bioscience scientists usually use DNA technology to splice genetic material into bacterial, yeast, or mammalian cells, which then produce proteins. A single molecule of these proteins may weigh one hundred times as much as a single molecule of the active ingredient in Lipitor (atorvastatin), the world's best-selling brand-name cholesterol-lowering drug manufactured by Pfizer. However, biopharmaceuticals are not made by chemical synthesis. Biopharmaceuticals are often made from Chinese hamster ovary cells (Jayapal et al., 2007) or an *E. coli* bacterium, through a very complex manufacturing route. It is the complexity of the production process, of coaxing live cells in a sterile, temperature-controlled environment to make biological matter, that makes biopharmaceuticals so expensive to produce.

Since biopharmaceuticals interfere with the way a disease causes damage, rather than treating the consequences of a disease, the risks of taking biopharmaceuticals are significant and often unpredictable. The hope is that biopharmaceuticals can, eventually, be individually tailored to the person taking the drug and that their benefits will generally outweigh their risks. At the current time, however, it must be said that personalized medicine is still out on the horizon in all but a few instances.

GLOBAL DRUG PRICING

Significant biopharmaceutical advances in treatments for Alzheimer's, cancer, diabetes, and other diseases are all but inevitable in the coming years. The biotechnology industry, however, is courting disaster with pricing policies that appear divorced from the economic benefits its drugs provide (Vagelos, 2004).

Research from the Wharton School at the University of Pennsylvania found that per capita spending on biopharmaceuticals is at least twice as high in the U.S. as in the other countries. This difference reflects primarily greater availability and use of new, relatively high-priced molecules and formulations. Prices for identical formulations are not higher on average in the U.S. The broader price indexes, which do not control formulation, are also not higher in the U.S., after adjusting for income. In summary, while the U.S. might spend more on biopharmaceuticals, prices are not noticeably higher (Danzon & Furukawa, 2006).

Problem: Drug Prices Unrelated to Value

Regulatory scrutiny of price controls or introduction of biosimilars is a possibility where economic standards are breached (Bouchard, 2007). For instance:

- Cancer drug that extends the life of patients by a few months but does not treat the underlying cancer, priced at hundreds of thousands of dollars
- Drug formulation of two separately available drugs that delivers a marginal improvement in effectiveness, but at double the price

Although high prices for drugs without profound medical value cannot be justified, the biotechnology industry continues to have vast potential to improve the health of individuals and society.

Moral Dilemmas

1. Should the free market dictate biopharmaceutical price points, or is it the government's fiduciary responsibility to ensure adequate patient access to these therapies?

Biopharmaceuticals Compared to Non-Treatment of Rare Orphan Diseases

Orphan diseases are so–called because no one was treating them before Congress enacted the Orphan Drug Act of 1983, 21 U.S.C.A. §§ 360aa *et seq.* (2009). Congress originally envisioned the development of drugs for rare orphan diseases as a sideline for the pharmaceutical industry to treat neglected diseases affecting small numbers of people; however, it has become a multibillion-dollar business for biotechnology companies.

Once the FDA certifies a drug with orphan status, companies have seven years of market exclusivity; in effect, companies are granted the same market protection as a drug patent would provide. Even after the seven-year exclusivity period expires, there is often no competition for drugs because there is no federal process for gaining approval of biosimilar versions of biotechnology drugs.

Orphan drug protection compares to pharmaceutical drug patents that have an average effective life of eleven years due to generic competition. While the law provides that drug patents have seventeen years of market exclusivity from the date of issue to twenty years from the date of application, with the longer of the two terms allowed for some drugs already on the market, the effective market exclusivity of drugs with sales over $100 million has been reduced to eleven years due to generic competition (Grabowski & Kyle, 2007). Another difference is that, unlike patents for new drug discoveries, a drug that has been on the market for other diseases or used in other countries can be given orphan drug status.

While competing patent claims often face lengthy court battles, orphan drugs are protected by the FDA, which is barred by law from approving another drug with the same active ingredient unless the new drug is proven clinically superior. The law also grants companies a 50 percent tax credit for research and development, grant money to defray the costs of clinical testing, and assistance in obtaining regulatory approval.

Similarities and Clinical Differences Between Innovator Biopharmaceuticals and Biosimilars

There is no federal process for gaining approval of biosimilar versions of innovator biopharmaceuticals. The term *biosimilars* is used in this text to refer to bio-generics, follow-on protein biologics, biocomparables, off-patent or multi-source biopharmaceuticals, or other terms for generic versions of biopharmaceuticals. FDA regulations for industrial laboratory manufacturing are distinct from regulations for production of therapeutic compounds produced by cellular processes.

Generic Versions of Traditional Pharmaceutical Drugs

For traditional pharmaceutical drugs, a generics manufacturer must merely show that its product has the same active ingredient, route of administration, dosage form and strength, and proposed labeling as the brand-name drug (*see* 21 U.S.C.A. § 355(j)(5)(B)(iv) (2008)). Furthermore, the generic producer must show bioequivalence to the original brand-name drug to win FDA approval. Bioequivalence is defined as "the absence of a significant difference in the rate and extent to which the active ingredient or active moiety in pharmaceutical equivalents or pharmaceutical alternatives becomes available at the site of drug action when administered at the same molar dose under similar conditions in an appropriately designed study."[LN3] *See* 21 C.F.R. §320.1(e) (2009).

Bioequivalence is very different from therapeutic equivalence or equivalence in how the human body metabolizes a drug. For instance, the active molecule in generic drugs may be a bioequivalent to the brand-name drug's active ingredients, but their absorption rates may vary by as much as 40 percent under provisions of the Hatch-Waxman law; this means their bioequivalency may be 20 percent more or 20 percent less than the brand-name drug. The critical distinction is that brand-name drugs also have this 20 percent range of bioequivalence; meaning a brand-name drug may be 20 percent more effective in some patients and 20 percent less effective in other patients. So, in effect, a bioequivalent generic drug may be 40 percent less effective than a brand-name drug if it is manufactured at the lower end of the bioequivalent curve, and the generic will still be termed equivalent.

There is no requirement that generics be exactly the same; there is no mandated actual therapeutic equivalence, as most consumers of health care believe there to be. Nor is there any requirement for bioequivalency in drug delivery mechanisms, meaning some generics may come with side effects not found in the brand-name drugs, such as:

- Headaches from dyes that make generics look similar to brand-name drugs
- Heartburn, acid indigestion, or upset stomach related to ingestion of lower quality capsule and tablet fillers
- Hives or other skin irritations from less expensive raw materials used in the formulation of generics
- Other physical discomforts or illnesses from contamination during the production and manufacturing of generics

(*See* Favole, 2008, for information on deaths from use of generic heparin)

The therapeutic effectiveness of generic drug delivery mechanisms varies from manufacturer to manufacturer.

Biosimilar Versions of Innovator Biopharmaceuticals

Currently, no regulations exist in the U.S. for evaluation, based on comparative, abbreviated applications or designations of therapeutic equivalence, and approval of biopharmaceuticals as generics. Similarly, there is no accepted or recognized definition for generics of biopharmaceuticals.

While the technical question about bioequivalence may not pose an insurmountable obstacle for biosimilar versions of innovator biopharmaceuticals that replace natural proteins in the body, no generic manufacturer has yet been successful in obtaining FDA approval for a biosimilar in the U.S. The FDA

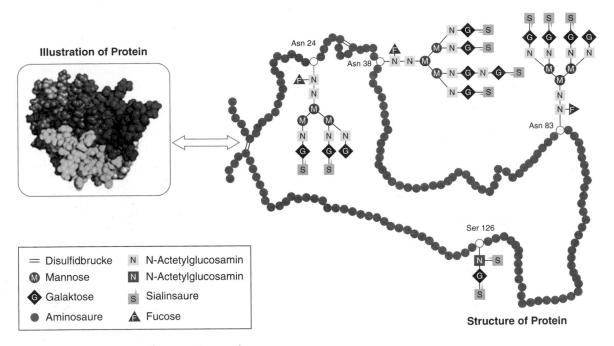

Illustration of Protein

Structure of Protein

= Disulfidbrucke	N	N-Actetylglucosamin
M Mannose	N	N-Actetylglucosamin
G Galaktose	S	Sialinsaure
Aminosaure	A	Fucose

FIGURE 18-2: Structure of Amgen's Erythropoietin

Delmar/Cengage Learning

has indicated that approval criterion for biosimilar versions of innovator biopharmaceuticals is a matter for Congress to determine; this is an acknowledgment that its model of drug development for pharmaceuticals is not suitable for approval of biosimilars. For instance, generic manufacturers have not been able to obtain regulatory approval of Amgen's Erythropoietin, as illustrated in Figure 18-2[LN4] and generally referred to as EPO. Erythropoietin is used for treating anemia resulting from:

- Chronic kidney disease
- Treatments for cancer
- Other critical illnesses

Many agree that current technology may present an insuperable barrier for the more complex biopharmaceuticals used to treat autoimmune diseases and cancer (Noah, 2006). The Biotechnology Industry Organization, a Washington, D.C., trade group, goes as far as to claim that it is not technologically possible to develop generic biopharmaceuticals without spending tens of millions of dollars for full clinical trials to obtain FDA approval. However, biosimilars have been approved in other countries, such as Japan. The Connors Group, a California-based trading firm, maintains that once a global standard has been established, it may become easier for U.S. regulatory authorities to recognize, adopt, accommodate, or modify international generic regulations for the biotechnology industry.

Credible Placebos

Some lower grade generic drugs could be compared to credible placebo drugs. Both types of drugs have a role in medical treatments. Credible placebos can help relieve and sometimes even cure physical and mental ailments (Wager, 2004) and depression (Ariely, 2009).

Placebo effects are now detectable with functional magnetic resonance imaging, where placebo effects account for both lower reported pain and reduced activity in pain-processing areas of the brain (Wager, 2004). Placebo effects are even detectable on the price of drugs; consumers of health care who buy cold medicine at discount prices report significantly worse medical outcomes than those who pay list price (Ariely, 2009). While placebo effects have long been shown to be pervasive, findings of pricing effects on physical ailments are relatively new. It should be understood, nevertheless, that the placebo effect is normally a short-term effect and only curative in rare examples.

With increasing evidence about the robustness of placebo effects, the American Medical Association recently issued an opinion against the use of placebos for clinical purposes (Kolber, 2007). More generally, a series of studies demonstrates a strong top-down effect of expectation on experience; if there is an expectation something will taste bad, the actual experience is worse than if there had been no biased expectation (Ariely, 2009). Recently, the connection between expectations and experience has been demonstrated at the neural level as well (Plassmann et al., 2007). The short-term nature of this placebo effect could confound the data derived from placebo-controlled clinical trials. Clearly, the placebo effect makes it difficult to use studies that test a new treatment side-by-side against an existing one and determine whether the new treatment works (Lynch, 2007). The question remains, can the therapeutic equivalence of generic and brand-name drugs be accurately tested?

Complexity of the Biotechnology Sector

While bioscience scientists struggle to understand the workings of the human body, biotechnology managers and investors are searching for ways to gain a greater understanding of the complexity in the biotechnology sector. The founding of Genentech in 1976 launched the biotechnology industry;[LN5] Genentech was the first company to successfully engineer drugs from living cells, instead of engineering drugs from chemicals in test tubes, which is the same process the pharmaceutical industry has used for more than 250 years.

Compared to other industries where few founders are academics, more than 40 percent of those founding biotechnology companies are academics, primarily from MIT and Stanford (Keusch, 2008). This movement of people has proved to be an important means for translating early-stage upstream research, characteristic of university-based bioscience, to product development and commercialization. Moreover, while this degree of movement of people from the academic to the corporate sector is unique to the biotechnology industry, it is consistent with the tendency for biotechnology companies to cluster around universities (Kesselheim, 2008). Academics are founders in companies mainly in the fields of biotechnology, pharmaceuticals, fine organic chemistry, and information and communications technology; however, the biotechnology industry is unique in the absolute number of academics that have founded biotechnology companies, as well as the percentage of the total industry that is comprised of former academics (Evans, 2008). A similar trend in England highlights the success of Cambridge Enterprise, the University of Cambridge's knowledge and technology transfer services company.

With between three hundred and four hundred public biotechnology companies, total sales revenue for the U.S. biotechnology industry exceeded $30 billion in 2007 (Mathews & Abboud, 2007). Further, despite advances in biotechnology, production of biopharmaceuticals via synthesis, tissue culture, or genetic manipulation often remains uneconomical for most companies (Frisvold & Day-Rubenstein, 2008).

While biotechnology may have the distinction of being the biggest money-losing sector of the health care industry (Pisano, 2006), and while the biotechnology sector is often described as an industry that hemorrhages money, biotechnology still attracts investors. Industry-university cooperation in biotechnology research and development is still advancing.

The nation's leading research universities have research and development departments, or knowledge transfer offices, as well as companies that provide commercialization services to the universities. The creation of research-owning companies provides medical research departments with the requisite legal capacity to enter into contracts for the development of medical products. With Genentech the exception to characterizations of this medical products sector, a sector more often than not characterized as having a steady flow of financial losses and a stream of high-profile failures, investors still hope to be a part of the "next" Genentech.

Inexplicable Future Possibilities

Bioscience differs from other medical technologies that have reconfigured the business landscape for the last two centuries in that the research underlying product development is far less easily understood (Huston, 2007). For instance, while the basic concept of coronary stents can be understood, what is happening in bioscience is more complex:

- Bioinformatics (using computers to create information databases that permit analyses of genomes, protein sequences, biomolecules, and other organic matter)
- Genomics (the study of genomes, including gene mapping, which involves figuring out the positions of genes on a DNA molecule)
- Proteomics (the cataloguing and analyzing of proteins in cells and tissue)

(Wharton, 2002)

Leading Biotechnology Companies in Dow Jones U.S. Biotechnology Index[LN6]					
	Market Cap (in billions)	Sales Revenue (in billions)	P/E Ratio	CAGR	ROI
Genentech	$45	$4	26	19%	21%
Amgen	$61	$15	15	13%	(32%)
Gilead Biosciences	$46	$4	25	34%	42%
Data derived from 2008 corporate reports to the U.S. Securities and Exchange Commission.					

Even scientists in the research and development areas of biotechnology companies are not completely certain what the future possibilities are for bioinformatics, genomics, and proteomics. The uncertainty factor is much greater in bioscience than with other medical technologies because there is much to understand and developments are occurring at a rapid pace. Also affected will be chemicals, agriculture (plant genetics), consumer products, information technology, and life and health insurers, where the potential use of genetic profiles to decide who gets coverage and at what cost has already generated debate. It is difficult to keep up with the stories about advances in biotechnology without feeling lost. Genomics, reprogenics, synthetic biology, and the rest of the biotechnology arsenal seem like something out of science fiction, but they are very real and potentially highly profitable (Wharton, 2006).

Moral Dilemmas

1. Should life and health insurers be permitted to use customers' personal genetic information in order to make coverage decisions?

Value-Added Medical Treatments

Most health care professionals, including physicians, are not trained in genomics, so they must also learn about the rapid advances in biopharmaceuticals for medical treatments. One way to look at genomics and the other biosciences is from the perspective of the value chain (Porter & Teisberg, 2006). A value chain is a set of activities that directly add value to a product or process.

In health care, bioscience research holds significant promise for patients facing serious illnesses, rare diseases, or life threatening conditions. The biotechnology industry, however, must understand and overcome the barriers to seeing that promise realized by rank-and-file health care professionals and the consumers of health care. Overcoming those barriers is how the biotechnology sector can add value to the health care industry and move forward within it.

In fact, today's biotechnology industry can be compared to the far-reaching changes ushered in by silicon chips, or, to go further back in time, petrochemicals and plastics. Fifty years ago, the microchip revolutionized the way the world computes, calculates, and communicates, ushering in the Information Age. These component materials remade society in pervasive and sometimes unexpected ways, forcing legal institutions to adapt old strategies to meet the new challenges. For instance, biotechnology did away with the traditional distinction between drugs and biologics; nanomedicine may do the same to the line separating devices and biologics. No one now would deny that regulatory agencies or courts have failed to appreciate these forces and design uniform responses (*see generally* Noah, 2006).

Moral Dilemmas

1. What will it take for traditional physicians and hospitals to use new biotechnologies in the diagnosis and treatment of patients with given diseases?

DRIVERS OF BIOSCIENCE

With about three hundred biopharmaceuticals in late-stage clinical trials, the long view of the biotechnology industry actually looks very promising (Mullen, 2007). Advancements in biology and chemistry have increased the volume and quality of potential drugs undergoing research, especially as the number of young biotechnology firms, aided by financing in the late 1990s, is growing (*compare* Zhang, 2009 regarding the effect of the recent economic recession on the biotechnology industry).

Seven key forces are driving this change in bioscience and in the biotechnology industry, in particular:

- Capital availability
- Market conditions, such as an aging population
- Maturing pharmaceutical sector
- Movement toward personalized medicine
- Ongoing consolidation and shakeout in the biotechnology industry
- Pricing pressure
- Value-creating innovations, such as predictive medicine and gene-guided drug development

(Day & Schoemaker, 2004)

One ongoing challenge is that of being able to manipulate the human genome, the genetic material in chromosomes (Wharton, 2002). Large-scale computers, greater than anything currently on the market, will eventually analyze gene structures and the flaws in them. When this technological challenge is met, genomics will allow for the advancement of personalized medicine with the ability to custom-tailor medicine to a patient's particular combination of genes and defects.

**Personalized Medicine
as a Major Wealth Creator**

As the scientific breakthrough of personalized medicine occurs and the world's medical community moves away from the trial-and-error approach to medical diagnostics and treatment, the biotechnology industry should become one of the major wealth creators in the U.S. Biopharmaceutical care is currently seeing greater customization to the unique needs of individual patients in targeted cancer treatments and the expansion of coordinated care programs for patients with specialized medical needs.

The importance of maintaining this leadership role is critical as the nation seeks to control health care costs and expand health insurance coverage. Advances in genetic testing will help physicians and other health care professionals predict the benefits and risks of drugs for each patient, so that decisions about drug selection and dosing can be more accurate and cost-effective (Medco, 2007).

In addition, the biotechnology industry is a key component of stability and future growth for the U.S. economy. U.S. biotechnology companies:

- Are net exporters in foreign trade, at a time when the U.S. is facing severe declines in its exportable products
- Capture most of the revenue in the U.S. from research, development, and manufacturing at a time when the nation is facing one of the highest trade deficits in the nation's history
- Have a highly educated, well-paid workforce, at a time of high unemployment of all socioeconomic classes

(Mullen, 2007)

With declining exports, massive trade deficits, and unemployment being national concerns, the immediate focus must be on the economic stimulus of U.S. industries that will contribute to future U.S. prosperity (Geithner, 2009). Closely related to this stimulus is reform of the regulatory regime of the U.S. health care system and supervision of large medical products companies by the various federal authorities.

Effects of a Stumble or Fumble

If the U.S. stumbles in its support of the biotechnology sector or fumbles regulatory overhaul of the nation's health care system, China, India, Singapore, and other emerging countries will gladly seize the leadership role in biotechnology and medicine. These countries are already actively courting global biotechnology companies, and offering a persuasive blend of financial incentives with lower corporate taxes, improving intellectual property laws, and a vast pool of scientific talent and expertise (Mathews & Abboud, 2007).

American "Canism"

While helping to maintain the economic leadership of the U.S., the biotechnology industry and new biosciences could significantly improve the lives of consumers of health care. The biotechnology industry should quickly mature as it gives birth to new

biosciences and innovative medical technologies. Innovations beyond anyone's imagination will develop and become reality. Further, the potential opportunity for real health care reform will present itself to innovative health care companies that are able to attract individuals trained to think outside their traditional roles.

There are those who think this sounds promising, yet very idealistic, considering the lack of equal access to health care in the U.S. at this time. They ask whether biotechnology will somehow help overcome this disparity in delivery of health care and whether the medical advances arising from the new biosciences will be affordable and accessible to the masses. Above all, they cannot envision how what is still a rather uneconomic enterprise could possibly transform health care.

Yet, the Renaissance, the Industrial Revolution, and the Information Age each represented great leaps forward in human potential; the genetic age promises another exponential increase in human knowledge and potential (Rifkin, 1998). Expanding on this prediction, many believe that once biotechnology has achieved this promise, all that must be done is to make U.S. biotechnology products and biopharmaceuticals accessible and affordable and provide them to the rest of the world.

EMERGING BIOSCIENCE TECHNOLOGIES

Today, advances in health information technology have led to industrialized methods of research where tens of thousands of experiments can be done simultaneously, such as:

- Computational biology, which applies the techniques of computer science, applied mathematics, and statistics to address phenomena in biology
- Microfluidics, which makes it possible to perform tasks such as analyzing DNA sequences by taking advantage of the chemical properties of liquids and gases with the electrical properties of semiconductors by combining them on a single microchip
- Ultra-high throughput screening that screens and analyzes thousands of genes or molecules at a time versus conventional screening that screens one gene or molecule at a time to see which items are active in particular conditions[LN7]

Bioscience has a confluence of multiple streams of technology, from gene sequencing to traditional molecular biology to information technology. Other medical technologies are just emerging into their own fields, such as:

- Stem cell research
- Reprogenics
- Synthetic biology

The announcement regarding mapping of the human genome made worldwide news. Whether more than a handful of bioscience scientists really understood what this meant at the time is unclear. For even though scientists have successfully sequenced the human genome, they still lack a clear picture of exactly how coding and non-coding DNA sequences function together, or how genomes evolve over time (Moran, 2009).

RNA Interference (RNAi)

At least three large global pharmaceutical companies have product development deals with biotechnology companies that support DNA-directed RNAi, the emerging area of bioscience research that involves blocking disease-causing proteins using technology in RNA interference. Such technology is used in developing treatments for diseases such as HIV/AIDS, hepatitis C, cancer, and autoimmune diseases (Wiegel, 2007). In cancer treatments, therapeutic RNA pairs up with cancer cell RNA, triggering an immune response that both destroys RNA strands and starves the cancer cell of necessary proteins (Mandel, 2008).

AstraZeneca, Merck, and Pfizer have records of accomplishment of making the right calls at the right time when acquiring and striking drug development deals with smaller biotechnology companies, so this bioscience technology should be monitored for opportunities. The fact that RNAi technology is also used to produce decaffeinated coffee plants is simply another business opportunity that helps pharmaceutical companies offset the cyclicality and risks of the drug industry (Ogita et al., 2003; Karnitschnig & Rockoff, 2009).

Telomerase Technology

Another emerging science, telomere biology, hints at the prospect of enhancing life spans. Parts of the human chromosomes called telomeres serve as a genetic clock for cellular aging. Telomeres shorten with each division of the cell and, at a certain length, they turn off the division process, which seems to lead to destructive effects. On the other hand, an enzyme called telomerase is capable of restoring telomere length, or resetting the clock, thereby increasing the lifespan of cells.

Geron, a California biotechnology company, has focused its telomerase technology on goals such as improved wound healing and cancer treatments. While Geron has never suggested its products will allow people to live forever, the National Science Foundation sees science quickly turning fiction into factual possibilities (National Science Board, 2009).

A company based out of New York City, TA Biosciences, licensed the single molecule that activates the telomerase gene from Geron and developed a nutraceutical to help manage aging. The downside is that the pill must be taken on an ongoing basis and costs about $23,000 a year, unless you are over forty and an employee of TA Biosciences. The company is also developing cosmeceutical products, which are new esthetician products emerging from the convergence of the cosmetic and pharmaceutical industries and directed at the high-end consumer market that purchases anti-aging skin treatments, body creams, and lotions.

CONVERGENT TECHNOLOGY

The National Science Foundation has taken a leadership role in determining how nanotechnology, biotechnology, information technology, and cognitive science can combine in what has been termed *convergent technology*. The driver in convergent technology is the life biosciences, where the focus is on enhancing both human performance and productivity (Johansen, 2003).

While some envision a time in the twenty-first century when death may become indefinite (Roco & Bainbridge, 2003), the immediate focus is on what is possible with regard to ability-enhancing technologies.[LN8] Many see the health care industry at the threshold of a renaissance in knowledge, based on the structure and behavior of matter from the nanoscale up to the complex system of the human brain (Wharton, 2006).

Examples of the revolutionary changes in health care might include:

- Advancing human capabilities for reproductive purposes
- Ameliorating the physical and cognitive decline common to the aging mind
- Developing highly effective communication techniques, including brain-to-brain interactions
- Early disease detection (Lieber, 2007)
- Enhancing individual sensory and cognitive capabilities
- Improving both individual and group efficiency
- Perfecting human-to-machine interfaces

Moral Dilemmas

1. When do technological advancements, which create the possibility of a virtual "fountain of youth," lead into ethical and moral concerns?

EMERGING AREAS OF BIOSCIENCE RESEARCH

Biopharmaceuticals have become some of the most important, and expensive, medical treatments in health care. Annual spending on biopharmaceuticals that treat small patient populations with chronic or life-threatening diseases represents a growing component of pharmacy spending.

For instance, Genzyme, a Cambridge-based biotechnology company, posts sales in excess of $1 billion annually on its drug for Gaucher disease, a rare, sometimes fatal disease that causes certain organs to swell and bones to deteriorate (Anand, 2005a; Lieber, 2007). Treating the average patient costs $200,000 annually, but the price of the drug at the highest dose levels (for patients who have used the drug for prolonged periods and developed a tolerance for its usual response) can run as high as $600,000 a year for adults on the higher of two recommended doses (Anand, 2005b).

The philosophy of the biotechnology industry has always been to create medicines to fill unmet needs and to recoup its research and development investment by obtaining patents and charging premium prices for its products and services. The National Science Board, however, is concerned with declining public support for expensive biopharmaceuticals. Over the past decade, there has been a decline in basic research funds from the federal government for biosciences research and development, as biosciences ran into political windstorms of ideology questioning the merits of advanced science (National Science Board, 2009).

Historically, biotechnology innovation in the U.S. has benefited from relatively free pricing. For instance, Genzyme follows an extremely disciplined *full price or free* strategy; it locates patients, donates its drug at first, and then pressures the government and private insurers to be paid the full retail price (Heuser, 2009). This invisible hand has allowed the biotechnology industry to attract investors to fund research projects that take approximately ten to fifteen years and more than $1 billion apiece to bring to market (Mullen, 2007).

PRICING OF BIOPHARMACEUTICALS

Biotechnology Industry Organization v. District of Columbia
[Biotechnology's Trade Association v. District]
496 F.3d 1362 (U.S. Court of Appeals for the Federal Circuit 2007),
rehearing en banc denied, 505 F.3d 1343 (U.S. Court of Appeals for the Federal Circuit 2007)

FACTS: The District of Columbia City Council adopted the Excessive Pricing Act (EPA), which prohibits any drug from being sold in the District for an excessive price. The operative section of the EPA reads: "It shall be unlawful for any drug manufacturer or licensee thereof, excluding a point of sale retail seller, to sell or supply for sale or impose minimum resale requirements for a patented prescription drug that results in the prescription drug being sold in the District for an excessive price." D.C. Code § 28-4553, held unconstitutional at the trial level by *Pharmaceutical Research and Mfrs. of America v. District of Columbia*, 406 F.Supp.2d 56 (U.S. District Court for the District of Columbia 2005). The Council determined that, since excessive drug prices were threatening the health of the District's residents, as well as the District government's ability to ensure its residents received basic health care, it was incumbent on the District to restrain the prices.

Evidence of excessive pricing was to be established where the wholesale price of a drug was over 30 percent higher than comparable prices in other high-income countries (like England, Germany, Canada, or Australia, where governments negotiate drug prices with the pharmaceutical and biotechnology companies). Once excessive pricing was shown, the burden shifted to the companies to prove that a given drug was not excessively priced given the costs of invention, development, production, global sales, profits, consideration of any government-funded research that supported development of the drug, and the impact of price on access to the drug by District residents. The EPA provided for an array of remedies, including injunctions, fines, treble damages, attorney's fees, and litigation costs.

ISSUE: Was the EPA pre-empted by federal patent law?

HOLDING AND DECISION: Yes, the EPA impermissibly attempted to regulate an area of law Congress intended to control.

(continues)

(continued)

ANALYSIS: The pharmaceutical and biotechnology companies sought to show that federal patent laws pre-empted the EPA in order to have the law declared unenforceable. The court determined that whether the EPA was actually enforced or not, its existence was likely to cause the companies to incur expenses in an effort to comply with it. While the EPA did not directly regulate prices, it regulated the company's activities, which could have resulted in more excessive drug prices.

Although there is no express provision in federal patent law to prevent regulation of drug prices, the EPA must yield to federal law if it obstructs the purpose of a federal law. This is the purpose of the Supremacy Clause in the U.S. Constitution. The pharmaceutical and biotechnology companies claimed the EPA offended Congress's intention to provide patent holders with the opportunity to secure the financial rewards that follow from the exclusive rights granted by drug patents.

The court found pharmaceutical and biotechnology companies undertake their research efforts with the expectation that they will be able to obtain a drug patent to protect the forthcoming financial rewards of their drug development efforts. A drug patent grants the companies exclusivity over their brand-name drugs, meaning generics are prohibited from copying brand-name drugs or selling them for a certain length of time. Encouragement of research and development is the fundamental purpose of drug patents, and is based directly on the right to exclude generics.

The court specifically recognized the importance of providing financial incentives to innovative drug companies to continue their costly development efforts. The court endorsed competition by determining that financial rewards during the period of patent exclusivity were the carrot to encourage investments, and that the marketplace should be the only limitation on the size of the carrot, rather than government regulation or judicial feats.

The court went on to explain why drug patents are granted for a limited time; once that time expires, drug prices will be lowered by competition. In this way, innovator drugs first benefit the patent-holder with profit exclusivity, and then benefit the public through liberated use, resulting in competition and lower prices. This is how Congress intended to resolve the tension between the interests of the pharmaceutical and biotechnology companies and the public's interests. The EPA was an attempt to shift the benefit away from the companies and toward the public earlier in the drug patent's lifetime than Congress intended and was thus void. The District impermissibly attempted to change federal patent policy within its borders.

RULE OF LAW: The EPA violated the Supremacy Clause of the U.S. Constitution by seeking to control an area of law that Congress intended to control, and was therefore pre-empted by federal patent law.

(*See generally* Lockwood, 2009; Ross, 2007).

Genomics and Reprogenics

In the field of genomics, a great deal of attention is focused on the emergence of new therapeutic drugs. However, advances in genomics also hold promise for other health care businesses as the source of future treatments is being developed. The companies that will make significant money in the short run are diagnostics companies and computer manufacturers serving the health information technology sector (Burns, 2005). As more individuals consent to genetic diagnostics and participate in biobanking, there will be a need to process and data-mine this information for use by the medical products industry. Therefore, while new personalized therapeutic drugs are promising in the long term, diagnostics companies and

computer manufacturers will bring in the revenue and profits in the short term.

Therapies to modify genes into building more muscle are another avenue of research. The University of Pennsylvania has been a leading institution in this effort. Through the use of a virus, leg muscle genes of mice have been altered to increase the amount of a substance called insulin-like growth factor I (IGF-1). IGF-1 activates so-called satellite muscle cells, which create new cells that repair muscle tissue. As the mice aged, the genetically enhanced leg muscles were the same size and strength as they were in young mice.

Research like this demonstrates the potential of gene therapy to enhance people in their prime.

In young adult mice, the gene treatment increased muscle strength by 15 percent versus untreated muscle. More recently, a hybrid mouse was created out of one strain with muscular dystrophy symptoms and another strain with high levels of IGF-1. The results were promising, with increases in muscle mass and muscle force, along with a reduction in muscle cell death (Parsons, 2007). Scientists at the University of Alabama at Birmingham School of Medicine have also shown that muscular mice result from blocking the gene for a growth regulator named myostatin (Bamman, 2008).

Genomic Esthetics: Nutraceuticals and Cosmeceuticals

Several consumer products companies, many of which are subsidiaries of global pharmaceutical companies, have changed the way they produce products because of their new knowledge in genomics. New aesthetic products in areas such as hair care, skin care, nutrition, and weight management are being introduced.

In the future, product design will be based on looking at consumers' genomes (Wharton, 2006). For instance, a person's genes will determine the design of skin care products. To address wrinkling, bioscience research is seeking to define what proteins can be managed within and between cells to cause certain effects that eliminate wrinkles. Some of the new wrinkle filler concentrates on the market are produced using nanotechnology and, while very expensive, are well-regarded in the high-end medical esthetician market. It is a matter of getting product development worked down to the level of impacting the cells, rather than relying on more surface-oriented empirical observations.

PHARMACEUTICAL AND BIOTECHNOLOGY REPOSITIONING AND RESTRUCTURING

Three to four hundred biotechnology companies are public entities. Most of the remaining 1,100 to 1,200 biotechnology companies are positioning themselves to survive until the day they go public or are acquired by a larger pharmaceutical or biotechnology company.

Merger of Pharmaceuticals and Biotechnology

There is a convergence of pharmaceuticals and biotechnology. Growing numbers of pharmaceutical companies are depending on biotechnology for:

- New products
- New technologies
- Scientific innovation

Biotechnology is also poised to reap the benefits of new medical technologies, including:

- Gene therapy
- Products from genomics and proteomics

While there has been some economic reward for the creation and use of biotechnology tools, the anticipated cash streams from the sale of drugs based on genomic and/or proteomics discoveries may take a decade or two longer than first anticipated (Burns, 2005). There is considerable debate about what direction the medical products industry will take in the next decade as it awaits these discoveries to come to fruition.

Some maintain that the recent trend toward consolidation of the biotechnology industry will continue as larger biotechnology companies seek to enhance their own pipelines and smaller firms hope to leverage a partner's expertise in regulatory procedure and marketing (Day & Schoemaker, 2004). Others suggest the consolidations in the medical products industry will only go so far; historically, waves of consolidation end when larger, healthier companies grow reluctant to take on troubled smaller firms (Treu, 2003). In past cycles, the consolidation process never fully played out; each time a wave of consolidation neared, the financing window opened up and saved all the biotechnology companies from the pain of merging with another company (Day & Schoemaker, 2004).

Strategic Alliances

Biotechnology companies are increasingly turning to global pharmaceutical firms, which have a need for new drugs to fill their vast marketing channels, particularly now that the biotechnology companies face a dearth of new products coming out of their own laboratories (Wharton, 2006). It has been noted that the:

- Biotechnology industry is opportunity long and capital short
- Pharmaceutical industry is capital long and opportunity short

(Treu, 2003)

Licensing

The pace of biotechnology-pharmaceutical licensing deals is slowing because many of the most promising projects have already been acquired. Some products will continue to become available as global pharmaceuticals merge and spin out compounds that do not fit with their larger corporate strategies. Moreover, smaller biotechnology companies can use partnerships with their larger corporate brethren or global pharmaceuticals as validation that their science is valuable.

GlaxoSmithKline (GSK), the world's second-largest pharmaceutical company, has made licensing a critical part of its research and development strategy. GSK licenses about ten potential drugs from other companies each year, preferring to buy late-stage products because of the lower risk. The corporate resources and its global sales force give GSK an advantage in competing for promising drugs, since size is very important in the medical products industry; success in final clinical development requires a worldwide infrastructure (Garnier, 2007).

Need for Capital Investments

One thing is certain: the nation's public and private biotechnology companies need vast amounts of capital. With combined assets of $43 billion in the nation's biotechnology industry, if all of them were to push a product through the clinical development pipeline, they would need more than $3.2 trillion ($3,200,000,000,000) (Frank, 2007). This is:

- Significantly less than the $9 trillion and counting for the bailout of the U.S. financial industry, only this would not be a bailout investment
- Equivalent to Germany's gross domestic product (*gross domestic product* is generally defined as the total cost of all goods and services produced within a country over a one-year period)
- A little more than the $2.8 trillion in total federal expenditures for all government activities in America in 2007

(CBO, 2007; Hilsenrath, 2008)

At this point, perhaps the National Science Board is correct and American taxpayers should be willing to loan trillions of dollars to the biotechnology industry (National Science Board, 2009); at least, the global population would have the possibility of better health. The investment might even ensure the U.S. retains its competitive standing as a global leader in biotechnology while acting as an economic engine of growth.

Venture Capital Investments

Global pharmaceutical companies have also acted as venture capitalists in the biotechnology industry to varying degrees over the past two decades. A few pharmaceutical companies, like Johnson & Johnson,[LN9] have been long-term players, while others step in and out of the role of venture backer, like Wyeth.

Pharmaceutical companies often begin by investing in venture capital funds. They then gain enough knowledge and confidence to make their own direct investments in biotechnology. Next, a management change determines it is not strategic, so they merge the biotechnology firm into their own research and development division, where interest in biotechnology flags, and the pharmaceutical exits the venture business (Wharton, 2006). The venture process then repeats itself in ten years (Day & Schoemaker, 2004).

Repositioning of Chemical Compounds

Another major trend bolstering the convergence of the pharmaceutical and biotechnology industries is the repositioning of chemical compounds by pharmaceuticals. Pharmaceutical companies eager to fill weak drug pipelines are going back into product portfolios to test old drugs for new uses (Wharton, 2006). Since the products have already been proven safe, development time and costs are reduced. Companies are also looking abroad for successful compounds that could be introduced in the U.S. market. Then there are always the serendipitous medical discoveries like Viagra, a drug originally developed to treat angina; while the clinical study participants reported little success with treating their angina, they did report an alternate pleasant surprise.

Moral Dilemmas

1. What will it take for developments in biotechnology to filter into everyday medical practice, and who is going to pay for it?

MANAGEMENT OF NEW SCIENTIFIC DEVELOPMENTS

Technological revolutions do not come in neat packages, and they defy simple attempts at management (Noah, 2006). The success of the biotechnology industry depends on many things, including the ability to be objective about what is possible and what remains as science fiction. Overall, scientists still do not recognize the full potential of the bioscience research surrounding genomics (Burns, 2005).

In fact, the FDA, accustomed to large clinical trials using a diverse subject population, and designed to test drugs with significant market potential along with its centralized manufacturing facilities and uniform labeling, must learn to deal with a radically altered model of drug development and use for biopharmaceuticals (Noah, 2006). Biopharmaceuticals rely on cutting-edge medical technologies that target similar subject populations.

Cutting-Edge Medical Technologies
- Protein drugs produced by splicing genes into bacteria, including:
  - Clotting factor for hemophilia patients
  - Erthropoietin to stimulate the production of red blood cells
  - Human growth hormone
  - Recombinant insulin
- Monoclonal antibodies (laboratory-made version of the naturally occurring protein that binds to and neutralizes foreign invaders) and interferons (proteins that interfere with the cell's ability to reproduce) are the basis of drugs for:
  - Chronic granulomatous disease
  - Genital warts
  - Hairy cell leukemia
  - Multiple sclerosis
  - Osteoporosis
- Gene therapies that augment normal gene functions or replace or inactivate disease-causing genes are being tested for:
  - Cancers
  - Heart disease
- Therapeutic vaccines designed to jump-start the immune system to fight disease are in development to treat:
  - Cancers
  - HIV/AIDS

Source: PhRMA, 2008.

The aggregate instincts of the biotechnology industry about how best to manage these new and emerging scientific developments may be erroneous. With the level of uncertainty so high in biotechnology, the normal reaction is to try to manage and control things, but this may be the wrong approach (Day & Schoemaker, 2004). With bioscience, the leading biotechnology companies continue to be flexible, riding the waves of entrepreneurship and developing corporate strategies for succeeding, no matter what their future brings.

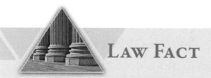 LAW FACT

BIOSCIENCE RESEARCH

How should the interests of patent holders, users of patented inventions, and the general public, all involved in a bioscience patent dispute, be balanced by the courts?

Both sides of the coin favor the users of patented biopharmaceuticals. Users are not required to break or terminate license agreements before seeking declaratory judgments in federal court that the underlying patents are invalid, unenforceable, or not infringed. On the one side, where patent disputes do not involve license agreements, patented biopharmaceuticals may be used in preclinical studies as long as there is a reasonable basis for believing that the experiments will produce the type of information that is relevant to an investigational new drug application or a new drug application under FDA regulations.
— *Merck KGaA v. Integra Lifesciences I, Ltd.*, 545 U.S. 193 (U.S. Supreme Court 2005).

On the other side, where patent disputes involve license agreements to research tools, courts must first determine whether the users of the patented invention are being coerced, either by the patent holder or the

(continues)

(continued)

> fear of losing business, to pay royalties under the licensing agreements. If coercion is found, the users of the patented research tool, the licensees, will be allowed to challenge the validity of the patented invention in court without being required to breach the licensing agreements first.
>
> —*MedImmune, Inc. v. Genentech, Inc.*, 549 U.S. 118 (U.S. Supreme Court 2007).
>
> Patent disputes where there are no licensing agreements will be controlled by the *Merck* decision; patent disputes involving license agreements will be controlled by the *MedImmune* decision.

CHAPTER SUMMARY

- The U.S. is the world's biotechnology leader, with about 75 percent of the industry's revenues.
- The biotechnology industry faces many of the same challenges as the pharmaceutical industry, but on a larger scale because the regulatory roles of the FDA and provider payers are unclear.
- Pharmaceutical drugs are made by synthesizing chemicals, while biopharmaceuticals are proteins made by living organisms.
- Although biotechnology continues to lose money through uneconomical production and failure to bring products to market, investors remain extremely interested in the industry.
- The full potential of the biotechnology industry, including that of bioinformatics, genomics, and proteomics, has yet to be realized; even scientists are unsure of its possibilities.
- Once the human genome is completely unlocked, the field will advance tremendously and scientists will be able to create personalized medical and cosmetic products; the science-fiction possibility of living forever may even become a reality.
- The life biosciences are the driver of convergent technology, which is the intersection of nanotechnology, biotechnology, information technology, and cognitive science.
- Although biotechnology has incredible medical technology possibilities, it is losing public support and funding; it currently relies on private investors to continue progressing and because of this, many biotechnology companies are either merging with each other or merging into the bigger pharmaceutical companies, where they risk falling by the wayside.
- Besides funding, one of the biggest challenges biotechnology faces, as an industry founded and run by academic scientists rather than business professionals, is developing corporate strategies to ensure sustainability and success.

LAW NOTES

1. One such surprise was BioMartin Pharmaceutical, a California biotechnology company. BioMartin raised $67 million in an initial public offering based on the promise of a single orphan drug still in clinical trials for Mucopolysacchardiosis I, a rare genetic disease affecting less than four thousand people and caused by a deficiency in an enzyme that leads to delayed mental development and impaired vision, among other symptoms. Within months of going public, BioMartin had a market capitalization of more than $1 billion. In a joint venture with Genyzme, BioMartin brought Aldurazyme (laronidase), an enzyme replacement therapy, to market in 2003 at an average cost of $175,000 per patient each year. The joint venture had sales in excess of $153 million in 2008 (Anand, 2005b).
2. Celegene, a New Jersey biotechnology company, licensed thalidomide in 1992, a drug that had been around for decades but had been off the market since the 1960s for causing birth defects. Orphan drug status was obtained for thalidomide's use in treating a side effect of leprosy in 1998, then later for multiple myeloma, a kind of cancer. Today, thalidomide is marketed under a tight distribution system under the trade name Thalomid. Celegene raised the price of a Thalomid pill from $6 in 1992 to about $53 today, in line with the price of other cancer drugs. The drug is so inexpensive to make that it is sold by other companies in Brazil for seven cents a pill (Anand, 2005b).
3. 21 U.S.C.A. § 355(j)(2)(A)(iv) (2008); 21 U.S.C.A. § 355(j)(8)(B) (2008) (defining bioequivalence); *see also* 21 C.F.R. § 320.1(e) (2009) (explaining that drug is bioequivalent if it shows comparable rate and extent that active ingredient is absorbed from drug and becomes available at site of action); Therapeutically Equivalent Drugs; Availability of List, 45 Fed. Reg. 72, 582 at 72,593 (1980) (discussing how bioequivalence requirement

ensures that generic drugs will perform with the same safety and effectiveness as their FDA-approved brand-name counterparts).

4. EGO is a glycoprotein that stimulates red blood cell production. It is produced in the kidney and stimulates the division and differentiation of committed erythroid progenitors in the bone marrow. EPO, a 165-amino acids glycoprotein manufactured by recombinant DNA technology, has the molecular weight of 30,400 Daltons and is produced by mammalian cells into which the human erthroprotein gene has been introduced. The product contains the identical amino acid sequences of isolated natural erthroproteins. EPO is formulated as a sterile, colorless liquid in an isotonic sodium chloride/sodium citrate buffered solution or a sodium chloride/sodium phosphate buffered solution with intravenous or subcutaneous administration (Amgen's Prescribing Information).

5. Genentech, based in South San Francisco, California, developed the first-ever genetically engineered human therapeutic to win FDA approval in 1977. Trading on the NYSE as DNA, Genentech began when venture capitalist Robert Swanson, in his mid-twenties, and biochemist Dr. Herbert Boyer agreed to invest $500 apiece to start a pharmaceutical company. Working with bioscience scientists from the Beckman Research Institute, a research facility affiliated with the City of Hope National Medical Center in Duarte, California, Genentech was the first to successfully express a human gene in bacteria to produce synthetic human insulin (Humulin). In partnership with insulin manufacturer Eli Lilly, a global pharmaceutical company headquartered in Indianapolis, Indiana, Humulin was licensed to and manufactured by Eli Lilly. Today, Genentech employs more than eleven thousand people and has sales revenue approaching $12 billion). Most of Genentech's shares are owned by Hoffmann-La Roche, a global pharmaceutical headquartered in Basel, Switzerland, with U.S. corporate headquarters in Nutley, New Jersey.

6. The Dow Jones U.S. Biotechnology Index is comprised of thirty-seven components: Advanced Tissue Biosciences, Affymetrix, Albany Molecular Resh, Alexion Pharmaceuticals, Amgen, Celgene, Cell Genesys, Cubist Pharmaceuticals, Curagen, CV Therapeutics, EntreMed, Enzo Biochem, Enzon, Genentech, Genzyme, Geron, Gilead Biosciences, Human Genome Biosciences, Immunomedics, Incyte Pharmaceuticals, Lexicon Genetics, Ligand Pharmaceuticals, Maxygen, Medarex, Myriad Genetics, Nabi Biopharmaceuticals, Neurocrine Bioscience, Northfield Labs, NPS Pharmaceuticals, Osi Pharmaceuticals, Pharmacyclics, Regeneron Pharmaceuticals, Techne, Trimeris, United Therapeutics, Vertex Pharmaceuticals, and Xoma.

7. Biotechnology companies are deploying platform technologies with high-throughput, automated technology aimed at a wide variety of disease conditions:
   - Affymetrix sells DNA microarrays, commonly called DNA chips, that consist of DNA implanted on wafers that allow bioscience researchers to analyze thousands of genes at a time to see which ones are active in particular conditions
   - Aurora Bioscience sells the Ultra-high Throughput Screening System Platform, which can screen more than 100,000 compounds a day with more than 2,400 re-tests, accessed from a store of over 1 million compounds
   - Celera Genomics industrialized gene sequencing with advanced instrumentation

8. Memory improvement is a target of several biotechnology firms. Axonyx, for instance, has the rights to a compound called Gilatide that is based on the saliva of the gila monster, a venomous lizard found in parts of the U.S. and Mexico. Other firms racing after memory improvement include Memory Pharmaceuticals and Helicon Therapeutics.

   While Genentech's recombinant human growth hormone was developed to treat growth hormone deficiency, athletes are suspected of using the hormone to boost their athletic performance. The International Olympic Committee has launched an effort to develop ways to detect biosynthetic growth hormone in athletes. Viagra also raises the therapy versus enhancement issue. Regularly providing sexual potency to eighty-year-olds may fix a malady, but it also endows them with unprecedented abilities, including geriatric paternity.

9. Johnson & Johnson Development Corp. (JJDC), a global venture capital group, has existed for almost forty years. JJDC views financial risk in two buckets, excluding early-stage seed investments. One is technology risk, and the other involves business risks, such as potential legal, financial, and management problems. JJDC looks at long-term investments to build its venture portfolio across different phases of product development, from the early pre-clinical stage through drug discovery and finally into clinical testing with a special focus on biotechnology and biopharmaceuticals. Since the venture capital fund is not primarily driven by its internal rate of return, JJDC can invest in biotechnology products that typically take fourteen years to develop, while most venture funds have a shorter time horizon. In addition, JJDP is a global investor with holdings

in Europe, Israel, and Canada. During the recent economic bubble, European nations offered subsidies to biotechnology companies, but many of them are struggling since the market has cooled; these same firms are now rationalizing and merging, creating new opportunity for JJDC (Nicholson et al., 2005). The parent company of JJDC, Johnson & Johnson, is one of the few global pharmaceutical companies with an active pipeline of drugs that have been developed in-house, compared to Pfizer, which is being forced to merge with Wyeth to obtain access to a farm of biopharmaceutical drugs (*see also* Croce, 2007).

CHAPTER BIBLIOGRAPHY

Anand, G. (2005, December 1). Support system: Through charities, drug makers help people and themselves: By donating money, firms keep patients insured and medicine prices high, Mrs. Gushwa's $2,000 pills. *Wall Street Journal*, p. A1.

___. (2005a, November 16). Uncertain miracle: A biotechnology drug extends a life, but at what price? For Ms. Lees, treatment bill now totals $7 million; Her bones keep crumbling, guilt of another $1,400 day. *Wall Street Journal*, p. A1.

___. (2005b, November 15). Lucrative niches: How drugs for rare diseases became lifeline for companies: Federal law gives monopoly for seven years, fueling surge in biotechnology profits, a teen's $36,000 treatment. *Wall Street Journal*, p. A1.

Ariely, D. (2009). *Predictably irrational: The hidden forces that shape our decisions* (revised expanded ed.). New York, NY: Harper (summarizing the latest research in the field of behavioral economics, the newest theoretical approach to law and economics).

Bamman, M. M. (2008). Regulation of muscle size in humans: Role of myostatin? *Journal of Musculoskeletal & Neuronal Interactions, 8* (4), 342-343.

Bouchard, R. A. (2007). Balancing public and private interests in the commercialization of publicly funded medical research: Is there a role for compulsory government royalty fees? *Boston University Journal of Science & Technology Law, 13*, 120-191.

Burns, L. R. (2005). *The business of healthcare innovation.* New York, NY: Cambridge University Press.

CBO (Congressional Budget Office). (2007). *The budget and economic outlook: An update.* Washington, DC: CBO.

Cotterill, R. (2008). *The material world* (2nd ed.). New York, NY: Cambridge University Press.

Cristianini, N., & Hahn, M. (2006). *Introduction to computational genomics.* New York, NY: Cambridge University Press (introduction to the profession of bioinformaticians: biologists fluent in mathematics and computer science and data analysts familiar with biology).

Croce, B., worldwide chairman, Johnson & Johnson (Cordis). (2007, February 15). 12th Wharton Health Care Business Conference. Philadelphia, PA.

Danzon, P. M., & Furukawa, M. F. (2006). Prices and availability of biopharmaceuticals: An international comparison: The U.S. might spend more on biologics, but prices are not noticeably higher than in nine other countries. *Health Affairs, 25* (5), 1353-1362.

Day, G. S., & Schoemaker, P. (2004). *Wharton on managing emerging technologies.* New York, NY: Wiley (based on six years of research from Wharton's Emerging Technologies Management Research Program, three areas are addressed: business models that are going to be successful and how they evolve over time; organization of firms through structure and financial incentives to take advantage of new technologies; and how companies can acquire and develop the capabilities to use bioscience to create new wealth).

Drahos, P. (2008). Trust me: Patent offices in developing countries. *American Journal of Law & Medicine, 34*, 151-173.

Evans, G. (2008). Strategic patent licensing for public research organizations: Deploying restriction and reservation clauses to promote medical R&D in developing countries. *American Journal of Law & Medicine, 34*, 175-223.

Favole, J. A. (2008, November 8). FDA seizes contaminated heparin. *Wall Street Journal*, p. A2.

Foster, R., & Kaplan, S. (2001). *Creative destruction: Why companies that are built to last underperform the market and how to successfully transform them.* Boston, MA: Currency (two McKinsey executives extensively document how today's biotechnology industry compares to earlier times in the semiconductor and pharmaceutical industries, based on the creative destruction concept first advanced in the 1930s and 1940s by economist Joseph Schumpeter; their research draws on the analysis of more than one thousand companies over four decades).

Frank, F., former vice chairman, Lehman Brothers. (2007, February 15). 12th Wharton Health Care Business Conference. Philadelphia, PA.

Frisvold, G., & Day-Rubenstein, K. (2008). Bioprospecting and biodiversity conservation: What happens when discoveries are made? *Arizona Law Review, 50*, 545-576.

Garnier, J-P., chief executive officer, GlaxoSmithKline (2007, February 15). 12th Wharton Health Care Business Conference. Philadelphia, PA.

Geithner, T., U.S. treasury secretary. (2009, January 21). Testimony before the U.S. Senate Finance Committee. Washington, DC.

Grabowski, H., & Kyle, M. (2007). Generic competition and market exclusivity periods in pharmaceuticals. *Managerial & Decision Economics, 28*, 491-502.

Heuser, S. (2009, June 14). One girl's hope, a nation's dilemma: A Cambridge firm's drug worked wonders, but was hugely costly, more than Costa Rica thought it could spend on one child among so many. *Boston Globe*, p. A1.

Hilsenrath, J. (2008, December 13-14). The big numbers behind the bailouts. *Wall Street Journal*, p. A3.

Huston, L., managing director, 4iNNO and former innovation officer, Procter & Gamble. (2007, June 27). Wharton

Executive Education Seminar: Full-spectrum innovation: Driving organic growth. Aresty Institute of Executive Education at the University of Pennsylvania, Philadelphia, PA.

Jayapal K. P. et al. (2007). Recombinant protein therapeutics from CHO cells—20 years and counting. *Chemical Engineering Progress Journal, 103* (7), 40-47 (noting "CHO" means *Chinese hamster ovary*).

Johansen, R., president, Institute for the Future. (2003, May 2). Wharton Conference on Peripheral Vision. Wharton School at the University of Pennsylvania, Philadelphia, PA.

Karnitschnig, M., & Rockoff, J. D. (2009, January 23). Pfizer in talks to buy Wyeth. *Wall Street Journal*, pp. A1 and A11.

Kesselheim, A. S. (2008). Think globally, prescribe locally: How rational pharmaceutical policy in the U.S. can improve global access to essential medicines. *American Journal of Law & Medicine, 34*, 125-139.

Keusch, G. T. (2008). When you reach a fork in the road, take it: Science and product development as linked paths. *Journal of Law & Medicine, 34*, 141-149.

Kolber, A. J. (2007). A limited defense of clinical placebo deception. *Yale Law & Policy Review, 26*, 75-78 (arguing that given current knowledge of placebo effects and patient preferences, the deceptive use of placebos should not be categorically prohibited).

Lerner, J. (2008). Intellectual property and development at WHO and WIPO. *American Journal of Law & Medicine, 34*, 257-277.

Lieber, C. M., professor of chemistry and chemical biology, Harvard University, and president, Nanosys. (2007, October 24). Lecture: Nanotechnology and the life biosciences: From ultrasensitive disease detection to hybrid "smart" materials. Nano/Bio Interface Center. University of Pennsylvania, Philadelphia, PA (Nanosys is a nanotechnology company involved in chemical and biological sensing).

Lockwood, C. E. (2009). *Biotechnology Industry Organization v. District of Columbia*: A preemptive strike against state price restrictions on prescription pharmaceuticals. *Albany Law Journal of Science & Technology, 19*, 143-181.

Lunshof, J. E. (2006). Personalized medicine: New perspectives—new ethics? *Personalized Medicine, 3* (2), 187-194.

Lynch, H. F. (2007). Give them what they want? The permissibility of pediatric placebo-controlled trials under the Best Pharmaceuticals for Children Act. *Annals of Health Law, 16*, 79-138.

Mandel, G. (2008). Nanotechnology governance. *Alabama Law Review, 59*, 1323-1384.

Mathews, A. W., & Abboud, L. (2007, March 14). For booming biotech firms, a new threat: Generics: Democrats' bills would clear way for copies; Preparations in Croatia. *Wall Street Journal*, p. A1.

McKnight, R. (2004). RNA interference: A critical analysis of the regulatory and ethical issues encountered in the development of a novel therapy. *Albany Law Journal of Science & Technology, 15*, 73-108.

Medco (Medco Health Solutions). (2007). *Drug trend report: Humanomics: Understanding the cost of cutting-edge healthcare*. Franklin Lakes, NJ: Medco.

____. (2006). *Drug trend report: Personalizing healthcare*. Franklin Lakes, NJ: Medco.

Meibohm, B. (ed.). (2007). *Pharmacokinetics and pharmacodynamics of biopharmaceuticals: Principles and case studies in drug development*. New York, NY: Wiley (covers biopharmaceuticals and explains bioequivalence).

Moran, N. A. (2009). The dynamics and time scale of ongoing genomic erosion in symbiotic bacteria. *Science, 323* (5912), 379-382.

Mullen, J. (2007, April 27). Gene therapy. *Wall Street Journal*, p. A17.

National Science Board. (2009). *Research and development: Essential foundation for U.S. competitiveness in a global economy*. Washington, DC: NSB.

Nicholson, S. et al. (2005). Biotechnology-pharma alliances as a signal of asset and firm quality. *Journal of Business, 78* (4), 1433-1464.

Noah, L. (2006). Managing biotechnology's revolution: Has guarded enthusiasm become benign neglect? *Virginia Journal of Law & Technology, 11*, 4-63 (describing difficulties with attempts to extend the FDA's authority to approve cheaper generics to biotechnology drugs).

Ogita, S. et al. (2003). RNA interference: Producing decaffeinated coffee plants. *Nature, 423* (6942), 823.

Parsons, S. A. (2007). Genetic disruption of calcineurin improves skeletal muscle pathology and cardiac disease in a mouse model of limb-girdle muscular dystrophy. *Journal of Biopharmaceutical Chemistry, 282* (13), 10068-10078.

Pauly, M. V. et al. (2005). Competition and new technology. *Health Affairs, 24* (6), 1523-1535.

PhRMA (Pharmaceutical Research and Manufacturing Association). (2008). *Biotechnology medicines in development: Biotechnology research continues to bolster arsenal against disease with 633 medicines in development*. Washington, DC: PhRMA.

Pisano, G. (2006). *Science business: The promise, the reality and the future of biotechnology*. Boston, MA: Harvard Business School Press (history of pharmaceuticals and biotechnology, beginning with Bayer's synthesis of willow tree bark in 1897 to make aspirin to today's biotechnology cancer drugs; categorizes "Big Pharma," with roots in the first half of the twentieth century, as companies that process naturally occurring compounds using organic chemistry, and compares them with biotechnology companies that synthesize and genetically engineer drugs in an attempt to fight disease).

Plassmann, H. et al. (2007). Orbitofrontal cortex encodes willingness to pay in everyday economic transactions. *Journal of Neuroscience, 27*, 9987-9988 (demonstrating activity in medial orbitofrontal cortex, which encodes people's willingness to pay during simple economic transactions).

Porter, M. E., & Teisberg, E. O. (2006). *Redefining health care: Creating value-based competition on results*. Boston, MA: Harvard Business School Press.

Rifkin, J. (1998). *The biotechnology century: Harnessing the gene and remaking the world*. Los Angeles: Tarcher/Penguin.

Roco, M. C., & Bainbridge, W. S. (2003). *Converging technologies for improving human performance: Nanotechnology, biotechnology, information technology and cognitive science*. New York, NY: Springer.

Ross, D. M. G. (2007). *Biotechnology Industry Organization v. District of Columbia*: The Federal Circuit expands its jurisdiction in order to extend preemption doctrine to state law restrictions on patent rights. *Tulane Journal of Technology & Intellectual Property, 10*, 339-351.

Stephenson, F. (2007). *DNA: How the biotechnology revolution is changing the way we fight disease*. New York, NY: Prometheus Books.

Treu, J., general partner, Domain Associates. (2003, February 23). 8th Annual Wharton Health Care Business Conference. Philadelphia, PA (Domain is a Princeton, New Jersey–based venture firm).

Vagelos, R, former chief executive officer, Merck (1985-1994). (2004, April 20). Leonard Davis Institute of Health Economics Seminar Series: Past and future of the pharmaceutical/biotech industry. Wharton School at the University of Pennsylvania, Philadelphia, PA.

Wager, T. D. (2004). Placebo-induced changes in MRI in the anticipation and experience of pain. *Science, 303*, 1662-1664.

Walsh, G. (2003). *Biopharmaceuticals: Biochemistry and biotechnology* (2nd ed.). New York, NY: Wiley.

Wharton (Wharton School at the University of Pennsylvania). (2006). Lawton Burns on the critical, and costly, role of companies that make healthcare-related products. *Knowledge@Wharton.*

___. (2002). From skin creams to life insurance to medical care, biosciences are the new frontier of business opportunity. *Knowledge@Wharton.*

Wiegel, P. (2007). Was the FDA exemption to patent infringement, 35 U.S.C. § 271(e)(1), intended to exempt a pharmaceutical manufacturer's activities in the development of new drugs? Boston College Law School Intellectual Property & Technology Forum at Boston College Law School. Boston, MA.

Zhang, J. (2009, July). The impact of the financial crisis on the pharma and biotech industries. *Life Science Leader.*

CHAPTER 19
MEDICAL DEVICES

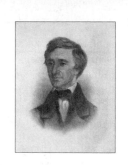

"Every man is the builder of a temple called his body."

—HENRY DAVID THOREAU (1817-1862), AMERICAN PHILOSOPHER, AUTHOR, AND POET

IN BRIEF

This chapter describes how the use of implantable medical devices to treat heart disease, orthopedic and ophthalmologic complaints, and other medical conditions is growing rapidly via advancing technology. This chapter focuses on the rationing of health care products and the increasing demand created by and for new device technologies. The premarket approval process is described in Chapter 2.

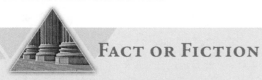

FACT OR FICTION

MEDICAL MONITORING

Do healthy patients have standing to sue device manufacturers if they face increased risks of harm from defective medical devices compared to those undergoing traditional surgery?

Michael Sutton sought to bring a class action lawsuit on behalf of about 50,000 patients who underwent cardiac bypass surgery using a medical device manufactured by St. Jude Medical, called the Symmetry Bypass System Connector device. Surgeons used this device during cardiac bypass surgery to attach vein grafts to the aortic surface of the heart without sutures. Sutton was implanted with the device during treatment for his heart condition.

    The device, however, led to severe and disabling medical conditions resulting from collapse and scarring of the graft in numerous patients, necessitating removal of the device and/or monitoring for further harm, including possible death. Sutton alleges St. Jude failed to use reasonable care, was negligent in designing the device, that the device was defective and unreasonably dangerous, and was sold and marketed without proper warnings. Although St. Jude had been informed of the adverse consequences associated with the device through incident reports from surgeons before Sutton had the defective device implanted in him, St. Jude continued to market and distribute the device without warnings. Sutton maintains he suffered economic losses and medical expenses when he had the defective device implanted and he now has a device in his body that increases his risk for cardiac occlusion and death. While future injuries are hypothetical, Sutton maintains his increased risk necessitates both current and future medical testing and monitoring.

    —*Sutton v. St. Jude Medical S.C., Inc.*, 419 F.3d 568 (U.S. Court of Appeals for the 6th Circuit 2005), rehearing en banc denied Jan. 23, 2006.

(See *Law Fact* at the end of this chapter for the answer.)

PRINCIPLES AND APPLICATIONS

Generally, a device is any medical product that does not achieve its principal intended purpose(s) by chemical action in or on the human body. Medical devices include instruments, apparatuses, machines, and implants that are intended for diagnosis or treatment of diseases or injuries, or that affect the structures or any function of the human body (*see* 21 U.S.C.A. § 321(h) (2007); FDA, 1984). With an estimated 35 million Americans suffering from conditions that can be treated by medical devices, and only some 2.5 million actually using them, there is an enormous capacity for absorbing medical device technology within the practice of medicine (Wharton, 2006a). Overall, the implantable technology market has U.S. sales of about $28 billion per year and has grown by 9 to 10 percent over the last five to seven years (Freedonia, 2007). The health care statistics in this chapter come from various components of the Centers for Disease Control's National Center for Health Statistics (NCHS) National Health Care Survey for 2006, unless otherwise cited.

    As illustrated in Figure 19-1, the device industry is by all measures one of the most productive and profitable sectors in health care. *Average operating profit margin* refers to earnings before taxes and interest relative to sales. The average operating profit margins for the larger device manufacturers have consistently been over 10 percent; four manufacturers are Fortune 500 companies: Johnson & Johnson, GE, Siemens, and Abbott Laboratories.

    The economic principle that demand falls as the price of goods rise does not seem to hold true for medical devices. In the medical device products industry, growth is sustainable because it is driven by:

- Demographic trends of age and obesity and the increasing demands from an aging and overweight population
- Continued prevalence of diseases
- Near infinite capacity for absorbing advanced medical technology within the practice of medicine
- Greater acceptance by physicians and patients of implantation as an alternative or a complement to medication

(Wharton, 2006a)

The use of implantable medical devices to treat heart disease, orthopedic problems, and other conditions is growing strongly. Consider the use of implantable defibrillators, which monitor the

	2007 Sales (in Billions)	Compound Annual Growth Rate (CAGR)	Operating Profit Margin (OPM)
Johnson & Johnson	$22.0	9%	27%
GE Healthcare	$17.0	13%	18%
Siemens Medical Services	$15.2	27%	45%
Medtronic	$12.3	14%	27%
Tyco Healthcare	$10.0	32%	N/A
Abbott Laboratories	$3.8 [(2005)]	14%	19%

FIGURE 19-1: U. S. Medical Devices Industry

Delmar/Cengage Learning
Data retrieved from: Corporate reports to the U.S. Securities and Exchange Commission.

heartbeat and give a potentially life-saving shock when needed. About 135,000 of these medical devices (House, 2006), costing approximately $68,300 to $101,500 each (Sanders, 2005), are implanted in patients in the U.S. each year. Stents are another example. About 1.2 million bare-metal stents were implanted in the U.S. each year after they were approved for use (Wharton, 2006a). Soon after, drug-coated stents were approved in 2003, designed to prevent the reclogging of arteries. They are considered a device/drug hybrid. By the end of 2006, over six million people worldwide had a drug-coated stent placed inside of a previously clogged artery to prop it open (Maisel, 2007), and approximately 130,000 stents are implanted each month in the U.S. (Wang, 2008). They cost about $3,000 each, which is triple the cost of plain stents, but neither patients nor their doctors object (Wharton, 2006a).

MEDICATION OVER SURGERY

Lifestyle choices seem to point to increased demand for medical devices. The increasing obesity of the U.S. population, notably among young people, suggests an enduring need for artificial measures such as coronary stents to keep clogged arteries from closing up altogether. The upbeat prospects have led stocks of leading device manufacturers to outperform the stock market as a whole (Wharton, 2006a).

However, growth is restrained by physicians' reluctance to use the technology until they see clear evidence of the benefits of medical device therapy, and by resistance from some patients who avoid implantation because it involves surgery. Until all parties are convinced, medication is likely to remain the first choice overall. Implants are almost always the therapy of last resort because they are invasive, involve surgical risk, and usually require monitoring

for the remainder of the patient's life. The device market is also prevented from reaching its potential by diagnoses that do not make a clear case for implantation. Hip replacements, for example, could in theory be performed on the estimated twenty million Americans with osteoarthritis. In some cases, the disease may not have progressed sufficiently to warrant hip replacement; in others, the patient may choose to defer the operation for as long as possible for personal reasons (Burns, 2006).

Physicians are understandably cautious about adopting new medical device technology. It sometimes takes a number of years to show how safe the latest innovative device technology is. The first cardiac pacemaker was developed in 1959 for just a few patients, and they have now become a multibillion-dollar market. Implantable defibrillators were initially seen as having a limited market and are now used for about half a million patients a year (NCHS, 2008). Together, pacemakers and implantable defibrillators now make up a $5 billion to $6 billion market (Pauly & Burns, 2008; Wharton, 2006a).

MARKET GROWTH

While cardiac stents can save lives if implanted during or shortly after a heart attack, the American Heart Association reports heart disease is still the leading cause of death in the U.S. and the number one reason for hospitalization among people over sixty-five. Five million people a year suffer from heart failure, half of whom will die within five years, and the incidence of heart disease is expected to double within the next five years because of increasing obesity rates and sedentary lifestyles (NCHS, 2008).

Growth in the market for implantable technology is also driven by an aging population, which requires more medical devices like pacemakers, defibrillators, artificial hips, and neurological medical devices (Jackson & Howe, 2008). The device industry is responding with smaller, more reliable, and less power-consuming equipment. More intelligent medical devices are constantly being developed, allowing medical problems to be better identified and dealt with in an appropriate and timely way (Burns et al., 2007).

Cardiology

A developing field is cardiac resynchronization therapy in which an implanted electronic medical device corrects the widespread tendency in heart failure patients for the heart chambers to contract at the wrong time, forcing the heart to work harder and increasing the risk of a heart attack. By achieving a resynchronization of the chambers, patients experience a remarkable improvement in quality of life. The patient not only has fewer symptoms, but tissue that has declined in efficiency then regains its effectiveness (Burns et al., 2007).

Among other sectors of the cardiac market, HealthCare Capital Advisors expects pacemakers to grow by 5 percent a year from the current $3 billion market. Medical devices designed to counter congestive heart failure are projected to surge 50 percent per year from a modest $1 billion base. Biodegradable stents, which treat blockages in coronary arteries and then degrade, are getting increased attention from the medical and investment communities.

Drug-Coated Coronary Stents

The Food and Drug Administration (FDA) approved drug-coated stents for use in 2003; since then, the U.S. market has grown to roughly $2 billion (Wang, 2008), while the global market is approaching $5 billion (Espicom, 2009). While standard stents are permanently inserted in a diseased coronary artery to keep it open, the new device builds on this platform by delivering a controlled flow of medication into the patient's bloodstream for a limited period to prevent the passageways from becoming reclogged by tissue buildup (Burns, 2006). Cardiologists quickly embraced the tiny mesh scaffolds; within a year, drug-eluting stents were used in almost all coronary interventions in the U.S. and today, several million have been implanted (NCHS, 2008).

Some are questioning what to do with device technologies that could be used in virtually everybody, even though they have only been studied in a minority of patients (Mathews & Winslow, 2006). The issue is really twofold: before a new medical device has the potential to reach blockbuster status, should it be subject to higher standards of safety and effectiveness prior to introduction into the marketplace, or should blockbuster devices be subject to closer post-marketing surveillance studies? The safety of drug-eluting

stents has not been established for relatively high-risk patients, a group that accounts for the majority of stenting procedures and for whom the new stents are not approved (Winslow & Mathews, 2006).

Some studies suggest the newer medical devices increase the risk of blood clots in high-risk patients compared with bare-metal stents (Westphal, 2005). Drug-coated stents are approved for use in patients with simple artery blockages, but more than half the procedures involving the medical devices are performed in patients with more complex conditions, such as:

- Heart attacks
- Multiple blockages requiring more than one stent
- Blockages in more than one branch of an artery

(Nussbaum, 2006)

The federal Agency for Healthcare Research and Quality found no conclusive evidence drug-eluting stents increase the risk of blood clots, heart attack, or death, compared with bare-metal stents when used within the scope of their FDA approval (Douglas & Sedrakyan, 2009). While off-label use of drug-coated stents appears to raise risks, it is unclear whether the increased risk is caused by the drug-coated stents or if it is a result of the poorer health of the higher-risk patients (Winslow & Mathews, 2006).

Moral Dilemmas

1. Should a patient who would have died or suffered greatly without a medical device and who had no alternative treatment options be permitted to sue for damages if the medical device does not perform as expected?

Implantable Cardiovascular Devices

The market for implanted defibrillators, medical devices about the size of a pager that shock the heart back to a normal rhythm when necessary, is expected to see sharp growth, with some 900,000 patients eligible to receive them (Burns et al., 2007). The value of the market could increase from $2.2 billion in 2007 to as much as $13.5 billion a year (Chow et al., 2007). The projected growth in implanted defibrillators is 14 percent annually for the next five years, although many consider this projection too conservative, and predict the true figure is likely to be about 22 percent (Wharton, 2006a).

The device industry's prospects are enhanced by the fact that implant technology saves the U.S. health care system money (Basile & Lorell, 2006). The potential of medical devices such as implantable defibrillators to save money will likely be the key to whether the insurance industry is willing to continue paying for them (Wharton, 2003). If they are proven to prevent heart attacks, or give early warning signs of problems that would otherwise be more expensive to treat if not detected until later, they will arguably be more attractive to insurers (Burns, 2006).

While implanted defibrillators are underutilized worldwide (Birnie et al., 2007), it is estimated as many as one-third of U.S. patients have defibrillators implanted into their chests needlessly (Chow et al., 2007). The overuse or inappropriate use of medical devices is a familiar theme, but defibrillators pose unique issues because they are increasingly used as a standard piece of safety equipment, like an air bag in an automobile, in an ever-growing number of heart patients whose individual need for the device is not clear (Pauly & Burns, 2008). Medical experts agree many, if not the majority, of defibrillator candidates are at a low risk of cardiac arrest (Basile & Lorell, 2006). The dilemma reflects a growing medical conundrum: groups at risk can be identified for use of advanced device technologies, but individual patients in those groups who are at higher risk cannot be identified.

Given their overuse in the U.S. it is difficult to determine whether implanted defibrillators actually reduce health care costs. However, if Medicare is willing to pay for a device, private health insurers often follow (McClellan & Tunis, 2005). The commercial potential of medical devices also depends on whether patients are willing to pay for them over and above their regular health insurance premiums (Burns, et al., 2007).

Defibrillator Recalls

Not all problems with medical devices are discovered before distribution. One of the most important sources of authority the FDA can exercise is the ability to force entities in the chain of distribution to notify the medical community that there is a problem with a medical device and to take other action (FDA, 2003).

The 2007 recall of about 268,000 defibrillator leads manufactured by Medtronic alerted the device industry of the need to improve information provided to patients and physicians about potential safety concerns in medical devices (Maisel, 2007). This lesson was learned from Guidant, which recalled an estimated 300,000 implantable cardioverter defibrillators because of the possibility the medical devices could malfunction (Steinbrook, 2005). Guidant was aware of the possibility of malfunction but did not notify physicians and patients about the potential problem (Berman, 2005) until after five patients' sudden deaths were linked to the device. Together the two massive recalls are the latest examples of the failure of device manufacturers and the FDA to provide patients and physicians with adequate information about potential safety concerns in medical devices.

Ophthalmology

Technology's advance has also reached into ophthalmology, where work is under way at Harvard Medical School to create an artificial retina with a chip inserted in the back of the eye. Medical device researchers are hoping to develop a camera the size of a pea that can be implanted within the eyeball, replacing natural tissue with artificial technology (Rose, 2008).

Neurology

In neuroscience, Medtronic has developed a technique known as Activa tremor control therapy. Activa can control trembling, such as occurs in Parkinson's disease, by using an implanted medical device that can deliver electrical stimulation to certain areas of the brain (Burns, et al., 2007).

Orthopedics

In orthopedics, the focus is on minimally invasive procedures in which physicians operate through ports into the body, particularly for hip and knee operations. At the same time, integrated medical products are increasingly used in orthopedic surgery. One such medical device used in spinal surgery involves a metal cage pre-packed with biologic drugs to promote bone growth (Wharton, 2006a).

Mandated Prosthesis Coverage

Amputees and device manufacturers of prosthetic limbs are urging states to introduce legislation that would require the health insurance industry to provide prosthesis coverage. Eight states currently have laws mandating prosthesis coverage similar to Medicare, and most states are considering similar legislation. The Amputee Coalition of America is lobbying to introduce federal legislation (Fuhrmans, 2008).

Medicare covers at least 80 percent of the cost of prostheses and allows regular replacement, generally every five years. Medicare also covers computer-assisted artificial limbs. As technological advancements have caused manufacturing and sales costs of the medical devices to rise, many health insurers have placed coverage limits of $2,500 or $5,000 annually on prosthetic medical devices, or restricted coverage to just one device per recipient in a lifetime. The cost for regular prosthetic limbs can range between $3,000 and $15,000, and costs can reach as high as $40,000 for more technologically advanced or computer-aided medical devices (Fuhrmans, 2008). Prosthetic medical devices, among the most expensive implants on the market, are one of the medical items most affected by efforts to contain rising health costs (Wharton, 2006a). It is not that there has been an increase in the need for prostheses, rather it is the cost of acquiring the most advanced prosthetic technology that is being met with resistance by health insurers.

Supporters of mandates maintain the additional coverage for prostheses would cost just pennies in monthly premium increases. Health insurers believe mandates collectively affect the affordability of health insurance.

Telemedicine and Remote Monitoring Technologies

Despite technological feasibility, leading-edge patient monitoring systems fall short on providing a comprehensive picture of chronic diseases to aid physicians. Moreover, there is fear among health care providers that with remote monitoring, they could incur legal liability for failure to recognize warning signals. Others predict the careful use of monitoring technologies could actually reduce liability (Feder, 2006).

In addition to the technological and legal challenges, health care providers face a pragmatic financial concern about gathering and reviewing remote data. Most health insurers are providing little or no reimbursement for such work. Reimbursement rates are in the range of $25 to $100 for each review of remote monitoring data. According to the Veterans Health Administration, most health insurance plans pay for physicians and nurses to check on patients in person, but not from a distance.

Many physicians currently rely on data collection services run by the device manufacturers and independent monitoring services to warn them of anomalies requiring prompt attention. For example, there is an implantable electrocardiogram (ECG) monitoring system comprised of a wireless medical device about the size of a dollar-coin, or the size of the smallest pacemakers, that can continuously gather data and then automatically and regularly forward it to a monitoring center operated by the manufacturer. There, certified cardiac technicians review the patient's information and send cardiac event data to the patient's physician. A significant advantage of remote monitoring technology is technicians at monitoring centers can automatically receive patient data, thereby allowing them to frequently review patient information for clinical irregularities.

Implant Devices

Implanted under the skin, the ECG loop recorder device monitors and records heart activity, allowing a physician to interrogate it non-invasively to check a patient's medical condition and detect any danger signs. The medical device is also used to treat epilepsy, following the discovery that a large number of epileptics actually have cardiac arrhythmia, or an irregular heartbeat, indicating they need a pacemaker rather than anti-seizure medicine. Another implanted medical device, a hemodynamic monitoring system, measures vital signs including blood pressure, pulmonary artery diastolic pressure, and heart rate. Its data can be downloaded to a physician's computer from the patient's phone line, facilitating timely decisions on treatment (Burns, 2006).

New device technologies could allow tens of millions of Americans with chronic diseases, such as heart failure, diabetes, and mental illnesses, to have their conditions constantly monitored, remotely and virtually, as they go about their daily lives (Monegain, 2006). The advanced technologies developed by Medtronic and Abbott Laboratories allow:

- Alerts to lung and/or circulatory problems
- Blood pressure, glucose, and weight monitoring
- Regulation of heart rate and delivery of shocks when necessary
- Wireless Internet communication between patients and physicians

Although data gathered by the newest devices reconstructs events that send patients to emergency rooms (Feder, 2006), the payoff for patients could be:

- Fewer and shorter hospital stays
- Longer stretches between routine visits to physicians' offices
- More effective use of drugs

According to a recent Department of Veteran Affairs (VA) study that followed seventy patients over three months, remote monitoring of their heart implants significantly reduced the time their physicians would have spent on office visits (Ferris, 2007).

Telehealth Monitors

An increased number of device manufacturers are competing in the market for telehealth monitors, which allow physicians and nurses to track the health of patients from remote locations. Use of telehealth monitors can keep patients comfortably at home and allow physicians and nurses to focus on the most serious cases, as well as save the expense and disruption hospital visits cause by catching signs of trouble before patients need an ambulance.

The VA is spending $20 million to install about 50,000 telehealth monitors in homes of veterans (Ferris, 2007). In addition, some home health care device manufacturers have begun to offer telehealth monitors to patients. Patients who require home health care, however, are unlikely to be able to navigate most systems and interfaces currently available in the market. Telehealth monitor manufacturers are beginning to address this concern (Kiplinger, 2006).

The cost is about $200 monthly to purchase and operate a telehealth monitor, compared with about $78 for a single nurse visit. In addition, telehealth monitors decrease health care costs through a reduction in hospitalizations. Predictions are the technology could reduce health care costs by one-third for patients who require home health care (Ferris, 2007).

Integrated Medical Products

Adapting existing regulations to fit novel technologies and medical products is not a new challenge for U.S. regulatory agencies or for the FDA specifically. There is, however, typically a lag between the development of innovative technologies, their adoption by the medical community, and the laws to oversee it.

Nevertheless, the century-old definitions for classifying medical products as drugs, devices, or biologics may be unsuitable for the convergence of devices combined with drug or biologics properties. A biologic is any product derived from a living organism (human, animal, or unicellular), such as gene therapies, vaccines, allergy shots, and blood products. Looking ahead, the trend toward integration is bound to increase as science and technologies advance (von Eschenbach, 2008).

Combination Devices

Combination drug/device and biologic/device products, which contain more than one regulated product, are rapidly advancing and may pose technological challenges for current FDA regulatory schemes (FDA, 2008). While devices and drugs have co-existed for decades, such as drug-eluting stents, antimicrobial catheters, and cell-matrix cartilage implants, devices and biologics, such as orthopedic repair using morphogenetic protein, are rapidly increasing.

Nanodevices

The area with the most potential to produce revolutionary scientific changes to health care is nanomedicine, particularly nanodevices (Fadern, 2007). Nanodevices are extremely small; a nanometer, one billionth of a meter, is about the size of a few atoms put together (Yeagle, 2007). By comparison, a human hair is about 80,000 nanometers wide. Most medical product companies are now following the example of nanodevice manufacturers and building from the molecular level downwards (Wharton, 2006a). The typical approach of device manufacturers has generally been top-down by taking existing medical devices and making them smaller.

The technology is moving forward and the market for nano-formulated devices is estimated to be $3 billion. Scientists are using silica spheres coated with gold to attack cancerous tumors; infrared light heats the gold, and the heat kills the cancer. Likewise, nanofilters are used to purify blood (Wharton, 2006a). Other medical device nanoproducts that have entered the market include Vitoss bone graft substitute, TiMesh tissue reinforcement and hernia repair, EnSeal tissue sealing, and hemostatis system for laparoscopic and open surgery (Paradise et al., 2008). Carbon nanosensors, made of tiny cylinders of graphite, with walls the width of a single carbon atom and a diameter of one to two nanometers, about the same size as

a strand of DNA, help emergency medical technicians monitor patients' breathing (Wharton, 2006a).

Perhaps the most recognized nanotech product is sunscreen. People no longer look like they are smeared with white paint because their sun block has been replaced by nanocrystalline sunscreens. Sunscreens formerly contained particles that reflected light; now the same particle compounds are nanosize and do not reflect light (Yeagle, 2007).

With the rising interest in nanodevices, a field with neither a single scientific definition nor a formal regulatory or statutory definition, attention is being drawn to the need for examining existing regulatory systems in terms of their applicability to nanoproducts (FDA, 2007). This is especially the case when nanodevices are regulated on the assumption that the toxicological profiles of nanoparticulate versions of compounds, like carbon or titanium, are the same as their larger chemically identical counterparts, for example, molecules (Yeagle, 2007). This regulatory assumption, however, is not necessarily true. One research study found fish swimming in water containing nanoparticles called buckyballs (soccer-ball shaped synthetic carbon molecules comprised of sixty atoms each) ended up with brain damage (Wharton, 2006a).

DIRECT MARKETING TO PHYSICIANS

Medical devices are marketed to a defined group of physicians who select the products for their patients. About 1.5 million stents are placed annually, yet only 6,200 interventional cardiologists do the brand selection. Hip implants are installed in hundreds of thousands of patients in the U.S. annually, but only 17,000 orthopedic surgeons do the procedures. Device manufacturers aim their marketing efforts directly at physicians, avoiding the expense of convincing patients one product is better than another (Wharton, 2006a).

Potential Conflicts of Interest

While the University of Pennsylvania Health System, for example, requires physicians to tell patients about any financial relationship with device companies, not all health systems have this professional restriction. Many physicians have financial ties to device manufacturers that are often not revealed to their patients or to hospitals. For example, forty surgical groups each received at least $1 million in payments from medical device manufacturers in 2007 (Patsner, 2009).

There is certainly the appearance of conflicts of interest when physicians use certain branded medical devices and also receive royalty payments or consulting fees from that brand company. While there are a myriad of reasons why device utilization has soared, questions arise as to whether financial ties between physicians and device manufacturers could be a factor in driving up spending on medical devices. An important FDA reform has been full disclosure by surgeon-consultants of their contracts with devices companies (FDA, 2007).

Another concern is the practice of sales representatives of device manufacturers often being present in operating rooms and helping physicians select medical devices. This custom increases the potential for conflicts of interest, because company representatives usually work on commission and can make as much from an operation incorporating the device as the surgeon does.

Kickbacks

In addition to conflicts of interest, the federal government is also focusing on kickbacks by the device industry. While kickbacks to physicians to recommend their products do not necessarily lead to higher Medicare spending since the government pays the same rate for a device regardless of the make, the anti-kickback law can be violated if a single bill is submitted for a procedure linked to a kickback.

While illegitimate payments to physicians have led to increased use of lower-quality medical devices in the spinal-implant market (Loyd, 2008), elimination of all such payments likely will prove difficult because they have become commonplace. Moreover, the anti-kickback law itself is insufficient to address the influence of money in the device industry because of the high burden of proof; prosecutors must generally meet a high specific intent standard, requiring proof defendants knew their conduct was unlawful and nevertheless engaged in the prohibited conduct (Altshuler et al., 2008). This requirement makes criminal convictions more difficult to obtain because of the need to prove intent to disobey the law.

Supporters of the consulting arrangements say they allow physicians and device manufacturers to collaborate, resulting in important advances in technology. Truthfully, most arrangements are quite legitimate compensation packages for research or product development, or royalties for products. The concern, however, is kickbacks might result in physicians opting for more expensive, lower-quality, or medically unnecessary medical devices for patients, which drives up health care costs, especially for Medicare. According to the federal Centers for Medicare and Medicaid, more than half of the nation's 700,000 hip and knee replacements are performed on Medicare beneficiaries. In theory, physicians use their best judgment about what is best for their patients, but to the extent they are given consulting arrangements, it could distort their incentives.

Artificial Joint Companies

Before 2007, pretrial diversion had been used in the health care fraud context in only two cases: the University of Medicine & Dentistry of New Jersey and Micrus Corp (Spivack & Raman, 2008). The University accepted a deferred prosecution agreement, which included the placement of a federal monitor to supervise all of its finances, or face indictment for federal fraud charges for overbilling, double-billing, and upcoding practices. The U.S. Department of Justice entered into a non-prosecution agreement with Micrus, a medical device company, in connection with its disclosure of $340,000 in bribes to physicians in France, Austria, Turkey, and elsewhere. Micrus agreed to pay a $450,000 fine, cooperate fully with the government's investigation, adopt a Foreign Corrupt Practices Act compliance program, and retain an independent compliance expert (DOJ, 2005).

Since 2007, there has been a notable increase of pretrial diversions in health care fraud involving violations of the:

- Anti-kickback law (42 U.S.C.A. §§ 1320a-7b (2006))
- Food, Drug, and Cosmetic Act (FDCA) 21 U.S.C.A. §§ 301 *et seq.* (2009))
- Health care fraud law (18 U.S.C.A. § 1347 (1996))

This marked increase in the use of deferred prosecution and non-prosecution agreements, also known as pretrial diversion agreements, is arguably the most profound development in corporate white-collar criminal practice over the past five years (Spivack & Raman, 2008).

The federal government reached settlements with the leading five artificial joint companies over kickbacks on hundreds of agreements under which physicians across the country received vacations and lavish meals. Some physicians accepted consulting fees as high as $200,000 from the firms in return for recommending their products. Biomet, Johnson & Johnson's DePuy Orthopaedics, Smith & Nephew, and Zimmer entered into deferred prosecution agreements and agreed to pay a combined $310 million to settle a federal investigation over allegations they paid about $800 million in kickbacks to physicians from 2002 to 2006. A fifth device company, Stryker, who cooperated early in the investigation, entered into a non-prosecution agreement and paid no fines. As part of the settlement, all five device manufacturers were required to make their consulting arrangements with physicians public and agreed to federal monitoring.

Kickback Settlements	
	(in millions)
Zimmer	$169.5
DePuy	$ 84.7
Smith & Nephew	$ 28.9
Biomet	$ 26.9
Stryker	-0-

Source: Spivack & Raman, 2008.

Stryker's non-prosecution agreement did not require the device company to admit to any facts or acknowledge any responsibility for its behavior. The other four device manufacturers did acknowledge responsibility and had criminal complaints filed against them generally outlining some of the relevant facts. In their civil settlements with the government, however, each of the four companies denied engaging in any wrongdoing and specifically denied any of the payments were illegal or resulted in any fraudulent claims. No physicians were identified or charged (Ridge & Baird, 2008; *see also* DOJ, 2007).

These 2007 diversion agreements were the first time companies were able to negotiate language affirmatively denying any wrongdoing. This major development is now commonly used in health care fraud contexts. This change reflects the belief that the principal role of the federal government in corporate criminal prosecution is to reform corporate cultures and effect widespread structural reform rather than to indict, prosecute, and punish (Spivack & Raman, 2008). Federal prosecutors, for example, declared the diversion agreements they negotiated with the orthopedic device sector were the "new" compliance standards for the device industry (DOJ, 2007).

Spinal Surgery

There is similar concern about device manufacturers in the $5.5 billion spinal-implant market (Loyd, 2008). In orthopedics in general, it has become almost as commonplace for surgeons to get money as device consultants, according to the Association for Ethics in Spine Surgery (Weiland, 2008). Yet, the federal Agency for Healthcare Research and Quality has little clinical evidence showing back surgery works for most patients, whether they get traditional fusion surgery or have a disk replaced (Martin et al., 2007).

Synthes, the third largest manufacturer of spinal implant devices, behind Medtronic and Johnson & Johnson, is facing a conflict of interest claim regarding surgeon-investigators who conducted a clinical trial of its artificial spinal disk, which the FDA approved in 2006. The surgeon-investigators claimed, in submissions to the FDA, the Synthes spinal disk worked much better than conventional surgery in which patients' vertebrae were fused (Abelson, 2008). This claim, however, became tainted when it was discovered the surgeon-investigators making the claims had hundreds of thousands of dollars invested with the New York investment company behind the device, Viscogliosi Brothers, according to information from a Philadelphia patient's 2007 lawsuit that settled for an undisclosed amount (Loyd, 2008). Additional lawsuits across the country are being filed against Synthes, as a growing number of patients experience problems with their spinal implants.

Device manufacturers have a legal obligation to inform the FDA of the financial interests of surgeon-investigators before they use a study's results for approval of their medical devices. While the FDA permits surgeons to have financial ties with manufacturers of the device they are studying, such relationships must be fully disclosed. When the FDA is aware of potential conflicts, it tends to subject the studies to a higher level of scrutiny. In addition, the FDA conducts on-site audits of clinical research study sites to detect chicanery; other times, simple data analysis reveals abnormalities requiring investigation of investigators. In the submissions by Synthes, the surgeons were found to have excluded an unusually high number of study participants with adverse outcomes from their study report to the FDA (Abelson, 2008).

Surgeon-investigators play a critical role in the FDA approval process for new medical devices. These surgeons are expected to act objectively in testing the safety and effectiveness of medical devices coming to market; however, when they stand to profit from FDA approval of the device they are testing, their professional objectivity is called into question. The investment interests of surgeons raise serious conflict of interest concerns about the integrity of clinical studies. Even though fusion surgery (surgically implanting an artificial vertebrae device onto the spine) continues to be the treatment of choice, there is substantial debate over how many patients actually benefit from it according to the Cochrane Collaboration, an international organization providing evidence-based research about the effects of medical treatments. Artificial spinal disks are now drawing the same skepticism from Medicare and most health insurers, who generally refuse to pay for artificial spinal disk surgeries.

Meanwhile, thousands of patients worldwide have received the spinal-implant devices manufactured by Synthes, which sell for about $10,000 in the U.S. The surgeon-investigators involved in the Synthes research, in the meantime, have moved on to study other medical devices by other device companies promoted by the Viscogliosi Brothers (Abelson, 2008).

Moral Dilemmas

1. How could neutral, unbiased, thorough testing of new medical devices be ensured?

PEDIATRIC DEVICES

The Institute of Medicine found pediatric devices are an example of where the FDA regulatory system does not work well for medical products where there are small numbers of widely varying patients. As defined by the FDA in connection with medical devices, a child is between the ages of two and eleven, up to twelve years of age. Physicians frequently jury-rig adult medical devices to fit in children's bodies, sometimes causing unexpected side effects. Yet the FDA lacks data on how medical devices affect children's growth and development or how the functioning of devices can be affected by the lifestyles and hormonal changes of children (Field & Tilson, 2005).

The FDA does not track post-market study commitments from the device industry involving children (21 U.S.C.A. § 360j(m)(8) (2007)). Agency regulators want extensive data before approving pediatric medical devices, yet there are few patients to acquire the data from because it is not feasible to conduct traditional regulated clinical trials on children. Moreover, when only a few children have a medical condition in need of a pediatric device, clinical trials and FDA approval of each device are impractical (Hall & Braun, 2008).

Pediatric Coronary Stents

There was little regulatory focus on the needs of children before the criminal investigation and misdemeanor conviction of the pediatric device company NuMED (Field & Tilson, 2005). NuMED has manufactured custom-made catheters, therapeutic balloons, and stents for children for more than forty years. NuMED's founder, president, and current chief executive officer pled guilty in federal court in Delaware on charges the company marketed unapproved stents for use in children, which resulted in a multimillion-dollar fine. The FDA and the U.S. Attorney's office in Wilmington, Delaware, took the position NuMED was using exceptions under FDA law to sell pediatric stents widely rather than to supply individual devices in cases of special need (Burton, 2007).

The FDA found NuMED had delivered more than thirty stents to pediatric surgeons at the DuPont Hospital for Children in Wilmington, Delaware, and concluded the hospital was using the medical devices too often for them to be considered custom medical devices, approved for use in emergencies. The FDA told NuMED it needed to obtain specific approvals each time it sold a device, which NuMED admits it did not do.

Currently, few U.S. companies make custom pediatric devices. The FDA has approved some pediatric devices for sale, most it has not. Some devices are used off label, meaning for a use the FDA has not specified; others are adult devices used off label for children. Still others are allowed by federal loopholes, including the custom device exemption, in which otherwise unapproved devices can be employed in emergency situations (Burton, 2007).

The case against NuMED offers a window into a crucial dilemma involving pediatric heart medical devices. While the FDA is not questioning the safety of NuMED's medical devices, pediatric surgeons worry the pediatric medical devices will become even harder to get with the new restrictions placed on NuMED. Pediatricians say treating infants and children with medical devices approved for use in adults is less safe than using the unapproved medical devices manufactured by NuMED. Without device manufacturers such as NuMED, children will need to go to Europe to receive pediatric cardiac medical devices. During the past two decades a number of pediatric catheterization devices, like the NuMED stents in question, have been developed in the U.S., approved, and used extensively and safely outside the U.S., but never approved for use inside the U.S. Many health care professionals blame cumbersome FDA policies and procedures that place children's safety over access to new pediatric devices that are needed by American children.

INSPECTIONS OF MEDICAL DEVICE MANUFACTURING FACILITIES

The reauthorized Medical Device User Fee Act provides almost $50 million for the FDA each fiscal year (von Eschenbach, 2008; see also Medical Device User Fee Amendments of 2007, 21 U.S.C.A. § 379j-1 (2007)). Yet, the resources and technology of the FDA are not enough to meet its regulatory responsibilities to oversee the device industry. For example, the General Accounting Office found the FDA cannot meet requirements for inspections of medical device manufacturing facilities in the U.S. or abroad. The FDA inspects U.S. facilities that manufacture the highest-risk medical devices once every three years and facilities that manufacture moderate-risk medical devices once every five years; both are supposed to be visited every two years (GAO, 2009).

NEGLIGENCE PER SE

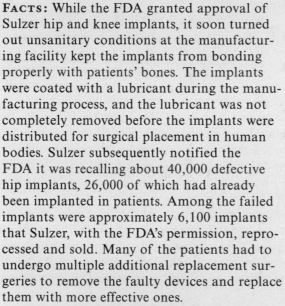

In re Sulzer Hip Prosthesis & Knee Prosthesis Liability Litigation
[Patients v. Medical Device Manufacturer]
455 F.Supp.2d 709 (U.S. District Court for the Northern District of Ohio,
Eastern Division 2006)

FACTS: While the FDA granted approval of Sulzer hip and knee implants, it soon turned out unsanitary conditions at the manufacturing facility kept the implants from bonding properly with patients' bones. The implants were coated with a lubricant during the manufacturing process, and the lubricant was not completely removed before the implants were distributed for surgical placement in human bodies. Sulzer subsequently notified the FDA it was recalling about 40,000 defective hip implants, 26,000 of which had already been implanted in patients. Among the failed implants were approximately 6,100 implants that Sulzer, with the FDA's permission, reprocessed and sold. Many of the patients had to undergo multiple additional replacement surgeries to remove the faulty devices and replace them with more effective ones.

To help compensate victims, Sulzer entered into a settlement agreement and established a research and monitoring fund for close to $1.0 billion. *In re Sulzer Hip Prosthesis & Knee Prosthesis Liability Litigation*, 2006 U.S. Dist. LEXIS 76009 (U.S. District Court for the Northern District of Ohio 2006). The settlement agreement is to terminate in 2012 even though Sulzer was purchased by Zimmer.

ISSUE: Are state claims premised on violation of FDA premarket approval requirements automatically pre-empted by the FDCA?

HOLDING AND DECISION: No, the FDCA automatically pre-empts state law claims for approved medical devices unless the device failed to conform with FDA premarket approval requirements.

ANALYSIS: The federal trial court began its analysis by affirming that FDA provisions on pre-emption pre-empt almost every type of state law claim that seeks to hold medical products

companies liable for approved medical devices. 21 U.S.C.A. § 360k(a) (1976). The only exception to this federal provision is claims that a medical device failed to conform to the FDA requirements prescribed by the premarket approval process.

To determine whether a particular state law claim is pre-empted involves a three-part inquiry: first, courts examine the general duties imposed by the state law causes of action; next, they consider the effect a successful lawsuit, asserting those state causes of action, would have on the FDCA; third, they determine whether the state claims threaten the federal premarket approval process requirements. Under this inquiry, state law claims of design defect are pre-empted. State law claims for failure to warn are also pre-empted, since the premarket approval process includes FDA scrutiny of the medical device's warning labels.

Implied warranty claims are based on the accepted standards of design and manufacture of medical devices. In the case of approved devices that have gone through the premarket approval process, these criteria are set by the FDA. Allowing breach of implied warranty claims would therefore create an irreconcilable conflict: a judgment for breach of implied warranty that rested on allegations about standards other than those permitted by the FDA would necessarily interfere with the premarket approval process and, indeed, would supplant FDA requirements. Accordingly, state claims for breach of implied warranty are also pre-empted by the FDCA.

RULE OF LAW: Approved medical devices that conform to FDA premarket approval requirements are not subject to state negligence design defect, failure to warn, or breach of warranty claims because they are preempted by the FDCA.

(*See generally* Valdeck, 2008).

While Sulzer lost its independence as a result of its failure to comply with generally accepted manufacturing practices and was purchased by Zimmer, this case demonstrates the lack of FDA regulatory enforcement of medical device manufacturers. Air emissions from medical device manufacturing facilities are routinely and arduously regulated by the federal Environmental Protection Agency, less any volatile organic compounds foul the nation's atmosphere (Approval and promulgation of air quality implementation plans; Control of volatile organic compounds from medical device manufacturing, 40 C.F.R. Part 52 (2007)).

FDA enforcement has been practically nonexistent for foreign medical device manufacturers. Though the FDA plans to conduct four hundred foreign site inspections in 2009, eleven inspections of foreign device manufacturers occurred between 2004 and 2008 (Crosse, 2008). Perhaps this historic level of inspection activity can be attributed to the fact that FDA computer systems cannot determine the number of medical device manufacturing facilities abroad that export products to the U.S. Nevertheless, even without knowledge of the number of foreign facilities exporting medical devices into the U.S., the FDA has estimated inspections of all medical device manufacturing facilities abroad would take twenty-seven years (GAO, 2007).

POST-MARKETING SURVEILLANCE

The FDA has suffered a string of regulatory failures with respect to medical devices, which is not necessarily unexpected, because it is difficult to test medical devices for safety and effectiveness (Valadeck, 2008). This difficulty explains why the statutory standard requiring a reasonable assurance of safety and effectiveness before approving medical devices is lower than the standard for drugs, which may receive approval only if shown to be safe and effective for their intended use. *Compare* 21 U.S.C.A. §§ 360c(a)(1) (2002), 360d(a)(2)(A) (1997) (providing the standard for medical devices) *with* 21 U.S.C.A. § 355(d) (2008) (providing the standard for new drugs). Moreover, the device industry is limited in its clinical testing of medical devices on healthy patients; thus, devices often receive approval on the basis of a single clinical trial. (21 C.F.R. § 814.20(b) (1997)). For this key reason, it is not uncommon for unforeseen risks to emerge after medical devices are approved for general marketing.

Furthermore, unless medical innovations are discontinued and medical devices are held to the status quo, it is a given that patients will be subject to some unforeseen risks in new treatments that come with the potential of improved care. Nevertheless, any serious failures are cause for concern. There have been massive recalls of pacemakers, heart valves, heart pumps, defibrillators, and hip and knee prostheses over the past two decades,[LN1] all of which have exacted a serious toll on the patients who faced removal and replacement surgeries (Vladeck, 2008).

While the FDA posts information about the status of medical device studies online to improve its procedures for regulating the studies, the agency still faces challenges in monitoring medical devices after they have been approved. The FDA has been challenged by:

- Competing interests of patient safety and approving new technology that could benefit patients
- Complexity of medical devices
- Growth in the device industry
- Increasing popularity of medical devices

(von Eschenbach, 2008)

As a growing number of medical devices with more and more technological complexities are approved by the FDA, there is less and less room for error. Yet, the FDA is confronted by administrative difficulties due to:

- Conflicting patient privacy and legal concerns
- Ongoing regulatory and/or criminal investigations of device manufacturers
- Inconsistent requirements for preserving trade secrets covering medical devices

Inadequate tracking and enforcement within the FDA has allowed several device manufacturers to avoid completing follow-up studies required as part of the approval of their products (FDA, 2007).

Moral Dilemmas

1. Does quickly approving new medical devices do more harm than good?

Internal Analysis of Follow-Up Studies

When an internal FDA task force recently examined approved medical devices where device manufacturers were required to complete follow-up studies, they found poor communication, a flawed safety reporting system, and inadequate enforcement within the agency. In addition, the task force found problems with medical devices are vastly underreported and most data submitted to the agency included incomplete and unreliable information (FDA, 2008). Specifically:

- More than half the device manufacturers' annual reports to the FDA lacked required post-marketing data
- Final results of post-marketing surveillance were overdue from most of the device manufacturers
- Follow-up results were unavailable for about one-fourth of the medical devices
- Information from reports to the FDA, or from FDA reviews of device manufacturers, were unavailable on approximately one-fifth of the medical devices
- The progress and results of follow-up surveillance studies by device manufacturers were not being monitored by the FDA
- Required follow-up studies for completion were not being tracked by the FDA, even though they were considered a condition of approval
- Device manufacturers were not being sanctioned for poor regulatory compliance

(FDA, 2007)

One in four of the FDA researchers, as well as an increasing number of outside experts (Field & Tilson, 2005), believe the agency lacks an effective system for monitoring the safety of approved medical devices. After shortfalls in the FDA's monitoring of medical devices were identified, several specific recommendations were made (Schultz, 2007). FDA researchers recommended the agency:

- Improve its tracking of studies done by device manufacturers after products are on the market
- Work with the private sector to improve device tracking methods, including the use of digital medical records
- Engage in less secrecy and more openness in the sharing of information about the benefits and risks of medical devices
- Collaborate with the National Institutes of Health to prioritize research on medical devices used on children, despite a lack of companies' studies in the pediatric field
- Collaborate with patients, health organizations, and the device industry to increase the reporting of safety concerns
- Create a public database indicating the status and findings of post-marketing surveillance studies
- Develop a unique tracking number for each medical device to serve as an identifier in the event of post-market concerns about a device

- Improve the way the FDA communicates with the public about recalled medical devices
- Integrate the medical device data maintained by other federal agencies including the VA and the Department of Defense
- Expand MedSun, a pilot program that collects safety reports from 350 hospitals in real time, and disseminate its findings to more medical professionals outside the network

(FDA, 2007; FDA, 2003)

Sentinel Initiative

The FDA always used voluntary self-reporting to discover adverse reactions from devices. However, self-reporting from health care providers revealed only an estimated one in ten problems (GAO, 2007; *see also* Liang, 2006). Device manufacturers and health care providers are required to report deaths or serious injuries resulting from the use of medical devices within ten business days to the FDA, and, if the manufacturer's identity is known, to the manufacturer as well; the device manufacturer must, in turn, investigate the event and provide additional information to the FDA within thirty calendar days (Medical device reporting: Manufacturer reporting, importer reporting, user facility reporting, distributor reporting, 21 C.F.R. Parts 803 and 804 (2000)). "Serious injury" is defined as any injury or illness that is life-threatening, results in permanent impairment to body function or permanent damage to body structure, or requires medical or surgical intervention to prevent such impairment or damage (*see* 21 C.F.R. § 803.3 (2008)).

Now, a new program, called the Sentinel Initiative, will allow the FDA and state regulatory agencies to mine electronic health records and claims data to identify patterns for possible problems with medical devices (von Eschenbach, 2008). Mining of this data will help ensure medical devices are safe for consumers after they enter the marketplace. Sentinel will access data from more than 25 million Medicare beneficiaries and 35 million members of WellPoint.

Sentinel could help reduce the $900 million spent on treating outcomes of adverse events each year. Data collected by Sentinel will also be used for comparative effectiveness research to compare the cost and effectiveness of different medical products.

Patient privacy will be preserved because the data will stay with Medicare and the private insurers. Personal information will not be used for Sentinel. What the FDA needs to know is what is happening in the population being treated by all these different medical devices. While the device industry is concerned Sentinel will raise unnecessary concerns because the analysis of data will not be as rigorous as clinical trials, it allows the FDA to move from reliance on voluntary reporting of adverse events to proactive monitoring of medical devices (von Eschenbach, 2008).

Reprocessed Medical Devices

There is increasing concern about reprocessed medical devices designated for single use, as the practice has developed into a $100 million market. Currently, the FDA requires reprocessors to register and obtain approval for each medical device they seek to reprocess. In addition, the FDA relies on physicians to report malfunctions of used medical devices, but this reporting is voluntary. While the FDA requires health care facilities to report patient deaths involving medical devices, there is no requirement to report device malfunctions.

Some U.S. hospitals reduce costs by recycling medical devices labeled for single use. Among the devices being reused are biopsy forceps (including those used for stomach and bowel surgery), membrane scrapers (often used in eye surgery), breast pump kits, surgical blades, and drill bits used to bore through bone. The FDA has approved the following reprocessed medical devices:

- Cardiovascular devices (angiography catheter, blood pressure cuff, cardiac guidewire, compressible limb sleeve, angiographic needle, intro-aortic balloon system, trocar, percutaneous transluminal coronary angioplasty catheter)
- Gastro/urology devices (endoscopic needles, urological catheters)
- General hospital devices (non-powered floatation therapy mattresses, mattress covers, surgical gowns, irrigating syringes)
- Obstetrics and gynecological devices (laparoscopic dissectors, scissors, endoscopic electrocautery and accessories, episiotomy scissors)
- Respiratory devices (short-term spinal needles, gas masks, breathing mouthpieces, tracheal tubes, oral and nasal catheters)
- Surgical devices (endoscopic blades, guidewires, blood lancets, disposable vein strippers, forceps, scalpel blades, pneumatically powered saws)

The practice is legal and well established as long as hospitals follow FDA regulations for reprocessing medical devices (see FDA, 2006). The policy rationale for permitting this practice is the belief that medical device manufacturers routinely designate devices single-use for economic, not safety reasons. Whether medical device companies would always escape liability if their single-use devices are recycled and lead to serious injuries remains to be determined.

While the practice of reprocessing devices in-house is fraught with risk and infection control, the process of shipping medical devices to reprocessing facilities to be cleansed, sterilized, and tested for reuse also raises safety concerns. Companies of the single-use medical devices say their medical products are not designed to withstand the strong chemicals and sterilization methods used at reprocessing plants. In addition, used medical devices with porous surfaces or small gaps may still contain traces of blood, tissue, or other bodily fluids that could transmit viral and bacterial infections (GAO, 2000).

Hospitals and reprocessing firms say reprocessed medical devices are just as safe as new single-use medical devices because of modern sterilization methods (Klein, 2005a). Supporters of the practice also say used medical devices cost 40 to 60 percent less. Estimates are the VA could save as much as $30 million a year by using reprocessed medical devices.

A GAO analysis of eight years of FDA data concluded there was no evidence reprocessed single-use medical devices increased health risks for patients. As many as one hundred single-use medical devices, or 2 percent of all single-use medical devices, are currently reprocessed for further use (GAO, 2009). The question arises whether this reprocessing industry could resemble the body parts industry addressed in a subsequent chapter. What actually happens to those ocular implant devices in the deceased?

Informed Consent for Use of Reprocessed Medical Devices

Device manufacturers are lobbying several states for legislation that would require hospitals and other health care providers to obtain informed consent from patients before reprocessed medical devices are used in medical procedures (Kerber, 2005). Currently, informed consent is not required for the use of reprocessed medical devices; patients are unaware used devices are being utilized by hospitals in their treatment. Theoretically, physicians know whether they are using reprocessed devices because of an FDA regulation requiring medical products to be marked as reprocessed.

Unregulated Internet Transactions

Auction Web sites are selling reprocessed medical devices designated for one-time use (e.g., Klein, 2005a). Where the Web sites are always getting their devices is unclear; are there established systems for collecting discarded devices from hospitals and medical clinics, or are there other sources? With the Internet sale of reprocessed medical devices unregulated, there is no reliable way of knowing:

- Where sellers obtained such used medical devices
- Who is authorized to purchase the used devices
- Whether the devices were first used by physicians or veterinarians (in human or animal patients)

- How used medical devices were handled and re-sterilized before being sold online
- What quality controls were utilized before the used medical devices are invasively used on patients

For example, eBay only requires sellers of regulated medical devices to add a disclaimer that no one should bid on the medical products unless they are authorized purchasers. One eBay seller offers laparo-scopic medical devices used in abdominal surgery, circumcision trays, catheters, and biopsy instruments, which are purchased by physicians, veterinarians, and hospitals. eBay claims no responsibility for items sold on its site; it views the site as a marketplace (Klein, 2005a). Alliance Medical, the largest U.S. reprocessor of medical devices, neither condones nor supports auction Web sites for the sale of reprocessed medical devices. ClearMedical, one of the five largest U.S. reprocessors, operates an eBay virtual storefront that sells non-invasive reprocessed medical devices, which do not enter the bloodstream when used on patients, such as pulse oximeter sensors and compression sleeves. Although ClearMedical does not confirm the identity of authorized purchasers, it is not concerned with who could buy its used medical devices.

Joint Device Registry

The FDA lags behind other countries' similar agen-cies when it comes to monitoring how people are faring with joint devices such as the metal hip socket from Zimmer. Zimmer suspended sales of the socket after physicians noticed patients who had received it were experiencing severe pain and needed another round of surgery to replace it. Problems with the medical device could have been detected sooner if the U.S., like most other countries, had a registry of patients who receive joint devices. The risk in the U.S. that a patient will need a replacement procedure because of a flawed product or technique can be up to double the risk in countries with such databases (Meier, 2009).

The federal Agency for Healthcare Research and Quality says the U.S. wastes billions of dollars annually on medical treatments that may not work; the financial and human consequences are also large when evidence exists but is not collected. The toll of early device replacement is magnified in the U.S. because of the sheer number of procedures that take place[LN2] (AAOS, 2009; Meier, 2009). Nearly one million hip and knee joint devices are used each year (NCHS, 2008).

The FDA does have a registry for some medi-cal products, for example, for patients on the acne medication Accutane, which can cause birth defects, but various hurdles block most product registries, including:

- Conflicting legal and privacy concerns
- A decentralized health care system where physi-cians often do not report problems with medical devices
- Lack of funding
- Irreconcilable differences regarding whether partici-pation should be mandatory
- Overwhelming number of medical devices to monitor
- Refusal by Medicare to gather registry data like private insurers

(Marinac-Dabic, 2007; Meier, 2009)

Two months after Congress introduced legislation to create a government-backed national device registry, the American Academy of Orthopaedic Surgeons formed the American Joint Replacement Registry, a nonprofit organization dedicated to collecting and reporting on hip and knee joint replacement proce-dures (AAOS, 2009).

Counterfeit Medical Device Transactions

Sophisticated, technologically savvy, and organized counterfeiters have entered the medical device mar-ket, especially the surgical supply sector (Cahoy, 2008). The process for counterfeit devices is virtually identical to problematic counterfeit pharmaceutical transactions with detection very much lacking due to underdeveloped and impractical technology by federal regulatory and law enforcement agencies. The FDA and international government authorities have warned counterfeit sales are linked to funding international criminal operations and terrorist activities, including those of Hezbollah and Al Qaeda (IACC, 2005). The World Health Organization estimates 10 to 15 percent of all medical devices in the world are counterfeit.

In one case, a U.S. company was convicted for introducing counterfeit surgical mesh, which it had purchased overseas and then resold to a domestic dis-tributor. The counterfeit surgical mesh was not only misbranded by virtue of being counterfeit, but was also adulterated as a result of unsanitary conditions. The company claimed it bought the product from an unnamed seller, mistakenly believing it was authentic (LaMendola, 2005).

Counterfeiters sell tainted, fake, and ineffective medical devices to unsuspecting health care providers, and they make a lot of money in the process. Passing off counterfeit devices is surprisingly easy because there is a general lack of suspicion in the medical community about fakes. Several interacting factors contribute to this reality:

- Providers have little, if any, suspicion a counterfeit medical device may be causing therapeutic failure associated with medical treatment

- Poor clinical responses are often attributed to human variation
- Providers rarely ask where medical devices were purchased to identify potentially problematic sources such as certain foreign countries or the Internet
- Penalties for counterfeiting are low

(Liang, 2006)

Medical Errors from Tube Misconnections to Devices

A small but steady number of tubes and catheters are being inadvertently connected to the wrong medical devices. Hospital errors each year involve misconnections, including:

- Intravenous lines connected to epidural lines
- Bladder irrigation solutions connected to central IV catheters
- Intravenous solutions sent through urinary tract, epidural, and kidney dialysis catheters

The Joint Commission on the Accreditation of Healthcare Organizations says misconnections generally are unreported and there is no accurate way to compare errors on a year-to-year basis, but they are a persistent and potentially deadly occurrence. According to the U.S. Pharmacopeia, more than three hundred misconnections occurred between 1999 and 2004, and it is likely that more than one thousand have occurred since 2004.

The main cause of misconnections is the universal connection system known as Luer fittings, which connect a broad range of medical devices, according to the U.S. Institute for Safe Medication Practice. Several hospital alliances and device manufacturers are working to address the problem. Premier, the purchasing alliance of 1,500 U.S. hospitals, is leading the most significant initiative by educating hospital staff about the errors and working with device manufacturers to redesign equipment so differing tube connectors are not compatible with each other. A system designed by Viasys Healthcare uses new connectors that are incompatible with Luer connectors and other tubes received FDA approval. Other groups are working to develop technical standards for use in designing safer tubing and connection systems.

STATE TORT CLAIMS AGAINST DEVICE MANUFACTURERS

Federal law makes no provision for damage suits against device manufacturers, and, as a result, injured patients have turned to state law and have won substantial awards. For years, the device industry maintained the FDA's authority pre-empted tougher state regulation. In 2004, longstanding federal policy on pre-emption was reversed; the FDA maintained that approved medical devices should override most claims for damages under state law, such as claims for defective design of devices, failure to warn, and negligence.

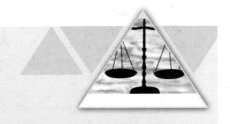

FEDERAL PRE-EMPTION

Riegel v. Medtronic, Inc.
[Patient v. Medical Device Manufacturer]
552 U.S. 312 (U.S. Supreme Court 2008)

FACTS: Charles Riegel experienced serious complications in 1996 when a balloon in a catheter manufactured by Medtronic burst in his severely blocked right coronary artery. Riegel and his wife filed a lawsuit against Medtronic in 1999 alleging the catheter had design flaws and a misleading label. Riegel died in 2004 of unrelated causes, but his wife pursued the lawsuit. Medtronic had received FDA approval to market the catheter in 1994. Two lower federal courts dismissed the lawsuit, based on the argument that companies who manufacture medical devices approved by the FDA are protected from product liability lawsuits filed in state courts.

ISSUE: Does FDA approval of medical devices protect companies from product liability lawsuits filed in state courts?

HOLDING AND DECISION: Yes, because product liability lawsuits filed against device manufacturers in state courts could undermine the balance between the benefits and risks of medical technologies as determined by the FDA.

ANALYSIS: The Court re-affirmed what most federal courts have regarded as settled law since the 1976 Medical Device Amendments were enacted; the FDA, rather than differing state

(continues)

(continued)

regulations and multiple conflicting jury verdicts, should determine the safety and effectiveness of medical technology. Congress gave the FDA pre-emptive authority for device approvals in 1976 and further review by state courts will not improve patient safety but will result in needless delays in patient access to essential medical technologies, more lawsuits, and ultimately higher health care costs. The pre-empted claims only address design and labeling (21 C.F.R. pt. 201 (2008)); device

manufacturers still could be held liable for other issues such as faulty manufacturing if something goes wrong.

RULE OF LAW: States cannot implement safety requirements for medical devices that differ from federal requirements.

(*See generally* Brennan, 2009; Bridy, 2009; Chemerinsky, 2009; Goldstein & Winograd, 2008; Troy & Wood, 2008).

The concept of pre-emption has its foundation in the U.S. Constitution, which provides that whenever there is a substantial conflict, federal law is superior to state law. Article VI of the Constitution provides that the laws of the United States "shall be the supreme Law of the Land;... any Thing in the Constitution or Laws of any state to the Contrary notwithstanding." Legislation has been introduced to overturn this Supreme Court decision whereby FDA approval of certain medical devices protects companies from product liability lawsuits filed in state courts. Opponents of the decision are concerned that if device manufacturers are not held liable, financial incentives will lead them away from ensuring the safety of their medical devices.

Supporters of the Supreme Court decision argue deferring scientific judgment from the FDA to the states would create a system where each state would have its own requirements, which would be cost prohibitive for device manufacturers. The medical products industries have contended for years the legal environment around their products has grown too restrictive and is stymieing innovation.

This Supreme Court decision applies only to medical devices that have undergone the FDA pre-market approval process, the most thorough process used by the agency. In 1996, the Supreme Court ruled that FDA approval of medical devices through other processes does not protect companies from product liability lawsuits filed in state courts. *See Medtronic, Inc. v. Lohr*, 518 U.S. 470 (U.S. Supreme Court 1996) (holding that the Medical Devices Act does not pre-empt state law claims that are equal to those imposed under federal law, or state law defective design claims); *see also Hillsborough County, Fla. v. Automated Medical Laboratories, Inc.*, 471 U.S. 707 (U.S. Supreme Court 1985) (holding that the FDA's authority in regulating blood banks was not sufficient to pre-empt local regulation). Most medical devices currently on the market underwent a process in which the FDA found them substantially equivalent to those marketed before the enactment of the 1976 Medical Device laws. Some

legal experts are recommending a government-run compensation fund be established for patients harmed by medical devices, similar to the fund for vaccines.

USE OF MEDICAL DEVICES FOR NON-MEDICAL OR ENTERTAINMENT PURPOSES

There is debate over the ethics and safety of using medical devices, such as ultrasound machines, for non-medical or entertainment purposes. In most states, there are gaping holes between federal and local oversight of ultrasound machine use.

Pregnant women can pay $160 to $295 at fetal imaging centers to receive high-resolution videos of moving images of their fetuses. The centers, which have operated in non-medical settings across the U.S. for several years, have caused concern because they are not regulated and because anyone with an ultrasound machine can open such a studio. While some believe the service is safe, the FDA and the American Institute of Ultrasound Medicine frown upon the practice. The FDA issued a statement in 2004 warning pregnant women against the fetal videos, saying it is an unapproved use of a medical device and people who perform ultrasounds for this purpose without physician oversight might be violating state or local laws. In addition, the agency says while there is no evidence of ultrasound scanning harming a fetus, casual exposure should be avoided because it can produce vibrations and increases the temperature of tissues. At the same time, device manufacturers maintain extra scans done purely for entertainment are not harmful, if the equipment is used properly.

Moral Dilemmas

1. What kinds of medical devices, if any, should patients not be entitled to reimbursement for?

FUTURE OF THE DEVICE INDUSTRY

Pharmaceutical company interest in acquiring medical device firms runs in cycles. The device industry goes through IPO boom and bust cycles. During each boom, most new entrants are not device manufacturers in the traditional sense; they have one product and probably should not go public. However, investors get caught up in the hype. During bust cycles, all but a few such one-product device manufacturers trade well below their offering price. Today, pharmaceuticals are starting to acquire device manufacturers to make them more diverse (Wharton, 2006a).

While the device industry does not have a tradition of spinning out or licensing products, there have been cases where larger device manufacturers bought entire firms for their products. An attractive option for venture capitalists and entrepreneurs is a sale to a large pharmaceutical or device company. Even though the public markets are currently shaky, device manufacturers with significant medical advancements have attractive valuations.

While prospects for the device industry are positive, the industry may be challenged in the long term by the ability and willingness of the nation's health care systems to pay for medical devices. With higher federal budget deficits, government spending on health care is unlikely to keep up with the demand created by and for new technologies. Unless the budget increases dramatically, the U.S. will have to start rationing medical technology.

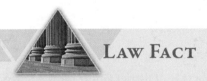

LAW FACT

MEDICAL MONITORING

Do healthy patients have standing to sue device manufacturers if they face increased risks of harm from defective medical devices compared to those undergoing traditional surgery?

An increased risk of future harm requiring ongoing medical monitoring due to an implanted cardiac medical device was sufficient to qualify as injury-in-fact to fulfill the first element of the standing to sue requirement. Standing may be conferred even though the device had not yet malfunctioned or caused any demonstrable physical injuries (*see* Schillaci, 2006; Clausen, 2006).
   —*Sutton v. St. Jude Medical S.C., Inc.*, 419 F.3d 568 (U.S. Court of Appeals for the 6th Circuit 2005) rehearing en banc denied Jan. 23, 2006.

CHAPTER SUMMARY

- The potential market for medical devices is enormous, as up to 35 million Americans have conditions that could be treated by them.
- The market is helped by the federal government, which quickly approves new medical devices and helps facilitate patient reimbursement.
- Physicians and patients, however, are slow to accept new medical device technology before it is proven safe and effective, especially as it usually requires invasive surgery to implant.
- It is difficult to test new medical devices for safety as there is often not a large pool of patients to test upon and patients' unique characteristics may affect the device's success or lack thereof; furthermore, the FDA lacks the resources to closely monitor testing, manufacturing, or results after approval, meaning problems are often largely undiscovered or unreported.
- Many medical devices require constant monitoring, and often insurance plans will not pay for remote monitoring, creating financial difficulties for both patients and health care providers; however, such devices can actually save insurers money, as they often allow the patient to receive treatment at the first sign of a problem, which usually costs less than receiving treatment after a problem has fully developed and sometimes even saves the patient's life.
- The FDA's regulations require updating in order to account for new hybrid devices that incorporate drugs and/or biologics.
- Nanodevices are the newest form of medical device technology and offer great promise; some are only the size of a few atoms.

- Children's medical devices are another area of the industry's market with the potential for further development.
- The medical device industry is wrought with conflict of interest problems, as doctors sometimes receive substantial kickbacks for utilizing certain brands and sometimes have financial ties to the investment companies funding device research and development.
- Reprocessed medical devices are another cause for concern as FDA standards are not always strictly adhered to, patients are not necessarily informed they are receiving a reprocessed device, and such devices are often obtained from unregulated sources, such as the Internet.
- Counterfeit medical devices also find their way into the market somewhat easily, as they are difficult to detect, the medical community does not have a high level of awareness of counterfeits, and the sanctions for counterfeiting are low.
- Debate over whether patients should be allowed to sue device manufacturers under product liability theories is ongoing; on one hand, it would encourage manufacturers to make their products safer; on the other, it would allow the FDA less control over product standards, possibly resulting in varying or conflicting standards between the states.
- As technology continues to allow for more advanced, and more expensive, medical devices, at some point, insurers may not be able to afford to reimburse every patient for every device.

LAW NOTES

1. *In re Guidant Corp. Implantable Defibrillators Product Liability Litigation* (U.S. District Court for the District of Minnesota, ongoing); *In re Sulzer Hip Prosthesis & Knee Prosthesis Liability Litigation*, 455 F.Supp.2d 709 (U.S. District Court for the Northern District of Ohio, Eastern Division 2006) (recall of hip and knee prostheses); *In re St. Jude Medical, Inc. Silzone Heart Valves Products Liability Litigation*, 2004 WL 45503 (U.S. District Court for the District of Minnesota 2004) (a heart valve's silver coating caused the valves to leak after they had been implanted in over 36,000 patients); *Horn v. Thoratec Corp.*, 376 F.3d 163 (U.S. Court of Appeals for the 3rd Circuit 2004) (a screw ring in the heart pump disconnected over time, causing death in some patients); *Goodlin v. Medtronic, Inc.*, 167 F.3d 1367 (U.S. Court of Appeals for the 11th Circuit 1999) (a Medtronic pacemaker was determined to be defectively designed; some patients died when the pacemaker's lead failed and other patients were forced to undergo open-heart surgery to replace the defective part), *rehearing denied*, 180 F.3d 276 (U.S. Court of Appeals for the 11th Circuit 1999); *Bowling v. Pfizer, Inc.*, 143 F.R.D. 141 (U.S. District Court for the Southern District of Ohio, Western Division 1992) (55,000 patients received defective heart valves).
2. During the life of the Swedish Hip and Knee Registries, the revision burden was reduced from 17 percent to 7 percent. In one year, the Australian National Joint Replacement Registry reported a 0.6 percent decrease in revision knee surgery at a savings value of $8.7 million. One estimate is that the American Joint Replacement Registry could result in a one-year savings of $30 million by simply reducing the number of revision surgeries and using more suitable medical products (Hayashi, 2008).

CHAPTER BIBLIOGRAPHY

AAOS (American Academy of Orthopaedic Surgeons). (2009, July 23). *Press release: American Joint Replacement Registry announced; American Academy of Orthopaedic Surgeons creates independent organization.* Rosemont, IL.

Abelson, R. (2008, January 30). Financial ties cited as issue in spine study. *New York Times,* p. A1.

Altshuler, M. et al. (2008). Health care fraud. *American Criminal Law Review, 45,* 607-663.

Basile, E. M., & Lorell, B. H. (2006). The Food & Drug Administration's regulation of risk disclosure for implantable cardioverter defibrillators: Has technology outpaced the agency's regulatory framework? *Food & Drug Law Journal, 61,* 251-272.

Berman, D. K. (2005, October 19). J&J is weighing its alternatives on Guidant deal. *Wall Street Journal,* p. A3 (Guidant failed to notify cardiologists of a malfunctioning device until after numerous patients had died).

Birnie, D. H. et al. (2007). Use of implantable cardioverter defibrillators in Canadian and US survivors of out-of-hospital cardiac arrest. *Canadian Medical Association Journal, 177* (1), 49-51.

Brennan, D. (2009). Federal preemption of all state law tort claims in *Riegel v. Medtronic*: A need to undo a serious wrong. *Western State University Law Review, 36,* 137-171.

Bridy, A. (2009). Trade secret prices and high-tech devices: How medical device manufacturers are seeking to sustain profits by propertizing prices. *Texas Intellectual Property Law Journal, 17,* 187-222.

Burns, L. R. et al. (2007). Assessment of medical devices: How to conduct comparative technology evaluations of product performance. *International Journal of Technology Assessment in Health Care, 23* (4), 455-464.

Burns, L. R. (2006). Dealing with innovation and costs in orthopedics: A conversation with Dane Miller. *Health Affairs.* 241-252 (an interview with the CEO of Biomet before he left the medical device manufacturer).

Burton, T. M. (2007, July 31). NuMED is guilty in FDA case. *Wall Street Journal,* p. B8.

Cahoy, D. R. (2008). Addressing the north-south divide in pharmaceutical counterfeiting. *Wake Forest Intellectual Property Law Journal, 8,* 407-432.

Chemerinsky, E. (2009). Twentieth annual Supreme Court Review: An overview of the October 2007 Supreme Court term. *Touro Law Review, 25,* 541-552.

Chow, T. et al. (2007). Microvolt t-wave alternans identifies patients with ischemic cardiomyopathy who benefit from implantable cardioverter-defibrillator therapy. *Journal of the American College of Cardiology, 49,* 50-58 (finding that one-third of the patients in two Ohio medical facilities had defibrillators implanted into their chests needlessly).

Clausen, J. C. (2006). Actual injury from medical device not required to confer standing in claim for medical monitoring: *Sutton v. St. Jude Medical, S.C., Inc.,* 419 F.3d 568 (6th Cir. 2005). *Suffolk University Law Review, 39,* 871-878.

Crosse. N., director of health care, General Accountability Office. (2008, January 29). Medical devices: Challenges for FDA in conducting manufacturer inspections. Testimony before the U.S. House Subcommittee on Oversight & Investigations, Committee on Energy & Commerce.

DOJ (U.S. Department of Justice). (2005, March 2). *Press release: Micrus Corporation enters into agreement to resolve potential Foreign Corrupt Practices Act liability.* Washington, DC: DOJ, Criminal Division.

Donohue, J. M. et al. (2007). A decade of direct-to-consumer advertising of prescription drugs. *New England Journal of Medicine, 357* (7), 673-681.

Douglas, P. S., & Sedrakyan, A., professors of medicine at Duke University. (2009, March 28). Clinical effectiveness of coronary stents in the elderly: Results from 262,700 Medicare patients in ACC-NCDR, American College of Cardiology's 58th Annual Scientific Session, Orlando, FL (comparative effectiveness study of drug-coated stents with bare metal ones on patients in the American College of Cardiology's National Cardiovascular Data Registry).

Espicom (Espicom Healthcare Intelligence). (2009). *The medical device market: USA.* Rockville, MD; Espicom, 2009 International.

Fadern, T. J., managing director, Office of Corporate Alliances, Mack Center for Technological Innovation. (2007, February 2). Panel discussion: Emerging technologies update day. Wharton School at the University of Pennsylvania, PA.

FDA (U.S. Food & Drug Administration). (2008). *Overview of the Office of Combination Products.* Washington, DC: FDA.

___. (2007, July 25). *Nanotechnology: A report of the U.S. Food & Drug Administration Nanotechnology Task Force.* Washington, DC: FDA.

___. (2006, November). *Report of the postmarket transformation leadership team: Strengthening FDA's postmarket program for medical devices.* Washington, DC: FDA Center for Devices & Radiological Health (CDRH).

___. (2004, June 1). *Guidance for industry and FDA staff: Medical Device User Fee and Modernization Act of 2002, validation data in premarket notification submissions (501k (s)) for reprocessed single-use medical devices.* Washington, DC: FDA CDRH.

___. (2003). *Guidance for industry: Product recalls, including removals and corrections.* Washington, DC: FDA Office of Regulatory Affairs/Office of Enforcement.

___. (2002, February 28). *Is the product a medical device?* Washington, DC: FDA CDRH.

Feder, B. J. (2006, September 9). Remote control for health care. *New York Times,* p. C2.

Ferris, N. (2007, October 31). Device manufacturers push Medicare reimbursement for remote patient care. *Government Health Information Technology Magazine: Solutions of State and Local Government,* Washington, DC (summarizes the medical device manufacturers' trade group report, "Telehomecare and Remote Monitoring: An Outcomes Overview" that reviewed evidence from the Veterans Health Administration, one of the most advanced users of telemedicine).

Field, M. J., & Tilson, H. (eds.). (2005). *Safe medical devices for children.* Washington, DC: Institute of Medicine.

Freedonia (Freedonia Group). (2007). *Implantable medical devices to 2011: Demand and sales forecasts, market share, market size, market leaders.* Cleveland, OH: Freedonia (analyzes the U.S. medical implant device industry).

Fuhrmans, V. (2008, March 11). Insurers pressed to pay more for prostheses. *Wall Street Journal,* p. D1.

GAO (General Accountability Office). (2009). *Medical devices: FDA should take steps to ensure that high-risk device types are approved through the most stringent premarket review process.* Washington, DC: GAO.

___. (2008). *Challenges for FDA in conducting manufacturer inspections.* Washington, DC: GAO.

___. (2007). *Medical devices: Status of FDA's program for inspections by accredited organizations.* Washington, DC: GAO.

___. (2006). *Improvement needed in FDA's postmarket decision-making and oversight process.* Washington, DC: GAO.

___. (2000). *Single-use medical devices: Little available evidence of harm from reuse, but oversight warranted.* Washington, DC: GAO.

Goldstein, T. C. & Winograd, B. (2008). Looking ahead: October Term 2008. *Cato Supreme Court Review,* 331-357.

Hall, R. F., & Braun, T. A. (2008). Leaving no child behind? Abigail Alliance, pediatric products and off-label. *Houston Journal of Health Law & Policy, 8,* 271-313.

Hayashi, A. (2008, March). Building a national joint replacement registry: Can the United States find its way? *AAOS Now, 2* (3), 7-10.

House, D. (2006). Access to justice: The economics of civil justice: Tort reform, what about the little guy? *Loyola of Los Angeles Law Review, 39,* 819-839 (examining the recall of defective medical heart devices).

IACC (International Anti-Counterfeiting Coalition). (2005). *White paper: The negative consequences of international intellectual property theft: Economic harm, threats to the public health and safety, and links to organized crime and terrorist organizations.* Washington, DC: IACC.

Jackson, R., & Howe, N. (2008). *The graying of the great powers: Demography and geopolitics in the 21st century.* Washington, DC: Center for Strategic & International Studies (summarizes research from the Global Aging Initiative on the global challenges of this emerging demographic revolution).

Kerber, R. (2005, October 19). Device makers fight reuse of surgical tools. *Boston Globe,* p. D1.

Kiplinger (Kiplinger Retirement Report). (2006, May). Gadgets to keep you safe and independent, pp. 12-13.

Klein, A. (2005, December 22). Used medical devices being sold on eBay; Refurbished items have little oversight. *Washington Post,* p. D1.

___. (2005a, December 11). Hospitals save money, but safety is questioned. *Washington Post,* p. A1.

LaMendola, R. (2005, July 18). Hollywood-area firms pleads (sic) guilty; Surgical mesh that company sold is not sterile, testing finds. *Sun-Sentinel* (Fort Lauderdale, FL), p. 2B.

Liang, B. A. (2006). Structurally sophisticated or lamentably limited? Mechanisms to ensure safety of the medicine supply. *Albany Law Journal of Science & Technology, 16,* 483-524.

Lindemann, D. J. (2006). Pathology full circle: A history of anti-vibrator legislation in the United States. *Columbia Journal of Gender & Law, 15,* 326-346.

Loyd, L. (2008, February 7). Spinal-disc maker gets subpoena from N.J.; Synthes Inc. is under inquiry for possible conflicts involving its spinal-implant devices. *Philadelphia Inquirer,* p. C2.

Maisel, W. (2007). Unanswered questions, drug-eluting stents and the risk of late thrombosis. *New England Journal of Medicine, 10* (356), 981-984.

Marinac-Dabic, D. et al. (2007). Medical devices post-approval studies program: Vision, strategies, challenges and opportunities. *Food & Drug Law Journal, 62,* 597-604.

Martin, B. I. et al. (2007). Reoperation rates following lumbar spine surgery and the influence of spinal fusion procedures. *Spine, 32* (3), 382-387.

Mathews, A. W., & Winslow, R. (2006, December 8). Panel supports drug-coated stents; FDA advisers give patients limited reassurance on use; A split over blood clots. *Wall Street Journal,* p. B2.

McClellan, M. B., & Tunis, S. R. (2005). Medicare coverage of ICDs. *New England Journal of Medicine, 352* (222), 285-287.

Meier, B. (2009, June 11). House bill would create artificial joints registry. *New York Times,* p. B3

Monegain, B. (2006, April 7). New study forecasts increased use of remote patient monitoring. *Healthcare IT News.*

NCHS (National Center for Health Statistics). (2008). *National Health Care Survey for 2006.* Atlanta, GA: Centers for Disease Control.

Nussbaum, S. chief medical officer, Wellpoint. (2006, April 17). Panel discussion: Assessing the value of expensive technology and treatments for chronic care. 3rd Annual World Health Care Conference. Washington, DC.

Paradise, J. et al. (2008). Exploring emerging nanobiotechnology drugs and medical devices. *Food & Drug Law Journal, 63,* 407-420.

Patsner, B. (2009). Problems associated with direct-to-consumer advertising (DTCA) of restricted, implantable medical devices: Should the current regulatory approach be changed? *Food & Drug Law Journal, 64,* 1-41.

Pauly, M. V. & Burns, L. R. (2008). Price transparency for medical devices. *Health Affairs, 27* (6), 1544-1554.

Ridge, R. J., & Baird, M. A. (2008). Unearthing corporate wrongdoing: Detecting and dealing with ethical breaches in the business world: The pendulum swings back: Revisiting corporate criminality and the rise of deferred prosecution agreements. *University of Dayton Law Review, 33,* 187-204.

Rose, D. (2008, April 22). Experimental surgery returns sight to blind. *Times* (London), p. 3.

Sanders, D. (2005). Cost-effectiveness of implantable cardioverter–defibrillators. *New England Journal of Medicine, 14* (353), 1471-1480.

Schillaci, S. W. (2006). Increased risk of future harm as injury in fact: Expanding or eroding standing? *Quinnipiac Health Law Journal, 10,* 1-43.

Schultz, D. (2007). Medical device safety: FDA's postmarket transformation initiative. *Food & Drug Law Journal, 62,* 593-595.

Spivack, P., & Raman, S. (2008). Regulating the "new regulators": Current trends in deferred prosecution agreements. *American Criminal Law Review, 45,* 159-190.

Srinivas, S. (2006, December 20). Rethinking the use of drug-coated stents; Panel says cardiologists are using the stents in complicated cases of heart diseases, for which the devices have not been tested in clinical trials. *Straits Times* (Singapore) (reporting on the World Health Congress).

Steinbrook, R. (2005). The controversy over Guidant's implantable defibrillators. *New England Journal of Medicine, 353,* 221-224.

Troy, D. E. & Wood, R. K. (2008). The business of the Court: Federal preemption at the Supreme Court. *Cato Supreme Court Review,* 257-283.

U.S. Attorney's Office-NJ. (2007, September 27). *Press release: Five companies in hip and knee replacement industry avoid prosecution by agreeing to compliance rules and monitoring.* Trenton, NJ: U.S. Attorney's Office.

Vandall, F. J. (2008). The criminalization of products liability: An invitation to political abuse, pre-emption, and non-enforcement. *Catholic University Law Review, 57,* 341-375.

Villarraga, M. L. et al. (2007). Medical device recalls from 2004 to 2006: A focus on Class I recalls. *Food & Drug Law Journal, 62,* 581-591 (summarizes the FDA recall process).

Vladeck, D. C. (2008). The FDA and deference lost: A self-inflicted wound or the product of a wounded agency? A response to Professor O'Reilly. *Cornell Law Review, 93,* 981-1002 (counter to the argument that the FDA's decline and the declining deference it receives from courts is the result of a handful of ill-considered, politically motivated decisions).

von Eschenbach, A. C. (2008). The FDA Amendments Act: Reauthorization of the FDA. *Food & Drug Law Journal, 63,* 579-584 (the text of prepared remarks by von Eschenbach, M.D., commissioner of the FDA, at the 51st Food & Drug Law Institute (FDLI) Annual Conference in Washington, DC, March 26, 2008, cosponsored by FDLI and FDA).

Wang, S. S. (2008, July 3). Abbott's drug-coated stent is approved. *Wall Street Journal*, p. B4.

Weiland, M. (2008, February 28). Drugs and devices: Senate Aging Committee hears support for physician payment disclosure proposal. *BNA Health Care Daily Report, 13* (9).

Westphal, S. P. (2005, October 21). Some doctors see long-term clot risk in stent patients. *Wall Street Journal,* p. B1.

Wharton (Wharton School at the University of Pennsylvania). (2006). The business of healthcare innovation: How new products come to market. *Knowledge@Wharton.*

___. (2006a). Personalized medicine and nanotechnology: Trying to bring dreams to market. *Knowledge@Wharton.*

___. (2003). An aging, fatter population drives demand for new medical devices. *Knowledge@Wharton.*

Winslow, R., & Mathews, A. W. (2006, December 9). How doctors are rethinking drug-coated stents; Safety concerns are altering treatment, narrowing use; FDA panel divisions emerge. *Wall Street Journal*, p. A1.

Yeagle, J. (2007). Nanotechnology and the FDA. *Virginia Journal of Law & Technology, 12,* 6-79.

CHAPTER 20

HEALTH INFORMATION TECHNOLOGY

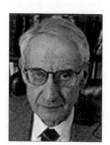

> *"Privacy is not simply an absence of information about us in the minds of others; rather it is the control we have over information about ourselves."*
>
> —CHARLES FRIED, HARVARD LAW SCHOOL PROFESSOR
> AND FORMER U.S. SOLICITOR GENERAL

IN BRIEF

Health information technology (IT) is reshaping how hospitals, physicians, patients, and payers interact with one another. E-health, electronic health records, information security, and privacy issues in this product sector are evolving and complex. Information technology and health Web sites are diverse and rapidly changing.

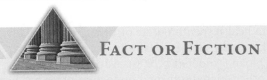

FACT OR FICTION

INTERNET PRESCRIBING

Can online questionnaires be substituted for face-to-face examinations or one-on-one conversations before approved drugs can be prescribed?

Dr. Thomas Hanny, a licensed physician for thirty years, began working for a health information company that sold prescription drugs over the Internet after his retirement as a surgeon. Hanny approved prescription requests based on a questionnaire completed by customers, but never reviewed the customers' health records. The Missouri Board of Medicine contacted Hanny and informed him that his actions constituted the illegal practice of medicine. When Hanny ignored this communication, the U.S. charged him with conspiring to distribute controlled substances outside the course of normal medical practice.

—*U.S. v. Hanny*, 509 F.3d 916 (U.S. Court of Appeals for the Eighth Circuit 2007).

(See *Law Fact* at the end of this chapter for the answer.)

PRINCIPLES AND APPLICATIONS

The health IT sector envisions a future with integrated networks sharing records that are completely electronic and accessible from anywhere, and where health care professionals enter orders on a computer, not on a medical chart. The goal is one of improving health care and reducing human errors and omissions. Over the next decade, of all the medical technologies that affect the health care experience, IT holds the greatest potential for positive change: more rapid and accurate diagnoses, less duplicative and more effective treatments, greater price and quality transparency, and reduction in the rise of costs (Goldsmith, 2005). It is estimated that a nationwide integrated health care network would save the U.S. health care system $77.8 billion a year (Walker, 2005).

ELECTRONIC HEALTH RECORDS SYSTEMS

The most important application of IT in health care is arguably the electronic health record (EHR). Since the 1970s, paper medical charts have been replicated in electronic form. Digitizing medical charts and creating mechanisms for making them usable at different points in the patient care process, from physician offices to diagnostic laboratories to operating suites to hospital rooms, has been a challenging technical aspiration.

Today, there are two forms of EHR transactions: Web-based personal health records (PHRs) that are individually controlled and potentially portable, and institutional health records that are used by hospitals to share lab results, X-rays, MRIs, CAT scans, medication history, and other information internally.

In this chapter, the term PHR includes continuity of care records (Kibbe, 2004). Computer physician order entry (CPOE) systems facilitate real-time information sharing by embedding medication orders and diagnostic procedures in EHRs, enabling medical professionals to respond directly to changes in a patient's status. This clinical process is further enhanced by computerized decision support (CDS) systems, which audit medical orders and flag decisions that might place patients at risk for adverse events.

These technologies come with a potential cost in information privacy and their own set of legal risks (Reiss, 2006). This chapter will review the health IT sector and look at the health law issues surrounding the adoption and use of these important medical information technologies. Privacy lacks a uniform definition and is not defined in the U.S. Constitution. Indeed, some scholars debate whether the Constitution actually confers a right to privacy, as that right is not explicitly set forth within its language. In this chapter, privacy is defined as the management and control of health information about identifiable patients and Internet users and its communication to other third parties.

Nationwide Interoperable Health Care Network

One principle of law is clear: information privacy should be addressed before intelligent record patterns are established and built into any national technology infrastructure (Gunter & Terry, 2005). CPOE and CDS systems will inevitably change both the clinical process and the division of administrative responsibilities within health care systems (Ash et al., 2007). With these changes, as many as a dozen distinct health care IT systems across the nation's clinical and administrative departments will be combined into a single patient care process. As disjointed health information domains are integrated, the patient care process itself is changing its inherent fragmentation, from a clinical system with tremendous variation in responses to diagnostic uncertainty, to a system with improved clinical performance and efficiency. The inconsistency in treatment, from patient to patient and hospital to hospital, is disappearing as IT grows in sophistication and better assists medical professionals in remaining current with the evolving state of medical knowledge as well as new medical product uses (Terry, 2007).

Whether the U.S. has the proper legal framework in place to proceed with building the nation's clinical information systems into one integrated nationwide network is a challenging question (Kreuser, 2007). Health laws are changing as health care systems move from supporting batch processing of health care transactions to adopting sophisticated, artificial-intelligence-assisted, real-time control of patient care processes (Goldsmith, 2005). Clinical services and administration will be reshaped as EHRs, diagnostic radiology picture archiving and communication systems, remote clinical management systems (*see* Herrmann, 2006), customized consumer-directed health insurance plans, and real-time claims management and payment systems increasingly expand over the next decade (Hillestad, 2005). New York City recently invested over $30 million to equip one thousand doctors' offices with EHR systems (Pizzi, 2007).

In early 2008, the Bush administration issued a legislative proposal that would require all U.S. health care providers to implement EHRs. A provision in the proposal requires the U.S. Department of Health & Human Services to develop and implement a nationwide interoperable health care network by 2020 (Executive Order No. 13335, 2004). The network would be required to make PHRs accessible to every Medicare beneficiary (Lueck, 2008). While the need is without dispute, the road to building this nationwide integrated health care network could be politically complex, and it could cost upwards of $400 billion (Klein, 2005).

Constraints on Adoption of Information Technologies

The U.S. is approximately a dozen years behind other industrialized countries in terms of adoption of health information technologies; these other countries' national governments have played major roles in establishing their national integrated health care networks, and health insurers there have paid most of the costs. Nevertheless, U.S. health spending per capita is almost two and a half times the median per capita health spending rate of other economically similar areas, such as Australia, Canada, Europe, and Japan (Anderson, 2006). Adoption of EHRs and other related information technologies has been minimal in the U.S. thus far, and is largely not a routine practice of medical providers (Wears & Berg, 2005). In fact, a recent study estimated that only one in four physicians use EHRs, while the use of CPOE and CDS systems is even lower among hospitals (Bender, 2005). Moreover, while EHRs have been deployed by many major health care systems, a single national standard still does not exist for sharing information between different neworks.[LN1]

Still, experts agree that the only way to reduce the number of medical errors along with duplicative and ineffective treatment services is widespread adoption of standardized IT (Hyman & Silver, 2005; Middleton et al., 2004). EHRs that can collect and share essential health information about patients and their care should ideally be linked to CPOE and CDS systems in a national network accessible by all health care organizations (Ebeler, 2007). Two of the main reasons for hesitancy to adopt health IT are cost and privacy concerns (Kaiser, 2008).

ONLINE CONTROL AND MANAGEMENT OF MEDICAL INFORMATION

The need for patients to have more control over their personal medical records and access to more relevant health information is largely driving this anticipated change. Health information companies, hospitals, health plans, and the government are all seeking to be part of this larger push to use IT to give patients more control over their online health records and access to their medical information. This IT push could in turn lower health care costs if access to more health information helps physicians and patients make better choices.

More than two hundred companies are involved in the online health market (Lawton, 2008). Among them are Aetna and WellPoint, which are building PHRs from billing and claims data, and newcomers like Google,[LN2] Microsoft,[LN3] and AOL, which are developing their own cyberspace ventures. A startup focused on Web-based personal genetic analysis, 23andMe, allows patients to pay about $1,000 for the opportunity to explore their own genomes. Some employers (including Intel, Wal-Mart, Pitney Bowes, British Petroleum, and Applied Materials) are also promoting PHRs in conjunction with group-sponsored health plans. These developments, and dozens of similar initiatives, are pushing the online sharing of identifiable medical information (IMI) into the mainstream (Mariner, 2007a).

Personal Health Records

In theory, PHRs could be a bridge between the various electronic records. Many institutional EMR systems provide a patient portal that views records and interacts with physicians in its health care network. The ideal would be a shared global repository under patient control with records stored on the Internet or a portable device. For instance, a patient could take a record from one health care network, store it on a Web-based service, and then share that information with other physicians or specialists of a different network anywhere in the world. However, the issue is that there is no agreement within the health care industry on where PHRs fit relative to other electronic records (Berner & Moss, 2005).

Another issue is how PHRs work with institutional EMR systems and how this information could be shared with other health care networks in an emergency. For instance, if patients were incapacitated, how would they provide access to their Web-based records in a different network? It is logical to expect PHRs to complement existing EMR systems. Further, there is no standard norm for Web-based health information. A partnership between the private sector and the government would be ideal. To achieve uniformity, it might help if there were tools endorsed by the federal government and professional associations. For complete accessibility, the government and the many companies in the health IT sector must cooperate in building a nationwide integrated health care network.

There is also a concern regarding quality of electronic records. Patients are probably not the best judge of what should be in their PHRs. Moreover, it is difficult to know how useful PHRs will be to physicians and other health professionals if they are not standardized and complete. Patients could record popular test results, such as a cholesterol score, but omit a lesser known detail, such as the triglyceride level. Patient-controlled health records are only as complete as the information entered. Selective disclosure could be a common problem and would hinder medical professionals' ability to render appropriate care using PHRs.

Online Sharing of Personal Health Records

Privacy issues are yet another major concern. Individuals' health records are personal and sensitive, but online PHRs are not yet covered by the Health Insurance Portability and Accountability Act (HIPAA), 18 U.S.C.A. §§ 24 et seq. (2009). HIPAA, passed in 1996, created minimum standards for disclosure, access, correction, and other elements of fair information practices, as well as addressed security and information privacy issues. Although HIPAA was passed in 1996, the security and privacy regulations did not become effective until 2003 (see 45 C.F.R. § 164.534 (2001)). It took ten years for the enforcement provisions to be finalized (see Federal Register,

2006). Under HIPAA, a patient's medical records and payment history cannot be linked together by an unauthorized person (see Pritts, 2002; Federal Register, 2000); Supplemental Information for 45 C.F.R. pts. 160-164, Standards for Privacy of Individually IMI (2009)). These rules, however, apply only to "covered entities," such as health care providers, health plans, health care clearinghouses such as billing services and information providers, and health care networks, rather than to the records themselves (Gellman, 2008).

No HIPAA Protection

Although HIPAA covers health care systems installing EHRs, regulations do not cover independent Web services that store PHRs online (see Brown, 2008). For instance, Microsoft's HealthVault records are individually controlled. In its "frequently asked questions" document, Microsoft outlines that individuals decide what information is stored in HealthVault, access is granted on a case-by-case basis, and health records are not used for commercial purposes unless authorized by opting-in. Genetic testing firms, like 23andMe, deCODE genetics, Navigenics, and other Internet-based companies, make similar promises, stating that it simply links patients to their genetic data and then stores and helps interpret the information (Abril, 2008). In addition, HIPAA does not prevent patients from uploading their PHRs and accepting terms of questionable online privacy agreements.

Still, there is the potential to restrict and tailor health plan benefits and employment from at-risk populations based on the information in online PHRs (Brown, 2008). At risk could be any number of factors from familial history to laboratory results to environmental exposures. Benefit coverage could be restricted unfairly or employment could be affected by medical history and at-risk variables with the online availability of IMI (Zarsky, 2003). This is important since not all states have privacy laws that apply to online PHRs, and most information privacy laws have yet to be tested in courts (Jean, 2004).

Moreover, any information privacy protection granted by Web sites could vanish at any time because most Web sites reserve the right to change their privacy policies without providing notice to their Internet users (Brown, 2008). There is a significant difference between Web sites legally covered by HIPAA versus sites that simply voluntarily comply with HIPAA. Voluntarily compliant Web sites are subject to this sudden change. While this is increasingly recognized as a privacy issue, legislation is required to regulate Web sites containing IMI (April, 2008).

While it may be idealistic to trust patients to maintain their own complete PHRs, third-party providers also present risks. Other parties, including the government, may have access to IMI under subpoena power. Web sites can promise privacy, but in reality, they may not be able to keep PHRs posted online private from third parties and the government.

While health information is typically considered more sensitive than financial data, there are similarities. Initially, financial data was largely paper-based and consumers were reluctant to share information electronically. Today, Web-based banking and financial transactions are commonplace. PHRs may soon follow the same path with information privacy safeguards in place.[LN4]

Public Health Monitoring of Chronic Diseases

One particular challenge facing health care providers is applying PHRs to those who may need it the most: patients with chronic diseases. This is a new role for most health care providers. While this role has traditionally been filled by public health agencies, the monitoring and management of patients with chronic medical conditions, such as diabetes, will eventually require integration of those patients' PHRs with disease management applications managed by hospitals or large physician clinics.

The New York City Department of Health and Mental Hygiene, for instance, currently maintains a public health registry on diabetics. Laboratories are required to submit electronic reports of blood sugar levels for diabetics by name and without patient consent (*see* New York City Health Code art. 13, § 13.04 (2005)). The City Health Department then intervenes and contacts patients at risk who are not controlling their blood sugar to encourage them to take medications properly, make better diet choices, and increase exercise (Mariner, 2007a).

With appropriate IT adaptations, public health laws authorizing this type of preventative health program could be expanded to include other chronic disease interventions. Cardiac instability, congestive heart failure, asthma, and chronic obstructive pulmonary diseases, for instance, could be monitored by public health agencies until the time that medical intervention is needed. More than three decades ago, a U.S. Supreme Court case established the foundation for this newly emerging type of public health monitoring.

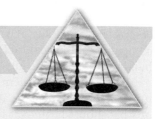

PERSONALLY IDENTIFIABLE MEDICAL INFORMATION

Whalen v. Roe

[State Commissioner of Health v. Patients and their Physicians]

429 U.S. 589 (U.S. Supreme Court 1977)

FACTS: State Health Commissioner Whalen sought review of a lower court decision that held that a New York State law which required a centralized filing system of all prescriptions written for controlled substances with the potential for abuse was unconstitutional. The law required physicians to report to the State all prescriptions written for drugs with both medical and recreational uses.

ISSUE: Can the government collect identifiable prescription records for certain drugs?

HOLDING AND DECISION: Yes, laws that require governmental collection of identifiable prescription records for certain drugs do not violate information privacy.

ANALYSIS: This decision upheld the creation of public health registries where personal health

records were released only to those having a legitimate interest in the health information. The U.S. Supreme Court reversed a lower court decision that held that the State could not record in a centralized computer file the identity of all prescribing physicians and patients who obtained prescribed drugs for Schedule II controlled substances for which there was both a lawful and an unlawful market. Challengers argued that this database infringed the right to information privacy because patients have a right to avoid disclosure of personal health matters. The Court rejected the challenge, but not before elaborating on the harm that disclosure of identifiable prescription records might cause.

The Court agreed that there was a constitutionally protected zone of information privacy that included the interest in avoiding disclosure of identifiable prescription records. It was suggested that individuals have a protected interest in making independent health

(continues)

(continued)

decisions. The Court did not reject the possibility that this right to information privacy might include the right to control access to one's health records.

The Court held the registry law adequately protected information privacy when it limited access to the IMI and built in protection from disclosure. Safeguards to prevent disclosure of identifiable prescription records were necessary, except when such disclosure was needed to stop illegal drug use. It was noted that the law created liability for anyone who failed to maintain proper security.

The Court also held that there was not sufficient evidence to establish that the law had affected any patients' decision-making abilities. It was noted that the requirement to report prescriptions was not distinguishable from other invasions of information privacy associated with health care, such as the requirements to report venereal disease, child abuse, injuries caused by deadly weapons, and certifications of fetal death. Requiring disclosures of identifiable prescription records to public health officials does not automatically amount to an impermissible invasion of privacy.

Finding that the law was the product of an orderly and rational legislative decision, the Court upheld the public registry law. The registry law was specifically designed to prevent individuals from obtaining Schedule II drugs from more than one physician or using stolen or altered prescriptions, prevent pharmacists from refilling inappropriate or dangerous prescriptions, and prevent physicians from over-prescribing drugs. If prevention failed, the health records would enable the State to identify, and possibly prosecute, those who were breaking the law. These goals were found to be reasonable. There was a reasonable expectation that the registry would have a deterrent effect on potential violators as well as aid in the detection and investigation of specific instances of apparent drug abuse.

RULE OF LAW: Identifiable prescription records are within the zone of information privacy and individuals have a protected interest in avoiding disclosure of personal health matters. Such records can be reported to a state registry, however, as long as proper privacy safeguards are maintained and there is a legitimate governmental purpose for reporting, such as preventing violations of the law. (*See generally* Dahl, 2008; Fleming, 2008; Hoffman & Podgurski, 2008; Kamm, 2005; Lawrence, 2006; Ogolla, 2008; Orden, 2005; Pottker-Fishel, 2007; Van Cise, 2005; Ward, 2008).

Interventions with Information Technologies

If patients with unstable health due to chronic diseases have implantable medical devices, advanced IT can monitor their medical conditions continuously. This remote IT monitoring and management is, in principle, no different than the IT applications used in telemetry units at hospitals or the observation units attached to emergency rooms. Rather than waiting to intervene until a catastrophic medical event occurs, IT interventions like this can take place and potentially avert the crisis. The earlier point of intervention might make the difference in the outcome of the situation (Lewis, 2006).

For instance, in 2000, the European Union approved insulin pump devices developed by Medtronic that can be implanted to alter insulin dosages continuously; while the French regulatory authorities approved distribution in France in 2003, the devices have yet to be cleared for use in the U.S. Through wireless IT, pump devices store and send information about an individual diabetic's status to a monitoring station as well as respond to external signals that can alter the insulin dosage. Pacemakers are being implanted in the same manner to monitor heart rhythms for cardiac patients and alert caregivers to the need for medical intervention when necessary (Boriani, 2008). Biometric sensor arrays are increasingly affordable. Sensor arrays can also be integrated with real-time, two-way voice communications, so that patients with implantable medical devices can be monitored with wireless connections, almost like a human OnStar™ safety system. Guidant and Boston Scientific have developed devices that are compatible with EHRs through wireless IT (Saxon, 2007).

Patients being monitored can span the health spectrum. Chronic diseases can be managed at home in the same way as critically ill patients are monitored in hospital intensive care units. For twenty years, hospitals with twenty-four-hour cardiology coverage have monitored critically ill patients in remote locations at smaller hospitals and clinics through electrocardiograph signals transmitted through telephone lines. Today, with biometric and IT advances, the physiological characteristics of patients in unstable health with a wide range of chronic clinical conditions can be monitored continuously from remote wireless locations (Madison, 2007).

Public Health Registries

The law on public health registries has involved two different kinds of information privacy interests. "One is the individual interest in avoiding disclosure of personal matters, and another is the interest in independence in making certain kinds of important decisions." *See Whalen v. Roe*, 429 U.S. 529 (U.S. Supreme Court 1977) (the seminal U.S. Supreme Court case concerning constitutional protection for control over information). Like all personal interests, though, the two are constrained and compete with the needs of the community at large.

So, when the federal agency that administers Medicare and Medicaid estimates that government spending on health care could increase by an additional $2 trillion by 2017 (Zhang, 2008), questions arise in communities nationwide as to why public health care spending is surging and what can be done to control the surge. Driven by the aging of the baby-boom generation and rising costs of new drugs and medical technologies, overall health care spending is projected to increase to $4.3 trillion, or nearly double the 2007 amount, by 2017 (Zhang, 2008). Given this dire warning, individual privacy interests may not prohibit public health agencies from taking action and making sure that chronic diseases are monitored and managed in their local communities.

The New York City public registry law merely reflects the current public health policy of collecting IMI about chronic diseases (New York City Health Code art. 13, § 13.04 (2005); *see also* Pizzi, 2007). Whether this policy shift is consistent with the autonomy to decide whether to accept medical care is uncertain and has not been addressed by the courts (Drexler, 2007). The U.S. Supreme Court has, however, found that this public health policy is consistent with making sure that the abuse of pharmaceutical drugs is monitored and managed and that unlawful diversion and use of legal drugs is minimized. Whether this public health policy on drug abuse will be extended to other health conditions, without informed consent, is a Machiavellian decision that Americans will have to soon decide upon.

The tradition of patient autonomy and information privacy in the U.S. can still be respected and is not mutually exclusive with the concept of identifying, monitoring, and managing patients with chronic diseases. At issue is not whether there is a right to individual privacy; rather, the issue is whether that right should be subverted to the importance of monitoring and managing chronic diseases, which may minimize health care costs. This is the focus of policy debates.

Computerized Physician Order Entry Systems

Experts agree that CPOE systems lie at the core of medicine's future (Goldsmith, 2005). The significance of CPOE is validated by the English Ministry of Health's action to devote nearly $6 billion (about $3.6 billion UK pounds) to implement CPOE for England's National Health Service (Burns, 2005). The federal Agency for Healthcare Research and Quality has estimated that CPOE systems alone have the potential to eliminate 200,000 adverse drug events in U.S. hospitals, saving the U.S. health care system more than $1 billion a year (Shekelle et al., 2006). The federal Agency for Healthcare Research and Quality, within the U.S. Department of Health & Human Services, was awarded $400 million in federal stimulus funding to support research to help build the technical and operational foundation of health IT in clinical settings.

Despite projected cost-savings, the investment in CPOE is often difficult to justify given the short-term cost pressures facing most American hospitals (Cutler et al., 2005; Kerr, 2007). The Leapfrog Group, a national coalition of major U.S. employers, advocates CPOE but notes that adoption has been "dismally slow" (Landro, 2005). Few U.S. hospitals have CPOE systems, in part because the IT can cost $500,000 to $14 million depending on hospital size (Lovelock, 2007), and in part because of some unplanned consequences of CPOE (Koppel et al., 2005).

A controversial study at Children's Hospital of Pittsburgh linking an increased death rate to the installation of a new computer system reinforced growing concern that CPOE, hailed as a panacea for medication errors and omissions, can actually slow down the delivery of care and trigger unintentional harm to patients if not carefully put into practice. A team of researchers from the University of Pittsburgh Medical Center described multiple technology glitches after CPOE was installed at Pittsburgh Children's Hospital over a six-day period:

- Physicians unable to pre-register critically ill children and then laboring to enter medication orders and tests electronically
- Nurses pulled away from the bedside to work with the technology, reducing the patient-to-staff ratio in pediatric critical care units
- System crashes that froze computers and delayed the delivery of vital medications

During the eighteen-month study period, the mortality rate for children admitted from other facilities more than doubled (Han et al., 2005; Landro, 2005; Taylor et al., 2008; Del Beccaro, 2006; Spooner & Council on Clinical Information Technology, 2007; Walsh et al., 2006; Wang et al., 2007).

Although the Pittsburgh study's findings quickly drew fire from IT experts and patient-advocacy groups, it highlighted the significant problems that can arise from activating CPOE (Bratton, 2006; Rosenbloom et al., 2006; Sittig et al., 2006). Although CPOE holds great promise as a tool to reduce human errors, there can be unintended adverse effects if hospitals do not carefully plan for implementation of advanced IT (Jacobs et al., 2006; Longhurst et al., 2006). The most common mistake was the lack of time and funding given to test CPOE. The Children's Hospital of Pittsburgh made its transition to CPOE in just six weeks, with much of the technology funding devoted to design and coding, rather than testing the new system. The lesson learned is that training, and efforts to reduce downtimes between the transitioning of old systems to the new, are necessary when implementing CPOE.

REMOTE MONITORING AND MANAGEMENT OF PATIENTS

All these concerns with controlling and managing electronic records could be resolved by further advances in IT. If PHRs were automatically shared between medical devices that test for chronic conditions, EMR systems, and Web-based services, there would be one integrated health care provider (Goldman, 2006). For chronic diseases, implantable devices could be linked to medical care providers and patients could be continuously monitored and managed. With IMI from continuously monitored patients, there would be:

- Ability to define health populations and subpopulations where medical products and services could be targeted, accessed, refocused, and improved
- Possibility to study health trends and endless hypotheses
- Potential to study the natural history of medical conditions and the health impact of different environmental or social circumstances, and then to identify at-risk populations
- Research opportunities to prospectively analyze the effectiveness of different treatments and diagnostic tests, from screening programs and prevention strategies, to the prognosis and the potential survival statistics associated with different conditions or different treatments

(Mariner, 2007)

Patient biosensors could conceivably transmit IMI into the information system that would populate their records.[LN5] As IT advances, biosensors could eventually enable medical professionals to monitor patients outside hospital and medical facilities on a continuous basis. Medical device companies such as Medtronic and the Cordis division of Johnson & Johnson are already developing intelligent implantable devices for virtually every organ system in the body. These implantable medical devices can continuously monitor and intervene to stabilize patients as necessary, as well as alert caregivers and monitoring centers if additional stabilization is required.

Remote monitoring of patients with chronic diseases has the potential to improve care and reduce hospitalizations, but it has been slow to catch on (Ferris, 2007). One might wonder why. One reason is that the federal Centers for Medicare and Medicaid Services and other payers have not adapted to this changing patient treatment approach. Medicare and most health plans still only reimburse for traditional patient care where patients are taken into physical custody for hands-on monitoring of their conditions. Without health insurers' acceptance of these new technological advances, medical providers are not reimbursed for care provided remotely.

ELECTRONIC MEDICINE

Just as the remote monitoring and management of patients is advancing through developments in IT, electronic medicine, or *E-medicine*, is also pushing into the mainstream. E-medicine is dividing along two lines: free general medical advice, such as the medlineplus program found on the Library of Medicine's patient Web site, and more time-consuming and personalized online consultations for which health care providers charge (Landro, 2003). Increasingly, health plans are reimbursing for online consultations, and the pressure is mounting for all payers to do so.

Patients are increasingly demanding electronic medical services beyond general medical advice and recommendations found on Web sites. Though more than one hundred million patients go online for health information every year, many actually want more online interaction with their health care professionals. While most physicians recommend Web sites to patients, few health care systems use e-mail to communicate with patients (Brooks & Menachemi, 2006). Again, one might ask why. For instance, are there justifiable concerns that physicians will be inundated with patient e-mails; or is it more efficient to have support staff screen patient issues rather than taking time for physicians to individually respond when they are not rendering direct clinical care? Moreover, what assurance would patients have that they are actually communicating with their physician as opposed to support staff?

Reimbursement remains a stumbling block to E-medicine. Professionals expect to be paid for their time. Medical groups have called on the federal Centers for Medicare and Medicaid Services, and all other payers, to work with providers to develop guidelines for reimbursement of online consultations (Ferris, 2007). Information benefits are just as important as drug benefits and would cost far less if provided electronically (Berner et al., 2005). Online consultations can more efficiently address non-urgent care, such as prescription refills, follow-up care for problems that have not worsened, reporting certain test results, and diagnosing common symptoms. They also can be used for continued personal counseling after an office visit.

For insured Americans facing higher out-of-pocket costs from their health plans, the idea of being able to get health information and advice from health care professionals without expensive, time-consuming, and sometimes unnecessary office visits is an attractive alternative, even if there is still a fee. Many health care systems let patients search online for physicians who use online consultations. As costs are increasingly shifted to patients, patients are looking for more efficient ways of obtaining quality care at an affordable price (Landro, 2003).

HEALTH SPACE

Related to E-medicine, and one of the more diverse segments of health IT, is the rapidly changing Web space dedicated to health care. For anyone with access to the Web, an array of drug and therapeutic offerings is easily found. The intricate global network of chemical and drug manufacturers, distributors, and buyers behind E-medicine and health care Web sites is challenging the ability of the U.S. Food and Drug Administration to provide its traditional public health safety net for Americans (Steinbock, 2006).

Health Web Sites

The proliferation of health information on the Web has the ability to positively affect health care. However, it is difficult to know if information on the Internet is updated and accurate. The Pew Research Center found that fully three-quarters of the health information seekers say they check the source and date "only sometimes," "hardly ever," or "never," which translates to about eighty-five million Americans gathering health advice online without consistently examining the quality indicators of the information they find (Fox, 2006).

As might be expected, there are gaps in the quality of online information. Information about physician credentials, training, and experience is available, but there is not much available regarding outcomes or quality (Kemper & Mettler, 2002). The fact that information is available in some form, however, means Internet users are becoming more involved in their own health care. The Pew Internet and American Life Project surveys Internet use in the U.S. and paints a picture of health care consumers who are researching physicians, paying attention to warnings about obesity and poor nutrition, considering entering clinical trials in greater numbers, and taking steps to better manage their health care costs.

Since the Pew survey started in 2002, the fastest growing topics of interest for Internet users include:

- Diet, nutrition, and vitamins
- Experimental treatments
- Health insurance coverage
- Information on physicians and hospitals
- Prescription and over-the-counter drugs

By reflecting Americans' shifting priorities in health care, the Pew findings may help provide a road map for employers, health plans, and patient advocates looking to provide better health information for patients in the future. Importantly, the survey also raises concerns about a new digital divide, between more educated and affluent Internet users with high-speed broadband access, about half of all Internet users at home, and less educated or older users with dial-up connections who are less likely to have sought various kinds of health information online. Health plans probably view this as a mixed blessing because it is likely to increase demand for new medical services and treatments. At the same time, it helps disseminate information on evidence-based medicine, which can then be used by patients and physicians to better understand the outcomes of certain treatments (Garg et al., 2005).

It is estimated that one million new Web sites go up each month (Fox, 2006). Some of the most frequented ones are health-related. Eighty percent of Internet users, including some 113 million Americans, access health care information online each year, and conducting searches for health care information is one of the most common reasons patients use the Internet (Fox, 2006). Online tools to evaluate and choose health care only scratch the surface; Web sites educate Internet users about their health, help them communicate with disease- and care-management professionals, and even help change unhealthy behaviors (Health2 Resources, 2006).

The value of these thousands of Web sites varies. Reputable Web sites, such as those of the National Institutes of Health and the Clinical Trials Database, are a public service. Many commercial Web sites mix accurate information with advertising, making it difficult to determine what is meaningful information, versus what is misleading and potentially harmful. Many health Web sites advertise heavily, but lack substance, or are even fraudulent (Terry & Francis, 2007). Some actually promote therapies that do not have a scintilla of truth behind them.

Social Networking Technologies

The health care industry has embraced the advanced IT that is part of the social networking revolution. Timely, personalized health information is readily available online. Patients who once connected mainly through e-mail discussion groups and chat rooms[LN6] have now built virtual communities to share information about their treatments with a network of online friends. The American Cancer Society and the Centers for Disease Control and Prevention have space on the Second Life Web site to determine whether social media can assist with publicizing issues such as nutrition awareness, cancer screening, and infectious disease prevention (see Shapiro, 2007). Second Life is a global, multi-player, online game where players create and control characters that live in an online community. Online support groups offer the most promise for patients with uncommon diseases or hard-to-diagnose symptoms. Frequently, the Internet has the broadest approach to issues arising from rare and orphaned diseases. The combined wisdom of these patients and caregivers is frequently deeper than single physicians can possibly develop in the time available, unless their entire careers have been devoted to the disease (Landro, 2003).

At the same time, traditional Web sites that once offered cumbersome pages of static data have developed blogs on Facebook or MySpace pages, podcasts, and customized search engines like WebMD and iVillage to deliver the most relevant information on health topics. Johnson & Johnson was one of the first pharmaceuticals in the blogosphere (Landro, 2007). Patients are constantly updated on relevant health news with personalized health awareness messages, reminders, and alerts delivered to their e-mail accounts, wireless devices, and mobile phones. Wikis allow patients to collaborate online on Web sites with photo albums and contact lists. Wikis are Web sites that users build together. One of the most renowned is the free encyclopedia Wikipedia. Communities even have Web sites to plan for public health emergencies such as flu pandemics.

Unprotected Communications Networks

Very little is known about these complex communications networks. One thing is certain, however: the health IT sector is actively monitoring all of this (Landro, 2006). What Internet users say online in discussion groups, chat rooms, health blogs, podcasts, virtual communities, and wikis is generally not protected information. To the extent that a private and confidential infrastructure is absent, these communications networks call for further study.

While remedies exist in the form of civil lawsuits if health advocacy groups, government agencies, and health care providers fail to adhere to their posted privacy policies, most health information companies maintain that if Internet users object to information privacy violations, they can simply not use those Web

sites whose policies they do not like. Some companies have, however, been sued for tracking Internet users without their permission. For instance, for several years, pharmaceutical companies contracted with Pharmatrak, a data-mining company that collected personal and identifying data on Internet users visiting pharmaceutical Web sites to learn about their drugs and to obtain rebates. When the tracking practice became public, American Home Products, Pharmacia, SmithKline Beecham, Pfizer, and Novartis terminated their IT contracts with Pharmatrak and litigation ensued. In no time at all, Pharmatrak went out of business. See Blumofe v. Pharmatrak, Inc. (In re Pharmatrak, Inc. Privacy Litigation), 329 F.3d 9 (U.S. Court of Appeals for the First Circuit 2003) (action under the federal Electronic Communications Privacy Act of 1986, which was adopted to protect the privacy of Internet communications).

Most Web sites do not disclose the use of Web bugs in their online privacy policies, even as it gets more and more difficult to block the bugs. Web bugs, also referred to as Web beacons, clear gifs, and pixel tags:

- Intercept personal information
- Obtain and collect the IP address, type of browser, and operating system of users
- Track Internet users' browsing patterns

(Ciocchi, 2007)

Moettreover, most Web sites do not strictly comply with their information privacy policies, and many regularly modify their policies without alerting users to the changes (DeMarco, 2006). In another example involving a pharmaceutical company, Eli Lilly promised in its privacy policy to maintain the confidentiality of information provided on its Prozac.com Web site. Yet, it sent Web site subscribers an e-mail with over 670 subscribers' addresses visible at the top of a drug alert (Spitzer, 2002). This meant that the recipients could potentially infer that all of the other recipients were being treated for depression, being advised to watch for suicidal thoughts, and were taking antidepressants, or at the very least, had an interest in Prozac.

While some states have mandatory regulations covering Web sites, they do not require any specific privacy policy terms.[LN7] The question is whether Internet users have an enforceable right, and therefore a legal remedy, when their information privacy is violated. Eli Lilly paid several states $160,000 to cover the costs of investigating its Web site policies, however, none of the 670 individual subscribers who had their e-mail addresses made public received compensation for violation of their privacy. Eli Lilly's response to violation of its information privacy policy is in line with the fact that companies have been unwilling to subject themselves to appropriate penalties when they violate their own privacy rules (Pollio, 2004). In addition, few Web sites have transparent information privacy practices or offer users choices about how the sites may use posted IMI (Wharton, 2000).

Protected Communications Network

Sermo, the nation's largest online physician community, is designed to redefine the way physicians in the U.S. and the health care industry work together to improve patient care. In collaboration with Pfizer and the American Medical Association, Sermo, which means "conversation" in Latin, is a Web-based community where more than 31,000 physicians share observations from daily practice, discuss emerging trends, and provide new insights into medications, devices, and treatments (Schmerken, 2008).

Internet Pharmacies

The traditional way in which drugs are dispensed in the U.S., that is, only by state-licensed health care practitioners, encompasses an important risk management system. Internet pharmacies are challenging long-established regulatory schemes and selling pharmaceuticals in confusingly diverse ways (*see Federal Register,* 2001). The U.S. Food and Drug Administration (FDA) classifies Internet pharmacies into five categories requiring different levels of scrutiny (Henney, 2000):

- Reputable, regulated Web sites that simply dispense approved drugs (state-licensed online pharmacies that require valid prescriptions for orders filled online)
- Unregulated Web sites that actually prescribe approved drugs, but circumvent traditional pharmacy safeguards
- Sites that provide drugs unapproved in the U.S., but approved in other countries (which may not necessarily be safe or effective for their intended use)
- Sites that provide drugs never approved anywhere, which are of questionable safety and effectiveness
- Sites offering other drug products and making unproven claims, such as those advocating miracle weight-loss drugs

The difference between regulated Web sites that dispense and unregulated Web sites that prescribe is noteworthy. Internet dispensing involves the delivery of prescription drugs by an Internet pharmacy. Internet prescribing arises when the Internet pharmacy prescribes the drug to patients without a physical examination.

Questions arise as to whether the Internet can substitute online medical questionnaires for live interaction with a health care professional. The courts are beginning to find that this substitution constitutes the unlawful practice of pharmacy and the FDA is shutting down such Internet pharmacies. Besides constituting unlawful, substandard health care, such questionnaires might jeopardize the confidentiality of health records. There are even online medical transactions in which medical professionals are completely absent: patients self-diagnose and treat themselves with the risk of negative outcomes such as harmful drug interactions, allergic reactions, or improper dosing, not to mention the risk of misdiagnosis and thus the failure to properly diagnose and treat the actual problem (Haight, 2006). It is important to note that in instances in which patients go online to order prescribed drugs, without a lawful prescription, they are breaking the law; their acts are the same as purchasing illegal drugs from a street drug dealer. The receipt of unlawful drugs is subject to prosecution, no matter how the drugs are obtained (*Federal Register,* 2001). One of the most recent examples of this is the unlawful obtaining of steroids by major league baseball players and other sports participants.

Lifestyle drugs are very popular on the Internet. For instance: Viagra, Levitra, and Cialis for erectile dysfunction; Propecia and Reviogen for hair loss; and Mediria, Xenical, and Reductil for obesity constitute a $28 billion market (Economist, 2007). While legal, they have dangerous side effects for certain patients, making their use without a prescription risky. Antihistamines and painkillers are also frequently ordered Internet pharmaceuticals. It appears some patients turn to the Internet when their physicians refuse to write additional prescriptions. Beyond simply wishing to circumvent physicians, many Americans shop for medical products online simply for the convenience, privacy as far as avoiding meeting face-to-face with a medical professional, and accessibility to product information (Clifton, 2004). Others use the Internet in hopes of finding better prices, but cost savings are generally a myth. Once all the charges are considered, the costs even out and sometimes increase, especially if patients cause further health troubles because of what they did or did not order (Haight, 2006).

The Internet's ability to cross state and international lines with anonymity and speed presents another regulatory issue for the FDA and law enforcement. Historically, states have had the authority to regulate both the practice of pharmacy and of medicine. However, most Web sites selling drug products are made up of multiple related sites and links that often cross state and country borders. Moreover, there are no international laws or treaties that regulate Internet drug sales from outside the U.S. to people located within the U.S. Through the World Health Organization, countries can share their regulations and monitor what is going on in other countries, but that is the only formal mechanism currently in place (Jerian, 2006).

INFORMATION PRIVACY

Information privacy is a significant issue for the health IT sector. An estimated 150 different individuals (from physicians and nurses, to technicians and billing clerks) have access to at least part of a patient's health records during a typical hospitalization (Foreman, 2006).[LN8] Self-regulation proposals from the IT sector, patient-advocacy groups intent on curbing online profiling, and various new health information companies aimed at helping patients protect their information privacy all have legitimate concerns.

At the same time, the health IT sector has a genuine commercial interest in the personalization of health information because it allows patients to receive information targeted to their personal health conditions. Furthermore, health information companies offer patients free access to information that would otherwise cost money, in return for the "cost" of allowing the health information companies to track the patient's personal health. Clearly, the boundaries of information privacy are uncertain.

Data-Mining

Should health Web sites be permitted to track internal data from browsers, if they guarantee they will not give IMI to anyone else? Unfortunately, there are many instances of IMI being sold to data brokers, drug and medical device manufacturers, or to private data collection agencies without the patient's knowledge or permission (Makdisi, 2004). Consent is often given for data-mining when, hypothetically, the request states that IMI "will be used to identify medical products and services that will better fit your needs." At this moment, secondary use of IMI is a multibillion-dollar business (Kizer, 2007; Patrick et al., 2008).

Put another way, most patients probably do not object to the practice of health plans and pharmacy benefit managers suggesting lab tests and drugs to them based on their health history. What they probably would object to, if they knew it was happening, is the way in which the health IT sector uses their IMI for things other than their individual health care. Some of these secondary uses include clinical research (Powell & Buchan, 2005), clinical audits, certification and accreditation of facilities, targeting of services (Mariner, 2007), and even marketing of products and services. IMI could certainly be used by predatory marketers to sell to populations using scare tactics. Information could be targeted to patients who are most likely to be susceptible to a sales pitch for bogus products.

While it is important that patients' needs are met (Bright, 2007), marketing and its use in health care commercial purposes is one place where the law is unclear.

Commercial Use of Identifiable Medical Information

At the time of its passage, New Hampshire's data-mining law was the first of its kind in the U.S. Now both Vermont and Maine have similar laws and numerous other states have proposed prescription information laws that are narrowly drawn around the states' interest in improving public health and mitigating health care costs. Vermont's prescription monitoring system restricts the sale of prescriber-identifiable data unless the prescriber (physician, nurse practitioner, physician assistant, mental health professional, or other health care professional authorized by state law to prescribe prescription drugs) opts-in to a program authorizing use of their prescribing records (*see* Protection and Disclosure of Information, 18 V.S.A. § 4284 (2005)).

Maine has an opt-out law that prohibits the sale of prescriber-identifiable data from prescribers who have filed for confidentiality protection (*see* Confidentiality of Prescription Drug Information, 22 M.R.S. § 1711-E (2008)). Patients are entitled to inspect the prescriber-identifiable data collected on themselves but have no control over who has access to their IMI.

Beneficial Uses of Identifiable Medical Information

The issues of privacy, confidentiality, and security must be viewed within the context of the very important and beneficial uses that go along with data-mining. When considering this issue, it is important to remember that data-mining is the analysis of health information for relationships that have not previously been discovered. Data could be used to look at state policy proposals and the cost-effectiveness of different medical products, as well as regional performance and quality improvement strategies. National studies could be done in ways that have never been done before (Powell & Buchan, 2005).

Few patients understand how easy it is to mine data, how much information is theoretically readily available, or how information that is collected can be saved forever. The reality is that as a result of IT, private space is shrinking and public space is increasing. Data-mining uses specialized software tools based on advanced electronic search and pattern recognition algorithms, multiprocessor computers, and comprehensive databases to develop measures that can investigate risk-related results and outcome comparisons, such as:

- Infections, such as viruses with the potential to become pandemics
- Medical errors and omissions
- Unnecessary diagnostic procedures
- Unwarranted medical treatments

SPSS's data-mining software, IBM's DB2 Intelligent Miner, and ACS's MIDAS+ Comparative Performance Measure System are being used to identify hidden problems, trends, and patterns that are fixable in health care systems (Solove, 2002).

Moral Dilemmas

1. If data-mining prohibitions increase the safe use of generic drugs and result in substantial cost savings, should data-mining laws be drawn for the purpose of mitigating health care costs?

Detrimental Uses of Identifiable Medical Information

What worries privacy advocates are the increasingly sophisticated methods, such as electronic tracking tags known as cookies and information transmitting devices known as Web bugs that are used to secretly track down individual information. Indeed, many Internet business models are based on the ability to aggregate and analyze IMI for a variety of profit-generating purposes. For instance, data brokers collect clickstream data to help construct computer profiles that are sold to Fortune 500 companies that regularly review this information before making hiring and advancement decisions (Solove, 2006).

Americans realize that on one level it is acceptable to sell information. The question now is whether this has gone too far in terms of the amount of processing going on and the correlation of health information back to one's physical identity. Even more disturbing is that individuals do not know how their IMI is being used and so have no way of tracking it, much less stopping it. One of the most notorious examples of violation of privacy policies involves ChoicePoint. ChoicePoint originally specialized in providing credit data to the insurance industry but it soon evolved into an all-purpose information broker by data-mining public records and then augmenting this information with:

- Conviction records
- Credit histories
- Employment histories
- Insurance claims
- Media reports
- Private investigations
- Social security numbers

Its database now contains information about nearly every American. Employers often hire ChoicePoint to conduct background checks on potential employees. Government agencies (including law enforcement) routinely use its database.

Prescriber-Identifiable Data

The use of prescriber-identifiable data is currently being litigated and one federal appellate court has recently decided that state laws can bar the data-mining industry from using prescriber-identifiable data for commercial purposes. It is certain that other federal and state courts will decide the same issue in conflicting ways. This health law issue has not been fully addressed by Congress or examined by the U.S. Supreme Court. The fundamentals are presently being debated by lower federal and state courts, Congress, and state legislatures. The *IMS Health* litigation outlined in this chapter draws attention to this emerging controversy as the facts of the data-mining industry are revealed in open courts of law.

IMPERMISSIBLE DATA-MINING

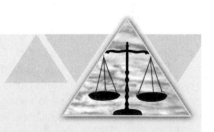

IMS Health Inc. v. Ayotte
[Health Information Companies v. State of New Hampshire]
550 F.3d 42 (U.S. Court of Appeals, 1st Circuit 2008),
U.S. Supreme Court certiorari denied, 129 S.Ct. 2864 (U.S. Supreme Court 2009)

FACTS: IMS Health and Verispan, the leading data-miners for the pharmaceutical and health care industries, filed suit to stop enforcement of a New Hampshire data-mining law restricting the commercial use of data on individual health care professionals.

ISSUE: Can state laws bar the data-mining industry from using prescriber-identifiable data for commercial purposes?

(continues)

(continued)

HOLDING AND DECISION: Yes, state laws can broadly restrict the data-mining of identifiable prescription data in pharmaceutical marketing.

ANALYSIS: The First Circuit held that a state law restricting the use of prescription data is constitutional under the First Amendment because it directly serves a substantial state interest and because the state law regulated conduct, not speech. The New Hampshire data-mining law prohibits prescription records containing patient IMI or prescriber IMI to be used for commercial purposes.

This prohibition directly impacts data-mining companies that purchase prescription data from pharmacies, match it with detailed information about individual prescribers, and sell the resulting prescriber "profiles" to interested parties. The revenue of data-mining companies derives nearly exclusively from sales to pharmaceutical companies that use the prescriber profiles to tailor their drug marketing efforts to individual physicians. IMS Health and Verispan claimed the law restricted their right to free speech under the First Amendment. The First Circuit disagreed.

The First Circuit held that the New Hampshire data-mining law directly advanced the State's legitimate interests in public health and cost containment. The court agreed with the State that the availability of prescription information renders pharmaceutical marketing more persuasive to prescribers and leads to increased prescribing of brand-name drugs. The court, however, rejected the idea that increased brand-name prescribing is necessarily injurious to public health and expensive to the health care system as a whole. The court noted that although some brand-name drugs, particularly those without generic equivalents, are the most appropriate medications for certain conditions, the data-mining law restricts the promotion of helpful and harmful brand-name drugs equally. The First Circuit found that the State demonstrated that the restriction of prescription data for use in marketing would directly promote public health and reduce costs without compromising patient care.

RULE OF LAW: State laws can restrict the use of prescriber IMI if the restriction directly serves the state's interests in promoting public health and containing health care costs.

(*See generally* Amar & Strumolo, 2007; Annual Review, 2008; Carver, 2008; Klein, 2008 for a discussion of the federal trial court decision and Dorfman, 2009 for a review of the First Circuit's decision).

Opting In or Out

The opting system is another controversy facing the health IT sector. One issue under debate is whether health Web sites should have to obtain opt-in permission from Internet users before using any IMI. This approach is favored by many patient-advocacy groups. The other option is whether users should be required to take steps to opt-out of any data collection process, an approach generally favored by the health IT sector.

Less than one-tenth of the health Web sites and less than fifty of the one hundred most popular health Web sites display an information privacy seal of reliability from the U.S. Food and Drug Administration (Bloom, 2006). One consistent barrier to the reliability of any opting system is that Web sites frequently revise their terms. These changes mean that the privacy permission Internet users initially granted could gradually become obsolete over time.

Numerous health information companies have chief privacy officers, apparently to articulate and enforce information privacy policies. A combination of government regulation and industry self-regulation are necessary to move forward (Hoffman & Podgurski, 2008). The health IT sector alone cannot completely address information privacy concerns, although it is certainly the preferred choice. Government can establish incentives for the IT sector to self-regulate, but at the same time, it should set minimum standards to ensure fair dealing for all involved.

Moral Dilemmas

1. Does self-regulation alone adequately protect the information privacy of online IMI health information, or is federal legislation needed to supplement self-regulatory efforts and guarantee basic protections?

Protection of Privacy Space

While patient advocacy groups are challenging the health information companies, new companies are emerging to offer protection against the growing variety of Web bugs that collect IMI in ever more sophisticated ways (Landro, 2007).[LN9] In this manner, as IT provides opportunities to violate information privacy, it also provides opportunities to protect IMI. Numerous fee-based services prevent tracking of IMI, an example of the market providing a solution to information privacy concerns. Users of social networks might ask themselves whether it is worth paying to try to stop the health information companies from doing what they are doing or whether resistance is futile.

The core questions raised by misuse of IMI are not new. They are related to the general way that health information companies use IMI that they can collect to advance their interests. The difference is the ease with which electronic health information can be collected and shared, and the ease with which it can be maintained for indefinite periods of time. In general, there has never been so much readily accessible IMI as there is today on the Internet (Knight, 2008).

Nonetheless, there is a difference between putting IMI on a purely public Web site and putting information on controlled, private sites available only to members. The question of who owns the IMI on these private Web sites is unclear. Most have policies declaring ownership of anything posted there, but clearly that does not grant the site's owners leeway to freely use the information as they see fit. These sites claim to have information privacy policies that impose limits on how they can use that IMI, but it is simply unclear under current law whether the posted health information actually belongs to the Internet users or the Web site owners.

In fact, with so much IMI available, it may all be considered a part of the public domain (Hirsch, 2006). It may not be legally public, but there is so much widely disseminated information and there are so many ways to access and collect it, that the issue of ownership may be a moot question. The real question is whether it is feasible to provide some information privacy protection in order to prevent all information about patients from being accessed by anyone and everyone. If that is not possible, how can individual privacy be protected at all? There are several critical questions with regard to the information privacy of IMI. Do patients expect their IMI to be private, and if so, are these expectations valid? Are patients aware of how high their expectations of privacy probably are, and that they might be impossible to meet?

Property or Privacy Rights

It is debatable whether it is more appropriate to view health records information as a form of property that is owned and therefore subject to property protections or to consider IMI protected by information privacy rights instead (Hylton, 2007). The debate

centers on whether the Internet and advances in IT over the last thirty years, from the time when the U.S. Supreme Court recognized a constitutional right to information privacy of IMI under certain circumstances, have made the property model arguably more suitable for protecting electronic health records and online IMI. *See Whalen v Roe*, 429 U.S. 589, 599-600 (U.S. Supreme Court 1977).

If the right to privacy of health records were similar to personal property rights, information privacy could be exchanged for other rights. Under the property model, information privacy belongs to individuals and it may be traded away in exchange for something of commensurate value, such as medical care, access to health information, or even payment (Ciocchetti, 2007). For instance, Internet users surfing the Web would be allowed to determine whether to submit requested pieces of IMI in return for free access to Web site content or pay to access a Web site containing similar information without having to submit any IMI. If the IMI requests are too intrusive, Internet users may always withhold their valuable IMI and move to a competitor's Web site that is less intrusive.

Under the privacy rights model, consent to medical care cannot be considered to include consent to any and all uses of IMI. The right to have health records information kept confidential includes the right to make certain kinds of important health care decisions. In this situation, HIPAA requires health care providers to state the intended use of any IMI collected for purposes other than personal health care, such as medical research and training (*see* 45 C.F.R. § 164.520(b)(1)(i) (2009)). Patients have a right to know how their IMI may be used and disclosed and how they can get access to this information before they decide to accept services from a particular health care provider. This includes the right to request restrictions on certain uses and disclosures of IMI (*see* 45 C.F.R. § 164.520(b)(1)(iv)(A-F) (2009) (HIPAA-covered entities are not required to honor such requests)).

Over time, the privacy rights model, rather than the property rights model, has emerged as the prism through which courts view rights to IMI. Under the privacy rights model, individuals have a fundamental right to maintain a sphere of privacy that should be protected from major invasions. However, with the growth of the health IT sector, this privacy rights model may not be as useful. The property model may be better suited to protect basic information rights given the ever-expanding Internet. It could be argued that IMI, like all other forms of information, should be treated as property (Posner, 2007). Arguably, IMI should be part of the protected sphere of privacy and should not be freely exchanged in an economic marketplace with information inequalities and differing power relationships stacked against the individual. Some Web sites advise users to check their privacy policy periodically for changes. Under this scenario, the party with the best knowledge that the changes have occurred and the extent of such changes requires the less-informed party to take the initiative to discover any modifications. The property model might be preferable in the health IT sector because transaction costs are extremely low; individuals can reach bargains that reflect their actual preferences for different levels of privacy.

Moral Dilemmas

1. Does the Fourth Amendment, the right to be free from unreasonable search and seizure, make information privacy of IMI a right or a privilege that needs basic protections?

2. Do the Internet and the advances in IT since the U.S. Supreme Court recognized a constitutional right to information privacy thirty years ago pose a danger to individual privacy rights?

Ownership of Personal Medical Information

The ownership model has not yet succeeded in health law. Essentially, whoever gathers the medical information owns it, whether it is the individual or not. For instance, courts have generally rejected arguments by patients who have challenged the ability of health care providers to use IMI collected from them. The notion that patients own their health records has been rejected by the courts; health records are the property of health care providers, not patients. Records taken by physicians and other health care professionals in their examination and treatment of patients become property belonging to the hospital or treating health care professionals.

Nevertheless, while health care providers and professionals own the actual health records and have primary custodial rights to the records of patients, patients have a property right in the information contained in the records. This property right is sufficient to give patients reasonable access to their records (Pritts, 2002).

Public Disclosure of Private Facts

There are limits to what one can say or post on the Internet without running the risk of being successfully sued. One limit is making money off the fame of someone else, such as a celebrity. Another is physical identity theft. However, for defamation by Web postings, truth is an absolute defense, meaning one cannot necessarily sue another solely for publicizing truthful information.

While an individual can sue someone for public disclosure of a private fact, this is difficult in the health IT sector. For one thing, the Web sites generally disclaim any liability for postings. For another, it is hard for patients to convince a court that they were harmed by information that they themselves posted or by true information about them posted by others. Nevertheless, for those wishing to go down this road, the tort of public disclosure of private facts consists of four elements:

- Public disclosure
- Private fact
- Objectionable and offensive to a reasonable person
- Not of legitimate public concern

Most courts have found that to support this theory of liability, widespread dissemination of information to the public must be proven (Standards for information transactions and data elements, 42 U.S.C.A. § 1320d-2 (1996)). This tort theory works mostly for cases involving publication through the media. In the context of HIPAA violations, however, health information will generally be delivered to interested parties (such as health care providers) rather than to the general public, and thus the tort of public disclosure of private facts will generally be inapplicable (Hoffman & Podgurski, 2008).

Assumption of Risk

E-mail also poses information privacy problems, especially due to the notion of assumption of risk. The risk that an e-mail might be forwarded is a risk assumed whenever an e-mail is sent, regardless of whether the information therein is considered private or confidential. If an e-mail is sent, the law considers that risk accepted.

When it comes to online consultations and e-mail messages between patients and medical professionals, patients tend to think of it as private correspondence, similar to a letter in a sealed envelope. However, e-mails are more like postcards. The administrators of e-mail servers are like the post office; e-mails are just files on the server. Most administrators have no reason to look at them, but they are there nonetheless. Are deleted e-mails gone? They may be gone from some places, but they could be backed up by the Internet service provider. It is nearly impossible to determine when, if ever, deleted e-mails are fully eradicated (Crist, 2006). One overarching concern is that patients are growing increasingly insensitive to their own information privacy interests. Many patients are indiscrete when it comes to IMI. It might be argued that if such personal indiscretion becomes the norm, then the need for information privacy protection rights might be lost. This is likely an outcome that not all patients would willingly accept.

Rethinking Social Norms on Information Privacy
Information privacy is only one issue regarding the amount of IMI available on the Internet in an age of increasingly universal connectivity. Health laws are gradually evolving to accommodate the Internet, mobile devices, wireless radio frequency identification tags, and other biosensors that can track individual activity (Hildner, 2006).

The reality is that a great deal of IMI is on the Internet. The reasons for this often have nothing to do with intentional efforts to convey IMI. Nevertheless, information privacy is probably not the best lens through which to examine IT management. Instead, there is a need to rethink what the health care industry considers the norm to be for IMI in a digital age. Information privacy is certainly important. There is IMI and PHR data that should not be disclosed. However, information privacy laws and policies tend to impose formalistic, legal labels and rules that may not be conducive to the Internet or other advanced IT (Trubek, 2006). The focus is slowly moving away from information privacy rights and toward industry norms. In a way, the small town is returning, where everyone knows about everyone else by virtue of the ever-expanding global information superhighway (McLaughlin, 2007).

Balancing Individual v. Community Needs
The information privacy issue raised with public health registries remains. Do patients have a right to expect that their health information will remain confidential? In this ongoing debate, information privacy is sometimes defended as an individual right. Patients, however, can and often must give up their information privacy for the public good. For instance, when children come into a hospital with signs of abuse, physicians set in motion investigations that violate the privacy of the family to protect the safety and welfare of children.

Most patients want their information privacy to be protected, but the other half of the equation is the need to give up privacy for the benefit of the community. The threat to information privacy is implicit in the accumulation of vast amounts of IMI in computerized data banks or other massive files. The collection of taxes, distribution of welfare and social security benefits, supervision of public health, management of the military, and enforcement of

criminal laws all require the orderly maintenance of IMI, much of which is potentially harmful if improperly disclosed.

Traditionally, the privacy battle was between personal interests and government intrusion. Today, there is a third factor: electronic cookies and other data-mining technologies that silently sweep up IMI and shuttle it from server to server. This is perhaps the broadest challenge to information privacy on the Internet (Rustad & Koenig, 2005).

It is difficult to determine the weight the right to information privacy ought to be given. In the case of drug store chains and drug manufacturers buying and selling IMI, information privacy may be eroded without benefiting the community, which is the traditional reason given to justify the invasion of privacy (Saul, 2006). Millions of health records are systematically mined for purposes that have nothing to do with the public good (Steinbrook, 2006). On the other hand, a decision by most states not to use blood taken from the heel of newborn children to test them for HIV may be a case in which information privacy is weighed too highly, sacrificing the rights of the newborn (Crossley, 1993). Should states require that newborns undergo HIV tests without parental consent if newborns could benefit from immediate treatment, even though information about the family may be revealed? The debate surrounding the family's right to privacy is again manifest when it comes to adolescents' medical care.

Adolescent Health Records
EMRs confront legal and technical challenges when balancing the rights of parents and adolescents in access to health records. Many adolescents depend substantially on the public sector rather than parents to help support their healthy sexual development and to protect them from sexual violence, disease, and pregnancy (Fine & McClelland, 2007). Laws setting the age of consent vary from state to state and are even different within the states themselves depending on the medical concern at issue (AAP, 2003). Various federal and state laws allow adolescents, between thirteen and seventeen years of age, to seek confidential family planning and mental health services without their parents' consent (Reddy, 2002). Such laws keep certain aspects of adolescents' health records private from parents. However, EMRs cannot always flag all confidential material and hide it from parents in the same way as paper records generally allow for. A further complication in most states is the inability of minors to enter into the security agreements required to grant access to their online PHRs, as most states only

allow minors to enter into contractual agreements under very limited circumstances.

Until providers can figure out how to give parents access to basic health care information for adolescents, without breaking confidentiality or other rules, many are leaving adolescents out of new electronic medical records systems altogether (Cohall & Vaugh, 2008). Other providers are revoking parental access to adolescent records as soon as a child turns thirteen (Gilbert, 2007).

Parents still have access to paper versions of an adolescent's non-confidential records, including immunizations, treatment for chronic conditions such as diabetes, and general medical care. Efforts are under way to find solutions, but policies of the American Academy of Pediatrics have not yet addressed electronic medical records issues (AAP, 2003). Meanwhile, software developers are working on more sophisticated records systems. Health plans modify adolescent online health records so parents can view standard non-confidential IMI, while letting adolescents confidentially refill prescriptions online and e-mail their physicians without parental access to either activity.

Assent and Disclosure Rules

Who should have access to adolescents' medical information is a difficult question. The laws are subtle, and do not always provide clear direction. Some states have laws regarding parental notification based on age and the specific medical problem (Ford et al., 2006). Other states leave many decisions about whether to notify parents up to the health care professionals.

Adolescents have wide confidentiality protection as part of an effort to reduce adolescent pregnancy rates and sexually transmitted diseases. Title X of the Public Health Service Act and the federal Medicaid statute both require all family planning clinics to offer confidential services to adolescents. The federal privacy law of 2002 extends additional protections to adolescents, including confidentiality of their medical records and health information. Most states allow minors to consent to treatments involving substance abuse, sexually transmitted diseases, and mental health counseling. Minors in most states can seek treatment for chemical dependency at age thirteen and seek contraception and reproductive health care at age fourteen, without parental consent or notification.

Health plans generally have parental access services, but parents lose access to an adolescent's online health records and services once the adolescent is thirteen years old. One of the nation's largest health plans, Kaiser Permanente, has a health care "proxy" agreement that allows adults to access health records of adult family members for whom they are caregivers, such as a sick spouse or elderly parent, as well as minor children. Specifically for adolescents, an advisory group is still trying to develop recommendations about how to proceed.

Efforts to come up with clear policies for adolescent health records are only likely to become more complicated. Examples of this are birth control and abortion, with most states mandating some sort of parental involvement (either consent or notice) before a minor can obtain abortion services, although several of those statutes are either permanently enjoined or currently being challenged. Advocates of more parental control continue to lobby to restore some parental rights. Some states have already considered repealing or modifying laws that allow minors control over reproductive health care decisions. In other states, adolescents must give explicit permission for their parents to review their health records, while still other states require assent for treatment from the adolescent combined with parental informed permission.

Eventually IT will make it possible for medical professionals to create health records that can automatically determine by age and state laws what information can be accessed by a parent. The guiding principle of information privacy for adolescents is that certain areas of care require that an adolescent be treated more as an adult than a child. Importantly, the goal is not to deter adolescents from seeking treatment for fear of disclosure of private information to their parents.

Moral Dilemmas

1. How should the information privacy rights of adolescents be assessed?

NEED FOR CLARIFICATION IN AN AGE OF RAPID TECHNOLOGICAL CHANGE

Although the right to information privacy is not absolute, there are ways to achieve common goals with little sacrifice of individual privacy. One way Congress and state legislatures have come to assess common goals is to use empirical studies, like Harris Interactive, to determine how Americans actually perceive issues:

- Do Americans perceive a need for information privacy of their IMI?
- What trade-offs might they accept for the public good?

It is not an absolute trade-off between individual rights and the public good. While the concept of the public good is often used to justify intrusions on individual rights, trade-offs are rarely simple. Moreover, the assertion of an absolute right to information privacy may fade as privacy expectations continue to erode.

Moreover, a public that is captivated by IT may have already desensitized itself to the need for information privacy. Facing rapid technological change, the need exists for Americans to further clarify privacy issues. Historically, it is worth remembering that technological developments continually outpace social and moral developments (Wharton, 2006).

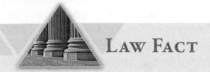 **LAW FACT**

INTERNET PRESCRIBING

Can online questionnaires be substituted for face-to-face examinations or one-on-one conversations before approved drugs can be prescribed?

No, licensed physicians cannot substitute online medical questionnaires for live consultations before prescribing approved drugs over Internet pharmacy Web sites. An Internet pharmacy cannot actively prescribe controlled substances online.

—*U.S. v. Hanny*, 509 F.3d 916 (U.S. Court of Appeals for the Eighth Circuit 2007).

CHAPTER SUMMARY

- Health IT holds great potential for positive change of the U.S. health care system by allowing for more rapid and accurate diagnoses, fewer human errors and omissions, and reduction in the rise of medical costs.
- A single global standard does not exist for sharing information between different EMRs, and there is no agreement within the health care industry on how PHRs work with other electronic records.
- A standard norm for Web-based health information is ideal so that PHRs can be compatible with institutional EMRs.
- Personal online health records are not currently covered by HIPAA.
- There is a significant difference between Web sites legally covered by HIPAA and Web sites that voluntarily comply with HIPAA; compliant sites could change their policies quickly and without notice.
- Disclosure of IMI to public health officials does not automatically amount to an impermissible invasion of information privacy.
- There are gaps in the quality of online information; data about the credentials, training, and experience of medical professionals is available, but information about outcomes or quality of care is limited.
- There are no international laws or treaties that regulate Internet drug sales from entities outside the U.S. to individuals located within the U.S.
- The issues of information privacy, confidentiality, security, and performance incentives must be viewed within the context of the very important and beneficial uses that go along with data-mining.
- Restrictions on identifiable prescription data are unconstitutional under the First Amendment because they stifle constitutionally protected commercial speech, which is not permissible unless the restriction directly serves a strong enough state interest, such as the promotion of public health or containment of health care costs.
- One consistent barrier to the reliability of any opt-in or opt-out system is that health Web sites frequently revise their policies, meaning that any permission Internet users initially grant regarding their information privacy might gradually become obsolete over time.
- What is posted on Internet discussion groups, chat rooms, health blogs, podcasts, virtual communities, and wikis is not protected information because it is in the public domain.
- Most health Web sites do not disclose the use of Web bugs in their information privacy policies or fully comply with their privacy policies, and they regularly modify their policies without alerting Internet users to the change.
- Whoever gathers an individual's health information owns it, whether it is the individual or not.

- The small-town model has returned to the health IT sector; everyone has access to everyone else's information by virtue of the continually expanding World Wide Web.
- Health care professionals must figure out how to give parents basic health information about their adolescent children without breaking confidentiality or other rules.

LAW NOTES

1. The University of Pennsylvania Health System (UPHS) uses an EMR by Epic Systems, one of the leading EMR corporations. While UPHS's EMR system yields benefits among its three Philadelphia hospitals (Hospital of the University of Pennsylvania, Penn Presbyterian Medical Center, Pennsylvania Hospital), three outlying facilities, and the PennCare primary care network, the electronic record ends if a patient goes to another health care network. For instance, if patients at UPHS go to the Main Line Health System in suburban Philadelphia, that hospital system has no information about them without phone calls, time, and faxing. This means that diagnostic procedures are often repeated with a consequent rise in duplicative costs (Burns, 2005).

2. Google has entered the online health care space with the Cleveland Clinic, a globally renowned academic medical center. Patients who already use the Clinic's PHRs can share prescriptions, conditions, and allergies between the Clinic and a Google online health profile, with patients controlling the information in their profile. The venture is intended to free IMI from EMRs so that patients can share IMI with health care providers, professionals, and pharmacies outside the Clinic's network. Since IMI is generally stored in institutional EMRs instead of in the hands of patients, this is a step in giving patients more control over their IMI (Lawton, 2008).

3. Microsoft's HealthVault is a free Web-based service that allows Internet users to store their health records online and eventually share them with physicians and medical professionals. One distinctive aspect of Microsoft's HealthVault is its number of project partners, including Allscripts (which provides EMR systems), the American Heart Association, Healthways (which provides wellness and disease prevention services), and various health care networks, such as the Mayo Clinic and New York Presbyterian Hospital. Other partners include medical device makers for monitoring various health conditions (Johnson & Johnson LifeScan for blood glucose, Microlife and Omron for blood pressure, and Polar for heart rate) (*see* Knight, 2008; Lawton, 2008; Walker et al., 2005).

4. The average victim of identity theft becomes aware only after about fourteen months have passed, but in some cases discovering the crime takes ten years or more. This chapter does not specifically address the theft of personal health information, which could be harder to discover than financial theft from credit cards or banks. For instance, it could be that only after someone is unexpectedly advised that they have met the lifetime level of insured coverage that they become aware that their medical identity has been stolen (Hoffman & Podgurski, 2008).

5. The Verichip, produced by Applied Digital in Florida, is the first implantable radio frequency identification device for humans. A glass casing, containing a chip about the size of a grain of rice, is placed beneath the skin. The whole procedure is often compared to getting a shot and is referred to as being "chipped" (Hildner, 2006). This monitoring system is described in its patent application as an:

   > Apparatus for tracking and recovering humans that utilizes an implantable transceiver incorporating a power supply and actuation system allowing the unit to remain implanted and functional for years without maintenance. The implanted transmitter may be remotely actuated, or actuated by the implantee. Power for the remote-activated receiver is generated electromechanically through the movement of body muscle. The device is small enough to be implanted in a child.

6. While not social networking sites per se, many Web sites take advantage of the phenomenon of connecting online to reach out to special audiences. The Wellness Community, a nonprofit group that provides free support and education to cancer patients and families, has a site that claims to reach more than 15 percent of the approximately fifty thousand adolescent cancer survivors in the U.S. With scheduled professionally moderated support groups, adolescents have access to message boards in a password-protected site. A comprehensive search engine allows adolescents to search for other adolescents with cancer by such criteria as age, location, or diagnosis. Another community site is Group Loop, where adolescents talk about more serious issues, like how their physical identity has changed as a result of cancer and their anxiety about the future (Landro, 2006).

7. Arizona Rev. Stat. Ann. §§ 41-4151 to -5152 (2009); Arkansas Code Ann. § 25-1-114 (Supp. 2003); California Gov't Code § 11019.9 (2002); Colorado Rev. Stat. Ann. §§ 24-72-501 to -502 (2009); Delaware Code Ann. Tit. 29, §§ 9017c-9022c (2009); Illinois Comp Stat. Ann. 5 §§ 177/1-177/15 (2009); Iowa Code § 22.11 (1984); Maine Rev. Stat. Ann. Tit. 1, §§ 541-542 (Supp. 2009); Maryland Code Ann., State Gov't § 10-624(4) (2008); Michigan Pub. Acts, Act 161 § 572(6) (2008); Minnesota Stat. Ann. § 13.15 (2003); Montana Code Ann. §§ 2-17-550 to -553 (2007); Neb. Rev. Stat. § 87-302(14)(2008) (prohibits knowingly making a false or misleading statement in a privacy policy published on the Internet regarding the use of IMI); New York (N.Y.S. Tech. Law §§ 201-207 (2002); 18 Pennsylvania Cons. Stat. Ann. § 4107(A)(10) (2005); South Carolina Code Ann. §§ 30-2-10 to -50 (Supp. 2009); Texas Gov't Code Ann. § 2054.126 (Supp. 2007); and Virginia Code Ann. §§ 2.2-3800 to -3803 (2009).

8. There is a real demand for medical information about public figures and celebrities. For instance, while former President Bill Clinton's quadruple bypass surgery was done under a pseudonym, there were multiple documented attempts to get into New York Presbyterian and Columbia Hospital to get information about his care. Another example is George Clooney's motorcycle accident and the unauthorized prying into his health records by more than two dozen staff members at Palisades Medical Center in North Bergen, New Jersey. More recently, several UCLA workers, including six physicians, were caught prying into Britney Spears's medical records (Ornstein, 2008).

9. Anonymizer technology companies such as Hushmail, IDcide, ZipLip, Disappearing, and Privacy Just Got Cool have emerged to protect "privacy space" (Lester, 2001). Zero-Knowledge, Intelytics, and Security Space have anonymizer programs that Internet users can use to spy on the spies. Their home pages promise Internet users that their software platforms can provide the protection to safely navigate through the increasingly unsafe channels of the connected cyberworld.

Chapter Bibliography

AAP (American Academy of Pediatrics), Committee on Pediatric Emergency Medicine. (2003). Consent for Emergency Medical Services for Children and Adolescents. *Pediatrics, 111,* 703-706.

Abril, P. S., & Cava, A. (2008). Health privacy in a techno-social world: A cyber-patient's bill of rights *Northwestern Journal of Technology & Intellectual Property, 6,* 244-277.

Amar, J., & Strumolo, A. R. (2007). Recent development in health law: Select recent court decisions. *American Journal of Law & Medicine, 34,* 703-708.

Anderson, G. F. et al. (2006). Health care spending and use of information technology in OECD countries, *Health Affairs, 25* (3), 819-831.

Annual review 2008: Privacy: Additional development. *Berkeley Technology & Law Journal, 23,* 783-785.

Ash, J. S. et al. (2007). The extent and importance of unintended consequences related to computerized provider order entry. Journal of the *American Medical Informatics Association, 14,* 415-423 (asserting unintended consequences of CPOE are widespread).

Bailey, M. E. C. (2006). The alpha subpoena controversy: Kansas fires first shot in nationwide battle over child rape, abortion and prosecutorial access to medical records. *University of Missouri-Kansas City Law Review, 74,* 1021-1041.

Barber, G. (2006). Personal information in government records: Protecting the public interest in privacy. *Saint Louis University Public Law Review, 25,* 63-121.

Bender, M. W. et al. (2005). What's holding back online medical data. *McKinsey Quarterly* (finding a national misalignment of incentives such that there is an inverse relationship between those required to invest in electronic health records and those who would benefit).

Berner, E. S., & Moss, J. (2005). Informatics challenges for the impending patient information explosion. *Journal of the American Medical Informatics Association, 12,* 614-617.

Berner, E. S. et al. (2005). Will the wave finally break? A brief view of the adoption of electronic medical records in the U.S. *Journal of the American Medical Informatics Association, 12,* 3-7.

Bloom, I. (2006). Freedom of information laws in the digital age: The death knell of informational privacy. *Richmond Journal of Law & Technology, 12,* 9.

Bodger, J. A. (2006). Taking the sting out of reporting requirements: Reproductive health clinics and the constitutional right to informational privacy. *Duke Law Journal, 56,* 583-609.

Boriani, G. et al. (2008). Telecardiology and remote monitoring of implanted electrical devices: The potential for fresh clinical care perspectives. *Journal of General Internal Medicine, 23* (1), 73-77.

Bratton, S. L. (2006). Unexpected increase in mortality associated with implementation of a computerized order entry system. *American Academy of Pediatrics: AAP Grand Rounds, 15* (3), 32-33 (response to Han research).

Bright, R. A. (2007). Strategy for surveillance of adverse drug events. *Food & Drug Law Journal, 62,* 605-616 (with data-mining of EHRs, a national drug safety system based on epidemiological principles could redress many of the surveillance deficiencies of the current system that relies on voluntary reporting of adverse events, inspection, and sampling).

Brooks, R. G., & Menachemi, N. (2006). Physicians' use of e-mail with patients: Factors influencing electronic communication and adherence to best practices. *Journal of Medical Internet Research, 8* (1), 2 (survey reporting only modest advances in the adoption of e-mail communication with patients by physicians).

Brown, T. R. (2008). Double helix, double standards: Private matters and public people. *Journal of Health Care Law & Policy, 11*, 295-376.

Burns, L. R. (ed.). (2005). *The business of healthcare innovation.* New York, NY: Cambridge University Press.

Carver, K. H. (2008). Analyzing the laws, regulations, and policies affecting FDA-regulated products: A global view of the First Amendment constraints on FDA. *Food & Drug Law Journal, 63*, 151-215.

Ciocchetti, C. A. (2007). E-commerce and information privacy: Privacy policies as personal information protectors. *American Business Law Journal, 44*, 55-126.

Clifton, L. B. S. (2004). Internet drug sales: Is it time to welcome "big brother" into your medicine cabinet? *Journal of Contemporary Health Law & Policy, 20*, 541-570.

Cohall, A., & Vaugh, R. (2008). *E-health: Adolescent medicine: State of the art reviews.* Elk Grove Village, IL: American Academy of Pediatrics.

Crist, M. P. (2006). Preserving the duty to preserve: The increasing vulnerability of electronic information, *South Carolina Law Review, 58*, 7-64.

Crossley, M. A. (1993). Of diagnoses and discrimination: Discriminatory non-treatment of infants with HIV infection. *Columbia Law Review, 93*, 1581-1667.

Cutler, D. M. et al (2005). U.S. adoption of computerized physician order entry systems. *Health Affairs, 24*, 1654-1663 (showing negative average net income per admission of hospitals in one study of hospitals who had adopted CPOEs; the operating margins among all U.S. acute care hospitals is less than two percentage points).

Dahl, T. (2008). Surveys in America's classrooms: How much do parents really know? *Journal of Law & Education, 37*, 143-192.

Del Beccaro, M. A. (2006). Computerized provider order entry implementation: No association with increased mortality rates in an intensive care unit. *Pediatrics, 118* (1), 290-295.

DeMarco, D. A. (2006). Understanding consumer information privacy in the realm of Internet commerce: Personhood and pragmatism, pop-tarts and six-packs. *Texas Law Review, 84*, 1013-1064.

Dorfman, H. L. (2009). The 2009 revision to the PhRMA code on interactions with healthcare professionals: Challenges and opportunities for the pharmaceutical industry in the age of compliance. *Campbell Law Review, 31*, 361-377.

Drexler, M. B. (2007). Privacy in medical research: A botched experiment. *Western New England Law Review, 29*, 535-569.

Ebeler, J. C. et al. (2007). *A letter report: Opportunities for coordination and clarity to advance the national health information agenda: A brief assessment of the Office of the National Coordinator for Health Information Technology.* Washington, DC: Institute of Medicine.

Economist. (2007). Billion dollar pills. *Economist-London, 382* (8513), p. 72.

Executive Order 13335 (2004, April 27). Incentives for the use of health information technology and establishing the position of the national health information technology coordinator. Washington, DC: The White House.

Federal Register. (2006, February 16). HIPAA administrative simplification enforcement. 71 FR 83 80-8391.

___. (2001, April 27). Dispensing and purchasing controlled substances over the Internet, 66 FR 21181-01.

___. (2000, December 28). Standards for privacy of individually identifiable health information. 65 FR 82462-01.

Internet, 66 FR 21181-01. Ferris, N. (2007). Device makers push Medicare reimbursement for remote patient care. *Government Health Information Technology* (summarizes the medical device manufacturers' trade group report, "Telehomecare and Remote Monitoring: An Outcomes Overview," that reviewed evidence from the Veterans Health Administration, one of the most advanced users of telemedicine).

___. (2006). Doctors want payment boost for using e-health records. *Government Health Information Technology* (detailing the American College of Physicians' call for Medicare to reimburse primary care physicians for using EHRs).

Fine, M., & McClelland, S. I. (2007). The politics of teen women's sexuality: Public policy and the adolescent female body. *Emory Law Journal, 56*, 993-1038.

Fleming, M. B. (2008). Feticide laws: Contemporary legal applications and constitutional inquiries. *Pace Law Review, 29*, 43.

Ford, E. et al. (2006). Predicting the adoption of electronic health records by physicians: When will healthcare be paperless? *Journal of the American Medical Informatics Association, 13*, 106-112 (concluding that universal EMR adoption will not be met by 2014; suggesting a conservative estimate that most physicians in small practices will be using EHRs by 2024).

Foreman, J. (2006, June 26). At risk of exposure: In the push for electronic medical records, concern is growing about how well privacy can be safeguarded. *Los Angeles Times*, p. F3.

Fox, S. (2006). *Online health search.* Washington, DC: Pew Internet and American Life Project (finding that most Internet users start at a search engine when looking for health information online; very few check the source and date of the information they find).

Garg, A. X. et al. (2005). Effects of computerized clinical decision support systems on practitioner performance and patient outcomes: A systematic review. *Journal of the American Medical Association, 293*, 1223-1236 (computer-driven decision-making improves guideline compliance but not necessarily patient outcomes).

Gellman, R. (2008). A legal and policy analysis: Personal health records: Why many PHRs threaten privacy. San Diego, CA: World Privacy Forum.

Gilbert, H. L. (2007). Minors' constitutional right to informational privacy. *University of Chicago Law Review, 74*, 1375-1409.

Goldman, D. (2006). I always feel like someone is watching me: A technological solution for online privacy, *Hastings Communications & Entertainment Law Journal, 28*, 353-407.

Goldsmith, J. C. (2005). The healthcare information technology sector in the business of healthcare innovation. In L. R. Burns (Ed.), *The business of healthcare innovation,* pp. 322-347. New York, NY: Cambridge University Press.

Gunter, T. D., & Terry, N. P. (2005). The emergence of national electronic health record architectures in the U.S. and Australia: Models, costs, and questions. *Journal of Medical Internet Resources, 14* (7), 1-3.

Haight, F. (2006). Illegal sales of pharmaceuticals on the Internet. *Albany Law Journal of Science & Technology, 16*, 565-570 (account of an eighteen-year-old student's death from prescription drugs dispensed over the Internet).

Han, Y. Y. et al. (2005). Unexpected increased mortality after implementation of a commercially sold computerized physician order entry system. *Pediatrics, 116* (6), 1412-1506 (finding an unexpected increase in mortality coincident with CPOE implementation at the Children's Hospital of Pittsburgh, suggesting the need to evaluate mortality effects and medication error rates for children dependent on time-sensitive therapies).

Health2 Resources. (2006). *How employers are using the Internet to increase employee health i-cue.* Washington, DC: Health2 Resources ("health i-cue" is a term used to describe consumer's ability to choose, use, and evaluate health care using IT).

Henney, J., former FDA commissioner. (2000, September 29). Health policy seminar series lecture: E-regulation and public health, FDA in the information age. Leonard Davis Institute of Health Economics at the University of Pennsylvania, Philadelphia, PA.

Herrmann, K. J. (2006). Cybersurgery: The cutting edge. *Rutgers Computer & Technology Law Journal, 32,* 297-323.

Hildner, L. (2006). Defusing the threat of RFID: Protecting consumer privacy through technology-specific legislation at the state level. *Harvard Civil Rights & Civil Liberties Law Review, 41,* 133-176.

Hillestad, R. et al. (2005). Can electronic medical record systems transform healthcare? *Health Affairs, 24,* 1103-1117 (reviews how patient processing inefficiencies in the U.S. health care system are one of the factors underlying medical tourism and explores the implications of this trend and the long-term effects that this could have on the U.S. health care and insurance industries).

Hirsch, D. D. (2006). Protecting the inner environment: What privacy regulation can learn from environmental law. *Georgia Law Review, 41,*1-64.

Hoffman, S., & Podgurski, A. (2008). Finding a cure: The case for regulation and oversight of electronic health record systems. *Harvard Journal of Law & Technology, 22,* 103-165.

___. (2007). In sickness, health, and cyberspace: Protecting the security of electronic private health information. *Boston College Law Review, 48,* 331-386.

Hylton, K. N. (2007). Property rules, liability rules, and immunity: An application to cyberspace. *Boston University Law Review, 87,* 1-39.

Hyman, D. A., & Silver, C. (2005). The poor state of healthcare quality in the U.S: Is malpractice liability part of the problem or part of the solution? *Cornell Law Review, 90,* 893-993 (discusses the error-reduction potential of EHRs).

Jacobs, B. R. et al. (2006). Perceived increase in mortality after process and policy changes implemented with computerized physician order entry. *Pediatrics, 117* (4), 1451-1452.

Jean, A. M. (2004). Personal health and medical information: The need for more stringent constitutional privacy protection. *Suffolk University Law Review, 37,* 1151-1173 (describing constitutional protections for IMI and advocating for increased protection).

Jerian, K. E. (2006). What's a legal system to do? The problem of regulating Internet pharmacies. *Albany Law Journal of Science & Technology, 16,* 571-597.

Kaiser Daily Health Policy Report. (2008, March 12). Health IT experts say incentives may be needed to encourage physicians to adopt electronic systems. Menlo Park, CA: Kaiser Family Foundation.

Kamm, N. (2005). HIV reporting in California: By name or by number? *National Association of Administrative Law Judges, 25,* 545-582.

Kemper, D. W., & Mettler, M. (2002). *Information therapy, prescribed information as a reimbursable medical service.* Boise, ID: HealthWise Center for Information Therapy (describes electronic information prescriptions, so-called information therapy, that is delivered to patients right before or after a physician visit, test, or surgery).

Kerr, R. A. (2007). The Patient Safety and Quality Improvement Act of 2005: Who should pay for improved outcomes? *Journal of Law & Medicine, 17,* 319-345.

Kibbe, D. C. et al. (2004). The continuity of care record. *American Family Physician, 70,* 1220-1223.

Kizer, K. (2007). Diagnosing the data. *Annals of Health Law, 16,* 323-334.

Klein, M. (2008). Recent development in health law: Select recent court decisions. *American Journal of Law & Medicine, 34,* 588-590.

Klein, S. (2005). *Quality matters: Who has $400 billion to build a national health information network?* New York , NY: Commonwealth Fund (overview of the potential cost-effectiveness of electronic records systems).

Knight, V. E. (2008). Health records may lack privacy. *Wall Street Journal,* p. D3.

Koehler, K. B. (2006). Medical: Toward implementation of electronic health records: Justifications, action, and barriers to adoption. *Journal of Law & Policy for the Information Society,* 651-682.

Koppel, R. et al. (2005). Role of computerized physician order entry systems in facilitating medication errors. *Journal of the American Medical Association, 293,* 1197-1203 (noting that computerized ordering of medication facilitated certain medication errors).

Kreuser, K. (2007). The adoption of electronic health records: Benefits and challenges. *Annals of Health Law, 16,* 317-322 (summary of the sixth annual Health Law and Policy Colloquium: Diagnosing the Data at Loyola University Chicago School of Law, Beazley Institute for Health Law and Policy in December 2006).

Landro, L. (2007, June 13). The growing clout of online patient groups. *Wall Street Journal,* p. D1.

___. (2006, December 27). Social networking comes to healthcare, online tools give patients better access to information and help build communities. *Wall Street Journal,* p. D1.

___. (2005, December 28). Tech glitches can slow patient care, new computers may deliver turmoil when they arrive; One study cites death rates. *Wall Street Journal,* p. D6.

___. (2003, July 17). Internet use for medical data shifts physician-patient roles. *Wall Street Journal,* p. D3.

___. (2003, May 22). "E-medicine" projects are gaining acceptance; What most patients really want is online interaction with physicians. *Wall Street Journal* (describes the Information Rx Project, a joint effort between the National Library of Medicine and the American College of Physicians-American Society of Internal Medicine that prescribes health information for patients).

Lawrence, S. E. (2006). Substantive due process and parental rights: From *Meyer v. Nebraska* to *Troxel v. Granville. Journal of Law & Family Studies, 8,* 71-117 (analysis of parental rights cases by the U.S. Supreme Court).

Lawton, C. (2008, February 21). Google and Cleveland Clinic form venture. *Wall Street Journal,* D3.

Lester, Toby (2001, March). The reinvention of privacy. *Atlantic Monthly, 287* (3), 27-39.

Lewis, C. E. (2006). My computer, my doctor: A constitutional call for federal regulation of cybermedicine. *American Journal of Law & Medicine, 32*, 585-609.

Longhurst, C. et al (2006). Perceived increase in mortality after process and policy changes implemented with computerized physician order entry. *Pediatrics, 117* (4), 1450-1451 (response to Han research).

Lovelock, J-D. et al. (2007). *Forecast: Healthcare IT spending, worldwide: 2006-2011*. Gartner Dataquest.

Lueck, S. (2008, February 18). Bush's Medicare plan likely to ignite partisan fight. *Wall Street Journal*, p. A4 (while the legislative proposal was allegedly dead-on-arrival, it highlights the role of health IT in the debate about how to deal with Medicare's rising costs).

Madison, K. (2007). Regulating health care quality in an information age. *University of California-Davis Law Review, 40*, 1577-1652.

Makdisi, J. M. Z. (2004). Commercial use of protected health information under HIPAA's privacy rule: Reasonable disclosure or disguised marketing? *Nebraska Law Review, 82*, 741-782.

Mariner, W. K. (2007). Extraordinary powers in ordinary times: Mission creep: Public health surveillance and medical privacy. *Boston University Law Review, 87*, 347-395.

___. (2007a). Medicine and public health: Crossing legal boundaries. *Journal of Health Care Law & Policy, 10*, 121-151 (discussion of the New York City regulation requiring laboratories to provide patient IMI to the Public Health Department).

McLaughlin, S. T. (2007). Pandora's box: Can HIPAA still protect patient privacy under a national health care information network? *Gonzaga Law Review, 42*, 29-60.

Middleton, B. et al. (2004). Accelerating U.S. electronic health records adoption: How to get there from here. Recommendations based on the 2004 American College of Medical Informatics Retreat. *Journal of the American Medical Informatics Association, 12*, 13-19.

Nadir, R. S. et al. (2006). Improving acceptance of computerized prescribing alerts in ambulatory care. *Journal of the American Medical Informatics Association, 13* (1), 5-11.

Naik, G. (2008, February 23-24). The gene police: In Britain, controversial DNA-tracing tactics are helping forensics experts crack unsolved crimes. *Wall Street Journal*, p. A1, A10 (explaining the rapid expansion of DNA databases in the U.S. and the FBI's plans to begin using familial searching and genetic surveillance).

Nath, S. W. (2006). Relief for the e-patient? Legislative and judicial remedies to fill HIPAA's privacy gaps. *George Washington Law Review, 74*, 529-552.

Ogolla, C. (2008). Will the use of racial statistics in public health surveillance survive equal protection challenges? A prolegomenon for the future. *North Carolina Central Law Review, 31*, 1-32.

Orden, J. F. (2005). DNA databases and discarded private information: "Your license, registration, and intimate bodily details, please." *North Carolina Journal of Law & Technology, 6*, 343-365.

Ornstein, C. (2008, March 15). UCLA workers snooped in Spears' medical records. *Los Angeles Times*, p. A1.

Patrick A. O. et al (2008, February 22). Reed buys ChoicePoint, opts to sell magazines. *Wall Street Journal*, p. B1 (announcing the purchase of ChoicePoint, the largest seller of personal data in the U.S. for $4.1 billion).

Pizzi, R. (2007, April 16). New York City brings EMRs to primary care providers. *Healthcare IT News*.

Pollio, M. C. (2004). The inadequacy of HIPAA's privacy rule: The plain language notice of privacy practices and patient understanding. *New York University Annual Survey of American Law, 60*, 579-620.

Posner, R. A. (2007). *Economic analysis of the law* (7th ed.). Amsterdam, Netherlands: Wolters Kluwer Law & Business (arguing that data privacy law is functionally "a branch of property law").

Pottker-Fishel, C. G. (2007). Improper bedside manner: Why state partner notification laws are ineffective in controlling the proliferation of HIV. *Journal of Law & Medicine, 17*, 147-174.

Powell, J., & Buchan, I. (2005). Electronic health records should support clinical research. *Journal of Medical Internet Research, 7* (1), 88-93.

Pritts, J. L. (2002). Altered states: State health privacy laws and the impact of the federal health privacy rule. *Yale Journal of Health Policy, Law & Ethics, 2*, 327-350.

Reddy, D. M. et al. (2002). Effect of mandatory parental notification on adolescent girls' use of sexual healthcare services. *Journal of the American Medical Association, 288*, 710-714 (finding that 59 percent of girls younger than eighteen seeking services at Planned Parenthood clinic indicated they would stop using all sexual health care services or delay treatment or testing for STDs if their parents were informed that they were seeking contraceptives).

Reiss, J. B. (2006). Going paperless: Electronic medical records come with own set of risks. *Food & Drug Law Institute*, 15-18.

Rosenbloom, S. T. et al (2006). Perceived increase in mortality after process and policy changes implemented with computerized physician order entry. *Pediatrics, 117* (4), 1452-1455 (response to Han research).

Rustad, M. L., & Koenig, T. H. (2005). The tort of negligent enablement of cybercrime. *Berkley Technology Law Journal, 20*, 1553-1611.

Saul, S. (2006). Doctors object as drug makers learn who's prescribing what. *New York Times*, p. A1 (describing computerized records with information concerning physicians and the drugs they prescribe that are used by drug sales representatives to influence physicians to write more prescriptions for drugs produced by their companies or fewer prescriptions for a competitor's drugs).

Saxon, L. A. (2007). Remote active monitoring in patients with heart failure (RAPID-RF): Design and rationale. *Journal of Cardiac Failure, 13* (4), 241-246.

Scardina, T. (2007). *Aid for Women v. Foulston*: The creation of a minor's right to privacy and a new preliminary injunction standard. *Denver University Law Review, 84*, 977-1000.

Schleiter, K. E. (2007). The dinosaur in the office: A consideration of the technical and ethical issues surrounding the adoption of digital medical data and the extinction of the paper record. *Annals of Health Law, 16*, 353-362.

Schmerken, I. (2008, December 1). Wisdom of the crowd; Bloomberg partners with online medical community to provide professional investors with access to thousands of practicing physicians. *Wall Street & Technology*, p. 17.

Shapiro, S. (2007, March 4). Finding your new self; In the online world of second life, let your avatar lead the way. *The Baltimore Sun*, p. 1N.

Shekelle, P. G. et al. (2006). *Costs and benefits of health information technology: Evidence report/Technology Assessment*

No. 132 (Prepared by the Southern California Evidence-Based Practice Center). Rockville, MD: Agency for Healthcare Research & Quality.

Sittig, D. F. et al. (2006). Lessons from unexpected increased mortality after implementation of a commercially sold computerized physician order entry system. *Pediatrics, 118* (2), 797-801 (response to Han research).

Solove, D. J. (2002). Access and aggregation: Public records, privacy, and the Constitution. *Minnesota Law Review, 86,* 1137-1218 (advocating increased access and use restrictions on health records and arguing such restrictions are constitutional obligations; notes that "[t]he threat to privacy is not in isolated pieces of information, but in increased access and aggregation, the construction of digital biographies and the uses to which they are put").

Solove, D. J. et al. (2006). *Information privacy law* (2nd ed.). Amsterdam, Netherlands: Wolters Kluwer/Aspen Publishers.

Spitzer, E. (2002, July 25). Press release: Major pharmaceutical company agrees to new safeguards for consumer data: Multistate settlement requires privacy safeguards to protect consumers. Albany, NY: Office of the New York State Attorney General.

Spooner, S. A., & Council on Clinical Information Technology. (2007). Special requirements of electronic health record systems. *Pediatrics, 119* (3), 631-637.

Steinbock, D. J. (2006). Designating the dangerous: From blacklists to watch lists. *Seattle University Law Review, 30,* 65-118.

Steinbrook, R. (2006). For sale: Physicians' prescribing data. *New England Journal of Medicine, 354,* 2745-2747 (reporting that during the last two decades, health information companies have routinely purchased electronic prescription records from pharmacies and elsewhere, which they then sold to drug manufacturers).

Taylor, J. A. et al (2008). Medication administration variances before and after implementation of computerized physician order entry in a neonatal intensive care unit. *Pediatrics, 121* (1), 123-128 (finding that while CPOE significantly decreases medication errors, errors still exceed 11 percent, suggesting that additional methods may be needed to improve neonatal patient safety).

Terry, N. P. (2006). To HIPAA, a son: Assessing the technical, conceptual, and legal frameworks for patient safety information. *Widener Law Review, 12,* 137-188 (documenting the media's reporting of lost, stolen, or hacked electronic health records).

___. & Francis, L. P. (2007). Ensuring the privacy and confidentiality of electronic health records. *University of Illinois Law Review,* 681-735.

Trubek, L. G. (2006). New governance and soft law in health care reform. *Indiana Health Law Review,* 3, 137-169.

Van Cise, M. L. (2005). The Georgia open records law electronic signature exception: The intersection of privacy, technology, and open records. *Journal of Intellectual Property Law, 12,* 567-595.

Walker, J. et al. (2005). The value of healthcare information exchange and interoperability. *Health Affairs,* 5-14.

Walsh, K. E. et al (2006). Medication errors related to computerized order entry for children. *Pediatrics, 228* (5), 1872-1879 (serious pediatric CPOE errors are uncommon, 3.6 errors per 1,000 patient-days; CPOEs can introduce new errors that are not typical of paper ordering systems).

Wang, J. K. et al. (2007). Prevention of pediatric medication errors by hospital pharmacists and the potential benefit of computerized physician order entry. *Pediatrics, 119* (1), 77-85 (clinical pharmacists effectively intercept inpatient prescribing errors but cannot capture potentially harmful administration errors; CPOEs unlikely to prevent administration errors, which pose the highest risk of patient injury).

Ward, K. A. (2008). A dose of reality: The prescription for a limited constitutional right to privacy in pharmaceutical records is examined in *Douglas v. Dobbs. Journal of Medicine & Law, 12,* 73-124.

Wears, R. L., & Berg, M. (2005). Computer technology and clinical work: Still waiting for Godot. *Journal of the American Medical Association, 293,* 1261-1263 (problems with medical software are not due to bugs, but rather due to poorly designed software with linear decisions being applied to complex decision-making scenarios).

Wharton (Wharton School at the University of Pennsylvania). (2006). Lawton Burns on the critical, and costly, role of companies that make healthcare-related products. *Knowledge@Wharton.*

___. (2000). Hunting snake-oil salesmen through cyberspace: The FDA vs. the Internet. *Knowledge@Wharton.*

Zarsky, T. Z. (2003). "Mine your own business!" Making the case for the implications of the data-mining of personal information in the forum of public opinion. *Yale Journal of Law & Technology, 5,* 1-56 (providing hypothetical situation in which employer terminates employee based on IMI it has purchased).

Zhang, J. (2008, February 26). Medicare spending to surge. *Wall Street Journal,* p. A3.

PART VIII

IMPROVING THE QUALITY OF HEALTH CARE

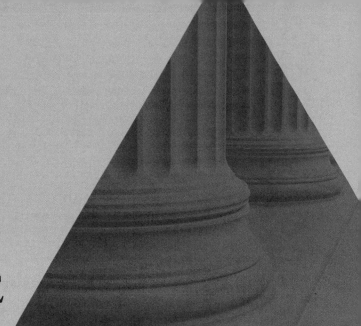

CHAPTER 21
DISEASE
MANAGEMENT

> "Moving into the next century, the most important breakthroughs will be in the form of clinical process innovation rather than clinical product improvement . . . the next big advances in health care will be the development of protocols for delivering patient care across health care settings over time."
>
> —J. D. KLEINKE, HEALTH CARE ECONOMIST AND AUTHOR OF *BLEEDING EDGE: THE BUSINESS OF HEALTH CARE IN THE NEW CENTURY*

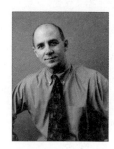

IN BRIEF

This chapter describes the demand for greater transparency regarding how physicians effectively treat patients and the concomitant drive to develop clinical information technology databases and other processes to assist health care professionals in making responsible medical treatment decisions.

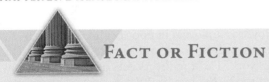

FACT OR FICTION

TRANSPARENCY OF PHYSICIAN EFFECTIVENESS

How should physicians' privacy interests be balanced against the public's need to monitor the cost and quality of health care provided under the Medicare program?

This lawsuit, explained in an earlier chapter on patient rights and responsibilities, is a key battle in the effort to reshape the nation's health care system. Consumer advocates, employers, and the health insurance industry maintain that access to Medicare claims filed by physicians could help independent groups monitor quality and wasteful health care; patients would not be identified. Physicians are worried such disclosures would violate their privacy, and that resulting ratings could portray some physicians' offices inaccurately.

The nonprofit Consumers' Checkbook, a ratings group, won a lower court ruling in 2007 directing the government to release the records under the federal Freedom of Information Act. The U.S. Department of Health and Human Services, joined by the American Medical Association (AMA), appealed over the issue of who should be allowed to see Medicare data on individual physicians.

—*Consumers' Checkbook, Center for the Study of Services v. U.S. HHS*, 502 F.Supp.2d 79
(U.S. District Court for the District of Columbia 2007), *reversed*, 554 F.3d 1046
(U.S. Court of Appeals for the District of Columbia Circuit 2009).
(See *Law Fact* at the end of this chapter for the answer.)

PRINCIPLES AND APPLICATIONS

Chronic disease management for common, preventable health conditions, such as hypertension and diabetes, is critical to containing health care costs. According to the Centers for Disease Control, approximately 1.7 million people die each year because of chronic disease. Estimates indicate ninety million people in the U.S. live with a chronic disease, the ongoing care for which amounts to 75 percent of the annual $2.5 trillion health care budget (CDC, 2004). The disconnect between reimbursing chronic health care initiatives and poor health outcomes has become an issue, not only for physicians and health care professionals, but for employers and third-party payers that ultimately play a major role in financing health care costs related to chronic diseases (Wolff & Boult, 2005).

Disease management is one of the reform strategies proposed to moderate health care spending growth and improve quality. Six key elements of disease management programs are:

- Evidence-based medicine guidelines
- Population identification processes
- Patient self-management education
- Collaborative practice models
- Process and outcomes measurement, evaluation, and management
- Routine reporting/feedback

(CBO, 2004; *see also* Birkemeyer & Dimick, 2004; Nicholson et al., 2005; Pentecost, 2006)

Although each of these components individually helps to achieve quality in health care, the impact of each is much more significant when combined. The extent to which a specific disease management program incorporates each component varies, but the most successful programs fully incorporate all six components (Wharton, 2005). An example of disease management initiatives at Merck and Dow Chemical, two corporate members of the highly successful Leapfrog Group, follows.

HEALTH CARE QUALITY

Many U.S. employers are investing in new disease management programs to improve the quality of health care for chronic health conditions (Wharton, 2005). Simultaneously, these employers are shifting more of the health care costs to their employees without understanding the implications on the amount and type of care employees will receive (Volpp, et al. 2009). Cost shifting to individuals with chronic health conditions, who need extensive care, does not constrain costs; in fact, it increases costs if employees cannot afford to pay for the cost shift and forego monitoring and preventive health care. These seemingly contradictory actions reflect the employer's inability to make an accurate assessment regarding how their decisions about providing health insurance to their employees affect their profits.

Like the cycle of poverty, the cycle of chronic health care continues indefinitely. Examples include employees with uncontrolled cholesterol who develop atherosclerosis, which leads to heart disease and strokes, and overweight employees who develop diabetes, which leads to kidney disease and renal failure, and eventually may result in the need for dialysis; uncontrolled diabetes is the number one reason adults need dialysis. When employees fail to monitor their chronic health conditions, they risk developing acute episodes; acute episodes often require emergency care and/or hospitalization. Health care delivered in an emergency setting, as well as general hospital care, almost always exceeds whatever it would have cost to monitor and take preventative measures in the first place. The end result, cost-shifting for chronic health conditions, is not cost-effective unless people can afford the shift in costs. Employers must:

- Determine how much should be invested in employee health
- Encourage appropriate use of health care by their employees
- Identify the best benefit designs to encourage appropriate health care delivery

(Nicholson, et al. 2008; Wharton, 2005)

One method, developed by Merck and Dow Chemical, improves employee health using estimates of the benefits of reducing absences and improving productivity. Employers benefit from:

- Decreased health care costs
- Improved on-the-job productivity
- Lower turnover
- Reduced absences

An employee who takes a sick day affects the entire workplace, with far-reaching financial consequences that go beyond the employee's individual duties, especially when the employee's team performs time-sensitive work. It is difficult, however, to measure the impact of employee absenteeism.

Job-by-Job Assessments

There are broad implications for job-by-job assessments. For instance, when the cumulative cost of productivity losses is calculated, estimates of the overall cost of health-related workforce absences increase by one-third. More importantly, the assessment can help justify spending more money to improve the quality of employer-provided health insurance. Disease management programs that help employees manage chronic health conditions, for instance, could pay for themselves by reducing absences and improving productivity, yet hard numbers are required to justify making these up-front expenditures. That is especially the case today when some employers are pushed by economics to drop health insurance altogether. Relative to healthy

employees, employees in poor health are more likely to be absent from work and less productive when they are at work. These indirect costs of poor health may actually exceed direct health care costs. The question is how employers can quantify the benefits of investing in employee health (Wharton, 2005).

Costs of Health-Related Absences from Work

The cost of health-related work absences often goes beyond salaries paid to absent employees. When perfect replacement employees are not available to substitute for an ill colleague, there are broader implications for productivity. As mentioned, this is especially true where employees work in teams and where team output is time-sensitive (Wharton, 2005).

For instance, many nurses serve as the physician's memory and legs by tracking patients and ensuring diagnostic tests and treatments are delivered in a timely fashion. When a nurse is absent, the loss in productivity can be large, as replacements struggle to learn about the absent nurse's workload. That is not as true, however, with the office phlebotomist. Because the phlebotomist tends to perform discrete, measurable tasks and works individually, medical practices do not face the same struggles in replacing a phlebotomist.

Salary Multipliers

Researchers at the Wharton School at the University of Pennsylvania put numbers to this concept of costs and identified thirty-five jobs in twelve industries involving different types of production functions. They then interviewed more than eight hundred managers to determine the financial consequences of employee absences. Based on the interviews, they estimated salary "multipliers" for each of the jobs. The multiplier reflects the costs of health-related absences from work as a proportion of the absent employee's daily salary. The median multiplier was 1.28, which means that for the median job, the cost of an absence was 28 percent higher than the employee's salary because of the impact on overall productivity (Wharton, 2005).

For instance, maintenance workers in hospitals and health care clinics were on the low end of the scale, with multipliers less than 1.1. Physicians were at the high end, with multipliers greater than 1.5. Employers with employees that have high multipliers would be more likely to invest in their employees' health, because the productivity impact of absenteeism is relatively high (Pauly, et al., 2008; Wharton, 2005). As illustrated in Figure 21-1, while most employers believe disease management programs are effective in containing health insurance costs, employers who account for salary multipliers when evaluating potential expenditures on employer-sponsored health insurance plans make very different decisions.

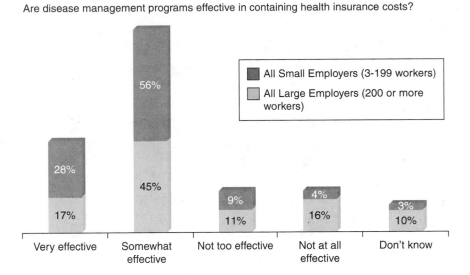

Are disease management programs effective in containing health insurance costs?

All Small Employers (3-199 workers)

All Large Employers (200 or more workers)

| Very effective | Somewhat effective | Not too effective | Not at all effective | Don't know |

28% / 17% · 56% / 45% · 9% / 11% · 4% / 16% · 3% / 10%

FIGURE 21-1: Perceived Effectiveness of Disease Management Programs

Delmar/Cengage Learning
Data retrieved from: Kaiser/HRET Survey of Employer-Sponsored Health Benefits, 2008.

Disease Management Programs

The extended hospital stay or major health complication for just one employee can be a huge financial burden for a small employer. To prevent such expenses, some small businesses are installing disease management programs staffed by nurses who work with employees to better manage and treat their chronic illnesses. Multinational corporations have used such programs for some time. Smaller employers are now finding the programs help employees reduce health complications, which leads to lower long-term health costs (Covel & Spors, 2008).

For instance, with disease management programs, nurses monitor employees with chronic health conditions to ensure they receive appropriate, timely health care. The programs do not generate enough of a return on investment simply in terms of health care costs they help employees avoid. Nor are the programs' net present values overwhelmingly positive when considering the salary value of the absences they help reduce. However, when employee salary values are weighted by salary multipliers, the scenario is different. The net present value of disease management programs over the first five years jumps nearly fourfold, making them a much easier sell (Wharton, 2005).

"Presenteeism"

Research at Dow Chemical took the salary multiplier concept one step further by looking at "presenteeism" (as opposed to absenteeism), or the impact of sickness on the productivity of those who come to work while ill (Pauly et al, 2008). When Dow asked about presenteeism issues in a survey on employee health, the survey found more than half of its employees reported having one or more chronic conditions. This generated a startling finding: while chronic ailments, such as diabetes, arthritis, and circulatory disorders, were responsible for the most direct health care costs, the costliest condition per employee overall, after factoring the costs of presenteeism, was depression. Such data helped Dow develop focused intervention strategies on specific conditions it would not have known about without the survey. Dow's strategy is now focusing more on:

- Prevention
- Quality of health care
- Value, with more sophisticated purchasing of health care, such as pay-for-performance programs that incorporate disease management

(Wharton, 2005)

EMPLOYER AMBIVALENCE ABOUT HEALTH INSURANCE

Theoretically, like Dow Chemical, employers could serve as catalysts for improving health care if they mobilized their purchasing power to compel the health industry to focus on safety and quality. In theory, U.S. employers have the power to drive change because they provide health insurance coverage for over 160 million people at a cost of nearly $2 trillion. Indeed, employers spent an average of $12,680 for a family and $4,704 for single-coverage health insurance premiums in 2008, above each employee's contribution (Kaiser & HRET, 2008). Collectively, employers have the market power to demand transparency and easy access to health care information. As illustrated in Figure 21-2, ambivalence on what strategy to pursue to change the U.S. health

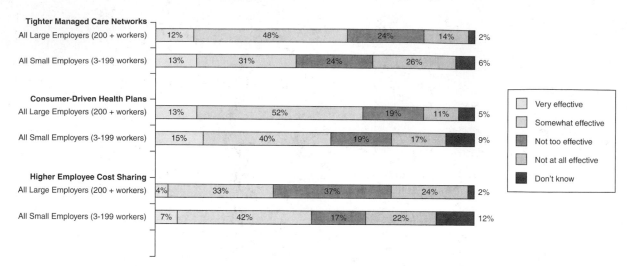

FIGURE 21-2: Perceived Effectiveness of Cost-Shifting Programs

Delmar/Cengage Learning
Data retrieved from: Kaiser/HRET Survey of Employer-Sponsorship Health Benefits, 2008.

care system appears to be thwarting this market force. Three current and seemingly contradictory trends in employer-provided health insurance suggest the American public is still ambivalent about the direction health care reform should take (*see generally* Baker & Delbanco, 2007; CBO, 2004; Wharton 2005).

Consumer-Driven Health Plans

More employers are shifting the costs of their health insurance plans to employees, partly because costs have ballooned more than 50 percent during the past six years (Kaiser, 2008). The highest profile example of this trend has been the move to higher deductible plans combined with health savings accounts (HSAs), championed as a way to combat health care inflation by giving health care consumers incentives to shop more astutely for care. The accounts also represent a way for employers to make employees more responsible for their own health care (Wharton, 2005).

Higher Employee Cost-Sharing

High-profile HSAs aside, cost-sharing can also be something as simple as increasing co-pays. Taken together, the expansion of consumer-driven health plans with higher employee cost-sharing illustrates that employers are struggling to make an accurate assessment about how health insurance decisions affect their bottom lines. The cost-sharing trend, in particular, comes at a time when information is lacking about whether:

- Short-term savings will lead to long-term health problems and costs because employees avoid primary care for financial reasons

- Employees will try harder to stay healthy in order to avoid paying more if they get sick

(Wharton, 2005)

Tighter Managed Care Networks

At the same time as employers are implementing consumer-driven cost-sharing programs, many are investing in disease management and pay-for-performance programs (P4P). In an attempt to control costs, employers more tightly manage the care networks employees can use so as to improve health care quality. The rationale is that if the quality of care improves by use of health care systems with less medical errors, less system defects, and a reduced level of unnecessary treatments, health care costs can be better controlled by the reduction in waste and inefficiencies caused by errors, misuse, and overuse of health care. While disease management is a system of coordinated interventions for populations with health conditions in which self-care is significant, another managed care intervention movement has emerged that involves adding an incentive component to disease management: P4P payments to health care providers based on meeting specific agreed-upon outcomes targets for each individual patient (*see generally* Baker & Delbanco, 2007).

Moral Dilemmas

1. Should disease management programs be supported if they have become merely a disguised framework for rationing care and addressing rising health care costs?

Leapfrog Group

The Leapfrog Group was formed in 1998 when a group of large employers expressed an interest in influencing the quality and affordability of health care. They recognized the dysfunction in the health care marketplace; they were spending billions of dollars on health care for their employees with no way of assessing its quality or comparing health care providers. The Institute of Medicine report, *To Err Is Human: Building a Safer Health System*, gave the Leapfrog Group its initial focus: reducing preventable medical mistakes. The report found that health care in the U.S. is not as safe as it should be and can be. In 1999, at least 44,000 people, and perhaps as many as 98,000 people, died in hospitals because of preventable medical errors (IOM, 1999).

At the time, more deaths were occurring in hospitals each year from medical errors than from vehicle accidents, breast cancer, and AIDS combined. The Institute of Medicine recommended that large employers provide more market reinforcement for the quality and safety of health care. The Leapfrog Group decided they could take "leaps" forward with their employees, retirees, and families by rewarding hospitals that implemented significant improvements in quality and safety (Moss, 2005).

Funding to set up Leapfrog came from the Business Roundtable and the Johnson and Johnson Foundation, as well as member employers.[LN1] Leapfrog members agreed to base their purchase of health care on principles that encouraged quality improvement among providers and consumer involvement. One of the Leapfrog Group's stated missions is to promote high-value health care through incentives and rewards. In 2005, it initiated a nationally standardized rewards program for participating hospitals and encouraged hospitals to adopt three practices to prevent medical errors:

- Computerized physician order entry (CPOE) systems for prescribing medications
- Evidence-based hospital referral
- Intensive care unit (ICU) staffing by physicians experienced in critical care medicine

Rewards in the form of bonus payments and higher reimbursement rates are given to hospitals that demonstrate excellence or show improvement. The Leapfrog Group has documented that:

- CPOE reduces serious prescribing errors in hospitals by more than 50 percent
- By referring patients needing certain complex medical procedures to hospitals offering the best survival odds based on scientifically valid criteria (such as the number of times a hospital performs these procedures each year), a patient's risk of dying can be reduced by 40 percent

- Staffing ICUs with physicians who have special training in critical care medicine (intensivists) reduces the risk of patients dying in the ICU by 40 percent

(Conrad & Gardner, 2005; Birkmeyer & Dimick, 2004)

The Leapfrog Group also focuses on measuring effectiveness and affordability in five clinical areas by having hospitals voluntarily establish system and process standards for:

- Acute myocardial infarction (acute MI)
- Coronary artery bypass graft (CABG)
- Obstetrical deliveries
- Percutaneous coronary intervention
- Pneumonia

Currently, more than 1,300 hospitals participate in this Leapfrog Group program and agree to adhere to the evidence-based standards. Participating hospitals, covering six out of ten hospital beds in the U.S., are surveyed on a regular basis and the results of the survey are made public.

Bridges to Excellence

Bridges to Excellence (BTE) is a national program initiated by employers with health insurers and individual physicians in response to the Institute of Medicine's 2001 report *Crossing the Quality Chasm: A New Health System for the 21st Century*, and, in particular, the report's recommendation to redesign reimbursement in order to effectuate quality improvement. General Electric worked for at least five years on this insurer-focused program to identify the higher-quality physicians used by its employees, thereby setting the stage for providing financial incentives for those employees who use better health care providers (Wharton, 2005).

The Leapfrog Group is involved in this insurer-focused effort, along with the National Committee for Quality Assurance. The three key principles guiding BTE are:

- Reengineering health care processes to reduce mistakes will require investments, for which employers and health insurers should create financial incentives
- Significant reductions in system defects (misuse, underuse, overuse) will help reduce waste and inefficiencies in U.S. health care
- Increased accountability and quality improvements will be encouraged by the release of comparative performance data on individual physicians, delivered to health care consumers

(Hanson, 2005)

In general, participating health insurers pay bonuses to individual physicians for program compliance.

Currently, BTE consists of health information technology programs that encourage physicians to become less reactive and more proactive in five areas:

- Cardiac care focused on hypertension, hyperlipidemia, coronary artery disease, and cardiovascular disease
- Diabetes care
- Spine care
- Depression care management
- Physician office management with development of medical homes for patients where specialist health care is coordinated, instead of individual patients receiving fragmented care from numerous unrelated health care providers

Medical Homes

Some patients have multiple chronic conditions, such as advanced diabetes or heart disease, that require disease management across many different specialties and one medical home, or one physician coordinating the patient's plan of care. Currently, when patients seek care for multiple problems, they often receive health care with little or no coordination between health care providers (Wharton, 2005). Specialty and primary care providers often administer parallel treatments with minimal ability to share information regarding a common patient. For instance, one patient may see a specialist, and then see their primary care physician, for the same condition. The primary care physician may be unaware of treatments, diagnostic tests, or medications prescribed by the specialist. This lack of coordination can lead to:

- Complication of ongoing treatment plans
- Jeopardizing patient safety, often resulting in conflicting medicines
- Loss of critical patient information
- Repeat of needless treatment procedures
- Treatment delays
- Unnecessary expenditures and administrative waste

Numerous factors drive this dislocation in care:

- Health insurance coverage
- Institutional and practice boundaries
- Professional behavior and staffing
- Technology availability to gather and exchange data

Successful and efficient patient outcomes require increased efforts to share patient information between health care providers, linked by health information technology programs. These coordinated efforts must be tied to best practices and clinical outcomes that can be measured and shared across clinic sites as standard treatment plans that define the acceptable level or type of care the patient should receive.

Employer Payoffs from Improving Employee Health

What is missing in this debate about health insurance, with both the Leapfrog Group and Bridges to Excellence, is:

- An accurate method to determine how much employers should invest in the health care of their employees
- Identification of the best health insurance designs to encourage appropriate health care delivery and use

When measuring the true cost of employee absences, employers should also accurately measure the payoffs that come from improving the health of their employees. Health care system improvements aside, how does this translate into lower health insurance premiums? Or does it?

EMERGENCE OF PAY-FOR-PERFORMANCE PROGRAMS

In recent years, the number of P4P programs has increased from the Leapfrog Group and BTE initiatives to about 160 different programs (Baker & Delbanco, 2007). While all these various P4P programs attempt to link health care spending to quality care, not all disease management is the same. The most important distinctions include:

- How performance is measured
- Who sponsors the program
- The level of involvement by physicians and other health care professionals
- How individual physicians and hospitals are compensated for quality or performance

Clinical and Non-Clinical Performance Measures

According to the National Committee for Quality Assurance, most P4P programs measure performance in both clinical and non-clinical areas. Patient satisfaction constitutes a common performance measure outside of the clinical realm.

Information Technology

Many P4P programs use information technology as the primary non-clinical measure. An adequate information technology structure is required for efficient collection and reporting of relevant measurement criteria. P4P programs may evaluate whether physicians have adequate information technology infrastructures and whether physicians are using those infrastructures. Since information technology is an integral component of P4P, the cost of information technology may be one of the major obstacles to widespread implementation of P4P programs. One independent physician association in California reported it paid $150,000 for technology to track claims, lab results, and prescriptions so it could report data in the Integrated Healthcare Association performance program (IHA, 2008).

Process of Care Targets

Clinical measurements can be categorized as process-oriented or outcome-oriented. P4P programs may measure several aspects of the process of care. For instance, the programs may review whether a physician uses a tracking system to remind patients to follow up on treatments, tests, or medication reviews. A program may also measure whether a physician uses any tools, such as education or resources, to assist patients in managing their own conditions. Programs typically measure whether the physician provides specific medications or diagnostic screenings to all patients with a certain disease. Finally, a major part of the process measures whether physicians follow clinical guidelines or evidence-based medicine for certain conditions.

Clinical Outcome Targets

Most P4P programs also measure clinical outcomes. For instance, a program may measure whether hypertension patients are within a range of acceptable blood pressure levels or diabetes patients are controlling their glucose levels. This is probably the most controversial aspect of performance measurement because outcomes are not entirely within the physician's control. A patient's clinical outcome depends on many factors unrelated to a physician's performance, and some argue this measurement fails to consider those factors.

Basic disease management standards are being jointly developed by the federal government, the health insurance industry, and professional physician groups. All health care providers should seek to meet certain clinical outcome targets, meaning their patient population should fall within certain percentage ranges, with outlier providers requiring further examination of their performance. For instance, one standard is that patients should be receiving an annual influenza vaccine; another standard is that patients with coronary artery disease should be prescribed lipid-lowering therapy. This is not to say that every patient should be vaccinated for influenza or that every patient with coronary artery disease should be prescribed lipid-lowering medicines; rather, there should be a clinical justification for patients not to be vaccinated, or for patients not to be prescribed lipid-lowering medicines.

Basic Set of Disease Management Standards

General Preventive Measures:
- Breast cancer screening
- Colorectal cancer screening
- Cervical cancer screening
- Tobacco use inquiry
- Smoking cessation advice
- Influenza vaccine
- Pneumonia vaccine

Coronary Artery Disease:
- Percentage of patients with coronary artery disease prescribed lipid-lowering therapy
- Beta-blocker treatment immediately after myocardial infarction
- Persistent beta-blocker treatment months after discharge

Heart Failure:
- Certain patients prescribed ACE inhibitor (pharmaceutical used primarily in treatment of hypertension and congestive heart failure) or ARB therapy (pharmaceutical given in combination with ACE inhibitors)
- Left ventricular failure assessment (classic site of myocardial infarction or heart attacks)

Diabetes:
- Perform one or more A1c tests (for glucose control or blood sugar)
- Percentage of patients with most recent A1c level greater than 9.0 percent (poor control)
- Percentage of patients with blood pressure below 140/90
- Percentage of patients with at least one LDL test
- Percentage of patients with most recent LDL less than 100mg/dL or 130 mg/dL
- Percentage of patients who received retinal or dilated eye exam by specialist

Asthma:
- Percentage of patients identified as having persistent asthma who were prescribed medications
- Percentage of patients prescribed preferred, long-term control medications or acceptable alternatives

(continues)

(continued)

Depression:
- Percentage of adults diagnosed with a new episode of depression treated with an antidepressant and who remained on medication during eighty-four-day acute treatment phase
- Percentage of adults who remained on antidepressant for six months

Prenatal Care:
- Percentage of patients screened for HIV during first or second prenatal visit
- Percentage of Rh negative patients who received anti-D immune globulin at twenty-six to thirty weeks
- Percentage of patients diagnosed with upper respiratory infection and who did not receive an antibiotic within three days
- Percentage of patients diagnosed with pharyngytis, prescribed an antibiotic, and received group A streptococcus test

Sources: Ambulatory Care Quality Alliance, American Academy of Family Physicians, American College of Physicians, America's Health Insurance Plans, and Agency for Healthcare Research and Quality.

Program Sponsorship by Health Insurers and the Government

Even though P4P programs vary, most can be categorized into a few common models:

- Employer-based initiatives: employers coordinate bonuses to individual physicians for each patient for achieving performance measures or improving performance; payments are usually true bonuses with the potential to change behavior
- Health insurer-based initiatives: insurers coordinate bonus payments to individual physicians for improved performance measures
- Government-based initiatives: more limited with respect to the conditions covered by the performance plan, which usually translates to smaller rewards for physicians

Health Insurer–Based Initiatives

Other than the BTE program, numerous health insurers have implemented their own individualized incentive programs to compel physicians' better use of evidence-based medicine and to cut down on over-treating and under-treating of chronic conditions.

Harvard Pilgrim Health Care

For instance, Harvard Pilgrim Health Care, a non-profit HMO serving Massachusetts, New Hampshire, and Maine, implemented an incentive program during negotiations for rate increases. The subsequently enacted rate increase included a portion that evaluated performance in specific areas, including adult diabetes, pediatric asthma, and inpatient utilization. In this program, health care providers receive the full amount of withheld funds if they demonstrate improved performance. Additionally, the Harvard Pilgrim Health Care plan withholds funds rather than

giving physicians a true bonus. In that program, if physicians do not meet performance measures, they will not receive the negotiated rate increase.

Integrated Healthcare Association

Similarly, in California, six health insurers (Aetna, Blue Cross of California, Blue Shield of California, CIGNA, Health Net, and PacifiCare Health Systems) have collaborated with a statewide initiative known as the Integrated Healthcare Association to establish a P4P program (Benko, 2006). Over $210 million has been paid out to physician groups who have met P4P quality measures in the first four years of the program (IHA, 2008).

Empirical Evidence of Effectiveness

While P4P programs have become standard features of health insurance design, there is thin evidence concerning their effectiveness (Mays et al., 2007; O'Kane, 2007; Smith, 2007).[LN2] Two systematic literature reviews found few empirical studies assessing the effect of explicit financial incentives for improved performance on measures of health care quality (CBO, 2004; Petersen et al., 2006).

Critics maintain the programs are nothing more than disguised withholding programs that managed care previously implemented to limit care, especially when bonuses are based on referral limitations and on physician productivity.[LN3] Humana was brought to task for this very criticism as described in the only lower state court trial case cited in this text; this case demonstrates one way attorneys are attempting to hold the health insurance industry accountable in the administration of its disease management programs.

Government-Based Initiatives

The Centers for Medicare and Medicaid Services (CMS) has implemented seven different demonstration efforts to evaluate P4P programs. Involving some

MISMANAGEMENT OF A P4P PROGRAM

Humana Health Plans of Texas, Inc. v. Smelik
[P4P Program v. Patient's Widowed Husband]
2006 WL 467987 (Court of Appeals of Texas, San Antonio 2006)
(vacated upon settlement of the parties)

FACTS: John Smelik sued his wife's physicians and Humana, a health maintenance organization, under the Texas HMO Act, the Texas Deceptive Trade Practices Act, and the Texas Insurance Code after she died from problems associated with kidney failure. Smelik claimed Humana breached its duty to supervise the quality of care provided to his wife. More specifically, Smelik claimed Humana did not properly inform his wife of her diagnosis and treatment options, furnish access to appropriate tests, provide a physician who specialized in kidney disease, or supply the proper Humana disease management programs her condition warranted.

The Texas Court of Appeals vacated the trial court's opinion at the parties' request once the parties reached a settlement. The case was dismissed with prejudice, meaning the parties are not permitted to later sue on the same claims again.

ISSUE: Did Humana mismanage its P4P program?

HOLDING AND DECISION: Yes, the trial court found Humana was negligent in the coordination and supervision of its enrollee's health care.

ANALYSIS: Smelik reached a confidential settlement with his wife's physicians prior to trial, but the suit against Humana proceeded to jury trial. The jury awarded $9 million in total damages to Smelik, of which Humana was responsible for $4.2 million. The jury determined Humana was 35 percent negligent, placing the remaining 65 percent of liability on the physicians and physicians' group. Following appeal of its $4.2 million judgment, Humana reached a confidential settlement with Smelik (*see* Mealey's Managed Care Liability Reporter, 2005).

This was a "mismanagement of managed care" case, not a "denial of benefits" case. Smelik did not claim Humana failed to pay for his wife's medical treatment, but instead argued Humana was negligent in the coordination and supervision of her care.

RULE OF LAW: The trial court found that HMOs must ensure that health care services are provided to enrollees under reasonable standards of quality of care that are consistent with prevailing standards of medical practice.

300,000 Medicare beneficiaries, each of thirty-five different programs has tied payment to quality of care and other evidence-based outcomes (Reschovsky & Hadley, 2007). While the programs include provider-based, third-party, and hybrid models, reducing costs sufficient to cover the costs of the disease management programs has proved particularly challenging. Final evaluations on twenty programs found three with evidence of quality improvement at or near budget neutrality, meaning the changes in delivery of health care brought about by use of disease management covered the costs of the disease management program. Interim monitoring on the remaining fifteen programs suggests four are close to covering their fees (Bott et al., 2009).

Physician Group Practice Demonstration Program

Ten large physician groups, each with over two hundred physicians from different communities across the U.S., are participating in the Physician Group Practice project. Reimbursement in that program is based on improving the quality and cost-efficiency of health care delivered to Medicare fee-for-service beneficiaries (Trisolin et al., 2008).

Premier Hospital Quality Incentive Demonstration Program

Another project, the Premier Hospital Quality Incentive Demonstration, helps to determine whether providing financial incentives to hospitals will improve patient outcomes and reduce costs. Participation is voluntary and hospitals receive bonuses in Medicare payments based upon performance of certain quality measures. Conversely, hospitals that do not perform well receive their standard Medicare fees without any incentive bonuses.

Premier collects a set of more than thirty evidence-based clinical quality measures from hospitals across the U.S. The quality measures track process and outcome measures in five clinical areas:

- Acute myocardial infarction
- Heart failure
- Coronary artery bypass graft
- Pneumonia
- Hip/knee replacement

Moral Dilemmas

1. Does the need for disease management programs indicate that physicians are not always motivated to achieve certain performance standards or strive for quality improvement, without financial incentives?

Physician Voluntary Reporting Program

CMS also implemented a Physician Voluntary Reporting Program (PVRP) in 2006. This is a simple P4P program without the payment incentive. Under PVRP, physicians may report certain patient care data to CMS. That data is then analyzed to measure physician performance. Currently, neither participation in the program nor the physician's performance results will affect reimbursement.

At first, CMS proposed the use of thirty-six performance measures under PVRP, but after receiving concerns from physician groups, reduced the number of initial performance measures to sixteen. Physicians in any specialty can participate in the program. CMS is analyzing and measuring each physician's performance.

Push-Back from the American Medical Association

The stated purpose of the government initiatives is to pay less for substandard health care. In order to do this, CMS will differentiate among physicians by attempting to address an inequity in the current Medicare system: paying physicians equally, regardless of who provides better care and who does not. CMS plans to implement its P4P program without any additional costs, which means payments to higher-performing physicians will come out of the pockets of lower-performing physicians. Some are concerned that the real goal of CMS is not to encourage physicians to achieve higher goals, but to eliminate lower-performing physicians. The concern is that lower-performing physicians are actually higher-skilled physicians seeing sicker patients (*contra* GAO, 2007). The fear is that the CMS system may result in some physicians refusing to treat the sickest patients with multiple disease conditions.

To address physician concerns, the AMA has developed five guiding principles in implementing P4P programs:

- Ensure quality of care: use evidence-based measures created by physicians and allow for variations based on sound clinical judgment
- Foster the patient-physician relationship: fair programs should support the relationship and recognize some obstacles, such as the patient's financial circumstances and compliance
- Participation should be voluntary: the programs should not adversely affect physicians who choose not to participate
- Use accurate data and fair reporting: physicians should be allowed to review, comment, and appeal the results
- Incentives should be fair: new funds should be provided for positive incentives

The AMA remains critical of the P4P initiatives and is prepared to oppose Medicare programs that do not comport with AMA principles and guidelines. Additionally, the AMA opposed PVRP prior to its implementation. One of the AMA's main concerns with PVRP is the manner in which physicians are required to report data with a new additional coding system that does not correlate to Medicare treatment codes. The AMA is also concerned the program will become mandatory, with a correlation between performance data and future reimbursement rates. Physicians cannot always control medical outcomes despite doing everything humanly possible; not every bad outcome is the result of poor health care.

TRANSPARENCY AND ACCESS TO HEALTH INFORMATION

The tussle between CMS and the AMA is a reminder of the relentless push and push-back highlighted at the start of this chapter in the Fact or Fiction case regarding patients' access to previously unavailable health information. While the AMA backs the ratings of physicians by the health insurance industry, the fear is Medicare data could be misinterpreted or oversimplified by ratings agencies without oversight by physicians and other health care professionals. However justified this concern, such interests are unlikely to stop the tide of groups seeking data to monitor the costs and quality of health care.

Moral Dilemmas

1. Is the public's interest in health care quality data and physician performance justified?

2. Is the AMA's interest against publishing data on physician performance justified?

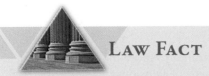

LAW FACT

TRANSPARENCY OF PHYSICIAN EFFECTIVENESS

How should physicians' privacy interests be balanced against the public's need to monitor the cost and quality of health care provided under the Medicare program?

The U.S. Court of Appeals refused to balance the physician's privacy interests against the public's need to monitor health care costs and quality of health care under Medicare, thereby rejecting a consumer group's bid to use Medicare records to rate the effectiveness of individual physicians.

—*Consumers' Checkbook, Center for the Study of Services v. U.S. HHS*, 502 F.Supp.2d 79 (U.S. District Court for the District of Columbia 2007), *reversed*, 554 F.3d 1046 (U.S. Court of Appeals for the District of Columbia Circuit 2009).

CHAPTER SUMMARY

- Disease management for common, chronic, and preventable health conditions is critical to containing health care costs because such diseases consume 75 percent of the nation's health care budget.
- Disease management standards encompass general preventive measures, as well as standards for treating coronary artery disease, heart failure, diabetes, asthma, depression, and prenatal concerns.
- The key elements of disease management include evidence-based medicine, population identification, patient self-management education, collaborative practice models, routine reporting/feedback, and process and outcomes measurement, evaluation, and management.
- Disease management is important to employers because it helps reduce health care costs and improve the quality of health care; when an employee is out sick, the financial impact on the employer goes beyond just the job that the sick employee performs, but it is difficult to concretely measure.
- Although chronic ailments, such as diabetes, are responsible for most of employers' direct health care costs, depression is actually the most costly condition overall when other costs, such as lower employee productivity, are taken into account.
- Employers are increasingly shifting health care costs onto employees. This is being done without knowing whether short-term cost-cutting might result in long-term increased costs due to health problems from employees choosing to avoid paying their own health care costs. Also not known is whether this will motivate employees to try harder to stay healthy in order to avoid paying their own health care costs.
- The Leapfrog Group was formed with the mission of reducing preventable medical mistakes, and its overall aim is to improve health care quality and safety, which it does through financial incentives.
- The BTE program has goals similar to those of the Leapfrog Group, which it aims to accomplish through encouraging investment in reengineering health care processes, reducing system defects, and increasing accountability and quality improvements; it also uses financial incentives.
- There are now approximately 160 such P4P programs, with varying ways of measuring performance, methods of sponsorship (employer, health insurer, or government), levels of health care provider involvement, and compensation for quality or performance.
- Such programs are voluntary because the costs to participate in the programs, especially with regard to improving information technology, are significant.
- P4P programs are increasingly common, but there is still little evidence regarding their effectiveness; critics argue they are actually ill-disguised withholding programs, modeled after managed care programs.
- The AMA is concerned that these programs will violate physician privacy and that performance data may come to determine reimbursement rates; it is also concerned that data may be misinterpreted or oversimplified if there is no appropriate oversight of its analysis.

LAW NOTES

1. Employers who are members of the Leapfrog Group provide health insurance to more than thirty-seven million employees in all fifty states: Alabama Power Company, Board of Pensions of the Presbyterian Church, Boeing, Chrysler, EMC, FedEx, General Motors Corporation, Goodwill Industries, IBM, Intel, Marriott, Motorola, Qwest, Sprint, Toyota, UPS, United Technologies, and municipal and state retirement plans in California, Ohio, and Maine.

2. Commonwealth Fund sponsored the first study to assess the effects of quality incentives in a large health insurance plan. Researchers examined disease management in a P4P program implemented by PacifiCare Health Systems (one of the nation's largest health plans) and found that a physician network that offered bonus payments outperformed another network that did not (Rosenthal et al., 2005). However, a year later, PacifiCare dropped out of the P4P program, citing rising costs (Benko, 2006).

3. Other insured-based programs have been disguised as P4P. The most infamous is likely the UnitedHealth program, implemented in the St. Louis area. UnitedHealth identified health care providers who had achieved quality and cost control and designated them as star providers. Enrollees who sought health care from non-star providers had to pay significant out-of-pocket expenses. Physicians and health systems had no input in the program and no warning prior to its implementation. Some quality measurements existed, but the star rating was largely based on costs. Originally, only about one of four physicians in the St. Louis area received a star rating. Shortly after the program began, the area's largest employer gave notice that it would terminate its contract with United Health, and the program was subsequently modified (Mays et al., 2007).

CHAPTER BIBLIOGRAPHY

Baker, G., & Delbanco, S. (2007). *Pay for performance: National perspective*. Washington, DC: Leapfrog Group & Leapfrog Group & San Francisco, CA: Med-Vantage.

Benko, L. B. (2006). Disease management strikes out; PacifiCare ends program early, CMS cites rising costs. *Modern Healthcare, 36* (4), 8-10.

Birkemeyer, J. D., & Dimick, J. B. (2004). *The Leapfrog Group's patient safety practices: The potential benefits of universal application*. Ann Arbor, MI: University of Michigan & Hanover, NH: Dartmouth Medical School.

Bott, D. M. et al. (2009). Disease management for chronically ill beneficiaries in traditional Medicare. *Health Affairs, 28* (1), 86-98.

CBO (Congressional Budget Office). (2004). *An analysis of the literature on disease management programs*. Washington, DC: CBO (literature review of empirical studies on P4P).

Commonwealth Fund. (2006). Quality matters: Pay-for-performance in Medicare. *Commonwealth Fund Newsletter 20*.

Conrad, D. A., & Gardner, M. (2005). *Updated economic implications of the Leapfrog Group patient safety standards*. Seattle, WA: University of Washington.

Cook, S. L. (2007). Will pay-for-performance be worth the price to medical employers? A look at P4P and its legal implications for employers. *Annals of Health Law, 16*, 163-212.

Covel, S., & Spors, K. K. (2008, June 26). Providing health insurance on a budget; Wellness programs, screenings and other services can help small firms rein in the rising cost of care. *Wall Street Journal*, p. B6.

Doran, T. et al. (2006). Pay-for-performance programs in family practices in the United Kingdom. *New England Journal of Medicine, 355*, 375-384 (P4P programs with respect to 146 quality indicators covering clinical care for ten chronic diseases, organization of care, and patient experience).

Douglas, M. E. (2008). Finally moving beyond the fiction: An overview of the recent state rally for health care reform. *Indiana Health Law Review, 5*, 277-336.

GAO (General Accountability Office). (2007). *Focus on physician practice patterns can lead to greater program efficiency*. Washington, DC: GAO.

Hanson, J. (2005, May 17). Testimony before the U.S. House Committee on Education and the Workforce Subcommittee on Employer-Employee Relations. *Examining pay-for-performance measures and other trends in employer-sponsored health care*. Washington, DC: 109th Congress.

Holmes, A. M. et al. (2008). The net fiscal impact of a chronic disease management program: Indiana Medicaid. *Health Affairs, 27* (3), 855-864.

IHA (Integrated Healthcare Association). (2008, February 27). *Press release: California health plans pay $65 million to improve performance in patient care*. Oakland, CA: IHA.

IOM (Institute of Medicine). (2002). *Crossing the quality chasm: A new health system for the 21st century*. Washington, DC: IOM.

___. (1999). *To err is human: Building a safer health system*. Washington, DC: IOM.

Kaiser (Kaiser Family Foundation) & HRET (National Opinion Research Center at the University of Chicago, Health Research & Educational Trust). (2008, September 24). *Employer health insurance survey (EHBS)*. Menlo Park, CA: Kaiser & Chicago, IL: HRET.

Kuhmerker, K., & Hartman, T. (2007). *Pay-for-performance in state Medicaid programs: A survey of state Medicaid directors and programs*. New York, NY: Commonwealth Fund.

Mays, G. P. et al. (2007). Convergence and dissonance: Evolution in private-sector approaches to disease management and care coordination. *Health Affairs, 26* (6), 1683-1691.

Mealey's Managed Care Liability Reporter. (2005, July 20). *Jury finds Humana negligent in care of enrollee: HMO to pay $4.2 million in damages.* Albany, NY: Mealey's.

Moss, R. (2005). *The future of learning: Building a bridge between competency and patient safety.* Denver, CO: Competency & Credentialing Institute.

Nicholson. S. et al. (2008). Getting real performance out of pay-for-performance. *The Milbank Quarterly, 86* (3), 435.

___. (2005). How to present the business case for health care quality to employers. *Applied Health Economics & Health Policy, 4* (4), 209-218.

O'Kane, M. E. (2007). Performance-based measures: The early results are in. *Journal of Managed Care Pharmacy, 13* (2S), S3-S6.

Pentecost, M. J. (2006). Health policy in focus: Pay-for-performance: At last or alas? *Permanente Journal, 10* (1), 77-79 (explaining the roles of the Leapfrog Group and BTE program in the emergence of P4P).

Petersen, L. A. et al. (2006). Does pay-for-performance improve the quality of health care? *Annals of Internal Medicine, 145*, 265-272 (systematic literature review of empirical studies on P4P).

Reschovsky, J., & Hadley, J. (2007). Issue Brief 108: Physician financial incentives: Use of quality incentives inches up, but productivity still dominates. Washington, DC: Center for Studying Health System Change.

Rosenthal, M. B. et al. (2005). Early experience with pay-for-performance: From concept to practice. *Journal of the American Medical Association, 294* (14), 1788-1793.

Sirota, D. (2008). *The enthusiastic employee: How organizations profit by giving employees what they want.* Philadelphia, PA: Wharton School Publishing.

Smith, A. L. (2007). Merging P4P and disease management: How do you know which one is working? *Journal of Managed Care Pharmacy, 13* (2S), S7-S10.

Trisolin, M. et al. (2008). *The Medicare physician group practice demonstration: Lessons learned on improving quality and efficiency in health care.* New York, NY: Commonwealth Fund.

Trude, S. et al. (2006). Health plan pay-for-performance strategies. *American Journal of Managed Care, 12*, 537-543 (review of twelve health plans investing in P4P programs).

Volpp, K. G. et al. (2009). P4P4P (Pay-For-Performance For Patients): An agenda for research on pay-for-performance for patients. *Health Affairs, 28* (1), 206-215.

Wharton (Wharton School at the University of Pennsylvania). (2005). Multiplier effect: The financial consequences of employee absences. *Knowledge@Wharton.*

Wolff, J. L., & Boult, C. (2005). Moving beyond round pegs and square holes: Restructuring Medicare to improve chronic care. *Annals of Internal Medicine, 493*, 439-445.

CHAPTER 22

EVIDENCE-BASED MEDICINE

> "The bottom line: all adults in the U.S. are at risk for receiving poor health care, no matter where they live; why, where, and from whom they seek care; or what their race, gender, or financial status is."
>
> —RAND CORPORATION, *THE FIRST NATIONAL REPORT CARD ON QUALITY OF HEALTH CARE IN AMERICA*

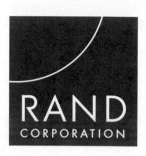

IN BRIEF

Evidence-based medicine (EBM), a philosophy of medicine that has been around for a little more than a decade, is at the top of the list of industry improvements in the U.S. to help rein in health care costs and provide more reliable medical treatment. This chapter provides an introduction to use of the best scientific evidence (current, valid, unbiased, clinically important medical research) to make decisions about the care individual patients should receive.

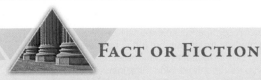

FACT OR FICTION

HORMONE REPLACEMENT THERAPY (HRT)

Is there any reliable evidence-based scientific research that combination HRT can cause breast cancer, heart disease, or dementia?

It is said that no other drugs in the history of medicine have been as consistently controversial as HRT. The debate began in the late 1800s, when physicians first began to feed pulverized cow ovaries to women, and continues to this day. In 2002, the National Institutes of Health warned women there were no safe HRT drugs. By the following year, some three thousand women in twenty-nine states claimed Wyeth's combination hormone therapy, estrogen-plus-progestin, had increased their risk of developing serious latent diseases and conditions. Women sued Wyeth claiming it failed to adequately test and sufficiently warn of the HRT drug's dangers and their breast cancer, heart disease, or dementia were caused by the failure to adequately test Prempro.

Reeves took prescription HRT because she was at high risk for osteoporosis and subsequently developed breast cancer. In 2003, Reeves sought class action status in a suit against Wyeth claiming negligence, design defect, consumer fraud, unfair competition, and failure to warn.

—*Reeves v. Wyeth (In re Prempro Products Liability Litigation)*, 2006 U.S. Dist. LEXIS 59049 (U.S. District Court for the Eastern District of Arkansas, Western Division 2006).

(See *Law Fact* at the end of this chapter for the answer.)

PRINCIPLES AND APPLICATIONS

One of the professional norms imposed on physicians by state licensing boards, quality of care organizations, medical associations, and health insurance plans is the use of EBM. EBM is among the professional norms physicians must adhere to, along with:

- Doing no harm
- Erring on the side of safety
- Referring patients to specialists when appropriate
- Staying current

(Powlowski, 2006)

DEFINITION OF EVIDENCE-BASED MEDICINE

Best defined as an attempt to apply epidemiological principles to clinical care, EBM promotes reliance on research data, particularly randomized controlled trials, in the practice of medicine (Dolinar & Leininger, 2006). EBM, which began in the early 1990s in Canada and the United Kingdom and developed later in the U.S., is a key component of disease management programs (Cohen et al., 2004).

Now, medical schools, government agencies, and the health industry are participating in the development of evidence-based practice guidelines, not only on how to treat common ailments such as asthma and upper respiratory infections, but also on how to perform surgeries and tackle serious diseases such as cancer.

With physicians unable to keep abreast of hundreds of clinical studies, make sense of conflicting scientific findings, and sift through available medical research for the most reliable and useful treatment conclusions, it is difficult to ensure they provide the best care to patients. EBM, which entails incorporating key scientific findings into medical practice and measuring the associated outcomes, provides a counterweight to this situation (Das, 2007).

In order to evaluate the limitations and criticisms of EBM, it is useful to provide a specific definition on which to base this analysis (Cohen et al., 2004). The 1995 editorial in the *British Medical Journal*, announcing the creation of the *Evidence-Based Medicine Journal*, gave this definition of EBM:

- Clinical decisions should be based on the best available scientific evidence
- The clinical problem, rather than habits or protocols, should determine the type of evidence to be sought
- Identifying the best evidence means using epidemiological and biostatistical ways of thinking
- Conclusions derived from identifying and critically appraising evidence are useful only if put into action in managing patients or making health care decisions
- Performance should be constantly evaluated

(Davidoff et al., 1995)

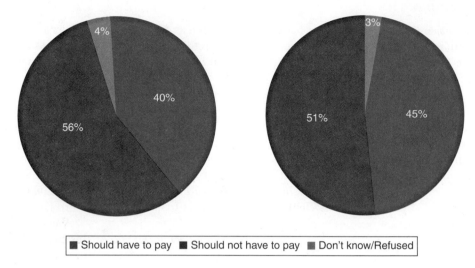

If an expensive new drug or medical treatment becomes available, but it has not been proven to be more effective than other, less expensive treatments, do you think insurance companies should or should not have to pay for the newer, more expensive treatment?

If a doctor recommends an expensive new drug or medical treatment, but it has not been proven to be more effective than other, less expensive treatments, do you think insurance companies should or should not have to pay for the newer, more expensive treatment?

■ Should have to pay   ■ Should not have to pay   ■ Don't know/Refused

FIGURE 22-1: Insurance Coverage of Treatments

Delmar/Cengage Learning
Data retrieved from: "Chartpack—The Public's Health Care Agenda for the New President and Congress" (#7854), The Henry J. Kaiser Family Foundation, January 2009.

While none of the later definitions are in disagreement with this definition, none of them are as complete. Most important, this definition contains the core set of issues historically and currently surrounding EBM (Cohen et al., 2004).

Paradigm Shift in Medicine

As illustrated in Figure 22-1, consumers of health care are ambivalent about EBM in terms of health insurance coverage. In spite of this public ambivalence, EBM has been characterized as a paradigm shift in medicine (Friedland, 2009). Today, a new mental model has evolved in the health industry that is changing clinical decisions from one point of view to a new one. The change is from a model of clinical decision-making based on traditional experience and authority-based clinical training to a model based on scientific evidence. This paradigm shift, where results from clinical trials rather than anecdotes, occurred when EBM discovered one-third of the nation's medical spending is devoted to health care services that do not improve health or the quality of care (*see* Fisher et al., 2003). There are undeniable outcome anomalies in traditional medical assumptions when one-third of the spending on health care may actually make things worse (Fisher et al., 2003). Dr. David Sackett, a pioneer of EBM, famously said, "Half of what you

will learn in medical school will be shown to be either dead wrong or out of date within five years of your graduation; the trouble is nobody can tell you which half—so the most important thing to learn is how to learn on your own" (Groopman & Hartzband, 2009). This responsibility to learn on one's own, along with making an effort to know what is going on with regards to one's health conditions, applies to the American consumer of health care, as well.

Traditional (Authority-Based) Assumptions

The traditional medical paradigm is comprised of four assumptions:

• Clinical experience and expertise in a given subject area is a sufficient foundation to enable physicians to understand and apply clinical practice guidelines
• Individual clinical experience provides the foundation for diagnosis, treatment, and prognosis
• Knowledge of pathophysiology, or changes and disturbances in human organs caused by disease, provides the foundation for clinical practice
• Traditional medical training and common sense are sufficient to enable physicians to evaluate new tests and treatments

(Friedland, 2009)

Evidence-Based Assumptions

EBM helps physicians make medical decisions with their patients systematically. The new EBM paradigm comprises a different set of assumptions:

- Knowledge of pathophysiology is necessary, but is insufficient for the practice of clinical medicine
- Understanding of certain rules of research and evidence is necessary to evaluate and apply the medical literature effectively
- When possible, physicians use information derived from systematic, reproducible, and unbiased studies to increase their confidence in the true prognosis, efficacy of therapy, and usefulness of diagnostic tests

(Friedland, 2009)

FAILURE TO USE EVIDENCE-BASED MEDICINE

Over the last few years, focus has been directed to costs and reliability in the U.S. health care system as a result of three forces:

- Number of reports from the Institute of Medicine about how well the U.S. health care system distributes medical technology
- Research about how the health care system is functioning
- Rising premiums for health insurance benefits

(IOM, 2001; RAND, 2006)

U.S. physicians and hospitals too often do not use the best scientific evidence available for treating even the most common medical conditions. There is a tremendous gap between what treatment is known to work and what treatment patients actually get because some physicians simply are not aware of what the most effective treatments are, or else have their own reasons for not using them. Examples of failures to use EBM include:

- Almost one-third of the surgeries performed on Medicare patients are unnecessary (Asch et al., 2006)
- Less than one-fourth of the people with hypertension have it under control with recommended blood pressure medications (RAND, 2006)
- One-third of medical spending is devoted to services that do not improve health or the quality of care, and may make things worse (Fisher et al., 2003)
- More than three-fourths of diabetics are not getting routine hemoglobin screening, which is essential to detect complications such as kidney failure (McGlynn et al., 2003)
- Adhering to EBM guidelines for treating hypertension alone could save at least $1.2 billion annually (Fischer & Avorn, 2004)

- Less than half of heart attack patients are on beta blockers, which cut the risk of premature death (McGlynn et al., 2003)
- A study in the *Journal of the American Medical Association* suggests brain cancer in adults is a dreaded diagnosis with few established treatment guidelines, resulting in wide variations in care that can make things worse for some patients (Chang et al., 2005)
- Nearly half of patients with brain cancer receive no chemotherapy, despite evidence that it can boost survival, anti-seizure drugs are widely used even though most patients do not have seizures, and while depression is common in people with brain cancer, more than 90 percent are never given antidepressants (Tanner, 2005); these findings stem from a survey of 788 adult brain cancer patients at fifty-two centers throughout the U.S. and Canada (Chang et al., 2005)

These statistics highlight a major shortcoming of the decentralized U.S. health care system: physicians treat common illnesses in a variety of ways, even though only one treatment has shown the most success.

Breakdown in Efficiency

The Commonwealth Fund recently published a score card on American medicine that established benchmarks for health care quality, access, equity, and outcomes. According to these measures of reasonably attainable levels of performance, an optimal score of 100 in each of these areas was actually being achieved, for international comparisons, by the average of the three best countries, or, for comparisons within the U.S., the best 10 percent of states. Overall, American health care earned a score of 66, otherwise commonly known in academia as a D. Some comparisons reinforce this point:

- Infant mortality rate in the U.S. is seven per 100,000 births, while the international benchmark is 2.7
- Sixty-year-old American men live 2.1 years less than the international benchmark
- Sixty-year-old American women live 2.9 years less than the international benchmark

(Schoen et al., 2006)

The efficiency of U.S. health care, or how much health Americans get for the money spent, earned a 51, otherwise commonly known in academia as an F. In other words, the U.S. wastes significant resources on suboptimal health care.

Halftime Estimate of Unnecessary Care

"Do no harm" is a bedrock principle of medicine. While needless tests and procedures provide no real benefit to patients and often cannot do anything but harm (Landro, 2007), they do enrich the health industry. RAND Corp., a California-based think tank, estimates people get the care they need, and only the care they need, less than half of the time (RAND, 2006). RAND's half-time estimate is supported by studies cited by the National Institute of Medicine that indicate as much as half of the care provided to Americans is unnecessary, including:

- Diagnostic tests that are repeated
- Drugs and treatment for which there is no evidence of benefit
- Medical procedures that do not do any good

(IOM, 2001)

Research from Dartmouth also supports the degree to which there are high variations in health care spending between specific regions of the country (Fisher et al., 2003).[LN1] There is accumulating evidence that excess quantity of care in the U.S. is actually overdosing Americans with respect to their health outcomes. More health care does not result in better health outcomes or higher satisfaction with care (Fisher et al., 2003).

RAND Corp. also released results from twelve major metropolitan areas supporting the Dartmouth research, saying all Americans are at risk for receiving poor health care, even from hospitals or physicians considered top notch (Kerr et al., 2004). The twelve metropolitan areas in this research included, among others, Boston, Cleveland, Greenville (South Carolina), Indianapolis, Lansing, Little Rock, Miami, Newark, Orange County (California), Phoenix, Seattle, and Syracuse. Substantial gaps between what physicians know works and the health care actually provided were revealed; these deficits persist despite initiatives by both the federal government and private health care delivery systems to improve care (RAND, 2005b).

- On average, residents received 50 to 60 percent of the recommended care for cardiac conditions and pulmonary problems; specifically, care for the following chronic conditions was unsatisfactory half the time: asthma, atrial fibrillation, chronic obstructive pulmonary disease, congestive heart failure, coronary artery disease, and hypertension
- Preventive care for sexually transmitted diseases, including human immunodeficiency virus, the virus that causes acquired immune deficiency syndrome, and substance abuse was consistently low
- The quality of preventive care for diabetes was consistently the worst in all twelve communities

(Kerr et al., 2004)

EVIDENCE-BASED MEDICAL PRINCIPLES WIDESPREAD

According to one estimate, more than one thousand practice guidelines are developed annually by quality of care organizations, medical associations, and health insurance plans (Timmermans & Mauck, 2005). The principles of EBM are already widespread among hospitals, medical groups, and health insurers in the U.S. In most cases, EBM guidelines are implemented as a computer-based care management or disease management program that provides physicians, nurses, and health plan case managers with a wide variety of information on accepted best practices for treating similar patients. Guidelines from the Agency for Healthcare Research and Quality (AHRQ) are authored by reputable and authoritative medical groups and often linked to financial incentives by health insurance plans (Saver, 2008).

Selected Agency for Healthcare Research and Quality Clinical Practice Guidelines
- Acute Low Back Problems in Adults
- Acute Pain Management
- Benign Prostatic Hyperplasia
- Cardiac Rehabilitation
- Cataracts in Adults
- Depression in Primary Care
- Early Alzheimer's Disease
- Early HIV Infection
- Heart Failure
- Management of Cancer Pain
- Otitis Media with Effusion
- Post-Stroke Rehabilitation
- Pressure Ulcer Prevention
- Pressure Ulcer Treatment
- Quality Mammography
- Sickle-Cell Disease
- Smoking Cessation
- Unstable Angina
- Urinary Incontinence in Adults

Sources: National Guideline Clearinghouse, an initiative of the AHRQ, U.S. Department of Health and Human Services, in partnership with the American Medical Association and the America's Health Insurance Plans.

These programs give providers an additional set of tools to analyze and evaluate potential care plans while maintaining the flexibility to deal with an individual patient's unique circumstances. The final medical decisions are still made by physicians and nurses consulting with their patients.

Point, Counterpoint on Evidence-Based Medicine

While over the last fifty years randomized clinical trials have produced relatively solid evidence, and their legitimacy and usefulness keeps growing, critics still claim EBM is not what it purports to be. The chief criticism is that many clinical guidelines are based on small trials with insufficient statistical power and nonrandomized studies. A second claim is that while EBM guidelines are indisputable in some areas, such as controlling diabetics' blood sugar levels, for many conditions, few reliable guidelines exist, or the evidence is contradictory, or new studies quickly emerge that undermine the original evidence (Landro, 2005).

Traditional Medical Culture

Patients typically trust their physicians are relying on experience and research when they are diagnosed and fail to ask about the cost-effectiveness of their treatment options. The option of simple surgical procedures over long-term drug use and its consequent side effects are seldom fully explained, so many patients never have the opportunity to make an informed individual choice.

For example, women experiencing stress incontinence seldom are offered the option of a retropubic suspension or suburethral sling; instead they are offered lifetime prescriptions for Pfizer's Detrol with the side effects of weight gain and mental confusion. Or, it is simply recommended they use pelvic floor exercises and adult diapers, rather than face the inherent dangers accompanying any surgical procedure. In this instance, even though one-third of women experience this condition as they age, reliable evidence on which to judge whether or not slings are better or worse than other surgical or conservative management is currently not available (Bezerra et al., 2005).

Why the resistance to EBM? Physicians simply do not want anyone advising them what is best for their patients when they believe a particular treatment works (Mendelson & Carino, 2005). Some physicians claim that results of clinical trials do not apply to their patients. Other physicians take a "show me" attitude, waiting to see if treating patients according to guidelines produces better outcomes. But treatment effects are often small, for instance, reducing future risk of heart attack by 25 percent; individual physicians typically have too few patients with any one illness or do not follow them long enough to detect such effects (Begley, 2003).

Time Commitment

Another obstacle to treating patients according to EBM guidelines is it takes time physicians claim they do not have. Proper treatment of diabetes, for instance, means blood tests, eye exams, meal plans, and more, much of which is poorly reimbursed by insurers. It also requires a team approach which some group practices,

let alone solo practitioners, cannot manage. Moreover, outside of the academic medical centers, hospitals often lack the information technology to let physicians electronically record information about patients and match it to best practices guidelines (Begley, 2003).

Spinal Fusion Controversy

One controversy, however, makes proponents of EBM question how many physicians believe in science-based care. When AHRQ issued a clinical guideline for lower back pain, which concluded spinal fusion surgery usually does no good, and suggested there were too many unnecessary back surgeries, orthopedic surgeons responded by lobbying Congress to punish the agency (Begley, 2003). Congress cut the group's budget and stripped its authority to make Medicare payment recommendations, crippling for years the very idea of EBM.

Today, a decade later, studies continue to challenge the overuse of spinal fusion surgery. There are:

- Excessive rates of complications
- High rates of reoperation
- Rapidly rising rates of surgery
- Wide variations in the rates of use

(Deyo et al., 2004)

All this indicates spinal fusion continues to be overused, with inpatient hospital patient care costs exceeding $12 billion year (AHRQ, 2007). All the while, surgical effectiveness for degenerative disk disease, the most common indication, still remains unclear. AHRQ and the Robert Wood Johnson Foundation are calling for a shift from examining how to perform fusion to examining who should undergo spinal fusion surgery (Deyo et al., 2004).

Best Practice Guidelines for Treatment

Clinical practice guidelines are one embodiment of EBM; in practice, the two terms are often used interchangeably. The complex history of clinical protocols can be traced back to the fourth century B.C. and has included repeated calls for EBM by such luminaries as Florence Nightingale and Abraham Flexner (Heimer, 2006).

With studies showing Americans get only half of the recommended health care, health insurers are increasingly using best practice guidelines drawn from EBM to make coverage decisions about drugs and treatments and to reward physicians who follow the rules. The National Business Group on Health, for instance, which represents large employers covering more than forty-five million workers, retirees, and their families, is developing recommendations for employers to use in designing health insurance plans that promote greater use of treatments and procedures supported by EBM. It is important for patients to understand the autonomy of their physicians is being very closely scrutinized (Landro, 2005).

Most EBM guidelines have been developed by medical schools, specialty medical groups, government agencies, or health care companies, and range from how to treat common ailments such as asthma and hypertension, to how to perform surgeries and tackle serious diseases such as cancer. But how good is the evidence behind the guidelines? Proponents of EBM say guidelines based on scientific studies are the best way to fix the health care system and ensure treatments are backed up by solid scientific proof they are effective from both a cost and quality standpoint (Landro, 2005). Consider clinical guideline resources from the:

- Minnesota Institute for Clinical Systems Improvement
- National Guideline Clearinghouse
- U.S. Preventive Services Task Force
- Medical specialty organization guidelines such as the American Association of Clinical Endocrinologists Clinical Guidelines and the American College of Cardiology Clinical Statements/Guidelines

Each of these groups explains and grades the quality of the research their recommendations are based on. Content aggregators like Medexact are another source of information.

Minnesota Institute for Clinical Systems Improvement

The Institute for Clinical Systems Improvement, comprised of fifty-three medical groups, including the Mayo Clinic in Rochester, Minnesota, develops EBM guidelines and hospital improvement programs for six Minnesota health insurers. Patient-friendly versions of its guidelines cover some sixty different diseases and conditions, including asthma, diabetes, and lower back pain.

National Guidelines Clearinghouse

The National Guidelines Clearinghouse was created by AHRQ in partnership with the American Medical Association and America's Health Insurance Plans. Summaries of current recommendations about a wide range of medical treatments are available based on AHRQ data.

Though primarily used by physicians and health care providers, patients can view the guidelines and updates on new evidence that should be considered in medical treatment. For instance, as soon as the Vioxx withdrawal was announced, all references to the drug in National Guidelines covering such conditions as arthritis, menstrual cramps, and joint pain were flagged, with a note adding the drug had been withdrawn from the market due to safety concerns about an increased risk of cardiovascular events.

POEMS

The patient-oriented evidence that matters system (POEMS) was developed in the mid-1990s specifically for primary care physicians (PCPs). It allows PCPs to disregard much of the medical literature and focus only on what is important to their medical practices, which simplifies EBM, a concept known as information mastery. POEMS entrusts to EBM experts the complicated, time-consuming task of searching the literature, filtering it for relevance using the POEMs criteria, and determining the validity of clinical studies (Slawson et al., 2007). It asks individual physicians to focus on finding useful information at the point of care that will assist them in caring for their patients (Rosser et al., 2004).

The theory behind POEMS can best be explained by analogy. For example, information mastery is the practical application of EBM, just like infectious disease practice is the practical application of microbiology. Knowledge of microbiology is necessary but not sufficient to treat people with infections. In the same way, EBM knowledge is necessary but not sufficient to practice medicine (*see* White, 2004).

U.S. Preventive Services Task Force

The U.S. Preventive Services Task Force is an independent panel of experts in primary care and prevention that systematically reviews the evidence of effectiveness and develops recommendations for clinical preventive services. Sponsored by AHRQ, the Task Force makes recommendations about which preventive services should be incorporated routinely into primary medical care in the U.S. and for which populations. It also identifies a national research agenda for clinical preventive care (*see generally* AHRQ, 2008).

Content Aggregators Such as MedExact

Given the amount of health care information in today's marketplace, there is a role for content aggregators, such as search engines, that summarize clinical content from reputable sources. MedExact offers centralized treatment information, on over six hundred medical conditions and disease states, from the National Cancer Institute, the National Institutes of Health, the American Diabetes Association, and other leading medical associations and institutions. Many leading academic health care systems offer portal-like blogs that tend to serve as content aggregators for health consumers by offering links to personal blogs, news stories, discussion threads, and other electronic content. Law and management textbook publishers are also having their authors develop personal blogs to provide updated headlines and news articles to sites that are of interest to their readers, including commentaries and recommendations compiled by the authors of their leading texts on health care.

Patient Registries

Diabetes registries have become prevalent in the past decade. The most renowned active diabetes registry in the U.S. is the Vermont Diabetes Information System (VDIS), sponsored by the National Institutes of Health (MacLean et al., 2006). The VDIS is primarily intended to improve adult diabetes treatment by monitoring patients and testing, but a secondary role is discovering new information for advancing diabetes management by providing researchers with access to collected data (Littenberg & MacLean, 2006; *see also* Krent etal., 2008).

There is a call for better evidence gathering to identify adverse effects and new risks, including the use of patient registries to track drug side effects once drugs or treatments are approved, and new information technology systems to synthesize data from clinical trials (Landro, 2005). There is also a need to track off-label use of drugs for clinical effectiveness. Similar to the diabetes registries, the FDA can require pharmaceutical and biotechnology companies to submit a Risk Evaluation and Mitigation Strategy (REMS) for their medical products based on the FDA's determination that a registry is necessary to ensure that the benefits outweigh the risks (OIG, 2006; *see* 21 U.S.C.A. § 355-1 (2008)).

Off-Label Use of Actimmune

The most recent instance of ineffective off-label drug use is Actimmune (Interferon gamma-1b), which had been prescribed off-label to patients with a potentially fatal lung condition, idiopathic pulmonary fibrosis (IPF). Actimmune is approved by the FDA to treat two other extremely rare diseases, but substantially all its sales (almost $100 million in 2006) came from the off-label use for IPF, which costs each patient about $50,000 per year. There was, however, no reliable evidence Actimmune was an effective treatment for IPF. In early 2007, InterMune abandoned its efforts to develop Actimmune as a treatment for IPF because clinical trials showed it failed to prolong lives and was no more effective than a placebo.

In late 2006, InterMune entered into a deferred prosecution agreement and paid nearly $37 million to resolve criminal charges and civil liability in connection with the illegal promotion and marketing of its drug Actimmune. InterMune also entered into a five-year Corporate Integrity Agreement with the Office of the Inspector General for the U.S. Department of Health and Human Services. Although a clinical trial in fact failed in 2002, InterMune issued a press release claiming the results of the trial established Actimmune helped IPF patients live longer. The former chief executive officer of InterMune was subsequently indicted on wire fraud and felony charges in 2008 for his role in the creation and dissemination of false and misleading information about the efficacy of Actimmune (Case #: CR 08-0164-CRB (Northern District of California 2008)).

FEDERAL AGENCY FOR HEALTHCARE RESEARCH AND QUALITY

AHRQ, which conducts research for federal health programs, has developed state-of-the-art information about the effectiveness of treatments, including prescription drugs, for the top conditions affecting Medicare beneficiaries, including:

- Arthritis
- Asthma
- Depression
- Diabetes
- Heart disease
- Pneumonia
- Stroke

The aim is to get better information on side effects and risks faster, and make it easier for physicians and patients to make informed decisions about health care. While there is a great deal of evidence and innovation in medicine, there is no effective way for patients to determine what medical treatments are right for them (Landro, 2005). AHRQ says the new studies of specific medical conditions will make it easier to speed up the adoption of treatments once they are proved effective. The good news about having some guidelines for care is they synthesize all of the information about medical evidence and tell physicians what they need to do. The next step is to make sure physicians have information at hand exactly when they need it. Medicare and AHRQ are sponsoring several pilot projects encouraging hospitals and physicians to use information technology, such as handheld prescribing devices and computerized decision support systems for quick access to EBM guidelines at the point of care where they need it most.

OVERUSED, UNDERUSED, AND MISUSED HEALTH CARE

Longstanding physician resistance to using EBM guidelines is often cited as a reason health care quality in the U.S. is not up to par with similar countries, especially considering how much is spent. Wide variations in how physicians treat patients with similar ailments are epidemic in American medicine, reflecting a large gap between medical knowledge and clinical practice. Many researchers and large purchasers of care consider EBM a critical factor in both cost and quality woes infecting the health care system. For instance, research shows health care is often overused, underused, or misused (Fisher et al., 2003).

Where there are more cardiac surgeons, for instance, there is greater utilization of their services; whether this is an overuse problem or simply the use of available resources is unclear. There is also an underuse problem in which physicians do not treat medical ailments as aggressively as best practices recommend. Individuals suffering myocardial infarctions are reportedly put on beta blockers only half the time (McGlynn et al., 2003). The use of EBM can reduce this variation on the supply side.

Pay for Quality

Linking financial incentives with EBM is controversial. Some question why physicians should be paid or incentivized to follow guidelines they should be adhering to already. Others say the financial incentive tactic is simply cost-containment disguised as EBM. Apart from the controversy, employers, health insurers, and government payers are experimenting with programs that reward adherence to EBM guidelines.

While few would argue against using medical evidence to treat patients, others worry going strictly by guidelines is akin to cookbook medicine and may interfere with physicians' intuition and experience when it comes to treating individual cases. A set-in-stone practice guideline for a specific disease or condition, they argue, does not allow physicians to use their medical experience and diagnostic skills fully. They also fear it could allow insurers to refuse to cover care that medical professionals might deem necessary for a patient if it does not follow exact guidelines.

Defenders insist, however, the guidelines do not exclude alternative treatments. They also stress clinical trials of so-called experimental procedures will always be important methods of gathering new evidence for the ever-evolving guidelines and they ask that all therapies be proven effective. Moreover, guidelines help physicians stay on top of the explosion in new data from clinical trials and medical research.

An instance of the tension between EBM and traditional medical intuitions is the medical basis for routine male genital alteration of newborns. In the 1970s, the American Academy of Pediatrics stated there was no medical need for circumcision. Then in 1989 it referred to potential medical benefits, and in 1999, it released a policy statement stating the practice does not have health benefits strong enough to warrant recommendation as a routine procedure (*see* Davis, 2001).

Treatment Effectiveness

Sound scientific evidence now exists for about half of the most prevalent medical conditions, but the gap between knowing what works best and the day-to-day provision of treatment services is wide, and continually expanding (Landro, 2007). One way to close this gap between knowledge and clinical practice is by insisting physicians' choice of treatment be backed by current evidence of a treatment's effectiveness. To budget billions for basic medical research by the National Institutes of Health and not get the benefits to patients is a huge, unnecessary waste (Begley, 2003).

Not all studies have speckled histories. Many uncover significant advances. Problems arise when studies are pursued to achieve economic goals, where political motivations seem to intrude on the design and conduct of the trials and bias not only how results are interpreted, but more especially, how they are reported. For instance:

- Antibiotics are over-treated
- Statins and beta blockers are under-treated
- Antidepressants are misused in the treatment of depressed children and adolescents

Antibiotics: Over-Treated

Another opportunity to save money is to eliminate the overuse of antibiotics, which account for 15 to 20 percent of the average hospital's drug budget (Landro, 2003). Overuse has caused microbe resistance to many antibiotics, leading to more medical complications and costs.

A study of eleven hospitals by the Veterans Health Administration found three common antibiotics used in patients with kidney failure or urinary tract infections were overused or unnecessarily used, based on clinical guidelines for their conditions (Asch, 2004). By using lower doses or less expensive drugs, the average 250-bed hospital found savings of $100,000 annually, which indicates more than $1 billion could be saved nationwide in all hospitals (*see* Landro, 2003).

Statins and Beta Blockers: Under-Treated

Treatment guidelines call for most patients with established heart disease to take aspirin as well as drugs to lower cholesterol and blood pressure, yet only about 25 percent of such patients are consistently taking the recommended regimen (Winslow, 2007). Money saved from the overuse of antibiotics could be redirected into proven care. For instance, the money spent on excess drugs used after surgery could give everyone a beta blocker to help control blood pressure after a heart attack (AHRQ, 2005).

After using its electronic records to identify people at risk for heart attacks, Group Health started eleven thousand previously untreated patients on cholesterol lowering drugs called statins. It based the move on evidence of the effectiveness of statins in the Heart Protection study, a five-year trial of more than twenty thousand patients. The decision cost $700,000 per year, but the expectation is it will save $5.0 million (Landro, 2003). Six years later, one-fourth of the outpatients at high cardiovascular risk continue to be undertreated as a result of a combination of physician underestimation of cardiovascular risk and barriers to implementation of EBM; the good news is three-fourths of the patients are now being successfully treated (Tsang et al., 2008).

Antidepressants in the Treatment of Depressed Children and Adolescents: Misused

The criterion of reliability of scientific evidence is whether study results are published, and therefore available to physicians, purchasers of health care, and policymakers. The classic instance here is the safety and efficacy of antidepressants in the treatment of depressed children and adolescents. In the scientific literature there were six articles, all showing these drugs to be safe and effective. Physicians had good reason to believe treatment of depressed children and adolescents with the new antidepressants was evidence-based care. What they did not know is that not six, but fifteen studies of the safety and efficacy of these drugs in children and adolescents were completed. The other nine unpublished studies had shown the drugs were neither effective nor safe, and that they doubled the rate of suicidal thoughts and behaviors. In fact, even among the six positive studies, the published claims in three were not confirmed after independent analysis (Abramson, 2006).

After the nine unpublished studies became public knowledge, in 2007 the FDA issued warnings that use of antidepressants posed a small but significantly increased risk of suicidal thoughts and behavior ideation for children and adolescents (FDA, 2004). Review of twenty-seven subsequent published studies found the benefits of antidepressants to be much greater than the risks, but called for continued clinical caution (Bridge, 2007). A 2009 study at the University of Pittsburgh Medical Center validated the scientific literature, and confirmed that the rate of suicidal thoughts and behaviors increases with antidepressants in the treatment of depressed children and adolescents and called for continued EBM study and reiterated the call for clinical caution (Brent et al., 2009). Nevertheless, the damage was done by misuse of scientific evidence: the reliability of antidepressants is now questioned, treatment with antidepressants has significantly dropped by 30 percent, and the annual suicide rate in children and adolescents has increased by 10 percent, or 3,040 more suicides are predicted as a direct result of this debacle (Gibbons et al., 2007).

ELIMINATION OF GEOGRAPHIC VARIATIONS

Another benefit of EBM would be to eliminate geographical variations in health care. Research shows physicians are not uniformly following EBM guidelines. If they were, there would not be six times as many angioplasties in Ohio per 1,000 Medicare-insured patients as there are in Pennsylvania. Nor would there be the national variability in breast cancer screening that exists.

The Institute of Medicine contends that even when there is a strong body of scientific evidence about new drugs and devices, it can take fifteen to twenty years for physicians and hospitals to incorporate them. Between the health care we have and the care we could have lays not just a gap, but a chasm (IOM, 2001). EBM could close it. The AHRQ is funding research at twelve medical centers in the U.S. and Canada with the aim of developing evidence reports on a wide variety of diseases and conditions.

Moral Dilemmas

1. Should public money be spent on researching the best evidence-based medicine available to treat preventable, self-inflicted ailments, such as those resulting from smoking or lack of healthy diet and exercise?

Shared Decision Making with Patients

The concern of EBM proponents is that patients waste valuable time and money on treatments that do not work. Patients also need to be made aware of the pros and cons of treatments so they can be involved in shared decision making with their physicians. Giving patients guidelines will also encourage them to follow treatment regimens and comply with physicians' orders, proponents say. Compliance is increasingly important to health insurers and employers eager to eliminate unnecessary tests and ineffective procedures, and to push patients to adopt healthier lifestyles, all of which help reduce medical bills in the long run.

Medical Technology Decisions

Increasingly EBM decisions are being used in every aspect of hospital operations, including questions such as whether it is necessary to use a high-priced medical device when a less-expensive one is available. At the same time, while EBM will offer guidance on a wide range of medical technologies, clinical evidence must be distinguished from the financial components of such decisions. The financial aspects of making a decision are important, as long as they are not disguised as science (*see* Goossens et al., 2008).

End-of-Life Care

One area where medical technology decisions are increasingly arising is in end-of-life treatment of terminal disease and illness. What factors define medically futile care for patients with terminal prognosis and should there be an expectation that insurers, including Medicare, will pay for it? Courts are increasingly faced with the struggles of families to compel the termination or to not stop the termination of an incompetent person's life-sustaining medical treatment. *See, e.g., Schiavo ex rel. Schindler v. Schiavo,* 403 F.3d 1289 (U.S. Court of Appeals for the 11th Circuit 2005).

Investigational Treatments and Medical Products

Another area where decisions arise is the right to access investigational treatments and medical products. Should terminally ill patients be able to access experimental medical technologies that have not completed the FDA approval process? Are there instances where individual rights should override scientific process and standards in determining the safety, efficacy, medical necessity, and medical appropriateness of medical technologies?

EVOLVING MEDICAL ADVANCEMENTS AND MEDICAL EFFICACY

By definition, EBM guidelines are developed in good faith based on the best available scientific evidence, whose performance is constantly evaluated. Unfortunately this is not always the case and this shortcoming must be acknowledged in any criticism of the medical profession's resistance to following clinical guidelines. The history of bias in development of guidelines is a real problem, from insurers as well as from government-sponsored medical research.

While the trend is to independently commission and evaluate medical research rather than relying solely on information presented by providers of medical products and services, federally-funded drug trials show it is unwise to develop guidelines in advance of or contrary to existing epidemiological and biostatistical evidence. Such trials include:

- Women's Health Initiative
- Antihypertensive and Lipid-Lowering Treatment to Prevent Heart Attack Trial (ALLHAT)
- Clinical Antipsychotic Trials in Intervention Effectiveness (CATIE)
- Macular Degeneration
- National Lung Screening Trial

Most importantly, government research must be transparent. Sometimes, government-funded outcome data is subject to secrecy for years following the comparative studies, as was the case with HRT research. Then, when the government data is finally released, often the results cannot be replicated and the government's initial conclusions are directly contradicted by independent studies. Such scenarios are not uncommon, however, with respect to pharmaceutical products or, indeed, any product or medical service that may implicate evolving scientific developments. The historical lack of scientific transparency in recent years, however, does make physician resistance to so-called EBM entirely understandable and valid. While the concept of EBM cannot be refuted, its implementation over the years raises serious concerns for the health care industry.

Women's Health Initiative

Prescriptions for HRT to treat the symptoms of menopause fell dramatically after interim results from a government study of the drugs showed they were causing heart attacks. However, follow-up studies based on the government data found many of the initial conclusions were:

- Clearly incorrect
- Not clear and not precisely defined
- Premature and without any link to the research data

While the $725 million Women's Health Initiative was well-intended, it was surrounded by fiscal and political disputes over the efficacy and cost of the HRT drugs. Unfortunately, this influenced not only how the findings were computed but also how they were received. When initial results appeared to confirm HRT drugs were overused, the data were widely disseminated, while subsequent efforts to test the initial conclusions were given little notice.

In the case of the HRT study, although the government initially said the findings applied to *all* women, regardless of age or health status, subsequent meta-analysis by the Mayo Clinic using the same data showed the age of a woman and the timing of hormone use dramatically changed the risk and benefits (Kahlenborn et al., 2006). In fact, the findings of these later studies directly contradicted some of the government's initial conclusions.

For instance, the World Health Organization recently classified ostmenopausal hormone replacement as a group one carcinogen. Yet, women in their fifties who took a combination of estrogen and progestin or estrogen alone had a 30 percent lower risk of dying from general causes than women who did not take hormones. Also, women in their fifties who regularly use estrogen alone show a 60 percent lower risk for severe coronary artery calcium, a risk factor for heart attack (Manson et al., 2003).

Antihypertensive and Lipid-Lowering Treatment to Prevent Heart Attack Trial

More than 60 percent of Americans sixty-five years of age and older have hypertension, while estimates of the cost of its treatment have ranged from $7 billion to $15.5 billion per year (Fisher et al., 2003).

ALLHAT was the largest clinical study of blood pressure treatments ever conducted in the U.S. With more than 42,000 patients ages fifty-five and older participating and followed over an eight-year period, ALLHAT was designed to test whether diuretics were as good as newer blood pressure drugs, or how calcium channel blockers compared to angiotensin-converting enzyme inhibitors. Federal researchers questioned the degree to which the newer pharmaceuticals improved upon older treatment options (NIH, 2003). The initial reports of the ALLHAT trial found older, inexpensive diuretic medications were just as good or better than costlier new drugs for treating high blood pressure.

The interpretation of ALLHAT results has subsequently been called into question by many leading experts. For instance, medical researchers, physicians, and patients currently are discussing and debating the meaning of two head-to-head studies of different hypertension medications, including a separate Australian study with contrary results (Hensley, 2003).

For one thing, as the ALLHAT study proved, detecting small clinical differences between two active drugs, such as whether one pill lowers blood pressure more than another, requires very large studies that often fail to capture all of the patient preferences and characteristics that go into real-world medical decisions (Hensley, 2003). Once the study is completed, determining whether small differences are clinically meaningful can take years of follow-up.

Clinical Antipsychotic Trials in Intervention Effectiveness

Meanwhile, the $40 million federally funded CATIE trial found older and less-expensive schizophrenia medications were just as good as newer, more expensive (and many believe far more tolerable) atypical antipsychotic drugs with fewer side effects (Siegel, 2008). The CATIE Study followed nearly 1,500 schizophrenic patients in fifty-seven cities across the country for eighteen months. It compared the efficacy of an older antipsychotic medication, perphenazine, with four newer atypical antipsychotics: olanzapine, quetiapine, risperidone, and ziprasidone (Siegel, 2008). Its result, however, has made little impact on real-world medical practice because few

physicians believe the study was credible (Liberman et al., 2005).

Incredibly, CATIE's complete safety data was released almost four years after the study was completed. Moreover, the drugs involved in these studies were for conditions where there is a great deal of individual variation in how people respond. Critics claim the government studies did not take measure of that.

Macular Degeneration Trial

Now the government is sponsoring a trial to test whether Avastin, a drug meant for injection into the veins to treat breast, colon, and rectal cancer, can also treat age-related macular degeneration in which vision is lost at the center of one's sight, a leading cause of blindness in people over age fifty (see Dimartino et al., 2008). Medicare reimburses providers for off-label use of Avastin for treatment of age-related macular degeneration, but most health insurers do not. In spite of this, Avastin's manufacturer, Genentech, developed a completely new drug called Lucentis, which is specifically designed to be injected into the eye and is better adapted to treat retinal degenerative diseases and blindness (Goldstein, 2007).

Since a single cancer infusion of Avastin contains a large volume of the drug, breaking the dose down into the small aliquots needed for the eye injections costs literally pennies on the dollar, making the government's study of it, when it was clearly not designed for eye treatments, a matter of cost containment. Surely if Avastin ends up harming those eyes, a plausible consequence of this off-label, if not illegally compounded use, it will not be the government on the hook with product liability damages, but Genentech. Genentech is directly or indirectly accepting funds from Medicare for off-label use (*see generally* CMS, 2009) and it is not providing a specific warning on the Avastin label warning of the dangers of periocular injections.[LN2] Medicare Part B claims use Health Care Common Procedure Coding System codes to capture patient information to permit an institution or provider to obtain payment from the Centers for Medicare and Medicaid Services (CMS) for biopharmaceutical products (Dimartino et al., 2008). Under the Medicare Modernization Act, CMS was authorized to assign a unique code to Avastin to facilitate separate payment with tracking to specific patients.

National Lung Screening Trial

In a dispute with broad implications for cancer treatment, controversy is surrounding the objectivity of the National Lung Screening Trial, a nine-year study that is tracking fifty thousand smokers at a cost of $200 million. The federal study is supposed to determine whether annual computed tomography

(CT) scans of smokers' lungs can save lives. However, charges of conflicts of interest and accusations the study has design flaws that could bias its outcome against screening (Armstrong, 2007).

Funded by the National Cancer Institute and due to be finished in 2009, the study is expected to have a major impact on whether regular CT scans for smokers will become a standard of care and whether tobacco companies could be forced to pay for them. The ninety million current and former smokers in the U.S. are all potential screening candidates, as are the millions exposed to secondhand smoke (family, workplace, and social). It seems virtually everyone could be a screening candidate (Armstrong, 2007). The economic justification, if any, of this medical monitoring is unclear.

The question under consideration in the study is a complex one. CT scanning is adept at detecting abnormalities that might be cancerous. Once they are detected, potentially risky lung biopsies are usually needed to confirm the presence of cancer in the lung. Often, the biopsies turn up no cancer. Skeptics say patients may suffer health problems as a result of universal screening, such as complications from biopsies or needless surgery, offsetting any gains from enhanced detection (*see* Armstrong, 2007). Critics also say fifty thousand patients are too few to detect a benefit.

A recent study of asymptomatic smokers found that while annual CT scans increased the rate of lung cancer diagnoses, there was no evidence CT screening reduced the risk of death due to lung cancer (Bach et al., 2007). The increase in diagnoses failed to reduce the death rate because the annual CT scans detected cancers that would not have grown sufficiently during the patient's lifetime to cause any harm. Yet the tenfold increase in the number of thoracic surgeries resulting from the additional diagnoses may well have caused harm because of the postoperative mortality rate of 5 percent and the frequency of serious complications, 20 to 44 percent. While another study found screening for lung cancer might be beneficial (Henschke et al., 2006), this study met with heavy criticism because it was based on survival rates rather than mortality rates and incorrectly assumed everyone with lung cancer would die of it without treatment, when the survival rate for lung cancer is 15 percent.

As a result, the position held by leading medical organizations that the costs of screening for lung cancer outweigh its benefits is unlikely to change. Unless the National Cancer Institute study releases significantly different information, there appears to be no pressing need to adopt a medical monitoring claim for asymptomatic smokers. Although medical monitoring is useful in some cases, the medical community

has cast significant doubt on the monitoring regime for lung cancer.

> *Moral Dilemmas*
>
> 1. Is it possible to conduct an entirely objective, accurate clinical study?

DRUG EFFECTIVENESS REVIEW PROJECT

The Drug Effectiveness Review Project (DERP) is a collaboration of fifteen states that commissions and uses systematic reviews of global research to inform drug purchasing decisions in an effort to compare the effectiveness of popular drugs (Gibson, 2006). The logic behind this effort is clear: to win FDA approval, a pharmaceutical company generally has to demonstrate a new drug is safe and more effective than a placebo. It does not, however, have to show how the new drug compares with other drugs already on the market. That is useful information, however, particularly when the new drug might cost significantly more than an over-the-counter alternative (Murray, 2004).

Formulary Restrictions

DERP has resulted in formulary restrictions that have reduced patients' access to medicines, according to a Kaiser Family Foundation report. The program distorts EBM to create a veil behind which the government and managed care organizations justify restrictions on patients' access to health care in order to reduce short-term drug costs. DERP fails to adequately take into account individual patients' medical needs and ways to contain health care costs overall in the long and short term (Wechsler, 2008).

Independent Comparative-Effectiveness Research

Better information about the effectiveness of drugs as well as their safety ought to be a starting point. Supporters of DERP challenge the pharmaceutical industry to take the lead in coming up with alternatives to their efforts. At issue is whether the pharmaceutical industry should be expected to do comparative research themselves. Others ask whether the U.S. needs a respected, independent organization, perhaps funded jointly by the health industry and government, to study the available evidence and, when necessary, commission further research.

Hierarchy of Scientific Research

The gold standard of evidence in EBM is a combination of double-blind, randomized, controlled trials and a systematic review of medical studies called meta-analysis (Dolinar & Leininger, 2006). EBM suggests that when a clinical problem arises, physicians should, in descending order of preference, look for guidance in:

- Systematic reviews of randomized controlled trials
- Results of individual controlled clinical trials
- Observational (uncontrolled) studies
- Anecdotal reports of clinical observations

(Bero, 2006)

This hierarchy implies a clear course of action for physicians addressing patient problems; they should look for the highest available evidence.

Confusion between Epidemiology and General Causation

The comparative effectiveness debate is clouded by epidemiological studies that can only go to prove a drug could have caused, but not that it actually did cause, a medical condition in a particular individual. There is often confusion in this regard; the incidence of disease in populations does not address the question of the cause of an individual's disease. This question, sometimes referred to as specific causation, is beyond the science of epidemiology. Epidemiology has its limits: at the point where an inference is made that the relationship between a drug and a disease is causal (general causation) and where the risk attributed to the drug has been determined. That is, epidemiology addresses whether a drug can cause a disease, not whether a drug really did cause a specific individual's disease (*see generally* Green et al., 2000). One recent case clarified the issue of general causation in drug liability lawsuits.

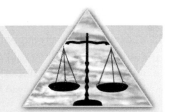

GENERAL CAUSATION IN DRUG PRODUCTS LIABILITY ACTIONS: DIFFERENTIAL DIAGNOSIS

Ruggiero v. Warner-Lambert Co.
[Widow v. Pharmaceutical Company]
424 F.3d 249 (U.S. Court of Appeals for the 2nd Circuit 2005)

FACTS: Anne Ruggiero is the widow of Albert Ruggiero who was diagnosed with Type 2 diabetes. Albert Ruggiero died of liver failure caused by cirrhosis fifteen months after he had started taking the diabetes medication Rezulin. Two years later, manufacturers and distributors of Rezulin halted its distribution in response to concerns Rezulin caused increased liver toxicity.

Ruggiero filed a federal product liability lawsuit against Warner-Lambert Co. and Parke Davis who manufactured and sold Rezulin. She claimed Rezulin caused her husband's death. The federal trial court dismissed the claim, holding Ruggiero produced insufficient evidence to show Rezulin was indeed capable of causing or exacerbating cirrhosis of the liver. Specifically, the court found the medical expert's differential diagnosis that Rezulin led to Mr. Ruggiero's death was insufficient to support general causation without a scientifically valid methodology for establishing the drug as a possible cause.

ISSUE: Can a differential diagnosis be used to show the use of Rezulin, an anti-diabetes drug, caused the death of Mr. Ruggiero by liver failure?

HOLDING AND DECISION: No, medical experts may not rely on differential diagnosis alone to corroborate that Rezulin was the cause of Mr. Ruggiero's liver failure; positive evidence from a scientifically valid methodology is required to support general causation.

ANALYSIS: The district court excluded the expert testimony of Dr. Douglas Dietrich, the sole evidence of general causation submitted by Ruggiero, because Dr. Dietrich's testimony failed to meet the standards required by the U.S. Supreme Court, the so-called *Daubert* principles, which suggest courts might consider:

- Whether a theory or technique has been and could be tested
- What its error rate was
- Whether scientific standards exist to govern the theory or technique's application

(continues)

(continued)

In addition, the Rules of Evidence require expert witnesses to:

- Base their testimony upon sufficient facts or data
- Use reliable principles and methods
- Apply the principles and methods reliably to the facts of the case

The court concluded Dr. Dietrich lacked a reliable basis for his opinion because he failed to reference any studies or anything else to suggest Rezulin could cause or exacerbate cirrhosis.

Dr. Dietrich employed a methodology known as differential diagnosis, which is a patient-specific process of elimination physicians use to identify the most likely cause of symptoms from a list of possible causes. In other words, physicians using differential diagnosis provide testimony countering other possible causes of the injuries at issue.

The court found this technique insufficient to support general causation. Differential diagnosis does not necessarily support an opinion on general causation because, as with any process of elimination, it assumes the final, suspected cause remaining after this process of elimination must actually have caused the injury. Furthermore, when an expert employs differential diagnosis to eliminate potential causes for a specific injury, he also must prove the suspected cause using scientifically valid methodology.

In *Daubert v. Merrell Dow Pharmaceuticals*, 509 U.S. 579 (U.S. Supreme Court 1993), the U.S. Supreme Court held a court may refuse to admit evidence if it concludes there is simply too great an analytical gap between the data and the opinion proffered. When expert testimony is based on data, a methodology, or studies that are inadequate to support the conclusions reached, *Daubert* and the federal Rules of Evidence mandate the exclusion of such unreliable opinion testimony.

Although differential diagnosis was not accepted as a valid methodology to support expert testimony on general causation in this case, the court cautioned that its ruling did not mean a differential diagnosis could never provide a sufficient basis for an opinion as to general causation. The court stated there may be instances where, because of the rigor of differential diagnosis performed, the expert's training and experience, the type of illness or injury at issue, or some other case-specific circumstance, a differential diagnosis is sufficient to support an expert's opinion on both general and specific causation. In other words, medical experts may not rely on differential diagnosis alone as a methodology to corroborate a particular drug is the cause of a specific illness in a patient. Instead, experts should be positive that evidence derived from a scientifically valid method supports general causation.

RULE OF LAW: Expert witnesses must produce positive evidence to establish general causation in drug products liability actions.

(See *generally* Choe, 2005).

PROBLEMS WITH AUTHORITY-BASED MEDICAL OPINIONS

Uncritical acceptance of authority-based medical opinions is pervasive in U.S. medicine, even though top authorities unsuccessfully predict what scientific knowledge will be preserved as fact (Guzelian & Guzelian, 2004). Reliance on expert medical opinions, which is not based upon an objective methodology, gives the status of knowledge to uncertainties (Sachkett et al., 2005). For instance, with infrequent medical complications, such as a patient who develops pneumonia following a heart-lung transplant, recommendations are sought, accepted, and applied from authorities in the relevant branch of medicine. When this health care is objectively appraised, some of it is effective, harmful, or useless, but in the traditional medical paradigm, there is no way to make sure which is which.

Vaccines and Childhood Autism

There is probably no better medical controversy to support the need for EBM than the dispute surrounding childhood autism, a neurodevelopment disorder marked by impaired social interactions, deficits in verbal and nonverbal communication, and restricted and repetitive patterns of behavior that persist throughout a person's lifetime. The debate over whether childhood vaccines cause autism ignited in 1998, when an NIH-sponsored study posited a connection (Courchesne et al., 1994). At the same time, the incidence of autism started increasing, with some figures estimating roughly 1 in 150 children suffers from autism (Johnson, 2009). One side of this controversy relies on anecdotal evidence to link the rising prevalence of autism to mercury-laden vaccines, the other side claims autism is simply better diagnosed and treatment services are better funded.

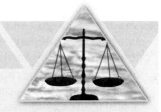

Remedies Available to Parents of Children with Vaccine-Related Injuries Under the National Childhood Vaccine Injury Act

Moss v. Merck & Co.
[Parents of Injured Child v. Manufacturers]
381 F.3d 501 (U.S. Court of Appeals for the 5th Circuit 2004)

FACTS: Scott and Janice Moss, the parents of a young child who developed autism after receiving vaccines containing mercury, pursued state law tort claims for injuries they suffered as a result of their child's medical condition. The Mosses filed a lawsuit against Merck, Aventis, Wyeth, and Eli Lilly. The federal trial court dismissed their claims on the grounds that the National Childhood Vaccine Injury Act precluded a tort remedy for a vaccine-related injury. *See* National Childhood Vaccine Injury Act of 1986, 42 U.S.C.A. §§ 300aa-2 *et seq.* (2009).

Federal law bars victims of a vaccine-related injury or death from seeking redress in court against a vaccine manufacturer unless the victims have first filed a claim for recovery in the specialized Vaccine Court. The term *vaccine-related injury or death* means an illness, injury, condition, or death associated with one or more of the vaccines set forth in the Vaccine Injury Table, except that the term does not include an illness, injury, condition, or death associated with an adulterant or contaminant intentionally added to such a vaccine. *See* 42 U.S.C.A. § 300aa-33(5) (2003). Congress designed the federal law to provide compensation to children injured by vaccines, while ensuring the nation's supply of vaccines was not unduly threatened by tort litigation.

To file a petition for compensation, there must be a vaccine-related injury. Legal representatives may file petitions for compensation on behalf of disabled or deceased children. If successful, acceptance of a compensatory award from the government causes the vaccine-injured children to waive any further tort rights. If a child declines the award, traditional tort relief may be available, but punitive damages are prohibited.

ISSUE: Can the parents of a child injured by a vaccine sue in federal court for their own injuries suffered as a result of their child's medical condition?

HOLDING AND DECISION: Yes, while the injured child may be precluded from suing for a vaccine-related injury, the parents are not.

ANALYSIS: On appeal to the Fifth Circuit, Eli Lilly argued federal law barred the Mosses' claims because Eli Lilly was a vaccine manufacturer. The Fifth Circuit held thimerosal was not a vaccine and Eli Lilly was not a vaccine manufacturer as defined in federal law. According to the court, thimerosal, when used as a preservative, is merely a component of a vaccine and, therefore, not the finished product itself. Federal health officials recommended that thimerosal be removed from vaccines in 1999, yet autism rates seem unaffected. Since 2001, thimerosal has not been used in routinely recommended childhood vaccines, with the exception of some flu shots (Johnson, 2009). Multiple EBM studies have failed to find any relationship between thimerosal exposure and autism (*see* Weeks, 2007). On its face, the statute only governs lawsuits filed against manufacturers of a completed vaccine shipped under its own label. Thimerosal is not sold as a vaccine; therefore, Eli Lilly is not a vaccine manufacturer, and is not entitled to federal protection.

In concluding federal law does not protect Eli Lilly from suit, the Fifth Circuit rejected Eli Lilly's argument that any injury arising from thimerosal is encompassed within the statutory definition of vaccine-related injury, and that those alleging an injury or death from the thimerosal preservative in vaccines are obligated to file their claim against a manufacturer of the vaccine in the Vaccine Court. Eli Lilly claimed victims of thimerosal-related injuries were obligated to pursue relief in the Vaccine Court. The Fifth Circuit disagreed with Eli Lilly, stating that

(continues)

(continued)

while a thimerosal-related injury is a vaccine-related injury, the inquiry does not end there. A claim is not barred unless the vaccine-related injury is filed against a vaccine manufacturer, which Eli Lilly is not.

Additionally, Eli Lilly argued federal law expressly barred the Mosses' claims of vaccine-related injury. The court determined federal law, does not protect non-manufacturers of vaccines and it does not apply to all tort claims having some connection to the administration of a vaccine. Rather, federal restrictions apply only to the claims of those who have sustained a vaccine-related injury or death. Because the Mosses never received a vaccine and did not personally sustain a vaccine-related injury or death, federal restrictions did not apply to them.

Eli Lilly also claimed literal application of federal provisions would impede the statutory goal of reducing the costs and risks of tort litigation. Relying on basic strict construction of federal law, the Fifth Circuit rejected Eli Lilly's argument, stating that because federal law neither provides a remedy nor openly bars the right of parents of vaccine-injured children to pursue remedies afforded by state tort law, the Mosses may pursue their claims.

RULE OF LAW: Because thimerosal, a mercury-containing preservative used in several childhood vaccines, is not a vaccine under the plain meaning of the statute, the manufacturer, Eli Lilly, is not entitled to the protections of the National Childhood Vaccine Injury Act.

(See *generally* Prussia, 2004; Sanders, 2006).

The courts are strictly construing federal law in vaccine-related tort litigation. No statutory protections are being extended to manufacturers of vaccine preservatives, such as thimerosal. Therefore, if victims are able to trace their injury to manufacturers of a vaccine preservative, there is nothing to prevent them from litigating their claims. This decision was the first time a federal appellate court found that parents of an injured child could sue vaccine manufacturers.[LN3] Considering the number of vaccine-related lawsuits brought against vaccine manufacturers, the implications of this decision are far-reaching. *See Aventis Pasteur, Inc. v. Skevofilax*, 914 A.2d 113 (Court of Appeals of Maryland 2007) (case dismissed due to inability of the Skervofilax family to obtain a medical expert to testify that their son's autism was caused by thimerosal used in pediatric vaccines).

Moral Dilemmas

1. Is it possible to definitively prove injury resulted from a vaccine or exposure to a chemical, and was not a result of another cause, such as a genetic defect, generally unhealthy lifestyle, or exposure to another toxin?

Side Effects of Vaccines

In rare cases, vaccines can cause shock, brain inflammation, and death, especially in children with allergies or compromised immune systems. The National Childhood Vaccine Injury Act recognizes specified side effects for each vaccine; autism is not among them. It allows parents to make claims for other side effects, but sets specific criteria they must meet to show blame. For instance, one recognized side effect of the Rubella virus-containing vaccine is chronic arthritis which is said to manifest in seven to forty-two days and an encephalopathy within five to fifteen days after administration of the vaccine. *See* 42 C.F.R. § 100.3(a) (2008).

In a settlement reached in the Vaccine Court, the federal government recently did concede that a young girl with autism had been damaged by vaccines. *See Poling v. Secretary of HHS*, 2008 WL 1883059 (U.S. Court of Federal Claims 2008). The case was not a precedent, however, because the child had rare genetic mitochondrial disorders that likely contributed to her autism. Mitochondria, the energy factories of cells, have their own genetic material that is passed directly from mother to child. Flaws in this material are relatively common. As those flaws multiply, they interfere with mitochondrial function. According to the Centers for Disease Control, as many as 700,000 people in the U.S. have flawed mitochondria, and in roughly 30,000 of them, the genetic flaws are expansive enough to cause disease.

Implications of Not Vaccinating

The availability of exemptions from compulsory vaccination requirements is a growing concern with 10 percent of the nation's children not being vaccinated with recommended pediatric vaccines. This represents about 7.4 million children (*see* Swartz, 2009).

Recent outbreaks of diphtheria, mumps (including a 2009 outbreak at Northeastern University), pertussis (whooping cough), polio, and rubella (measles) have confirmed the continued threat of vaccine-preventable diseases.[LN4]

When people decide to forgo vaccination, they threaten the entire public health care system. They increase their own risk and the risk of everyone else, including infants too young to be vaccinated and people with immune systems impaired by disease or chemotherapy. Of course, it is the very success of modern vaccines that makes exemptions possible. In previous generations, when epidemic diseases swept through communities, it was easy to persuade everyone that the small risks associated with vaccination were worth it. Now that infectious disease epidemics have stopped, because of widespread vaccinations, it is easy to forget the world of microbes is still dangerous.

THE FUTURE OF EBM

As the debate on EBM continues, many agree the current health care system covers too few, costs too much, and does not deliver consistently high-quality health care. The question is how to ensure patients receive quality, affordable health care. Without ensuring quality, access to health care may be meaningless. Without addressing costs, health care becomes inaccessible. By building EBM into reform measures, Americans might get the right health care at the right time.

LAW FACT

HORMONE REPLACEMENT THERAPY (HRT)

Is there any reliable evidence-based scientific research that combination HRT can cause breast cancer, heart disease, or dementia?

Class action status was denied; each individual case must be tried separately. Reeves could not overcome the problems with individual issues of law and fact as to what caused each individual's medical condition.

—*Reeves v. Wyeth (In re Prempro Products Liability Litigation)*, 2006 U.S. Dist. LEXIS 59049 (U.S. District Court for the Eastern District of Arkansas, Western Division 2006.)

CHAPTER SUMMARY

- Evidence-based medicine is the application of epidemiological principles to clinical health care; it entails incorporating key scientific findings into medical practice and measuring the associated outcomes.
- The traditional way of practicing medicine focused more on the doctor's individual experience, familiarity with and observation of the patient, and common sense.
- EBM encourages the use of reliable studies based upon scientifically sound rules of research and evidence.
- Although EBM can help pinpoint which treatments are best for which conditions, patients often still do not receive the best available treatment because health care professionals are not aware of the best treatment or have their own reasons for not using the recommended treatment.
- The fact that EBM has not been thoroughly implemented in U.S. health care is likely one reason why American health care falls short of international benchmarks despite its high cost.
- A chief criticism of EBM is it is extremely difficult to design a study that accurately determines exactly what the best course of care is or what the cause of a medical problem is; related to this problem is the criticism that studies often emerge contradicting other studies.
- Another chief criticism of EBM is studies are too easily tainted by any number of causes, including bias, financial concerns, lack of transparency, and failure to consider all factors affecting the outcome; the gold standard of evidence in EBM is a combination of double-blind, randomized, controlled trials and a systematic review of medical studies called meta-analysis.
- Some physicians are resistant to implementing EBM because they want to be sure it will work for their patients and it is better than the treatments they currently offer; also, to fully implement EBM is cost- and time-prohibitive for many conditions.

- Practitioners are also resistant to relying solely upon EBM because they feel it interferes with their autonomy and intuition.
- There are several organizations attempting to collect and condense the most reliable EBM studies for both health care insurers' and providers' use.
- EBM can help identify which courses of care are overused, underused, and misused, which could help allocate health care dollars more efficiently.

LAW NOTES

1. Dartmouth Medical School's Center for the Evaluative Clinical Sciences analyzed variations in medical spending in all 306 Medicare regions in the U.S. Each state has ten to fifty Medicare regions to maximize Medicare insurance plan participation and the availability of plans to Medicare beneficiaries (*e.g.*, CMS, 2009). The description of the 306 regions is complex, confusing, and impossible to understand, let alone use to implement insurance plans without violating some other regulations. The study found patients living in the highest spending regions received 60 percent more care than patients living in the lowest spending regions, and these differences were not explained by age, sex, or disease burden (Fischer & Avorn, 2004). They then looked at how patients with three distinct disease entities were treated according to the level of spending in their Medicare region:
   - First broken hip
   - First heart attack
   - Initial diagnosis of colon cancer
      Patients in the higher spending regions had no:
   - Better access to health care
   - Greater patient satisfaction with care
   - Higher quality of care

   (Fischer & Avorn, 2004)

      Based on this data, the Commonwealth Fund subsequently determined that if all Medicare-insured patients with these three medical conditions had received the quality of care provided in the best performing Medicare regions, better health outcomes would have been achieved for significantly less money:
   - 8,400 lives could be saved each year
   - $900 million in unnecessary health care costs could be saved annually

   (Schoen et al., 2006)

2. Specifically, the off-label use is one that is not provided for on Avastin's FDA-approved labeling. In this instance, the off-label use involves using an injectable drug for treatment to a patient group other than those for whom the FDA approved it. Even though Genentech developed Lucentis expressly for this patient group, it still has a continuing duty to warn of related risks from Avastin since it knows it is being used as substitute for Lucentis based on the price differential. Genentech has a duty to warn patients and physicians of the possible dangers and must share this information with them by means of warnings. In this situation, Genentech is aware of the risks associated with periocular injection of Avastin and is also aware the drug is being administering in this fashion as an off-label use. Consequently, Genentech has a legal obligation to warn about the risks of periocular injection of Avastin, and its failure to do so could make Avastin defective and unreasonably dangerous (*see generally* Ausness, 2008). *Compare Proctor v. Davis*, 682 N.E.2d 1203 (Appellate Court of Illinois, 1st District, 5th Division 1997) (involving periocular injections of Depo-Medro manufactured by Upjohn Pharmaceutical), *appeal denied*, 689 N.E.2d 1146 (Supreme Court of Illinois 1997).

3. A special master in the U.S. Court of Federal Claims ruled that routine childhood immunizations are not linked to autism, handing down the first decision from the Vaccine Court since hearings began in 2007 in the controversy over whether vaccines can cause autism. The court denied damages to three families who claimed the thimerosal found in the measles, mumps, and rubella vaccine (the so-called MMR vaccine) made in the U.S. by Merck led to their children's autism. *See Cedillo v. Secretary of HHS*, 2009 WL 331968 (U.S. Court of Federal Claims 2009), *reconsideration denied*, 2009 WL 996299 (U.S. Court of Federal Claims 2009). The Vaccine Court found the anecdotal evidence did not support a connection between vaccines and autism, noting numerous EBM studies performed by scientists worldwide have agreed.

   Some five thousand families are seeking damages from the federal Vaccine Injury Compensation Fund program to compensate children allegedly harmed by vaccines. *See* 26 U.S.C.A. § 9510 (2000) (establishing a

Vaccine Injury Compensation Trust Fund in the Treasury of the U.S. States); *see also* 26 U.S.C.A. § 4131 (1997) (imposing a tax of 75 cents per dose of vaccine). As of January 2009, there was approximately $ 2.7 billion in the trust fund (Johnson, 2009). Each of the test cases represents different theories for how vaccines could cause autism:

- Measles vaccine causes a low-level measles infection that affects children's brains
- Mercury-containing vaccine preservative, thimerosal, poisons the brain, causing autism
- Vaccines may cause or contribute to an underlying mitochondrial disorder, which in turn causes autism
    New hypotheses rapidly replace those that are scientifically refuted. EBM studies have discredited the connection between vaccines and autism, but parents have continued to argue for a link, with some accusing the government and medical communities of a cover-up.

4. The symptoms of these vaccine-preventable diseases are noteworthy because many people have forgotten how horrible these diseases are:

- Diphtheria: a highly contagious upper respiratory tract illness characterized by sore throat and fever, it causes the progressive deterioration of myelin sheaths in the central and peripheral nervous system, leading to degenerating motor control and loss of sensation.
- Mumps: characterized by a painful swelling of the salivary glands and sometimes a rash; in teenage males, testicular swelling often results in infertility.
- Whooping cough: people experience spasms of coughing involving up to a dozen coughs before they can catch their breath. Such coughing spasms may occur up to fifty times a day. The cough produces large amounts of mucus and vomiting of mucus and food is common during the coughing spasms. Complications include choking, which may lead to convulsions, cerebral hemorrhage, brain damage, and death. Hernias of the rectum or abdomen also occur and bleeding from small ruptured blood vessels of the eye, face, and neck are common. Inhaled secretions into the lungs during the coughing spasms can cause lung complications including pneumonia and collapse of the lungs.
- Polio: an acute viral infection where most people develop non-paralytic meningitis, headaches, and pain in the neck, back, abdomen, and extremities, fever, vomiting, and lethargy. Some cases progress to paralytic disease, in which the muscles become weak and finally completely paralyzed.
- Measles: characterized by a mild pinpoint rash, swollen and tender glands, and fever with joint pains that can last up to a month. Complications may include infection of the brain tissues (encephalitis). Almost all fetuses exposed to rubella develop syndromes that generally result in serious, incurable birth defects, including hearing impairment, cataracts, glaucoma, and other eye problems, heart defects, brain problems, mental and physical retardation (stunted growth), and bone disease.

(See *generally* Atkinson et al., 2006.)

CHAPTER BIBLIOGRAPHY

Abramson, J. (2006). The reliability of our medical knowledge as a product of industry relationships. *Hofstra Law Review, 35* (69), 691-704 (research results presented in respected, peer-reviewed journals are not always based upon an unbiased analysis of the data that are consistent with the pre-specified outcome measures of benefit and harm identified in the original research designs).

AHRQ (Agency for Healthcare Research and Quality). (2008). *Guide to clinical preventive services: Recommendations of the U.S. Preventive Services Task Force.* Rockville, MD: AHRQ.

___. (2007). *Hospital stays involving musculoskeletal procedures: Healthcare cost and utilization project (HCUP) statistical brief.* Rockville, MD: AHRQ.

___. (2005). *Fact sheet: Beta-blockers for acute myocardial infarction.* Rockville, MD: AHRQ.

ALLHAT Officers and Coordinators for the ALLHAT Collaborative Research Group. (2002). Major outcomes in high-risk hypertensive patients randomized to angiotensin-converting enzyme inhibitor or calcium channel blocker vs. diuretic: The Antihypertensive and Lipid-Lowering Treatment to Prevent Heart Attack Trial (ALLHAT). *Journal of the American Medical Association, 288* (23), 2981-2997 (erratum in: (2004 May) and (2003, January), *Journal of the American Medical Association, 289* (2), 178-191).

Armstrong, D. (2007, October 8). Critics question objectivity of government lung-scan study tobacco companies paid key researchers as expert witnesses. *Wall Street Journal,* p. B1.

Asch, S. M. et al. (2006). Who is at greatest risk for receiving poor-quality health care? *New England Journal of Medicine, 354* (11), 1147-1156.

___. (2004). Comparison of quality of care for patients in the Veterans Health Administration and patients in a national sample. *Annals of Internal Medicine, 141* (12), 938-945 (patients from the VHA received higher-quality care according to a broad measure).

Atkinson, W. et al. (eds.). (2006). *Epidemiology and prevention of vaccine-preventable diseases* (9th ed.). Washington, DC: Centers for Disease Control & Prevention.

Ausness, R. C. (2008). "There's danger here, Cherie!" Liability for the promotion and marketing of drugs and medical devices for off-label uses. *Brooklyn Law Review, 73*, 1253-1326.

Bach, P. B. et al. (2007). Computed tomography screening and lung cancer outcomes. *Journal of the American Medical Association, 297*, 953-961.

Begley, S. (2003, September 26). Too many patients never reap the benefits of great research. *Wall Street Journal*, p. B1.

Bero, L. (2006). Evaluating systematic reviews and meta-analyses. *Journal of Law & Policy, 14*, 571-593 (explaining the need for systematic unbiased reviews of EBM; national meta-analysis showed HRT had no effect).

Bezerra, C. A. et al. (2005). Traditional suburethral sling operations for urinary incontinence in women. *Cochrane Database of Systematic Reviews*, Issue 3.

Brent, D. A. et al. (2009). Predictors of spontaneous and systematically assessed suicidal adverse events in the treatment of SSRI-resistant depression in adolescents (TORDIA) study. *American Journal of Psychiatry, 166*, 418-426.

Bridge, J. A. (2007). Clinical response and risk for reported suicidal ideation and suicide attempts in pediatric antidepressant treatment: A meta-analysis of randomized controlled trials. *Journal of the American Medical Association, 297* (15), 1683-1696.

Cerminara, K. L. (2005). Dealing with dying: How insurers can help patients seeking last-chance therapies (even when the answer is no). *Journal of Law & Medicine, 15*, 285-328 (describing how decisions of whether to cover last chance therapies arise only in cases in which experimental or investigational treatments are of unknown efficacy, at best, and when lifesaving options supported by evidence-based authorities are lacking).

Chang, S. M. et al. (2005). Patterns of care for adults with newly diagnosed malignant glioma. *Journal of the American Medical Association, 293* (5), 227-235.

Choe, J. (2005). Expert testimony: Expert witnesses must be prepared to produce positive evidence to establish general causation in drug products liability action. *American Journal of Law & Medicine, 31*, 529-532.

Clamon, J. B. (2006). Insurance law annual: Does my health insurance cover it? Using evidence-based medicine and binding arbitration techniques to determine what therapies fall under experimental exclusion clauses in health insurance contracts. *Drake Law Review, 54*, 473-508 (exploring the use of EBM to decide what is and is not covered by health benefit plans).

CMS (Centers for Medicare and Medicaid Services). Covered medical and other health services. (2009). In *Medicare benefit policy manual:* (chapter 15). Washington, DC: CMS.

Cochrane, A. (1972). *Effectiveness and efficiency: Random reflections on health services.* London, England: Royal Society of Medicine Press (classic text by the pioneer of EBM that laid the foundation for the worldwide task of the Cochrane Collaboration in preparing, maintaining, and disseminating systematic reviews of the effects of health care).

Cohen, A. M. et al. (2004). A categorization and analysis of the criticisms of evidence-based medicine. *International Journal of Medical Informatics, 73* (1), 35-43 (reviewed the medical literature and found five recurring criticisms of EBM: overreliance on empiricism as a philosophical basis for medicine; restrictive definition of evidence; lack of evidence of efficacy; limited usefulness for individual patients; and threats to the autonomy of the physician/patient relationship; despite these criticisms, they recommended EBM be incorporated into individual patient care).

Cook, S. L. (2007). Will pay for performance be worth the price to medical providers? A look at pay for performance and its legal implications for providers. *Annals of Health Law, 16*, 163-212 (considers the legal implications of P4P programs mainly from the perspective of health care providers).

Coulter, I. D. (2007). Evidence-based complementary and alternative medicine: Promises and problems. *Forsch Komplementarmed, 14* (2), 102-108 (examining the experience of establishing a center for evidence-based complementary and alternative medicine (EBCAM) practice while recognizing the demand for EBM from allopathic medicine may simply be part of the continuing medical opposition to CAM intended to perpetuate their dominance in health care).

Courchesne, E. et al. (1994). Cerebellar hypolasia and hyperplasia in infantile autism. *Lancet, 343*, 63-64.

Das, A. (2007). The asthma crisis in low-income communities of color: Using the law as a tool for promoting public health. *New York University Review of Law & Social Change, 31*, 273-314.

Davidoff, F. et al. (1995). Editorial: Evidence based medicine. *British Medical Journal, 310*, 1085 (announcing creation of the *Evidence Based Medicine Journal*).

Davis, D. S. (2001). Male and female genital alteration: A collision course with the law? *Journal of Law & Medicine, 11*, 487-570 (examining the history of the withdrawal of medical support for routine circumcision in the U.S.).

Davis, K. et al. (2008). Aiming high for the U.S. health system: A context for health reform. *Journal of Law, Medicine & Ethics, 36* (4), 629-643.

Deyo, R. A. (2007). Back surgery: Who needs it? *New England Journal of Medicine, 356,* (22), 2230-2243.

Deyo, R. A. et al. (2004). Spinal-fusion surgery: The case for restraint. *New England Journal of Medicine, 350*, 722-726.

Dimartino, L. D. et al. (2008). Using Medicare administrative data to conduct post-marketing surveillance of follow-on biologics: Issues and opportunities. *Food & Drug Law Journal, 63*, 891-900.

Dolinar, R., & Leininger, S. L. (2006). Pay for performance or compliance? A second opinion on Medicare reimbursement. *Indiana Health Law Review, 3*, 391-420 (reviews the Medicare Value Purchasing Act, which would implement pay for performance in the Medicare program by tying physician payments to compliance with EBM).

Eddy, D. (2005). Evidence-based medicine: A unified approach. *Health Affairs, 21* (1), 9-17.

FDA (U.S. Food and Drug Administration). (2004). *FDA news: FDA launches a multi-pronged strategy to strengthen safeguards for children treated with antidepressant medications.* Bethesda, MD: FDA.

Fischer, M. A., & Avorn, J. (2004). Improvements in prescribing medications for elderly patients with high blood pressure could result in better outcomes and cost savings. *Journal of the American Medical Association, 291*, 1850-1956.

Fisher, E. S. et al. (2003). The implications of regional variations in Medicare spending, part 2: Health outcomes and satisfaction with care. *Annals of Internal Medicine, 138* (4), 288-298 (researchers from Dartmouth Medical School's

Center for the Evaluative Clinical Sciences looked at the variations in medical spending in the 306 Medicare regions around the U.S.).

___. (2003). The implications of regional variations in Medicare spending, part 1: The content, quality, and accessibility of care. *Annals of Internal Medicine, 138* (4), 273-287.

Fox, D., & Greenfield, L. (2006). Helping public officials use research evaluating healthcare. *Journal of Law & Policy, 14*, 531-550 (review of EBM's history and progress in systematically reviewing treatment outcomes).

Friedland, D. J. (2009). *Evidence based medicine: A framework for clinical practice.* New York, NY: Prentice-Hall Health (clinical introduction to EBM).

Garber, A. (2005). Evidence-based medicine guidelines as a foundation for performance incentives. *Health Affairs, 24* (1), 174-179.

Gibbons, R. D. et al. (2007). Early evidence on the effects of regulators' suicidality warnings on SSRI prescriptions and suicide in children and adolescents. *American Journal of Psychiatry, 164*, 1356-1364.

Gibson, M. (2006). Science for judges: Techniques for evidence-based medicine: When good information truly matters: Public sector decision makers acquiring and using research to inform their decisions. *Journal of Law & Policy, 14*, 551-568 (explains DERP).

Goldstein, J. (2007, October 31). Genentech delays move on Avastin use. *Wall Street Journal,* p. D8.

Goossens, A. et al. (2008). Physicians and nurses focus on different aspects of guidelines when deciding whether to adopt them: An application of conjoint analysis. *Medical Decision Making, 28*, 138-145.

Green, M. D. et al. (2000). *Reference manual on scientific evidence.* Eagan, MN: West Group Publishing.

Groopman, J., & Hartzband, P. (2009, April 8). Why "quality" care is dangerous. *Wall Street Journal,* p. A13.

Guzelian, P. S., & Guzelian, C. P. (2004). Authority-based explanation. *Science, 303* (5863), 1468-1469.

Haas, J. S. et al. (2006). Changes in newspaper coverage about hormone therapy with the release of new medical evidence. *Journal of General Internal Medicine, 21* (4), 304-309.

Heimer, C. A. (2006). Responsibility in health care: Spanning the boundary between law and medicine. *Wake Forest Law Review, 41*, 465-507.

Henschke, C. I. et al. (2006). Survival of patients with stage I lung cancer detected on CT screening. *New England Journal of Medicine, 355*, 1763-1771.

Hensley, S. (2003, February 13). Hypertension report disputes earlier study. *Wall Street Journal,* p. B1.

Higashi T, et al. (2005). Quality of care is associated with survival in vulnerable older patients. *Annals of Internal Medicine, 143* (4), 274-281 (linking poor quality and patient outcomes; after three years, 28 percent of those who had received an average of 44 percent of recommended care had died, compared with 18 percent of patients who had received on average about 62 percent of recommended care).

Houck, J. A. (2006). *Hot and bothered: Women, medicine and menopause in modern America.* Cambridge, MA: Harvard University Press.

IOM (Institute of Medicine). (2001). *Crossing the quality chasm: A new health system for the 21st century.* Washington, DC: IOM (criticizes the U.S. health care system's failure to rely on EBM as standards for clinical practice and faults providers for failing to systematically record and report treatment outcomes).

___. (1999). *To err is human: Building a safer health system.* Washington, DC: IOM (44,000 to 98,000 deaths occur annually in the U.S. due to errors in hospital care, more due to error-prone institutional systems than mistakes by individuals).

Johns, M. Z. (2007). Informed consent: Requiring physicians to disclose off-label prescriptions and conflicts of interest. *Hastings Law Journal, 58*, 967-1024.

Johnson, A. (2009, February 13). U.S. court rejects vaccine connection to autism: Rulings deny notion that mercury preservative interacts with other childhood inoculations to cause the disorder. *Wall Street Journal,* p. A3.

Kahlenborn, C. et al. (2006). Oral contraceptive use as a risk factor for premenopausal breast cancer: A meta-analysis. *Mayo Clinic Proceedings, 81*, 1290-1302 (review of original data from thirty-four research studies worldwide).

Kerr, E. et al. (2004). Profiling the quality of care in twelve communities: Results from the CQI study. *Health Affairs, 23* (3), 247-256 (analyzing the Community Quality Index (CQI) study, a comprehensive examination of how effectively care was delivered in twelve metropolitan areas; finding room for improvement in quality of preventive, acute, and chronic care with no community being consistently best or worst).

King, J. S., & Moulton, B. W. (2006). Rethinking informed consent: The case for shared medical decision-making. *American Journal of Law & Medicine, 32*, 429-493 (EBM requires both patients and physicians to contribute information and participate in the medical decision-making process).

Kleinman, D. L. et al. (2005). *Controversies in science and technology: From maize to menopause.* Madison, WI: University of Wisconsin Press.

Krent, H. J. et al (2008). Whose business is your pancreas? Potential privacy problems in New York City's mandatory diabetes registry? *Annals of Health Law, 17*, 1-37.

Landro, L. (2007, May 16). Better ways to treat back pain; insurers, employers target excessive scans and surgeries to improve patient outcomes. *Wall Street Journal,* p. D1.

___. (2005, January 26). Are treatment guidelines reliable? *Wall Street Journal,* p. D4.

___. (2003, December 22). Who gets health care? Rationing in an age of rising costs; dose of prevention: Six prescriptions to ease rationing in U.S. health care; getting wired; using research; changing pay; managing disease; fixing ICUs; patient: Educate thyself. *Wall Street Journal,* p. A1.

Lerner, J., & Robertson, D.C. (2006). When there are no randomized controlled trials: A case history of a controversial procedure for metastatic breast cancer. *Journal of Law & Policy, 14*, 597-616 (reviewing observational studies on the ineffectiveness of bone marrow transplants to treat advanced cases of breast cancer and the lawsuits by women denied insurance coverage).

Lieberman, J. A. et al. (2005). Effectiveness of antipsychotic drugs in patients with chronic schizophrenia. *New England Journal of Medicine, 353*, 1209-1223.

Littenberg, B., & MacLean, C. D. (2006). Passive consent for clinical research in the age of HIPAA. *Journal of General Internal Medicine, 21* (3), 207-211.

MacLean, C. D. et al. (2006). Diabetes decision support: Initial experience with the Vermont Diabetes Information System. *American Journal of Public Health, 96* (4), 593-595.

Manson, J. E. et al. (2003). Estrogen plus progestin and the risk of coronary heart disease. *New England Journal of Medicine, 349* (6), 523-534.

Massie, A. M. (2004). In defense of the professional standard of care: A response to Carter Williams on evidence-based medicine. *Washington & Lee Law Review, 61* (1), 535-552.

Mathews, A. W. (2005, May 10). Worrisome ailment in medicine: Misleading journal articles. *Wall Street Journal*, p. A1.

McGlynn, E. et al. (2003). The quality of health care delivered to adults in the U.S. *New England Journal of Medicine, 348* (26), 2635-2645 (summarizing a RAND Corp. study that found Americans receive only about 55 percent of recommended care for a variety of common conditions).

Mendelson, D., & Carino, T. (2005). Evidence-based medicine in the U.S.: De rigueur or dream preferred? *Health Affairs, 24* (1), 133-136 (advocating that medical judgments must incorporate all relevant factors and available EBM).

Murray, A. (2004, November 30). Politics & policy; trade group's fight against drug review is self-defeating. *Wall Street Journal*, p. A4.

NAAG (National Association of Attorneys General). (2005). *Presidential report: Addressing the costs and benefits of prescription drugs*. Washington, DC: NAAG.

Neumann, P. J. Emerging lessons from the drug effectiveness review project. *Health Affairs, 25* (4), 262-271.

NIH (National Institutes of Health). (2003). *News release: NHLBI study finds traditional diuretics better than newer medicines for treating hypertension*. Bethesda, MD: NIH.

Noah, L. Medicine's epistemology: Mapping the haphazard diffusion of knowledge in the biomedical community. *Arizona Law Review, 44* (2), 373-468.

OIG (Office of Inspector General) & HHS (U.S. Department of Health & Human Services). (2006). *FDA's monitoring of post-marketing study commitments*. Washington, DC: OIG-HHS.

Parker-Pope, T. (2007). *The hormone decision: Untangle the controversy—understand your options—make your own choices*. Emmaus, PA: Rodale.

Peirce, J. C. et al. (2006). In response: Regional variations in health care intensity and physicians' perceptions of care quality. *Annals of Internal Medicine, 145* (10), 788.

Powlowski, M. (2006). The regulation of traditional practitioners: The role of law in shaping informal constraints. *North Carolina Journal of International Law & Commercial Regulation, 32* (2), 195-258.

Prussia, K. (2004). Recent development in health law: Select recent court decisions: Vaccine Act: Fifth Circuit reinstates action against thimerosal manufacturer: *Moss v. Merck & Co.,* 381 F.3d 501 (5th Cir. 2004). *American Journal of Law & Medicine, 30,* 565-567.

RAND Corp. (2006). *First national report card on quality of health care in America (the community quality index study)*. Santa Monica, CA: RAND (largest and most comprehensive examination of U.S. health care quality, in assessing the extent to which recommended care was provided to over 14,000 adults in twelve metropolitan areas; found that all were at risk for receiving poor health care, even from the best hospitals and physicians).

___. (2005). *Challenges in systematic reviews of complementary and alternative medicine topics*. Santa Monica, CA: RAND.

___. (2005a). *Profiling quality of care: Is there a role for peer review?* Santa Monica, CA: RAND.

___. (2005b). *Consumer use of information when making treatment decisions*. Santa Monica, CA: RAND.

___. (2004). *Systematic reviews for evidence-based management: How to find them and what to do with them*. Santa Monica, CA: RAND.

Rosser, W. W. et al. (2004). *Information mastery: Evidence based family medicine* (2nd ed.). Shelton, CT: PMPH (Physicians Medical Publishing House).

Sackett, D. L. (1985). *Clinical epidemiology: A basic science for clinical medicine*. Boston, MA: Little Brown (classic text that expanded upon the work of Cochrane by applying the principles of epidemiology to the clinical practice of patient care).

Sackett, D. L. et al. (2005). *Evidence-based medicine: How to practice and teach evidence-based medicine* (3rd ed.). Oxford, England: Elsevier: Churchill Livingstone (provides introduction to EBM).

___. (1996, January). Evidence based medicine: What it is and what it isn't. *British Medical Journal, 312,* 71-72 (calling for the systematic review of all available randomized controlled trials).

Sackett, D. L., & Evidence-Based Medicine Working Group. (1992). Evidence-based medicine: A new approach to teaching the practice of medicine. *Journal of the American Medical Association, 268* (17), 2420-2425.

Sage, W. (2006). Pay for performance: Will it work in theory? *Indiana Health Law Review, 3,* 303-324 (P4P can promote EBM; scientific best practices exist that need to be more widely applied to clinical care).

Sanders, C. P. (2006). A roadmap for vaccine injury litigation in Tennessee. *Tennessee Bar Journal, 42,* 22-24.

Saver, R. S. (2008). In tepid defense of population health, physicians and antibiotic resistance. *American Journal of Law & Medicine, 34* (4), 431-491.

Schoen, C. et al. (2006). U.S. health system performance: A national scorecard. *Health Affairs, 56,* 457-475.

Schwartz, J. L. (2009). Unintended consequences: The primacy of public trust in vaccination. *Michigan Law Review, 107,* 100-104.

Seaman, B. (2005). *The greatest experiment ever performed on women*. New York, NY: Hyperion.

Siegel, D. M. (2008). Involuntary psychotropic medication to competence: No longer an easy sell. *Journal of Medicine & Law, 12,* 1-16.

Slawson, D. et al. (2007). *Essential evidence: Medicine that matters*. Maiden, MA: Wiley-Interscience.

Tanner, L. (2005, February 1). Study says brain cancers vary. *Wall Street Journal*, p. A1.

Timmermans, S., & Mauck, A. (2005). The promises and pitfalls of evidence-based medicine. *Health Affairs, 24* (1), 18-28.

Tsang, J. et al. (2008). Discordance between physicians' estimation of patient cardiovascular risk and use of evidence-based medical therapy. *American Journal of Cardiology, 102* (9), 1142-1145.

Wechsler, J. (2008). Healthcare reform proposals challenge manufacturers. *Pharmaceutical Technology, 32* (6), 32-36.

Weeks, E. A. (2007). Using torts to promote public health. *Journal of Health Care Law & Policy, 10,* 27-59.

White, B. (2004). Making evidence-based medicine doable in everyday practice. *Family Practice Management, 11* (2), 51-58.

Williams, C. (2004). Evidence-based medicine in the law beyond clinical practice guidelines: What effect will evidence-based medicine have on the standard of care? *Washington & Lee Law Review, 61*, 479-533 (advocating replacement of the medical standard of care with a professional judgment-based standard that would recognize EBM).

Winslow, R. (2008, November 10). Cholesterol drug cuts heart risk in healthy patients. *Wall Street Journal*, p. B1.

___. (2007, January 23). Opening arguments—the case against stents: New studies hint at overuse; defenders say devices for heart disease give quick symptom relief. *Wall Street Journal*, p. A1.

CHAPTER 23

IMPROVING PATIENT SAFETY AND QUALITY OF HEALTH CARE

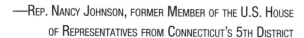

"These are complicated issues, … It is important we resolve them right because there is only one goal here: patient care and doctor power. That's what has made America's health care system great. And that's where we have to end up. And if it takes a day or two longer, if it takes a week or two longer, if it takes a month longer, that is not the issue."

—REP. NANCY JOHNSON, FORMER MEMBER OF THE U.S. HOUSE
OF REPRESENTATIVES FROM CONNECTICUT'S 5TH DISTRICT

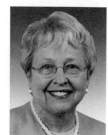

IN BRIEF

This chapter reviews programs targeting patient safety that are meant to prevent dangerous lapses in quality care, such as when health care professionals fail to explain and monitor medical product use, deliver test results, or schedule follow-up care.

FACT OR FICTION

PATIENT SAFETY

Can a hospital suspend a physician's clinical privileges without a pre-suspension hearing, where there are reasonable grounds for assuming that patient safety is at risk?

When the chairman of the Department of Radiology informed the Medical Executive Committee (MEC) at Midland Memorial Hospital and Medical Center that Dr. P. V. Patel, a board-certified cardiologist, had an unusually high rate of "catastrophic outcomes" among his recent interventions, the MEC conducted a peer review of his cases. The internal peer review prompted the MEC to revoke Dr. Patel's clinical privileges. A subsequent outside peer review found evidence that suggested poor medical judgment and Dr. Patel was suspended from the practice of medicine at Midland.

Dr. Patel requested a full hearing, at the conclusion of which the hearing committee found that while Dr. Patel was not a danger to his patients, his inadequate documentation had contributed to the questionable appearance of his cases. The hearing committee also held that there were reasonable grounds for the action taken by the physicians who had reviewed Dr. Patel's cases prior to the suspension. After his clinical privileges were restored, Dr. Patel filed suit against Midland and its physicians, claiming they violated his due process rights by failing to provide him with a pre-suspension hearing. Dr. Patel also filed antitrust and defamation claims against Midland and the physicians.

Midland and the physicians claimed they were immune from due process, antitrust, and defamation claims under the Health Care Quality Improvement Act of 1986 (HCQIA) 42 U.S.C.A. §§ 11101 *et seq.* (2009). They maintained they had immunity from damages to Dr. Patel because they were participating in a professional review action that met statutory requirements. The federal district court granted a summary judgment against Dr. Patel and he appealed.

—Patel v. Midland Memorial Hospital & Medical Center, 298 F.3d 333 (U.S. Court of Appeals for the 5th Circuit 2002), *U.S. Supreme Court certiorari denied,* 537 U.S. 1108 (U.S. Supreme Court 2003); *see also* Montero, 2003. (See *Law Fact* at the end of this chapter for the answer.)

PRINCIPLES AND APPLICATIONS

An important development in health law over the last decade has been the growing emphasis on patient safety, quality of health care, and the availability of information about provider safety and quality for consumers. After decades of inattention to the problem of medical injuries, patient safety is now occupying a prominent place on the health policy agenda and garnering renewed regulatory interest (Mello et al., 2005). When most people think of patient safety, they think of the Institute of Medicine (IOM) study *To Err Is Human,* which estimated the numbers of deaths due to medical error. That study found that forty-four thousand to ninety-eight thousand people die each year because of medical errors; the annual cost of medical errors, including the expense of additional care, lost income, and disability, was estimated to be between $17 and $29 billion (IOM, 1999). Those numbers remain frequently quoted to this day, even though the numbers are based in part on the experiences of hospital patients in the 1990s.

While the financial pressures in the U.S. health care system are very real, an arguably more important issue is patient safety and the quality of health care services. Evidence suggests that Americans receive lower-quality care than the residents of other industrialized nations:

• The U.S. spends more per capita on health care than any other country, yet Americans' health status lags far behind that of other nations
• Out of thirteen comparably industrialized countries, the U.S. ranks an average of twelfth on sixteen health indicators such as years of potential life lost and age-adjusted mortality
• The U.S. ranks seventy-second in the world on the World Health Organization's index of how efficiently health systems translate expenditures into health as measured by disability-adjusted life expectancy

(WHO, 2008)

Medical Malpractice Framework

Today, when a hospital's quality management committee learns that a medical error or adverse event has occurred, they question:

- What is the appropriate course of action?
- Who needs to know?
- What are the implications for reimbursement?

(Mattie & Webster, 2008)

The IOM highlighted the failure of the medical malpractice framework, which is primarily designed to apportion blame to individual health care providers, to adequately address patient safety problems (IOM, 1999). For example, medical malpractice lawsuits allow patients to recover only if they can prove a causal connection between a health care professional's lapse in applying treatment protocols and their resulting injury. Some have suggested moving toward an enterprise liability model, in which financial liability is imposed on hospitals rather than individual health care professionals, although a professional's breach of duty would remain a predicate for liability (Baker, 2005; Mello et al., 2005).

The IOM report argued that the root cause of medical error is poorly designed systems. The tremendous complexity of health care delivery systems makes hospitals highly susceptible to both technological and human error (Deutsch, 2008). The IOM argued that hospitals should strive to create a culture of safety in which systems are designed to cooperatively keep patients safe from harm, rather than blaming individual health care professionals for adverse outcomes. Faulting individuals for errors generated by systems only discourages health care professionals from candidly identifying and addressing medical errors (IOM, 1999). Since its publication, *To Err Is Human* has produced a rough consensus that bad systems, not careless health care professionals, are responsible for most medical errors (Leape & Berwick, 2005).

The IOM followed up in 2001 with *Crossing the Quality Chasm*, which analyzed the multiple levels at which the health care system should be reconfigured to improve patient care. In response, Congress appropriated $50 million annually for patient safety research to be conducted by the federal Agency for Healthcare Research and Quality (AHRQ). Subsequently, a joint report by the U.S. Federal Trade Commission and the U.S. Department of Justice called for competition in the health care market as a way to push patients to choose better health care systems as their providers of choice (*see* FTC & DOJ, 2004).

National Database for Patient Safety Research

The AHRQ grants funding for research on:

- Health information technology
- Patient safety
- Pharmaceutical outcomes
- Prevention and care management

Just as the National Institutes of Health (NIH) steers national research on the best ways to treat specific health conditions, the AHRQ's role is to identify prescriptions for health care processes.

Health Information Technology

Health information technology initiatives are the only health care reform proposals to gain bipartisan support in recent years (Deutsch, 2008). The AHRQ has prioritized digitized personal health data as a means for improving patient safety and reducing bureaucratic costs (HHS, 2004).

Joint Commission on the Accreditation of Healthcare Organizations

The Joint Commission on the Accreditation of Healthcare Organizations (JCAHO) could implement a system for reporting medical errors. JCAHO currently requires reporting of sentinel events, which are not the same as preventable medical errors. A sentinel event is defined as an unexpected incident or risk of an unforeseen occurrence that involves death or serious physical or psychological injury to an individual patient (JCAHO, 2007).

Hospitals that do not comply with JCAHO requirements risk losing Medicare funding, so JCAHO could therefore enforce mandatory, confidential reporting as a condition of accreditation. However, JCAHO is generally reluctant to actually withdraw accreditation, making any requirements somewhat ineffective (Lauth, 2007). JCAHO's existing policy on sentinel events is widely regarded as futile; it has not resulted in the aggregation of national patient safety data (Harrington, 2005).

Disclosure of Medical Errors

Today, more than half the states have some form of mandatory disclosure law for medical errors (Nicholson & Mitchel, 2008). For instance, in Pennsylvania, the State Health Care Cost Containment Council:

- Imposes penalties for failures to report medical errors
- Requires reporting of serious events to both the state and to patients directly affected by the medical error
- Requires hospitals to disclose specific hospital-acquired infections

- Publishes each hospital's rate of infection

(Medical Care Availability and Reduction of Error (MCARE) Act of 2002, 40 P.S. §§ 1303.101 *et seq.* (2009))

Pennsylvania also protects whistleblowers by allowing health care employees to anonymously report events, as well as immunizes documents provided to the state from discovery in most litigation (*see* Peng et al., 2006). With a few exceptions, patient safety work product is not subject to discovery or subpoena in state, federal, civil, or criminal proceedings, nor is it admissible in disciplinary proceedings conducted by state professional bodies (Liang, 2005). The federal government also encourages voluntary reporting by shielding providers from legal liability related to patient safety data. *See* Patient Safety and Quality Improvement Act of 2005 (PSQIA), 42 U.S.C.A. §§ 299b-21–299b-26 (2005).

A national public-private partnership aimed at increasing voluntary hospital reporting of quality data is premised on consumer use of health care data to select high-quality providers (*see Federal Register,* 2008). When the Healthcare Infection Control Practices Advisory Committee (HICPAC), which advises the U.S. Department of Health and Human Services and the Centers for Disease Control on infection control, recently evaluated mandatory reporting statutes, however, it found no evidence that public disclosure of infection rates was effective in reducing hospital-acquired infections (McKibben et al., 2005). The health insurance industry is, nonetheless, selecting health care providers that will be included in managed care networks based on this quality data.

While there are no nationwide standards applicable to patient safety reporting regarding mandatory versus voluntary reporting and disclosure issues, the consensus appears to support the states in mandating reporting. Mandated reporting of quality data is both a way to provide information to health care consumers and a means designed to collect information for analysis to prevent medical errors from occurring in the first place.

Patient Safety Organizations

In an effort to minimize medical errors and prevent adverse events from occurring at all, Congress has proposed that health care providers use independent third parties to monitor and evaluate their provision of care in terms of patient safety. Consequently, patient safety organizations (PSOs) have arisen to contract with health care providers to review and analyze patient safety reports and make recommendations for improving the quality of health care, which includes:

- Collecting and analyzing patient safety work product
- Developing and disseminating information to improve patient safety (recommendations for system improvements, protocols, and best practices)
- Maintaining procedures to preserve the confidentiality and security of patient safety work product
- Utilizing patient safety work product to encourage a culture of safety by health care providers
- Providing feedback and assistance to minimize patient risks and medical errors

(42 U.S.C.A. § 299b-21(5) (2005))

Reimbursement Incentives

Several private health insurers, such as Aetna and WellPoint, have moved to end reimbursements to hospitals for treatment resulting from serious medical errors. The insurers also will not allow their members to be billed for hospital errors. Similarly, Medicare will no longer reimburse hospitals for the treatment of bed sores, falls, and other preventable conditions that occur in the facilities. Nor will hospital-acquired infections, blood clots in legs and lungs, and pneumonia contracted from a ventilator be reimbursed.

In hospital contracts, Aetna includes a provision that ends reimbursements for twenty-eight "never events" outlined by the National Quality Forum (Mattie & Webster, 2008). In Virginia, WellPoint tested a policy that ends reimbursements for four "never events" before expanding the policy to eight states (Connecticut, Georgia, Maine, Massachusetts, New Hampshire, New York, Rhode Island, and Vermont). UnitedHealth Group and Cigna have similar policies. Providers of private health insurance are now banning reimbursements for only the gravest of mistakes, such as:

- Administration of incompatible blood
- Infants discharged to the wrong person
- Medication errors that result in death or disability
- Surgeries on the wrong limbs

(NQF, 2007)

It is most likely only a matter of time before the health insurance industry also stops paying for some of the more common and less clear problems that Medicare is tackling. Medicare is refusing to make payments for:

- Air embolisms
- Blood poisoning arising from incompatibility
- Hospital-acquired injuries
- Hospital-acquired urinary tract infections associated with catheters
- Objects left behind in surgery
- Pressure ulcers

- Surgical site infections (such as mediastinitis after coronary artery bypass graft surgery)
- Vascular catheter-associated infections

(CMS, 2007)

While not every negative care outcome is a result of negligence, or even an entirely preventable error, providers of health insurance maintain that the no-pay policies will help improve patient safety and reduce health care costs (Avery & Schultz, 2007). Some hospitals have raised concerns that the new strategy could drive up medical costs in other ways as hospitals absorb or pass on the expense of introducing the safety and screening procedures needed to help avoid mistakes (O'Brien & Anderson, 2007).

Moral Dilemmas

1. Is denying health care providers reimbursement for costs associated with an adverse medical event that was not preventable and did not result from negligence appropriate?

Evidence-Based Guidelines

The lack of standardized, universally accepted treatment guidelines, firmly supported by scientific evidence, is a significant obstacle to the prevention medical errors (McNeill et al., 2005). Since 2000, it has been recognized that physicians' expertise should be applied in a manner consistent with information from scientific research. Processes that support more accurate identification of what treatment is appropriate for each patient can have profound implications for decreasing adverse events and containing the escalating costs of health care (Eden et al., 2000). For instance, one of the largest and most expensive components of U.S. health care is the intensive care units (ICUs) in acute-care hospitals:

- Representing approximately 30 percent of the nation's acute-care costs
- Costing over $180 billion annually
- Serving more than 5 million patients each year
- Nearly every ICU patient suffers at least one potentially life-threatening adverse event

(Pronovost & Goeschel, 2005)

Nearly all of these adverse events could be prevented with simple clinical processes in place. Evidence suggests that using chlorhexidine to clean the skin prior to placing a central venous catheter can cut the risk of catheter-related bloodstream infections in half with minimal, if any, increase in costs. Yet it is infrequently used (Pronovost & Goeschel, 2005). Many commentators ask why patient safety procedures such as this are not mandated by states and accreditation organizations.[LN1]

Moral Dilemmas

1. Should the federal government support the states and begin mandating the use of generally accepted clinical procedures approved by the AHRQ in all acute-care hospitals, not just those receiving Medicare funding, in an effort to decrease health care costs?

Pharmaceutical Outcomes

Every five to ten years, major legislation addresses pressing issues concerning the federal Food and Drug Administration (FDA). A decade ago, reform was motivated by the perception that the FDA was not getting new drugs to market as efficiently as possible. Today, the leading concern is that the FDA is not protecting the public from the risks of drugs as effectively as it might.

Rofecoxib, or Vioxx, started the drive for tougher drug safety laws and an overhaul of FDA oversight. An exhaustive analysis of drug safety data recently conducted by researchers at MIT and the University of Chicago concluded, among other things, that congressional efforts in the 1990s to speed up FDA review times did not fuel a drug safety crisis; rather, the data indicates that about 2 to 3 percent of approved drugs continue to be withdrawn, which is the same rate as before passage of these reforms (Grabowski & Wang, 2008).

A very careful balance exists at the FDA that looks at the benefits and risks of potential treatments to determine if they should be approved. It is not a perfect system. Then again, in the real world, patients' appetite for risk depends in large measure on the disease from which they suffer. In fact, every day patients make this risk-risk assessment. They decide whether the potential risk of a therapeutic option outweighs the risk of a given disorder. Thus, cancer patients are willing to tolerate chemotherapy in an attempt to rid themselves of their disease.

Risk-Risk Calculus

This risk-risk proposition was evident when Elan Pharmaceutical withdrew Tysabri, a multiple sclerosis therapy, from the market because of a rare and serious potential side effect. Multiple sclerosis patients with limited therapeutic options organized, made their voices heard, and demanded a return of Tysabri to the market. Today, Tysabri is back on the market in no small measure because of the efforts of patients with multiple sclerosis. While patients want to be warned of known risks, they also understand their disease and want, even demand, the right to choose their own therapies.

A key incident in raising such concern was the 2004 withdrawal by Merck of Vioxx, because of an apparent increased risk of serious cardiovascular events. The withdrawal came amid questions about the FDA's handling of a possible association between selective serotonin-reuptake inhibitors and suicidal ideation in adolescents. Further concerns were raised about the agency's handling of staff disagreements about these and other drugs. In this context, the FDA sought a review from the IOM.

The IOM's 2006 report included a broad range of recommendations (Baciou et al., 2006), and the FDA has issued an action plan (FDA, 2007). Based on these documents, Congress developed a more systematic approach to improving drug safety and effective use (*see* Food and Drug Administration Amendments Act of 2007 (FDAAA), 21 U.S.C.A. §§ 350f *et seq.* (2009); 42 U.S.C.A. § 247d-5a (2007)). However, the steps intended to enhance safety also increase costs and reduce access to beneficial drugs. Over-warning, just like under-warning, can similarly have a negative effect on patient safety (FDA, 2007). *See* 21 C.F.R. Parts 201, 314, and 601.

The tools available for learning about drugs and their effectiveness include:

- Drug coverage, including tiered benefits by the health care industry based on proven effectiveness (*i.e.*, patients may have access to medications that their physicians believe are more efficacious in treating their particular medical conditions, but if therapies are not supported by evidence-based studies as the most cost-effective means of treatment, patients will be required to pay more out of pocket for selecting such medications)
- Drug utilization management programs that influence prescribing (alerting to under- and over-prescribing, as well as patient adherence to drug therapies)
- Electronic data on prescription use and patient outcomes (controlling for adverse reactions to incompatible drugs, as well as attempting to minimize the use of drug cocktails, where patients are taking dozens of medicines that counteract one another)
- Internet resources for health care consumers to understand their use of medications

(McClellan, 2007a)

INSTITUTE OF MEDICINE AND FOOD AND DRUG ADMINISTRATION REFORMS

The reforms recommended by the IOM and proposed by the FDA fall into four main categories:

- Need to balance industry users' fees and federal appropriations
- Balancing drug safety against access to innovative treatments
- Post-marketing drug surveillance
- More effective use of prescribed drugs

The Prescription Drug User Fee Act of 1992 (PDUFA), 21 U.S.C.A. §§ 379g, 379h (2007), provides for user fees to be paid by the pharmaceutical and biotechnology industries for review of new medicines.

Need to Balance Industry Users' Fees and Federal Appropriations

Total user fees were nearly $400 million in 2008, accounting for less than 40 percent of FDA resources for drug regulation (FDA, 2007). While FDA critics claim this has affected drug safety, the rate at which drugs have been withdrawn from the market has not increased since user fees were implemented (McClellan, 2007a). In addition, the increase in FDA resources has resulted in important public health benefits, including a reduction in drug review time, which is estimated to have saved 180,000 to 210,000 lives (Philipson et al., 2006). While critics claim this level of industry user fees fuels a perception that the FDA is beholden to the industry it regulates, others assert that regulated industries should cover the costs required to help regulate and monitor their conduct in the marketplace.

Balancing Drug Safety Against Access to Innovative Treatments

The FDA has authority to help assure drug safety, including the ability to:

- Impose special requirements for prescribers, such as documentation of laboratory testing that would be monitored by the FDA
- Limit direct-to-consumer marketing
- Mandate post-marketing studies
- Require special medication guides for patients
- Restrict which physicians can prescribe a drug, for instance, restricting certain therapeutic classes to oncologist or cardiologist prescribers

Critics believe such steps strengthen the FDA's enforcement authority. Although the agency can already remove drugs from the market for noncompliance with marketing or labeling recommendations, it rarely takes this extreme step. However, others counter that the liability and adverse publicity facing companies that fail to act on FDA drug safety findings already compel compliance. Some also argue that increased reliance on special, drug-by-drug regulatory steps is burdensome and confusing, leading to access problems, the substitution of less safe or effective treatments, and medical errors (McClellan, 2007a).

Post-Marketing Drug Surveillance

A fundamentally better system for post-marketing surveillance could help avoid increased costs and reduced access due to drug-by-drug regulation, with the development of better risk information based on actual experience with every new drug. Many high-profile safety problems have resulted not from the FDA's inadequate authority to regulate drugs on the basis of known risks, but from post-marketing delays in determining whether suspected adverse events were causally related to drug use.

One reason drugs may be used for years by millions of Americans before risks become evident is that the U.S. has no active drug surveillance system. While the U.S. obtains innovative drugs two to three years ahead of its European counterparts, Europe has a compulsory drug surveillance system. The FDA relies on its Adverse Event Reporting System (AERS), which involves the investigation of voluntary adverse event reports from health care providers, pharmaceutical companies, and consumers of health care. While AERS is important, unfortunately it captures only a fraction of adverse events (McClellan, 2007a).

With almost all prescriptions now processed electronically, and with the availability of increasingly detailed data on health care utilization and outcomes for insured Americans, a routine, systematic approach to active population-based drug surveillance could be implemented that could identify potential safety problems much more effectively and relatively inexpensively (McClellan, 2007a). For instance, with a data network, including information on one hundred million patients, a statistically significant signal of serious cardiovascular risk could have been detected after less than three months of experience with Vioxx (Platt, 2007). Such an electronic surveillance network could also help in targeting follow-up clinical studies to determine:

- Causality, or the causal relationship between drug use and adverse events, when necessary
- Follow-up actions on adverse events causally related to drug use, to influence future prescribing

(McClellan, 2007a)

More Effective Use of Prescribed Drugs

While it has been proposed that a regulatory entity be formed that is separate from the FDA pre-marketing review process, the IOM rejected this possibility. The IOM concluded that achieving a balanced approach to the assessment of risks and benefits would be greatly complicated, or even compromised, if two separate agencies were working in isolation from one another (Baciu et al., 2006).

Ideally, a more systematic approach to post-market monitoring of drugs needs to be implemented. More effective use of drugs could be promoted by augmenting FDA resources with the rapidly growing array of electronic resources related to drug use. Such an approach could help to minimize the safety problems and scientific disagreements that accompany drug use when evidence is limited, without pushing the pendulum toward excessive restrictions on access to valuable drugs (McClellan, 2007a).

PREVENTION OF MEDICAL ERRORS AND ADVERSE EVENTS

While some still claim adverse events are an inherent risk in receiving health care, the consensus is that medical errors should not be tolerated. States are increasingly requiring health care professionals to report adverse events, with harsh penalties for non-reporting; transparency and public disclosure of medical errors are gradually becoming mandatory. The financial disincentives for medical errors also are becoming more significant, as Medicare and the health insurance industry refuse to compensate care associated with adverse events. It is becoming imperative that health care providers develop health information systems for tracking adverse events so they are prepared to make mandatory reports, are able to track the costs of care associated with medical errors and adverse events, and, ultimately, take action to prevent medical errors from happening to begin with (O'Brien & Anderson, 2007).

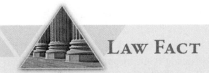

LAW FACT

PATIENT SAFETY

Can a hospital suspend a physician's clinical privileges without a pre-suspension hearing, where there are reasonable grounds for assuming that patient safety is at risk?

Although the U.S. Court of Appeals for the Fifth Circuit upheld the summary judgment, it avoided deciding the issue of Midland's immunity under the HCQIA. Until courts are willing to enforce the HCQIA, hospitals and other health care providers will remain reluctant to rely solely on its protections when suspending or denying clinical privileges to physicians that are perceived to be a danger to patients' safety. In *Patel*, the court passed up the opportunity to provide such an incentive by avoiding the issue of immunity altogether, thus frustrating Congress's intent to reduce this type of litigation.

—*Patel v. Midland Memorial Hospital & Medical Center*, 298 F.3d 333
(U.S. Court of Appeals for the 5th Circuit 2002), *U.S. Supreme Court certiorari denied*, 537 U.S. 1108 (U.S. Supreme Court 2003); *see also* Montero, 2003.

CHAPTER SUMMARY

- Several thousand patients die each year because of medical errors; medical errors result in billions of dollars in costs annually.
- Evidence suggests Americans are likely to receive lower quality care than residents of other countries.
- One shortcoming of the health care industry is that it tends to apportion blame for patient safety problems rather than address their root causes, which are often poorly designed systems rather than individual health care professionals.
- Competition within the health care industry is meant to encourage patients to choose better health care systems, but it is difficult for consumers to do this due to the lack of a comprehensive set of relevant data, such as treatment success or failure for a particular condition.
- At least half of the states have laws mandating disclosure of medical errors; there are no nationwide standards for disclosure.
- Patient safety organizations are third parties that contract with health care providers to monitor patient safety and recommend ways to improve the quality of health care.
- Many private health insurers, as well as Medicare, will no longer reimburse health care providers for costs resulting from medical errors, even though not all such errors result from negligence or are necessarily entirely preventable.
- Many adverse medical events could be prevented with the implementation and use of evidence-based guidelines; many question why they are not mandated.
- Although some patients are willing to tolerate higher risks than other patients due to their particular medical conditions, there is still substantial concern over whether the FDA is effectively protecting the public from drug risks, particularly after drugs are approved for marketing.
- Proposed FDA reforms include balancing industry users' fees and federal appropriations, balancing drug safety against innovation, better post-marketing drug surveillance, and more effective use of prescribed drugs.

LAW NOTES

1. Five procedures in the Keystone intervention developed by Johns Hopkins University for use in ICUs are hand-washing, using full barrier precautions when inserting catheters into central lines, cleaning the skin with chlorhexidine, avoiding the femoral vein, and removing catheters as soon as they became clinically unnecessary. For instance, ICUs in Michigan eliminated catheter-related bloodstream infections in their ICUs with these straightforward, simple procedures (Pronovost & Goeschel, 2005).

CHAPTER BIBLIOGRAPHY

Avery, G., & Schultz, J. (2007). Regulation, financial incentives, and the production of quality. *American Journal of Medical Quality, 22* (4), 265-273.

Baciu, A. et al. (2006). *The future of drug safety: Promoting and protecting the health of the public.* Washington, DC: Institute of Medicine, Committee on the Assessment of the U.S. Drug Safety System.

Baker, T. (2005). *The medical malpractice myth.* Chicago, IL: University of Chicago Press.

Brennan, T. A. et al. (2005). Accidental deaths, saved lives, and improved quality. *New England Journal of Medicine, 353,* 1405-1409.

Carpenter, D. et al. (2008). Drug-review deadlines and safety problems. *New England Journal of Medicine, 358,* 1354-1361.

Deutsch, R. (2008). The federal role in reducing hospital-acquired conditions: Are Medicare reimbursement incentives enough? *Columbia Journal of Law & Social Problems, 42,* 1-41.

Eden, J. et al. (2000). *Commission on reviewing evidence to identify highly effective clinical services: Knowing what works in health care.* Washington, DC: Institute of Medicine.

FDA (U.S. Food and Drug Administration). (2007). *The future of drug safety: Promoting and protecting the health of the public: FDA's response to the Institute of Medicine's 2006 report.* Rockville, MD: FDA.

FTC (U.S. Federal Trade Commission) & DOJ (U.S. Department of Justice). (2004). *Improving health care: A dose of competition.* Washington, DC: FTC & DOJ.

GAO (General Accountability Office). (2006). *VA health care: Patient safety could be enhanced by improvements in employment screening and physician privileging practices.* Washington, DC: GAO.

Grabowski, H., & Wang, Y. R. (2008). Do faster Food and Drug Administration drug reviews adversely affect patient safety? An analysis of the 1992 Prescription Drug User Fee Act. *Journal of Law & Economics, 51,* 377-404.

Harrington, M. (2005). Revisiting medical error: Five years after the IOM report, have reporting systems made a measurable difference? *Journal of Law & Medicine, 15,* 329-382 (discussing the lack of a uniform definition of medical error and the disincentives for disclosure embedded in many reporting systems).

HHS (U.S. Department of Health and Human Services). (2004). *Harnessing information technology to improve health care.* Washington, DC: HHS.

IOM (Institute of Medicine). (2007). *Challenges for the FDA: The future of drug safety.* Washington, DC: IOM.

____. (1999). *To err is human: Building a safer health system.* Washington, DC: IOM.

Jacobson, P. D., & Tunick, M. R. (2007). Consumer-directed health care and the courts: Let the buyer (and seller) beware. *Health Affairs, 26* (3), 704-714.

JCAHO (Joint Commission on the Accreditation of Healthcare Organizations). (2007). *Sentinel event policy and procedures.* Chicago, IL: JCAHO.

Kerr, R. A. (2007). The Patient Safety and Quality Improvement Act of 2005: Who should pay for improved outcomes? *Journal of Law & Medicine, 17,* 329-345 (noting that the PSQIA does not provide funding for PSOs, and prevents HMOs from sponsoring PSOs; proposes that the pharmaceutical industry fund PSOs).

Lauth, L. A. (2007). The Patient Safety and Quality Improvement Act of 2005: An invitation for sham peer review in the health care setting. *Indiana Health Law Review, 4,* 151-172.

Lavine G. (2008). Pharmacists can play active role as hospitals prepare for CMS rule changes. *American Journal of Health Systems Pharmacies, 65* (7), 595-596.

Lawrence, D. (2007). Costly infections. A new CMS hospital-acquired infection mandate is putting hospitals on the alert. *Healthcare Informatics, 24* (11), pp. 10, 12, 14.

Leape, L. L., & Berwick, D. M. (2005). Five years after *To Err Is Human*: What have we learned? *Journal of the American Medical Association, 293* (19), 2384-2390.

Liang, B. A. (2005). Collaborating on patient safety: Legal concerns and policy requirements. *Widener Law Review, 12,* 83-105 (discussing how legal liability deters health care providers from sharing quality and safety information, and the function of the PSQIA).

Mattie, A. S., & Webster, B. L. (2008 Centers for Medicare and Medicaid Services' "never events": An analysis and recommendations to hospitals. *Health Care Manager, v27* (4), 338-349.

McClellan, M. (2007). Drug safety reform at the FDA: Pendulum swing or systematic improvement? *New England Journal of Medicine, 356* (17), 1700-1702.

____. (2007a, March 14). Testimony before the U.S. Senate Health, Education, Labor, and Pensions Committee: *Fundamental improvements in drug safety for the 21st century: Time for a systematic, electronic infrastructure.* Washington, DC 110th Congress..

McKibben, L. et al. (2005). Guidance on public reporting of health care-associated infections: Recommendations of the Healthcare Infection Control Practices Advisory Committee. *American Journal of Infection Control, 33* (4), 217-226.

McNeill, D. et al. (2005). Beyond the dusty shelf: Shifting paradigms and effecting change. In *Advances in patient safety: From research to implementation.* Washington, DC: AHRQ.

Mello, M. M. et al., (2005). Fostering rational regulation of patient safety. *Journal of Health Politics, Policy & Law, 30* (3), 375-426 (discussing the inadequacy of tort law to address patient safety due to courts' lack of health care expertise and insufficient evidence that the tort system deters health care professionals' errors).

Montero, G. A. (2003). Protecting public health abrogates due process requirement for suspension proceedings. *Journal of Law, Medicine & Ethics, 31,* 167-170.

National Academy for State Health Policy. (2008). *State patient safety centers: A new approach to promote patient safety.* Portland, ME: National Academy.

Nicholson, D. C., & Mitchel, L. A. (2008). A medical error happened: Now what? The implications for medical errors heat up. *Journal of Health Care Compliance, 1,* 5-14.

NQF (National Quality Forum). (2007). *Serious reportable events in healthcare: Update.* Washington, DC: NQF.

____. (2002). *Serious reportable events in healthcare: A consensus report.* Washington, DC: NQF.

O'Brien, K., & Anderson, J. (2007). High quality, efficient care for Medicare beneficiaries – but at what cost? *Compliance Health Care Association, 2007* (11), 11-13.

Peng, M. M. et al. (2006). Adverse outcomes from hospital-acquired infection in Pennsylvania cannot be attributed to increased risk on admission. *American Journal of Medical Quality, 21* (6), 17S-28S.

PHCCC (Pennsylvania Health Care Cost Containment Council). (2007, October 5). Press release: Pennsylvania's health care system in "critical condition." Harrisburg, PA: PHCCC.

___. (2006). *Measuring the quality of Pennsylvania's commercial HMOs.* Harrisburg, PA: PHCCC.

Philipson T. J. et al. (2006). *Assessing the safety and the efficacy of the FDA: The case of the Prescription Drug User Fee Acts.* Cambridge, MA: National Bureau of Economic Research.

Platt, R. (2007). *The future of drug safety: Challenges for the FDA.* Washington, DC: IOM Forum.

Pronovost, P., & Goeschel, C. (2005, March/April). Improving ICU care: It takes a team. *Healthcare Executive,* 15-22.

Sipkoff, M. (2007). Hospitals asked to account for errors on their watch: CMS and states may stop paying for specific hospital-acquired conditions. Will health plans follow suit? *Managed Care, 16* (7), pp. 30, 35-37.

Wachter, R. (2007). *Understanding patient safety.* New York, NY: McGraw-Hill Professional.

WHO (World Health Organization). (2008). *The world health report: Primary health care: Now more than ever.* Geneva, Switzerland: WHO.

PART IX

OUR HEALTH CARE SYSTEM'S RESPONSE TO ILLNESS

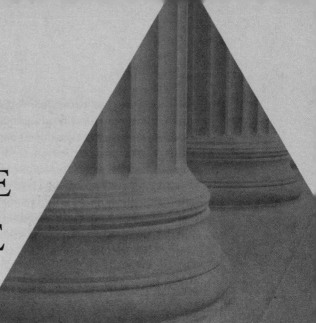

CHAPTER 24

HUMAN BODY PARTS INDUSTRY

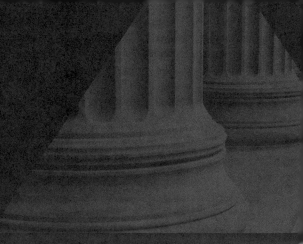

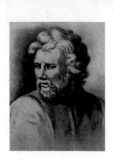

"*You are a little soul carrying around a corpse.*"

—EPICTETUS (55-135 A.D.), GREEK PHILOSOPHER

IN BRIEF

This chapter describes the procurement side of the billion-dollar human body parts industry and how it is intertwined with the U.S. health care system. Willed body programs, the marketing and commoditization of human cadavers, property rights, and the implications of publicized scandals involving the illicit sale and resale of donated human body parts are examined.

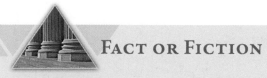

FACT OR FICTION

WILLED BODY PROGRAMS

Can body parts lawfully obtained from cadavers that are donated to universities for medical research be subsequently sold to third parties?

Henry Reid, Director of the willed body program at the University of California–Los Angeles (UCLA) Medical School, was arrested and charged with grand theft for allegedly selling hundreds of cadavers donated to UCLA. Reid charged Ernest Nelson more than $1 million over a five-year period for the sale of 496 cadavers that had been donated to the University. Nelson, a body broker and former mortuary worker associated with Empire Anatomical Services in Los Angeles, was arrested and charged with receipt of stolen property. About twice a week, Nelson entered the UCLA Medical Center with a saw and collected tissue, organs, tendons, bones, joints, limbs, hands, feet, torsos, and heads culled from the dead; he then sold the body parts to a number of medical research companies, including a Johnson & Johnson subsidiary, DePuy Mitek. Massachusetts-based Mitek manufactures medical devices that treat soft tissue injuries.

The UCLA program, the oldest willed body program in the country, receives donated cadavers for use by its researchers and medical students. Reid, hired after claims in 1996 that the UCLA program had mishandled and improperly disposed of donated remains, allegedly drew from and sold the program's surplus materials for about $1,400 per body. Nelson maintains that his role in the reselling of cadavers and body parts received from Reid was legal because he had no reason to believe that he was in receipt of stolen goods, and because he did not sell the remains for a profit. Johnson & Johnson admitted that Mitek purchased dismembered human remains from Nelson, but claimed ignorance as to their stolen origin.

A class-action lawsuit filed against Johnson & Johnson, Mitek, Empire, and associates claims fraud, negligence, and intentional infliction of emotional distress caused by buying, selling, and reselling whole and dismembered human remains. The remains were obtained from bodies donated to the University for medical research and educational purposes. At issue is whether the parties lawfully obtained body parts from cadavers donated to UCLA.

—See e.g., *Cohen v. NuVasive, Inc.,* 79 Cal.Rptr.3d 759 (Court of Appeal, 2nd District, Division 3, California 2009); *see also* Goodwin, 2006; Goodwin, 2006a (See *Law Fact* at the end of this chapter for the answer.)

PRINCIPLES AND APPLICATIONS

Human material is used to develop medical devices and cosmetic products, as well as in most surgeries. Multinational corporations, such as Johnson & Johnson, Bristol-Myers Squibb, Stryker, and Medtronic, rely on human remains to guide them in developing medical products. Other consumer product corporations such as L'Oréal, Max Factor, and Revlon use body tissues to create cosmetics. Physicians use body parts to:

- Plump up lips and eliminate wrinkles
- Repair bones
- Replace heart valves
- Treat burn victims

(*see* Cheney, 2006)

It is estimated that the human body parts industry in the U.S. generates $500 million annually in the

procurement side of the industry alone; some attribute a significantly higher dollar figure to the entire domestic industry given the cash transfers involved in many of the sales transactions (Wharton, 2006). By some estimates, more than eight thousand donated cadavers are sold annually in the U.S., some of which are closely tied to major medical research organizations (Cheney, 2006).

MISCONDUCT IN THE HUMAN REMAINS MARKET

American medicine has always struggled to procure enough cadavers for research and education. Since the late eighteenth century, when dissection became an essential component of medical training, the demand

MEDICAL PRODUCTS LITIGATION

In Re Human Tissue Products Liability Litigation
[Decedents' Relatives v. Human Material Processing Corporations]
2007 WL 4165688 (U.S. District Court for the District of New Jersey 2007)

FACTS: This is a class action comprised of forty-two lawsuits in sixteen states (Alabama, California, Florida, Georgia, Indiana, Iowa, Kentucky, Louisiana, Minnesota, New Jersey, New York, Ohio, Pennsylvania, South Carolina, Tennessee, and West Virginia) against companies that harvested human tissue from corpses without obtaining proper consent and without following proper procedures. The scheme by Medical Tissue Services and its ringleader, former oral surgeon Dr. Mastromarino, involved procuring human tissues from funeral homes and crematoria without the proper consents and then selling the tissue to tissue banks, tissue processing companies, and multinational medical products firms, who processed the tissue without checking or following procedures to determine the origin, nature, or suitability of the tissue for human transplantation. Moreover, it is alleged that the tissue processors engaged in flawed procedures that did not properly cleanse the received tissue and then distributed the tissue.

Dr. Mastromarino made between $6 million and $12 million over a four-year period selling tissue and bone illicitly carved from corpses. Following almost three years of legal proceedings and a criminal investigation by the Brooklyn District Attorney, Mastromarino had his dental license revoked and agreed to a prison sentence of eighteen to fifty-four years after pleading guilty to charges of body stealing, forgery, grand larceny, and enterprise corruption in 2007.

More than a thousand civil suits from tissue recipients have been filed against Mastromarino, his tissue harvesting company, Medical Tissue Services Ltd., and three tissue-processing companies that sold Mastromarino's human material to hospitals and other health facilities. First headquartered in Brooklyn, New York, and then Fort Lee, New Jersey, Mastromarino paid funeral directors $1,000 per corpse. He then divided each corpse and sold the bone and tissue for at least $13,000 per corpse to tissue-processing companies, who then resold the body parts to hospitals for many times that amount. Body parts included sheets of skin for burn victims and cosmetic operations, bone for dental implants, tendons and ligaments for orthopedic replacement procedures, and cardiac valves for those with heart problems.

With a crew of cutters, including several nurses, Mastromarino harvested more than 1,600 bodies from funeral homes without consent. Mastromarino and his assistants forged consent forms and death certificates to conceal the fact that many of the corpses died from hepatitis, cancer, AIDS, or other dangerous ailments. Under federal regulations, transplants from such corpses are prohibited. They routinely falsely lowered the ages of the deceased to make the stolen specimens appear more desirable.

ISSUE: Are organs and tissue from human corpses being harvested without obtaining proper consents?

HOLDING AND DECISION: While litigation is ongoing, this case demonstrates one way attorneys are attempting to hold the body parts industry accountable for the administration of its illegitimate body harvesting programs.

ANALYSIS: This criminal enterprise case will proceed to trial or settlement. Separate criminal proceedings related to the harvesting of body parts are ongoing in state courts.

RULE OF LAW: This litigation will likely result in changes to regulation of the human body parts industry as new rules of law emerge to address this controversy.

(*See generally* Struve, 2008).

---

for cadavers has far exceeded the supply. Back then, the solution was the robbing of graves. Entrepreneurs could make a tidy profit digging up freshly interred bodies and delivering them, under cover of night, to medical men willing to pay handsomely for them. People also used to obtain bodies from orphanages, poor houses, and insane asylums. These were good sources of bodies since disease was often rampant there and society never questioned what happened to orphans, the indigent, or the insane (Roach, 2004).

Today, body brokers are not robbing graves; they are violating corpses before they ever get to the grave. There are two distinct forms of misconduct in the human remains market (Cheney, 2006). The first is the procurement, harvesting, and sale of body parts taken from the dead who never consented to be donors.

The second, more complicated form of misconduct involves the illicit trade in the bodies of people who have donated themselves to science.

The Underground Market in Human Body Parts

As the host of Public Broadcasting Services' long-running *Masterpiece Theater*, Alistair Cooke represented American taste and refinement at its best. Since his death in 2004, Cooke has also become the symbol of a little known market termed "the human body parts industry," America's underground market that illegally sells corpses and body parts.

Unbeknownst to his family, Cooke's bones were cut out of his body before he was cremated and his bones were sold for $7,000 by Regeneration Technologies, a Florida-based tissue processor that did $19 million in business in 2007, and Florida-based Tutogen Medical Inc., a manufacturer of biological implant products with $8 million in revenue in 2007. While Cooke's fate was gruesome, what is perhaps most disturbing is that it was not unusual. The Cooke scandal raised concerns about the marketing and commoditization of human bodies, property rights, and the implications for medical research that are arising from publicizing this illicit sale and resale of body parts (Cheney, 2006; Goodwin, 2006a).

Fraud and Negligence in the Illicit Sale of Human Body Parts

Fraud and negligence issues surround the sale of human corpses and body parts, as well as the medical research industry. Liability for the fraudulent receipt of stolen goods is a factual issue determined by the courts, considering all relevant evidence. In the case of Cooke, the difficulty with holding anyone liable is proving a buyer's knowledge that the body parts were stolen.

The Uniform Anatomical Gift Act prohibits the sale of body parts and was adopted by the states in order to protect corpses. Congress subsequently set a minimum standard of care for the sale of body parts when it adopted the National Organ Transplant Act (*see* Uniform Anatomical Gift Act (UAGA) of 1968, Uniform Laws Annotated; National Organ Transplant Act (NOTA), 42 U.S.C.A. §§ 274-274e (2009)). Negligence may arise when either of these statutes is violated, resulting in injury to a corpse. Corpses are a statutorily protected group.

Negligence per se arises as a matter of law. Courts are not free to decide what a reasonable person would have done under the circumstances and a breach of duty owed the victim is not required, unlike in a regular negligence action. For instance, the UCLA scandal at the start of this chapter involved the negligent sale and receipt of cadavers. A reasonable person might have accepted the cadavers and body parts, believing that they were not stolen and sold, but that is irrelevant. Federal statutes were violated and whoever accepts the stolen body parts may be liable. In other words, when Johnson & Johnson admitted that Mitek purchased dismembered human remains from Nelson, it could not claim ignorance as to their stolen origin and subsequent sale. Their error in judgment in dealing with suspect body brokers is irrelevant; they may be determined to have been negligent per se. The same rationale applies to Regeneration Technologies and Tutogen Medical, two companies intertwined in the class action products liability litigation described all through this chapter on this very issue. *See In Re Human Tissue Products Liability Litigation,* 435 F.Supp.2d 1352 (Judicial Panel on Multidistrict Litigation 2006).

Moral Dilemmas

1. What is the ethical justification underlying laws that restrict accepting or offering payment for human corpses and body parts?

Billion-Dollar Global Industry

The true prevalence of the illicit sale of discarded body parts is anyone's guess. Legitimate sales of human body parts are a billion-dollar global industry (Buck, 2007). The answer to the question about the level of corruption is in the details; with one harvested corpse worth $200,000 on the black market, the temptations are great and the oversight almost non-existent (Wharton, 2006). To further complicate the issue, there are legitimate sales that use illegitimate means, such as lack of consent.

As multidistrict litigation, described throughout this chapter, proceeds in the federal courts on an international body parts operation involving Medical Tissue Services and Mastromarino, the global pervasiveness of the illegal harvesting of body parts may be brought to light. Criminal proceedings related to this operation are also ongoing in state courts nationwide.

Some commentators think about 15 percent of the billion-dollar global body parts industry could be illegitimate, or about $150 million. This estimate is extrapolated from a comparative analysis of the $4.5 trillion retail industry, where an estimated $30 billion is illegitimate due to organized crime, exclusive of shoplifting. Keep in mind, just one body broker, Dr. Mastromarino, harvested more than 1,600 bodies in the U.S. before he was caught in 2007. From the body broker scandals that have been uncovered, prosecutors cannot assign an accurate sales figure to the clandestine operations they investigated for years. Sales are speculated to be in multimillion-dollar ranges for each case. What we do know is there appears to be no shortage of reportable cases and scandals for this scarce commodity of human materials.

ILLEGAL HARVESTING OF BODY PARTS

Graves v. Biomedical Tissue Services (In Re Human Tissue Products Liability Litigation)

[Decedents' Relatives v. Human Material Processing Corporations]

2007 WL 3396414 (U.S. District Court for the District of New Jersey 2007)

FACTS: This lawsuit was brought by the immediate family of Graves, who died from complications arising from cancer in 2005. Following the death of Graves, his family contracted with a funeral home for funeral arrangements and cremation services. After the funeral home took possession of Graves's body for cremation, it allowed a tissue bank to remove bones and tissue from Graves's body for medical research and implantation. Neither Graves nor his family consented to the harvesting of the body parts and the funeral home never disclosed that such harvesting would occur.

ISSUE: Did the tissue banks fail in their legal duty to obtain proper consents and did they willfully disregard regulations regarding the procedures for harvesting human organs?

HOLDING AND DECISION: The issue was never addressed in this part of the lawsuit; summary judgment was granted and the complaint was dismissed without prejudice against one of the five tissue banks that had no records of receiving any human organs or tissue from the funeral home that handled Graves's cremation; the remaining four tissue banks remain involved in this ongoing class-action litigation. The plaintiffs failed to meet their burden to provide affirmative evidence of the particular tissue bank's involvement in the harvesting or processing of Graves's body or body parts.

ANALYSIS: This case was certified as part of the class action, *In Re Human Tissue Products Liability Litigation,* and will proceed to trial or settlement. Separate criminal proceedings related to the harvesting of body parts are ongoing in state courts.

RULE OF LAW: There must be records indicating that a tissue bank received or processed organs and tissue from the specific funeral home that handled Graves's cremation; the remaining four tissue banks did have such records.

GENERAL UNAWARENESS OF CORRUPTION

There is general unawareness and lack of knowledge about how pivotally positioned health care professionals may exploit the dead and endanger the living. Given that the demand for human cadavers consistently exceeds supply, the allocation of scarce body parts is an issue of great value with no easy solutions. Moreover, there is no political consensus on whether:

- A legalized market for buying and selling cadavers would decrease illicit transactions;
- More explicit rules and regulations should be adopted for the sale of body parts; or
- Society is so opposed to the commoditization of the human body that such a market would be incomprehensible.

As seen in the UCLA willed body program at the start of this chapter, athough cadavers were stolen then bought and sold and resold, the dismembered body parts were ultimately used in medical research. While the lack of an open market for body parts may be stifling medical research and challenging the potential lifesaving authority of the human body parts industry, perhaps the societal value of assuring funeral rights for the families of loved ones is a more important value until a political consensus can be reached about the value of human materials (Calandrillo, 2004).

COMMODIFICATION OF HUMAN MATERIALS

Dead human bodies are the cornerstone of the lucrative and important business of advancing scientific knowledge and improving medical techniques. Human body parts underwrite both cutting-edge research and everyday medical procedures. Medical researchers rely on human cadavers to hone surgical techniques.

Yet, there is no consensus about the possibility of commodifying body parts:

- How much independence should universities have in determining the uses of donated cadavers?

- Should donors begin to explicitly define the roles regarding the future use of their bodies?
- If so, what rights should donors have in this regard, if any?

Many leading commentators on the human body parts industry (including Annie Cheney, Michele Goodwin, Nancy Scheper-Hughes, Lesley Sharp, and Catherine Waldby) claim that the business of saving human lives will thrive if cadaveric body parts can be permitted to enter an open marketplace and the sale of cadavers properly regulated. The argument is that a regulated trade would be preferable to existing black market organ dealings, which can be exploitative and unsafe (Handwerk, 2004). The case of an

MEDICAL RESEARCH

Washington University v. Catalona

[Medical Research Institution v. Medical Researcher]

490 F.3d 667 (U.S. Court of Appeals for the 8th Circuit 2007), U.S. Supreme Court certiorari denied, 128 S.Ct. 1122 (U.S. Supreme Court 2008)

FACTS: This case involved a dispute between Washington University and Dr. Catalona, a medical researcher, who left his position at Washington University and took a position at a new institution. Catalona wanted to take with him the tissue samples he had collected from his patients for his prostate cancer research. He maintained the samples belonged to his patients and that they had consented to let him take their parts with him to his new institution. Washington University maintained that because it had developed, paid for, and maintained a substantial repository of tissue samples for prostate cancer research, and that because the initial consent forms were made out in the name of Washington University, not Dr. Catalona personally, the University owned the tissue samples.

ISSUE: Once patients sign an informed consent form donating their tissue, blood, DNA, or other body parts for research purposes to a University, who has the right of ownership?

HOLDING AND DECISION: Patients surrender all rights of ownership to direct the use and transfer of their body parts once they consent to donate; they could not come back later and direct a new use or ownership.

ANALYSIS: The court was ambiguous as to whether the patients ever had a property interest in their tissue samples. On the one hand, they potentially had such an interest, but lost it when they donated their tissue for research. On the other hand, they never had such an interest.

The court equated the University's possession and control over the tissue samples with ownership under state law and concluded that the University owned and controlled the removed samples. In reaching its conclusion, the court relied on the case, *Moore v. Regents of the University of California,* and one subsequent case, *Greenberg v. Miami Children's Research Institute (see* 793 P.2d 479 (Supreme Court of California 1990), and 264 F.Supp.2d 1064 (U.S. District Court for the Southern District of Florida, Miami Division 2003), respectively). In the *Moore* case, Moore underwent supposedly necessary medical treatment at a university medical center where his physician and others used human body parts extracted from him for medical research without his permission. In *Greenberg*, families with a rare genetic disorder believed they had an agreement with researchers that, in return for their donation of tissue and other samples with genetic materials, the researchers would develop a genetic test that would be made widely available to the families. The researchers, however, gained a patent over the genetic test and disagreements arose between the patent holders and the families as to the manner in which the tests would be made broadly available and affordable. The families sued, claiming that their property had been unjustly used to enrich the researchers and alleging conversion of property. The lower court, citing *Moore,* found that the families had no property rights in their donated tissue and DNA.

RULE OF LAW: Once a patient donates body parts for research, regardless of what relationship or legal interest the individual had prior to the donation, the body parts become an object, similar to equipment, brick and mortar, or intellectual property, in which title and ownership vests with the institution conducting the research.

(*See generally* Blue, 2008; Clamon, 2008; Moses, 2008).

Moral Dilemmas

1. What legal and ethical distinctions are there between selling human body parts versus human tissue, blood plasma, ova, or sperm?

inmate on death row selling his body parts through an eBay auction is just one bizarre example of the current system (Stepanak, 2000).

Limited Property Interest in Human Material

Corpses and human material have characteristics similar to property in the law. Most courts refuse to overturn traditional notions of a limited property interest in the human body.

Sometimes, the U.S. health care system fails to carry out donors' wishes, and puts patients at risk because health care providers are complacent about what actually happens to corpses and discarded body parts or products. Few ask the body brokers where the human material that sustains this enormous industry comes from. Johnson & Johnson never asked, nor did the U.S. Army as discussed later in this chapter. The National Organ Transplant Act regulates the procurement of organs and transplantable tissue, but it does not regulate human remains used for medical research or medical education.

Through ongoing lawsuits, questions are proliferating about the entire human body parts industry. Unanswered are questions about the liability and benefits of the various willed body programs in the medical schools running such programs, and about the legal status of the medical research community itself. While it is legal to gift body parts to a specific person or entity in private through one's last will and testament, in general, people cannot place restrictions on the gift. As the courts review the human body parts industry and the need for cadavers in medical research and education, the rationale behind the criminality of body parts sales may come under scrutiny, and perhaps undermine the ideals behind willed body programs and medical research on cadavers in general.

Over the past decade, the growth in the human tissue processing market has raised concerns about the transfer of disease during orthopedic and neurosurgical operations. Dr. Mastromarino contributed to those concerns by acknowledging that he sold several tissue samples that were cancerous or infected with the human immunodeficiency virus (HIV) and/or hepatitis, but disguised those facts through fake documentation. The body parts were used in disk replacements, knee operations, dental implants, and other surgical procedures performed by unsuspecting doctors across the U.S. More than ten thousand people received tissue supplied by Medical Tissue Services; the Food and Drug Administration recalled thirteen thousand pieces of tissue.

According to the UAGA, it is illegal to buy and sell the dead. The UAGA provides that a "person may not knowingly, for valuable consideration, purchase or sell an organ for transplantation or therapy, if removal of the organ is intended to occur after the death of the decedent." *See* § 10(a), 8A U.L.A. 58

International Body Broker

Anyone could have found James Cohan, of Sun Valley, California, on the Internet selling organ transplant brokering services. His stated fee was $140,000 for a kidney and $290,000 for a heart, liver, or lung. These fees included hospital and surgeon charges, and flights and accommodations to a network of fifteen or so transplant hospitals he claimed to have cultivated in China, India, the Philippines, South Africa, Singapore, Pakistan, and South America. Cohan's sales pitch was that the quality of the organs was more important than the choice of the physician performing the transplant surgery, and he claimed that he knew how to get fresh organs quickly from healthy, young donors.

Cohan spent several months in an Italian jail in the late 1990s on ultimately unsubstantiated allegations that he was buying and selling organs from South Africa, following an article published in the British medical journal, *Lancet*, that was similar to the articles in *Forbes Sunday Times* (London), and *The Globe* (Canada). In all the interviews, Cohan claimed that his body brokering service, in existence for more than twenty years, was entirely legal; he was simply pairing customers facing certain death if they did not procure organ transplants with hospitals that were equipped to provide organ transplants in the developing world. Cohen claimed that his customers came in at the rate of one a week from all over the Western world. All information about his international business quickly disappeared as soon as the light of day exposed his operation. *See, e.g.*, Morais, 2007.

For a decade after the FBI searched his Hollywood, California, home in 1998 and said his body broker scheme was a fantasy because they could not locate any victims (*e.g.*, Associated Press, 1998), Cohen's international body brokerage operation was repeatedly described in news reports in the U.S., Canada, England, and Scotland. *See, e.g.,* Jones, 2007; Harlow & Bagenal, 2007; Macaskill, 2007.

(2006). However, according to NOTA, it is legal to recuperate "costs" involved in securing, transporting, storing, and harvesting human body parts. NOTA excludes "reasonable payments associated with... the expenses of travel, housing, and lost wages incurred by the donor of a human organ in connection with the donation of the organ" from the definition of *valuable consideration* (42 U.S.C.A. § 274e(c)(2) (2007)). *Costs* is an expansive term; it can mean whatever the body brokers want it to represent. In practice, the loopholes in the UAGA and NOTA mean that bones, tissue, organs, joints, limbs, heads, and even entire torsos are scarce commodities in an international marketplace where the demands of medical researchers, product developers, and physicians far exceed the supply.[LN1] Heads currently sell for upwards of $900, legs for close to $1,000, and hands, feet, and arms for several hundred dollars apiece. According to Organs Watch, a live donor kidney typically trades for:

- $1,500 in the Philippines
- $2,700 in Moldova and Romania
- $7,500 in Turkey
- $10,000 in Peru
- $30,000 in the U.S.

Fully dismembered and eviscerated, a human corpse can generate close to $200,000 on the open market (Wharton, 2006). For the body brokers who supply materials to corporations, research centers, tissue banks, and other health care clients, the profit motive is strong and government oversight is weak. Many families now wonder whether their loved ones may have been sold and resold into the hands of large multinational corporations or used as gruesomely by the U.S. military. The cremation and burial in which they participated may have only been an illusory gesture.

At this point in time, the body parts scandals may discourage donation of cadavers, or cause contracts to be rescinded by those who have willed their corpses to medical research. How all this will affect the manner in which willed body programs function and how medical research companies go about obtaining research subjects in the future cannot be determined. One thing is certain: the issues highlighted in this chapter are what keep many people from signing up to become organ donors, and thus many lives are lost while waiting for a transplant.

Illegal Procurement and Sale of Body Parts

The lawful, as well as the unlawful, procurement and sale of body parts is a complex and confusing interplay of:

- Economic opportunity
- Legal loopholes
- Moral limits
- Scientific innovation

In the absence of medical and moral clarity about the interchange of human biological material, people are left with the corrupting promise of unlimited economic opportunity in exchanging superfluous body parts, and a legal system that is ill equipped to cope with the kind of ethical dilemmas raised by scientific innovation. The disposition of a decedent's remains is a largely unregulated area. While there are federal regulations concerning the funeral industry, there are none dealing with the disposition of remains in particular (Murphy, 2007). Sometimes, body parts are illicitly taken from corpses during autopsies or in morgues and funeral homes before burial in the ground, internment in a vault, or cremation.

Few states inspect crematoria or require crematorium workers to be certified. Regulation in some parts of the country is weak; some states have no regulations at all, and except for Environmental Protection Agency regulations governing emissions from the amalgam fillings in teeth of the corpses (Baga, 2007), many crematoria are unregulated. Cremation services, another thinly regulated business intertwined with the U.S. health care system, are of vital importance to those working in the euthanasia underground or in those states where physician-assisted death is banned. When corpses are cremated, it eliminates the possibility of police, coroners, or other investigatory agencies finding out what drugs were in the patient's body at the time of death (Murphy, 2007).

One California crematorium owner made hundreds of thousands of dollars illicitly dismembering cadavers meant for cremation and then selling the body parts to the highest corporate bidders; he was convicted for mutilation of human remains and embezzlement (Cheney, 2006). The assistants who help pathologists with autopsies and manage morgues are also well positioned to covertly sell body parts. So are undertakers. Often morticians replace the stolen body parts with pieces of plastic or metal pipe, as was done to Alistair Cooke's body, mentioned at the start of this chapter, in order to cover the damage for open casket funerals.

The sale of caskets is more heavily regulated in the U.S. than the state licensing of morticians and funeral home owners (Ellig & Agarwal, 2006). Some states even limit who may sell a casket, which can preclude families from purchasing caskets through entities such as Costco.

Illegal Sale of Cadavers Through University Willed Body Programs

The second, more complicated, form of misconduct involves the trade in corpses from university willed body programs. Donors will their corpses to science,

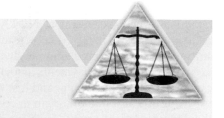

UNAUTHORIZED MUTILATION OF CADAVERS

Gudo v. Administrators of the Tulane Education Fund
[Family Members of Donated Cadavers v. University]
966 So.2d 1069 (Louisiana Court of Appeal, 4th Circuit 2007)

FACTS: The cadavers in question had been sent to the willed body programs at Tulane University's Health Sciences Center for the purpose of medical research and training. Because more bodies were collected than were needed, they were sold to other entities without informing the family members.

The University acknowledged that the U.S. Army acquired cadavers donated to them. Cadavers were allegedly given to New York–based National Anatomical Service, a national distributor of donated cadavers, which then sold them to the Army for between $3,600 and $4,300 per body, according to the Army's Medical Research and Materiel Command in Fort Detrick, Maryland. The cadavers were then blown up in land mine experiments at Fort Sam Houston in San Antonio, Texas. Family members contended that their loved ones' donated cadavers had not been used properly.

ISSUE: Can donated cadavers be used in a manner not authorized by the surviving family members?

HOLDING AND DECISION: The statutory definition of what encompasses an action for the unauthorized desecration and mutilation of a cadaver is broad enough to cover cadavers being blown up in land mind experiments.

ANALYSIS: This case was certified as a class action and will proceed to trial or settlement. The courts will most likely be asked to consider whether the U.S. Army believed surviving family members donated their family members' corpses for this kind of research, or whether this constituted medical research or training.

RULE OF LAW: In order to maintain an action for the unauthorized mutilation of cadavers, the unauthorized mutilation must be negligent or wanton and the surviving family members must have suffered emotional distress as a direct result upon becoming aware of the unauthorized mutilation.

expecting that their cadavers will be delivered to the anatomy laboratories of medical schools, and that, in being dissected, they will help train the next generation of physicians. Most do go this route, but not all.

Louisiana State University, Tulane University, and UCLA were all implicated in the underground traffic of cadavers. They were caught selling body parts to brokers and suppliers who then resold them to independent buyers. All three universities are now involved in ongoing class action lawsuits with regards to their willed body programs.

For years, military researchers bought corpses through this market to use in research involving explosive devices. In the past several years, the U.S. Army has used cadavers to determine safe standoff distances from explosives in tests to determine how to build the best blast shelters, and to improve combat helmets. Along the way, these cadavers make a lot of money for the brokers, suppliers, and vendors who handle them. Needless to say, donors' families are neither informed of that profit nor invited to share in it.

Moral Dilemmas

1. What legal and ethical considerations underlie willed body programs and the human body parts industry itself?

Sale and Transplantation of Contaminated Body Tissue

These two types of misconduct, the illegal procurement and sale of corpses and body parts and the improper use of corpses donated for medical research and training, blur together in another health care problem of systemic proportions: the harvesting of contaminated ligaments, tendons, bones, and other valuable body tissues. Cases of contaminated tissue are rare, but they are making headlines more often. Tissue from one contaminated donor can go to dozens of patients.

The UAGA bans the sale of transplant tissue and the U.S. Food and Drug Administration (FDA) forbids the transplanting of cancerous tissue. The

ILLEGAL TISSUE HARVESTING

Michelli v. Medical Tissue Services (In Re Human Tissue Products Liability Litigation)

[Decedents' Relatives v. Human Material Processing Corporations]

255 F.R.D. 151 (U.S. District Court for the District of New Jersey 2008)

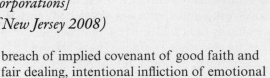

FACTS: Elizabeth Michelli filed a class-action lawsuit against funeral homes and several publicly traded U.S. medical technology companies: Medical Tissue Services, a New Jersey–based human tissue recovery firm; Regeneration Technologies, a Florida-based manufacturer of allograft and xenograft implants formerly affiliated with the University of Florida Tissue Bank; Medtronic, a multinational corporation headquartered in Minnesota; and Spinal Graft Technologies, a Medtronic subsidiary. All are alleged to have harvested tissue for transplant from her husband's corpse without her knowledge or consent.

Michelli's lawsuit is against the for-profit side of the human body parts industry that processes the tissue, as well the nonprofit side that is comprised of the competing mix of tissue banks that make up the backbone of the industry. The lawsuit seeks damages on behalf of the thousands of people whose family members have suffered similar illegal tissue harvesting. She alleges breach of contract, mishandling and desecration of corpses, breach of implied covenant of good faith and fair dealing, intentional infliction of emotional distress, and negligence.

ISSUE: Is the medical products industry lawfully obtaining human body parts from cadavers?

HOLDING AND DECISION: Although litigation is ongoing, this case demonstrates how the pharmaceutical, biotechnology, and medical devices industries are interconnected with the harvesting of human body parts.

ANALYSIS: This case was certified as part of the class action *In Re Human Tissue Products Liability Litigation,* and will proceed to trial or settlement.

RULE OF LAW: New rules of law will emerge as this class action proceeds through the court system, encompassing many of the issues addressed in this chapter.

FDA Center for Biologics Evaluation and Research has a regulatory framework for Human Tissue and Cellular and Tissue Based Products (HCT/Ps) that is designed to prevent the introduction, transmission, or spread of communicable diseases by HCT/Ps. Commercial human tissue recovery firms are required to screen and test donors for relevant communicable disease agents and diseases, and to ensure that HCT/Ps are processed in a way that prevents communicable disease contamination and cross contamination. However, the reality is that the regulations governing donor screening and record-keeping practices are seldom enforced (Buck, 2007):

- Death certificates maintained by human tissue recovery firms often do not match state death certificates regarding the cause of death
- Donors are not always screened for risk factors or clinical evidence of disease agents and diseases
- HCT/Ps are often recovered in a manner that causes contamination

The FDA does not have the investigation or enforcement staff to stop corrupt body brokers who simply change the cause of death on the certificate in order to circumvent the one restriction on transplant tissue, while simply ignoring the other restriction forbidding commercial sales. One untrustworthy operator, using one set of sources to get tissues, can skew the whole regulatory system.

Today, medical technology can transform tissue from cadavers into a variety of skin graft or bone chip implants. Surgeons use implants to repair a wide variety of bone and other tissue defects, including spinal vertebrae repair, musculoskeletal reconstruction, fracture repair, joint repair, and reconstruction for sports medicine injuries. More than a million Americans every year undergo medical procedures that use skin tissue or bone harvested from cadavers (Wharton, 2006). Contaminated and cancerous tissue transplants, however, can injure, infect, and even kill. The corrupt world of global body brokering threatens the health of everyone who receives such transplants.

Laundering of Corpses

When corpses have been sold and resold, it is unclear when the charge of receipt of stolen body parts may be dropped, or if such charges should ever be dropped. When the purchase of body parts is highly separated from the act of theft (for instance, when a large medical research corporation purchases stolen body parts that have already been sold and resold numerous times), can the purchasing corporation be absolved of the earlier crimes, or would this simply encourage a longer chain of transfers before stolen body parts would ever reach the medical research corporation?

The legal principle of *caveat emptor* states that buyers must be aware that what they purchase may be accompanied with legal baggage, but the principle of good faith also excuses those who, even with due diligence, claim ignorance to the stolen nature of their purchase. It is unclear how far each of these legal principles can or should be extended to purchasers of stolen body parts, particularly when many of the middlemen in the procurement chain are linked to large U.S. medical technology corporations or the U.S. military.

Criminal and Civil RICO Liabilities

The federal RICO legislation, originally passed to control organized crime, may create both criminal and civil liabilities against individual health care providers and medical research corporations involved in the underground human body parts industry. RICO does not specifically prohibit the sale of human materials, but rather prohibits the means used to achieve fraudulent ends.

Fraud refers to the deception of another for the purpose of obtaining money or property from them. The UCLA scandal involved the fraudulent sale and receipt of stolen body parts. In other words, at the start of this chapter, Reid sold Nelson cadavers that had been donated to UCLA for medical research and training, who sold the stolen dismembered body parts to Empire for harvesting, who then resold the remains to Mitek for medical research; this chain of business transactions constitutes fraud. While RICO does not deal with the specific business transactions in the body parts industry and does not address the legal and medical questions confronting the sale of human materials, prosecutors are beginning to use this law in an attempt to address some of the scandals in the body parts industry.

If the government proves criminal liability, all parties may be compelled to forfeit any property or money used in the criminal acts or derived from them. This could potentially include all revenue derived from the sale of medical products developed from improperly obtained cadavers. Forfeitures from the sale of medical devices and cosmetics could easily exceed the value of this billion-dollar human body parts industry. This has never occurred, but theoretically, a prosecutor might be able to convince a court that this is what should happen.

RICO also creates civil liability. In theory, donors' families could seek treble damages from both individuals and corporations for violating RICO. In other words, a judgment could conceivably be rendered for three times the harm actually suffered, plus legal fees. This is the part that frightens the middlemen and makes them turn over information on the big medical technology corporations to law enforcement.

One might ask what could constitute a RICO violation in the human body parts industry. Hypothetically, it could be argued that RICO prohibits using two or more racketeering acts to accomplish:

- Acquiring legitimate body parts that were stolen from donated cadavers
- Maintaining tissue processing organizations and medical research organizations through acceptance of stolen body parts
- Operating a body parts business with resold body parts that never should have been commoditized

A two-step process could be used to prove that individuals and corporations violated RICO, whether it would be a criminal prosecution or a civil lawsuit.

First, it would have to be shown that two or more racketeering acts were committed, which would be any of a list of specified criminal acts, including theft, sale, and receipt of stolen property, and fraud. Thus, if stolen body parts were accepted from one donated cadaver, and later additional body parts are sold from another donated cadaver, that commercial exchange would constitute two racketeering acts.

Second, it must be shown that the racketeering acts were used to accomplish one or more of the above three purposes. If stolen corpses were sold to a body broker, who brokered a sale for harvesting of the body parts, who then resold the remains for medical research, this would violate RICO.

Moral Dilemmas

1. What legal and ethical considerations are behind the criminality of human body parts sales?

2. Is the trading of human body parts different from slavery and prostitution? If so, what is the distinction?

MEDICAL RESEARCH AND DEVELOPMENT OF MEDICAL TECHNOLOGIES

This chapter is more than an inquiry into criminal law and the resale of stolen property for medical research and development of new medical technologies. It raises concerns about the purpose and value behind organ procurement and transplantation and the role of the U.S. medical research community.

Though the idea of placing a price on corpses and body parts as products may be objectionable to some people, this commoditized value must be weighed against the intangible value of human lives. Although cadavers are bought and sold as commodities, this commodity market is used for the benefit of the living.

Cadavers and body parts, though they may be illegally bought and sold, are often ultimately used in medical research. However, as new medical technologies are continually developed, more and more human tissues, such as skin, bones, heart valves, embryos, and stem cell lines, are being stored and distributed for therapeutic and research purposes in a hidden market with few regulations and great opportunities for financial gain. It is arguably unfair that neither the decedents' estates nor their families are receiving any of this profit.

The health law issue that must be addressed is whether the lack of an open, free market for cadavers and body parts affects medical research and its potential lifesaving ability. Right now, several class-action lawsuits are focusing on those that deal in cadavers and body parts: the body brokers who supply materials to medical technology corporations, research centers, tissue banks, and other health care clients; the companies that process tissue and parts for sale; and the hospitals that do business with all these players. There is no oversight of hospitals involved in the human body parts industry; it remains to be seen what, if any, sanctions will be imposed on hospitals involved in the *Human Tissue Products Liability Litigation* described throughout this chapter.

It should be remembered that physicians and dentists treat patients frequently with medical products made from these cadavers and dismembered

The Challenge to Think About the Societal Costs of Ignoring the Body Parts Industry

In Claire Denis's 2005 film *L'Intrus*, the protagonist is an active man who has lived an isolated existence on the French-Swiss border. As he ages and becomes ill with a weak heart, he begins to recognize his own physical vulnerability and decides to purchase a new heart (and transplant surgery) from the international black market in organs and organ transplants. He travels to Geneva, Switzerland, to pay for the transplant, where he meets a woman in a hotel room, to whom he gives his order for a young heart. Scenes of him moving with ease through a number of countries in order to accomplish his project are intercut with scenes of attempts at illicit border crossings, both by individuals engaged in illegal imports smuggling and undocumented immigrants.

The film, however, does not operate only at the level of the story of the purchase of a heart; the heart transplant is a symbol of the effects of the human body parts industry. It highlights the inequalities that exist in an open market through which the privileged can move with ease and can benefit and challenges us to think about what it means to take from others for our own personal benefit. This challenge is presented in the film through two images. First, Denis presents the image of the heart as an intruder in the host body, as she forces us to ask:

• Does the new heart, as such a dominant organ, change the old person?
• Is identity, the sense of self, changed?
• Will the new heart be willing to operate as part of the old body?
• Will the old body refuse the new heart?

Second, Denis presents the cost of such a transaction through the image of the contract for the new heart. Having paid the full price demanded for the heart, the protagonist in the film is thrown off balance when he realizes the woman to whom he paid the money keeps reappearing at different locations; it seems that she is following him. When he confronts her, reminding her that he has already paid the price for the heart, she tells him that he will never finish paying. She has become not only a continual reminder of his heart transplant, but also his own memory of that which he can never escape; she is now as much a part of him as his transplanted heart. In the final moments of the film, when the credits roll on the screen, her role is named as the "angel of death."

—L'Intrus (Ognon Pictures 2005). This film was inspired by Jean-Luc Nancy's 2000 meditation on his own heart transplant, also entitled *L'Intrus*.

body parts. As medical researchers continue to push the frontiers of science, it will become even more critical to strike a balance between stronger legal scrutiny of transactions involving corpses on the one hand and, on the other hand, allowing medical research corporations the freedom to develop lifesaving technologies without the burden and cost resulting from excessive regulation.

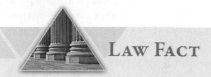

LAW FACT

WILLED BODY PROGRAMS

Can body parts lawfully obtained from cadavers that are donated to universities for medical research be subsequently sold to third parties?

Truth be told, it is an open secret. Only university willed body programs dispose of the human materials, without calling the transaction a sale, and then collect procurement, transport, and storage costs. The legal and financial repercussions of designating body parts as medical waste, then recycling the human material for medical research, is a subject that is just beginning to come under investigation. In what has come to be known as part of the body parts scandal, the problems at the UCLA willed body program are drawing attention to complex issues surrounding cadaver donation and the sale of human body parts, as well as the medical research industry generally. Indications are that the UCLA incident is part of a larger problem in the procurement sector of the human body parts industry, which is certainly not limited to the U.S. The *Human Tissue Products Liability Litigation* outlined in this chapter will draw attention to this emerging controversy as the facts of the underground body parts trade are revealed in open courts of law.

—*See e.g., Cohen v. NuVasive, Inc.,* 79 Cal.Rptr.3d 759 (Court of Appeal, 2nd District, Division 3, California 2009); *see also* Goodwin, 2006; Goodwin, 2006a.

CHAPTER SUMMARY

- Human body parts and products are used for medical research, medical teaching, medical treatment, consumer product testing, and for military purposes.
- There is a billion-dollar body parts and products industry; some experts estimate that the underground market is worth at least $150 million.
- The NOTA regulates the procurement of human organs and transplantable tissue, but it does not regulate human remains used for research and education.
- The UAGA prohibits the buying and selling of corpses and bans the sale of human transplant tissue.
- While people can donate their bodies or body parts to a specific person or entity, they cannot place restrictions on the gift's uses.
- It is legal to recuperate costs involved in securing, transporting, storing, and harvesting human body parts.
- There are two distinct forms of misconduct in the human body parts industry: the procurement, harvesting, and sale of body parts from the dead who never consented to be willed donors, and the trade in corpses of willed donors who did consent, but not to that particular purpose.
- Recently, several scandals have come to light involving harvesting body parts from the dead without consent from either the deceased's last will and testament or the surviving family members, and then sold for profit; all of the pieces of a corpse combined can generate up to $200,000.
- The other kind of scandal that has recently emerged involves universities selling corpses or body parts and products that were donated with the intent of being used for research or teaching purposes, rather than being sold for profit.

- The FDA forbids the transplanting of human tissue contaminated with cancer or other communicable diseases; one major problem with the underground trade of such products is that they are often contaminated.
- The theory of *caveat emptor* states that buyers must be aware that what they purchase may be accompanied by legal problems.
- When the ultimate purchase is highly separated from the initial act of theft, purchasers may be absolved of procurers' earlier crimes.
- In commercial sales, the principle of good faith excuses buyers who, even with due diligence, can claim ignorance to the stolen nature of their purchase.
- RICO creates both criminal and civil liabilities, with the potential of being assessed treble damages.
- In theory, if the government proves criminal liability under RICO, all parties involved may be compelled to forfeit any property or money used in the racketeering acts or derived from them.
- The lack of an open free market for human cadavers and body parts hinders medical research and its potential lifesaving ability.
- A legalized market for body parts and products may minimize the underground trade, but ethical concerns surrounding the commoditization of the human body have hindered progress toward such a market.

LAW NOTES

1. Despite the regulatory schemes under the UAGA and NOTA, organs are bought and sold on black markets. Traffic in organs from executed Chinese prisoners or the poor in Brazil, Russia, India, and other less developed, poor nations is well documented. The Institute of Medicine's report on organ donation discusses a study of individuals in Chennai, India, who sold kidneys to pay off debt. Ultimately, these organ transplants resulted in poor outcomes for all involved. There were complications, including sepsis, hepatitis B, and liver cirrhosis, as well as other complications in those who received the organs, and there were no long-term benefits to the donors, as their health deteriorated without adequate follow-up care. *See e.g.*, Cheney, 2006; Childress & Liverman, 2006; Goodwin, 2006, 2006a.

CHAPTER BIBLIOGRAPHY

Associated Press. (1998, November 7). FBI agents' searches alleged organ broker's Hollywood home.

Baga, K. M. (2007). Taking a bite out of the harmful effects of mercury in dental fillings: Advocating for national legislation for mercury amalgams. *Journal of Law & Health, 20,* 169-197.

Blue, A. E. (2008). Redefining stewardship over body parts. *Journal of Law & Health, 21,* 75-121.

Buck, L. A. (2007). Regulating human tissue banks. *St. Thomas Law Review, 20,* 121-153.

Calandrillo, S. P. (2004). Cash for kidneys? Utilizing incentives to end America's organ shortage. *George Mason Law Review, 13,* 69-133.

Cheney, A. (2006). *In body brokers: Inside America's underground trade in human remains.* New York, NY: Broadway (a chronicle of how corpses are procured, processed, marketed, and used in the U.S.; of the human body parts industry that lacks oversight; of the limited supply of corpses and the endless demand for body parts; and of body brokers and the altruistic donors that hospitals, physicians, and scientists take advantage of).

Childress, J. F., & Liverman, C. T. (2006). *Organ donation.* Washington, DC: Institute of Medicine.

Clamon, J. B. (2008). Tax policy as a lifeline: Encouraging blood and organ donation through tax credits. *Annals of Health Law, 17,* 67-99.

Ellig, J., & Agarwal, A. (2006). Buried online: State laws that limit e-commerce in caskets. *Elder Law Journal, 14* (2), 283-330 (discussing variations in state casket sales laws).

Goodwin, M. (2006). *Black markets: The supply and demand of body parts.* New York, NY: Cambridge University Press (case law is used to describe how the willed body system, based on altruistic donations, has failed to meet the need for body parts).

___. (2006a). Formalism and the legal status of body parts. *University of Chicago Legal Forum, 26,* 317-388 (examines whether there is a remedy for stealing body parts, an answer that is dependent on whether body parts are defined as property, products, mere possessions, borrowed vessels belonging to the state, or services).

___. (2004). Altruism's limits: Law, capacity, and organ commoditization. *Rutgers Law Review, 56,* 305-406 (medical corporations heavily invest in body parts in order to obtain their own intellectual property rights).

Handwerk, B. (2004, January 16). Organ shortage fuels illicit trade in human parts. *National Geographic.*

Harlow, J., & Bagenal, F. (2007, January 28). NHS patients buy organs from Third World. *The Sunday Times (London),* p. 27.

Harris, J. (2003). Organ procurement: Dead interests, living needs. *Journal of Medical Ethics, 29,* 130-134 (notes that while cadaveric interests deserve some respect, such interests are weak when compared with the interests of the living persons who will be harmed in person by neglect of their interests).

Harrison, C. H. (2002). Neither *Moore* nor the market: Alternative models for compensating contributors of human tissue. *American Journal of Law & Medicine, 28,* 77-105 (explores the financial discrepancies in the human body parts industry and notes how medical researchers and medical products companies gross substantial profits from the remains of donated cadavers, but the donors rarely see any of these proceeds).

Haustein, S.V., & Sellers, M.T. (2004). Factors associated with (un)willingness to be an organ donor: Importance of public exposure and knowledge. *Clinical Transplant 18,* 193-200.

Jones. D. (2007, March 25). Organ failure. *The People* (London), p. 16 (claims that one-third of the patients who have organ transplants overseas either die or suffer donor organ failure as opposed to a one-in-ten failure rate in England).

Kahn, J. P., & Delmonico, F. L. (2004). The consequences of public policy to buy and sell organs for transplantation. *American Journal of Transplantation, 4* (2), 178-180 (the business of saving lives can thrive if tissues and cadaveric organs enter an open marketplace where commercial transactions are regulated).

Macaskill, M. (2007, May 20). Scots fuel & pound. *The Sunday Times* (London), p. 16.

Mayne, J. (2005, July 1). Foreign bodies in the films of Claire Denis. *Chronicle of Higher Education,* p. 10.

Mitford, J. (2006). *The American way of death revisited.* New York, NY: Knopf (classic investigative research that served as the catalyst for the Federal Trade Commission's passage of a regulation entitled Funeral Industry Practices, commonly known today as the Funeral Rule).

Moses, L. B. (2008). The applicability of property law in new contexts: From cells to cyberspace. *Sydney Law Review, 30,* 639-662.

Morais, R. C. (2007, January 29). Desperate arrangements. *Forbes, 1* (2), 72.

Murphy, A. M. (2007). Please don't bury me down in that cold ground: The need for uniform laws on the disposition of human remains. *Elder Law Journal, 15,* 381-471.

Roach, M. (2004). *STIFF: The curious lives of human cadavers.* New York, NY: W. W. Norton & Company (describing the University of Tennessee Forensic Anthropology Facility that studies the decomposition and insect infestation of decaying bodies to better enable law enforcement to identify bodies and establish times of death and causes of death).

Scheper-Hughes, N. (2007). Kidney kin: Inside the transatlantic transplant trade (underground markets). *Harvard International Review, 27,* 62-66 (exposes the global trade of body brokers, citing the names of towns in Asia known as kidney zones, where the sale of human body parts is legal, and where many locals bear scars marking the removal of their organs for American and European transplant patients).

Scheper-Hughes, N., & Wacquant, L. (2003). *Commodifying bodies.* Thousand Oaks, CA: Sage Publications (covers the cultural disposal and media treatment of corpses; the biopolitics of cells, sperm banks, and eugenics; the international trafficking of kidneys; and the development of transplant tourism).

Sharp, L. A. (2006). *Strange harvest: Organ transplants, denatured bodies, and the transformed self.* Berkeley, CA: University of California Press (focuses on the issue of body commoditization from an anthropological perspective).

___. (2006a) *Bodies, commodities, and biotechnologies: Death, mourning, and scientific desire in the realm of human organ transfer.* New York, NY: Columbia University Press (three essays on organ transplantation, procurement, and donation).

Stepanak, M. (2000, November 20). Making a killing online. *Business Week,* p. B84 (reporting that an inmate on death row sold parts of his body through an auction on eBay).

Struve, C. T. (2008). Greater and lesser powers of tort reform: The primary jurisdiction doctrine and state-law claims concerning FDA-approved products. *Cornell Law Review, 93,* 1039-1073.

Veatch, R. M. (2003). Why liberals should accept financial incentives for organ procurement. *Kennedy Institute of Ethics Journal, 13,* 19-36 (explains why it is unethical for society to withhold the assistance needed by many poor people, while depriving them of the ability to market the one valuable commodity they possess).

Waldby, C., & Mitchell, R. (2006). *Tissue economies: Blood, organs, and cell lines in late capitalism.* Durham, NC: Duke University Press (examines the ethical and social implications of tissue transfers and the networks in which such transfers occur; draws a distinction between tissue as a gift, to be exchanged in transactions that are separate from commercial markets, and tissues that are commodities, that are to be traded for profit).

Wharton (Wharton School at the University of Pennsylvania). (2006). The billion-dollar body parts industry: Medical research alongside greed and corruption. *Knowledge@ Wharton.*

CHAPTER 25

ORGAN AND TISSUE PROCUREMENT AND TRANSPLANTATION

"Our bodies are our gardens to which our wills are gardeners."

—WILLIAM SHAKESPEARE (1564-1616), ENGLISH POET
AND PLAYWRIGHT, FROM *OTHELLO*

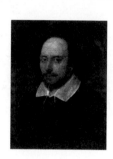

IN BRIEF

This chapter describes the process of organ and tissue transplantation as it relates to donors and recipients. Organs represent one of the most highly regulated and cumbersome fields involving human biological materials, as well as one of the more publicly visible uses of body parts. Regulation of the tissues industry lacks this public visibility and, consequently, consistent oversight. This chapter explains the principles and flaws of organ and tissue transplantation. Proposals to increase the number of patients receiving organ transplants are also reviewed. The legal process itself and its accompanying ethical arguments for and against the sale of donated organs and tissues are discussed.

Presumed consent, directed donations, commodification, and xenotransplantation, or the transplantation of cells, tissues, and whole organs across species, offer future alternatives for enhancement of the supply of body parts. Xenotransplantation poses greater risk to human health and is far too premature to guarantee success. None of these alternatives is without controversy.

FACT OR FICTION

MEDICAID COVERAGE FOR A LIVER TRANSPLANT: CURE OR DISEASE MANAGEMENT?

Must a state's taxpayers pay for a liver transplant to cure a hereditary disease if the disease can be treated by dietary management?

Physicians at the Children's Hospital of Pittsburgh determined an eight-year-old child with a genetic disorder known as Maple Syrup Urine Disease (MSUD) could only be cured with a liver transplant. The Missouri Medicaid program declined to cover the liver transplant and maintained the child's MSUD had been well-managed by diet. Children with MSUD are unable to metabolize essential amino acids used by the body to build proteins. As a result, children with the disease must restrict their intake of natural proteins, replacing them with daily intake of a special MSUD amino acid formula. When affected children become ill with a routine viral or bacterial illness or are unable to maintain their special diet, they are at risk for severe metabolic decomposition with neurological deterioration, brain swelling, coma, permanent brain injury, and death. Even with dietary management, metabolic decomposition can occur.

The medical community was split over the medical necessity of a liver transplant when a child's condition was well-managed with dietary treatment. Given the risks associated with a liver transplant, there was disagreement over the possible outcomes of the child's treatment.

—*J.D. v. Sherman*, 2006 WL 3163053 (U.S. District Court for the Western District of Missouri, Central Division 2006).

(See *Law Fact* at the end of this chapter for the answer.)

PRINCIPLES AND APPLICATIONS[LN1]

The primary need for human body parts is for the transplantation of organs, tissues, and cells into humans. A secondary need for human body parts is for medical research in regenerative medicine, especially in stem cell and gene-based therapy (HHS, 2006). Human organ transplantation can be used to treat diseases of the heart, lungs, liver, kidneys, and pancreas, which are some of the most common causes of infirmity and death. Organ failure and tissue loss account for almost $400 billion in U.S. health care costs today, particularly among older adults (GIA, 2008). This cost covers approximately eight million surgical procedures to treat these disorders, as well as recurring treatments for related chronic diseases and their subsequent complications (HHS, 2006).

Treatment needs for organ failure and tissue loss are expected to increase as the average age of the population increases (Platt et al., 2004), including the need for:

- Transplantations
- Surgical reconstructions
- Mechanical devices (mechanical kidneys rather than dialysis machines)

While each of these treatments has its own limitations, of the three treatments, transplantation of organs and tissues has the greatest potential to treat:

- Gross organ failure, such as renal failure
- Chronic conditions like diabetes (through regeneration of insulin-producing tissue) and Parkinson's disease
- Congenital conditions such as hemophilia
- Acquired conditions such as cancer (by replacing the removed cancerous tissue with externally grown healthy tissue)

Organ transplantation is often the only treatment for end-stage organ failure, such as liver and heart failure.

TYPES OF TRANSPLANTATION AND LIMITATIONS

There are three types of transplantation: autotransplantation, allotransplantation, and xenotransplatation. The first two are used extensively; the third is developing amidst rigid regulations.

Autotransplantation

Autotransplantation is a process through which human material is harvested and subsequently transplanted from one part of an individual's body to another. The limitations associated with autografts (the material used in autotransplantation) include the availability of human material as well as donor site diseases.

The most litigated issue in this type of transplant involves insurance coverage for bone marrow autotransplants in the mid-1990s (Jagger, 2006). For more than a decade, the medical community generally thought bone marrow transplants produced remissions in advanced breast cancer patients unresponsive to conventional therapy. While some states mandated coverage, insurers often excluded coverage of the bone marrow transplant procedure as experimental treatment or as medically unnecessary. After a decade of controversy, medical studies concluded the procedure was in fact ineffective and even potentially harmful (Jacobson, 2007).

Allotransplantation

Allotransplantation occurs where human material is harvested from one individual and subsequently transplanted to another individual. The challenges associated with allogeneic grafts (cells, tissues, or organs involved in allotransplantation) covered in this chapter include:

- Donor-recipient blood type compatibility
- Donor-recipient physical compatibility (organ size, capacity, and lifespan)
- Damage to donor organs and tissue during the transport process
- Transmission of donor site diseases to recipients (human immunodeficiency virus (HIV), as well as hepatitis B and C viruses)
- Rejection of immunologically incompatible organs and tissues
- Use and long-term cost of immunosuppressive drugs to circumvent transplant immunorejection
- Shortage of organs and tissue

(Brody, 2007)

Xenotransplantation

Xenotransplantation is the use of animal materials to replace human cells, tissues, or organs. A central limitation is the risk of transmission of novel viral and microbial pathogens from donor xenografts to human recipients, known as xenozoonoses. For instance, diseases that began in non-human animals, but that now affect humans include mad cow disease, HIV/AIDS (from monkeys), hantavirus pulmonary syndrome (from

mammals), avian flu (from chickens, ducks, and geese), the influenza virus of 1918 (from birds), swine flu (from pigs), swine flu (from pigs), Ebola, herpes, hepatitis B and C, and rabies. Not surprisingly, rejection is a more significant issue with interspecies transplantation. While litigation is just beginning to emerge for these transplants, the Campaign for Responsible Transplantation has been engaged in the federal courts since the late 1990s for freedom-of-information demands for proprietary information about the FDA's regulation of xenotransplantation.

ORGAN TRANSPLANTATION

The law addressing organ transplantation is vast, contradictory, and complex. How to treat organ transplants is far from obvious, as case law and regulations are to a large extent conflicted over the best approach to apply in allocating a scarce resource (Buck, 2007). Each potential framework for organ transplants offers appealing aspects, but each also has difficulty in meeting all of the concerns surrounding the use of human biological material.

Organ transplantation is not a new scientific concept, although several important medical advances have occurred recently, allowing for more successful transplants in terms of recipient survival and improved quality of life. Eighteenth-century experimentation with animal organ transplants led to the early human organ transplants. The first actual documented human organ transplants began to occur with some regularity in the 1950s and 1960s.

Tissue typing dramatically improved the survival odds for transplant patients. Organs that can be transplanted from corpses include kidneys, skin, corneas, livers, hearts, pancreata, lungs, intestines, bone marrow, heart valves, and connective tissue. Living donors can donate part of the liver, part of the lung, a kidney, and bone marrow (Meckler, 2007c). Over three-quarters of transplants come from people who indicate their desire to be organ donors after death by either signing a directive or directing their personal representative to allow for donation (Truog, 2005).

Current Context

The remarkable potential for saving lives with organ transplantation is severely constrained by the failure of regulatory policy to keep pace with technological advances in medicine (Buck, 2007). Cadaveric organ procurement policies in the U.S. and other countries have failed to effectively

Important Transplant Developments

- 1869—first tissue transplant
- 1911—first human-to-human organ transplant was conducted in the U.S.
- 1954—first "successful" human-to-human organ transplant was performed in the U.S. (a living donor donated his kidney to his identical twin)
- 1968—first heart transplant
- 1968—Uniform Anatomical Gift Act (UAGA) legalized donating tissues and organs (*see* Uniform Anatomical Gift Act (UAGA) of 1968, U.L.A. §§ 1-11 (1968); UAGA of 1987, U.L.A. §§ 1-17 (1987); UAGA of 2006, §§ 1-27 (2006) (every state has adopted its own version of the 1968 UAGA; some states later adopted newer versions of the UAGA))
- 1983—FDA approval of the first anti-rejection drug, cyclosporine, a drug that helps stop transplant organ or tissue rejection from the recipient's body and thus improves the recipient's chance of survival
- 1984—National Organ Transplantation Act (NOTA), which rendered it unlawful to "knowingly acquire, receive, or otherwise transfer any human organ for valuable consideration for use in human transplantation if the transfer affects interstate commerce" (*see* National Organ Transplant Act of 1984, 42 U.S.C.A. §§ 274-274e (2009) (§ 274e is named for Charlie W. Norwood, the late congressman from Georgia (1941-2007), who underwent a lung transplant and who was an avid advocate of patients' rights))
- 1986—Congress established the Organ Procurement and Transplantation Network (Organ Network), which sets standards and regulates organ transplant centers across the country; the Organ Network establishes the process and policies for allocating organs through the federal contractor that operates the network, the United Network for Organ Sharing (NOTA § 274)
- 1988—Joint Commission on Accreditation of Healthcare Organizations (JCAHO) sets donor standards and requires hospital policies and procedures for organ and tissue procurement
- 1996—Congress authorized the dissemination of organ donation information along with income tax refunds to approximately seventy million households to increase awareness and encourage organ donation; state tax agencies followed the federal example soon after
- 1999—Organ Network Final Rule (*see* 42 C.F.R. §§ 121.1-121.12 (2007))
- 2000—Children's Health Act established the National Center on Birth Defects and Developmental Disabilities (*see* Children's Health Act of 2000, 42 U.S.C.A. § 247b-4 (2003))
- 2004—Organ Donation and Recovery Improvement Act to provide funding for transplant centers and qualified organ procurement organizations to increase the rate of organ donations (*see* Organ Donation and Recovery Improvement Act of 2004, 42 U.S.C.A. §§ 273a, 274f-1-274f-4 (2004))
- 2007—Norwood Living Organ Donation Act (Norwood) codified a U.S. Justice Department ruling intended to increase the number of patients receiving paired kidney transplants by ensuring that criminal penalties do not apply (NOTA § 274e)

Sources: HHS, 2005; Kaserman, 2007.

respond to the growing demand for transplantable organs that has resulted from significant strides achieved in immunosuppressive therapy (Kaserman, 2007).

The result of this regulatory policy failure has been a chronic and growing shortage of human organs available for transplantation (Brody, 2007). As of late 2009, there were over 105,000 people awaiting organ donations on the Organ Network's candidate waiting list. Competing ideals surround the entire process of organ procurement and transplantation. Current legislation regulating the process is unable to reconcile practical necessities

with ethical considerations, resulting in a demand for transplantable organs that far exceeds the available supply.

Of all transplantable organs, the shortage of kidneys is the most acute (Brody, 2007). More than three-quarters of the wait list population is comprised of people suffering from renal failure, also called end-stage renal disease (ESRD). Over eighty-two thousand people are waiting for kidneys. Presumably, a central financial authority could pay for these kidney transplants from tax revenues, such as Medicare's ESRD Program for dialysis and transplant services. Recent analysis suggests that taxpayers could save money with this approach so long as the cost was less than $90,000 (Brennan, 2007).

Another 16,500 people or so are waiting for livers (Barshes, 2007). The rest are waiting for pancreata, intestine, heart, or lung transplants. Many people are waiting for more than one kind of organ. Over 450,000 transplants have been performed in the U.S. to date. The number of people who need transplants is growing at about five times faster than the rate of donations.

About 6,700 Americans die waiting for transplant operations each year. Only about fifteen thousand people a year die under circumstances that would make them suitable donors for lifesaving transplants. However, these deaths could help *more* than fifteen thousand people live because each person can donate multiple needed organs. Patients generally wait five years for donated organs, and on average, seventeen of them die each day.

Although most Americans claim to approve of organ donation and transplantation, only about one in four expressly declare themselves organ donors. Clearly the demand for organs far exceeds the supply and much could be done to alleviate the shortage, such as relaxing the restrictions on who can donate, clarifying the misunderstandings surrounding organ donation, and perhaps even compensating donors or their families (Brody, 2007). Whatever approach is chosen, it is worth keeping in mind that the U.S. is among eleven countries listed by the World Health Organization as organ importers, meaning that a relatively high number of citizens get organs from someone from another nation.

Moral Dilemmas

1. Can we confine our arguments about health care efficiency to organ transplants, or can one argue that other types of medical treatments and health care services are also scarce?

2. Is the shortage of organs available for transplantation one health care problem that could be solved by unlimited funding of the health care system?

In Theory: How Organ Procurement and Transplantation Occur

The federal Health Resources Services Administration oversees the transplantation of human organs. To address the nation's critical organ donation shortage and improve the organ matching and placement

process, Congress passed NOTA. NOTA makes it illegal to sell human organs and tissues and imposes fines and imprisonment for doing so.

Congress went on to institutionalize a complex system of nonprofit organizations solely responsible for collecting and allocating all transplantable organs. NOTA provided for the establishment of the Organ Network, which administers the retrieval, distribution, and transplantation of organs. All U.S. transplant centers and organ procurement organizations must be members of the Organ Network in order to receive any funds through Medicare. Currently, there are about 200 transplant centers for kidney transplants (NKF, 2008), 150 for heart transplants, and 100 for liver transplants.

The Organ Network also standardizes the criteria for placement on distribution lists and maintains a national registry for organ matching. The U.S. Department of Health and Human Services (HHS) established the Organ Network and contracted its management out to the United Network for Organ Sharing (UNOS), a private, nonprofit entity. UNOS maintains a secure, Web-based computer system that stores the nation's organ transplant waiting list and matches recipient and donated organ characteristics. The organ matching and placement process is facilitated by a fully staffed Organ Center, which operates twenty-four hours a day.

Despite all this legislation and accompanying regulatory oversight, there are still many problems with the Organ Network (Buck, 2007). Some of the criticisms are that it fails to detect or fix problems at some transplant centers, and when there is a problem, the investigation is slow and its findings are kept secret. Problem transplant centers are almost never sanctioned, or very weak sanctions are imposed. Furthermore, the Organ Network is unable to police itself because it is essentially a network based on membership, with no overarching supervision. Transplant centers are able to find ways around transplant rules, and patients are often not informed about a particular center's transplant policies or outcomes. The federal government has previously sued the Organ Network and has threatened to become more involved in its oversight. In response to some of the criticisms, the Organ Network maintains it is better to privately resolve conflict in order to better protect the public's interests.

Several studies have revealed that nearly every organ procurement organization is in violation of at least one UNOS policy on the distribution of organs (Childress, 2006). In response, more regulations were adopted allowing the federal government additional control and further limitations over how organs are allocated. Any new policies UNOS proposes must be approved by HHS, and it often takes a decade or more for policy changes to become effective. The 1999 regulations that became effective fifteen years after NOTA was adopted by Congress sought to establish a standardized method of distributing donated organs to patients on transplant waiting lists and also made organ transplant data more available to the public.

Prior to 1999, organs were retained in the geographic area where they were obtained if a transplant patient was also waiting in that area. This meant the waiting time for organs varied widely between geographic regions, and patients with a more urgent need or with a better chance of survival often were denied organs. For example, the waiting time for a liver in one region was as low as 20 days, while in another region, it was as high as 443 days. The thinking behind this policy was that organs could be better preserved and patient costs could be kept to a minimum if transplants remained localized. The 1999 regulations allocated organs based on medical urgency and patient appropriateness, with the goal of making wait times more even across the country.

There are many different people on a patient's transplant team. Clinical transplant coordinators oversee patient evaluation, treatment, and follow-up care. Transplant physicians manage patient medical care, tests, and medications. Transplant surgeons perform the actual transplant surgery and follow-up medical care. Financial coordinators organize and clarify the financial aspects of patient care before, during, and after the transplant. Finally, social workers help patients and their families cope with the issues associated with the transplant, including any illness or side effects.

Moral Dilemmas

1. What is the justification underlying laws restricting accepting or offering payment for transplant organs?

2. What legal distinction is there between selling human organs versus human tissues, blood plasma, ova, and sperm?

3. What practical considerations support or detract from legally regulating organ procurement and transplantation?

United Network for Organ Sharing

The first step in the transplant process is that the physician and transplant center decide whether and when to place a patient on the UNOS computer registry. According to the Scientific Registry of Transplant Recipients, located at the University of Michigan,

statistics show age is by far the biggest factor predicting how long someone will live after a transplant.

Organs are currently allocated based on a point system that considers how long the patient has been on the donor list and how urgent the patient's medical status is. For kidneys, it is proposed that time on the donor list be substituted with time on dialysis; time on the donor list would be a secondary factor in allocating kidneys, particularly for the best quality kidneys. This regulatory change would favor healthier patients over those who may be too ill to benefit from the transplantation, a change that has already been adopted for livers, hearts, and lungs.

Under the proposed scenario, the healthiest kidneys would be distributed through a formula relying largely on net benefit, while the formula for kidneys coming from older or sicker donors would give greater weight to time on dialysis. Already, kidneys from donors under age thirty-five are automatically offered first to children under eighteen if any are on a waiting list (Meckler, 2007b).

Many factors affect how long a patient may be on the organ transplant waiting list, such as the:

- Patient's blood type, tissue type, height, and weight
- Size of available organs
- Transplant center's criteria for accepting donated organs
- Number of organs available for donation

While potential donors who die in a hospital have the best chance of donating viable organs (because organs have to be harvested almost immediately after death), alternatives are arising to address this issue. New York City has special organ recovery ambulances that travel to the homes of people who die suddenly (Goldstein, 2008). With improved medical technologies, Cold Ischemic Times have been extended to allow for truly national allocations. Cold Ischemic Time is the time interval that begins when an organ is cooled with a solution after organ procurement surgery and ends when the organ is implanted.

Moral Dilemmas

1. Would it be permissible to remove the organs of healthy, deceased prisoners to save the lives of five to eight others who need organ transplants?

2. Under what circumstances might palliative sedation facilitate organ transplants?

Factors that do *not* affect the waiting time are gender, religion, financial status, and the willingness of recipients to someday donate their own organs.

The patient's physician has a considerable amount of discretion in deciding how to list the patient on the registry. The federal government has previously investigated listing practices at major hospitals, such as the University of Chicago and the University of Illinois, where physicians were accused of exaggerating their patients' medical urgency status. The hospitals denied the allegations and settled with the government.

There are no uniform criteria for deciding when to list patients for transplantation or for identifying patients' medical urgency status. Moreover, medical criteria differ with each organ; certain organs require extensive prescreening to find a positive match for a patient, while different organs remain viable before transplant for different periods of time. In addition, UNOS encourages physicians to consider non-medical factors such as whether patients have:

- Organ failure caused by their own behavior (diseases tied to smoking, drinking, or unhealthy diet and exercise patterns, among other lifestyle factors) (Platt et al., 2004)
- Complied with and adhered to their treatment regimen
- Received prior organ transplants
- Had or might have success with treatment other than a transplant (adults with MSUD, for example)

The UNOS Ethics Committee suggests non-medical factors used to evaluate transplant candidates should be monitored and updated to reflect changes in technology and medicine, and to minimize subjectivity. For example, African Americans are much more likely than Caucasians to have blood type B, but there are not as many B organ donors, a major obstacle for African Americans waiting for kidney transplants (NKF, 2008). To resolve this disparity, it is proposed that certain blood type A kidneys, which work effectively in both A and B patients, be made available to patients with blood type B.

Non-Governmental Networks

There is an ideological and practical divide between UNOS and the medical community concerning the procedures and criteria for allocating organs, as well as the procedures for reviewing the organ allocation system. The root of this disagreement appears to be how to deal with scarcity. Regulatory policy decisions determining who receives the limited number of organs have crucial consequences for patients. These are medical decisions that might better be made by the medical community rather than the government. It should be noted this does not imply UNOS is ineffective, but only suggests that commercial networks may better allocate scarce organs on a competitive basis.

Recently, Aetna developed the national Cofinity Institute of Excellence network comprised of facilities that manage heart, lung, simultaneous heart/lung, kidney, liver, pancreas, simultaneous kidney/pancreas, small bowel/intestinal, bone marrow, and stem cell transplants. All of the facilities in the Aetna network have met quality, volume, and outcomes standards through Aetna's credentialing process and external quality guidelines, such as those established by organizations such as Medicare and UNOS. Commercial developments like this may produce a change in how organ procurement and transplantation occur and more closely parallel the rapid advances occurring with tissue transplantations.

Donation Criteria

Non-directed donations, or donations by strangers, account for less than 1 percent of live kidney donations in the U.S. (Lobas, 2006). Donors themselves must usually be eighteen years of age or older, unless a parent or guardian of a deceased minor consents to donation. Donors must have written documentation of their wish to donate, such as a signed donor card or indication on their license. If a deceased person did not consent to donation prior to their death, a spouse, adult child, parent, adult sibling, grandparent, or legal guardian can consent to donation.

Even when people did consent to donation prior to death, their relatives may still be asked for permission, and in some cases, the relatives may deny permission (Mishra, 2007). This is one example of the many factors resulting in a shortage of organs available for donation. In fact, less than 50 percent of families give permission to donate a relative's organs after death, even if the decedent previously consented. One reason for this is because some cultures and religions forbid donating organs after death. Even if a culture or religion does not expressly forbid organ donation, some are under the false impression that their culture or religion does forbid it.

This falsehood seems to be particularly rampant among the Jewish community, many of whom believe organ donation is "a desecration of the body," although Jewish religious law is, in reality, more nuanced than that. All four branches of Judaism (Orthodox, Conservative, Reform, and Reconstructionist) support and encourage donation. Moreover, the Rabbinical Council of America (Orthodox) requires approved organ donations from brain-dead patients.

Harvesting of Body Parts

Carey v. New England Organ Bank
[Parents of Tissue Donor v. Organ Bank]
843 N.E.2d 1070 (Supreme Court of Massachusetts 2006)

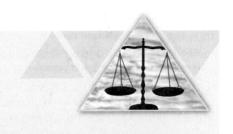

Facts: A sixteen-year-old boy was mortally injured in a vehicle mishap. About two hours after his death, his parents consented to tissue donation; however, their son's cornea and blood vessels were harvested and his tissues were unusable following saline infusions in the hospital emergency room before his death.

Issue: Were the boy's organs improperly harvested when his parents only consented to donate the tissues of their deceased son for transplantation?

Holding and Decision: No, organ and tissue banks are not required to harvest and allocate body parts according to the donor's wishes.

Analysis: The court reviewed the UAGA and acknowledged time is always very limited for obtaining consent and procuring body parts. Once consent for a post-mortem gift is received, organ and tissue banks are not required to disclose that the donation may be unusable for specified purposes. While a cause of action may arise when organs are harvested beyond the scope of consent, the UAGA's good faith immunity provision often protects organ banks. Moreover, improper harvesting claims address the right to prevent the harvesting of corpses without consent; there is no requirement that banks harvest and allocate body parts according to the donor's wishes.

Rule of Law: The UAGA may provide grounds for a donor's family to sue when donated body parts are used for a purpose other than their specified purpose of transplantation, although organ and tissue banks may be excused from liability by good faith protections.

Repeal of the Zero Antigen Mismatch Rule

The question of how to distribute scarce organs presents a classic conflict between utility, which seeks to provide the greatest good for the greatest number, and equity, which seeks fairness for all individuals. The changes now under way are the most significant since a national allocation policy was first developed twenty years ago. A new UNOS allocation policy is likely to scrap rules automatically sending organs to anyone who is a perfect match on six antigens relevant to transplantation. Already, the notion that exact matching should be the only prescribed course of treatment for bone marrow transplants has been rejected.

One factor consistently overriding all other factors was whether there was a zero antigen mismatch between the transplant patient and the donated organ. A zero antigen mismatch meant the antigens all matched up, meaning the transplant patient's body was much less likely to reject the organ; in short, it was akin to a perfect match between organ and patient. If there was a patient who had zero antigen mismatch to an available organ, that patient automatically had top priority in receiving the available organ. If there were no patients with zero antigen mismatches to the available organ, the organ went to a patient with a partial antigen match. All these zero mismatch trumps would be eliminated under the UNOS new allocation policy.

This so-called zero antigen mismatch rule accounts for how about one-fifth of the donated kidneys are distributed in the U.S. Because more Caucasians donate organs than any other race, this has resulted in more Caucasians receiving organs because there is more likely to be zero antigen mismatches when the donor and transplant patients are of the same race. Because of this disparity, UNOS relaxed its zero antigen mismatch policy in 2003, which allowed more minorities to receive donated organs. In reality, the rule does little to improve kidney transplant outcomes because of advanced anti-rejection drugs in use today (NKF, 2008). This is another example of incongruous regulatory policy failing to rapidly adapt to technological advances in medicine.

Limited Property Interest in Human Biological Material

Regardless of all these regulatory changes, and even as scientific advances lead to increased use of and demand for human organs, the body continues to take on the functional characteristics of property in the law. Most courts refuse to overturn traditional notions of a limited property interest in the human body, as demonstrated in the *Colavito* case.

In Reality: How Organ Procurement and Transplantation Occurs

Historically, organs were recovered from people who suffered cardiac death (meaning the victim was no longer breathing, had no pulse, and the heart could not be revived). This often meant that by the time their organs could be transplanted, they could no longer be used because they had been without a blood

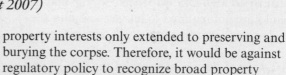

PROPERTY RIGHT IN DONATED, CADAVERIC ORGANS

Colavito v. N.Y. Organ Donor Network, Inc. (NYODN)
[Recipient of a Designated Kidney v. State Network for Organ Sharing]
486 F.3d 78 (U.S. Court of Appeals for the 2nd Circuit 2007)

FACTS: A widowed wife made a directed kidney donation to Colavito. While awaiting implantation of the first kidney, the attending surgeon discovered the kidney had been damaged by aneurysms. Therefore, a staff member called to request the second kidney be airlifted for transplantation. However, the NYODN informed the party that the second kidney had already been implanted in another recipient; as it turned out, the kidney was not transplanted until three days later. Instead of Colavito receiving both kidneys, one kidney was successfully transplanted in another donee. Colavito brought suit, alleging fraud and conversion in the kidney donation, and alleging the NYODN violated organ donor laws. As it turned out, the donated kidneys were incompatible with Colavito's immune system, although Colavito refused to concede that he could not have derived a medical benefit from the transplant regardless.

ISSUE: Does either the donor or next-of-kin have a property right in regards to a cadaveric organ donated for transplantation?

HOLDING AND DECISION: No, neither the donor nor next-of-kin has any property rights to a donated incompatible organ.

ANALYSIS: The court found corpses were not recognized as property in common law, and that property interests only extended to preserving and burying the corpse. Therefore, it would be against regulatory policy to recognize broad property rights in the body of a corpse.

The court reasoned there was no consensus that body parts are excluded from conversion actions, noting that the existence of property rights in body parts is a new question with very little authority and commentary (Appel Blue, 2008). The court concluded Colavito may have been able to maintain a cause of action had the organ been compatible because, as a human organ recipient, the suit was not brought for control of the corpse and its parts but rather for the deprivation of a working organ (Mishra, 2007). In short, the court argued Colavito may have had a legal claim based on the loss of a functioning organ, if the organ would have otherwise medically benefitted him.

In its resolution, the court adhered to the common law rule and refused to identify or forecast the circumstances in which someone might have actionable rights in the corpse or organ of a deceased person.

RULE OF LAW: No one can have a property right in a corpse; next-of-kin only have a common law right to possess the corpse for the purposes of burying it and a corresponding duty to do so.

(See Morris 2009.)

and oxygen supply for so long they would be unlikely to function in the recipients.

In 1968, the medical community redefined death to include brain death, which occurs when the brain is no longer functioning, despite the body being sustained by drugs and machines. This means organs can be transplanted earlier, or before they suffer blood and oxygen deprivation, making them much more likely to be viable.

The concept of brain death was recently described as "at once well settled and persistently unresolved" (Truog, 2007). Use of brain death has, however, led to the rampant misunderstanding that patients who might otherwise survive might be "killed" for their organs, something unconditionally prohibited. Although organs transplanted from a brain-dead patient are more likely to be useful, only 1 to 2 percent of patients who die in hospitals are declared brain dead.

Until recently, deaths occurring outside of a hospital setting almost never resulted in useable transplant organs. This is because organs need a continuous supply of blood and oxygen in order to be transplantable. Some transplant centers still do not consider transplanting organs from patients who are older than sixty-five or who have high blood pressure. This is so even though studies have shown organs from these "less than perfect" patients can be successfully transplanted. All these factors further contribute to the short supply of useable transplant organs.

This is also why the transplant community wants to do more for living donors, such as providing insurance and reimbursing them for lost time at work. At the same time, there is significant disagreement about how far medicine should go in encouraging people to donate organs, whether living or post-mortem donations.

Access to Organ Transplantations

As illustrated in Figure 25-1, organ transplants are expensive procedures, available only to those who have health insurance, government-provided health care, or private funds. Many health insurance policies do not cover the full cost of transplantation of organs, which must then be paid out of pocket.

Transplant	Procurement	Hospital	Physician	Evaluation	Follow-up	Immuno-suppressants	Total
Heart Only	$89,900	$383,300	$40,300	$22,900	$93,000	$29,400	$658,800
Single Lung Only	$40,371	$209,329	$33,200	$20,000	$65,600	$30,500	$399,500
Double Lung Only	$81,742	$257,558	$52,600	$31,600	$104,100	$29,800	$557,400
Heart-Lung	$152,900	$502,900	$56,800	$26,400	$105,400	$30,700	$874,800
Liver Only	$59,100	$248,100	$66,900	$25,900	$88,500	$31,100	$519,600
Kidney Only	$58,300	$74,500	$21,500	$14,600	$48,000	$29,500	$246,400
Pancreas Only	$66,200	$107,100	$24,600	$14,700	$48,300	$36,400	$297,300
Kidney-Pancreas	$124,500	$120,300	$24,600	$14,700	$48,300	$36,200	$368,600
Intestine Only	$75,449	$602,451	$87,100	$41,700	$78,500	$23,400	$908,600
Liver-Intestine	$134,549	$674,551	$87,100	$41,700	$88,500	$31,700	$1,058,100
Liver-Pancreas-Intestine	$200,749	$587,751	$87,100	$41,700	$88,500	$35,100	$1,040,900
Pancreas-Intestine	$141,649	$586,751	$87,100	$41,700	$78,500	$35,400	$971,100
Kidney-Heart	$148,200	$419,200	$40,300	$22,900	$93,000	$35,100	$758,700
Liver-Kidney	$117,100	$321,100	$66,900	$25,900	$88,500	$37,200	$657,000

FIGURE 25-1: Estimated U.S. Average First-Year Billed Charges per Transplant

Delmar/Cengage Learning

Data retrieved from: Hauboldt, (2007) (Based on data from the: Organ Procurement and Transplantation Network, Scientific Registry of Transplant Recipients, United Network for Organ Sharing, National Marrow Donor Program, International Bone Marrow Transplant Registry, Analogous Blood and Marrow Transplant Registry, and Eye Bank Association of America).

Kidney Transplants

Kidney transplantation is the most frequently performed organ transplant in the U.S. (Brennan, 2007). This can be expected, since the diseases with a high predisposition to ESRD are diabetes mellitus and arterial hypertension, diseases tied to the epidemic of weight-related conditions. A typical twenty-five-year-old diabetic will gain an extra 8.7 years of life from a transplant, while a typical fifty-five-year-old diabetic will gain only 3.6 extra years.

Regardless of age, most individuals with ESRD are covered under Medicare. The cost of lifetime dialysis or, for individuals who receive kidney transplants, the costs of the transplants and three years of follow-up care including immunosuppressive drugs needed to sustain the transplants, are covered by Medicare. Although ESRD can be treated through other renal replacement therapies, kidney transplantation is generally accepted as the best treatment both for quality of life and cost-effectiveness (NKF, 2008).

Medicare has been paying in excess of $32 billion in ESRD-related costs each year, or about $65,000 per person. A debatable issue is whether Medicare should continue paying for most adult kidney transplants in the U.S. when the underlying diseases leading to the need for transplants are usually caused by lifestyle choices. This question is directly related to the high incidence in transplant failures from one year to three years due to treatment noncompliance and continued unhealthy behavior.

As discussed, a new UNOS policy is expected to rely significantly, though not exclusively, on the concept of net benefit, which seeks to give kidneys first to those who will benefit most from them. This would favor recipients who have more years to gain from a new organ, meaning individuals with healthier lifestyles who have demonstrated compliance with health care treatments.

Heart Transplants

Every year, about five hundred people on the transplant wait list die before a heart is made available. Thousands more die because they are considered too old or sick to get on the list to begin with. Many of these people could be saved if transplant centers were less particular about the quality of donor hearts. In response to this need, more hospitals are starting alternate heart programs that provide lower-quality hearts to older and sicker patients.

While about two thousand hearts are transplanted each year, an additional three thousand were offered by families of the deceased that were rejected, according to the Scientific Registry of Transplant Recipients. These three thousand hearts were often rejected because they were not top quality, and the hearts were consequently buried or cremated with their original owners. Estimates are that half the rejected hearts are suitable for transplanting.

One limitation to establishing alternate heart programs is that insurers scrutinize success rates at each transplant center to decide whether they will cover transplant operations performed there. If a transplant center accepts too many sick recipients or individuals over the age of sixty-five, its success rate will go down and it may lose its reimbursement status. Heart transplants, which cost patients upwards of $600,000, are a profit generator at many hospitals. This is one reason alternate heart programs are usually found at major teaching hospitals like the UCLA Medical Center, which can afford to accept donor hearts that either require bypass surgery prior to transplantation or originate from older donors.

While UCLA was the nation's first alternate heart program to offer transplantation to seniors with end-stage heart failure, other teaching hospitals have developed similar programs (Satel & Hippen, 2007). Alternate heart recipients do somewhat worse than top-quality heart recipients, but still do fairly well in comparison to how they would have done with no heart transplant at all.

UNOS will often find no takers for alternate hearts, and that is where UCLA and other transplant centers with alternate donor lists come in. After everyone else says no, UNOS will call an alternate heart program and look for a patient to accept the lower quality heart. Patients on the alternate list must agree they will not ordinarily be eligible for a heart from the regular list. This leaves another dilemma for the medical community: how far should transplant centers go in using lower quality organs?

Anencephalic Neonates

One of the early controversies surrounding organ donation involved anencephalic neonates.[LN2] Anencephalic neonates are babies who are born nearly entirely brain dead, with the exception of minor electrical activity. They have no possibility of living a life beyond the vegetative state within which they are born, and are permanently unconscious. They do not feel pain due to the lack of cerebral function. Most, in fact, die within days of birth.

In order to donate organs, there must be either total brain death or cardiopulmonary death (Truog, 2007). An anencephalic neonate cannot be declared dead either way. If their life support machines are turned off and death occurs naturally, their organs are no longer useable because of the time it takes death to occur and the damage to their fragile organs in the meantime. The American Medical Association was originally of the opinion that it was ethically acceptable to transplant the organs of such infants even before they were technically dead, as long as there was parental consent and certain other safeguards were followed, but it was forced to withdraw that opinion due to controversy.

HIV-Positive Transplant Candidates

Additionally, there is public controversy over whether HIV-positive transplant candidates should receive organs, even if they have no symptoms and are not in the end stage of the disease. While positive HIV status was once thought to be a relative or even absolute contraindication to transplantation, UNOS policy does not bar HIV-positive patients from receiving organs. HIV-positive patients argue their status is at least equal to other transplant patients who previously received transplants, but whose bodies rejected the organs, or transplant patients with other diseases, such as hepatitis or diabetes, or elderly transplant patients. With the advent of antiretroviral drugs, those infected with HIV are now living longer and dying from illnesses other than AIDS. Recent studies have demonstrated results comparable to those of recipients without HIV infection (Pelletier et al., 2004). Still, a number of issues persist regarding ethics, patient selection, postoperative management, and drug interactions between antiretroviral and immunosuppression agents (Ciuffreda et al., 2007). Some transplant centers often refuse to list HIV-positive patients in the national registry of those waiting for organs; this is so even though some HIV-positive patients have the disease through no fault of their own, such as those who were born with the disease or who contracted it through violence or medical error.

These and other controversies over the way organs are allocated have led to the suggestion that potential survivability should be the only criteria for selecting transplant recipients. Some states have gone as far as to reject the 1999 HHS regulations and have enacted their own state legislation in an attempt to maintain local geographic preferences for organ transplants by restricting organ donors from donating their organs out of state.

Alternative Procurement of Organs

Before resorting to xenotransplantation, several alternatives are immediately available to enhance organ procurement and increase organ supply. In the U.S., federal and state governments are considering alternatives, such as mandated choice, which would force everyone to choose whether or not they want to be a donor, or presumed consent, which would assume everyone wants to be a donor unless they indicate otherwise.

While stem cell therapies and xenotransplantation also offer future alternatives for organ enhancement or supply, neither is without controversy (Munzer, 2007). Both alternatives pose greater risk to human health since they are both emerging medical procedures without guaranteed success.

Further controversy surrounds how organs for transplantation are sometimes obtained. Many states have statutes allowing any organ to be removed from a cadaver without consent as long as an attempt was made to contact the family. California and Idaho are two such states. Other states allow for the removal of specified items as long as no objection is actually known, whether or not an attempt to notify the family was made. Missouri, Arkansas, and Colorado are three such states. The UAGA allows a donor to specify a recipient, a regulatory policy adopted to encourage more donations.

Presumed Consent or Opt-Out

Presumed consent systems, common in Europe and Eastern Asia, provide that organs will be automatically donated at death, unless stated otherwise (Clamon, 2008). This method is often called an opt-out plan because persons who do not wish to donate their organs upon death must opt-out during life. The advantage of this system is an increase in the available supply of organs (Statz, 2006). However, there is some opposition to the practice of silence as consent.

Mandated Choice

Mandated choice is very similar to presumed consent, except that under mandated choice, individuals must either op-in or opt-out; there is no presumption of opting-in. The advantage of this system is greater autonomy, the lack of which is the main criticism of presumed consent. Similar to the presumed consent method, it places the burden on individuals to think about organ donations. The largest criticism of mandated choice is the cost of coordinating a national system, since everyone's organ donation preference would have to be recorded and followed.

Internet Solicitation

Another approach to organ procurement involves communication between potential donors and recipients through Internet-based chat rooms and Web sites (Steinbrook, 2005). The Web site MatchingDonors.com and a free message board at livingdonorsonline.org have allowed individuals in need of organs to meet and chat with others who are willing to be living organ donors. The idea remains controversial because it raises questions about potential commercialism and donor compensation.

MatchingDonors.com, created in 2004, is a for-profit Internet business charging $595 per month for a person in need of an organ (or $25 per month if the recipient applies for a credit card to cover medical expenses that carries a variable interest rate pegged at the prime rate + 14.99%). The Web site claims over 5,100 recipients are registered; several hundred recipient profiles are from the U.S. Potential donors determine who the most deserving person is for their organ based on information provided by potential recipients.

Live Organ Swaps and Paired Living Donations

There are also organizations, such as LifeSharers, designed to improve transplant candidates' chances of receiving an organ by requiring members to agree to donate organs to other members before the general public. LifeSharers has over nine thousand members (Clamon, 2008). These organizations argue it is not fair to give organs to patients who have not also agreed to donate their own organs should the opportunity arise. LifeSharers points out that organ donors themselves receive only about 30 percent of donated organs in the U.S., whereas the remaining 70 percent go to non-donors (Statz, 2006).

The medical community is beginning to experiment with new ways to get organs to transplant patients more quickly. "Kidney swaps" are one newly popular but complex method for doing so. Also known as "kidney-paired donation," the process connects an incompatible donor-recipient pair, such as a husband and wife or parent and child, with another incompatible donor-recipient pair. The healthy member of each pair donates a kidney to the person who is the medical match in the other pair, and the surgeries are performed simultaneously so the healthy donor cannot back out after their partner receives a kidney. Sometimes the swaps involve as many as five pairs. The first swap of this kind actually occurred in 2000, and several hundred have occurred since then. At least three paired kidney organizations foster this method of allocating kidneys: the Alliance for Paired Donation, the North American Paired Donation Network, and the New England Organ Bank (Meckler, 2007a).

Regulatory Changes

In 2003, UNOS determined that paired organ donations do not violate the prohibition against organ selling. Paired organ donations do not create any additional risks to organ donors and encourage more donations because the chance of compatibility increases with more willing participants (Lobas, 2006). As long as all parties follow the appropriate procedures for informed consent, paired organ exchanges are encouraged.

The slow initial growth of this approach partly reflected concerns that trades might violate a federal ban on selling organs. However, Congress passed Norwood in 2007, clarifying that such arrangements are legal. It is estimated there could be as many as four thousand kidney exchanges per year (NKF, 2008), a big addition to the kidney transplants performed every year involving living donors. Still, this is not nearly enough organs to satisfy the UNOS wait list for kidney transplants.

As interest in kidney swaps grows, logistical, medical, ethical, and legal questions are emerging. One of the fundamental issues is who should get priority on a match. A donor with blood type O, for instance, can give to patients of any blood type and might match with hundreds of pairs.

In the early days of kidney swaps, transplant surgeons matched pairs using a pen and paper or by moving magnetic pieces around on a board. Today, computer experts, working with economists and clinical researchers, are optimizing matches to enable the greatest number of organ transplants. Mathematical techniques from major league baseball schedules, airline departures, and online driving directions are being used. The days when UNOS regulations allocated scarce organs based on a list of evolving technical criteria are over. The goal of many is to develop a national paired kidney network.

Federal and State Innovations

The federal government established a program to reimburse living donors for expenses including travel, lodging, and meals. States are also experimenting with how to increase cadaveric and live donor rates with more than a dozen states offering tax deductions to help defray expenses.

Wisconsin gives state tax breaks of up to $10,000 to benefit organ donors for expenses such as travel, hotel bills, and lost wages. Pennsylvania has a fund from voluntary donations when state residents apply for driver's licenses or vehicle registration; the fund provides up to $3,000 per cadaveric donor to help with hospital, medical, and funeral expenses. In both instances, the expenses are paid directly to providers to avoid conflicting with the ban on payment for organs.

Some states propose mandates requiring all organ donors to have lifetime insurance coverage; others propose that Medicare cover all organ donors. Both proposals are medically responsible and could serve as an inducement. Most recently, South Carolina introduced legislation that would shorten the term of a prisoner's sentence if he or she chose to donate an organ.

Other ideas include tax credits, tuition vouchers, deposits in retirement accounts, and recognition of tax deductions for charitable contributions. All these could be offered in a regulated environment overseen by tax authorities. The savings from dialysis could be used to underwrite the various types of compensation. According to the Congressional Budget Office, Norwood alone will save almost $500 million in Medicare costs over ten years.

Compelled Donations

Advances in immunology and the growing ability to circumvent rejection of transplanted organs are slowly replacing the need for compelled donations (Brennan, 2007). Today, the focus has turned to anonymous donations, which again brings to the fore the place where strangers go to transact business: the market.

Still, every year, organs are harvested from minors and mentally incompetent adults who neither voluntarily donate their organs nor consent to the surgical procedure (Schenberg, 2007). Compelled living donations from children and incompetent persons are the least desired forms of organ donation (Nygren, 2006). Since living donations generally involve kidneys, part of a liver, or bone marrow, donation does not involve serious physical harm to donors. However, the physical pain or risks to the donor should not be minimized, especially in the case of kidney or liver donations, which are major surgeries involving general anesthesia. Also, in the case of kidney donation, the donor is left with only one kidney, which puts him or her at a greater risk for kidney complications in the future. Siblings are usually the best donors, for reasons including matching blood types and relative ages of the donor and recipient. Therefore, sometimes the best possible match, and maybe the only possible match, will be the recipient's incompetent sibling.

Incompetency is defined as a lack of legal ability in some respect. Looking to a variety of factors, courts determine whether a person is legally incompetent. Generally, organ donations from living minors are only permitted if the donor is above the age of twelve or thirteen (Hebert, 2008). Children under the age of eighteen are generally considered legally incompetent.

Cognitively impaired children are considered legally incompetent if born severely cognitively impaired or if born healthy, but become severely cognitively impaired before age eighteen. Legal competency is disputable if a child is close to eighteen before becoming severely cognitively impaired.

Incompetence can vary among persons from severe and profoundly impairing, to mild and less impairing. When incompetence is severe, individuals will have limited awareness of their surroundings and will often have serious medical conditions. The severity of incompetence can therefore vary significantly and should be considered (Nygren, 2006).

Generally courts use substituted judgment reasoning to determine whether the best interests of potential donors are being met (Schenberg, 2007). Most family requests are resolved at the lower court level in favor of donation with few decisions appealed, thus the paucity of reported cases. In an attempt to address donor coercion, organ transplant teams have long allowed potential donors to opt-out of donation by providing blameless medical excuses, which are intended to shield donors from external pressures, real or perceived, to donate.

Creation of Child Donors Through Assisted Reproductive Technologies

Parents sometimes conceive another child for the purpose of donating bone marrow to an older sibling in need of a human leukocyte antigen (HLA) match. Whether this is legally or ethically sound remains unclear. It is clear that there is no legal obligation for siblings to donate.

The practice of procuring tissue and organs from children drastically changed when it became possible to use assistive reproductive techniques (ART) primarily for the purpose of a child becoming an organ donor. Preimplantation genetic diagnosis (PGD) and in vitro fertilization (IVF) can be used to conceive a child who is a perfect HLA match for an older sibling. Stem cells from the ART child's umbilical cord blood can be harvested from the newborn at birth and transplanted into the older sibling.

This controversial technique has been used in only about two thousand children worldwide since 2000 because:

- The procedure is expensive ($15,000 per each of the mother's menstrual cycles)
- There are only about fifty reproductive centers worldwide offering the technique
- The process is time consuming
- Cord blood is in short supply

Despite the limited use of this procedure, it is likely to be used extensively in the near future to conceive child donors as the costs decrease and technological advances in ART are made, and the number of reproductive centers offering the procedure increases. Just as the history of organ donation has rapidly evolved, so likely will the use of ART to create child donors. Healthy cord blood donors hold great promise to treat those with Fanconi anemia, leukemia, thalassemia, Hurler syndrome, and other diseases causing the immune system and bone marrow to fail.

What is perhaps more worrisome than using ART more extensively in the future to create perfectly HLA-matched child donors is the fact that younger siblings might be asked to donate their bone marrow if the stem cell transplants are unsuccessful. If a bone marrow transplant fails for any reason, they may be asked to donate other tissues and organs. In fact, children conceived via ART combined with IVF and PGD for HLA-matching could be asked to serve as donors for their ailing siblings throughout their entire lives.

Procurement Protections for Compelled Donors

The current legal framework under which compelled donations occur may not adequately protect children and the cognitively impaired unless several standards are followed. Most important, a guardian ad litem should always be appointed to look out for the interests of compelled donors with respect to their donation. Many courts require family and independent counseling to ensure parents understand the dynamics and depth of their actions and the potential long-term consequences. Often, independent physicians are appointed for the prospective compelled donors to avoid conflicts of interest. Ideally, a statement should be issued to the court from the donor as to why they desire to participate as an organ or tissue donor.

Restricting compelled donations may reduce the pool of viable organs, and other solutions may have to be sought. However, limiting the pool of incompetent donors will necessitate and hopefully force a reconsideration of the altruistically-based procurement regime (Goodwin, 2007).

Lengthening Post-Transplant Organ Survival

A variety of techniques prevent injury that results from temporary arterial blockage and restoration of blood flow to transplanted organs. Rejection of the donor organ or tissue is also preventable through the use of a variety of tissue and molecular manipulations before the transplant occurs.

Medicare pays for most organ transplants in the U.S. However, coverage of immunosuppressant drugs ends thirty-six to forty-four months after transplant surgery or when the patient reaches adulthood. Many patients, especially young adults, cannot afford to pay for these maintenance drugs without health insurance. For individuals who have employer-sponsored and private health insurance, coverage ends once a patient reaches a lifetime maximum amount. Transplant patients who lose their insurance coverage are more likely to stop taking necessary anti-rejection drugs, and not taking the drugs increases the risk of losing the transplanted organs due to organ failure or other complications.

Immunosuppressive drugs that prevent organ rejection can exceed $13,000 per year. This represents a significant financial burden for families, even if insured, because of co-payment obligations. If families cannot afford medicine, it can mean losing the transplanted organ or even death. Outcomes for children whose families are uninsured are very poor (Schnitzler, 2007). Young adults also face great risk, as one-third of this age group lacks medical coverage.

The cost of failed organ transplants is also high. Functioning transplants are ten times less expensive to maintain than the costs involved in the year following a failure: $14,000 in maintenance costs for a successful transplant recipient, compared to the cost of returning to dialysis after transplant failure at $140,000 (Schnitzler, 2007). This is one reason proposals are emerging to require lifetime health care coverage for organ transplant recipients; it would be cost-effective and would prolong patients' longevity and their productivity.

Sure enough, there are black market drugs available through an underground network run by transplant patients with the cooperation of sympathetic health care workers, and overlooked by law enforcement. They simply give drugs away to patients who cannot afford immunosuppressant drugs. Their sources include patients who have changed drug regimens and contribute their old medicines, some drug manufacturers, and drugs scavenged and unused from the dead and passed on to the underground. There is probably an illicit underground in every major metropolitan area (Lobas, 2006).

TISSUE TRANSPLANTATION

Human tissue is anything donated from the human body that is not a vital organ. Blood vessels, bone, bone marrow, connective tissues such as tendons and cartilage, corneas, heart valves, and skin are common types of tissues used for transplants to help patients in many different types of surgeries. Transplantation of musculoskeletal tissues is the most common medical procedure, including skin tissue replacements to treat burns, bone to facilitate spinal fusions, and tendons to reconstruct knee ligaments and repair joint and limb injuries. It also includes implantation of dura mater, hematostem/progenitor cells derived from peripheral and cord blood, oocytes, and semen.

U.S. Navy Tissue Bank

The first tissue bank was established by the U.S. Navy in 1949 and remained the primary tissue bank in the U.S. for almost thirty years. Scientists at the

Navy Tissue Bank pioneered many of the commercial standards followed today:

- Identification of appropriate donor criteria for tissue donation
- Procurement and processing methods
- Establishment of a graph register
- Documentation and clinical evaluation of tissues
- Cryopreservation, freeze drying, and irradiation sterilization of tissue
- Immunological principles of tissue transplantation, including cadaveric bone marrow recovery and immunosuppressive protocols

The Navy was also instrumental in establishing the National Marrow Donor Program and the American Association of Tissue Banks. Although the Navy Tissue Bank ceased operations after fifty years, it pioneered the establishment of regional tissue banks. Similar to blood banks, they provided the human tissue necessary to meet the demands of their local communities.

Current Context

Tissue transplantation has grown quickly and its visibility and ability to escape government over-regulation has allowed it to separate itself from organ transplantation. This new visibility has come with the rise of for-profit tissue banks, which highly process, transform, package, and store tissue for years before distribution for transplantation, unlike organs that are transported quickly and rarely change form before getting to a recipient.

With the growth of tissue transplantations, it has been easy for human tissue to be commodified and turned into valuable medical products. As the market expanded, the regional tissue banks began to distribute outside of their local communities. The 1990s saw an expansion and consolidation in the tissue industry as the large for-profit tissue banks moved to control more than half of the tissue bank business.

Today, the typical tissue donation chain is as follows:

- Procurement agencies meet with the donor's family in order to get consent for tissue removal and then procure the tissue at a hospital (most of the recoveries occur in hospital operating rooms) or morgue (FDA, 2006); recoveries are often made at multiple sites
- Procurement agencies then give the recovered tissue to a processor and collect recovery fees
- Tissue processors process the transplantable tissue into marketable tissue products
- Tissue processors then distribute the processed tissue products to marketing agencies and collect processing fees
- Marketing agencies market and sell the processed tissue products to hospitals and physicians for transplantation and collect distribution fees
- Hospitals and physicians then transplant the processed tissue products into patients and collect medical fees

Some of the most important technological advances in the tissue industry have occurred because of for-profit tissue processors. Over the course of two decades, the tissue industry has evolved from a $20 million industry to a multibillion-dollar industry with double-digit growth.

Kinetic Concepts, Inc. (KCI), a publicly traded company in San Antonio, Texas, specializing in tissue repair, had sales revenue of $1.6 billion in 2007 and employed over 6,500 people. In mid-2008, KCI doubled its size when it acquired Life Sciences Corporation, a tissue processor specializing in repair of damaged tissue in hernias and breast reconstruction, in a deal valued at $1.7 billion.

Another large tissue processor is Florida's RTI Biologics, Inc. (RTI), a publicly traded company with sales revenue of $94 million in 2007 and employing over five hundred people. RTI makes use of natural tissues and technologies to produce orthopedic, cardiovascular, and other surgical implants that repair and promote the natural healing of human bone and other human tissues. RTI processes human musculoskeletal and other tissue, including bone, cartilage, tendon, ligament, dermal, and cardiovascular tissue, in producing its allograft. RTI also processes bovine tissue to produce its Sterling xenograft line of transplantable products. These tissue products meet the highest standards of purity through irradiation sterilizations that virtually eliminate the risk of transmission of xenozoonoses.

Regulatory Oversight of Human Tissue

When the tissue bank industry emerged, federal regulations were non-existent. Even though tissue transplantations are similar to organ transplantations, the two entities are treated completely differently. Traditionally, organs have been thoroughly regulated by the federal government and individual state governments. The same cannot be said for human tissue (Williams, 2005).

Until 1993, the idea of regulating the tissue industry was foreign. The government did not have regulations for tissue banks until the 1990s, when it was discovered there was a need to protect the public from the possibility of transmitting disease through tissue transplants. Even with this pressing need, it still took years to enact regulations.

Today, human tissue is regulated by the Center for Biologics Evaluation and Research (CBER) (*see* 21 C.F.R. §§ 1270-1271 (2009)). The federal regulations act as a base for the state regulations to stand on. The regulations created by the states require that tissue banks comply with federal regulations, but often the state regulations appear more specific and better enforced. The states appear to give more protection and instructions to tissue banks than the federal regulations. Florida, New York, Maryland, and California have enacted their own state regulations and standards for tissue banks that operate in their states. Further, the American Association of Tissue Banks (AATB) has its own voluntary regulations and accreditation guidelines for all tissue banks. In order to legally comply with CBER regulations, tissue banks must register with the FDA. Many do not, and thus exist under the radar of the FDA.

American Association of Tissue Banks

AATB accredits tissue banks with higher standards than the FDA or state laws require. Created in 1976, AATB works through regional and local tissue banks to ensure the availability of a safe, adequate, and economical supply of tissues and cells for medical procedures and research, as it seeks to:

- Ensure quality standards
- Encourage human tissue donation
- Create a forum for scientific exchange
- Promote ethical standards throughout the tissue industry
- Secure an adequate supply of transplantable human tissue

While most of the major U.S. tissue banks are accredited by the AATB, less than one hundred of the two thousand tissue banks registered with CBER are actually accredited. When a tissue bank is in the process of accreditation, inspectors visit the bank and review its onsite operations and procedures. Tissue banks that do not meet the AATB standards are denied accreditation.

Tissue banks are accredited for three years. In addition, employees who are certified specialists participate in continuing education units (CEUs), programs aimed at continuing education of tissue bank employees. Categories for CEUs include basic science, medical and social issues, medical practices, and ethical, moral, and legal aspects of tissue banking.

The AATB develops technical standards for recovery and preservation of human tissues. Specific areas cover screening for communicable diseases, tissue labeling, qualification of tissue bank personnel, safety practices, equipment testing, and facilities for tissue storage. The AATB and the CBER work together to address tissue bank donor selection criteria, quality processing, and record-keeping in an attempt to keep infectious tissue out of circulation. Neither the AATB nor the CBER concerns itself with distribution issues in the tissue industry; allocations are market-driven.

Biosynthetic Tissues

Biosynthetic tissues, including synthetic skin and bone substitutes, are viable alternatives to traditional human transplantation materials. Numerous restrictions, however, such as the technical limitations associated with engineering complex tissues so as to duplicate their innate functions, currently limit their use outside major teaching hospitals.

XENOTRANSPLANTATION

It is estimated only 5 percent of the human organs needed are actually made accessible for transplantation (Cascalho et al., 2004). This disparity between need and availability has led medical researchers to consider the possibility of animal-to-human transplants, or xenotransplantation. Strictly regulated by the FDA, xenotransplantation involves any procedure that transplants, implants, or infuses into a human either:

- Live cells, tissues, or organs from a non-human animal source
- Human body fluids, cells, tissues, or organs that have had contact with live non-human animal cells, tissues, or organs

(*Federal Register,* 2003)

A medical practice first endorsed by the President's Council on Bioethics in 2004, xenotransplantation is used to treat certain diseases such as neurodegenerative disorders, liver failure, and diabetes, where human body parts are not usually available. While the transplantation, implantation, or infusion into a human recipient of cells, tissues, or organs from a non-human animal source has been occurring in some fashion for over one hundred years, it often results in rejection by the recipient's immune system (HHS, 2004).

In order to minimize the rejection of xenotransplants, the possibility of using part-human organs, tissues, and cells, such as pig hearts containing human DNA, for transplantation is actively being explored. Xenotransplantation, developed in the late twentieth century simultaneously with the use of artificial organs, calls into question the once clear distinction between human and animal life (Westphal, 2006). As human genes are introduced into mammals such as pigs to make the animals' organs more acceptable to the human body for the purposes of organ transplantation, this scientific development blurs distinctions. These technologies are expensive and have lower success rates than human organ donation, so they are unlikely to comprise many organ transplantations in the near future.

Oversight of Safety and Effectiveness

For over twenty years, the National Institutes of Health's Recombinant DNA Advisory Committee publicly disclosed summary safety and effectiveness data for studies related to xenotransplantation (HHS, 2004). In 2001, proposed rules were made to extend this same level of disclosure to the FDA's regulation of xenotransplantation, given the concerns about protecting animals and humans from cross-species diseases, known as zoonoses. However, the rules were never finalized (*Federal Register,* 2001). *See* Availability of Public Disclosure and Submission to FDA for Public Disclosure of Certain Data and Information Related to Human Gene Therapy or Xenotransplantation. 66 *Federal Register* 4688-01 (Jan. 18, 2001). The concern is that communicable diseases, or the infectious agents that cause them, might move from animals to humans through xenotransplantation (Spillman & Sade, 2007).

An edifice of exemptions has protected confidential commercial information about xenotransplantation from disclosure to the public. At the same time, the larger question of whether commercial interests should automatically take priority over public health concerns is strongly debated (Lurie & Zieve, 2006).

Most current xenotransplantation research focuses on the pig as an organ donor because of its size and commonalities with humans in some physiological pathways. New strategies are being examined for their ability to prevent rejection of organ allograft. The goal of preventing rejection of donor tissue is to selectively suppress the immune response to the organ while retaining normal immune response to pathogens. Techniques to accomplish this selective immune suppression are expected to improve in the future as medical researchers gain and apply new knowledge about immune function from the results of the Human Genome Project (Sykes et al., 2004). A number of potential methods are under consideration and are being pursued. These include:

- Transplantation of bone marrow (as a source of precursor donor T cells)
- Organ, clonal T-cell deletion
- Modification of the donor to increase its compatibility with the recipient

(FDA, 2006)

The latter is considered the most successful medical treatment, with transgenic techniques used to introduce genes for recipient surface antigens. Efforts to produce transgenic animals, such as pigs altered with human DNA, are under way in the hopes of tricking the human body into accepting the animal organ. The goal is to create partially humanized pig organs to use as spare parts for humans (HHS, 2004). A number of additional issues must be overcome before xenotransplantation becomes widespread. For example, organs and tissues from animal sources may carry endogenous retroviruses, which must be identified and removed (FDA, 2003). Additionally, the ethics surrounding the use of animals for human benefit must be explored and resolved. Nevertheless, xenotransplants of nervous tissue are currently used to treat patients with Parkinson's disease.

Xenotransplant Tourism

One resulting problem is xenotransplants occurring in countries with no regulatory oversight. Patients seeking xenotransplantation procedures visit countries like Mexico, Cambodia, Laos, and Myanmar for controversial treatments that can be exceedingly dangerous (Cortez, 2008). Moreover, xenotransplant tourism by patients willing to pay for unproven interventions in countries without adequate controls risks global dissemination of new pathogens and may undermine this fledgling field just as it is emerging (WHO, 2008).

ALTERNATIVE STRATEGIES FOR DEVELOPING ORGAN AND TISSUE REPLACEMENTS

Current research efforts can be divided into four areas:

- Methods for improving organ and tissue preservation during transport from donor to recipient
- Procedures for lengthening post-implantation survival of the organ and the recipient
- Improvement in medical devices to replace organs or organ functions
- Development of new organs, taking advantage of advances in stem cell biology (Munzer, 2007), genetic engineering, and tissue engineering

While engineering of replacement tissues now uses large-scale tissue cultures, research is extending relatively crude current cell and tissue culture techniques to better determine the conditions required to create organ systems in vitro. Matrices and factors controlling tissue architecture outside the human body are continuously enhanced.

Research laboratories and companies around the world are actively trying to create skin, blood vessels, cartilage, bone, and corneas through similar tissue engineering techniques. Other efforts in less advanced stages include windpipe, kidney, pancreas, liver, and heart tissue. Tissue engineering has seen a number of ups and downs in the twenty years since its inception.

Initial success at growing tissues in labs and in small animals led people to declare success too early. As soon as the same tissues were tested in larger animal models, it became clear that size is one of the significant limiting factors in tissue engineering; the thicker the tissue one aims to grow, the harder it is to create.

Use of undifferentiated pluripotent stem cells and other undifferentiated cells is extending the possibilities for tissue culture. Further research is occurring on stem cell isolation and culture, while identification of cell surface markers allows for easier isolation of stem cells. In addition, the conditions required for stem cell differentiation are being identified, including signaling pathways, transcription factors, and gene activation sequences.

MOVING ALTRUISM FORWARD

Competing legal and social interests surround the transplantation of human organs in the U.S. Unfortunately, as medical advances have made organ transplants easier and more successful, more and more thorny bioethical questions arise as to who should receive the limited supply of transplantable organs.

Which patient should be the priority when an organ becomes available: the sickest and the one suffering the most, or the healthiest and the most likely to survive? The one who has been waiting the longest? Are living donations ethical? Should donors be compensated similarly to those who donate plasma or reproductive material?

The fair and equal access to few, if any, other goods or services in the U.S. is as highly controversial as health care access, particularly access to transplantable organs. Health care is perhaps the only service Americans view as something beyond a commodity. Rather, health care is viewed as something everyone should have access to.

The question becomes, then, if basic economic concepts are not an appropriate way to distribute scarce transplantable organs, what is the best way to do so?

Now that Congress has clarified NOTA through Norwood, the next move might be to change the prohibition against rewarding donors who decide to donate their organs or families who donate the deceased's organs. The current procurement system demands altruism as the sole legitimate motivation for donation of human biological material. However, altruism is not producing the number of organ donors necessary to keep pace with the ever-increasing number of wait-listed patients, many of whom die while waiting. The current altruistic system of organ procurement, which relies primarily on cadaveric donors, does not take into account today's technological advances.

Organ procurement policies based on a transplant system relying exclusively on living related donors has evolved into a system that now relies heavily on cadaveric organs and living unrelated donors. No-sale policies are now one of the principal causes of the ongoing organ shortage (Meckler, 2007). At the end of the day, transplant policies have not kept pace with medical technology or the realities of the marketplace.[LN3] While altruistic procurement of organs is not meeting the[LN1] growing demand for transplantable organs (Goodwin, 2004), there is not sufficient moral certainty to warrant allowing marketplace approaches to organ transplants (Engelhardt, 2007).

The idea of combining organ donation with material gain can make some people uneasy, yet the mix of financial and altruistic motives is common. Few object to tax credits for charitable contributions. An increase in the supply of organs could prevent needless suffering and death. It could be argued this is more important than whether an organ has been given freely or for material gain.

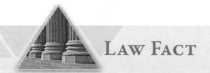

LAW FACT

MEDICAID COVERAGE FOR A LIVER TRANSPLANT: CURE OR DISEASE MANAGEMENT?

Must a state's taxpayers pay for a liver transplant to cure a hereditary disease if the disease can be treated by dietary management?

The harm to an individual life and health clearly outweighs any fiscal harm a state may suffer. Notwithstanding the fact that lifelong dietary management is an option for MSUD sufferers, UNOS ranks children with classical MSUD as high-priority liver transplant candidates because of the neurological burden and risks of the disease.
—*J.D. v. Sherman*, 2006 WL 3163053 (U.S. District Court for the Western District of Missouri, Central Division 2006.)
(See *Law Fact* at the end of this chapter for the answer.)

CHAPTER SUMMARY

- Organ transplantation dates back to the late 1800s, although more recent scientific advances have made the process much more likely to be successful and have expanded the kinds of transplantations that can be accomplished, leading to a higher demand for transplantable organs across the board.
- The demand for transplantable organs far exceeds the supply. Of the over one hundred thousand people awaiting organ donations, approximately 70 percent are awaiting kidneys. This is leading the federal and state governments to consider incentivizing donations.
- Patients wait an average of five years for a transplant, and many of them die waiting. Despite the fact that most Americans approve of organ donation, only about 25 percent expressly declare themselves donors.
- NOTA makes it illegal to sell human organs and established the Organ Network, which administers the organ transplantation process. However, other methods of allocating organs have appeared, such as Life-Sharers, paired-kidney swaps, and making use of lower quality donor organs.
- Although the Organ Network makes the recipient patient selection process more fair and equitable through the establishment of standardized criteria, it has been criticized for not regulating transplant centers more closely in order to ensure they adhere to the regulations.
- Organs are allocated based upon a point system that considers how long the patient has been on the list and the urgency of the patient's medical status, as well as criteria matching an available organ to a patient on the list, such as blood types.
- Organ donations come from those with written documentation prior to death of their wish to donate, or those whose family members consent to donation after death. Even when there is written documentation of a desire to donate, in some states family members may withdraw permission after death and prevent donation. In other states, donation will proceed as long as there is no known objection. New methods of procurement are under consideration, including presumed consent, opt-out, and mandated choice.
- Before organs can be removed from a body, the person must be declared dead either by cardiopulmonary or brain death. This regulation excludes some potential donors, such as anencephalic infants.
- There are many ethical controversies over how organs are allocated, such as whether HIV-positive patients should receive organs, or whether patients who have not declared themselves donors should receive organs.
- The UAGA prohibits the sale of human organs, but there are loopholes allowing practically everyone involved in the trade of human organs, except for the donors and their families, to profit. This has led to support for financial incentives for donation, as has the argument that financial incentives would increase the number of donors.
- Those against financial incentives argue it demeans the human body and may exploit the poor to the advantage of the rich.
- Demand for organs is so high that Americans have resorted to visiting other countries in order to receive transplanted organs, and sometimes organs transplanted from animals, because the wait time is too long in the U.S.
- Tissue transplantation appears much less controversial than organ transplantation, and is treated entirely differently. The tissue industry is comprised of for-profit tissue banks and is run according to basic market principles of supply and demand. Further, it appears to be more highly regulated by states and other organizations, rather than the federal government.
- Xenotransplantation is emerging as one possible solution to the shortage of human organs. However, much research must be done in order to ensure safety and effectiveness before it can become widely accepted or supported by government assistance or private health insurance funds.

LAW NOTES

1. The data reported in this chapter was prepared by the Scientific Registry of Transplant Recipients (SRTR), a national database of transplantation statistics at the University of Michigan, unless otherwise stated. Founded in 1987, data in the registry are collected by the OPTN from hospitals and organ procurement organizations across the country. The SRTR contains current and past information about the full continuum of transplant activity, from organ donation and waiting list candidates to transplant recipients and survival statistics.

2. In a high profile case in the early 1990s, parents of an anencephalic newborn sought a Florida Supreme Court declaration stating their child was "dead" so they could donate its organs (see In re T.A.C.P., 609 So.2d 588 (Florida Supreme Court 1992)). The newborn had a fatal birth defect in which the child was born with only a brain stem but otherwise lacked a brain. In this case, the back of the skull was entirely missing. Anencephalic newborns can sometimes survive several days after birth because their brain stem

has a limited capacity to maintain autonomic bodily functions such as breathing and heartbeat; this ability soon ceases, however, in the absence of regulation from the missing brain. The parents found out about the child's condition during the mother's eighth month of pregnancy, but on the advice of physicians expressly continued the pregnancy in the hopes they could donate the child's organs and save the lives of other children. After the child's birth, however, health care providers refused to declare the child dead for donation purposes out of fear they would incur civil or even criminal liability. The child died while court proceedings were ongoing, thereby preventing the donation of any organs, as child organs are too fragile to be sustained after cardiopulmonary death. The court denied the parents' request to declare their newborn "dead" for several reasons:

- It was uncertain whether anencephalic newborns could provide viable organs to be successfully transplanted to other children in need
- The medical community's opinions on the ethical considerations were in flux
- The court was reluctant to possibly create further legal or constitutional issues without any consensus on the merits of using anencephalic newborns as organ donors

3. Until recently, outright sales of human organs have remained a largely unpopular subject. However, at the 2008 annual meeting of the American Society of Transplant Surgeons, most were in favor of studying incentives for living donors, and the fastest growing source of transplantable organs is now living donors (Satel & Hippen, 2007). The American Medical Association is now calling for pilot studies of incentives for organs (AMA, 2009). The public seems receptive as well, according to a new Gallup poll on attitudes toward donation of organs. The most striking results were among eighteen- to thirty-four-year-olds, wherein 34 percent said that incentives would make them more likely to donate, while 6 percent said less likely.

CHAPTER BIBLIOGRAPHY

AMA (American Medical Association). (2009). *Financial incentives for organ donation*, Policy E-2.15, AMA Policy Database. Washington, DC: AMA.

Appel Blue, E. E. (2008). Redefining stewardship over body parts. *Journal of Law & Health, 21*, 75-121.

Barshes, N. R. (2007). Justice, administrative law, and the transplant clinician: The ethical and legislative basis of a national policy on donor liver allocation. *Journal of Contemporary Health Law & Policy, 23*, 200-230.

Becker, G. S., & Elías, J. J. (2007). Introducing incentives in the market for live and cadaveric organ donations. *Journal of Economic Perspectives, 21* (3), 3-24.

Brennan, T. (2007). Markets in health care: The case of renal transplantation. *Journal of Law, Medicine & Ethics, 35*, 249-255.

Brody, J. E. (2007, August 28). The solvable problem of organ shortages. *New York Times*, p. F7.

Buck, L. A. (2007). Regulating human tissue banks. *St. Thomas Law Review, 20*, 121-153.

Carlson, P. D. (2006). The Organ Donation Recovery and Improvement Act: How Congress missed an opportunity to say "yes" to financial incentives for organ donation. *Journal of Contemporary Health Law & Policy, 23*, 136-166.

Cascalho, M. et al. (2004). Xenotransplantation and the future of renal replacement. *Journal of the American Society on Nephrology, 15*, 1106-1112.

Childress, J. F., & Liverman, C. T. (eds.). (2006). *Organ donation: Opportunities for action*. Washington, DC: Institute of Medicine Committee on Increasing Rates of Organ Donation.

Ciuffreda, D. et al (2007). Effects of immunosuppressive drugs on HIV infection: Implications for solid-organ transplantation. *Transplant International, 20* (8), 649-658.

Clamon, J. B. (2008). Tax policy as a lifeline: Encouraging blood and organ donation through tax credits. *Annals of Health Law, 17*, 67-99.

Cortez, N. (2008). Patients without borders: The emerging global market for patients and the evolution of modern health care. *Indiana Law Journal, 83*, 71-132.

Delmonico, F. L. (2004). Exchanging kidneys: Advances in living-donor transplantation. *New England Journal of Medicine, 350*, 1812-1814.

Deschamps, J. Y. (2005). History of xenotransplantation. *Xenotransplantation, 12* (2), 91-109.

Dunham, C. C. (2008). "Body property": Challenging the ethical barriers in organ transplantation to protect individual autonomy. *Annals of Health Law, 17*, 39-65.

Engelhardt, H. T. (2007). The injustice of enforced equal access to transplant operations: Rethinking reckless claims of fairness. *Journal on Law, Medicine & Ethics, 35* (2), 256-264 (addresses questions of justice and fairness in decisions by organ transplant selection committees and argues that there is no need to address moralities in our essentially secular society, so there is no warrant to prohibit free exchanges between willing traders; regulation is coercive and thus immoral).

Federal Register. (2003, October 23). Federal infectious disease issues in xenotransplantation. 68 F.R. 60697-02.

____. (2001, January 18). Availability of public disclosure and submission to FDA for public disclosure of certain data and information related to human gene therapy or xenotransplantation. 66 F.R. 4688-01.

FDA (U.S. Food & Drug Administration). (2006). *Xenotransplantation action plan*. Bethesda, MD: FDA, Center for Biologics Evaluation & Research.

____. (2003). *Guidance for industry: Source animal, product, preclinical, and clinical issues concerning the use of xenotransplantation products in humans: Final guidance.*

Bethesda, MD: FDA, Center for Biologics Evaluation & Research.

GIA (Global Industry Analysts). (2008). *Organ and tissue transplantation.* San Jose, CA: GIA.

Gitter, D. M. (2006). Am I my brother's keeper? The use of preimplantation genetic diagnosis to create a donor of transplantable stem cells for an older sibling suffering from a genetic disorder. *George Mason Law Review, 13,* 975-1035.

Goldstein, J. (2008, June 6). New York to test "rapid-organ-recovery" ambulance. *Wall Street Journal,* p. D2.

Goodwin, M. (2007). New frontiers in private ordering: The body market: Race politics & private ordering. *Arizona Law Review 49,* 599-636.

___. (2007a). My sister's keeper? Law, children, and compelled donation. *Western New England Law Review, 29,* 357-404.

___. (2004). Altruism's limits: Law, capacity, and organ commoditization. *Rutgers Law Review, 56,* 305-406.

Gross, J. A. (2008). E pluribus UNOS: The National Organ Transplant Act and its postoperative complications. *Yale Journal of Health Policy, Law & Ethics, 8,* 145-252.

Hauboldt, R. H. (2007). *2007 U.S. organ and tissue transplant cost estimates.* Brookfield, WI: Milliman. (Based on data from the: OPTN, Scientific Registry of Transplant Recipients, UNOS, National Marrow Donor Program, International Bone Marrow Transplant Registry, Analogous Blood and Marrow Transplant Registry, and Eye Bank Association of America).

Hebert, N. (2008). Creating a life to save a life: An issue inadequately addressed by the current legal framework under which minors are permitted to donate tissue and organs. *Southern California Interdisciplinary Law Journal, 17,* 337-379.

HHS (U.S. Department of Health & Human Services). (2006). *2020: A new vision—a future for regenerative medicine.* Washington, DC: HHS.

___. (2005). *Significant milestones in organ donation and transplantation.* Washington, DC: HHS.

___. (2004). *Consent in clinical research involving xenotransplantation.* Washington, DC: HHS. (emphasizing the necessity of continued, periodic testing for potential diseases or cancers).

HHS Secretary's Advisory Commission on Xenotransplantation. (2004). *Report on the state of the science in xenotransplantation.* Washington, DC: HHS.

Holland, J. A. (2006). The "catch-22" of xenotransplantation: Compelling compliance with long-term surveillance. *Houston Journal of Health Law & Policy, 7,* 151-182 (arguing xenotransplantation, a promising therapy using animal-to-human transplants, comes with numerous risks necessitating that xenotransplant recipients consent to long-term surveillance).

Jacob, M-A. (2003). On silencing and slicing: Presumed consent to post-mortem organ "donation" in diversified societies. *Tulsa Journal of Comparative & International Law, 11,* 239-242 (articulating a communitarian perspective on organ giving, suggesting that when individuals die, their legacy is best served by organ donations).

Jacobson, J. P. (2007). To pay or not to pay, that is the question: Coverage disputes between health plans and members. *Hamline Journal of Public Law & Policy, 29,* 445-462.

Jagger, S. F. (1006). *Health insurance: Coverage autologous bone marrow transplantation for breast cancer.* Washington, DC: U.S. General Accounting Office.

Johannes, L. (2005, April 14). Double standard: For some transplant patients, diseased hearts are lifesavers: Surgeons enlist elderly sick to receive inferior organs; the new ethical issues facing a risk of hepatitis C. *Wall Street Journal,* p. A1.

Jonsen, A. (2007). The God squad and the origins of transplantation ethics and policy. *Journal of Law, Medicine & Ethics, 35* (2), 238-240 (discussion of how mid-twentieth-century renal dialysis and transplantation functioned and how technology always held sway over human dignity).

Kaserman, D. L. (2007). Fifty years of organ transplants: The successes and the failures. *Issues on Law & Medicine, 23,* 45-69.

Katz, R. A. (2006). The re-gift of life: Who should capture the value of transplanted human tissue? *Health Lawyer, 18,* 14-43.

Lobas, K. (2006). Living organ donations: How can society ethically increase the supply of organs? *Seton Hall Legislative Journal, 30,* 475-507.

Lurie, P., & Zieve, A. (2006). Sequestered science: The consequences of undisclosed knowledge: Sometimes the silence can be like the thunder: Access to pharmaceutical data at the FDA. *Law & Contemporary Problems, 69,* 85-97.

McKeefery, M. J. (2007). A call to move forward: Pushing past the unworkable standard that governs undocumented immigrants' access to health care under Medicaid. *Journal on Health Care Law & Policy, 10,* 391-419.

McLean, S., & Williamson, L. (2005). *Xenotransplantation.* Rochester, MN: Mayo Clinic (provides a systematic account of the law and ethics of xenotransplantation).

Meckler, L. (2007, November 13). Kidney shortage inspires a radical idea: Organ sales: As waiting list grows, some seek to lift ban; Exploiting the poor? *Wall Street Journal,* p. A1.

___. (2007a, October 15). Kidney swaps seen as way to ease donor shortage. *Wall Street Journal,* p. A1.

___. (2007b, March 10). Picking winners, more kidneys for transplants may go to young: Policy to stress benefit to patient over length of time on wait list. *Wall Street Journal,* p. A1.

___. (2007c, January 30). What living organ donors need to know: Even as transplants surge, data on long-term impact on givers remain scant. *Wall Street Journal,* p. A1.

Mishra, D. (2007). Tis better to receive: The case for an organ donee's cause of action. *Yale Law & Policy Review, 25,* 403-414.

Morris, B. (2009). You've got to be kidneying me!: The fatal problem of severing rights and remedies from the body of organ donation law. *Brooklyn Law Review, 74,* 543-580.

Munzer, S. R. (2007). Human-nonhuman chimeras in embryonic stem cell research. *Harvard Journal of Law & Technology, 21,* 123-178.

NKF (National Kidney Foundation). (2008). *25 facts about organ donation and transplantation.* New York, NY: NKF.

Nygren, S. L. (2006). Organ donation by incompetent patients: A hybrid approach. *University of Chicago Legal Forum, 2006,* 471-502.

Pelletier, S. J. et al. (2004). Review of transplantation in HIV patients during the HAART era. *Clinical Transplants,* 63-82.

Platt, J. L. et al. (2004). Fusion of approaches to the treatment of organ failure. *American Journal of Transplantation, 4,* 74-77.

President's Council on Bioethics. (2004). *Reproduction and responsibility: The regulation of new technologies.* Washington, DC: PCB

Satel, S. L., & Hippen, B. E. (2007, January). When altruism is not enough: The worsening organ shortage and what it means for the elderly. *Elder Law Journal, 15,* 153-204.

Schenberg, B. A. (2007). Harvesting organs from minors and incompetent adults to supply the nation's organ drought: A critical review of the substituted judgment doctrine and the best interest standard. *Indiana Health Law Review, 4,* 319-359.

Schnitzler, M. (2007). Teens may lose transplanted organs when insurance runs out: Drugs that prevent organ rejection often too expensive for uninsured families. *Pediatric Transplantation, 11,* 127-131.

Spillman, M. A., & Sade, R. M. (2007). Clinical trials of xenotransplantation: Waiver of the right to withdraw from a clinical trial should be required. *Journal of Law, Medicine & Ethics, 35,* 265-272. (describing how the FDA requires lifelong surveillance of xenotransplant recipients because of the risks to public health posed by xenogeneic infectious diseases).

Statz, S. E. (2006). Finding the winning combination: How blending organ procurement systems used internationally can reduce the organ shortage. *Vanderbilt Journal of Transnational Law, 39,* 1677-1709.

Steinbrook, R. (2005). Public solicitation of organ donors. *New England Journal of Medicine, 353* (5), 441-444.

Sykes, M. et al. on behalf of the IXA Ethics Committee. (2004). Position paper of the Ethics Committee of the International Xenotransplantation Association. *Transplantation, 78* (8), 1101-1107.

Truog, R. D. (2007). Brain death, too flawed to endure, too ingrained to abandon. *Journal of Law, Medicine & Ethics, 35* (2), 273-281 (questions the integrity of policies that allow declarations of death in persons who are not actually dead with definitions of death driven more by politics than by ethical arguments, a dispute that will be settled only when human organs are no longer needed because of the clinical emergence of xenotransplantation).

____. (2005). The ethics of organ donation by living donors. *New England Journal of Medicine, 353* (5), 444-446.

Westphal, S. P. (2006, April 4). Bladders built in the lab: Cells, plastic shell combine to make the nearest thing yet to a fully man-made organ. *Wall Street Journal,* p. D1.

WHO (World Health Organization). (2008). *WHO guidance on xenogeneic infection/disease surveillance and response: A strategy for international cooperation and coordination.* Geneva, Switzerland: WHO

Williams, J. L. (2005). Patient safety or profit: What incentives are blood shield laws and FDA regulations creating for the tissue banking industry? *Indiana Health Law Review, 2,* 295-328.

CHAPTER 26
HIV/AIDS PANDEMIC

> *"No State, no matter how powerful, can by its own efforts alone make itself invulnerable to today's threats."*
>
> —Kofi Annan, former United Nations Secretary-General

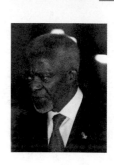

IN BRIEF

This chapter describes the devastating global Human Immunodeficiency Virus/Acquired Immune Deficiency Syndrome (HIV/AIDS) pandemic and examines the efforts of the U.S. to deal with this disease within its own borders. Attention is increasingly focused on the global pharmaceutical companies holding patents and controlling prices for antiretroviral drugs (ARVs) and AIDS drugs. Bowing to a variety of forces, the pharmaceutical industry now offers key drugs to resource-limited countries and low-income Americans at prices far below market prices. Rather than ending debate about the role and responsibility of the pharmaceutical industry in addressing the AIDS pandemic, however, the industry's moves have spurred further demands on pharmaceutical companies to address additional threats to global public health.

The HIV/AIDS pandemic has led to a critical examination of the U.S. Food and Drug Administration's system for oversight of developing and marketing new drugs in the U.S. and has also intensified the call to address the long-term health care needs of the chronically ill, including Americans living with HIV/AIDS. One policy issue under debate is whether a profit-oriented economic scheme is the most effective system for dealing with public health issues like the HIV/AIDS pandemic.

The effort of the U.S. to deal with the HIV/AIDS pandemic is described in this chapter within the context of the global fight against HIV/AIDS. This chapter focuses on three economically vulnerable populations:

- Low-income citizens in the U.S. who do not have access to medical treatment until they are disabled and become eligible for government medical benefits
- Newborns in the U.S.
- Resource-limited countries that do not have the manufacturing resources to supply their citizens with essential ARV/AIDS drugs or the resources to import them

Opinions about the HIV/AIDS pandemic are highly charged. The debate is emotional, opinionated, and thorny because it elicits reactions that are often religiously based about:

- Abortion
- Gay, lesbian, bisexual, and transgender (GLBT) people
- Government-funded abilities to deliver essential health services
- Morality
- Rights to freedom of speech and association
- Women's rights to self-determination and dignity

482

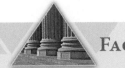

FACT OR FICTION

EARLY DETECTION OF HIV

Is there a heightened duty to routinely test high-risk patients for HIV infection?

In mid-1997, Armando Lopes, a gay man in Philadelphia, began treatment at Thomas Jefferson University Hospital for regular checkups and sick visits, including at least three routine blood screenings between 1997 and 2004. Lopes never requested a test for HIV, the virus that causes AIDS, at any time during the eight times he presented himself to the Department of Internal Medicine complaining of fatigue, anxiety, weight loss, memory loss, and dizziness during the summer of 2004. It was not until referral to a neurology resident after his eighth visit that Lopes underwent an HIV test, which came back positive. In 2006, Lopes filed a malpractice suit claiming his referring physician knew or should have known of his sexual orientation and that since he was at high risk for HIV, an HIV test should have been performed before his HIV infection progressed to symptomatic AIDS. Lopes maintained that if his HIV status had been detected earlier, his HIV infection could have been managed with ARVs, which could have slowed the disease's progression.

—*Lopes v. Shpigel,* 965 A.2d 311 (Superior Court of Pennsylvania 2008)
(affirming Court of Common Pleas' decision).
(See *Law Fact* at the end of this chapter for the answer.)

PRINCIPLES AND APPLICATIONS

HIV/AIDS is the foremost preventable disease worldwide. As a result, the HIV/AIDS pandemic is one of the most pressing threats to global public health in the present day (WHO, 2008). This chapter refers to HIV/AIDS as a pandemic, rather than an epidemic, because it more accurately describes the destructiveness of the incidence of this communicable disease. Epidemics are defined as communicable disease outbreaks that spread more quickly and extensively among groups of people than expected. Epidemics become categorized as pandemics when, like the HIV virus that causes AIDS, the disease occurs over a wide geographic area and affects large numbers of people (Kaiser, 2008). Often, the terms *pandemic* and *epidemic* are used interchangeably; this chapter, however, only uses the term *epidemic* in reference to tuberculosis (TB).

Moral Dilemmas

1. Should HIV/AIDS be treated as a routine communicable disease in the U.S.?

LEADING COMMUNICABLE DISEASE KILLER WORLDWIDE

The global impact of HIV/AIDS has been described as no less destructive than war (Ferreira, 2002). AIDS is the leading communicable disease killer worldwide, with TB second, and malaria close behind (WHO, 2008).

By definition, HIV and AIDS are simply two different stages of the same disease, hence the use of the term *HIV/AIDS* throughout this chapter. Basically, the HIV virus destroys certain white blood cells called CD4+ T cells, which are cells critical to the normal functioning of the human immune system by defending the body against illness. When HIV weakens the immune system, a person becomes more susceptible to developing a variety of cancers and infections from viruses, bacteria, and parasites (CDC, 2007d). People who test positive for HIV are diagnosed with AIDS when laboratory tests show their immune system is severely weakened by the virus or when opportunistic infections develop, which are diseases that might not affect people with normal immune systems but that take advantage of damaged immune systems (CDC, 2007a).

There is no cure for HIV/AIDS at this time, and a widely disseminated preventive vaccine or curative medicine is likely years away (IAVI, 2006). Once people are infected with HIV, they either control the damaging progression of the virus with ARV drugs before infections appear; or they become symptomatic with AIDS and face imminent death from multiple cancers and infections. ARVs can slow down the rate at which HIV weakens the immune system to the point of being diagnosed with full-blown AIDS.

There are also other medical treatments that can prevent or cure some of the infections associated with AIDS, but not AIDS itself. The simple, but essential, fact is that most of the deaths due to the disease could be prevented if people everywhere had access to information and medical treatment for preventing and treating HIV infection (WHO, 2004).

It is important to understand that HIV can be managed as a chronic lifelong disease, *if* the HIV infection is detected early enough and *if* the infected person has access to medical treatment to treat the opportunistic infections. It is these two "ifs" that make the HIV/AIDS pandemic such a global tragedy. Once a person is infected with HIV, they remain infected for life. HIV infections, however, do not have to lead to AIDS, if infected persons have access to ARVs.

With access to essential health care, AIDS deaths need not occur: 5,700 people need not die every day from AIDS and 800 children need not die from AIDS every single day because they lack access to the necessary health care (UN, 2007). This chapter uses the internationally accepted definition of children as those under the age of fifteen, which is also the definition used by most global health organizations. This is the primary reason why so much attention is being directed to AIDS: millions of people, including children, are dying from this preventable disease.

Key Public Health Statistics

One out of every twenty people worldwide is infected with HIV/AIDS (World Bank, 2008). It is difficult to imagine 33.2 million people being infected with HIV/AIDS worldwide (Kaiser, 2008). Imagine all the undergraduate college students between the ages of sixteen and twenty-four in the U.S. and then multiply this number by three; this statistic represents about 33.2 million people, which is almost one-tenth of the U.S. population, or only about 3.3 million less than California's population (BLS, 2008). Statistics like this are important, but they can also be numbing and desensitizing. They can make one forget an important fact: each of these numbers represents a person, not just a faceless, anonymous statistic.

The extent of the continuing HIV/AIDS epidemic in the U.S. is illustrated in Figure 26-1. According to the Centers for Disease Control, there are approximately 1.3 million people living with HIV/AIDS in the U.S., or slightly less than Hawaii's population. Of the total infected with HIV/AIDS worldwide, 2.5 million are children, which would represent slightly less than Nevada's population. Almost half of all new adult infections occur among the age group of fifteen to twenty-four years old (UNAIDS & WHO, 2007).

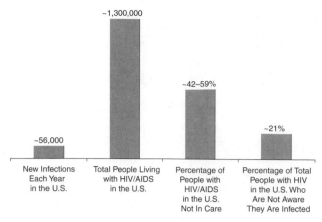

Figure 26-1: Continuing HIV/AIDS Epidemic in the U.S.

Delmar/Cengage Learning
Data retrieved from: Hall et al., 2008.

Key HIV/AIDS Statistics: U.S. and Globally

- New HIV infections annually: 56,000 in the U.S. (153 per day) and 2.5 million globally (6,800 per day)
- Annual deaths from HIV/AIDS and related illnesses: 14,000 in the U.S. (approximately 38 per day) and 2.1 million globally (over 5,700 per day)
- Children dying annually from HIV/AIDS and related illnesses: 18 in the U.S. (1 to 2 per month) and 300,000 globally (over 800 per day)
- People on ARVs: 10,000 in the U.S. and 2.1 million globally

Sources: CDC, 2008; UNAIDS & WHO, 2007; WHO, 2008; and NCHHSTP, 2008.

The question is: who should fund the staggering cost of treating this global pandemic? Who is responsible for addressing a pandemic combining a disease process that is still not completely understood and a pandemic with no known cure? The answers to both questions really depend upon how much leaders in the health care industry choose to engage this issue.

Successive Waves of the AIDS Pandemic

One thing is certain: the impact of HIV/AIDS is still not fully understood, particularly when the long term is considered. The HIV/AIDS pandemic appears to come in successive waves in different geographic areas. The first wave is HIV infection. This is followed several years later by a wave of opportunistic diseases, and then a wave of AIDS illnesses. Last, there is a wave of preventable deaths.

UNAIDS believes Africa is just entering the second wave of the HIV/AIDS pandemic (WHO, 2007). Africa has about 22.5 million people living with HIV/AIDS. Nearly 90 percent of all HIV-positive children live in sub-Saharan Africa, one of the poorest places in the world. Sub-Saharan Africa is comprised of the eight countries of Botswana, Lesotho, Mozambique, Namibia, South Africa, Swaziland, Zambia, and Zimbabwe. Botswana is said to have not yet been hit by the peak of the third wave, and has not advanced very far into the fourth wave (Guzik, 2007). Almost all of these HIV-positive children were born with the virus. Compared to the rest of the world, Africa accounts for almost 70 percent of the total HIV/AIDS cases worldwide (UNAIDS & WHO, 2007).

The U.S. has not successfully quarantined itself from Africa's first wave of HIV infection. In the mid-1970s, HIV crossed the shorelines of the U.S. Clearly, public health contagion is no longer restricted by country boundaries, if infectious disease waves ever were constrained by geographic boundaries. Today, no nation exists in isolation; the HIV/AIDS pandemic is a global phenomenon.

Global Interdependence

Beyond doubt, the HIV/AIDS pandemic has made the world more globally interdependent. While this trend is not new, the U.S. has reached a degree of more personal interdependence that Americans have never experienced before: what happens on one continent today affects those on another continent tomorrow.

The National Institutes of Health acknowledges the 1999 research finding that a subspecies of chimpanzees native to West Equatorial Africa was identified as the original source of the HIV virus (Gao et al., 1999). The virus most likely was introduced into the human population when hunters were exposed to the infected blood of non-human primates (Weis & Wrangham, 1999; NCHHSTP, 2007). The HIV/AIDS infection crisis is just the latest instance of the global phenomenon facing leaders in the health care industry. Virus infections in Africa infect people in the U.S., and vice versa. Interdependencies in public health are the direct consequence of globalization; it is also the recognition that we all live in a continually shrinking global village (Wharton, 2006a).

Emerging Epidemic of Tuberculosis

There is no need to look further than the airborne infectious disease of TB to fully grasp the global nature of public health today. There are over fourteen million TB cases worldwide, with almost ten thousand cases in the U.S. (CIA, 2007). HIV weakens the cells in the immune system needed to fight TB; up to half of all those living with AIDS eventually develop TB and it is the leading killer among patients who are HIV-positive (WHO, 2008a).

The seriousness of this emerging epidemic becomes obvious when the epidemiological data of this disease is analyzed. Worldwide, more than 9.2 million new TB cases appear each year with about 1.7 million deaths, of which about 700,000 cases and 200,000 deaths are AIDS-related (WHO, 2008a). The connectivity of communicable diseases is most evident with the HIV/AIDS pandemic, with HIV/AIDS being largely responsible for the growing number of TB cases in Asia and Africa.

Most significant is the fact that multi-drug-resistant TB appeared in the U.S. in December 2007. This is a TB that WHO describes as virtually incurable. The fear is that the present global caseload of TB infections may eventually be replaced by patients with multi-drug-resistant TB. Roughly half the multi-drug-resistant cases are in India and China. Moreover, data on drug resistance is available in only six countries in Africa where TB has tripled in the past fifteen years along with the rise of AIDS (WHO, 2008a). The biggest single factor driving up resistance of TB to drugs is irregular use of antibiotics, often a result of infrastructure breakdowns in the delivery of antibiotics to patients. HIV/AIDS, however, is aggravating and contributing to the spread of the TB problem (WHO, 2008a).

By contrast, although ARVs can treat HIV infections as a chronic disease, treatment for multi-drug-resistant TB works for only about 30 percent of those infected, even when essential health care is available. With communicable diseases like TB, bacteria is spread from person to person through the air; someone in Africa can cough at an airport, the bacteria contaminates a plane, and the plane heads to the U.S. filled with people who have been exposed to the bacteria. Clearly, it really does matter what happens outside the U.S.

THE DUAL ROLE OF GOVERNMENTS AND THE GLOBAL PHARMACEUTICAL INDUSTRY

While critics claim the global pharmaceutical industry is excessively profitable, there is no compelling evidence one way or the other. During the past five years, pharmaceutical stocks have under-performed in the overall market. The AMEX Pharmaceutical Index, composed of the fifteen largest pharmaceutical firms, has given investors returns below the Standard and Poor's 500 Index, a gauge of the broad market. All of the major HIV/AIDS drug manufacturers are in the AMEX Index, which has seen a decline in growth over the past decade. Still, there are suggestions the HIV/AIDS pandemic is a special disease state, one so serious the pharmaceutical industry has a moral obligation to provide essential ARVs and AIDS drugs to ameliorate this preventable disease, a moral obligation that should come before profits.

Calls for the global pharmaceutical industry to do more to meet the needs of people living with HIV/AIDS, however, are not limited to HIV/AIDS activists. WHO, along with almost every advocate of world economic reform, is demanding more action from the global pharmaceutical industry (*see e.g.*, Gostin, 2008; Lewis, 2006).

At the same time, it should not be forgotten that governments worldwide have responsibility for providing essential health care, including lifesaving ARVs and AIDS drugs, to their citizens. The U.S. and Europe, in particular, greatly benefit from their immense pharmaceutical resources. The HIV/AIDS pandemic obliges both the global pharmaceutical industry and governments worldwide, but especially governments in the high-income nations that benefit the most from the pharmaceutical industry, to ask how they can help correct things for those infected by HIV/AIDS (Wharton, 2006a).

Individual Entitlement to Health

The dual responsibility of the global pharmaceutical industry and governments worldwide to take action arises from the universal human rights founded in international law and the principles of moral obligation. The individual right to health is emphasized in customary international laws (WHO, 2007a). For instance, the International Covenant on Economic, Social, and Cultural Rights acknowledges the universal right to enjoyment of the highest attainable standard of health. The Academy of European Law goes so far as to argue that this means those infected with the HIV virus are entitled to ARVs to prevent their disease from progressing to full-blown AIDS (*see e.g.*, Goldschmidt, 2007).

Access to Essential Health Care

Closely related to this individual entitlement to health is a government's minimum obligations to its citizens, one obligation of which is the provision of access to essential health care (Yamin, 2003). The debate over what constitutes access (who has the right to make use of what medical innovations) and what comprises essential health care is unresolved; what is clear is that there is no consensus on either question.

One argument is that lack of early access to ARVs to slow down the rate at which HIV weakens the immune system is the difference between life and death for some people. Therefore, there is a right of mutually affordable access to ARVs. In this instance, the universal right to benefit from medical progress applies to medical treatment and the provision of ARVs as well as other essential AIDS drugs.

How these dual obligations to individual citizens, the entitlement to health and the right of access to essential health care, are being met is the topic of the next part of this chapter. The focus is on the role of governments and the global pharmaceutical industry in their fight against HIV/AIDS on the world stage.

THE FIGHT AGAINST HIV/AIDS IN THE U.S.

This section focuses on the fight against the HIV/AIDS pandemic in the U.S. Since the first case of AIDS was documented in the U.S. in 1981 (it was an additional two years before the HIV virus was identified), the pandemic has changed dramatically. At the same time, some attitudes have remained unchanged. The onset of the HIV/AIDS pandemic set the tone for blatant stigma and discrimination in the U.S. People with HIV/AIDS were:

- Evicted from their homes
- Excluded from schools
- Routinely fired from their jobs
- Shunned by family members
- Threatened with violence

(Schalman-Bergen, 2007)

Without existing treatment, people with HIV had little hope of survival in the 1980s and much of the 1990s. A positive HIV test result meant social isolation along with an inevitably painful death.

At the onset of the HIV/AIDS pandemic, HIV infection was primarily limited to three risk groups:

- Hemophiliacs
- Homosexual men
- Injection drug users[LN1]

Accordingly, public health policies and laws were targeted to those specific high-risk groups. HIV testing was offered only to persons who engaged in specific risk behaviors (*see generally* Schalman-Bergen, 2007).

Counseling and testing were available only for high-risk groups and for those in health care settings with high HIV prevalence (CDC, 2006). This approach lasted until the late 1990s, as more than forty thousand Americans became newly infected with HIV each year. Many Americans regarded the high-risk groups of HIV/AIDS victims as evidence the disease was a curse, and therefore it was proper to shun and even punish those who became HIV-infected (Hilzendeger, 2003).

Two-Pronged Approach to Health Care

In the late 1990s when ARVs first became widely available, the law and health care policies began to change. Today, there are two prongs of the approach to the HIV/AIDS pandemic in the U.S. The first prong is early detection and treatment of HIV. The second prong is containment (Bond, 2005). In an effort to contain the spread of HIV, the U.S. has:

- Criminal sanctions in place for the knowing transmission of HIV (Gallery & Pinkerton, 2006)
- Mandatory reporting requirements of HIV/AIDS infections
- Strict entry controls into the U.S. for persons with HIV/AIDS

Changing Demographics of the Disease

Both approaches to the HIV/AIDS pandemic in the U.S. are influenced by the changing demographics of the disease. While one-third of the new HIV infections are still among injection drug users, a trend that appears to have remained constant since the early 1980s (CDC, 2007a), the remaining two-thirds of those newly infected with HIV fall into groups not traditionally associated with HIV/AIDS:

- African Americans (Fenton et al., 2007)
- Heterosexual men and women (Kaiser, 2008a)
- Persons living outside of urban areas, many of whom do not believe they are at risk for HIV (Marks et al., 2006; CDC, 2003)
- Persons under the age of twenty (Chesson et al., 2004; Weinstock et al., 2004)

Disparate Impact of the Disease

African Americans make up about 47 percent of the total HIV-positive population and more than half of new HIV cases in the U.S., despite making up only 12 percent of the population (NCHHSTP, 2008).

- African American teenagers account for most of the new HIV cases reported (Kaiser, 2008a)
- AIDS is one of the top causes of death for African Americans (NMAC, 2006)
- African American women are nineteen times more likely to contract HIV than Caucasian women (CDC, 2007c)

This racial disparity is attributed primarily to high-risk heterosexual contact between African Americans who are unaware of their HIV status. Other contributing explanations are barriers to early diagnosis of HIV and poor access to quality health care (CDC, 2006c).

Late Testers

Unfortunately, most people in the U.S. are tested only after HIV/AIDS symptoms appear, which may be ten years or more after being infected (Feachem, 2007). These late testers are more likely to be African American or Hispanic, and are more likely to have contracted HIV through heterosexual contact (Schalman-Bergen, 2007). A debate is emerging in the U.S. over whether the concentrated attention upon the HIV/AIDS pandemic in resource-limited countries may inadvertently have caused the decline of HIV/AIDS detection in the U.S. (Yeun, 2007).

One of the most important factors linking poverty to HIV/AIDS in the U.S. is the lack of access to medical treatment. More than one-quarter of the unemployed and most low-wage earners in the U.S. lack health benefits. Over 15 percent of full-time workers and 20 percent of part-time workers are uninsured largely because they are concentrated in sectors in which their employers do not provide health benefits. The incomes of many low-wage earners make them ineligible for Medicaid and those who have employer-provided benefits often delay accessing health care due to high deductibles and other cost-sharing mechanisms in their benefit plans (NCHHSTP, 2008).

In part because of barriers to access, economically vulnerable populations often postpone treatment until they have full-blown AIDS (Yamin, 2003). Even when they are aware of their HIV status during the early stages of infection, they do not have access to ARVs or to comprehensive treatment to manage and monitor medical complications associated with HIV (Bartlett et al., 2004). This lack of access inevitably fuels a downward cycle of poverty. Individuals with HIV/AIDS who are unable to obtain treatment are forced to abandon the labor force due to illness and infection and are pushed further down the economic ladder as they seek to attend to their basic needs (NCHHSTP, 2008). Over one-third of Americans living with HIV/AIDS delayed or did not obtain needed health care because of food and housing needs (Ryan, 2004), while one-third to one-half are either homeless or in imminent danger of losing their homes (HUD, 2009). Homelessness and loss of homes is due to compounding factors, such as increased medical costs and limited incomes or reduced ability to keep working due to HIV/AIDS and related illnesses.

Moral Dilemmas

1. If HIV is a chronic, manageable disease when ARVs are taken early and consistently, why are so many Americans being tested for HIV only after the disease has progressed and symptoms appear?

First Prong: Detection and Treatment of HIV/AIDS

Angered by apparent intolerant reactions to individuals with HIV/AIDS, activists have demanded greater confidentiality and anti-discrimination protections for this vulnerable population (UCSF & National HIV/AIDS Clinicians' Consultation Center, 2008). Federal legislation and few states, however, afford adequate protection against discrimination for individuals with HIV/AIDS. This lack of comprehensive protection may be related to concerns regarding the potential costs of accommodating the 1.3 million people living with HIV/AIDS in the U.S., especially if such accommodation occurs from the time of their infection.

Current restrictions on discrimination against individuals with HIV-positive status mirror existing social norms (Selmi, 2006). While enactment of the Americans with Disabilities Act (ADA) in 1990 represented a consensus in the U.S. that there should be a comprehensive national mandate for the elimination of discrimination against individuals with serious disabilities, there is little support for extending anti-discrimination laws to those who appear undeserving of protection. Thus, there is generally broad support for protecting individuals with serious disabilities at the end stage of AIDS, but there is little support for extending protections to asymptomatic HIV-infected individuals.

Routine HIV Testing and Detection in the U.S.

The good news is with improvements in treatment and the advent of some confidentiality protection, as illustrated in Figure 26-2, HIV testing is slowly becoming a more constructive tool in the fight against HIV/AIDS (Schalman-Bergen, 2007). In 2006, the federal government revised its guidelines for HIV testing and detection (CDC, 2006b). Routine testing of everyone between the ages of thirteen and sixty-

four is now recommended, regardless of individual risk factors.

While HIV testing remains voluntary, it is usually offered on an opt-out basis. Separate, written informed consent is no longer needed. Consent is part of the general informed consent for health care. In addition, counseling is no longer required with HIV testing. Routine HIV screenings should identify persons with unrecognized infections in the same way as screening and diagnostic tests for high cholesterol or some sexually transmitted diseases do. Today, HIV tests are increasingly treated the same as cholesterol tests and Pap smears, standard diagnostic tests routinely administered.

Early HIV diagnosis is crucial because early intervention leads to slower disease progression. When ARVs are taken early and consistently, HIV is a chronic, manageable disease that generally does not develop into full-blown AIDS because of the low maintained level of virus in the bloodstream (Bartlett et al., 2004). Opportunistic diseases arising from the HIV infection can generally be individually treated with other curative drugs. ARVs also significantly reduce the transmissibility of HIV by lowering the amount of virus in the bloodstream of those infected (Montaner et al., 2006).

HIV Testing Among Pregnant Women

Federal guidelines recommend HIV testing for all pregnant women since perinatal transmission of HIV is substantially reduced by the administration of ARVs to HIV-infected pregnant women and their newborns (CDC, 2007). Transmission of HIV can be managed during the period surrounding

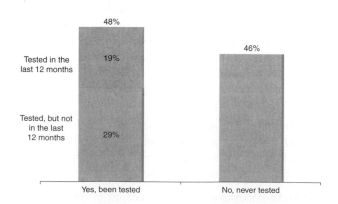

FIGURE 26-2: The U.S. Public's Experience with HIV Testing

Delmar/Cengage Learning
Data derived from Schalman-Bergen, 2007.

childbirth, which is around week twenty-eight of an HIV-infected mother's pregnancy to around one month after the birth (Anderson & Sansom, 2006). Nonetheless, and in spite of this available health care, HIV testing is not routinely offered to pregnant women on a standard basis in the U.S. Yet, with proper prenatal treatment, the risk of an HIV-positive pregnant woman passing HIV to her newborn child is less than 1 percent (McKenna & Hu, 2007).

Repeat HIV screening in the third trimester is recommended for high-risk women and for women in areas with elevated rates of HIV infection among pregnant women (CDC, 2007). High-risk women are most likely to be under thirty years of age (Branson et al., 2001) and have:

- A sexual partner who has HIV
- A sexual partner who may have had sex with other men
- Shared needles or other equipment with injection partners
- Unprotected sexual intercourse with multiple sex partners (male or female)
- Used or has a sexual partner who has used injection drugs in the past ten years

It is recommended pregnant women receive preventive information including a description of interventions that can reduce HIV transmission from mother to infant, such as not breastfeeding, and the meanings of positive and negative test results, such as that test results may not appear positive until three months after infection (CDC, 2006b).

Newborn HIV Testing

Much work remains regarding testing pregnant women. Between one hundred and two hundred infants are infected with HIV each year in the U.S. (CDC, 2008). Many of these newborn infections involve women who were not treated early enough in pregnancy or who did not receive detection services or information on preventing transmission (CDC, 2007b).

Perinatal HIV transmission is the most common route of HIV infection in children and is now the source of almost all HIV/AIDS cases in U.S children (CDC, 2007). Children born HIV-positive who go without treatment usually develop HIV-related infections within the first year (Yeun, 2007). Without treatment, children infected with HIV progress very rapidly towards AIDS and die within a few years. However, medications can prevent children with HIV from developing AIDS.

Newborn testing is generally mandatory if a mother's HIV status is unknown or test results are not available. If the mother's HIV status is unknown prior to the onset of labor and rapid HIV testing is not done during labor, rapid HIV testing of the infant immediately post-partum is routinely done with or without the mother's consent (CDC, 2006a).

Minors' Right to Consent to HIV Testing and Treatment

Since the first HIV/AIDS case was reported in the U.S., states have expanded minors' authority to consent to health care without parents taking part in the decisions, including care related to sexual activity. The age of majority is generally accepted as eighteen years in this chapter, as distinguished from the international definition of children as those under the age of fifteen. All states allow most minors, generally beginning at twelve to fourteen years of age, to consent to HIV testing (AGI, 2008).

While all states permit minors to consent to HIV/AIDS treatment, some states allow physicians to inform parents if a minor is seeking or receiving treatment. Iowa is the only state that requires parental notification in the case of a minor's positive HIV test; in Colorado, physicians may inform parents of a minor's decision to consent to HIV/AIDS medical services if the minor is younger than sixteen.

Access to Medical Treatment

HIV testing should ideally be coordinated with treatment, which raises the issue of access to health care in the U.S. Early medical treatment significantly improves the health of HIV-positive patients while also greatly reducing transmissibility of the disease. Therefore, early access to health care is crucial to the success of widespread HIV testing. Unfortunately, early access in the U.S. is unobtainable for most people with HIV, especially those without access to private health care (Yamin, 2003).

Medicaid, the federal and state medical assistance program, represents the largest source of health care coverage for Americans living with HIV/AIDS. Almost half of the individuals living with HIV/AIDS are enrolled in Medicaid; 20 percent are uninsured (NASTAD, 2008). However, in order to qualify for Medicaid, most HIV-positive people must be both low income and disabled. Most symptomatic individuals with AIDS qualify for Medicaid because they are Supplementary Security Income (SSI) beneficiaries, both disabled and low income. The SSI income standard is 74 percent of the Federal Poverty Level, which is $10,830 annually for an individual in 2009 (74 *Federal Register* 4199-04).While all states are required to provide Medicaid to the disabled, people with HIV do not qualify as disabled without an AIDS diagnosis in most states (Kaiser, 2006). The cruel irony is Medicaid requires persons to manifest symptoms of the disease before providing the ARV drugs that would have prevented the symptoms. This means treatment is withheld for most low-income Americans until it is too late for preventative health care (Montaner et al., 2006).

States have limited discretion to structure their own Medicaid programs (NASTAD, 2007a). Currently only Massachusetts, Maine, and the District of Columbia have received waivers from the federal government to permit HIV-positive patients to access Medicaid before they are certified disabled by AIDS. Ironically, most state Medicaid eligibility rules are not in line with the federal government's guidelines of the standard of care for treating HIV/AIDS (PricewaterhouseCoopers, 2003).

Federal legislation would enable state Medicaid programs to offer early coverage for pre-disabled, low-income persons living with HIV; the Early Treatment for HIV Act (ETHA) has not been approved by Congress since it was first introduced in 2004 (Anderson & Sansom, 2006). Such legislation might help address the limited access to medical treatment for HIV-infected individuals in many parts of the U.S.

Second Prong: Containment
of HIV Infections

The second prong of the U.S. approach to containment is reporting and contact notification of HIV infections. Numerous health laws come into conflict on this debate, including:

- Entitlement to know of risks
- Right of confidentiality and privacy
- Protection against discrimination
- Duty to warn
- Obligation to protect the public health

Coupled with these conflicts is the tension between public health agencies with their duty to the greater good of the community and physicians with their duty towards their individual patients.

Partner Notification Requirements

Both physicians and laboratories are required to report the names of newly diagnosed HIV patients to state communicable disease registries. A controversial issue is whether physicians should also disclose the HIV status of their patients to known sexual partners, such as spouses, to whom HIV is likely to be transmitted (Pottker-Fishel, 2007).

The failure to warn does not give rise to liability if the known sexual partner simply fears becoming infected, but physician liability could arise if the known sexual partner is not notified and subsequently becomes HIV-positive (Lin & Liang, 2005). At the same time, physicians of HIV-infected patients are not required to investigate and notify third parties about their risk of contracting HIV.

The confidentiality requirements of the Health Insurance Portability and Accountability Act (HIPAA), and various confidentiality laws that vary by state, all add to the confusion. Most states have duty-to-warn laws requiring sexual partners to be informed of their HIV exposure; other states require that if a newly diagnosed HIV patient refuses to report a partner to the state who may have been exposed, physicians must report any partner of whom they are aware (Lin & Liang, 2005). Some states also have laws mandating a duty to warn and requiring notification by physicians to third parties known to be at risk for future HIV transmission from patients known to be infected.

In general, states have one of three types of partner notification laws:

- Physicians are mandated to report the partner's name and the state then notifies the partner
- Physicians may either report the partner's name or notify the partner directly
- Reporting is optional

Obviously, all information regarding HIV status must be reported on a need-to-know basis; otherwise, health care providers may face liability for publicly and needlessly disseminating personal information. Both the ADA and a number of court decisions treat HIV status as a private fact whose disclosure is highly offensive (Strahilevitz, 2008). Health care providers may be assessed punitive damages for wrongful disclosure of HIV status in violation of HIPAA and state confidentiality statutes if such information is disclosed to anyone without the need to know.

Wrongful Disclosure of HIV Status

Individuals with HIV, whose status was made public to someone without the need to know, have found limited relief in attempts to protect the privacy of their HIV status (Hilzendeger, 2003). One obstacle to finding liability for wrongful disclosure is that the definition of publicity in many states is disclosure and release of information to a large group of people. Communication of facts, such as HIV status, to a single person or even to a small group of persons is not wrong under many state confidentiality statutes unless a special relationship exists, such as the relationship between a patient and health care professional or between employee and employer.

> ## Moral Dilemmas
>
> 1. Should health care providers be required to disclose the status of their newly diagnosed HIV patients to their patient's known sexual partner(s) to whom HIV is likely to be transmitted?
>
> 2. What about their employer(s) if HIV infection poses a risk in the patient's work place, such as someone who works in health care?

Criminal Statutes

Many states have criminal laws that in effect discourage HIV testing. For example, most states will prosecute persons with HIV who engage in various sexual activities without first disclosing their HIV-positive status to prospective sex partners (Gallery & Pinkerton, 2006).

All states have criminal laws that punish HIV-positive individuals for sexual behaviors posing some risk of HIV transmission, even if no transmission occurs. Most states have laws criminalizing sexual contact by persons with HIV unless they:

- Abstain from unsafe sex
- Disclose their HIV status to their partners
- Obtain consent from their partners

Most states find the knowing transmission of HIV to be a felony. Alabama, Kansas, Montana, and New York are the only four states to recognize transmission as a misdemeanor crime (ACLU, 2008). Whether these contrasting laws influence high-risk sexual behaviors is debatable (Burris et al., 2007).

Federal immigration policies also pose significant disincentives to voluntary testing, as anyone living in the U.S. without legal status may be removed if they are found HIV-positive (Schalman-Bergen, 2007). In addition, strict controls against entry into the U.S. are in place for people with HIV/AIDS; anyone found bringing ARVs or AIDS drugs into the U.S. will be arrested and placed on a flight back to their country of origin.

Mandatory Testing of Sexual Offenders

Mandatory HIV testing is generally required for anyone arrested for a crime involving sexual intercourse or sexual contact. Most states require accused sex offenders to submit, in response to a court order or a request by the alleged victim, to HIV testing and follow-up testing if the initial test is negative. Some states require that an indication of potential viral transmission take place, such as the exchange of bodily fluids, before testing is required.

HIV as Another Communicable Disease

In the U.S., HIV is technically treated no differently from other communicable diseases (Fairchild et al., 2003). There are two sides to this policy. One side maintains the current privacy and anti-discrimination laws at the federal and state levels sufficiently protect persons living with HIV/AIDS. Proponents of this view accept routine HIV testing and do not see any significant existing stigma associated with HIV/AIDS (Bayer & Fairchild, 2006).

The other side maintains there is ongoing stigma, discrimination, and distrust of the health care system in many high-risk communities in the U.S. Proponents of this view are concerned with civil rights and privacy protections of those in society at the greatest risk of discrimination. They want to treat HIV/AIDS differently from other afflictions. Both sides of this debate agree on the need for a national, coordinated public health response to the HIV/AIDS pandemic in the U.S. (CDC, 2006; Rajkumar, 2007; *see generally* Schalman-Bergen, 2007).

Adequacy of Protection from Stigma and Discrimination

One central disagreement over routine HIV detection, testing, and reporting is whether current anti-discrimination laws adequately protect against the stigma of HIV/AIDS. Though both state and federal confidentiality and anti-discrimination protections exist, state statutes vary widely, many without fully protecting persons living with HIV/AIDS (Schalman-Bergen, 2007).

HIV Discrimination Under the Americans with Disabilities Act

At the federal level, persons with HIV/AIDS do not enjoy guaranteed protection against discrimination under the ADA. Courts, including the U.S. Supreme Court, usually insist only a narrow set of deserving individuals with HIV-positive status qualify for protection. For the first time, in *Bragdon v. Abbott*, the U.S. Supreme Court had the opportunity to address the issue of whether HIV/AIDS infection itself constituted a disability.

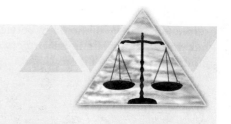

HIV INFECTION AS A DISABILITY

Bragdon v. Abbott

[Dentist v. HIV Patient]

524 U.S. 624 (U.S. Supreme Court 1998)

FACTS: Sidney Abbott, after being refused in-office treatment by her dentist due to her HIV-positive status, sued under the ADA. Abbott refused to pay $185 for a hospital procedure that would cost only $35 at her dentist's office.

ISSUE: Did a dentist's refusal to treat an HIV-infected patient constitute disability discrimination?

HOLDING AND DECISION: Yes, HIV-positive status, from the moment of infection, constitutes a disability under the ADA if the HIV infection substantially limits a major life activity.

ANALYSIS: The Supreme Court applied a three-part test to determine whether Abbott was disabled and found that her HIV-positive status constituted a disability under the ADA. The Court held Abbott was disabled because of reproduction concerns. Abbott's decision not to have children was motivated by her HIV diagnosis. Therefore, her HIV infection was an impairment that substantially limited the major life activity of reproduction.

First, the Court decided HIV-positive status constituted an impairment under the ADA. The Court was influenced by the fact that HIV follows a predictable and unalterable course. The Court assumed HIV was non-treatable; HIV-positive status was characterized as being constant and permanent.

Second, the Court determined HIV-positive status affected the major life activity of reproduction. The possibility that an individual's HIV status might affect other major life activities was left open.

Finally, the Court found Abbott's HIV-positive status substantially limited her ability to reproduce; the risks of HIV transmission to a male sexual partner, and the risks of perinatal transmission of HIV to a newborn constituted substantial limitations on reproduction. While the use of ARV treatment to lower the risk of perinatal transmission was considered, the Court did not find the reduction in risk affected the limitations on reproduction. HIV was characterized by the Court as a dreadful and fatal disease.

The Court conceded reproduction may be possible for women infected with HIV, but found the danger to public health resulting from such reproduction constituted a substantial limitation on procreation. To support this conclusion, the Court considered the negative economic and legal consequences of the decision of HIV-infected women to have children, including the costs of treating a newborn with HIV and the criminality of sexual activity for individuals with HIV/AIDS in most states.

RULE OF LAW: The Court held that an individual's HIV infection must substantially limit a major life activity to be considered a disability for purposes of ADA protection, and declined to decide whether HIV/AIDS infection was a per se disability under the ADA.

(*See generally* Bucholtz, 2005; Burgdorf, 2008; Gersen, 2006; Kaufman, 2006; Keshishyan, 2008; Rosenthal, 2006; Rothstein, 2008; Whitebread, 2006).

The U.S. Supreme Court remanded the case to the First Circuit to determine whether filling the dental cavity of an asymptomatic HIV patient posed a direct threat to a dentist. The First Circuit subsequently ruled that universal precautions sufficiently reduced the risk of infection in a dentist's office. The *Bragdon* decision that HIV infection is not by itself a per se disability remains controversial (Christie, 2007). The Supreme Court remains very hesitant to open the door to a non-traditional disability such as a communicable disease. However, the aim of recent amendments to the Americans with Disabilities Act is to restore its original purpose of protecting the disabled (*see* 42 U.S.C.A. § 12101 (2009)).

HYGIENIST'S HIV INFECTION AS A DISABILITY

Waddell v. Valley Forge Dental Associates, Inc.

[Dental Hygienist v. Dental Clinic]

276 F.3d 1275 (U.S. Court of Appeals for the 11th Circuit 2001),

U.S. Supreme Court certiorari denied, 535 U.S. 1096 (U.S. Supreme Court 2002)

FACTS: Spencer Waddell, an HIV-positive dental hygienist, sued Valley Forge Dental Associates, his employer, alleging *inter alia* he was discriminated against in violation of the ADA when his employer refused to allow him to continue treating patients due to his HIV-positive status.

ISSUE: Was an HIV-positive dental hygienist discriminated against in violation of the ADA?

HOLDING AND DECISION: No, because the hygienist posed a significant risk of transmitting his disease to patients, he was not a qualified individual under the ADA.

ANALYSIS: The court concluded that several factors, when taken together, indicated the hygienist posed a significant risk to others in the workplace:

- Possibility of an inadvertent bite or other accident during a dental cleaning
- Risk that hygienists will be stuck or pricked while using an instrument
- Routine patient bleeding during dental work

- Statements of the hygienist and his medical experts acknowledging there was some risk, even if theoretical and small, blood-to-blood contact between hygienist and patient can occur
- Use of sharp instruments by dental hygienists

The court noted that "the Supreme Court declined to address whether asymptomatic HIV is a per se disability, arguably suggesting, at least implicitly, that the preferred method is to address whether an impairment causes a substantial limitation upon a major life activity on a case-by-case, individualized basis."

RULE OF LAW: The hygienist, because he was infected with HIV, was a direct threat to his workplace, and, therefore, was not a qualified individual under the ADA.

(*See generally* Gupta, 2005).

Review of subsequent court decisions finds individuals with HIV-positive status are continually failing to present the necessary evidence to obtain protection from discrimination.[LN2] Any further restriction in the U.S. Supreme Court's interpretation of ADA law could have significant repercussions for HIV-infected people (Metnick, 2003).

Moral Dilemmas

1. Would defining HIV or AIDS as a disability increase the stigmatization of people with HIV/AIDS?

Confidentiality of HIV Status

Virtually every state collects the names of individuals who test positive for HIV. Many states also require physicians to report private information, such as drug use and sexual history about anyone who tests positive (ACLU, 2008). While public health reporting actions are a valid exercise of the state's police powers and are not viewed as an impermissible intrusion into personal privacy, the collection of identifiable HIV test results is still strongly debated. Despite the U.S. Supreme Court's ruling on medical privacy issues, the privacy arguments in *Whalen* are being repeated in battles over HIV reporting (Richards, 2007; *see Whalen v. Roe*, 429 U.S. 589 (U.S. Supreme Court 1977)).

The debate over whether states are required to report new cases of HIV infection by full names rather than by codes is another aspect of the argument over whether to treat HIV as a routine communicable disease in the U.S. One side of the debate claims name-based reporting is essential for epidemiological purposes, while the other side claims the practice is unnecessary and dissuades some persons from being tested out of concern for their confidentiality (Stoto, 2008).

Preventing Occupational HIV Transmission

The HIV Post-Exposure Registry documents about sixty cases of occupational exposure among health care professionals in the U.S. This means about three health care professionals become infected with HIV each year. To prevent HIV transmissions, health care professionals should assume the blood and other body fluids from all patients are potentially infectious. They should therefore follow infection control precautions at all times (CDC, 2002). These universal precautions include:

- Routine use of barriers such as gloves and/or goggles when anticipating contact with blood or body fluids
- Washing hands and other skin surfaces immediately after contact with blood or body fluids
- Careful handling and disposing of sharp instruments during and after use

While safety devices have been developed to help prevent needle-stick injuries, they must be used properly to reduce the risk of exposure to HIV. Most infections are related to sharps disposal. Although the most important strategy for reducing the risk of occupational HIV transmission is to prevent occupational exposures to blood-borne pathogens, risk plans for post-exposure should be in place in all health care settings (CDC, 2001).

THE GLOBAL BLOOD SUPPLY

HIV tests currently in use are highly accurate, but still cannot detect HIV 100 percent of the time in donated blood (FDA, 1992). This is especially true as HIV sometimes cannot be detected until three months after infection took place.

Blood Safety in the U.S.

Today, the blood supply in the U.S. is one of the safest in the world, with stringent donor selection practices and numerous diagnostic screenings. Since 1984, gay men have been banned from the donation of blood (FDA, 1992; see 21 C.F.R. § 640.3). This federal policy is one of the few government policies that makes any differentiation based on sexual orientation (Pulver, 2008).[LN3] Additionally, the improvement of collection and processing methods for blood products has reduced the number of HIV infections resulting from the use of these products. Currently, the risk of infection with HIV through receiving a blood transfusion or blood products is extremely rare in the U.S. and has become progressively lower, even in geographic areas with high HIV rates (CDC, 2006a).

Nearly everyone infected with HIV through blood transfusions received those transfusions before 1985, the year HIV testing began for all donated blood (FDA, 1992). The Institute of Medicine found many organizations shared blame for the compromised U.S. blood safety at the onset of the AIDS pandemic in the 1980s:

- American Red Cross
- Blood and plasma collection agencies
- Blood product manufacturers
- Centers for Disease Control and Prevention
- Community blood banks
- National Hemophilia Foundation
- National Institutes of Health
- U.S. Food and Drug Administration

Specifically, blood banks and fractionation companies were criticized for not initiating surrogate laboratory testing and for accepting blood donations from gay men (Leveton et al., 1995).

As a result of the contaminated blood supply in the 1980s, HIV-infected transfusion recipients received compensation awards and financial settlements. The federal Ricky Ray Hemophilia Relief Fund Act of 1998 authorized $750 million in payments to more than 6,200 hemophiliacs who had received HIV-infected clotting concentrate (see 42 U.S.C.A. § 300c-22 note (2000)). Four drug companies subsequently completed a financial settlement with the Committee of Ten Thousand, a group of ten thousand HIV-infected hemophiliacs. It authorized individual payments of $100,000 to about 8,700 HIV-infected hemophiliacs and to individuals they had infected (Pulver, 2008).

This settlement involved a nationwide group of HIV-positive hemophiliacs who sued four drug companies that manufactured blood solids, claiming that the negligence of the companies caused the plaintiffs' infections. First identified in 1981, AIDS was diagnosed in hemophiliacs beginning in 1982, and by 1984 the medical community agreed that the virus was transmitted by blood as well as by semen. That year it was demonstrated that treatment with heat could kill HIV in the blood supply and in the following year a reliable test for the presence of the virus in blood was developed (unfortunately, the cure for HIV/AIDS cannot be resolved by a something like a dialysis of people's blood who are HIV-positive; HIV is a virus that attacks the body's cells). By this time, however, a large number of hemophiliacs had become infected. HIV-positive hemophiliacs who could prove they had not engaged in high-risk behaviors received compensation from the settlement since it was more likely than not that contaminated blood caused their HIV infections.

Blood Safety in Resource-Limited Countries

It is estimated that up to 10 percent of the global HIV infections result from transfusion of contaminated blood or blood products (Walker, 2007). Blood safety continues to be a global concern, as almost half the donations in resource-limited countries are unscreened for HIV. Moreover, resource-limited countries do not routinely screen for the hepatitis B virus or the hepatitis C virus (Weinberg, 2002).

LACK OF ACCESS TO HEALTH CARE

HIV/AIDS remains a death sentence for most low income adults in the U.S. and for those in resource-limited countries. While HIV has become a serious, but manageable, chronic condition for those with the resources to gain access to health care, lack of early access to care is the difference between life and death from AIDS (WHO, 2007a).

THE GLOBAL HIV/AIDS CRISIS AND PHARMACEUTICALS

The search for new health care models to help the world's poorest populations is perhaps most evident in sub-Saharan Africa, where the HIV/AIDS crisis has drawn international attention to the suffering of millions who live without essential health care. While the HIV/AIDS pandemic has focused largely on the development of drugs, it has raised awareness about the lack of essential health care systems to deliver health care in poverty-ridden developing countries.

Coupled with the debate about global responsibility for the HIV/AIDS pandemic is the question of how to address it in the U.S. While recognizing the nature of the global pandemic, HIV/AIDS could enable broader health care development in the U.S. (Mukherjee, 2007). All the money and attention being directed to this particular disease segment could be used to build a foundation for universal primary care and comprehensive high-quality disease management of chronic conditions (Wharton, 2006a).

Federal Government Expenditures on HIV/AIDS Programs since 2001
- More than $108 billion:
  - $89 billion for treatment
  - $18 billion for research
  - $1 billion for testing
- About $1.5 million per hour

Source: The White House Office of National AIDS Policy, Special Data Request (2009).

The federal Ryan White Comprehensive AIDS Resources Emergency Act of 1990 (CARE) is one of the largest sources of funding for HIV/AIDS health care and covers both uninsured and underinsured persons living with HIV/AIDS (*see* 42 U.S.C.A. § 300ff-33 (2006)). In addition, CARE specifically addresses care for families and children with provisions for ARV treatment and both prenatal and postnatal care of HIV-positive pregnant mothers (White House, 2006).

Access to ARVs and AIDS Drugs

The public perception of the HIV/AIDS pandemic and pharmaceuticals situation is that there needs to be an immediate procurement of drugs. However, the problem with access to medical treatment is not necessarily the cost of drugs like it was in the earlier years of the outbreak (Mukherjee, 2007). Instead, it is now the multifaceted difficulty of finding the workers to provide health care in resource-limited countries (Philips & Moffett, 2005) and the struggle of obtaining early access to medical treatment.

These difficulties are intertwined with the willingness of those infected to accept responsibility for adherence to their drug regimes (Tsai, 2007), as well as the responsibility not to knowingly infect others. HIV treatment requires a high degree of adherence to taking ARVs. With the advent of combination drug therapies, regimen compliance for HIV/AIDS patients is particularly complex. In the past, some of the ARVs were unpleasant, debilitating, and lifestyle limiting, but this is no longer the case for most brand drugs. Nevertheless, ARV therapy should be part of an integrated package of interventions that includes care and support activities, all of which complement and reinforce adherence to ARV drug regimes.

Persons living with HIV who take less than 95 percent of their medications run the serious risk of developing resistance and failing therapy. Additionally, there is the very real danger non-compliance will lead to transmission of resistant viruses to others, a phenomenon that is already emerging. On the other hand, the virulence of the HIV virus decreases if ARVs are taken as prescribed. Transmission of the HIV virus is always possible with someone who is HIV-positive, but with safe sex practices such as condom use, transmission of the disease is less likely. Nevertheless, once infected with HIV, individuals are infected for life; there is no curative treatment for HIV infections (IAVI, 2006).

Humanitarian Tradition of the Pharmaceutical Industry

The global pharmaceutical industry does, contrary to widespread belief, have a humanitarian tradition. Pharmaceutical employees believe their corporations are different from other multinational corporations. While there is a longstanding norm in the U.S. for industry to engage in philanthropic activities, the most effective and appropriate contributions are those that draw on a company's core business expertise.

At the same time, discounting ARVs and AIDS drugs in resource-limited countries is not entirely altruistic. For one thing, the pharmaceutical industry is not giving up many sales at higher prices, since these countries are too poor to pay otherwise. The industry also needed a public relations boost in the U.S., as it became clear the HIV/AIDS crisis was reaching catastrophic proportions worldwide, partly because of the industry's early failure to supply needed drugs to resource-limited countries (Ferreira, 2002).

Competitive Threats from Generics

The pharmaceutical industry also faces serious competitive threats from generics. Cipla, a generic drug manufacturer in India, asked the South African government for permission to sell cheaper copies of eight ARVs and AIDS drugs, including those on which Merck holds patents. A South African law allows the government to give such permission in an emergency. The Brazilian and Thailand governments are also threatening to permit use of generic versions of patent-protected drugs. For the pharmaceutical industry, discounting the prices of ARVs and AIDS drugs is better than surrendering the market to generics. This is a problem that could spill over to other drugs.

Pricing of ARVs and AIDS Drugs

As publicly- traded companies, the pharmaceutical industry is obligated to seek profits for shareholders. Like any profit-seeking company, they are free to charge the highest prices the market will bear. Consider though, is the pharmaceutical industry really like other for-profit businesses when it comes to the HIV/AIDS pandemic?

ARVs and AIDS drugs are not like most consumer products. For example, Apple may have a monopoly on iPhone technology, but if it charges too much, customers can choose Samsung or Sony Ericsson instead, or can choose to purchase nothing at all. Pharmaceuticals, on the other hand, can charge patients $10,000 to $15,000 a year for drugs costing only a few hundred dollars to make. Most patients do not have the option of not buying most lifesaving drugs; they either pay the retail price or go without the drug treatment. Where a generic drug is available, patients may have the option of choosing a cheaper drug, but this is another misnomer when it comes to the pharmaceutical industry: not all generics are cheaper. In countries where drug prices are regulated, there is no substantive difference in the price of generic drugs. However, any debate about profit margins is an unsuitable way to describe how drugs are

priced because it is based on an incomplete picture of the industry.

Manufacturing costs alone do not reflect the hundreds of millions of dollars that have gone into discovering, testing, and marketing new ARV and AIDS drugs. Three pharmaceutical companies, Merck, Bristol-Myers Squibb, and Gilead Science, have stepped up research to produce a new combination drug AIDS patients can take in one daily dose. The goal is to make treatment for the disease easier and less costly, crucial elements in the effort to help millions of AIDS victims in Africa and other regions of the world (Wharton, 2004). This needed innovation would probably never happen if the pharmaceutical industry was in a price-regulated market worldwide. The U.S. is the only country that does not regulate drug prices, and there is much debate on whether price regulation would affect pharmaceutical innovation.

The pharmaceutical industry maintains most ARVs and AIDS drugs under study since 1981 never made it to market. They turned out to be ineffective, burdened by side effects, and/or too expensive to produce and disseminate. Therefore, a few successful drugs must recoup the research and development costs of all the failures under the current global regulatory scheme for drugs. Again, the HIV/AIDS pandemic has forced examination of the entire regulatory scheme and how to best price drugs.

Price Discrimination

At present, the global pharmaceutical system relies on its relatively wealthy markets to subsidize the research and development costs of both its successful and unsuccessful ARVs and AIDS drugs. Wealthy markets subsidize poorer ones, just as the affluent in theory pay more taxes (Danzon & Furukawa, 2003). The best way to get ARVs and AIDS drugs to resource-limited countries is to have wealthier countries pay more for them (Whobrey, 2007). This kind of price discrimination is what the pharmaceutical industry already does and, with regards to ARVs and AIDS drugs, it is probably best for everyone it does this.

Not only are ARVs and AIDS drugs cheaper in resource-limited countries, they are cheaper in many developed ones as well, frequently because of price regulation. Bargain rates come at a cost, though: less money spent on researching and developing new ARVs and AIDS drugs.

Some argue Americans pay for most of the new drugs coming out all over the world, not just ARVs and AIDS drugs. However, even within the U.S., different HIV/AIDS patients are charged different prices for the same drug. HIV/AIDS patients who join an HMO, which can negotiate volume discounts, are likely to pay less than if they are uninsured or otherwise pay out-of-pocket. Other industries do this, too. An airline passenger forced to fly on short notice may pay significantly more than one who reserved an identical seat weeks in advance.

Price discrimination is both equitable and efficient; without it, seizing patents might be a legitimate, justified action for resource-limited countries (Ferreira, 2002). The pharmaceutical industry has research and development costs which, as a whole, are worth incurring, and which have to be dispersed. Somebody has to pay them. Many economists would argue these costs should be paid by those who are most able and willing to pay them.

Access as an Insurance Problem, not Simply a Drug Pricing Problem

In recent years, the pharmaceutical industry's long-standing price discrimination system has come under pressure. The uninsured and those with inadequate prescription benefit plans have discovered they are paying much more for ARVs and AIDS drugs than HIV/AIDS patients in the rest of the world. Low-income patients in the U.S. complain about being denied access to ARVs that can prevent their immune systems from being weakened to the point where they are disabled by full-blown AIDS (Yamin, 2003).

However, this may not be simply price discrimination. The problem of obtaining access to ARVs is also an insurance problem, not simply a problem due to drug prices. Individuals who are HIV-positive need health benefit plans with reasonable prescription coverage, meaning co-payments that are at an affordable level and plans that provide coverage for needed drugs without unnecessary restrictions and barriers to access.

The pharmaceutical industry is reluctant to sell large quantities of drugs at low prices in resource-limited countries for fear some will flow back to the U.S., known as compounding access. Underground drug markets will undermine the high prices being charged in high-price markets (Yu, 2007). Still one must ask why patients living with HIV/AIDS in resource-limited countries are being provided access to ARVs at three times the rate of infected Americans (WHO, 2006).

HIV/AIDS statistics can, however, be misleading (Ustun et al., 2005). Are some HIV/AIDS patients in the U.S. being denied access to care due to price, or is there another statistical explanation for this disparity in rates of access?

Pricing Incentives

At the onset of the HIV/AIDS pandemic, the pharmaceutical industry erred by not quickly reaching an agreement to provide lifesaving ARVs and AIDS drugs cheaply to African nations. It did so only after massive public pressure and as the number of people who have been, or

are, directly affected by this pandemic approached one hundred million worldwide (WHO, 2008).

A radical change occurred as more than sixty-five million people contracted HIV over time since 1981. Five years ago, the pharmaceutical industry looked at risks in isolation. More and more pharmaceutical companies now recognize the risks' interdependencies when mapping their vulnerabilities (Wharton, 2007). More than twenty-five million people have died of AIDS since 1981 (UNAIDS & WHO, 2007; WHO, 2008), many deaths due to the lack of access to drugs in sub-Saharan Africa in the early years of the pandemic. This fact alone significantly damaged the reputation of the global pharmaceutical industry and made governments worldwide scrutinize the industry in all other respects.

To critics of the pharmaceutical industry, any effort to keep the prices of ARVs and AIDS drugs high seems immoral in the face of the seriousness of the pandemic. It was not difficult for activists to argue the industry has a debt to society. At issue was whether the pharmaceutical industry was meeting its corporate obligations in return for the government benefits it was receiving. What was society obtaining for the billions of dollars in government-financed (that is, taxpayer-financed) research? Also, what was society receiving in return for governments providing patent protection with up to twenty-five years of monopoly?

When tens of millions of people died as a direct result of lack of access to available ARVs and AIDS drugs, the pharmaceutical industry suddenly faced different pressures than other industries enjoying similar government benefits. While parallels can be made to demands placed on the oil industry whenever Americans face the rising costs of energy, there is a stark difference between pricing lifesaving drugs and pricing a gallon of gasoline. Both examples, however, go to show whenever the balance between public expectations of a fair price for a product and the price set by an industry dramatically differ, the vulnerabilities of industry players come into play. Be it the price of drugs or the price of a gallon of gasoline, the value dynamics are the same.

While incentive policies are meant to encourage drug development, HIV/AIDS activists question whether the rewards for the pharmaceutical industry are higher than they should be. Similar questions are being directed to research universities and their commercialization activities. Ideally, society would find the exact point at which the financial incentives are just strong enough to cause needed drugs to be developed, and no stronger. It is very difficult to know when an incentive is too much, or at what point it generates windfall profits or benefits.

The calls to the pharmaceutical industry for assistance are widespread and come from both activists and advocates of world economic reform. As an example, the pharmaceutical industry has been asked for:

- Reduction in the price of ARVs and AIDS drugs to levels affordable for populations of resource-limited countries (Yamin, 2003)
- Removal of all conditions from concessionary price reductions (Yu, 2007)
- Permission for governments to employ compulsory licensing, parallel importing, and other mechanisms to protect public health (Yu, 2007)
- Guarantees for an uninterrupted supply of donations to all developing countries without arbitrary time limitations (Mukherjee, 2007)

It is not possible to gauge the right level of incentive with mathematical precision. It is, however, obvious that as the HIV/AIDS pandemic tears through the world, new incentive policies need to be developed to overcome the failure of the pharmaceutical industry and governments worldwide to help the millions of people suffering from HIV/AIDS and lack of access to essential health care.

Price Discounting

It is clear the pharmaceutical industry is under siege by political forces that are threatening to revoke intellectual property rights, which are the foundation of the pharmaceutical industry's profit structure (Guzik, 2007). The issues surrounding patents, licensing, and knowledge management are not unique to pharmaceuticals; however, the same intellectual property questions face many industries worldwide. The focus in this chapter is simply on how intellectual property affects the prices of ARVs and AIDS drugs.

Intellectual property threats are based on concerns the pharmaceutical industry is using its patent protections to prevent generics from offering ARVs and AIDS drugs to the global marketplace (UN, 2007). This is not to say the current twenty-five-year protection length is exactly right for these drugs, but any judgment about the system's effectiveness would necessarily involve subjective views of whether the

world is getting the ARVs and AIDS drugs it needs. For example, in South Africa, a low-cost, generic, three-drug ARV treatment costs $2,000 per person each year at private-sector wholesale prices and $750 per person per year for the public sector. However, the median yearly household income in South Africa is only $1,000, much too little to afford complete ARV treatment (Collins-Chase, 2008).

Without treatment, HIV-positive individuals develop AIDS and die within five to ten years. With partial ARV treatment, HIV-positive individuals frequently develop resistance to existing ARVs and AIDS drugs and the virulence of the HIV virus is enhanced more often than not. Highly virulent strains of HIV more rapidly weaken the immune systems of individuals, eventually leading to full-blown AIDS. The higher the viral load, the shorter the time to develop AIDS and the shorter the survival rate.

Compulsory Licensing

If financial incentives are too strong, the world gets more drugs than it needs and prices are too high. If incentives are too weak, the world gets cheaper drug prices, but misses out on valuable innovations. This is a concern for current and future HIV/AIDS patients, and indeed the global population at large.

A Canadian company, Apotex, was granted the first compulsory license under WTO rules by the Canadian government in 2007 to provide ARVs and AIDS drugs to Rwanda under the emergency WTO provision. Thailand issued six compulsory licenses since 2006, but continues to negotiate with Merck over domestically produced copies of Merck's Efavirenz, an HIV/AIDS drug (Savoie, 2007). Brazil, which also issued a compulsory license for Efavirenz, has not started to import it, but is rather using the threat of doing so as a tool to force Merck to lower its prices. Abbott Laboratories did not discount pricing as Merck did in Botswana and has not muted HIV/AIDS activists' calls in Thailand.

Discounting of Drugs in Botswana

How can pharmaceutical companies be encouraged to produce new drugs?

Merck sells its ARVs and AIDS drugs at a discounted price to resource-limited countries and is involved in a joint project with the Gates Foundation and the government of Botswana to provide detection, education, and ARVs in the country, which has an HIV infection rate of over 40 percent of its population. Taking such steps in Botswana muted calls for an overthrow of Merck's patents on its drugs.

Source: Odindo, 2007.

Compulsory Licensing of ARV Drugs in Thailand

How can pharmaceutical corporations be incentivized to produce new ARV drugs?

HIV/AIDS activists asked Thailand's Administrative Court to evaluate a Thai government decision to not file suit against Abbott Laboratories for violating trade laws when the company canceled registration of its new ARV, Aluvia, with the country's Food and Drug Administration. This request ensued after the Thai government had issued a compulsory license to produce a lower cost generic version of Abbott's ARV, Kaletra. Abbott offered to sell Aluvia, an updated version of Kaletra, at a reduced price in Thailand on the condition the government agreed not to allow generic versions of Aluvia into the Thai market.

A compulsory license for Aluvia was issued by the Thai government after a price agreement could not be reached with Abbott. Thailand's Food and Drug Administration then registered a generic version of Aluvia for use under the government's compulsory licensing program. The generic version, a non-branded, lower quality drug, is manufactured by an Indian generic pharmaceutical company, Matrix Laboratories. Abbott canceled registration of Aluvia in Thailand after the Thai government issued a compulsory license for the drug.

Source: Yu, 2006.

There are a lot of small companies looking for new ARVs and AIDS drugs, and a lot of research and drug development by established pharmaceutical firms in response to the effectiveness of the current incentives (Lazo, 2007). Whether there is too much or too little research and development is difficult to tell. Even when a new HIV/AIDS drug comes to market, it is often impossible to gauge its value precisely.

When is a new HIV/AIDS drug worth the research and development costs if it is provided royalty-free? Bristol-Myers Squibb and Merck agreed to license to the International Partnership for Microbicides four experimental ARV treatments to be formulated and tested as microbicides to help prevent infection among women by preventing HIV from entering the immune system cells it normally invades (Russell, 2005). The licenses, which are royalty-free, provide the Partnership with the rights to distribute the compounds in developing countries. This is the first time the pharmaceutical industry has helped develop gels, films, sponges, and other products to help prevent the sexual transmission of HIV and other sexually transmitted diseases in women.

THE UNRELENTING STIGMA OF AIDS

Returning to the discussion earlier in this chapter, the paradox of our time is that although AIDS causes more than 5,600 deaths each day worldwide, in many ways the HIV/AIDS pandemic remains hidden (UNAIDS & WHO, 2007). With thirty-eight deaths per day in the U.S., the HIV/AIDS pandemic is not seen as a devastating issue to most Americans.

There is no simple solution for eliminating HIV/AIDS. A complex set of intertwined factors present significant challenges (Yamin, 2003), including:

- Denial
- Discrimination
- Homophobia
- Limited access to health care
- Poverty
- Racism
- Stigma
- Misinformation
- Fear

Each of the factors further complicates efforts to comprehensively address the HIV/AIDS pandemic (CDC, 2007a).

Moral Dilemmas

1. What factors should be considered when encouraging pharmaceutical corporations to develop needed ARVs and AIDS drugs, without generating windfall profits?

2. Is the HIV/AIDS pandemic so catastrophic and overwhelming that the ordinary rules of doing business should be set aside?

3. If so, do pharmaceutical corporations have a moral obligation that should override best business practices?

In many parts of the U.S., the stigma from testing HIV-positive today is not substantially different from testing positive in the 1980s:

- Anti-discrimination protections in many states are inadequate
- Many low wage jobs do not provide private health insurance
- No laws can address the stigma that alienates HIV-positive persons from their families and communities
- The medical assistance program, Medicaid, is structured as a disability care system rather than a health care system that prevents diseases and illness

What should be accomplished before the HIV/AIDS pandemic could possibly devastate the health of communities worldwide? What can the global community do, in addition to everything already being done? Suggestions include:

- Comprehensively contain communicable diseases acquired from birth, accidents, violence, or lifestyle choices
- Continue funding comprehensive public health programs to address communicable diseases worldwide

- Find a way to weigh and then balance civil liberties protection with routine HIV testing
- Provide palliative care to persons experiencing AIDS-related end-stage illnesses

THE SECOND WAVE OF HIV/AIDS

Almost 600,000 Americans have died from AIDS since the first case was documented in the U.S. in 1981; 1.3 million people are currently living with the disease in the U.S. (UNAIDS & WHO, 2007).

The world has begun to accept responsibility. Worldwide, between about 250,000 and 350,000 deaths were averted in 2005 as a result of increased treatment access. All the same, almost two hundred nations agree HIV/AIDS is both a local and worldwide issue of the highest priority (UNAIDS & WHO, 2007). As the second wave of the HIV/AIDS pandemic begins to hit Africa with a wave of opportunistic infections, the question is whether we are taking too long to learn from the lessons of the recent past (Wharton, 2007). To paraphrase a question put by Archbishop Desmond Tutu, former President of South Africa, at the University of Washington: when will we come to learn we are not our brother or sister's keeper, we are our brother's brother, and our sister's sister?

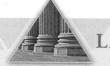

LAW FACT

EARLY DETECTION OF HIV

Is there a heightened duty to routinely test high-risk patients for HIV infection?

High-risk patients themselves make conscious decisions to knowingly engage in a lifestyle that carries fatal risks affecting their health; it is this participation alone that places them at higher risk for contracting HIV, not any delay in detection and treatment for HIV/AIDS infections. There is no heightened duty to test high-risk patients for HIV infections simply because of their sexual preference.

—*Lopes v. Shpigel*, 965 A.2d 311 (Superior Court of Pennsylvania 2008)
(affirming Court of Common Pleas' decision.)
(See *Law Fact* at the end of this chapter for the answer.)

CHAPTER SUMMARY

- An HIV infection is a serious, but manageable, chronic condition if detected and treated early and if patients have access to comprehensive lifelong medical treatments that treat opportunistic infections associated with a weakened immune system.
- HIV/AIDS remains a fatal illness for those in resource-limited countries and for most low-income adults in the U.S. without early access to medical treatment.
- Almost half of all new adult HIV infections in the U.S. occur among young people fifteen to twenty-four years of age.

- Perinatal HIV transmission is the source of almost all HIV/AIDS cases in children under fiteen years of age in the U.S.
- HIV/AIDS treatment requires a very high degree of adherence to drug regimes; non-compliance leads to the serious risk of developing resistance, which may lead to transmission of resistant HIV strains to others.
- The current problem with access to medical treatment is not necessarily the cost of ARVs and AIDS drugs as it was in earlier years of the outbreak; instead, it is the multifaceted difficulty of finding health care in resource-limited countries and of obtaining early access to high quality care in the U.S.
- Manufacturing costs alone do not reflect the hundreds of millions of research and development dollars that go into discovering, testing, and marketing new ARVs and AIDS drugs.
- Drug price discrimination enables the pharmaceutical industry to provide low priced, high quality innovative ARVs and AIDS drugs to resource-limited countries.
- The global pharmaceutical system relies on its relatively wealthy markets to subsidize poorer ones; the most efficient way to get ARVs and AIDS drugs to resource-limited countries is to have more wealthy countries like the U.S. pay more for them.
- Intellectual property regimes are the foundation of the pharmaceutical industry's current profit structure.
- There are two prongs of the approach to the HIV/AIDS pandemic in the U.S.: early detection and treatment of the HIV infection and containment of the disease.
- The government recommends everyone in the U.S. between the ages of thirteen and sixty-four be routinely tested for HIV, regardless of individual risk factors; at this time, HIV testing remains voluntary on an opt-out basis.
- The government recommends all pregnant women be tested for HIV because perinatal transmission of HIV can be reduced to less than 1 percent by the administration of ARVs to infected mothers and their newborns.
- Most minors can consent to testing and treatment of HIV/AIDS.
- Only Massachusetts, Maine, and the District of Columbia have received waivers from the federal government to permit HIV-positive individuals to access Medicaid before they are certified disabled; in all other states, symptoms must be manifest before medical treatment is provided that would have prevented the symptoms in the first place.
- Both physicians and laboratories are required to report the names of newly diagnosed HIV patients to government communicable disease registries, along with personally identifiable information about drug use and sexual history of persons infected.
- In the absence of state duty-to-warn laws, a physician's failure to warn the known sexual partner(s) of a newly diagnosed HIV patient does not generally give rise to liability.
- All states have criminal laws punishing HIV-positive individuals for sexual behaviors that pose a risk of HIV transmission, even if no transmission occurs; such behavior is usually a felony.
- Federal legislation provides that any non-citizen found importing ARVs or AIDS drugs into the U.S. will be arrested and placed on a flight back to their country of origin.
- HIV-infected individuals do not enjoy guaranteed protection against discrimination under the ADA.
- Health care professionals should follow universal infection control precautions at all times to prevent exposure to blood-borne pathogens.
- Since 1984, gay men have been banned from donating blood in the U.S.
- Almost half the blood donations in resource-limited countries are unscreened for HIV. Therefore, one in ten HIV infections is the result of tainted blood or blood product transfusions.

LAW NOTES

1. Injection drug use is a disturbing transmitter of HIV infections. At the start of every injection, blood is introduced into the needle and syringe. Therefore, a needle and syringe that someone who is HIV-positive uses can contain blood that contains the virus. The reuse of a contaminated needle or syringe by another drug injector carries a high risk of HIV transmission because infected blood can be injected directly into the bloodstream. Sharing other drug equipment also can be a risk for spreading HIV. Infected blood can be introduced into drug solutions through using blood-contaminated syringes to prepare drugs; reusing water; reusing bottle caps, spoons, or other containers used to dissolve drugs in water and to heat drug solutions; or reusing small pieces of cotton or cigarette filters used to filter out particles that could block the needle (CDC, 2002a).

2. The U.S. Supreme Court held Bragdon was disabled because her HIV substantially limited her major life activity of reproduction. The Court found Bragdon's decision not to have children was motivated by her HIV diagnosis. Given that many HIV persons have never considered having children, and given that current therapies make the risk of mother-to-child transmission negligible today, the protections extended in *Bragdon* are far from comprehensive. Further, because personal choice is almost always a factor in a decision to reproduce, the Court set the ADA standard of what constitutes a disability excessively high, requiring specific evidence HIV status is the sole reason for a decision not to procreate. *See Blanks v. Southwestern Bell Communications, Inc.*, 310 F.3d 398, 401 (U.S. Court of Appeals for the 5th Circuit 2002) (declining to classify an HIV-positive man as disabled because his wife had undergone a tubal ligation and he had no plans to have more children; therefore, the activity of reproduction was not considered a major life activity for him).

3. Advocacy around the ban against gay men donating blood has been limited and no litigation has been filed to repeal the government policy. Nonetheless, college and university students continue to engage in acts of advocacy calling for change, labeling the ban as absurd (Culhane, 2005), discriminatory (Hemingway, 2006), and even unconstitutional (Belli, 2003). Student-based campaigns have ranged from the 2006 "Fight to Give Life" campaign, where student groups at campuses nationwide led gay male students to blood centers, where they attempted to give blood, to individual campus protests at community blood drives.

CHAPTER BIBLIOGRAPHY

ACLU (American Civil Liberties Union). (2008). *State criminal statutes on HIV transmission*. New York: ACLU.

___. (2006, September 21). *Press release: ACLU says new CDC HIV testing recommendations raise health and civil liberties concerns*. New York, NY: ACLU.

AGI (Alan Guttmacher Institute). (2008). *Minors' access to STI services: State policies in brief*. New York, NY: AGI.

Anderson, J. E., & Sansom, S. (2006). HIV testing among U.S. women during prenatal care: Findings from the National Survey of Family Growth. *Maternal & Child Health Journal, 10* (5), 413-417.

Bartlett, J. G. et al. (2004). *A guide to primary care of people with HIV/AIDS*. Washington, DC: Health Resources and Services Administration.

Bayer, R., & Fairchild, A. L. (2006). Perspective: Changing the paradigm for HIV testing: The end of exceptionalism? *New England Journal of Medicine, 355*, 647-649.

Belli, M. C. (2003). The constitutionality of the "men who have sex with men" blood donor exclusion policy. *Journal of Law & Society, 4*, 315-375 (finding the gay ban policy fails to meet rational basis scrutiny).

BLS (Bureau of Labor Statistics). (2008, April 25). *News: College enrollment and work activity of 2007 high school graduates*. Washington, DC: U.S. Department of Labor (special data request from the U.S. Census Bureau's Current Population Survey, a monthly survey conducted for BLS of about sixty thousand households).

Bond, L. (2005). HIV testing and the role of individual- and structural-level barriers and facilitators. *AIDS Care, 17* (2), 125-140.

Branson, B. M. et al. (2001). Revised guidelines for HIV counseling, testing and referral and revised recommendations for HIV screening of pregnant women in health care settings. *Morbidity and Mortality Weekly Report (MMWR), 55*, 1-17. Atlanta, GA: Centers for Disease Control and Prevention.

Bucholtz, B. K. (2005). Rules, principles, or just words? The interpretive project and the problem of legitimacy. *Texas Wesleyan Law Review, 11*, 377-397 (explaining how arguments that a law cannot go beyond its text can be confronted by the opposing argument that to effect its purpose a law may be implemented beyond its text; legitimacy resides in the persuasiveness of the reason for choosing a particular interpretation, rather than the law itself).

Burgdorf Jr., R. L. (2008). Restoring the ADA and beyond: Disability in the 21st century. *Texas Journal on Civil Liberties & Civil Rights, 13*, 241-365.

Burris, S. et al. (2007). Do criminal laws influence HIV risk behavior? An empirical trial. *Arizona State Law Journal, 39*, 467-517.

CDC (Centers for Disease Control and Prevention). (2008). *HIV/AIDS surveillance report*. Atlanta, GA: U.S. Department of Health and Human Services, CDC.

___. (2007). *Public Health Service Task Force recommendations for use of antiretroviral drugs in pregnant HIV-infected women for maternal health and interventions to reduce perinatal HIV transmission in the U.S.* Atlanta, GA: U.S. Department of Health and Human Services, CDC.

___. (2007a). *HIV prevention strategic plan: Extended through 2010*. Atlanta, GA: U.S. Department of Health and Human Services, CDC.

___. (2007b). *CDC Questions and answers: CDC's clinical studies of pre-exposure prophylaxis for HIV prevention*. Atlanta, GA: U.S. Department of Health and Human Services, CDC.

___. (2007c). Update to racial/ethnic disparities in diagnoses of HIV/AIDS: 33 states. *Morbidity and Mortality Weekly Report, 56* (09), 189-193.

___. (2007d). *CDC Questions and answers: How does HIV cause AIDS?* Atlanta, GA: U.S. Department of Health and Human Services, CDC.

___. (2006). Comprehensive HIV prevention: *Essential components of a comprehensive strategy to prevent domestic HIV.* Atlanta, GA: U.S. Department of Health and Human Services, CDC.

___. (2006a, October 20). *How safe is the blood supply in the U.S.?* Atlanta, GA: U.S. Department of Health and Human Services, CDC.

___. (2006b). Revised recommendations for HIV Testing of adults, adolescents, and pregnant women in health care settings. *Morbidity & Mortality Weekly Report, 55* (14), 1-17.

___. (2006c). Racial/ethnic disparities in diagnoses of HIV/AIDS. *Morbidity & Mortality Weekly Report, 55* (05), 121-125.

___. (2003). Behavioral risk factor surveillance system, HIV testing. *Morbidity & Mortality Weekly Report, 52* (23).

___. (2002). *Preventing occupational HIV transmission to healthcare personnel.* Atlanta, GA: U.S. Department of Health and Human Services, CDC.

___. (2002a). *Drug-associated HIV transmission continues in the U.S.* Atlanta, GA: U.S. Department of Health and Human Services, CDC.

___. (2001). Updated U.S. Public Health Service guidelines for the management of occupational exposures to HBV, HCV, and HIV and recommendations for post-exposure prophylaxis. *Morbidity & Mortality Weekly Report, 50* (142).

Chesson, H. W. et al. (2004). The estimated direct medical cost of sexually transmitted diseases among American youth. *Perspectives on Sexual & Reproductive Health, 36* (1), 11-19.

Christie, S. R. (2007, October). AIDS, employment, and the direct threat defense: The burden of proof and the circuit court split. *Fordham Law Review, 76,* 235-282.

CIA (Central Intelligence Agency). (2007). *World factbook.* Langley, VA: CIA.

Collins-Chase, C. T. (2008, Spring). The case against TRIPS-PLUS protection in developing countries facing AIDS epidemics. *University of Pennsylvania Journal on International Law, 29,* 763-802.

COTT (Committee of Ten Thousand) et al. (2007, November 29). *An open letter on safety to the manufacturers of clotting factor products and the government agencies who regulate them.* Washington, DC: COTT, National Hemophilia Foundation, Hemophilia Federation of America.

Culhane, J. G. (2005). Bad science, worse policy: The exclusion of gay males from donor pools. *St. Louis University Public Law Review, 129,* 131-148.

Danzon, P., & Furukawa, M. (2003). Prices and availability of pharmaceuticals: Evidence from nine countries. *Health Affairs,* 521-536.

Fairchild, A. L. et al. (2003). The myth of exceptionalism: The history of venereal disease reporting in the twentieth century. *Journal of Law, Medicine & Ethics, 31,* 624-637 (noting the similarity between HIV/AIDS policy and venereal disease policy to demonstrate AIDS has not been treated so differently from all other diseases).

FDA (U.S. Food and Drug Administration). (2007, May 23). *FDA policy on blood donations from men who have sex with other men.* Bethesda, MD: FDA.

___. (1992, April 23). *Revised recommendations for the prevention of Human Immunodeficiency virus (HIV) transmission by blood and blood products.* Bethesda, MD: FDA.

Feachem, R. (2007, January 27). Long-term plan is needed to fight HIV/AIDS spread. *Wall Street Journal,* p. A10.

Federal Register. (2009, January 23). Annual Update of the HHS Poverty Guidelines, 74 F.R. 4199-04.

Feldman, E. A. (2000). Blood justice: Courts, conflict, and compensation in Japan, France, and the U.S. *Law & Society Review, 34,* 651-698.

Fenton, K. et al. (2007, June). *A heightened national response to the HIV/AIDS crisis among African-Americans.* Atlanta, GA: Centers for Disease Control and Prevention.

Ferreira, L. (2002). Access to affordable ARV/AIDS drugs: The human rights obligations of multinational pharmaceutical corporations. *Fordham Law Review, 71,* 1133-1179.

Gallery, C. L., & Pinkerton, S. D. (2006). Conflicting messages: How criminal HIV disclosure laws undermine public health efforts to control the spread of HIV. *AIDS & Behavior, 10,* 451-461 (noting few laws require that actual exposure occurs and none requires transmission).

Gao, F. et al. (1999). Origin of HIV-1 in the chimpanzee Pan troglodytes troglodytes. *Nature, 397,* 436-441.

Gersen, J. E. (2006). Overlapping and underlapping jurisdiction in administrative law. *Supreme Court Review, 2006,* 201-247 (examining how decision-making authority should be allocated among political institutions).

Goldschmidt, J. E. (2007). Reasonable accommodation in EU equality law in a broader perspective. *ERA Forum, 8* (1), 39-48.

Gostin, L. O. (2008). Global health: Meeting basic survival needs of the world's least healthy people: Toward a framework convention on global health. *Georgetown Law Journal, 96,* 331-392.

Gupta, M. (2005). Occupational risk: The outrageous reaction to HIV positive public safety and health care employees in the workplace. *Journal of Law & Health, 19,* 39-73.

Guzik, B. (2007, Spring/Summer). Botswana's success in balancing the economics of HIV/AIDS with TRIPS obligations and human rights. *Loyola University of Chicago International Law Review, 4* (2), 255-271.

Hall, I. et al. (2008). Estimation of HIV incidence in the United States. *Journal of the American Medical Association, 300* (5), 520-529.

Hilzendeger, K. J. (2003). Unreasonable publicity: How well does tort law protect the unwarranted disclosure of a person's HIV-positive status? *Arizona State Law Journal, 35,* 187-218.

Hemingway, S. (2006). UVM blood drives to continue. *Burlington Free Press,* p. 1B (discussing discrimination charges brought relating to blood drives at the University of Vermont).

HUD (U.S. Department of Housing & Urban Development's). (2009). Special Data Request. Washington, DC: Office of HIV/AIDS Housing.

IAVI (International AIDS Vaccine Initiative). (2006). *Imagining a world without AIDS: A history of the International AIDS Vaccine Initiative.* New York, NY: IAVI.

Kagan, E. T. (2007). Morality v. reality: The struggle to effectively fight HIV/AIDS and respect human rights. *Brooklyn Journal on International Law, 32,* 1201-1226.

Kaiser (Kaiser Family Foundation). (2008). *HIV/AIDS policy fact sheet: Black Americans and HIV/AIDS.* Menlo Park, CA: Kaiser.

___. (2008a, April). *State health facts.* Data Source: Centers for Disease Control and Prevention, Division of HIV/AIDS Prevention-Surveillance and Epidemiology, Special Data Request. Menlo Park, CA: Kaiser.

___. (2006, October). *HIV/AIDS policy fact sheet: Medicaid and HIV/AIDS.* Menlo Park, CA: Kaiser.

Kaufman, E. (2006). Seventeenth annual Supreme Court review: October 2004 Supreme Court term: Discrimination Cases in the October 2004 Term. *Touro Law Review, 21*, 829-847.

Keshishyan, H. (2008). We shall overcome . . . if the courts allow us: The United States Supreme Court's decisions regarding mitigating measures, and its connection to the circuit split on whether life accomplishments should be considered in determining disability under the ADA. *Southwestern Law Review, 38*, 357-393.

Lazo, J. A. (2007). The Life-Saving Medicines Export Act: Why the proposed U.S. compulsory licensing scheme will fail to export any medicines or save any lives. *Brooklyn Journal of International Law, 33*, 237-276.

Leveton, L. B. et al. (1995). *HIV and the blood supply: An analysis of crisis decision-making: U.S. Institute of Medicine Committee to study HIV transmission through blood and blood products*. Washington, DC: IOM.

Lewis, S. (2006). *Race against time: Searching for hope in AIDS-ravaged Africa (CBC Massey lecture)* (2nd ed.). Toronto, Ontario: House of Anansi Press.

Lin, A., & Liang, B.A. (2005). Striking the balance between legal mandates and medical ethics. *Ethics Journal of the American Medical Association, 7* (10), 1-6.

Marks G. et al. (2006). Estimating sexual transmission of HIV from persons aware and unaware that they are infected with the virus in the USA. *AIDS, 20* (10), 1447-1450.

McKenna, M. T., & Hu, X. (2007). Recent trends in the incidence and morbidity associated with perinatal human immunodeficiency virus infection in the U.S. *American Journal of Obstetrics & Gynecology, 197* (3) (supplement 1), S10-S16.

Metnick, J. M. (2003). Evolving to asymptomatic HIV as a disability per se: Closing the loophole in judicial precedent. *DePaul Journal of Health Care Law, 7*, 69-104 (discussing the failure of *Bradgon* to provide comprehensive ADA protection for persons living with HIV).

Montaner, J. S. et al. (2006). The case for expanding access to highly active antiretroviral therapy to curb the growth of the HIV pandemic. *Lancet, 368*, 531-536 (citing studies that find a significant reduction in HIV transmission for patients on highly active ARV therapy and arguing for expanded access to ARVs).

Mukherjee, G. N. (2007). Improving the pharmaceutical industry: Optimality inside the framework of the current legal system provides access to medicines for HIV/AIDS patients in sub-Saharan Africa. *Journal of Transnational Law & Policy, 17*, 121-150.

NASTAD (National Alliance of State and Territorial AIDS Directors). (2008). *National ADAP monitoring project annual report*. Washington, DC: NASTAD & Menlo Park, CA: Kaiser Family Foundation.

___. (2007). *Early Treatment for HIV Act (S 860)*. Washington, DC: NASTAD & Menlo Park, CA: Kaiser Family Foundation.

___. (2007a). *Report on findings from an assessment of health department efforts to implement HIV screening in health care settings*. Washington, DC: NASTAD & Menlo Park, CA: Kaiser Family Foundation.

NCHHSTP (National Center for HIV/AIDS, Viral Hepatitis, STD, and TB Prevention). (2008). Health disparities in HIV/AIDS, viral hepatitis, sexually transmitted diseases and tuberculosis in the U.S.: Issues, burden and response. In *Update: NCHHSTP health disparities report*. Washington, DC: U.S. Department of Health and Human Services.

___. (2007). *Where did HIV come from?* Washington, DC: U.S. Department of Health and Human Services.

NMAC (National Minority AIDS Council). (2006). *African Americans, health disparities and HIV/AIDS: Recommendations for confronting the epidemic in black America*. Washington, DC: NMAC.

Novotny, T. E. (2007). Global governance and public health security in the 21st century. *California Western International Law Journal, 38*, 19-40.

Odindo, C. chief executive officer, International Development & Policy Corp. (2007, October 8). Fifteenth Annual Wharton Africa Business Forum: Africa rising: The new dawn of trade and investment. Wharton School at the University of Pennsylvania. Philadelphia, PA.

Phillips, M. et al. (2008). Task shifting for antiretroviral treatment delivery in sub-Saharan Africa: Not a panacea. *Lancet, 371*, 682-684 (responding to the health worker crisis, the international community collectively created the Global Health Workforce Alliance in 2006).

Phillips, M., & Moffett, M. (2005, May 2). Brazil refuses U.S. AIDS funds, rejects conditions. *Wall Street Journal*, p. A3.

Pottker-Fishel, C. G. (2007, Winter). Improper bedside manner: Why state partner notification laws are ineffective in controlling the proliferation of HIV. *Journal of Law & Medicine, 17*, 147-179.

PwC (PricewaterhouseCoopers). (2003). *An analysis of the Early Treatment For HIV Act, prepared for the Treatment Access Expansion Project (TAEP)*. Washington, DC: TAEP.

Pulver, A. R. (2008). Gay blood revisionism: A critical analysis of advocacy and the gay blood ban. *Law & Sexuality, 17*, 107-130.

Rajkumar, R. (2007). A human rights approach to routine provider-initiated HIV testing. *Yale Journal of Health Policy, Law & Ethics, 7*, 319-378.

Ray, J. A. (2007). A social disability? The medical realities and social implications of classifying asymptomatic HIV as a disability under the Americans with Disabilities Act. *Loyola Law Review, 53*, 257-289.

Richards, E. P. (2007). Public health law as administrative law: Example lessons. *Journal of Health Care Law & Policy, 10*, 61-88.

Rosenthal, L. D. (2006). Reasonable Accommodations for individuals regarded as having disabilities under the Americans with Disabilities Act? Why "no" should not be the answer. *Seton Hall Law Review, 36*, 895-969.

Rothstein, L. (2008). Strategic advocacy in fulfilling the goals of disability policy: Is the only question how full the glass is? *Texas Journal on Civil Liberties & Civil Rights, 13*, 403-412.

Russell, S. (2005, November 1). Four drugs hold promise for new HIV preventive; Goal is to create a topical cream. *San Francisco Chronicle*, p. A5.

Ryan, C. (2004). *Reducing barriers to care*. Washington, DC: Health Resources and Services Administration, U.S. Department of Health & Human Resources.

Savoie, B. (2007, Fall). Thailand's test: Compulsory licensing in an era of epidemiologic transition. *Virginia Journal of International Law, 48*, 211-248.

Schalman-Bergen, S. (2007). CDC's call for routine HIV testing raises implementation concerns. *Journal of Law, Medicine & Ethics, 35*, 223-225.

Selmi, G. (2006). Interpreting the Americans with Disabilities Act: Why the Supreme Court rewrote the statute, and why Congress did not care. *George Washington Law Review, 76*, 522-575.

Starr, D. P. (1998). *Blood: An epic history of medicine and commerce.* New York, NY: Alfred A. Knopf.

Stoto, M. A. (2008, January). Public health surveillance in the twenty-first century: Achieving population health goals while protecting persons' privacy and confidentiality. *Georgetown Law Journal, 96*, 703-719.

Strahilevitz, L. J. (2008). Symposium: Surveillance: Privacy versus antidiscrimination. *University of Chicago Law Review, 75*, 363-381.

Tsai, J. T. (2007). Not tripping over the pebbles: Focusing on overlooked TRIPS Article 66 for technology transfer to solve Africa's AIDS crisis. *Michigan State University Journal of Medicine & Law, 11*, 447-476.

Tutu, D. M. (2002). HIV/AIDS and the global community: We can be human only together. *Seattle Journal of Social Justice, 1*, 253-254.

UCSF (University of California-San Francisco) & National HIV/AIDS Clinicians' Consultation Center. (2008). *State HIV testing laws compendium.* San Francisco, CA: UCSF.

UN (United Nations). (2007). *World mortality report.* New York, NY: UN, Department of Economic and Social Affairs, Population Division.

UN Secretary-General. (2004). *A more secure world: Our shared responsibility: Report of the high-level panel on threats, challenges and change.* New York, NY: United Nations General Assembly.

UNAIDS & WHO (World Health Organization). (2007, December). *2007 AIDS Pandemic Update.* New York. NY: Joint United Nations Programme on HIV/AIDS (the Joint U.N. Programme on HIV/AIDS (UNAIDS) is comprised of ten U.N. system organizations: The Office of the U.N. High Commissioner for Refugees, the U.N. Children's Fund, the World Food Programme, the U.N. Development Programme, the U.N. Population Fund, the U.N. Office on Drugs and Crime, the International Labour Organization, the U.N. Educational, Scientific and Cultural Organization, the World Health Organization, and the World Bank).

Ustun, T. B. et al. (2005). Quality assurance in surveys: Standards, guidelines and procedures. In *Household sample surveys in developing and transition countries.* New York, NY: UN.

Walker, E. M. (2007). The HIV/AIDS pandemic and human rights: A continuum approach. *Florida Journal of International Law, 19*, 335-419.

Weinberg, P. D. (2002). Legal, financial, and public health consequences of HIV contamination of blood and blood products in the 1980s and 1990s. *Annals of Internal Medicine, 136*, 312-319.

Weinstock, H. et al. (2004). Sexually transmitted diseases among American youth: Incidence and prevalence estimates. *Perspectives on Sexual & Reproductive Health, 36* (1), 6-10.

Weis, R. A., & Wrangham, R. W. (1999). From Pan to pandemic. *Nature, 397*, 385-386.

Wharton (Wharton School at the University of Pennsylvania). (2007). View from Dalian, China: The new risk architecture and our growing interdependence. *Knowledge@Wharton.*

___. (2006). Pandemics in an integrated global society: An economist's view. *Knowledge@Wharton.*

___. (2006a). Raising money to treat the world's sickest persons isn't the problem: Spending it is. *Knowledge@Wharton.*

___. (2004). Roy Vagelos talks about leadership and the need for new drug pricing policies. *Knowledge@Wharton.*

Whitebread, C. H. (2006). The 2005-2006 term of the United States Supreme Court: A Court in transition. *Whittier Law Review, 28*, 3-173.

White House, The (2009). Special Data Request. Washington, DC: Office of National AIDS Policy.

___. (2007, November 30). *Press release: President's HIV/AIDS initiative.* Washington, DC: Office of the Press Secretary.

___. (2006, December 19). *Press release-fact sheet: The Ryan White HIV/AIDS Treatment Modernization Act of 2006.* Washington, DC: Office of the Press Secretary.

Whobrey, B. (2007). International patent law and public health: Analyzing TRIPS' effect on access to pharmaceuticals in developing countries. *Brandeis Law Journal, 45*, 623-642.

World Bank. (2008). *Global economic prospects 2008.* Washington, DC: World Bank.

World Health Organization (WHO). (2008). *World health statistics.* London, England: WHO.

___. (2008a) *Global tuberculosis control—surveillance, planning, financing.* London, England: WHO.

___. (2007, June 25). *WHO report of the regional director on tuberculosis and HIV/AIDS: A strategy for the control of a dual epidemic in the WHO African region.* London, England: WHO.

___. (2007a, April 17). *Progress report. Towards universal access: Scaling up priority HIV/AIDS interventions in the health sector.* London, England: WHO.

___. (2006). *Understanding the latest estimates of the 2006 report on the global AIDS epidemic.* London, England: WHO.

___. (2004). *Antiretroviral drugs for treating pregnant women and preventing HIV infection in infants: Guidelines on care, treatment and support for women living with HIV/AIDS and their children in resource-constrained settings.* London, England: WHO.

Yamin, A. E. (2003). Not just a tragedy: Access to medications as a right under international law. *Boston University International Law Journal, 21*, 325–371.

Yeun, M. (2007). HIV testing of pregnant women: Why present approaches fail to reach the desired objective & the unconsidered option. *Cardozo Journal on Law & Gender, 14*, 185-210.

Yu, P. K. (2007). The international enclosure movement. *Indiana Law Journal, 82*, 827-909.

___. (2006, February 3). Director of Intellectual Property Law Center at Drake University Law School at the Saving Profits, Saving Lives Symposium: A comprehensive discussion of the social, legal, and economic implications of reverse engineering and parallel importing on the pharmaceutical industry at the University of North Carolina School of Law. Chapel Hill, NC.

CHAPTER 27

MENTAL HEATH

> "Statistics on sanity are that one out of every four Americans is suffering from some form of mental illness. Think of your three best friends. If they are okay, then it is you."
>
> —RITA MAE BROWN, AMERICAN WRITER AND POLITICAL ACTIVIST

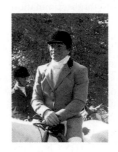

IN BRIEF

This chapter focuses on the U.S. health care system's response to mental illness. This epidemiological approach reveals the magnitude of mental illness and ranks depression as more of a burden to the U.S. health care system than any other illness. A significant number of new mental health issues were recently judicially addressed by the highest federal legal authorities; therefore, five case decisions are presented in this chapter.

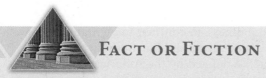

FACT OR FICTION

COVERAGE FOR ACUTE MENTAL HEALTH TREATMENT

Following a pre-certification approval, can an insurer retrospectively deny coverage for ensuing treatment of a severe mental illness, when the patient is completely dysfunctional and suicidal?

The State of Vermont contracted with Merit to provide mental health care benefits to state employees under the state's medical benefit plan. By providing these benefits, Merit functioned as a review agent. For its part, Merit contracted with Austen Riggs, a mental health care facility, to be one of its mental health care service providers under the state plan. Austen Riggs specialized in the care of severely ill, treatment-resistant patients. Under its contract with Merit, Austen Riggs agreed to cooperate with pre-certification and concurrent review procedures and policies.

Jane Doe, a state employee covered under the state's plan, was referred to Austen Riggs for treatment of a long-term mental disorder. Doe was in the midst of a major depressive episode of the illness, which had proven resistant to various attempts at treatment over the years, including short-term hospitalization, residential/day treatment, aggressive medication therapy, cognitive-behavioral therapy, and electroconvulsive treatment. After Doe's pre-certified admission to Austen Riggs, a dispute arose between Merit and Austen Riggs over Doe's treatment plan. The conflict centered around inconsistencies between Austen Riggs's policy of having patients stay a minimum of thirty days once they were found to be appropriate candidates for treatment and Merit's policy of requiring daily review to ensure continued residential mental health care services were medically necessary.

Shortly after Doe was admitted to Austen Riggs, Merit's medical director informed Austin Riggs he could not conduct concurrent review of Doe's treatment because Austen Riggs's treatment plan did not fit Merit's method of managing inpatient treatment. Merit's medical director noted Austen Riggs did not share Merit's assumptions that each day needed to be reviewed and a patient should be discharged or at least stepped down to a lesser level of care as soon as clinically appropriate. Merit claimed it had been misled about Austen Riggs's willingness to work with its system of review and length of stay for admitted patients, while Austen Riggs claimed Merit knew of its policies, including its minimum stay policy, when Merit contracted with it to be one of its mental health care providers. In the end, Merit informed Austen Riggs it would approve Doe's initial six-day stay and consider her claim for further treatment after retrospective review of her medical record.

Several days later, Merit informed Doe it had authorized payment for her initial stay at Austen Riggs, but would determine the medical necessity of Doe's treatment after her discharge. Austen Riggs also sent Doe a letter stating that because Merit had declined its request for approval of a further medically necessary stay, she would have to guarantee payment for treatment herself if she decided to stay at Austen Riggs. She agreed to do so, and remained at Austen Riggs for the next several months.

After her discharge, Doe sought reimbursement from Merit for her treatment at Austen Riggs. Merit denied Doe's claim because available documentation did not support the medical necessity of her level of care. Doe appealed to the Independent Panel of Mental Health Care Providers, a statutory body established to promptly consider adverse decisions made by review agents. Following a hearing, the independent panel concluded Doe's treatment at Austen Riggs was medically necessary and therefore covered under the state's plan. Merit appealed the Independent Panel's coverage decision.

—*Merit Behavioral Care Corp. v. State Independent Panel of Mental Health Providers*, 845 A.2d 359

(Supreme Court of Vermont 2004).

(See *Law Fact* at the end of this chapter for the answer.)

PRINCIPLES AND APPLICATIONS

The population of those with severe mental disorders has less access to treatment and receives poorer quality of treatment than persons without mental illness (Horvitz-Lennon et al., 2006). While mental illness is the leading disease burden on the U.S. health care systems (WHO, 2008), it takes tragedies such as the school massacre at Virginia Tech to focus public attention on the nation's response to what many view as one of the most overlooked disease states in the U.S., similar to HIV/AIDS.

While the National Institute on Mental Health estimates only a small percentage of the forty-four million Americans suffering from mental illness has a severe mental disorder, it is the mentally ill population at imminent risk of causing harm that should concern everyone. At Virginia Tech, twenty-three-year-old Seung Hui Cho's strange behavior indicated more than a year before the shootings that he was at imminent risk of causing harm; when finally ordered by a judge to seek counseling, outpatient treatment was recommended (Bernstein, 2008). Under the imminent danger standard in Virginia, mentally ill individuals who had not committed an overt act were free from involuntary commitment (Pfeffer, 2008). Rather than focus on whether a mentally ill individual has committed an overt act or deteriorated to an extreme degree, courts tend to regard the severity and type of symptoms of an individual's mental illness, including self-destructive behavior, as indicative of whether involuntary civil commitment is warranted. Virginia has taken the crucial step of amending its prior involuntary civil commitment law in the wake of the Virginia Tech tragedy. As a result, it serves as a primary example to Georgia, Hawaii, Montana, and Ohio, which all have imminent danger standards in need of reform (Pfeffer, 2008).

Less than a year after it was recommended he receive treatment in a less restrictive environment than an inpatient psychiatric hospital, thirty-two students and faculty were murdered and twenty-five injured by Cho in two related campus incidents before Cho commit suicide (Kaine, 2007). A key contributor to mass school shootings, like Virginia Tech, is the disconnection in the health care system that provides most of the care for the severely mentally ill. There was no continuum of quality care for Cho as an outpatient mental patient in the community, and no one felt responsible for monitoring his medication regime.

KEY TERMS

The law has rarely doubted the existence of mental illness, but has struggled with its definition and its disposition (Erickson, 2008). While mental health and mental illness are points on a continuum, the first Surgeon General's report ever issued on the topic set forth the most accepted definition of mental health as a condition of successful performance of mental function, resulting in:

- Productive activities
- Fulfilling relationships with other people
- Ability to adapt to change and cope with adversity

(U.S. Surgeon General, 1999)

Mental illness, in contrast to mental health, was broadly defined as all diagnosable mental disorders, as defined by the American Psychiatry Association, which developed the *Diagnostic and Statistical Manual of Mental Disorders*, currently in its fourth edition and known by mental health professionals as *DSM-IV. DSM-IV* contains diagnostic codes and detailed descriptions for all recognized mental illnesses. Although there may not be biological tests to diagnose different mental illnesses, fairly standard methods of diagnosis exist (DSM-IV, 2000). Mental disorders, in turn, may be defined as biologically-based health conditions characterized by:

- Alterations in thinking, mood, or behavior
- Distress, defined as mental anguish and misery characterized by feelings of grief, anxiety, and unhappiness (DSM-IV, 2000)
- Impaired mental functioning, characterized by a heightened risk of death, pain, disability, or loss of freedom (DSM-IV, 2000)

As public stigma would have it, mental disorders are not character flaws, but legitimate illnesses that respond to specific treatments, just as other physical health conditions respond to medical interventions (*see* Erickson, 2008; Gostin & Gable, 2004; Horvitz-Lennon et al., 2006). The shame and disgrace attached to mental disorders indicates that, in the twenty-first century, mental illnesses are still regarded by many as socially unacceptable health conditions.

While most definitions of what constitutes a mental disorder are expansive, different mental illnesses range in severity and treatment. Some of the more severe mental illnesses include:

- Alzheimer's disease, a mental disorder marked by alterations in thinking, especially forgetting
- Bipolar disorder
- Borderline personality disorder
- Major depression, a mental disorder largely marked by alterations in mood
- Obsessive compulsive disorder
- Panic disorder
- Post-traumatic stress disorder
- Schizophrenia

(DSM-IV, 2000)

Although less severe, attention deficit disorder (ADD) and attention deficit and hyperactivity disorder (ADHD), often diagnosed in children (mental disorders largely marked by alterations in behavior (over-activity) and/or thinking (inability to concentrate)), are considered within the definition of mental illness (DSM-IV, 2000).

EPIDEMIOLOGY OF MENTAL ILLNESS

Even though mental disorders are widespread in the population, the main burden of severe mental illness is concentrated in a much smaller proportion (Tovino, 2009). The National Alliance on Mental Illness estimates:

- About 6 percent, or one in seventeen Americans, suffers from a severe mental illness
- Mental illness affects one in five families in the U.S.

All the same, treatments for severe mental illnesses today are highly effective; between 70 and 90 percent of individuals have significant reduction of symptoms and improved quality of life with a combination of pharmacological and psychosocial treatments and support. Without treatment, the consequences of mental illness for the individual and society are staggering:

- Homelessness
- Inappropriate incarceration
- Co-occurring substance abuse
- Suicide
- Unemployment
- Unnecessary disability
- Wasted lives

(U.S. Surgeon General, 1999)

Individuals with co-occurring substance abuse suffer from both mental illness and substance abuse. This chapter does not address substance abuse alone or the abuse of alcohol and drugs in the absence of mental illness. While spending on mental health and co-occurring substance abuse treatment is expected to increase to $239 billion by 2014, it is anticipated to fall as a share of all health spending (Levit et al., 2008). While the federal Mental Health Parity Act mandates that health insurers treat mental illness in the same manner as physical illness, public funds to treat mental illness are declining and in many instances, simply disappearing. The U.S. is increasingly facing a shortage of treatment slots, publicly funded and private treatment facilities are generally running at full capacity with growing wait lists. The result of this treatment shortage is that while spending on mental health and co-occurring substance abuse treatment is increasing, the number of individuals being treated remains the same, but only the most serious cases are being accepted to receive treatment (House Report, 2007). Non-serious cases are left to be dealt with by the general health care system, including by physicians not trained to treat either mental health illnesses or co-occurring substance abuse and by the nation's emergency rooms.

Global Burden of Disease Study

The Global Burden of Disease Study, originated in the early 1990s by the World Health Organization in collaboration with the World Bank and Harvard University, was the first effort to systematically look at mortality and other dimensions of ill health. The overall burden of disease was assessed using the disability-adjusted life year (DALY), a time-based measure that combines years of life lost due to premature mortality and years of life lost due to time lived in states of less than full health (WHO, 2008). By focusing not just on causes of death but also charting the costs of living with a disease or disability, the study reveals the magnitude of health issues such as mental illness (Helliker, 2007). For instance:

- Mental illness is the second leading cause of premature mortality
- Four of the ten leading causes of disability in the U.S. are mental disorders
- Mental disorders collectively account for more than 15 percent of the overall burden of disease from *all* causes and slightly more than the burden associated with all forms of cancer
- By 2020, major depressive illness will be the leading cause of disability for women and children as the rate of this disease state continues to grow

(WHO, 2008)

Major depressive disorders are more common in people who have a history of trauma, sexual abuse, physical abuse, bereavement at a young age, alcoholism, and insufficient family structure. These are common psychosocial and environmental factors in many parts of the world for most people, and descriptive of the largest parts of America's inner cities and areas of the country at the bottom of the nation's economic pyramid.

Homelessness and Mental Illness

There is a high incidence of mental illness among the homeless. Published estimates vary from 23,500 to 43,400 at the low end of the range to 211,500 to 390,600 mentally ill homeless Americans on any given day (HUD, 2007). Knowledge of this number of people without shelter, whichever range is selected, is enough to identify a major health care problem in need of attention (Charles, 2009). What these numbers would be but for the $1.5 billion in federal assistance to address homelessness every year since 2001 is debatable. *See* Stewart B. McKinney Homeless Assistance Act of 2000, 42 U.S.C.A. § 11301(b)(2)-(3) (2004) (also establishing the Interagency Council on Homelessness). While there is no definitive estimate of the percentage of homeless who suffer from mental illness, the National Coalition for the Homeless points out that while government estimates varied from 10 to 90 percent, they ultimately settled on one in three as a reliable number of mentally ill individuals among the homeless, or 78,000 to 145,000 people.

Most homeless persons with mental illness do not need to be institutionalized, but can live in the community with appropriate supportive housing options. However, many mentally ill homeless people are unable to obtain access to supportive housing or other treatment services. Consequently, they are more than ten times more likely to be incarcerated than the general population (Greenberg & Rosenheck, 2008).

Incarceration and Mental Illness

The involuntary commitments by the courts and a safety conscious society have left the prisons and jails in the U.S. unable to control their inflow and outflow (Erickson, 2008). Government acquires obligations when it imprisons people, even when it does so for good reason; significant obligations are acquired when it decides to imprison over 2.3 million Americans (BJS, 2008), a higher percentage of the general population than any other country in the world (Walmsley, 2009). Almost half of the world's prison population is held in the U.S., followed by China (1.6 million sentenced prisoners), then Russia (0.9 million), three countries that account for just over a quarter of the world's population. The U.S. has the world's highest prison population rates; incarcerating seven people out of one thousand, which is higher than Russia and China (Walmsley, 2009). By comparison, other industrialized nations have universal health care coverage with better mental health care options and significantly lower rates of incarceration (*see* Brink, 2005).

Prison Population Rate per 100,000/National Population

U.S. 738
Russia 611
China 184
England 148
Australia 126
Canada 107
France 85
Japan 62

Source: Walmsley, 2009.

When over 400,000 incarcerated people in the U.S. have a severe mental illness (NAMH, 2006), a grave health care problem is likely being ignored

(McNeil et al., 2005). The surge in imprisonment of people with mental illness appears to be a phenomenon caused by the failure of the nation's community mental health sector combined with criminal sentencing processes that increase penalties for quality of life and drug offenses while reducing the exculpatory effects of mental illness (Santarelli, 2007). Quality-of-life offenses include public nuisance offenses such as disorderly conduct, urinating in public, and noise violations. Today, it seems the nation's largest mental health facilities are in urban jails:

- About one out of every five prisoners has a severe mental illness
- An estimated 700,000 people with severe mental illness are placed in American jails each year, about three-quarters of whom also have co-occurring substance abuse disorders
- The incidence of schizophrenia in state prisons is three to five times higher than in the general population, and two to three times higher in local jails than in the general population
- Imprisoned adolescents are about ten times more likely to suffer from severe mental illnesses and psychosis than their peers

(BJS, 2008; Brink, 2005; Fazel, 2008; Helliker, 2007)

While this data on the prevalence of mental illness among prisoners may be contested in their specifics, it is clear that severe mental disorders among the incarcerated are a significant health problem that defies simple explanation and resolution.

Self-Defeating Cycle of Delusion

Prisoners commonly suffer from delusional disorder, a psychiatric diagnosis denoting a psychotic mental illness that involves holding the fanciful delusion that they are unfairly imprisoned or that if a judge or someone in the criminal justice system would simply understand what happened to them, they would no longer need to be incarcerated. Though these false beliefs are pathological, many prisoners hold these extremely unreasonable beliefs with absolute conviction of their certainty. Moreover, many prisoners are incorrigible, no compelling counterargument or proof to the contrary could ever convince them to accept responsibility for the actions that led to their incarceration. While these prisoners think that the more appeals they file, the more likely they will be released, the judiciary becomes convinced the prisoners are precisely where they should be and sees their endless appeals as a failure to accept responsibility for their criminal behavior and considers them just another instance of a vicious self-perpetuating cycle of illnesses within the nation's health care system (*see generally* Brink, 2005).

Constitutional Rights of Prisoners
with Severe Mental Illness

While the constitutional rights of prisoners with
severe mental illness may be violated by the nation's
systemic failure to provide adequate treatment before,
during, and after their imprisonment, the courts have
repeatedly indicated that government has an affirmative duty to act. It is an obligation state and local
governments have largely demoted, after the federal
government essentially stopped its funding of the
nation's criminal justice system, notwithstanding constant arguments and court orders to the contrary.[LN1]

States facing limited financial resources for social
programs prefer to allocate taxpayer funds to the community's economic development, education, or health
care, rather than to its criminal justice system
(Bernstein, 2008). Even when the criminal justice
system does receive government funding, when a
choice has to be made between allocating funds for
law enforcement or corrections, funds generally go to
the police rather than to jails or prisons (Brink, 2005).
Without federal mandates and oversight, the nation's
correctional system may continue to deteriorate; while
the rights of prisoners with severe mental illness will
continue to be recognized by the judiciary, remedies
for violation of prisoners' rights will be denied without
federal funds to meet the affirmative duty of state and
local governments to act.

Perhaps treatment of the incarcerated population
with severe mental illness should be advanced pursuant
to selfish interests based on the potentially devastating
effects on the public health of the general population
flowing from poor prison care. Most of the 400,000
mentally ill prisoners incarcerated today will eventually be released to their communities (Helliker, 2007).
The failure of prisons to provide adequate treatment
for mental illnesses, not to mention the variety of sexually transmitted and communicable diseases, threatens
those communities to which prisoners are released with
physical and financial harm, infection, and illness. Such
public health arguments might have the potential to
move society to pay the costs for mental health care in
prisons out of clear self-interest, where heretofore the
public has been unwilling to do so as a matter of justice
or morality (*see generally* Helliker, 2007).

MENTAL ILLNESS WITHIN SPECIFIC POPULATIONS

Three particular populations will be addressed in this
chapter:

- College-age adults
- Health care professionals
- Returning combat veterans

College-Age Adults

Mental illnesses usually strike during adolescence
and young adulthood. All ages are susceptible, but
college-age adults are especially vulnerable because
their lives are generally characterized by rapid intellectual and social development (Ruan et al., 2008).
The National Institute on Alcohol Abuse and Alcoholism recently released the National Epidemiologic
Survey on Alcohol and Related Conditions, a nationwide longitudinal survey of alcohol and drug use and
associated psychiatric and medical co-morbidities. The
survey looked at the nineteen- to twenty-five-year-old
college-age adult population in the U.S. and found:

- The most common disorder is alcohol abuse
- One in five has a severe disorder that disrupts their
  daily lives
- Less than one in four with severe mental illness
  actually seeks treatment (5 percent of the total
  college-age adult population seeks treatment)

(Blanco et al., 2008)

While these incidence numbers may be increasing, the
increase may be partly because:

- The stigma attached to mental illness is fading
- New medications are allowing college-age adults
  to function better while acknowledging that
  they are having difficulties adjusting to life on
  their own

(Bernstein & Koppel, 2008)

These findings underscore the importance of treatment and prevention interventions by health care
professionals serving this population cohort (Grant,
2008). The overall rate of mental health disorders is
not different between college-attending individuals
and their non-college-attending peers (Blanco et al.,
2008). At the same time, college-attending individuals
cannot be forced to obtain mental health treatment.
While schools often decline to reach out to parents
or share information about students' behavior, citing
the federal Family Educational Rights and Privacy
Act (FERPA), 20 U.S.C.A. § 1232g (2002), this law
only protects student health and academic records
(White, 2007). Moreover, students can sign a FERPA
waiver allowing information to be shared with
their parents, something more schools are offering
(Bernstein, 2008).

FERPA also has loopholes whereby schools may
alert parents and authorities. While FERPA protects
student academic records, it allows schools to break
confidentiality and notify parents or authorities in
the case of a health or safety emergency, or a drug
or alcohol violation involving students under age
twenty-one. Schools can also share information with

parents who claim students as dependents on their tax returns. Further, if a potential danger stems from behavior that is not part of academic records, schools do not have to apply the privacy law at all. While state laws protect the privacy of medical records, including mental health counseling records, these laws allow mental health professionals to share information with police or other authorities, or even call for forced hospitalization, if there is a risk of imminent harm (*see* Bernstein, 2008).

Moral Dilemmas

1. How much access and influence should parents have when it comes to college-age students, particularly if parents are paying the student's tuition?

2. Should colleges and universities offer student privacy waivers to their students so parents can have more oversight of their behavior, or should schools encourage parents to take a hands-off approach?

Health Care Professionals

Given the health care community's access to and ability to prescribe drugs, it has always been assumed health care professionals have higher rates of drug abuse than other similar professionals. There is no credible research, however, to support this assumption about the culture in the nation's health care community. Plus, while the health care industry continues to be accused of not prioritizing mental health within its four walls (Hampton, 2005; Monahan, 2003; Center et al., 2003), health care professionals seem to have rates of substance abuse similar to the general population, no higher and no lower:

- 10 to 15 percent of all health care professionals misuse drugs during their career
- 6 to 8 percent of physicians have substance use disorders
- About 14 percent of physicians have alcohol use disorders

(Baldisseri, 2007)

Although the use of drugs and alcohol is slightly higher for some medical specialties, such as emergency medicine, psychiatry, anesthesiology, and high stress nursing specialties (Mavrofour et al., 2006), the recovery rates of health care professionals as a group are higher compared with the general population (Baldisseri, 2007).

Returning Combat Veterans

Since October 2001, close to two million U.S. troops have been deployed in Afghanistan and Iraq. Early evidence suggests the mental toll of these deployments, many involving prolonged exposure to combat-related stress over multiple deployments, may be disproportionately high compared with the physical injuries of combat (Tanielian & Jaycox, 2008). Preventing suicides and treating post-traumatic stress disorder (PTSD), traumatic brain injury (TBI), and depression among returning veterans will be an increasing problem for the U.S. Department of Veterans Affairs (VA) and the U.S. health care system.

A class action lawsuit was filed in the U.S. Court of Federal Claims in Washington, D.C., in late 2008, alleging that the U.S. Department of Defense illegally denied medical and disability benefits to veterans of the wars in Iraq and Afghanistan who were diagnosed with post-traumatic stress disorder. The lawsuit claims individuals were discharged from duty after Army review boards concluded they had experienced PTSD and were unable to serve; however, following their discharge, the Veterans Administration ruled they did not qualify for medical coverage to treat their PTSD because their disorders were not rated severe enough.

With almost two million U.S. armed services personnel deployed around the world as part of the U.S. efforts to combat global terrorism, countless thousands have been exposed to traumatic events during combat, and many have returned home with a variety of psychological and mental injuries (O'Brien, 2008). A decision needs to be made whether veterans who are discharged from service for PTSD are entitled to medical coverage for treatment of the disorder that led to their discharge. The VA, the President's Commission on Care for America's Returning Wounded Warriors, as well as the RAND Center for Health Policy Research, an independent review group, have estimated the magnitude of severe mental illness in returning veterans from Afghanistan and Iraq:

- About one in three, or about 300,000, returning veterans have severe mental health disorders, generally PTSD or major depression
- More than one in five returning veterans have TBI
- Roughly half of the returning veterans who need treatment for PTSD, TBI, or depression seek it, but only slightly more than half obtain quality, evidence-based care
- The number of returning veterans diagnosed with PTSD is growing by about eight thousand per year

(Tanielian & Jaycox, 2008)

VA specialty mental health services serve an average of 37,000 veterans per year, including more than 22,000 per year with PTSD from prior wars and conflicts, as well as those returning from Afghanistan and Iraq.

LIABILITY FOR DEATHS A MENTALLY ILL VETERAN CAUSED AFTER DISCHARGE FROM TREATMENT

DeJesus v. U.S. Department of Veterans Affairs
[Parents of Murder Victims v. VA]
479 F.3d 271 (U.S. Court of Appeals for the 3rd Circuit 2007)

FACTS: Alejandro DeJesus, an unemployed, homeless Vietnam veteran suffering from mental illness and a co-occurring substance abuse disorder with a history of domestic violence, voluntarily entered a VA inpatient program where he was diagnosed with intermittent explosive disorder, a condition characterized by repeated violent outbursts. He was prescribed medications to control his condition. Later, DeJesus was diagnosed with only mild depression. In response to this depression diagnosis, the VA assigned DeJesus to psychotherapy and substance abuse counseling.

After a few months of inpatient treatment, the VA recommended DeJesus for a transitional residence program that provided mental and physical health care to homeless veterans. The VA failed to inform the program about his intermittent explosive disorder and did not release his inpatient records, even though the records would have alerted the program that DeJesus suffered from violent outbursts and suicidal ideations. While in the transitional residence program, DeJesus threatened another resident with a knife, leading the VA to recommend his discharge. The transitional residence program acknowledged it dismissed DeJesus because of the VA's recommendation.

Before DeJesus left the transitional residence program, he gave away all his possessions and shredded his clothing. Despite the fact that this behavior indicated suicidal intentions, none of the staff who participated in DeJesus's discharge followed involuntary commitment procedures or internal emergency psychiatric intervention procedures. Eighteen hours after leaving the transitional residence program, DeJesus charged into his estranged wife's apartment and shot and killed two of their children and two other children before turning the gun on himself.

His wife and the mother of the other deceased children filed a federal claim against the VA alleging that by negligently discharging and subsequently failing to recommit DeJesus, even when he overtly posed an imminent threat, the VA caused the wrongful deaths of their children. Further, they claimed the VA negligently failed to warn them about DeJesus's mental state.

ISSUE: Is the VA liable under the Federal Tort Claims Act of 1946 (FTCA) for the wrongful death of four children that were killed eighteen hours after DeJesus was released from a transitional residence program for homeless veterans while severely mentally ill?

HOLDING AND DECISION: Yes, the VA is liable under the FTCA for the wrongful death of the four children; it breached the standard of care established by state law and was grossly negligent in deciding DeJesus should be discharged from a transitional residence program, and in its failure to involuntarily recommit him. *See* 28 U.S.C.A. §§ 1291 *et seq.* (2009) (permitting private parties to sue the federal government in federal court for torts committed by persons acting on behalf of the government).

ANALYSIS: The Third Circuit looked to Pennsylvania law and common law to determine the standard of care for federal agencies under the FTCA. The court noted that if a state's highest court has not spoken on an issue, a federal court must predict how it would decide in light of:

- Holdings in related areas
- Intermediate state court decisions
- Federal cases interpreting state law
- Case law from other jurisdictions

First, the court addressed the failure-to-warn claim, and analyzed whether the VA had a duty to warn third parties about DeJesus's mental health status. Mental health workers have an affirmative duty to warn an intended victim if a patient poses a severe danger of violence. However, this duty does not extend to a situation involving no specific threat of immediate harm to a readily identifiable victim.

The court then considered whether the VA was grossly negligent. Here, a state mental health

(continues)

(continued)

law provided the source of state law necessary to hold the government liable under the FTCA. The state mental health law provided immunity to health care providers for treating and discharging mentally ill patients from treatment, in the absence of willful misconduct or gross negligence. While this state law generally protects providers from liability, it also imposes an affirmative duty to refrain from gross negligence in the treatment and discharge of mentally ill patients. In the present case, DeJesus received inpatient treatment at a VA facility and the VA participated in the decision to discharge him from a transitional residence program for homeless veterans, thus imposing on the VA a duty to refrain from gross negligence in DeJesus's treatment and discharge.

In evaluating the gross negligence standard, the court looked at the definition of gross negligence: a form of negligence where the facts support substantially more than ordinary carelessness, inadvertence, laxity, or indifference. Here, several actions demonstrated the VA's gross negligence:

- DeJesus's complete medical history, including his diagnosis as having an intermittent explosive disorder, was never transmitted to his treatment

providers, either while he was receiving inpatient or outpatient treatment at VA facilities
- VA failed to recognize DeJesus's violent outbursts leading up to the shootings as consistent with his particular mental illness
- VA failed at both preventing DeJesus's release and effecting his recommitment, despite his suicidal tendencies

Simple negligence involves significantly less egregious breaches of the standard of care. Finding the VA's actions met the standard for gross negligence, the VA was liable for breaching its duty under the state mental health law, and thus was liable for DeJesus' post-discharge actions.

RULE OF LAW: The FTCA overcomes sovereign immunity and makes the federal government liable for tort claims in the same manner and to the same extent as private parties under like circumstances; a federal agency's duty under the FTCA stems from state law, which the VA violated by discharging and failing to recommit DeJesus after his release from a transitional residence program for veterans.

(See generally Martin, 2007).

This decision could potentially impact the mental health sector of the U.S. health care system. It reinforces the fact that VA providers must be familiar with the law in the states in which they practice. While the duty owed to returning veterans differs by state, state laws written to protect mental health providers from liability can be broadly read as imposing an affirmative duty to refrain from negligence in the treatment and discharge of mentally ill patients. Accordingly, providers may be liable for the actions of mentally ill patients they release; discharging a severely mentally ill patient from treatment is a potential danger, not only to the patient but to others. Given this heightened standard, providers should exercise due care in treating and discharging patients (Martin, 2007).

INTELLECTUALLY DISABLED

Intellectually disabled persons are one of the most socially stigmatized groups health care providers encounter when dealing with mental illness (Stein & Stein, 2007). This is so because their disability renders

them less able either to assert their rights or to protect themselves with regard to medical decisions (Gostin & Gable, 2004).

Medical Decision Making

There is a critical shift occurring in the perspective of what is referred to as intellectual disability. For example, the major association concerned with the rights of intellectually disabled persons, the American Association on Intellectual and Developmental Disabilities (AAIDD), was founded in 1878 as the Association of Medical Officers of American Institutions for Idiotic and Feebleminded Persons; in 1906, that name was changed to the American Association for the Study of the Feebleminded; then to the American Association of Mental Deficiency in 1933; in 1987, the name was changed again to the American Association on Mental Retardation; then most recently to the AAIDD in 2007. During this transition, courts are struggling with providing medical care for intellectually disabled persons. One of the most recent cases to tackle this issue was a class action lawsuit in the District of Columbia.

MEDICAL DECISIONS ON BEHALF OF INTELLECTUALLY DISABLED PERSONS

Doe ex rel. Tarlow v. District of Columbia
[Incompetent Intellectually Disabled Persons v. District Mental Health Agency]
489 F.3d 376 (U.S. Court of Appeals for the District of Columbia 2007)

FACTS: This is a class action comprised of a class of intellectually disabled persons who live in District of Columbia facilities and receive medical services from the District. They have never had the mental capacity to make medical decisions for themselves. The policy at issue was adopted to regulate the medical care of intellectually disabled persons in the District. For intellectually disabled persons who have always lacked the mental capacity to make informed medical decisions, the policy authorized the District mental health agency to make medical decisions on behalf of them if:

- Two licensed physicians have certified in writing that the proposed treatment is in the best interests of the intellectually disabled person
- Attempts were made to provide an explanation of the proposed treatment to the intellectually disabled person
- No guardian, family member, or other close friend or associate is available to consent or withhold consent

The Health Care Decisions Act, the District of Columbia law alleged to be inconsistent with the medical care of intellectually disabled persons policy, provides that in making a medical decision on behalf of an incompetent person, the decision must be based on the known wishes of the incompetent person or, if the wishes of the person are unknown and cannot be ascertained, on a good faith belief as to the best interests of the incompetent person.

ISSUE: Do the wishes of incompetent, intellectually disabled persons, who have never had the mental capacity to make medical decisions for themselves, need to be considered?

HOLDING AND DECISION: No, the policy was consistent with the Health Care Decisions Act.

ANALYSIS: The court began its statutory analysis by observing that the Health Care Decisions Act implicitly distinguishes between two categories of persons who lack mental capacity, those who:

- Once possessed the mental capacity to make medical decisions (such as those in a coma)
- Have always lacked the mental capacity to make medical decisions

For persons who once had the mental capacity to make medical decisions, medical decisions must be based on the "known wishes" of the person, if those wishes can be ascertained. For patients who have never had the mental capacity to make medical decisions, medical decisions must be based on the "best interests" of the patient.

The court then held that the policy regulating the medical care of intellectually disabled persons did not infringe upon either procedural or substantive due process rights. While acknowledging the policy did not consider the wishes of persons who have never possessed the mental capacity to make a medical decision, the court held that this does not violate procedural due process because acting on the wishes of such persons could result in erroneous medical decisions, with harmful or even deadly consequences. Persons who have always lacked the mental capacity to make medical decisions do not have a constitutional right to have their wishes considered.

RULE OF LAW: The rights of incompetent persons who once possessed the mental capacity to make medical decisions are distinct from the rights of intellectually disabled persons who never had such capacity.

(*See generally* Amar & Strumolo, 2007).

While the known wishes and the best interests standards are almost always guaranteed to result in the same outcome for competent adults, this is not the case for incompetent persons. Incompetent

persons may wish to make decisions that have harmful consequences or that are even deadly; they lack the ability to know what is in their best interests. Therefore, the court logically determined that persons who never met a competency standard were incapable of knowing what decisions were in their best interests.

Defining Intellectual Disability

The term *intellectually disabled* does not define a distinct class of persons; in fact, individual abilities may differ widely and there is no recognized assessment method firmly grounded in scientific evidence (Weithorn, 2008). This chapter uses the term *intellectually disabled* to describe what has historically been referred to as *mentally retarded*. The term *intellectually disabled* focuses on intellectual capabilities instead of mental functions and properly categorizes the condition as a disability. Current clinical definitions of the intellectually disabled, as recognized by the U.S. Supreme Court, require not only sub-average intellectual functioning, but also significant limitations in adaptive skills to care for themselves and diminished capacities to:

- Understand and process information
- Communicate
- Abstract from mistakes and learn from experience
- Engage in logical reasoning
- Control impulses and act pursuant to a premeditated plan
- Understand the reactions of others
- Self-direct themselves (in group settings they are followers)

(*See Atkins v. Virginia*, 536 U.S. 304 (U.S. Supreme Court 2002) (holding death is an inappropriate criminal sentence for intellectually disabled persons, but leaving it to the states to determine who is intellectually disabled))

Today, most Americans could quickly identify public figures that fit the broad clinical definition recognized by the U.S. Supreme Court; at least one commentator has suggested adding "diminished capacity to appreciate the merits of term limits" to this list of adaptive limitations.

The American Association on Intellectual and Developmental Disabilities defines significant sub-average intellectual functioning as an IQ standard score of approximately 70 to 75 or below (Edwards & Luckasson, 2002). While such intellectual deficiencies diminish the personal culpability of intellectually disabled persons for their actions while they are undergoing treatment, it also leads to confusion as to what constitutes a disability when health care providers are facing questions such as:

- Informed consent for life-threatening medical treatments
- End-of-life care
- Involuntary commitments and hospitalizations

The general consensus is that people are intellectually disabled when they fail to achieve minimal functional capability levels (Stein & Stein, 2007).

INVOLUNTARY CIVIL COMMITMENTS

There are at least two divisive issues confronting health care providers as they provide treatment to mentally ill persons with severe mental disorders:

- Involuntary commitment procedures for the mentally ill, especially for persons suffering from dangerous mental disorders
- Conditional releases of mentally ill persons from involuntary commitment

Involuntary civil commitment is a process governed by state law that allows for mentally ill persons to be committed to a hospital on an involuntary basis. The two major phases of the process are the petition and pre-hearing detention period, and the involuntary civil commitment hearing. Mentally ill persons enter the process through an emergency court order requiring they be taken into custody and examined. Following the evaluation, they are either released or detained for additional evaluation and treatment under a temporary detention order. Courts may order involuntary civil commitments only if there is clear and convincing evidence that the individual poses a danger to self or others, or is largely incapable of caring for themself and no less restrictive alternative treatment is available (Pfeffer, 2008).

Dangerous Mental Disorders

While the insanity defense dates back at least to the days after the Norman conquest of 1066 when the English common law began developing, the law continues to struggle with involuntary commitment procedures for persons who are dangerous to themselves and to society. The U.S. Supreme Court has addressed this double-edged issue in at least five decisions (*see* Barth, 2007).[LN2]

While this Second Circuit opinion allows New York to continue recommitting certain persons at a lower evidentiary standard, it is not clear this policy will remain in place indefinitely. Because the Second Circuit does not foreclose the possibility that other persons may raise a constitutional objection to New York's recommitment procedure, or seek relief through other legal means, it appears likely this issue is not settled and other cases may have the opportunity to challenge the New York law in the future (Erickson, 2008).

Conditional Releases

Absent public safety concerns or the need for mental health treatment, involuntary confinement cannot be justified; mental illness alone cannot justify involuntary confinement of a person indefinitely against their will (*see O'Connor v. Donaldson*, 422 U.S. 563 (U.S. Supreme Court 1975)). For instance, a person cannot be involuntarily confined because of an antisocial personality absent a showing of dangerousness because the behavior is not a recognized mental disease or defect (*see Foucha v. Louisiana*, 504 U.S. 71 (U.S. Supreme Court 1992)).

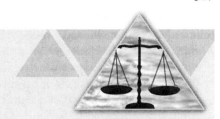

INVOLUNTARY COMMITMENT OF MENTALLY ILL PERSONS

Ernst J. v. Stone

[Mentally Ill Patient v. State Commissioner of Mental Health]

452 F.3d 186 (U.S. Court of Appeals for the 2nd Circuit 2006)

FACTS: Ernst suffered from chronic schizophrenia. During a psychotic episode where he heard voices and thought an elderly man was the devil, Ernst attacked the man, leaving him with severe bite wounds to his hand and genitalia. Ernst was charged with assault in the first degree, assault in the second degree, and burglary in the second degree. Ernst pleaded "not responsible by reason of mental disease or defect" (NRRMDD) to assault in the second degree. In accordance with criminal procedure, psychiatrists examined Ernst and determined that although he suffered from schizophrenia, at the time of the examination he was not suffering from a dangerous mental disorder, nor was he mentally ill. The psychiatrists recommended Ernst be required to obtain psychiatric treatment in an outpatient setting. The court agreed with the psychiatrists' recommendation and designated Ernst a track three NRRMDD person. The court ordered that he be conditionally discharged, subject to a five-year order of conditions. One of the conditions was that Ernst was required to remain in outpatient treatment five days per week for his ongoing mental illness.

Two years later, Ernst was arrested for criminal trespass and harassment. He pleaded guilty to harassment in the second degree and was sentenced to conditional discharge.

The following year, Ernst was arrested again for criminal trespass, although he was not prosecuted for this offense. As time passed, Ernst's behavior became increasingly violent.

A year later and within days of the expiration of his five-year order of conditions, Ernst, while living in a residential treatment center, took a female social worker hostage and threatened to sexually assault her. After this incident, he was transferred to the custody of Interfaith Hospital on an emergency basis. Soon after, Ernst's order of conditions was extended and his involuntary commitment was extended.

A month later, Ernst was transferred to Kingsboro Psychiatric Center where he continued his violent behavior. Kingsboro requested a three-month period of retention upon clear and convincing evidence Ernst was mentally ill and posed a substantial threat of physical harm to himself and others. Additionally, his order of conditions was extended for the second time, this time for an additional period of three years. After three months of treatment, Kingsboro determined Ernst had developed a dangerous mental disorder and sought a court order for him to be committed to a secure psychiatric facility.

Ernst moved to dismiss the application for recommitment, arguing the Fourteenth Amendment of the U.S. Constitution prohibited New York from recommitting him under the lower evidentiary standard of a preponderance of the evidence, rather than the higher clear and convincing evidence standard required for an original determination of involuntary commitment. Ernst claimed that because at the initial commitment hearing the court found him mentally ill but not afflicted with a dangerous mental disorder, there was no basis to subject him to a lower standard of proof for the recommitment proceedings.

ISSUE: Can New York law have one set of administrative procedures for the involuntary civil commitment of persons suffering from mental illness who are not dangerous and a different set of procedures for mentally ill persons determined to be dangerous?

HOLDING AND DECISION: Yes, a lower standard of proof may be used to involuntarily hospitalize persons suffering from a dangerous mental disorder who are determined to be NRRMDD, as opposed to the higher standard required for mentally ill persons who are not dangerous.

ANALYSIS: Certain protections exist for involuntary civil commitment, such as requiring clear and convincing evidence that a mentally ill person poses a danger to themselves or others.

(continues)

(continued)

Extensive evidence must be presented to show the mentally ill person is substantially more likely than not to engage in dangerous behavior. Mentally ill means:

- Currently suffering from a mental disease or defect
- Treatment in an inpatient psychiatric center is essential to the person's welfare
- Person's judgment is so impaired they are unable to understand the need for such treatment

Courts must first order a psychiatric examination to determine the person's current mental condition, followed by a hearing as to their appropriate treatment. Pursuant to the findings at the hearing, the person is placed in one of three NRRMDD tracks based on a preponderance of the evidence. The tracking decision requires a lower standard of proof than the commitment decision. Evidence is merely required to show a mentally ill person is more likely than not to demonstrate one of three behaviors:

- Track one persons are determined to suffer from a dangerous mental disorder and must be committed to a secure psychiatric facility
- Track two persons are determined not to be suffering from a dangerous mental disorder, but are nonetheless mentally ill
- Track three persons are neither mentally ill nor suffering from a dangerous mental disorder

Track two NRRMDD persons are remanded to the custody of the state mental health agency subject to an order of conditions. An order of conditions means a court order directing a mentally ill person to comply with their prescribed treatment plan, or any other condition the court determines to be reasonably necessary or appropriate. Orders of condition are valid for five years, except for good cause shown; the court may extend the period for an additional five

years. Their commitment is then governed by the civil commitment provisions of the state mental hygiene law.

Track three NRRMDD persons are either discharged unconditionally or discharged subject to an order of conditions, which generally requires them to enroll in outpatient psychiatric treatment. State law recognizes the possibility a track two or track three NRRMDD person may, during the course of outpatient care, develop a dangerous mental disorder and require commitment in a secure psychiatric facility. For a court to order recommitment, the NRRMDD person must have a dangerous mental disorder. Dangerous mental disorder means:

- Person currently suffers from a mental illness
- Because of such condition, they currently constitute a physical danger to themselves or others

In civil commitment proceedings, states must prove the elements of mental illness and dangerousness by no less than clear and convincing evidence (*see Addington v. Texas*, 441 U.S. 418 (U.S. Supreme Court 1979)). This evidentiary standard concerns only the initial confinement of mentally ill persons, and does not specifically address the standard of proof applicable to recommitment or release proceedings (*see Jones v. U.S.*, 463 U.S. 354 (U.S. Supreme Court 1983)). States may not, consistent with the Fourteenth Amendment, continue to confine in a psychiatric facility persons who remain dangerous but who no longer suffer from any mental illness (*see Foucha v. Louisiana*, 504 U.S. 71 (U.S. Supreme Court 1992)).

RULE OF LAW: It is not unreasonable for New York to provide for the recommitment of mentally ill persons who pleaded NRRMDD under the low preponderance of the evidence standard; this mental health policy does not violate either due process or the equal protection clause of the Fourteenth Amendment.

(*See generally* Erickson, 2008).

Other circuit courts have added non-medical conditions to the conditional release of mentally ill patients from involuntary commitment, if the patients had been found NRRMDD, or insane. The NRRMDD defense is also referred to as "not guilty by reason of insanity."

This chapter uses the former term. The Eighth Circuit extended this policy with respect to persons in federal custody for other mental health related reasons and then went one step further by providing for recommitment as a permissible mechanism for enforcing such conditions.

CONDITIONAL RELEASE FROM INVOLUNTARY COMMITMENT

U.S. v. Franklin

[Federal Government v. Involuntarily Committed Patient]

435 F.3d 885 (U.S. Court of Appeals for the 8th Circuit 2006)

FACTS: Gordon Franklin was involuntarily committed for twelve years due to mental disease. When he was released due to improvement in his mental condition, his release was subject to seven conditions requiring him to comply with a prescribed treatment regime. In addition, he was required to comply with the standard conditions of probation.

A year following his release, Franklin called the probation office and first spoke to a receptionist, and then to his probation officer, Mark Davy. Davy told Franklin he should discuss his issues with Davy or Davy's supervisor rather than with the receptionist. In response, Franklin became agitated and upset with Davy and made death threats directed toward Davy, Davy's supervisor, and the judge who had ordered his commitment, such as "I will blow your brains out" and "the judge who messed me up needs to be killed."

Franklin's conditional release was immediately revoked on the grounds that he violated the required conditions of his release and he was recommitted. Franklin then filed a motion for his release and requested a mental examination. A clinical psychologist examined him and concluded he continued to suffer from bipolar disorder and met the criteria for involuntary commitment. A risk assessment report compiled by a panel of mental health experts found that despite Franklin's reported compliance with his prescribed treatment regime, his mental condition had deteriorated to a point where his medications were no longer adequate. The report concluded that because Franklin had resisted increasing the dosage level of his medications, his release would pose a substantial safety risk to himself and others. Franklin testified he regretted his comments to Davy, that he was coping with his mental disease, and that he would not pose a danger to himself or others as long as he continued taking his prescribed medications.

The court determined that although there was no direct evidence Franklin did not follow his prescribed treatment regimen, his sudden behavioral change supported that conclusion. Franklin's conditional release was revoked and he was involuntarily committed.

ISSUE: May the release of a mentally ill patient from hospitalization be conditioned upon fulfilling requirements, other than the requirement to comply with a prescribed treatment regime?

HOLDING AND DECISION: Yes, the conditional release of a mentally ill patient from hospitalization may be revoked and the patient may be involuntarily recommitted for failure to comply with requirements other than the requirement to follow a prescribed treatment regime.

ANALYSIS: Franklin claimed there was insufficient evidence to conclude he violated the requirements of his release by failing to take his prescribed medications. The government maintained Franklin violated his probation by breaking the law when he threatened Davy, Davy's supervisor, and the judge who had ordered his commitment. Franklin countered he could not be recommitted on these grounds, because federal law only allows the revocation of a conditional release when a person fails to comply with their prescribed treatment regime.

The court held that when a person suffering from mental disease or defect is released from hospitalization, additional conditions may be imposed that are ancillary to the prescribed medical regimen, such as probation, as long as the additional conditions are related to the person's mental illness and reasonably necessary to protect the safety of others. In addition, a conditional release may be revoked for violation of a non-treatment-related condition, at least when the violation flows from the person's mental disease and demonstrates that continued release presents a danger to others.

A conditional release may be revoked after determining that a person failed to comply with their prescribed treatment regimen if their

(continues)

(continued)

continued release would create a substantial risk to the safety of others (*see* 18 U.S.C.A. § 4246(f) (1997)). Although federal law does not specifically mention what recourse is available when a released person violates a non-treatment-related condition, the court reasoned that Congress must have contemplated a mechanism for enforcing violations of non-treatment-related conditions. Otherwise, the released person could blatantly violate such conditions and courts would be powerless to revoke their release, even if the violations demonstrated the person posed a danger to the public.

Applying these principles to this situation, the court found the condition of probation was related to Franklin's illness and was reasonably necessary to ensure his safety and the safety of others, at least as far as it required Franklin to refrain from violating probation standards by threatening the lives of his probation officers and the judge who had ordered his commitment. The court revoked Franklin's conditional release, finding his violation of probation flowed directly from his mental disease and demonstrated a threat to himself and others.

RULE OF LAW: When mentally ill persons are released from an involuntary commitment, additional conditions may be imposed on their release that are unrelated to compliance with their prescribed treatment regime; their release may be subsequently revoked and they may be recommitted for violating such non-medical conditions.

This decision raises several unanswered questions regarding mentally ill persons. For instance, can mentally ill persons be required to waive their right to confidentiality regarding their mental health treatment to allow sharing of information with their probation officers, as a condition of their release from hospitalization? Is this waiver reasonably necessary to protect the community's safety? Regardless of the answers to these questions, health care providers serving mentally ill persons should be aware of this court's holding and its potentially broad reach.[LN3]

PROTECTION AND ADVOCACY FOR INDIVIDUALS WITH MENTAL ILLNESS

Congress created the national Protection and Advocacy for Individuals with Mental Illness program (PAIMI) to curb abuse and neglect of the mentally ill, primarily in institutions (*see* 42 U.S.C.A. §§ 247a *et seq.* (2009)). Beginning in the 1960s and 1970s, many abuses were uncovered at hospitals, where patients were inappropriately physically restrained, neglected, or overmedicated. Today, some physicians, hospital administrators, and mental health workers claim patient advocates endanger the mentally ill by too often fighting for their right to refuse treatment when the patients actually present a danger to themselves and the public. Proponents of patient advocates say they are essential to protecting

Moral Dilemmas

1. While clear and convincing evidence is required for involuntary commitment of mentally ill persons, what standard of proof should be used for recommitment or release proceedings?

2. What standard of proof should be used to determine whether a mentally ill person has in fact developed a dangerous mental disorder?

3. Should courts be permitted to force antipsychotic medications on a mentally ill person so they can stand trial for a criminal offense or should the person always be committed involuntarily?

the rights of the mentally ill from inappropriate incarceration and homelessness. The National Disability Rights Network, which provides lobbying and other services for the patient-advocacy system, maintains patient advocates play a critical oversight role (Yen, 2008).

In recent years, there has been a wave of legislative efforts, many inspired by violent crimes, to make it easier to mandate treatment for the mentally ill who pose a substantial risk of harm to themselves or others. Patient advocates have blunted those efforts in California, New Mexico, and Michigan.

VIOLATION OF PATIENT RIGHTS

Davis v. Rennie

[Mentally Ill Patient v. Mental Health Staff]

*264 F.3d 86 (U.S. Court of Appeals for the 1st Circuit 2001), U.S. Supreme
Court certiorari denied,* 535 U.S. 1053 (U.S. Supreme Court 2002)

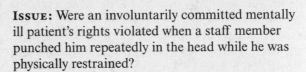

FACTS: Jason Davis, a mentally ill patient involuntarily committed at Westborough State Hospital, suffered from schizo-affective and bipolar disorders. Davis and another patient violated hospital rules by leaving the grounds without permission. Greg Plesh, a police officer from the hospital, found the patients consuming alcohol behind a local liquor store and brought them back to the hospital. The hospital staff found both patients to be loud and demanding, and the unit's head nurse, Joyce Wiegers, decided to place Davis in an isolation room. According to Davis, two mental health staff workers, Michael Hanlon and Paul Rennie, remained outside the isolation room and taunted him. Davis tried to do a double drop kick, and it is disputed as to whether Davis intended to kick one of the guards, or just aimed toward the wall. According to Davis, Rennie then entered the room, choked Davis, and threw him to the ground with deadly force. Rennie disputes this account and contends he merely physically restrained Davis and did not injure him.

At this point, Wiegers summoned several more staff and Plesh to lead Davis out of the room. Davis alleges Rennie continued to taunt him, and Davis kicked Rennie in the stomach. The staff wrestled Davis to the ground, with one on each limb. Davis testified another staff member, Phillip Bragg, punched him repeatedly in the head. Plesh testified that since no one intervened, he did and pushed Bragg away while the others rolled Davis onto his stomach. Bragg denied punching Davis and the other mental health staff denied seeing Bragg punch Davis. Davis also testified Wiegers taunted him while Plesh handcuffed him for transport to another room. After Plesh secured Davis in another room, he arrested Bragg for assault and battery.

Medical evidence introduced at trial showed Davis suffered serious physical injuries from the assault. Davis sued multiple mental health staff workers involved for the use of excessive force during the two instances of physical restraint. Davis also sued the staff for failing to intervene to prevent Bragg's use of excessive force during the second restraint and for violating Davis's right to freedom from unreasonable bodily restraint. The jury returned a verdict against seven of the staff.

ISSUE: Were an involuntarily committed mentally ill patient's rights violated when a staff member punched him repeatedly in the head while he was physically restrained?

HOLDING AND DECISION: Yes, the mental health staff used excessive force, violated Davis's right of freedom from unreasonable bodily restraint, and failed to intervene when a staff member repeatedly punched him.

ANALYSIS: Davis's constitutional rights were violated; therefore, he was entitled to $100,000 in compensatory damages and $1.55 million in punitive damages. The damage award was based on a fourfold analysis:

- Failure to intervene when Davis was attacked while restrained
- Mental health staff violated the Massachusetts Civil Rights Act by coercively abusing Davis with the use of excessive force to restrain him and then threatening more abuse after the restraint
- Qualified immunity is negated when an affirmative duty to intervene is disregarded
- Evil motives, lying, and attempts to cover up wrongdoing justify punitive damages

Davis's claim is based on the Fourteenth Amendment's protection against state action depriving an individual of life or liberty without due process of law. There is a duty to protect those who are involuntarily committed for mental disease or defect. Failures to act may create a due process violation because the confinement of mentally ill patients prevents them from being able to help themselves. Although Davis was drunk and potentially threatening, once he was restrained, the situation no longer required the use of force. Moreover, patients who are involuntarily committed are entitled to more considerate treatment than criminals; the conduct of mental health staff is held to a higher standard than prison guards or police officers.

The mental health staff maintained there was no evidence Bragg punched Davis. The court noted there was sufficient evidence to reasonably

(continues)

(continued)

infer the staff witnessed the attack. In addition, the court found there was time and opportunity to intervene based on testimony, which created a possible inference the staff was nearer to Davis than Plesh when Plesh intervened. Thus, the court found the staff failed to intervene to protect Davis as he was repeatedly punched in the head while restrained.

The court next held the actions of the mental health staff in continuing to hold Davis down was a form of acquiescence to Bragg, who clearly intended to violate Davis's rights, and the restraint was coercion under the Massachusetts Civil Rights Act. Furthermore, the court found Rennie's use of excessive force in the first physical encounter was intimidating and coercive in itself. Finally, the court found Wiegers threatened Davis with more abuse after the restraint. Therefore, the court found liability against all of the staff under the Massachusetts Civil Rights Act.

In addition, the court defined qualified immunity as a protection for state actors from liability for civil damages arising from their conduct as long as the actors did not violate some clearly established right a reasonable person would have known. With regard to this situation, the court held that the mental health staff should have known they had a legal duty to intervene when Bragg used excessive force against Davis. Specifically, the court found Wiegers had a duty to stop Bragg, or at least to attempt to stop Bragg by calling out rather than physically interfering. The

qualified immunity defense of the mental health staff failed because they were reasonably expected to know Bragg's attack created an affirmative duty to intervene.

Finally, while the mental health staff denied harboring any ill will toward Davis, the court found there was sufficient evidence to support a finding of evil motive toward Davis. Rennie taunted and provoked Davis and then used excessive force to restrain him, the staff held Davis down knowing Bragg was punching him, and Wiegers did nothing to protect her patient. Furthermore, the court found the staff attempted to cover up their wrongdoing by filing inaccurate reports and lying when they testified. Thus, the court held punitive damages were appropriate due to the reprehensible conduct of the staff.

RULE OF LAW: Patients who have been involuntarily committed must be given extra protections from abuse because they may be unable to help or control themselves; mental health staff, therefore, have an affirmative duty to prevent any excessive force from being applied to patients to restore order. This affirmative duty also applies to observers, such as supervisory nurses, to prevent excessive force, even if the observers do not directly participate in any of the physical restraining. Furthermore, mental health staff does not have the same freedoms police officers or prison guards have to use force to restore order.

(See generally Talley, 2009).

Nevertheless, the mental health sectors are being given greater leeway to disclose patient information to those who may be affected by the conduct of the mentally ill. Further, it is becoming easier to medicate involuntarily committed patients (Yen, 2008).

SEX ADDICTION AND HUMAN TRAFFICKING FOR THE PURPOSE OF SEXUAL EXPLOITATION

When does a pattern of behavior become a mental disorder? In the case of sex addiction, this question has been debated for decades. Sex addiction was added to the *DSM-III* in 1980, dropped from *DSM-IV* in 1994, and now the debate is over whether to restore sex addiction for *DSM-V*. The official

position of the Society for the Advancement of Sexual Health, an advocate organization in San Diego, California, for the treatment of sexual addictions and compulsivity, is that sexual behavior becomes a mental disorder when it adversely affects a person's life and the lives of others.

The blend of humor and pathos in the fictional portrayal of sex addiction, as evidenced by the Showtime comedy *Californication* and by the movie *Choke*, implies a collective ambivalence of Americans toward sex disorders (Beck, 2008).[LN4] Ambivalence aside, the U.S. Department of State finds that the magnitude of human trafficking for the purpose of sexual exploitation by persons with sex addictions has exploded in the U.S. in the past decade (U.S. Department of State, 2007).

The U.S. Department of State estimates 14,500 to 17,500 people (including men) are trafficked into the U.S. every year (U.S. Department of State, 2007), but other sources estimate the number may be as high as 50,000 to 100,000 women and children alone (Yen, 2008). Trafficking for sex is a sophisticated underground industry that generates billions of dollars in profit every year, yet destroys the lives of innocent victims. Many of the trafficked victims are impoverished children and young women from economically depressed countries who are forced to work as prostitutes under brutal conditions in the U.S. Sometimes they are tricked into the trade. One example is when a victim applies for what they think is an au pair position, only to be enslaved upon arrival in the U.S.

To date, the legislative and law enforcement attention has focused on the supply side of the sex trafficking equation in the U.S., namely, the traffickers and the victims. Little focus has been directed to the demand side of the problem, namely the sex-addicted patrons of the prostitutes. The demand for commercial sexual services sustains and grows the sex trafficking industry. If sexual addiction is again recognized as a mental disorder in *DSM-V*, the U.S. could possibly take a more demand-oriented approach to fighting sex trafficking. The issue under debate is whether offenders who participate in sex trafficking should be involuntarily committed like pedophiles or face extreme penalties more befitting their behavior.

Moral Dilemmas

1. If pedophilia is a recognized mental disorder for purposes of involuntary commitment, should the *DSM-V* also add sexual addictions that harm others?

SEX ADDICTION AND INTERNET PORNOGRAPHY

The number of Americans who are active users of Internet pornography is having a devastating effect on marriages and relationships. In addition, there is a huge problem with Internet pornography in the workplace (*see* Bertagna, 2008). While the research continues to grow and demonstrates a serious mental health condition, whether Internet pornography is a mental disorder or an excuse to behave badly remains to be determined (Beck, 2008). One thing is certain, Internet pornography is a growing industry, generating over $12 billion a year in revenue. Moreover, while many believe that viewing online pornography is a harmless expression of sexual curiosity, its effects are often more profound. For 15 percent of the online porn habitués, viewing pornography develops

into compulsive behavior that disrupts their lives (Mitchell, 2007).

BIBLIOTHERAPY

While bibliotherapy has been around since the 1930s, most self-help books are reminiscent of the market for elixirs, oils, and pills before the advent of federal regulation. Today, however, bibliotherapy is gaining credibility from evidence-based research showing some self-help books can actually improve mental health. U.S. revenue for self-help books exceeds $600 million according to Simba Information, a market research firm in Stamford, Connecticut (Helliker, 2007). In the United Kingdom, where the wait for mental health services can stretch to six months, the national health system has embraced bibliotherapy as the first line of intervention for non-emergency cases. The national health system in Britain prescribes self-help books for people seeking medical attention for mood disorders. The program varies, but in most parts of the country, health officials have stocked about 30 approved books at local libraries. Seekers of non-emergency mental health services receive book prescriptions enabling them to check out books for at least three months (Anderson et al., 2005; *see also* Bernstein & Koppel, 2008).

Now, mental health professionals in the United Kingdom, the U.S., and elsewhere are determined to distinguish the most proven offerings. The aim is to recommend books shown to be successful in published clinical trials conducted and peer-reviewed by reputable, independent researchers. Evidence-based trials are conducted in much the same way as clinical research is done for drugs, comparing patients' symptoms before and after bibliotherapy, compared with patients who did not undergo the book therapy (Floyd et al., 2006). In the U.S., no official list of bibliotherapy treatments exists. Nevertheless, over three thousand mental health professionals have contributed to a self-help manual ranking more than one thousand self-help books, autobiographies, and popular films according to their clinical effectiveness, based on clinical trials and clinical experience (Norcross et al., 2003).

Bibliotherapy, when used as an adjunct therapy for depression, works best on mild to moderate symptoms. While not regarded as a replacement for conventional treatments, the most recent reviews of the published research on bibliotherapy concluded it could successfully treat depression, mild alcohol abuse, and anxiety disorders (Norcross et al., 2008), but was less effective with smoking addiction and severe alcohol abuse (Floyd et al., 2003). Research suggests bibliotherapy is most effective when used in conjunction with conventional therapy or while waiting for conventional therapy to begin (*see* Bernstein & Koppel, 2008).

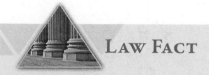

LAW FACT

COVERAGE FOR ACUTE MENTAL HEALTH TREATMENT

Following a pre-certification approval, can an insurer retrospectively deny coverage for ensuing treatment of a severe mental illness, when the patient is completely dysfunctional and suicidal?

No, insured persons are entitled to the assurance of timely notification concerning approval and reimbursement; reviewing agents and mental health care providers are required to make timely decisions, thereby giving the insured the security of focusing on their true task: rehabilitation.

—*Merit Behavioral Care Corp. v. State Independent Panel of Mental Health Providers,* 845 A.2d 359 (Supreme Court of Vermont 2004.

CHAPTER SUMMARY

- Mental illness is the leading disease burden on the U.S., with forty-four million sufferers, but it receives very little public attention.
- A healthy psyche is indicated by engaging in productive activities, fulfilling relationships with other people, and an ability to adapt to change and cope with adversity.
- Mental disorders are characterized by alterations in thinking, mood, or behavior, distress, and impaired mental functioning.
- Mental disorders are legitimate illnesses that respond to specific treatments, just as other physical health conditions respond to medical treatment.
- About 6 percent of Americans suffer from severe mental illness, meaning the sufferers risk harming themselves or others.
- There is a particularly high incidence of mental health disorders among the homeless, the incarcerated, college-age adults, and returning combat veterans.
- State laws written to protect mental health providers from liability can be broadly read as also imposing an affirmative duty to refrain from negligence in the treatment and discharge of mentally ill patients.
- The intellectually disabled are a subset of people with mental disorders; they are characterized by sub-average intellectual functioning and significant limitations in the ability to care for themselves.
- Involuntary commitments require future dangerousness coupled with a mental illness as the basis for the imposition of commitment and mental health treatment.
- Absent public safety concerns or the need for mental health treatment, involuntary commitment is not permitted for a mental illness alone.
- When mentally ill persons are released from an involuntary commitment, various conditions may be imposed upon their release and they may be recommitted for violating such conditions.
- Although patient advocates may play a critical role in overseeing the treatment of the mentally ill, some argue that the rights of the mentally ill to refuse treatment should not take precedence over the patient's or others' safety.
- Mental health care workers are subject to a higher standard of care than police officers or prison guards when using force to maintain or restore order.
- One subset of mental disorders currently receiving much public attention is sexual disorders, particularly because they result in pedophilia and fuel widespread human trafficking for sexual exploitation purposes.
- Bibliotherapy is slowly gaining credibility from evidence-based research showing some self-help books can actually improve mental health for those with mild to moderate disorders.

LAW NOTES

1. Established by the Omnibus Crime Control and Safe Streets Act, the federal Law Enforcement Assistance Administration (LEAA), within the U.S. Department of Justice, administered federal funding to state and local governments, and funded state and local planning agencies to oversee the nation's criminal justice

system (*see* 5 U.S.C.A. § 7313 (1968); 18 U.S.C.A. §§ 921 *et seq.* (2009)). Structured like the Medicaid insurance system's Federal Medical Assistance Percentages (FMAP), the federal share of LEAA spending was determined by the amount of federal matching funds for states. When the agency was abolished in 1982, many local crime initiatives were shut down and the nation's reform of its criminal justice system came to a virtual halt but for private funding schemes. As society matures into acceptance of the philosophical justification of distributive justice and more fully understands the economic impact of LEAA-type programs, agencies like LEAA will again return to meet the needs of the most disadvantaged (*see* Brink, 2005). For almost fourteen years, LEAA led prisoner reform efforts in the U.S. and the rest of the world noted the nation's reputation for fairness and respected its criminal correctional system (Santarelli, 2007).

2. Civil commitments regard future dangerousness when coupled with a mental illness as a legitimate basis for the imposition of involuntary commitment and treatment for violent offenders (Pfeffer, 2008). *See, e.g., Kansas v. Crane*, 534 U.S. 407 (U.S. Supreme Court 2002) (requiring proof of a serious difficulty in controlling behavior in order to involuntarily commit a sexual offender); *Kansas v. Hendricks,* 521 U.S. 346, 358 (U.S. Supreme Court 1997) (finding of dangerousness alone is ordinarily not a sufficient ground upon which to justify indefinite involuntary commitment; civil commitment laws may be sustained when proof of dangerousness is coupled with proof of some additional factor, such as a mental illness or mental abnormality); *Heller v. Doe,* 509 U.S. 312, 314-15 (U.S. Supreme Court 1993) (sustaining Kentucky law permitting commitment of mentally ill and dangerous individual); *Allen v. Illinois,* 478 U.S. 364, 366 (U.S. Supreme Court 1986) (sustaining Illinois law permitting commitment of mentally ill and sexually dangerous individual); *Minnesota ex rel. Pearson v. Probate Court of Ramsey County*, 309 U.S. 270, 271-72, (U.S. Supreme Court 1940) (sustaining Minnesota law permitting commitment of dangerous individual with psychopathic personality).

3. Keep in mind that a non-mentally ill person's parole would likely be revoked (meaning they would return to jail) for making threats such as these; a general condition of parole is that it will be revoked if the parolee breaks the law. Also, parole conditions not related to the original crime may be imposed, such as that the parolee obtain their GED or secure stable housing.

4. *Choke*, a 2008 Sundance movie, is about Victor Mancini, a sex-addicted medical school dropout who devises a complicated scam to pay for elder care for his Alzheimer's-afflicted mother in an expensive private hospital by pretending to choke on food while dining in upscale restaurants. Victor then allows himself to be saved by wealthy patrons, who, feeling parasitically responsible for his life, go on to send checks to support him and his mother. When Victor is not pulling his choking stunt, he cruises sex addiction recovery workshops for sexual partners (Beck, 2008).

CHAPTER BIBLIOGRAPHY

Amar, J., & Strumolo, A. R. (2007). Medical decision on behalf of incompetent patients: Federal court upholds law allowing medical decisions for incompetent patients: *Doe ex rel Tarlow v. District of Columbia. American Journal of Law & Medicine, 33,* 703-708.

Anderson, L. et al (2005). Self-help books for depression: How can practitioners and patients make the right choice? *British Journal of General Practice, 55* (514), 387-392.

Baldisseri, M. R. (2007). Impaired healthcare professional. *Critical Care Medicine, 35,* S106-S116.

Barth, A. S. (2007). A double-edged sword: The role of neuroimaging in federal capital sentencing. *American Journal of Law & Medicine, 33,* 501-522.

Beck, M. (2008, September 30). Is sex addiction a sickness, or excuse to behave badly? *Wall Street Journal,* p. D1.

Bernstein, E. (2008, October 16). How new law boosts coverage of mental care. *Wall Street Journal,* p. A1.

Bernstein, E., & Koppel, N. (2008, August 16). Death in the family, aided by advocates for the mentally ill, William Bruce left the hospital only to kill his mother. *Wall Street Journal,* p. A1.

____. (2007, April 27). Delicate balance, colleges' culture of privacy often overshadows safety, laws allow disclosure of troubling behavior but many schools resist. *Wall Street Journal,* p. A1.

Bertagna, B. R. (2008). The Internet: Disability or distraction? An analysis of whether internet addiction can qualify as a disability under the Americans with Disabilities Act. *Hofstra Labor & Employment Law Journal, 25,* 419-481.

BJS (Bureau of Justice Statistics). (2008). *Correctional surveys (the National Prisoner Statistics Program, Annual Survey of Jails, Annual Probation Survey, and Annual Parole Survey).* Washington, DC: U.S. Department of Justice, BJS.

Blanco, C. et al. (2008). Mental health of college students and their non-college-attending peers: Results from the national epidemiologic study on alcohol and related conditions. *Archives of General Psychiatry, 65* (12), 1429-1437 (surveying more than five thousand nineteen- to twenty-five-year-old young adults) .

Braddock, D. L. (2008). *State of the states in developmental disabilities.* Washington, DC: American Association on Intellectual & Developmental Disabilities.

Brink, J. (2005). Epidemiology of mental illness in a correctional system. *Current Opinion in Psychiatry, 18* (5), 536-541 (establishing that the prevalence of psychiatric illness in correctional settings is significantly elevated).

Burnam, N. A. et al. (2009). *Improving mental health care for returning veterans.* Santa Monica, CA: RAND Center for Health Policy Research.

CBO (Congressional Budget Office). (2008). *H.R. 1424, Paul Wellstone Mental Health and Addiction Equity Act of 2008.* Washington, DC: CBO.

Center, C. et al. (2003). Confronting depression and suicide in physicians: A consensus statement. *Journal of the American Medical Association, 289,* 3161-3166 (concluding that the culture of medicine does not give a high priority to physician mental health, noting the barriers to treatment).

Charles, J. M. (2009). "America's lost cause": The unconstitutionality of criminalizing our country's homeless population. *Boston University Public Interest Law Journal, 18,* 315-348.

DSM-IV (Diagnostic and Statistical Manual of Mental Disorders). (2000). *American Psychiatric Association: Diagnostic and statistical manual of mental disorders.* (4th ed.). Arlington, VA: American Psychiatric Publishing, Inc.

Edwards, W., & Luckasson, R. A. (2002). *Mental retardation: Definition, classification, and systems of supports.* Washington, DC: American Association on Intellectual & Developmental Disabilities.

Erickson, S. K. (2998). The myth of mental disorder: Trans-substantive behavior and taxometric psychiatry. *Akron Law Review, 41,* 67-121.

Fazel, S. (2008). Mental disorders among adolescents in juvenile detention and correctional facilities: A systematic review and metaregression analysis of 25 surveys. *Journal of the American Academy of Child & Adolescent Psychiatry, 47* (9), 1010-1019.

Floyd, M. et al. (2006). Two-year follow-up of bibliotherapy and individual cognitive therapy for depressed older adults. *Behavior Modification, 30* (3), 281-294.

___. (2003). Bibliotherapy as an adjunct to psychotherapy for depression in older adults. *Journal of Clinical Psychology, 59* (2), 187-195.

Friedman, R, A. (2006). Uncovering an epidemic, screening for mental illness in teens. *New England Journal of Medicine, 355* (26), 2717-2719.

Gostin, L. O., & Gable, L. (2004). The human rights of people with mental disabilities: A global perspective on the application of human rights principles to mental health. *Maryland Law Review, 63,* 20-121.

Grant, B. F. (2008). Sociodemographic and psychopathologic predictors of first incidence of DSM-IV substance use, mood, and anxiety disorders: Results from the Wave 2 National Epidemiologic Survey on Alcohol and Related Conditions. *Molecular Psychiatry, 10,* 1038-1079.

Greenberg, G. A., & Rosenheck, R. A. (2008). Jail incarceration, homelessness, and mental health: A national study. *Psychiatry Services, 59* (2), 170-177.

Hampton, T. (2005). Experts address risk of physician suicide. *Journal of the American Medical Association, 294* (10), 1189-1191 (discussing prevention of physician suicide and barriers to prevention).

Helliker, K. (2007, July 31). Bibliotherapy: Reading your way to mental health. *Wall Street Journal,* p. D1.

Horvitz-Lennon, M. et al. (2006). From silos to bridges: Meeting the general health care needs of adults with severe mental illnesses. *Health Affairs, 25* (3), 659-669.

House Report No. 110-374 (2007). Paul Wellstone Mental Health & Addiction Equity Act of 2007. U.S. House Committee on Education & Labor. Washington, DC: U.S. House of Representatives.

HUD (U. S. Department of Housing & Urban Development). (2007). *The annual homeless assessment report to Congress.* Washington, DC: HUD.

Kaine, T. M. (2007). Review Panel to Governor Kaine of the Commonwealth of Virginia. (2007). *Mass shootings at Virginia Tech.* Richmond, VA.

Levit, K. R. et al. (2008). Future funding for mental health and substance abuse: Increasing burdens for the public sector. *Health Affairs, 27* (6), 513-522.

Martin, K. R. (2007). Third Circuit holds federal agency liable for deaths mentally-ill patient caused after negligent discharge from treatment program: *DeJesus v. United States Department of Veterans Affairs. American Journal of Law & Medicine, 33,* 527-530.

Mavrofour, A. et al. (2006). Alcohol and drug abuse among physicians: A review of the literature. *Journal of Medicine, 25* (4), 611-625 (indicating higher incidence among anesthesiologists, possibly because of easier access to certain drugs; discussing factors that may relate to drug and alcohol abuse).

McCurran, K. (2008). Mental health screening in schools: An analysis of recent legislative developments and the legal implications for parents, children and the state. *Quinnipiac Health Law Journal, 11,* 87-143.

McNeil, D. E. et al. (2005). Incarceration associated with homelessness, mental disorder, and co-occurring substance abuse. *Psychiatry Services, 56,* 840-846.

Mitchell, J. (2007). Sex, lies, and spyware: Balancing the right to privacy against the right to know in the marital relationship. *Journal of Law & Family Studies, 9,* 171-188.

Monahan, G. (2003). Drug use/misuse among health professionals. *Substance Use & Misuse, 38,* 1877-1881.

NAMH (National Alliance on Mental Illness). (2006). *Grading the states: A report on America's health care system for severe mental illness.* Arlington, VA: NAMH.

NCH (National Coalition for the Homeless). (2008). *Why are people homeless?* Washington, DC: NCH.

Norcross, J. C. et al. (2008). *Clinician's guide to evidence based practices: Mental health and the addictions.* New York, NY: Oxford University Press.

___. (2003). *Authoritative guide to self-help resources in mental health (the clinician's toolbox).* New York, NY: Guilford Press.

O'Brien, J. C. (2008). Loose standards, tight lips: Why easy access to client data can undermine homeless management information systems. *Fordham Urban Law Journal, 35,* 673-699.

Pew Center on the States. (2008, February 8). *One in 100: Behind bars in America 2008.* Washington, DC: Pew.

Pfeffer, A. (2008, September). "Imminent danger" and inconsistency: The need for national reform of the "imminent danger" standard for involuntary civil commitment in the wake of the Virginia Tech tragedy. *Cardozo Law Review, 30,* 277-312.

Ruan, W. J. et al. (2008). The Alcohol Use Disorder and Associated Disabilities Interview Schedule-IV (AUDADIS-IV): Reliability of new psychiatric diagnostic modules and risk factors in a general population sample. *Drug & Alcohol Dependence, 92,* 27-36.

Santarelli, D. E., chairman, National Committee on Community Corrections & president, Center for Community Corrections. (2007, October 30). International Community

Corrections Association 15th Annual Research Conference, San Diego, CA.

Stein, M. A., & Stein, P. J. S. (2007). Beyond disability civil rights. *Hastings Law Journal, 58*, 1203-1240.

Talbott, J. A. (2004). Deinstitutionalization: Avoiding the disasters of the past. *Psychiatric Services, 55*, 1112-1115.

Talley, K. O. (2009). Independent protection and advocacy: The role of counsel in institutional settings. *New York Law School Law Review, 53,* 55-76.

Tanielian, T., & Jaycox, L. H. (2008*). Invisible wounds of war: Psychological and cognitive injuries, their consequences, and services to assist recovery*. Santa Monica, CA: RAND Center for Health Policy Research (comprehensive study of the post-deployment mental-health-related needs associated with Iraq and Afghanistan veterans, the health care system in place to meet those needs, gaps in the care system, and the costs associated with these conditions and with providing quality health care to all those in need).

Tovino, S. A. (2009). Neuroscience and health law: An integrative approach? *Akron Law Review, 42*, 469-517.

U.S. Department of State. (2007). *Trafficking in persons report*. Washington, DC: U.S. Department of State.

U.S. Surgeon General. (1999). *Mental health: A report of the Surgeon General*. Rockville, MD: U.S. Department of Health & Human Services, Office of the Surgeon General.

Walmsley, R. (2009). *World prison population list* (8th ed.). London, England: King's College, International Centre for Prison Studies.

Weithorn, V. L. (2008). Conceptual hurdles to the application of *Atkins v. Virginia. Hastings Law Journal, 59*, 1203-1234.

White, B. (2007). Student rights: From in loco parentis to sine parentibus and back again? Understanding the Family Educational Rights and Privacy Act in higher education. *Brigham Young University Education & Law Journal, 2007*, 321-350.

WHO (World Health Organization). (2008). *The global burden of disease*. Geneva, Switzerland: WHO.

Yen, I. (2008). Of vice and men: A new approach to eradicating sex trafficking by reducing male demand through educational programs and abolitionist legislation. *Journal of Criminal Law & Criminology, 98*, 653-686.

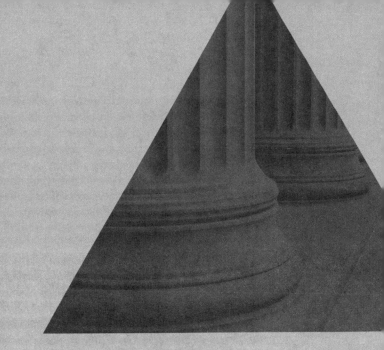

PART X

END-OF-LIFE HEALTH CARE

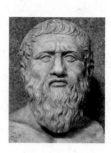

> *"Now death is not the worst that can happen to men . . ."*
>
> —PLATO (B.C.), GREEK PHILOSOPHER

IN BRIEF

Hospice occupies a specialized and growing niche in the health care economy. With more than two out of every five of the nation's deaths occurring in Medicare-certified hospice programs, it has been demonstrated that hospice care improves quality of life for patients and families. Hospice is that rare situation in the U.S. health care system through which quality of life is improved while costs may be reduced.

This chapter focuses first and foremost on hospice care as it relates to the elderly. Many children and young adults, however, also qualify for hospice care, including accident victims and those who have Acquired Immune Deficiency Syndrome (AIDS), fatal birth defects, muscular degeneration, spinal cord injuries, and strokes. Perinatal hospice is also available for families where the fetus has a lethal condition.

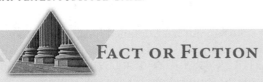

FACT OR FICTION

ACCEPTANCE OF PATIENTS INTO HOSPICE CARE

Should hospices face litigation from family members disappointed with a valid state court order mandating a patient's transfer to their care?

Terri Schiavo, age twenty-seven, suffered cardiac arrest as a result of a potassium imbalance brought about by the eating disorder of bulimia. Her husband, Michael Schiavo, called 911, and Terri was immediately rushed to a hospital, but she never regained consciousness. For ten years, Terri lived in nursing homes with constant care, where she was fed and hydrated by tubes. She had numerous health problems, but none were life-threatening. The evidence was overwhelming that Terri was in a permanent or persistent vegetative state (PVS).

   After ten years of futile health care, Michael sought judicial authorization to terminate Terri's life-prolonging procedures and permit her entry into hospice. Following a five-day trial, the trial court ordered that Terri's artificial nutrition and hydration be removed and that she be transferred to a hospice where her natural death process could take its course. Years of litigation followed Terri's transfer to hospice care, beginning in the Florida state courts and ending in the Eleventh Circuit U.S. Court of Appeals five years later. All the while, Terri's artificial nutrition and hydration were maintained in a hospice.

—In re Guardianship of Schiavo, 780 So.2d 176 (District Court of Appeal of Florida, Second District 2001), *Supreme Court of Florida review denied*, 789 So.2d 348 (Supreme Court of Florida 2001). (See *Law Fact* at the end of this chapter for the answer.)

PRINCIPLES AND APPLICATIONS

The pattern of life and death has shifted dramatically in the last century in developed economies and for the billion people in the top 15 percent of the economic pyramid. The average life span of Americans has nearly doubled, from just forty-nine years in 1900 to nearly eighty years today. Lifetimes have increased by about three months every year since the mid-nineteenth century as a direct result of improved health care (RAND, 2004). At the same time, the pattern of life and death in developing economies and for people in the bottom 85 percent of the economic pyramid (the remaining 5.8 billion people in the world) is what it was in North America and Western Europe in the mid-seventeenth century (Prahalad, 2006). For most of the world's population, health care has not improved in the last century; half the people in the world die of acute causes by the age of twenty from severe diseases that quickly result in death. The leading diseases that cause death in developing economies are perinatal conditions (including birth asphyxia, birth trauma, and low birth weight), lower respiratory infections, diarrheal diseases commingled with undernourishment, HIV/AIDS, malaria, and tuberculosis (Lopez et al., 2006).

DEMOGRAPHICS OF LIFE AND DEATH

While people at the top of the economic pyramid live longer, healthier lives, most of them will spend their last few years living with disabilities or chronic illnesses. Relatively few Americans die of acute causes or accidents anymore. Instead, most Americans die from lingering and often complex or combined illnesses that eventually prove fatal. Dementia and frailty shape the last years of life for a large part of the population in developed economies (RAND, 2004). By 2030, the baby-boom generation of the 1950s born after World War II will begin to turn eighty-five, an age when most people are showing evidence of frailty. In 2000, approximately four million Americans were eighty-five or older. In 2030, this number is projected to be over nine million (NHPCO, 2007; NHO, 2006).

OVERVIEW OF HOSPICE CARE

Hospice is not a place; rather, it is a philosophy of palliative care that provides pain management, symptom control, psychosocial support, and spiritual care to patients and their families (NHPCO, 2007). In most cases, hospice is provided in the patient's home, but care can also be given in freestanding centers, hospitals, nursing homes, and other long-term care facilities. With roughly one in three older Americans using hospice services to cope with the dying process, hospice has evolved from a purely nonprofit mission into a growing health care business (Wharton, 2006). Four out of six hospice patients are sixty-five years of age or older, and one-third are eighty-five years of age or older. As the baby-boom generation of some seventy-six million (the largest population cohort in U.S. history) ages, the number of persons aged sixty-five and older is thus expected to grow (NHPCO, 2007).

The death-with-dignity movement and its accompanying hospice philosophy started in England and came to the U.S. in the early 1970s.[LN1] The movement did not gain widespread recognition until Medicare began to pay for hospice services and the Joint Commission on Accreditation of Healthcare Organizations (JCAHO) initiated hospice accreditation criteria. While JCAHO is not an official governmental regulatory agency, it is instrumental in developing and maintaining standards of quality in hospice care, and accreditation is an indication that a hospice program maintains a certain standard of care. Today, the National Hospice and Palliative Care Organization (NHPCO) reports that more than 1.3 million Americans received hospice care in 2006. This represents a steady increase of about 100,000 new patients using hospice in each of the past several years, a growing trend that is expected to continue as an aging generation of baby-boomers faces end-of-life situations for themselves (Taylor, 2007).[LN2]

A handful of publicly held companies provide hospice care along with hundreds of smaller private companies and well-established nonprofit ventures. Medicare currently funds more than three-quarters of the cost of hospice care.

From the late 1980s to the mid-1990s, hospital managers believed the health care industry's future would expand to include offering integrated services to patients. They began buying physician practices and other health service organizations, including hospices, thereby spurring interest in the hospice business. For-profit programs now provide care for 35 percent of hospice patients. Nonprofit groups provide care for 56 percent, while government and other types of organizations help the remaining 9 percent (Wharton, 2006).

STATE LICENSING REGULATIONS

Under current state laws, most hospice facilities must be licensed as hospitals, nursing facilities, assisted living facilities, or in-home services agencies. While most states do not have detailed hospice licensing regulations, several states apply the federal regulations (42 C.F.R. §§ 418.1-418.405 (2009)) for certification of hospices: Connecticut, Delaware, Hawaii, Idaho, Kansas, Louisiana, Maryland, Massachusetts, Montana, New Hampshire, New Jersey, New Mexico, New York, North Dakota, Oregon, South Carolina, Texas, Vermont, Virginia, Washington, and West Virginia.

Some have raised concern about the relevance of assisted living facility and in-home services regulations to hospices. To address this concern, states are developing new regulations specific to hospice facilities that are not inpatient facilities and are currently licensed as assisted living facilities or in-home services agencies.[LN3] For instance, regulations for nutrition services, treatments for infections, and plans of care are particularly unique to hospice care.

Nutrition Services

Artificial nutrition and hydration through intravenous administration or by putting a tube in the stomach is available for patients who are very sick and receiving curative treatments or recovering from surgery. However, the service is rarely used for hospice patients whose bodies are beginning to stop functioning and instead require comfort treatments.

When hospice patients with a serious, life-limiting illness are no longer able to eat or drink, it usually means that their bodies are beginning to stop functioning. Artificial nutrition and hydration will not bring them back to a healthy state. Most physicians agree that artificial nutrition and hydration can increase suffering in hospice patients who are dying and no longer have the ability or interest to eat food and drink liquids themselves. Artificial nutrition and hydration can add more discomfort to a dying patient's physical symptoms such as: bloating, swelling, cramps, diarrhea, and shortness of breath. It is important to remember that the body is beginning to shut down because of disease and the dying process, not because of the absence of foods and liquids. There are ways to ensure comfort at the end of life; hospice and palliative care professionals are experts in providing comfort treatments (Caring Connections & NHPCO, 2005).

Treatments for Infections

Treatable infections are generally treated for patients who are also receiving other curative treatments. With hospice patients at the very end-stage active phase of dying, where treatment for an infection would not be effective, treatment may be declined by a patient or health care representative.

Plans of Care

Hospice regulations provide for interdisciplinary teams to develop and monitor plans of care for hospice patients, including a:

- Doctor of medicine or osteopathy
- Pastoral or other counselor
- Registered nurse
- Social worker

By regulation, plans of care must be reviewed and updated at specified intervals; hospice teams usually meet for one or two hours, two to four times a month to review patients' care, status, and needs.

HOSPICE'S FINANCING STRUCTURE

Payment for hospice treatment can lead to legal concerns. Questions about the availability of Medicare benefits can pose additional legal questions, as can eligibility under Medicaid and private health care plans. Medicaid helps terminally ill patients under age sixty-five who meet low-income criteria and cannot afford health care to cover some or all of their medical expenses.[LN4] Increasingly, this group includes patients with inadequate health care plans and the uninsured.

Medicare initiated the hospice benefit in response to families who wanted a way to cover the expenses of caring for patients who chose to die at home (Wharton, 2006). Since then, three out of every four hospice patients die in a private residence, nursing home, or other residential facility versus acute-care hospital settings; this exceeds the rate seen in the general population, about half of whom die in hospitals (Werth, 2007).

Another measure of the increased acceptance of hospice as a viable treatment option is the fact that many third-party payers (Medicare, Medicaid, and most private insurance and managed care plans) extend coverage for hospice care. The Medicare hospice benefit, however, is the dominant source of payment to hospice providers and is very different from other health care reimbursement programs.

Medicare's Six-Month Restriction

Some barriers to hospice referral arise from Medicare's hospice eligibility requirements, which is an instance of statutory provisions driven by budgetary scorekeeping. Congress, concerned that large numbers might choose the Medicare hospice benefit as an alternative to home care, added the six-months-to-live requirement to address this cost concern.

These barriers will be difficult to eliminate without major changes to hospice organization and financing (Casarett & Quill, 2007). To enter hospice, a patient's physician must certify that they believe their patient could die if the illness runs its normal course (Byock et al., 2001). The Medicare hospice benefit is available only to patients who:

- Are eligible for insurance coverage under Medicare Part A
- Have been certified by their physicians that their expected mortality is less than six months
- Understand the nature and purpose of palliative care
- Agree that by selecting hospice, they waive their right to certain other Medicare services

(CMS, 2005; Medicare and Medicaid programs: Hospice conditions of participation, 70 *Federal Register* 30,840 (2005, May 27); 42 C.F.R. § 418 (2009))

Hospice care was at first controversial because of the waiver requiring patients and their physicians to forgo further efforts at finding a cure (Rutkow, 2005). Medicare legislation clearly structured hospice as an alternative to conventional care. For example, regulations require explicit and careful consent from patients, acknowledging that they are giving up curative treatment (Lynn, 2004). The hospice philosophy, however, neither hastens nor postpones death (NHO, 2006).

Medicare's Per Diem Reimbursement Schedules

The Medicare Benefit Policy Manual explains Medicare's reimbursement schedules. Most hospice payments are based on an all-inclusive per diem rate, except for physician services, which are mostly paid for in the conventional manner.[LN5] When hospices were first established, Medicare covered virtually every service required, with the possible exception of long-term assistance by an aide. Today, the Medicare hospice benefit is paid at one of four rates for custodial care:

- Continuous attendance at home
- Inpatient respite care and general inpatient care
- Inpatient symptom management care
- Routine home care

For qualified patients, hospice benefits include:

- Durable medical equipment and supplies
- Home health aide and homemaker services
- Nursing care
- Nutrition and dietary counseling
- Physical therapy, occupational therapy, and speech/language pathology services
- Physician services (if that physician is part of the hospice team)
- Prescription drugs related to the terminal illness
- Short respite care in an inpatient facility
- Social services, including bereavement counseling

Additional covered hospice services are defined as any other item or service covered by Medicare, which is indicated as necessary for the treatment of the terminal illness or related conditions.

Medicare Part A will reimburse a hospice for two ninety-day periods and then repeated sixty-day periods during a patient's lifetime. Hospice coverage is unlimited so long as the patient remains eligible; meaning that the expected prognosis of the patient's medical condition if it took its standard course would be a mortality of less than six months. Services must be provided through an interdisciplinary team that assesses the needs of each patient and the patient's family and then develops and implements an appropriate care plan (*see generally* CMS, 2007).

Medicaid Restrictions

In recognition of the fact that Medicaid insures the poorest Americans, Medicaid protects hospice patients from the out-of-pocket costs typically imposed by private health plans. While Medicare has always imposed substantial premiums, deductibles, and co-payments, Medicaid prohibits states from imposing any enrollment fees or cost-sharing on Medicaid recipients for hospice services (*see* 42 U.S.C.A. § 1396o (2006); 42 C.F.R. § 447.53 (1986)). States are specifically prohibited from imposing enrollment fees for hospice services (*see* 42 U.S.C.A. § 1396o(a)(1) (2006)).

GROWTH INDUSTRY

Since the first program opened in 1974, approximately 4,500 hospice programs are now operating in the U.S. Medicare reimbursement for hospice care has grown from around $68 million in 1986 to almost $10 billion in 2006, with spending projected to increase by slightly over 9 percent by 2012 (NHPCO, 2007).

By 2030, as baby-boomers enter their eighties and beyond, hospice spending is expected to climb to almost $46 billion, according to data supplied by the Centers for Medicare & Medicaid Services (CMS, 2008), which administers hospice benefits within the Medicare program. In addition to the aging of the population, there is room for hospice programs to grow to accommodate medical conditions beyond cancer, traditionally the illness that has been most often associated with hospice care (Wharton, 2006). Hospice is increasingly caring for patients in the final stages of chronic diseases (NHPCO, 2007), such as:

- Acquired Immune Deficiency Syndrome (AIDS)
- Amyotrophic lateral sclerosis (ALS), often referred to as Lou Gehrig's disease
- Alzheimer's disease
- Diabetes
- Emphysema

- Heart disease and strokes
- Neuromuscular, kidney, and liver disease
- Other life-limiting conditions

Growth is also likely to occur by geographic region. In ten states, including Arizona, Texas, and Florida, more than 40 percent of deaths occurring in the population over age sixty-five were under hospice care. By contrast, in thirteen states, including Massachusetts, New York, and also Washington, D.C., hospice deaths occur in only 20 percent of the same population group (Connor, 2007).

While hospice care is gaining acceptance, its growth remains hampered by physicians who are reluctant to recommend it. Physicians are trained to do all they can to prolong life. There is a fundamental, almost philosophical, conflict between the way physicians are trained and the goals of hospice (Wharton, 2006). A physician must concede that a patient's illness is terminal and that the patient will not recover before the patient can enter into hospice care. Many physicians find that difficult to do (CMS, 2005). One might question whether it is time to change medical education of U.S. physicians regarding end-of-life care.

While advocates for hospice argue it is primarily a compassionate way to make it easier for people to die quietly at home, some research indicates the service can also reduce costs for Medicare (Wharton, 2006). The routine Medicare hospice benefit costs are in the range of $125 per day, compared to daily inpatient payments of more than $3,000 (CMS, 2007).

Moral Dilemmas

1. Does the large number of patients with terminal prognoses, such as cancer or multi-organ system failure, dying in intensive care settings as opposed to hospice care indicate that there is a systemic failure in meeting patients' needs and expectations?

2. Considering medical technology's ability to prolong near-death life longer and longer, should economic reasoning ever be used to stop treatment?

3. Should the compassionate administration of life-shortening analgesia in hospices be unlawful?

CONFLICTING PERSPECTIVES

The largest portion of hospital expenses is incurred during the last few weeks of a patient's life. One could argue that if it were possible to make relatively accurate judgments about when an illness is terminal, and if legitimate hospice services can be provided to the patient, cost savings would result. If a patient is terminally ill, why spend money to prolong life for one week or three weeks (Wharton, 2006)? Why spend money on increasingly desperate attempts at curative treatment? While this arguably does not appear to be money well spent, some patients and their families want to do everything possible to prolong life. So there is a potential conflict on the surface of hospice between cost-containment and potential legal disputes with the family. There is no conflict, however, if patients and their families want to pay for medically futile care for patients with terminal prognosis and there is no expectation that insurers, including Medicare, will pay for ineffective health care. The problem with all this is that there is no legal or ethical consensus as to what futile health care means.

Nevertheless, hospice patients are distinctly less likely to have surgery, hospitalization, resuscitation, or other technological interventions, although these services are not explicitly precluded by Medicare regulations (CMS, 2008). Perhaps, the growing interest in hospice care versus high-technology curative care for an additional few weeks of living with a terminal illness may demonstrate a growing recognition in the U.S. that death is part of life and should not be resisted at every turn (Poblenz & Richard, 2006).

Informed Consent

Hospice care brings various legal issues to the forefront. From a health law perspective, informed consent for hospice treatment is one of the most important concerns. If the patient is competent, or has signed an advance directive and/or a power of attorney giving someone else the authority to make their medical decisions, the patient's wishes should be determined prior to admission to hospice care (Casarett & Quill, 2007).

Hospices that are Medicare and Medicaid providers are required to give patients, at the time of their enrollment, information about their rights under state laws, including their rights to:

- Direct their own health care decisions
- Accept or refuse treatment
- Prepare an advance directive
- Get information on the hospice's policies that govern rights

(42 U.S.C.A. §§ 1395cc (2008))

While the law of informed consent favors a patient's right of preference, the potential for serious legal issues arises when patients are not legally competent and have no advance directive. Every hospice

struggles with what to do with patients who, at the time of potential entry to hospice, lack the capacity to make end-of-life medical decisions.

Legal Competency

The question of when a patient is determined to be competent to make end-of-life decisions is very different from competency in general. Legal competency is often defined as the ability to make clear and definite decisions (Black's, 2009). In this instance, it is the ability to choose and make up one's mind about stopping curative treatments for a terminal illness without too much wavering, after considering the other possible choices of palliative care and entry to hospice.

While mature minors have been determined to be competent and mature enough to make their own medical decisions, the American Academy of Pediatrics maintains the criteria should be the same for determining whether a child is competent to accept entry to hospice (AAP, 2000). Most likely this will be a court determination if the parents disagree with the child's decision about hospice care.

Best Interests Standard

When making decisions about entry to hospice for those adults who lack decision-making capacity and have no discernable preferences, the "best interests" standard is generally used (Kopelman, 2007). The same standard for entry into hospice care is recommended for minors by the American Academy of Pediatrics (AAP, 2000).

This standard means the best available care will be administered to the patient. This care is not necessarily for the purpose of extending biological life for the longest time, but to offer comfort and pain control (Lynn, 2007; Faull et al., 2005; Doyle et al., 2005; NHO, 1993).

Legal problems arise with hospice patients who are in a PVS; they also arise where patients suffer from various forms of dementia, in cases of severe mental illness, and in situations where curative treatment itself interferes with mental capacity. Each state has had to resolve what to do in such situations; there is no overriding federal legislation. The result has been an array of state statutes and regulations dictating how hospice decisions are to be made, and how the wishes of patients are to be determined in such uncertain situations.[LN6]

Moral Dilemmas

1. Does inappropriate use of curative treatment deprive patients of their fundamental right to dignity and humane treatment?

One Hospice's Debacle

This chapter opened with the Terri Schiavo case to illustrate what hospices face when they accept patients who cannot make their own end-of-life decisions (Greene, 2005). This case was one of the most bitter and protracted civil actions regarding end-of-life medical treatment ever in U.S. jurisprudence, with hospice care at the center of the debate (Caplan et al., 2006). There was a disagreement within the family that presented legal difficulties resulting in a legal challenge to hospice care (Hook & Mueller, 2005).

Basically, the debate centered on the right to die in accordance with the true wishes of a patient on life support. Family members simply disagreed about what the wishes of the patient were and had differing levels of understanding relative to the medical condition and prognosis of someone in a PVS. Consequently, one side was not allowed to make a decision to disconnect her life support, while the other side was not allowed to make a decision to maintain her life support.

This family dispute could have been avoided if an advance directive (popularly known as a living will) and a health care proxy had been in place. As it turned out, after Schiavo's cardiac arrest stopped her heart and killed her brain in 1990 (Solloway et al., 2005), she received artificial nutrition and hydration for fifteen years before she died. The following federal decision from the Eleventh Circuit U.S. Court of Appeals finally resolved this controversy.

DISCONTINUANCE OF LIFE SUPPORT

Schiavo ex rel. Schindler v. Schiavo

[Parents of Daughter v. Hospice and Husband (Son-in-Law)]

403 F.3d 1289 (U.S. Court of Appeals for the 11th Circuit 2005),
rehearing denied, 404 F.3d 1282 (U.S. Court of Appeals for the 11th Circuit 2005)

FACTS: This is the highly publicized court battle between Terri Schiavo's parents and Michael Schiavo, her husband and legal guardian, regarding the removal of life-prolonging procedures. Terri was a PVS patient in a hospice in Florida and her parents were seeking an injunction to require that she be transported to a hospital for restoration of nutrition and hydration and for medical treatment.

In a PVS, Terri Schiavo was not in a coma; she had cycles of apparent wakefulness and apparent sleep without any cognition or awareness. As she breathed, she often moaned; her hands, elbows, knees, and feet were severely contracted. Over the span of ten years, her brain deteriorated from the lack of oxygen it suffered at the time of her heart attack. By mid-1996, CAT scans of her brain showed that most of her cerebral cortex was gone and had been replaced by cerebral spinal fluid (*see* Caring Connection & NHPCO, 2005).

ISSUES: Do hospices violate the Americans with Disabilities Act (ADA) and the Rehabilitation Act when they withhold artificial nutrition and hydration from PVS patients (*see* Rehabilitation Act of 1973, 29 U.S.C.A. § 701 (1998) (protects the right of the disabled to be free from discrimination); Americans with Disabilities Act of 1990,

42 U.S.C.A. § 12101 *et seq.* (2009) and 47 U.S.C.A. § 225 (1996) (provides additional protections to the disabled))? Must an incapacitated patient's wishes be proven by clear and convincing evidence prior to hospice care in order to comport with the Due Process Clause? Does hospice care constitute cruel and unusual punishment under the Eighth Amendment?

HOLDING AND DECISION: No. The Eleventh Circuit rejected all claims, based on statutory and constitutional arguments, holding that denial of a temporary restraining order was proper where the parents of a severely brain damaged patient sought to restore life support that had been removed in compliance with a state court order following eight years of litigation.

ANALYSIS: The court addressed each of the five counts of the parents' complaint.

The first claim alleged that Michael Schiavo and the hospice were acting in violation of the ADA. The court found that Michael was neither a public entity nor a public accommodation, nor was he acting under color of state law, as required for a claim under the ADA to proceed. Turning to the claim against the hospice, the court noted that

(continues)

(continued)

if the hospice was a place of public accommodation, the withholding of nutrition and hydration was not done on the basis of Terri's disability, but in compliance with a valid court order. The court further observed that the ADA was never intended to provide an avenue for challenging judicial orders in termination of care cases.

The next claim alleged that the hospice violated the Rehabilitation Act by refusing treatment to Terri on the basis of her disability. The court found that the case was not within the scope of the Rehabilitation Act because Terri would not have had any need for a feeding tube to deliver nutrition and hydration but for her medical condition. The court noted that, like the ADA, the Rehabilitation Act was not meant to deal with end-of-life medical treatment.

The third claim alleged that an incapacitated patient's wishes must be proven by clear and convincing evidence prior to admission to hospice and termination of curative care in order to comport with the Due Process Clause. There are three standards of proof used in different legal contexts in U.S. courts to prove that something is true:

- Lowest standard: preponderance of evidence; a finding that more than half the persons would find something to be true
- Middle standard: clear and convincing evidence; a finding that more than half the persons would find something to be true, but not everyone would find to be true
- Highest standard: proof beyond a reasonable doubt; a finding that any reasonable or rational person would find something to be true

The court found this argument to be without merit for two reasons. First, the court noted that states may apply a clear and convincing standard of review in termination of care proceedings, but they are not required to do so. Second, the state courts in this case had already applied a broad clear and convincing standard of review rather than a high standard.[LN7]

Fourth, the court held that the claim of cruel and unusual punishment under the Eighth Amendment was without merit. This constitutional provision applies only to punishments inflicted after conviction for crimes, not to life support or medical treatment decisions.

The fifth and final claim was that the Fourteenth Amendment Due Process Clause was violated when the hospice deprived Terri of nutrition and hydration against her wishes. However, the court noted that eight years of litigation was procedural due process in abundance. Turning to substantive due process, the court noted that substantive due process does not require a state to protect its citizens against injury by non-state actors; therefore, since neither the husband nor the hospice were state actors, the claim of violation of substantive due process was without merit.

RULE OF LAW: Hospice care does not violate the ADA or the Rehabilitation Act, nor is it considered cruel and unusual punishment under the Eighth Amendment. In termination of care proceedings, a clear and convincing standard of review may be used by states, but is not required.

(*See generally* Allen, 2006; Boozang, 2006; Burt, 2005; Dubofsky, 2007; Hartnett, 2005; Kreimer, 2007; Perry, 2006; West, 2009).

Moral Dilemmas

1. What rights do family members have to weigh in on decisions about hospice care?

2. How should hospice programs balance the liberty interests of PVS patients to refuse life-saving hydration and nutrition alongside the right to self-determination at the end of life?

In the wake of the Schiavo case, the American Medical Association adopted a policy opposing state legislation that presumes incapacitated patients want life-sustaining treatment unless they have clearly stated otherwise. This policy was in response to proposed model legislation from the National Right to Life Committee requiring physicians and hospitals to presume that all patients unable to speak for themselves would want to continue to receive hydration and nutrition, unless the patients had clear living wills stating otherwise (Snead, 2005). Looking beyond Schiavo, policy proposals are beginning to emerge in several states that would create a presumption mandating life-sustaining treatment. Against this trend, current case law supports self-determination at the end-of-life decision-making stage (Lynn, 2007). Every competent adult has liberty interests over their person, notwithstanding attempts by the National Right to Life Committee to restrict and limit these natural rights inherent to death-with-dignity (Hook & Mueller, 2005), including the accepted rights of:

- Choosing a health care proxy
- Executing an advanced health care directive (AHCD)
- Refusing medical intervention
- Using hospice to ease pain and increase comfort level at the end of life

HEALTH CARE DECISION LAWS

Decision-making of patients in hospice care is affected by:

- AHCDs
- State surrogate laws
- Health care proxies
- Do-not-resuscitate protocols (DNRs)
- Physician orders for life-sustaining treatment (POLSTs)
- Anatomical gifts

Advance Health Care Directives

The National Hospice and Palliative Care Organization reports that most Americans emphatically agree they should have the power to make their own health care decisions, but do not take the necessary steps to ensure their wishes are known or honored. There are approximately two million deaths annually in the U.S., and AHCDs were executed less than 50 percent of the time (Gruber, 2007). An AHCD, also commonly known as an advance decision or living will, provides instructions about what health care actions should be taken in the event of an individual's illness or incapacity and they are no longer able to make their own decisions. A health care proxy, another part of the AHCD, allows individuals to appoint someone to make health care decisions on their behalf if they cannot speak for themselves.

State Surrogate Laws

Without a health care proxy or health care power of attorney, state surrogate laws determine who will make decisions on behalf of a person when they are incapacitated. Laws vary by state, but generally have a priority list that begins with family members.

Health Care Proxies

Health care proxies (a/k/a durable powers of attorney for health care, medical powers of attorney, health care agents, or authorized surrogates) grant authority to give substituted consent for decisions regarding another person's health care. All states permit pre-identified proxies to make decisions about life-sustaining treatment if a person is incapacitated.

Some states limit the proxy's authority to medical precondition requirements. For instance, the proxy could make decisions about medical complications arising from pre-existing Parkinson's disease but would not be authorized to make decisions if the same person were involved in a life-threatening auto accident. Iowa is the only state to require that a witness be present when a proxy consents to forgo life-sustaining treatment (Hickman et al., 2008).

Do-Not-Resuscitate Protocols

DNRs exist by statute or regulation in all but four states: Minnesota, Mississippi, Missouri, and North Dakota (Hickman et al., 2008). Most DNRs must be signed by patients along with their attending physician; some states also require one or two witnesses.

Physician Orders for Life-Sustaining Treatment

Increasingly states are adopting POLSTs, medical orders for life-sustaining treatment, and medical orders for sustaining treatment as an alternative to DNRs (see ABA, 2008).[LN8] POLSTs are similar to DNRs, in that they outline an individual's wishes regarding health care as an illness or disease advances, such as:

- Antibiotics
- Hospitalization
- Nutrition and hydration
- Resuscitation
- Ventilation

While similar to AHCDs, POLSTs do not replace them (AMA, 2007). Rather, POLSTs combine AHCDs and surrogate decision-making into a single document.

Anatomical Gifts

A source of confusion arises when people execute organ donation documents and advance health care directives. Which document controls? Under the Uniform Anatomical Gift Act of 2006, mandated choice has been adopted by all but four states (ABA, 2008). When individuals are incapacitated, their health care proxies make decisions about organ donation (Revised Uniform Anatomical Gift Act § 21 (2006)).

Three states, Arkansas, Idaho, and Montana, still require affirmative donations (opt-in rules) by individual donors (Arkansas Code Ann. § 20-17-1221 (2009); Idaho Code Ann. § 39-3422 (2007); Montana Code Ann. § 72-17-216 (2007)). Donor procurement agencies in Indiana face a six-hour time restriction on finding evidence of individual donor intent, after being notified of a potential organ donation, to determine the eligibility of donors on life support (Indiana Code Ann. § 29-2-16.1-20(b) (2007)).

EMERGING INDUSTRY CONSOLIDATION

The U.S. hospice market remains fragmented, with the top five publicly held hospice companies collectively controlling less than one-fifth of the market (CMS, 2007):

- Vitas of Miami, Florida, the nation's largest hospice company, is a subsidiary of Chemed serving more than twelve thousand patients per day
- Beverly Enterprises of Ft. Smith, Arkansas, was recently acquired by a private equity firm and subsequently delisted in March 2006
- ManorCare of Cleveland, Ohio, operates hospice divisions as part of their larger health care operations
- Odyssey HealthCare of Dallas, Texas, is publicly traded
- VistaCare of Scottsdale, Arizona, is also publicly traded

There are a number of hospice start-ups that have occurred in the last few years and, like other industry growth, a natural consolidation is occurring. Private equity has already moved into the hospice sector (*see generally* Wharton, 2006).

Unique Challenges of For-Profit Hospices

Even though hospice is heavily reliant on Medicare funding, Congress seems intent on keeping hospice well-funded. While Medicare mandates much of what hospice companies must provide and what they will be paid, there are ways for companies to run profitably. It is really about the ability to get a toehold in local markets. The public companies point to well-run nonprofits as their major competitors in many markets because they have been there longer and have better name recognition (Wharton, 2006). For-profit corporations with better access to funding and economies of scale, however, will be able to compete effectively against local nonprofits.

Profit margins for the major companies range from 6 percent to nearly 15 percent. Meanwhile, personal and home care aides earn less than $10 per hour, without health benefits (BLS, 2007).

All the same, running a for-profit hospice offers some unique challenges. For example, hospice care is a highly regulated industry in which federal oversight of the quality of care and payment rates are a major part of the business model. As in so many other industries, the hospice business is likely to be transformed as the baby-boom generation ages and confronts death (Wharton, 2006).

Another constant challenge is finding good direct care workers. While the labor shortage for nurses has improved over the past several years (BLS, 2007), there remains a shortage of home care workers (HHS, 2007). This shortage is crucial, since most hospice care is provided by home care workers, variously known as:

- Home health aides
- Homemakers
- Personal care aides
- Personal care attendants

(Smith, 2007)

Home care workers number about three million; most face continued marginalization in the U.S. because of laws that do not always regulate their wages, hours, health, or safety (Kaye et al., 2006).

REGULATION OF HOME CARE WORKERS' WAGES AND HOURS

Long Island Care at Home, Ltd. v. Coke
[Hospice Worker v. Hospice Provider]
551 U.S. 158 (U.S. Supreme Court 2007)

FACTS: Evelyn Coke, a home care worker who provided companionship services, sued Long Island Care at Home, alleging that she had not been paid the minimum wages and overtime wages to which she was entitled under the Fair Labor Standards Act (FLSA). *See* Fair Labor Standards Act of 1938 (FLSA), 29 U.S.C.A. §§ 201-204, 206, 207, 209-219 (2009).

(continues)

(continued)

Issue: Are home care workers entitled to federal minimum wages and overtime?

Holding and Decision: No, home health care workers are not entitled to federal minimum wages and overtime.

Analysis: A unanimous Supreme Court rejected Coke's claim for wage protection, upholding a U.S. Department of Labor (DOL) regulation exempting home care workers from federal minimum wage and overtime rules. While the FLSA clearly exempted home care workers hired directly by patients, it was unclear whether home care workers hired by an agency were also meant to be exempt from the minimum wage and overtime provisions.

The DOL's most recent regulation exempted such workers from the wage protections and the question in this case was whether that regulation was consistent with the FLSA. The Court found the federal regulation was entitled to deference because Congress had left a definitional gap in the statute, and the DOL's interpretation was reasonable.

Rule of Law: Direct health care workers employed by hospice agencies to work in patients' homes are exempt from federal minimum wage and overtime protections.

(*See generally* Bobroff, 2008; Brunsden, 2008; Horton, 2008; Kaufman, 2008; Light, 2008; Miller, 2008; Pearlstein, 2009; Ruckelshaus, 2007; Whitebread, 2007; Wildermuth, 2008).

This U.S. Supreme Court decision was severely criticized by labor unions and women's groups that pointed to the fact that home care workers, the majority of whom are low-income African American women, provide indispensable services to the terminally ill. Without a doubt, any concerted labor actions on a state or national level regarding wage protections, would erode operating margins of hospice operators.

In addition to these unique challenges, Medicare states that hospice operators must include volunteer workers in their operations, an unusual requirement for any industry. Today, U.S. hospice programs have about 500,000 volunteers, although most contribute only a few hours overall (NHPCO, 2007). It would be beneficial to everyone if hospice programs could persuade one-time volunteers to continue their involvement with the industry rather than simply being used as a government mandated statistic.

Cost Analysis

Medicare has not done a cost-benefit study of hospice but recognizes that this would require taking into account many variables, including the cost of treating conditions not related to the underlying terminal illness. However, if costly hospitalizations are relinquished in return for palliative care at home, it is reasonable to expect cost savings (Wharton, 2006).

Hospices have been expected to reduce health expenditures since their addition to the Medicare benefit package in the early 1980s, but the literature on their ability to do so has been conflicting (Taylor, 2007). In the early days of the Medicare benefit, hospice benefits were designed around the disease trajectory

for cancer, in which patients followed a fairly predictable course (CMS, 2005). At that time, in-home hospice care appeared to be a major cost savings, but more recent reports have shown mixed results (*e.g.*, Campbell et al., 2004; Connor, 2007; Solloway et al., 2005; RAND, 2004; and Taylor, 2007).

According to a Harvard Medical School study, hospice care reduces the costs of caring for many terminally ill patients with various forms of cancer. The savings, however, are not as clear for other diagnoses, including dementia and advanced stage organ system failures, such as advanced chronic congestive heart failure and chronic obstructive pulmonary disease, increasingly part of the hospice treatment mix (Conner et al., 2007). Among the patient populations studied, the mean survival was about a month longer for hospice patients than for non-hospice patients. In other words, patients who chose hospice care lived an average of one month longer than similar patients who did not choose hospice care (Connor et al., 2007).

The most recent research study, conducted by the RAND Corporation, found that while expenses were marginally higher for the last year of life among patients who used hospice services compared to similar patients who received traditional health care, hospice reduced Medicare costs by an average of $2,309 per hospice patient:

- Average costs were 11 percent higher for hospice patients who died from illnesses other than cancer.
- Cancer patients who chose hospice care were only slightly less expensive for Medicare to treat
- Savings were as large as 17 percent for patients with aggressive tumors, such as those related to lung cancer

While hospice use beyond these periods cost Medicare more than conventional care, more effort needs to be put into increasing short stays as opposed to focusing on shortening long ones (Taylor, 2007).[LN9]

PREVENTION VERSUS ADD-ON COSTS

Hospice programs offer unique benefits for patients nearing the end of life and their families, and growing evidence indicates that hospice can provide high-quality care. Despite these benefits, many patients do not enroll in hospice, and those who do enroll generally do so very late in the course of their illness (Smolensky, 2006). This delay is often attributable to the fact that physicians, while doing their best to predict a disease's course or the length of time someone has until their death, are often inaccurate (Glare et al., 2003).

The higher medical costs for hospice patients are a result of delays in patients entering the program. For years, the average length of stay has held steady at about two months. Only a third of those who die under hospice care are in the program seven days or less (Wharton, 2006). Medicare costs would be reduced for most hospice patients if hospice were used for a longer period of time (Taylor, 2007), in contrast to having patients use futile intermittent hospitalizations at the end of life. In other words, given the length of hospice use observed in the Medicare program, increasing the length of the hospice stay for most Medicare hospice users earlier in their terminal disease states would increase savings (CMS, 2005). Clearly, the biggest problem is that patients receive hospice care for too short a time. Hospice adds value by providing quality care and preventive medicine. If the patient is in hospice seven days or less, it is too late to prevent that final hospitalization and hospice care becomes an add-on cost at that point (Wharton, 2006).

Moral Dilemmas

1. Should insurers, including Medicare, refuse to pay for medically futile care for patients with terminal prognoses?

While hospitals do earn substantial revenue providing services to patients in their dying days, treating those patients also results in high costs that can exceed what Medicare and other insurers cover. In addition, Medicare regulations prevent reimbursement for providers that attempt to push unnecessary services to generate profits (Wharton, 2006). While Medicare tries hard to set payment rates to avoid unusually high profits, its payment system does not reward health providers who find ways to keep patients out of the hospital (OIG, 2007).

Moral Dilemmas

1. What is the distinction between medically unnecessary care and futile care for terminally ill patients?

PERINATAL HOSPICE

Six thousand to ten thousand of all live births each year are afflicted with defects severe enough to cause neonatal death, and there are also significant numbers with conditions severe enough to cause intrauterine demise (CDC, 2008). Thus, there are a significant number of children who are candidates for perinatal hospice in the U.S., a compassionate intervention for which there seems to be an unmet demand (D'Almeida et al., 2006). A Washington University School of Medicine study found up to 20 percent of the parents with a fetus with known severe chromosomal or anatomic anomalies chose to continue their pregnancy (Schechtman et al., 2002). Experience with perinatal hospice finds that more than 80 percent choose hospice when it is offered in a supportive environment (D'Almeida et al., 2006).

MEDICAL FUTILITY

Hospice might be most valuable for families who want extra assurance that physicians will not use heroic measures to prolong a patient's life for only a short, and often painful, period of time. Given the hospital culture of trying to save patients no matter what, hospice is a way to signal to the health care system, more strongly than a living will, that a patient is ready to let go rather than continue treatments that have a small probability of success, are costly, and can seem inhumane. The advent of new lifesaving medical technology has made it more difficult for physicians to resist attempting to save a terminally ill patient (Wharton, 2006). Because the technology for heroic measures now exists, the technology tends to be used, not from a financial point of view, but from a cultural point of view (Lynn, 2004).

Consequently, hospices often face a double-edged sword when treating terminally ill patients (Hilliard, 2007). The law requires that hospices provide treatment to the best of their ability or potentially face heavy fines. At the same time, physicians do not want to be investigated for over-prescribing medication to terminally ill patients. It is alleged that recent federal regulatory oversight hinders effective palliative care to terminally ill patients (Trehan, 2007), at a time when most pain associated with severe illness can be relieved if well-established palliative care guidelines are followed (Quill & Meier, 2006).

The law is clearer than the cultural views in this regard. Physiological medical futility determinations have been accepted by the courts as a legitimate reason for withdrawing care; physicians have no duty to continue life-sustaining treatment once it becomes futile (Feldhammer, 2006). Despite the popular misconception that people try everything when finally faced with death, the Multisociety Task Force finds that patients and their families generally accept death when the time actually arrives.[LN10]

PRE-HOSPICE PALLIATIVE CARE

Patients who are terminally ill and seeking palliative care often choose hospice care. While palliative care may be offered to any seriously ill patient, hospice care is offered only to a patient with a life expectancy of months, rather than years.

When the U.S. hospice community was established in the 1970s, cancer patients made up the largest percentage of hospice admissions, but today cancer diagnoses account for fewer than half of all hospice admissions. In fact, less than a quarter of U.S. deaths are now caused by cancer, with the majority of deaths due to other chronic conditions. The top four chronic conditions served by hospice include heart disease, unspecified debility, dementia, and lung disease (Miniño et al., 2007).

Hospitals are increasingly adding pain management and other non-curative treatments to their business models. Some hospitals are developing innovative programs for palliative care that serve as pre-hospice care for patients in need of pain and symptom management, but who are not quite ready for hospice care (Wharton, 2006). There is a synergy developing between hospice and hospitals that may yet improve quality of care while reducing health care costs (Help the Hospices, 2007).

Moral Dilemmas

1. What kind of new end-of-life or curative technology developments do you envision occurring during your lifetime that might present further ethical challenges?

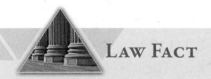

LAW FACT

ACCEPTANCE OF PATIENTS INTO HOSPICE CARE

Should hospices face litigation from family members disappointed with a valid state court order mandating a patient's transfer to their care?

The hospice faced years of litigation when it accepted into its care the transfer of a PVS patient. Interested parties may challenge decisions of a proxy or surrogate concerning discontinuance of life support to a PVS patient in hospice. In Florida, if the evidence of the patient's wishes is conflicting, it must be assumed that the patient would choose to defend life.

—*In re Guardianship of Schiavo*, 780 So.2d 176 (District Court of Appeal of Florida, Second District 2001), *Supreme Court of Florida review denied*, 789 So.2d 348 (Supreme Court of Florida 2001.)

CHAPTER SUMMARY

- Hospice is a philosophy of palliative care that provides pain management and symptom control at the end of life.
- The Medicare hospice benefit is available only to patients eligible for Medicare Part A and who are expected to live less than six months.
- Medicare hospice benefits cover all-inclusive per diem rates for routine home care, continuous attendance at home, inpatient respite care, or general inpatient symptom management care.

- Covered hospice services must be necessary for the treatment of terminal illnesses and related conditions provided in the patient's home, freestanding centers, hospitals, nursing homes, or other long-term care facilities.
- Medicare will reimburse a hospice for two ninety-day periods and then repeated, unlimited sixty-day periods during a patient's lifetime.
- The largest portion of hospital expenses is incurred in the last few weeks of life.
- The law of informed consent favors a competent adult's right to choose between forms of end-of-life care, but an advance directive, or living will, and health care proxy should be in place before entry to hospice care.
- When making decisions about entry to hospice for adults lacking decision-making capacity and having no discernable preferences, the "best interests" standard prevails, meaning the best available care that will control pain will be provided to the patient.
- A collection of state laws protect hospice patients with limited mental capacity, such as those in a permanent vegetative state and those suffering from dementia or mental illness.
- Hospice care does not violate the Americans with Disabilities Act or the Rehabilitation Act, nor is it considered cruel and unusual punishment under the Eighth Amendment, despite the fact that it does not include curative care.
- Current laws support self-determination at the end of life, with the right to refuse medical intervention.
- Hospice care is a highly regulated industry in which the federal Centers for Medicare and Medicaid Services and corresponding state agencies oversee the quality of care and payment rates.

LAW NOTES

1. Dr. Cicely Saunders started the death-with-dignity movement in 1967 when she founded St. Christopher's Hospice in London. Hospice in the U.S. was cultivated by the influences of Dr. Saunders, Florence Wald, former dean of the Yale School of Nursing, and Dr. Elisabeth Kubler-Ross, a psychiatrist who studied and wrote extensively on the psychology of end-of-life issues. The first congressional legislation for hospice care failed in 1974; however, Congress took the program more seriously after the U.S. Department of Health, Education and Welfare reported that hospice might reduce overall health care costs. By 1983, hospice became a valid health care option in the U.S. when Congress approved the Medicare hospice benefit.

2. In the late 1960s as hospice was first appearing in the U.S., early versions of the mechanical respirator called the "Bird," invented by a California physician named Forrest Bird, looked like a glass lunch box on a metal stand. Lacking an automatic switch, nurse's aides (like one of the authors of this textbook when she was a pre-medical student) would sit with the patient and the machine in shifts, flipping the Bird switch every couple of seconds to shoot air into the patient's body. No one thought about whether extended use of this medical technology was appropriate; either patients breathed on their own after a few days, or they died. Thirty years later, an article in the journal *Nature* appeared about a doctor in New York City doing robotic gallbladder surgery on a patient in France. The so-called Lindbergh operation (named after the first transatlantic plane flight by Charles Lindbergh, who contributed to the invention of the artificial heart), manipulated a robot's arms with signals that went under the ocean on transatlantic cable (Marescaux et al., 2001). If the U.S. health care system has moved from the Bird respirator to the Lindbergh operation in thirty years, what kind of end-of-life choices are going to be available in the next thirty years?

3. Eighteen states with licensing statutes specifically for hospices have adopted laws that correspond to the federal certification regulations: Alabama Code §§ 420-5-17 to 420-5-25: Hospice (2009); Alaska Stat. §§ 18.5 to 18.490: Hospice and Home Care Programs (2009); Florida Stat. Ann. §§ 58-A-2 Hospice (2009); Illinois Comp. Stat. §§ 77-1-B, 280 Hospice Administrative Code and 210 ILCS 60: Licensing (2009); 755 Indiana Code. Ann. §§ 16-25-3: Licensure of Hospices and 16-25-4 (2009); Iowa Ann. Code §§ 481-53 Inspections and Appeals-Hospice Licensing Standards (2009); Kentucky Revs. Stat. Ann. §§ 907-1:1330 Hospice (2009); Maine. Revs. Stat. Ann. tit. 10 §§ 144-120: Hospice (2009); Minnesota Stat. Ann. §§ 4668.0210: Provider Hospice (2009); Mississippi Code Ann. §§ 41-85-1 to 41-85-25 Hospice (2009); Ohio Revs. Code Ann. §§ 3701-19: Hospice Care Programs (2009); Oklahoma Stat. Ann. tit. 310 §§ 661: Hospice Licensing (2009); Pennsylvania Cons. Stat. §§ 1130.1 to 1130.101 (2009); Rhode Island Gen Laws §§ 23-17: Hospice (2009); South Dakota Codified Laws §§ 44.04 (2009); Tennessee Code Ann. §§ 1200-8-27-01 to 1200-8-27-01: Standards for Homecare Organizations Providing Hospice Services and §§ 1200-8-15-01 to 1200-8-15-15: Standards for Residential Hospices (2009); Utah Code Ann. §§ 432-16: Hospice Inpatient Facility Construction and §§ 432-750: Hospice (2009); Wisconsin Stat. Ann. §§ 131.11 to 131.64: Hospices (2009).

4. Individuals may be eligible for both Medicare and Medicaid to cover their hospice costs. Medicare is a federal insurance program available primarily for individuals age sixty-five or older, but is also available to anyone with disabilities or End Stage Renal Disease (permanent kidney failure requiring dialysis or a transplant). Medicaid, on the other hand, is a federal-state medical assistance program available to:
   • Low-income individuals
   • Those who fit into eligibility groups recognized by federal and state law (pregnant, disabled, blind, or aged)
   • Those with excessive medical expenses
   Each state sets its own eligibility guidelines for Medicaid services. States are entitled to receive federal matching funds for optional services such as hospice.

5. The attending physicians of hospice patients bill Part B of Medicare (covering outpatient health care expenses including physician fees). The hospice physicians who meet the general medical needs of hospice patients to the extent that they are not met by the attending physicians may not bill Part B for what would normally be Part B services. Rather, the hospice bills Part A (covering inpatient hospital expenses) and reimburses the hospice physician. *See* 42 C.F.R. § 418.304 (2006). However, if the attending physician is unable to continue rendering services to a hospice patient, then the hospice physician must provide direct care and is brought in as a consultant, and physician visits are covered under Part B. *See* 42 C.F.R. § 418.58 (2008).

6. All fifty states have enacted statutes that relate to a competent adult's right to make decisions regarding entry to hospice case, as well as a surrogate's decision-making capacity: Alabama Code §§ 22-8A-1 to 22-8A-10 (2009); Alaska Stat. §§ 13.26.332-13.26.358, 18.12.010-18.12.100 (2009); Arizona Revs. Stat. Ann. §§ 36-3201 to 36-3210, 36-3221, 36-3261 to 36-3262 (2009); Arkansas. Code Ann. §§ 20-17-201 to 20-17-218 (2009); California. Health & Safety Code §§ 7185-7195 (2009); California. Prob. Code §§ 4600-4806 (2009); Colorado Revs. Stat. §§ 15-14-503 to 15-14-509, 15-18-101 to 15-18-113 (2009); Connecticut. Gen. Stat. Ann. §§ 19a-570 to 19a-580c (2009); Delaware Code Ann. tit. 16, §§ 2501-2518 (2009); District of Columbia Code Ann. §§ 6-2401 to 6-2430 (2009); Florida. Stat. Ann. §§ 765.201-765.205, 765.301-765.310 (2009); Georgia. Code Ann. §§ 31-32-1 to 31-32-12, 31-36-1 to 31-36-13 (2009); Hawaii. Revs. Stat. §§ 327D-1 to 327D-27, 551D-2.5 (2009); Idaho Code Ann. §§ 39-4501 t-o 39-4509 (2009); 755 Illinois Comp. Stat. §§ 35/1-10, 45/4-1 to 45/4-12 (2009); Indiana. Code. Ann. §§ 16-36-4-1 to 16-36-4-21, 30-5-2-4 to 30-5-2-5, 30-5-5-16 to 30-5-5-17, 30-5-6-5 to 30-5-7-6, 30-5-9-10 (2009); Iowa Code Ann. §§ 144A.1-11, 144B.1 to 144B.12 (2009); Kansas Stat. Ann. §§ 58-625 to 58-632, 65-28, 101-109 (2009); Kentucky. Revs. Stat. Ann. §§ 311.621-311.643 (2009); Louisiana. Revs. Stat. Ann. §§ 40:1299.58.1-40:1299.10 (2009); Maine. Revs. Stat. Ann. tit. 18A, §§ 5506, 801-817 (2009); Maryland. Code Ann., Health-Gen. §§ 5-601 to 5-618 (2009); Massachusetts. Gen. Laws Ann. ch. 201D, §§ 1-17 (2009); Michigan Comp. Laws Ann. § 700.496 (2009); Minnesota Stat. Ann. §§ 145B.01-145B.17, 145C.01-145C.15 (2009); Mississippi Code Ann. §§ 41-41-101 to 41-41-121, 41-41-151 to 41-41-183 (2009); Missouri Revs. Stat. §§ 404.800B404.865, 404.872, 459.010-459.055 (2009); Montana Code Ann. §§ 50-9-101 to 50-9-111, 50-9-201 to 50-9-206 (2009); Nebraska Revs. Stat. §§ 20-402 to 20-416, 30-3401 to 30-3432 (2009); Nevada Revs. Stat. Ann. §§ 449.535 to 449.690, 449.800 to 449.860 (2009); New Hampshire Revs. Stat. Ann. §§ 137-H:1-16, 137-J:1B137-J:16 (2009); New Jersey Stat. Ann. §§ 26:2H-53 to 26:2H-78 (2009); New Mexico Stat. Ann. §§ 24-7A-1 to 24-7A-18 (2009); New York Pub. Health Law §§ 2980-2994 (2009); North Carolina Gen. Stat. §§ 32A-15 to 32A-27, 90-320 to 90-322 (2009); North Dakota Cent. Code §§ 23-06.4-01 to 23-06.14, 23-06.5-01 to 23-06.5-18 (2009); Ohio revs. Code Ann. §§ 1337.11-1337.17, 2133.01-2133.15 (2009); Oklahoma Stat. Ann. tit. 63, §§ 3101.1-3101.16 (2009); Oregon Revs. Stat. §§ 127.505-127.585, 127.605-127.660 (2009); Pennsylvania Cons. Stat. §§ 5401-5416 (2009); Rhode Island Gen. Laws §§ 23-4.10-1 to 23-4.10-12, 23-4.11-1 to -14 (2009); South Carolina Code Ann. §§ 44-77-10 to 44-77-160, 62-5-504 (2009); South Dakota Codified Laws §§ 34-12D-1 to 34-12D-22, 59-7-2.1, 59-7-2.5 to 59-7-2.8, 59-7-8 (2009); Tennessee Code Ann. §§ 32-11-101 to 32-11-112, 34-6-201 to 34-6-216 (2009); Texas Health & Safety Code Ann. §§ 672.001-672.021; Texas Civs. Prac. & Rem. Code Ann. §§ 135.001-135.018 (2009); Utah Code Ann. §§ 75-2-1101 to 75-2-1119 (2009); Vermont. Stat. Ann. tit. 14, §§ 3451-3465, tit. 18, §§ 5251-5262 (2009); Virginia Code Ann. §§ 54.1-2981 to 54.1-2993 (2009); Washington Revs. Code Ann. §§ 70.122.010-70.122.920 (2009); West Virginia Code Ann. §§ 16-30-1 to 16-30-13, 16-30A-1 to 16-30A-20 (2009); Wisconsin Stat. Ann. §§ 154.01 to 154.15, 155.01 to 155.80 (2009); Wyoming Stat. Ann. §§ 3-5-201 to 3-5-213, 35-22-101 to 35-22-208 (2009).

7. The third appellate trial court opinion summarized the evidence of Terri Schiavo's wishes in In *re Guardianship of Schiavo,* 800 So.2d 640 (District Court of Appeal of Florida, Second District 2001) as follows:
   • Her prognosis was the type of end-stage medical condition that permits the withdrawal of life-prolonging procedures (the trial court determined on the basis of expert testimony that Terri was in a PVS; the only disputed issue was whether she had a small amount of isolated living tissue or no living tissue in her cerebral cortex)

- She did not have a reasonable medical probability of recovery so that she could make her own decision to maintain or withdraw life-prolonging procedures
- The trial court had the authority to make such a decision when a conflict within the family prevented a qualified person from effectively exercising the responsibilities of a proxy (Terri's husband sought the removal of her feeding tube many years after her initial collapse, while Terri's parents fought against the removal)
- Clear and convincing evidence at the time of trial supported a determination that Terri would have chosen in February 2000 to withdraw the life-prolonging procedures

8. *See* California Probate Code §§ 4780-4785 (2009) (requires health care surrogates to consult with treating physicians before modifying an individual's POLST); Idaho Code § 39-4510 (2007); Maryland Health Care Gen. 70 § 5-602 (2007); New York Public Health Law § 2977 (2008); North Carolina Gen. Stat. § 90-21.17 (2007); Oregon Laws Ch. § 697; Utah St. §75-2a-1101-1123 (2009); Washington Revised Code § 43.70.480 (2009); West Virginia Code §§ 16-30C-3(k), 64-48-1116-30C-6(f), 16-30C-7 and 16-30C-13 (2008).

9. Hospice use reduced Medicare program expenditures during the last year of life by an average of $2,309 per hospice user. Expenditures after initiation of hospice were $7,318 for hospice users compared to $9,627 for controls. Maximum cumulative expenditure reductions differed by primary condition. The maximum reduction in Medicare expenditures per user was about $7,000, which occurred when a patient had a primary condition of cancer and used a hospice for their last 58 to 103 days of life. For other primary conditions, the maximum savings of $3,500 occurred when a hospice was used for the last 50 to 108 days of life (Campbell et al., 2004).

10. This observation is a matter of common knowledge. *See, e.g.*, Benson, 2005 ("Every day, ventilators are shut off and feeding tubes are removed in hospitals and hospices...."); Leven, 2005 ("Every day, throughout the U.S., people decide, as they legally can, to have feeding tubes removed or not inserted in the first place..."); *see also* Orentlicher & Callahan, 2004 ("The literature reports data on the number of feeding tubes inserted, but we do not have data on the number of patients for whom feeding was discontinued or never started."); Meisel & Cerminara, 2004 ("A presumption against judicial review of decisions made by properly designated surrogates to forego life-sustaining treatment began to emerge beginning with the earliest end-of-life cases....This presumption is now well solidified"). *See also* Saunders, 2004.

CHAPTER BIBLIOGRAPHY

AAHPM (American Academy of Hospice and Palliative Medicine). (2007). *Policy on physician-assisted death.* Glenview, IL: AAHPM (policy replacing a policy adopted in the 1990s that used the term *physician-assisted suicide*).

AAP (American Academy of Pediatrics). Committee on Bioethics. (2000). Ethics in the care of critically ill infants and children. *Pediatrics, 98* (1), 149-152.

ABA (American Bar Association). (2008). *Summary of health care decision statutes enacted in 2008.* Chicago, IL: ABA.

AHLA (American Health Lawyers Association). (2005). *A guide to legal issues in life limiting conditions.* Washington, DC: AHLA.

Allen, M. P. (2006). Justice O'Connor and the "right to die": Constitutional promises unfulfilled. *William & Mary Bill of Rights Journal, 14*, 821-841.

AMA (American Medical Association) House of Delegates. (2007). *Resolution-hospice services in the nursing facility.* 708 (A-07) 1-2. Washington, DC: AMA.

APHA (American Public Health Association). (2005). *Supporting public health's role in addressing unmet needs at the end of life.* Washington, DC: APHA.

Benson, L. (2005, April 4). Schiavo story blown far out of proportion. *Deseret Morning News*, p. B1.

Black's Law Dictionary. (2004) (8th ed.). Eagan, MN: Thomson Reuters West Publishing Co.

BLS (Bureau of Labor Statistics). (2007). *Occupational outlook handbook, nursing, psychiatric, and home health aides.* Washington, DC: U.S. Department of Labor, BLS.

Bobroff, R. (2008). The early Roberts Court attacks Congress's power to protect civil rights. *North Carolina Central Law Review, 30*, 231-266.

Boozang, K. M. (2006). End of life decision makng: The right to die?: Divining a patient's religious beliefs in treatment termination decision-making. *Temple Political & Civil Rights Law Review, 15*, 345-360.

Brunsden, A. C. (2008). Hybrid class actions, dual certification, and wage law enforcement in the federal courts. *Berkeley Journal of Employment & Labor Law, 29*, 269-310.

Burt, R. A. (2005). The Schiavo case: A symposium: Family conflict and family privacy: The constitutional violation in Terri Schiavo's death. *Constitutional Commentary, 22*, 427-455.

Byock, I. R. et al. (2001). Beyond symptom management: Physician roles and responsibilities in palliative care. In Lois Snyder & Timothy E. Quill (Eds.). *Physician's guide to end-of-life care* (pp. 56-71). Philadelphia, PA: American College of Physicians & American Society of Internal Medicine.

Campbell, D. E. et al. (2004). Medicare program expenditures associated with hospice use. *Annals of Internal Medicine, 140*, 269-277 (RAND study of 250,000 elderly Medicare fee-for-service beneficiaries who received thirty-six months of continuous Part A and B coverage before their death during 1996 to 1999).

Caplan, A. et al. (Eds.). (2006). *The case of Terri Schiavo: Ethics at the end of life*. Amherst, NY: Prometheus Books (details the chronology of the Schiavo litigation, both state and federal, including a compilation of edited documents and other materials relevant to the case).

Caring Connections & NHPCO (National Hospice and Palliative Care Organization). (2005). *Artificial nutrition and end-of-life decision making*. Washington, DC: Caring Connections & NHPCO (provides information about the use of artificial nutrition and hydration, how it is given, and some of the legal and ethical issues that may arise).

Casarett, D. J., & Quill, T. E. (2007). I'm not ready for hospice: Strategies for timely and effective hospice discussions. *Annals of Internal Medicine, 146*, 443-449 (describes a structured strategy for effectively discussing hospice with patients).

CDC (Centers for Disease Control & Prevention). (2008). Infant, neonatal, and postneonatal annual mortality rates in the U.S. *MMWR* (*Morbidity Mortality Weekly Report*), *57* (14), 377. Atlanta, GA: U.S. Department of Health and Human Services, CDC.

CMS (Centers for Medicare and Medicaid Services). (2008). Coverage of hospice care under hospital insurance. *In Medicare benefit policy manual* (Ch 9, § 10). Washington, DC: CMS.

___. (2007). *Medicare reimbursement rates: Update to the hospice payment rates, hospice cap, hospice wage index and the hospice prices for fiscal year 2008*. Washington, DC: CMS.

___. (2005) *Medicare hospice benefits: A special way of caring for people who have a terminal illness*. Washington, DC: CMS.

Colby, W. H. (2007). *Unplugged: Reclaiming our right to die in America*. New York, NY: American Management Association (the Schiavo case galvanized millions to think about end-of-life decision-making and question when life ends and how to define a good death; Colby, the lawyer for Nancy Cruzan, whose 1988 case was one of the first to raise such questions, asserts that the right to die is a new subject because of the technology that allows patients to be alive indefinitely is recent; Colby also discusses the evidence of Terri's medical condition).

___. (2006). Conference on the law of death and dying: From Quinlan to Cruzan to Schiavo: What have we learned? *Loyola University Chicago Law Journal, 37*, 279-296.

Connor, S. R. (2007). Geographic variation in hospice use in the U.S. *Journal of Pain & Symptom Management, 34* (3), 277-285.

Connor, S. R. et al. (2007). Comparing hospice and non-hospice patient survival among patients who die within a three-year window. *Journal of Pain & Symptom Management, 33* (3) 238-246 (analysis of the difference in survival periods of 4,493 terminally ill patients with either congestive heart failure or cancer of the breast, colon, lung, pancreas, or prostate between those who received hospice care and those who did not).

D'Almeida, M. et al. (2006). Perinatal hospice: Family-centered care of the fetus with a lethal condition. *Journal of the American Physicians & Surgeons, 11*, 52-55.

Doyle, D. et al (2005). *Oxford textbook of palliative medicine* (3rd ed.). New York, NY: Oxford University Press (considered the definitive book on hospice and palliative care).

Dubofsky, J. E. (2007). Judicial performance review: A balance between judicial independence and public accountability. *Fordham Urban Law Journal, 34*, 315-342.

Faull, C. et al. (2005). *Handbook of palliative care* (2nd ed.). Hoboken, NJ: Blackwell Publishing.

Feldhammer, J. D. (2006). Medical torture: End-of-life decision-making in the United Kingdom and U.S. *Cardozo Journal of International & Comparative Law, 14*, 511-556 (New York is the only state to statutorily define medical futility; it has done so in the context of DNR orders: "'Medically futile' means that cardiopulmonary resuscitation will be unsuccessful in restoring cardiac and respiratory function or that the patient will experience repeated arrest in a short time period before death occurs").

Ganzini, L. et al. (2003). Nurses' experiences with hospice patients who refuse food and fluids to hasten death. *New England Journal of Medicine*, 349-365 (numerous reports by hospice nurses caring for terminally ill patients dying by dehydration indicate that their patients do not experience much, if any, discomfort; patients who stop eating or drinking experience comfortable and peaceful deaths).

Glare, P. et al. (2003). A systematic review of physicians' survival predictions in terminally ill cancer patients. *British Medical Journal, 323*, 195-200 (found that "doctors' predictions for terminally ill cancer patients, a population very close to death with a median survival of approximately four weeks, were inaccurate—they were correct to within a week in only 25 percent of cases and off by more than four weeks in a similar number").

Greene, L. (2005, March 26). Medicine, money, and Terri Schiavo: Q&A. *St. Petersburg Times*, p. 8A (stating that Terri Schiavo was enrolled in the Florida Medicaid medically needy program, which paid approximately $200/month for her medication costs, with the Hospice of Florida Suncoast paying for most of Schiavo's care for about two years).

Gruber, W. (2007). Life and death on your terms: The advance directives dilemma and what should be done in the wake of the Schiavo case. *Elder Law Journal, 15*, 503-532.

Hartnett, E. A. (2005). The Schiavo case: A symposium: Congress clears its throat. *Constitutional Commentary, 22*, 553-583.

Help the Hospices. (2007). *Access to pain relief: An essential human right*. London, England: Help the Hospices (the U.S.-based National Hospice & Palliative Care Organization works collaboratively with Help the Hospices, the UK's national hospice charity, and the World Health Organization to advance global efforts to improve end-of-life care).

HHS (U.S. Department of Health & Human Services). (2007). *Nursing aides, home health aides, and related health care occupations: National and local workforce shortages and associated data needs a guide to legal issues in life limiting conditions*. Washington, DC: HHS. (the supply of health care workers, while continuing to grow, has been slipping relative to demand, a situation likely to continue well into the future; questions whether there will be adequate supply of workers in these occupations to meet the expected increase in demand).

Hickman, S. E. et al. (2008). The POLST (physician orders for life-sustaining treatment) paradigm to improve end-of-life care: Potential state legal barriers to implementation. *Journal of Law, Medicine & Ethics, 36*, 119-140.

Hilliard, B. (2007). The politics of palliative care and the ethical boundaries of medicine: *Gonzales vs. Oregon* as a cautionary tale. *Journal of Law, Medicine & Ethics, 35*, 158-171.

Hook, C. C., & Mueller, P. S. (2005, November). The Terri Schiavo saga: The making of a tragedy and lessons learned. *Mayo Clinic Procedures, 80*, 1454-1455 (in the Schiavo case, the question of whether to continue or halt medical treatment was complicated by the issue of who was the best person to serve as Terri's proxy).

Horton, D. (2008). The uneasy case for California's "Care Custodian" statute. *Chapman Law Review, 12*, 47-69.

Kalen, S. (2008). The transformation of modern administrative law: Changing administrations and environmental guidance documents. *Ecology Law Quarterly, 35*, 657-720.

Kaufman, E. (2008). Nineteenth annual Supreme Court review: Civil rights and related decisions. *Touro Law Review, 23*, 855-888.

Kaye, H. S. et al. (2006). The personal assistance workforce: Trends in supply and demand. *Health Affairs, 25*, 1113-1114 (observing that low wages, scarce health benefits, and irregular work schedules make it problematic to attract and retain qualified workers).

Kopelman, L. M. (2007). The best interests standard for incompetent or incapacitated persons of all ages. *Journal of Law, Medicine & Ethics, 35*, 187-194.

Kreimer, S. F. (2007). Rejecting "uncontrolled authority over the body": The decencies of civilized conduct, the past and the future of unenumerated rights. *University of Pennsylvania Journal of Constitutional Law, 9*, 423-455.

Kubler-Ross, E. (2007). *On death & dying*. London, England: Taylor & Franci (original 1969) (classic on the hospice movement and developing the five stages of death).

Kubler-Ross, E., & Kessler, D. (2006). *On grief and grieving: Finding the meaning of grief through the five stages of death*. New York, NY: Simon & Schuster: Scribner (written right before Kubler-Ross's own death, this text applies the five stages of death—denial, anger, bargaining, depression, and acceptance—to the grieving process).

Leven, D. C. (2005, October 3). Oregon assisted-dying law should stand. *Journal News*, p. 4B.

Light, A. (2008). *A servant of one's own: The continuing class struggle in feminist legal theories and practices: Mrs. Woolf and the servants: An intimate history of domestic life*. New York, NY: Bloomsbury Press.

Lopez, A. D. et al. (2006). *Global burden of disease and risk factors*. Washington, DC: World Health Organization.

Lynn, J. (2004). *Sick to death and not going to take it anymore: Reforming health care for the last years of life*. Berkeley, CA: University of California Press (reviewing the prolonged period of progressive illness and disability before death).

___. & Adamson, D. (2006). *RAND research brief: Redefining and reforming health care for the last years of life* (pp. 1-5). Santa Monica, CA: RAND (summarizes findings on hospice actions that can be taken to cost-effectively improve the U.S. health care system).

___. & Adamson, D. (2003). *RAND white paper: Living well at the end of life: Adapting health care to serious chronic illness in old age* (pp. 1-26). Santa Monica, CA: RAND.

___. & Harrold, J. (2001). *The Center to Improve Care of the Dying Handbook for mortals: Guidance for people facing serious illness*. New York, NY: Oxford University Press (excellent practice guidance for end-of-life issues for caregivers and the dying).

___. et al. & Palliative Care Policy Center. (2007). *The common sense guide to improving palliative care*. New York, NY: Oxford University Press (practical advice for administrators).

___. (2007). *Improving care for the end-of-life: A sourcebook for health care managers and clinicians*. New York, NY: Oxford University Press (result of a research project, sponsored by the Center to Improve Care of the Dying and the Institute for Healthcare Improvement, that included more than four dozen health care organizations).

Marescaux, J. et al. (2001). Transatlantic robot-assisted telesurgery. *Nature, 413*, 379-380.

Meisel, A., & Cerminara, K. L. (2004). *The right to die: The law of end-of-life decision making* (3rd ed.). New York, NY: Aspen Publishers (this law text reviews liability issues regarding acceptance of hospice and the decisions to forgo curative care, as well as right-to-die issues).

Miller, S. D. (2008). Atrophied rights: Maximum hours labor standards under the FLSA and Illinois law. *Northern Illinois University Law Review, 28*, 261-346.

Miniño, A. M. et al. (2007). Deaths. *National vital statistics report, 55* (19). Hyattsville, MD: National Center for Health Statistics.

NHO (National Hospice Organization). (2006, October 3). *Press release*. Alexandria, VA.

NHPCO (National Hospice & Palliative Care Organization). (2007). *Facts and figures: Hospice care in America*. Arlington, VA: NHPCO.

OIG (Office of Inspector General) U.S. Department of Health & Human Services. (2007, December 21). *Regulatory alert: OIG report on hospice care in nursing facilities*. Washington, DC: OIG (compares hospice care in nursing facilities and beneficiaries in other settings).

Orentlicher, D., & Callahan, C. M. (2004). Feeding tubes, slippery slopes, and physician-assisted suicide. *Journal of Legal Medicine, 25*, 389-402.

Perry, J. E. (2006). Biblical biopolitics: Judicial process, religious rhetoric, Terri Schiavo and beyond. *Journal of Law & Medicine, 16*, 553-630.

Pearlstein, L. C. (2009). Employment-related crimes. *American Criminal Law Review, 46*, 429-469.

Poblenz, N. T., & Richard, G. E. (2006). Hospice: The emerging way to care for terminally ill patients. *Houston Lawyer, 43*, 54-57.

Prahalad, C. K. (2006). *The fortune at the bottom of the pyramid: Eradicating poverty through profits*. Philadelphia, PA: Wharton School Publishing.

Quill, T. E., & Meier, D. E. (2006). The big chill: Inserting the DEA into end-of-life care. *New England Journal of Medicine, 354*, 1-2.

RAND Corp. (2004, February 16). *News release: RAND study finds choosing hospice care raises Medicare costs for the last year of life*. Santa Monica, CA: RAND.

Ruckelshaus, C. K. (2007). The Supreme Court's 2006-2007 term employment law cases: A quiet but revealing term. *Fordham Urban Law Journal, 35*, 373-406.

Rutkow, L. (2005). Optional or optimal? The Medicaid hospice benefit at twenty. *Journal of Contemporary Health Law & Policy, 22*, 107-142.

Saunders, C. (2004). A hospice perspective. In K. Foley & E. Hendin (Eds.), *The case against assisted suicide: For the right to end-of-life care*. Baltimore, MD: Johns Hopkins University Press.

Schechtman, K. B. et al. (2002). Decision-making for termination of pregnancies with fetal anomalies: Analysis of 53,000 pregnancies. *Obstetrics & Gynecology, 99*, 216-222.

Smith, P. R. (2007). Aging and caring in the home: Regulating paid domesticity in the twenty-first century. *Iowa Law Review, 92*, 1835-1900.

Smolensky, K. R. (2006). Defining life from the perspective of death: An introduction to the forced symmetry approach. *University of Chicago Legal Forum*, 41-84.

Snead, O. C. (2005). The (surprising) truth about Schiavo: A defeat for the cause of autonomy. *Constitutional Commentary*, 22, 383-404 (describing the parents' legal and moral aspects of their daughter's case).

Solloway, M. et al. (2005). A chart review of seven hundred eighty-two deaths in hospitals, nursing homes, and hospice/home care. *Journal of Palliative Medicine, 84* (4), 789-796 (finding that approximately one-third of people who die require some form of alternate decision-making process at the end of their lives due to their lack of capacity to make health care decisions at that critical time).

Taylor, D. H. Jr. (2007). What length of hospice use maximizes reduction in medical expenditures near death in the U.S. Medicare program? *Social Science & Medicine, 65* (7), 1466-1478 (retrospective case study of Medicare decedents (National Long Term Care Survey screening sample) comparing 1,819 hospice decedents with 3,638 controls matched via their predicted likelihood of dying while using hospice; variables used to create matches were demographic, primary medical condition, cost of Medicare financed care prior to the last year of life, nursing home residence, and Medicaid eligibility).

Trehan, A. B. (2007). Fear of prescribing: How the DEA is infringing on patients' right to palliative care. *University of Miami Law Review, 61*, 961-995.

Werth, J. L. (2007). The Schiavo case: Interdisciplinary perspectives: Some personal aspects of end-of-life decision-making. *University of Miami Law Review, 61*, 847-860.

West, L. R. (2009). Judicial independence: Our fragile fortress against elective tyranny. *Oklahoma City University Law Review, 34*, 59-73 (keynote address at the 2008 Oklahoma Bar Association Rule of Law Conference at Oklahoma City University School of Law).

Westmoreland, T. (2007). Standard errors: How budget rules distort lawmaking. *Georgetown Law Journal, 95*, 1555-1610.

Wharton (Wharton School at the University of Pennsylvania). (2006). The business of hospice care. *Knowledge@Wharton*.

Whitebread, C. (2007). The conservative Kennedy Court: What a difference a single justice can make: The 2006-2007 term of the United States Supreme Court, *Whittier Law Review, 29*, 1-145.

Wildermuth, A. J. (2008). What Twombly and Mead have in common. *Northwestern University Law Review Colloquy, 102*, 276-284.

CHAPTER 29

MATURE MINOR RIGHTS TO REFUSE LIFE-SUSTAINING MEDICAL TREATMENT

"Neither youth nor childhood is folly nor incapacity. Some children are fools and so are some old men."

—WILLIAM BLAKE (1757-1827), BRITISH POET AND ARTIST

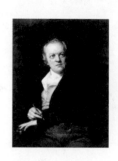

IN BRIEF

This chapter is focused on the question of whether mature minors have the right to refuse life-sustaining medical treatment (LSMT). In this chapter, a *mature minor* is defined as a child, generally an adolescent, who has decision-making capacity. The state's interest in preserving life and in protecting the health and welfare of children is greatest when a child desires to refuse LSMT. Depending on one's view of life support, the term *death-prolonging* could be substituted for *life-sustaining*.

FACT OR FICTION

WITHDRAWAL OF LIFE-SUSTAINING MEDICAL TREATMENT

When, if ever, should LSMT be withdrawn from a stable and completely alert minor with a progressive terminal disease?

H, a fourteen-year-old boy, suffers from Hunter syndrome, a rare but progressive and ultimately fatal genetic disorder for which there is no known cure. The buildup of complex carbohydrates that occurs in Hunter syndrome eventually causes permanent damage affecting appearance, mental development, organ function, and physical abilities. The Mayo Clinic describes Hunter syndrome as an enzymatic defect with a buildup of complex carbohydrates in the connective tissue. Patients suffer from various defects in bone, cartilage, and connective tissue, as well as seizure disorders and congenital heart disease. The defects in their aortic and mitral valves are eventually fatal. Patients also suffer from enlarged livers and spleens as well as characteristic body features, including a short stature with an enlarged head. The disease affects the airways, trachea, and large bronchial tubes, in that the structural support disappears and they collapse (*see* Wraith et al., 2008).

H was admitted to University Medical Center with breathing difficulties; within a day, he was placed on a ventilator to enable him to breathe, trached in order to stop aspiration, and had a feeding tube inserted into his stomach. H's condition is now stable and he is completely alert. Generally, H is not in pain, although he experiences pain whenever he is moved, washed, or suctioned since water fills his connective tissues. H is slowly but progressively becoming more rigid and anatomically malformed as his disease progresses. He is generally not on any pain medication due to the fleeting nature of his pain when he moves.

H has requested removal of the ventilator and palliative care while his dying process occurs; he clearly understands this action will hasten his death. H is informed of his medical condition and rationally acknowledges he is aware he is becoming deaf and losing his sight. At the court hearing to determine H's level of maturity to make this decision, H's parents testified they agreed to the withdrawal of H's life-sustaining treatment; they felt it was in their son's best interests to be weaned from the ventilator in an effort to end his discomfort and suffering. The hospital medical ethics committee supported the parents' decision. However, the director of pediatric critical care and H's pediatrician testified they would feel very uncomfortable removing the ventilator from H because he was an awake and alert minor who was nowhere near terminal. Both testified they were involved in removing ventilators from other minors, but they were always comatose with no quality of life.

H is to be transferred to a nursing home where his parents cannot visit and care for him very day. While H's parents have provided care for H in their home since his diagnosis of Hunter syndrome at the age of three, they can no longer care for him on artificial life support. Everyone agrees H could be kept alive another two to three years through artificial means without any hope of recovery or cure as his disease progresses and his heart fails from the progressive thickening of his heart's valves. H's parents are concerned their son will not receive the monitoring and care during his final years of his life that they have provided to him at their home.

—Case synopsis based on *In re Gianelli*, 834 N.Y.S.2d 623
(Supreme Court of New York, Nassau County 2007).
(See *Law Fact* at the end of this chapter for the answer.)

PRINCIPLES AND APPLICATIONS

In order to understand precisely what this chapter is about, it is crucial to define LSMT, a term that refers to advanced medical technologies, such as:

- Dialysis
- Feeding tubes to provide artificial hydration and nutrition
- Intravenous medicines that maintain blood pressure
- Mechanical ventilators and respirators

Although LSMT forestalls the moment of death, by definition LSMT can only sustain life. It cannot save life or improve a patient's condition. This is a crucial distinction because medical treatment at the end of life at best can only prolong the inevitable slow deterioration and predictable death. *See In the Matter of Karen Quinlan*, 355 A.2d 647, 663 (Supreme Court of New Jersey 1976), *U.S. Supreme Court certiorari denied*, 429 U.S. 922 (U.S. Supreme Court 1976).

Its potential benefit can only be measured in relation to the patient's personal values. *See Cruzan v. Director, Missouri Department of Health,* 497 U.S. 261, 309 (U.S. Supreme Court 1990) (Brennan, J., dissenting) ("The right to be free from unwanted medical attention is a right to evaluate the potential benefit of treatment and its possible consequences according to one's own values and to make a personal decision whether to subject oneself to the intrusion."). The decision to accept or refuse LSMT determines not only the time of one's death, but also the manner in which death occurs. Thus, a denial of a mature minor's autonomy to refuse LSMT is a denial of the right to decide whether the medical prolongation of life, as it transforms into a prolongation of death, is worth the high physical and psychological burdens that will have to be endured, including:

- Embarrassment and humiliation
- Emotional suffering
- Intractable pain
- Invasive and/or inhumane interventions designed to sustain life
- Irremediable disability or helplessness
- Other activities that severely detract from the quality of life as viewed by the patient

(AAP, 2007)

Parental Autonomy

As a rule, only parents can grant or decline permission for medical treatment of their children. The exception is that a state may seek to override parental choices that jeopardize a child's welfare. The power of parents to make decisions regarding medical treatment of their children does not require any assessment of the child's level of maturity, nor does it allow for any degree of autonomy for the child. *See Troxel v. Granville,* 530 U.S. 57 (U. S. Supreme Court 2000) (explaining that because of the presumption that fit parents will act in the best interests of the child, there is usually no reason for a state to become involved in the private realm of the family to decide what is in the best interests of the child). The emerging exception, however, is for mature minors (Cohan, 2006).

In the U.S., adolescents and pre-adolescents constitute the largest class of patients of questionable or borderline competence for the health care decisions they commonly face (Austin, 2007). The consensus is that some minors have sufficient maturity to understand and appreciate the benefits and risks of proposed medical treatment of all kinds, and thus those mature minors should have the right to give or decline to give informed consent regarding all health care decisions. Since the 1960s, states have recognized that

mature minors may enjoy many of the adult rights of medical consent. States have passed laws allowing minors to bypass the parental consent tradition and to consent to a narrow range of medical treatments:

- Care related to a sexual assault
- Contraceptive services
- Drug and alcohol abuse and dependency treatment
- Emergency treatment where parents are not immediately available
- Mental health care
- Pregnancy-related care
- Treatment for sexually transmitted diseases (STIs, HIV, or other reportable diseases)

(Dickens & Cook, 2005)

Adolescents, defined by the World Trade Organization as ten to nineteen years old, can give independent consent for reproductive health services if their capacities for understanding have sufficiently evolved.

Although not every state has laws covering minors in each of the status categories listed above, every state has provisions for some of them (Ford et al., 2004). Courts have recognized the mature minor doctrine as one of at least seven exceptions to the requirement for parental consent in medical treatment of minors. The state laws recognize some measure of autonomy for certain types of treatment and allow minors to give informed consent on their own. Such consent is to be:

- Informed, with the ability to understand conflicting advice
- Rational, showing evidence of clear thinking and sensible judgment based on reason rather than emotion
- Voluntary and intentional

(English & Kenney, 2003; Kuther, 2003)

Criteria for Determining Maturity of Minors

Whether a minor has the capacity to consent to medical treatment depends upon the totality of the circumstances and the facts of each case. Criteria to be considered include:

- Age
- Conduct and demeanor of the minor at the time of the incident involved
- Degree of maturity or judgment
- Education and training (whether the minor is a high school graduate)
- Life experiences (such as whether the minor is emancipated, married, pregnant, a parent, or is living apart from the parents)

- Ability to appreciate risks and consequences
- Nature of the treatment

(Austin, 2007; English & Kenny, 2003; Vukadinovich, 2004)

Adoption of the mature minor exception to the common law rule is not a general license to treat minors without parental consent. There is always the problem of deciding whether minors are in fact mature enough to make their own medical decisions.[LN1]

In other contexts, states have developed standards for determining whether minors have the capacity to formulate the necessary intent to commit crimes so as to be tried as adults. For instance, most state Juvenile Court Acts and the federal Juvenile Justice and Delinquency Prevention Act presupposes a sliding scale of maturity in which minors can be mature enough to be tried and convicted as adults (*see* 18 U.S.C.A. §§ 4351 *et seq.* (2009)). When a minor is mature enough to have the capacity to formulate criminal intent, minors are generally treated as adults. The concept of legal competency, used in criminal law and in determining the capacity of minors to testify as witnesses, applies the common law rule of sevens, under which minors:

- Under the age of seven are not presumed to be competent or mature
- Between seven and fourteen are not presumed to be competent or mature, but may be proved otherwise
- From fourteen to twenty-one are presumed to be competent and mature

Clear and Convincing Standard of Maturity

There are so many factors to be considered when determining whether a minor is mature that a well-reasoned uniform standard has failed to emerge (Slonina, 2007). Evidence must demonstrate, with the highest level of persuasion, that a minor is mature enough to:

- Appreciate the consequences of their choices and actions
- Exercise the judgment of a competent adult
- Make personal health care choices

Is it more likely than not that a mature minor can make the decision to refuse LSMT? If the evidence is clear and convincing, then the mature minor doctrine affords mature minors the common law right to consent to or refuse medical treatment. While judicial proceedings are generally necessary to assess the minor's maturity in order for a minor's medical choices to be valid (when a temporary guardian is not appointed), in some situations a minor is so seriously ill or injured, recourse to the courts is impractical. In these situations, considerable emphasis is generally placed on whether the parents actually agree with their child's decision.

Many interesting questions emerge. For example, a fourteen-year-old minor, presumed to be mature under common law, has a baby. The baby is on life support with no chance of recovering from some terminal illness. Would anyone question the fourteen-year-old mother's right to make decisions for her baby? Would it not be strange if she were allowed to make that kind of decision for her own baby but not for herself, assuming she lives in a state that would not consider her a mature minor, regardless of her life experience of being a parent?

COMMON LAW PRINCIPLE OF SELF-DETERMINATION

The international Convention on the Rights of the Child, almost universally ratified, limits parental powers and duties by a minor's evolving capacities for self-determination (Dickens & Cook, 2005). While the U.S. Supreme Court recognized the right of adults to refuse LSMT, this right was never extended to mature minors. In the U.S., the mature minor doctrine is generally a creature of case law that extends the common law principle of self-determination to minors (Cohan, 2006). The doctrine recognizes decision-making capacity increases with age. There is usually no chronological age of consent for medical care, but rather a condition of consent, meaning the capacity for understanding (Dickens & Cook, 2005). This capacity is best assessed on a case-by-case basis.

Even though parents may authorize do-not-resuscitate (DNR) orders for their children, health care professionals should obtain the consent of mature minors before administering or withholding treatment to avoid the possibility of wrongful death or other tort suits when a child dies. Professionals have an affirmative duty to find out whether their patients are mature enough to consent to DNR orders and, by implication, other kinds of protocols before authorizing them.

If health care professionals conclude a minor is mature, then the minor's choices must be followed notwithstanding the objections of the parents. While this places a professional in the difficult position of determining the minor's maturity, and while a professionals decision on the maturity level of a minor will often be second-guessed, nonetheless the decision should be made using the professional's best medical judgment (Cohan, 2006). Professionals who make good-faith determinations about the maturity of a minor are not generally liable for failing to obtain parental consent if the parents disagree with the minor's decision (Slonina, 2007).

States have enacted legislation codifying these principles and reflecting policy judgments that certain minors have attained a level of maturity or autonomy that makes it appropriate for them to make their own medical decisions (Ford et al., 2004). For instance, West Virginia's legislation provides:

> If the minor is between the ages of sixteen and eighteen and, in the opinion of the attending physician, the minor is of sufficient maturity to understand the nature and effect of a do-not-resuscitate order, then no such order shall be valid without the consent of such minor. In the event of a conflict between the wishes of the parents or guardians and the wishes of the mature minor, the wishes of the mature minor shall prevail. For purposes of this section, no minor less than sixteen years of age shall be considered mature.
>
> W. Va. Code § 16-30C-6(d) (2002)

In other states, minors, regardless of their maturity, may not refuse unwanted medical care. *See, e.g.,* Code of Laws of South Carolina 1976 Annotated § 44-78-50(b) (1994); Tennessee Code Annotated § 68-11-224(a) (2004). This policy approach, in limiting the rights of mature minors, is opposed by the Society for Adolescent Medicine (Morreale et al., 2004).

Moral Dilemmas

1. Could there ever be justification for a medical team to withhold individualized prognosis or treatment plan information from a mature minor?

2. What is the proper balance between a parent's right to choose or refuse LSMT for their child over a mature minor's rights?

RIGHT TO REFUSE LIFE-SUSTAINING MEDICAL TREATMENT

At issue is whether and when, if ever, mature minors have the right to refuse LSMT. This is particularly controversial when treatment is refused based on religious beliefs and when treatment would most likely achieve remission of a disease or illness (Chen, 2007). Generally, hospitals seek to have the courts appoint a temporary guardian with authority to consent or refuse consent of all medical treatment required (*see generally* Teaster et al., 2007).

State interests may be greater than the interests of mature minors or their parents in refusing to consent to medical treatments if the treatment options and their risks, side effects, and benefits are negligible (such as is often the case for refusing blood transfusions for religious reasons). In these situations,

parents who support their child's right to refuse LSMT risk being charged with neglect if death results from the minor's refusal of treatment.

Moral Dilemmas

1. Should the First Amendment's Free Exercise Clause entitle a mature minor to decline medical care because it contravenes sincerely held religious beliefs?

2. When should a state intervene, if ever, when the failure of parents to accept and begin LSMT endangers a child's life?

3. What should determine the proper balance between the rights of mature minors and parental rights when the minor requests protection of the state to begin or end LSMT?

4. Does a state have the fiscal ability or responsibility to pay for a child's medical treatment of a life-threatening condition when a parent refuses traditional medicine?

Common Law Right to Refuse Medical Treatment

Still, mature minors have a common law right to consent to or refuse medical treatment. Like adults, mature minors enjoy confidentiality and the right to treatment according to their wishes rather than their best interests. Minors capable of self-determination may grant or deny assent to treatment regardless of whether parents or guardians provide consent (Dickens & Cook, 2005). Emancipated minors' self-determination may also be recognized in some contexts, such as on marriage or default of adults' guardianship.

Since most states do not have absolute eighteen-years-old age barriers prohibiting minors from consenting to medical treatment, age is not a barrier that necessarily precludes minors from exercising medical rights normally associated with adulthood. Thus, unless expressly prohibited by state law, mature minors may refuse medical treatment, even if this refusal results in their death.

Common law rights are not, however, absolute and, as with adults, must be balanced against state interests, such as:

- Maintaining the ethical integrity of the medical profession
- Preserving human life
- Preventing suicides
- Protecting the interests of third parties

(*See generally Vacco v. Quill*, 521 U.S. 793 (U.S. Supreme Court 1997))

The most significant of the four interests is the preservation of life, which is particularly compelling when dealing with minors. If parents oppose a mature minor's refusal to consent to LSMT, this opposition weighs heavily against the minor's right to refuse.

WITHDRAWAL OF LIFE-SUSTAINING MEDICAL TREATMENT

When deciding whether to withdraw LSMT, the best interests of the child rather than a substituted judgment standard applies. A substituted judgment standard permits a surrogate to make decisions regarding medical care based on what a person would have chosen had they been competent (Schneider, 2003). As for clear and convincing evidence of a child's best interests, courts generally consider such factors as:

- Benefits from treatment versus the burdens to the child
- Degree of humiliation, dependence, and loss of dignity resulting from the condition and treatment
- Likelihood pain or suffering from withholding or withdrawal of treatment could be avoided or minimized
- Motivations of the family in advocating a particular course of treatment
- Nature and degree of physical pain or suffering resulting from the medical condition
- Opinions of the family
- Pain, suffering, or serious complications caused or that may be caused by the treatment
- Physical, sensory, emotional, and cognitive capacities of the child
- Preferences of the child, if they can be ascertained
- Quality of life, life expectancy, and prognosis for recovery with and without treatment
- Suffering to the child if treatment is withdrawn
- Treatment options and their risks, side effects, and benefits

(*See generally In re Christopher I,* 131 Cal.Rptr.2d 122 (Court of Appeal, Fourth District, Division 3, California 2003); Canter, 2005; Schneider, 2003)

This modified approach, while often problematic, appears to provide the best solution for making medical decisions for mature minors regarding life-sustaining decisions.

Moral Dilemmas

1. Who should determine what is in the best interests of mature minors regarding the value of their life and the end of their life?

WORDS OF CAUTION FOR HEALTH CARE PROVIDERS

Health care providers face complicated issues with regard to LSMT for minors. Since legitimate public concerns underlie this evolving controversy over the right to refuse medical care, providers should obtain and document informed consent from all appropriate, authorized legal representatives, including the parents and the mature minor, and any other authorized persons (Vukadinovich, 2004). To be valid, any consent must be informed and must be given by a person with the requisite legal capacity. Thus, a physician who proceeds with a treatment in conformity with a mature minor's request and a signed agreement still might be proceeding without legal consent because the minor may lack capacity due to age. On the other hand, if a physician proceeds at the parents' request in conformity with the best interests of a mature minor, the physician might be proceeding without legal consent because the minor may have legal capacity due to maturity.

Providers should be particularly attentive when treating mature minors; mature minors need to understand the nature of their medical treatment, its risks and benefits, and alternatives, so their decisions, along with their parents' decisions, are truly informed. Determining the maturity of minors is essential to legal compliance, protecting against liability, and ensuring children receive the best end-of-life care possible.

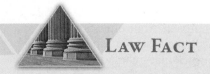

LAW FACT

WITHDRAWAL OF LIFE-SUSTAINING MEDICAL TREATMENT

When, if ever, should LSMT be withdrawn from a stable and completely alert minor with a progressive terminal disease?

Since the 1960s, the technological innovations of science and medicine have had a significant impact on life and death and blurred the line between the two. Members of our society now enjoy a healthier and longer life. The symptoms of some rare diseases that at one time would have resulted in certain early death in children are now treatable, but the child's discomfort and suffering become indescribable. Medical treatment can keep children with progressive terminal diseases alive without any hope of recovery, cure, or even improvement in their condition. The ability of the medical community to artificially keep bodies alive has given rise to many ethical and moral dilemmas and arguments, with no clear answers.

The court found that the minor lacked the capacity to make reasoned decisions concerning his treatment and that his parents' request to discontinue his treatment was premature and not in the minor's best interests. However, the court recognized the parents' right to work with the medical community to reach a medically appropriate decision concerning their son. The court found no reason for the state to become involved in the private realm of this family; the parents could decide, with their son's treating physician, what was in the best interests of their son.

—Case synopsis based on *In re Gianelli*, 834 N.Y.S.2d 623
(Supreme Court of New York, Nassau County 2007).

CHAPTER SUMMARY

- Generally, parents have the responsibility of deciding upon medical treatment for their children; the state may only intervene when the parents' choice may jeopardize the child's welfare.
- An exception to parents' complete control of medical decision-making regarding their children is emerging for mature minors; the consensus is that mature minors should be able to consent to or decline treatment.
- In many states, minors can now make medical treatment decisions without their parents' input regarding mental health, drug and/or alcohol dependency, sexually transmitted diseases, pregnancy, contraception, sexual assault, and emergency treatment.
- The criteria for minors to give informed consent are generally the same as for anyone else; the consent must be based on the ability to understand conflicting advice, it must be voluntary and intentional, and it must be based upon rationality rather than emotion.
- Criteria for determining whether a minor is mature include the minor's age, life experiences, education, demeanor, and the minor's ability to appreciate the risks and consequences of consenting to or declining treatment; the standard for determining whether a minor is mature is clear and convincing.
- If health care professionals determine that a minor is mature, then the minor's choices take precedence over the parents' choices; in some states, minors may not refuse medical treatment regardless of their maturity.
- In some states, parents may be charged with neglect or even manslaughter if death results from the minor's refusal of treatment, especially if the refusal was made for religious reasons and the treatment's risks or side effects would have been negligible compared to the treatment's benefit.
- Unless expressly prohibited by state law, mature minors may refuse lifesaving medical treatment.
- The reason states get involved in minors' medical care is to protect the states' interest in preserving human life, preventing suicides, protecting third parties, and maintaining the ethical integrity of the medical profession, the strongest of which is the preservation of human life.
- When deciding whether to withdraw life-sustaining treatment from a minor, a "best interests of the child" standard is applied, taking into account many factors, such as the child's quality of life, treatment options, degree of pain and suffering, and family opinions.
- Determining and documenting a minor's maturity is essential for medical care providers to protect themselves from liability and to ensure the minor receives the best care possible.

LAW NOTES

1. While developmental psychologists define as mature anyone who responds to circumstances in a socially appropriate manner, determining the maturity of minors has proven to be complicated. Medical literature questions the validity of the concept of legal competency and the rule of sevens in minors (Braddock et al., 2008). While developmental theorist Jean Piaget's four-stage model of development proposes that most minors begin to employ mature thinking processes between the ages of eleven and fifteen (Piaget, 2001), critics question whether Piaget's developmental stages take into account the social and environmental pressures affecting the decision-making capability of minors when faced with the intense stress of life-threatening medical conditions (Paterick, 2008). Some studies show fourteen-year-olds possess the same maturity and decision-making capability as adults (Schwartz & Meslin, 2008). Other developmental research claims minors and adults have very different perspectives on the world. Minors generally:

   - Are more susceptible to peer pressure
   - Have impaired judgment when facing the possibility of death regardless of their age
   - Make riskier choices
   - Tend to focus on immediate rather than long-term consequences

   (Braddock et al., 2008)

   Modern cognitive theory has not yet defined the interaction between personal characteristics and maturity; focused research has not identified the personality traits or individual behaviors that could be used to define the maturity of minors. In recognition of the fact that some minors are more mature than some adults will ever be, the concept of maturity in general requires better definition in the social context of LSMT.

CHAPTER BIBLIOGRAPHY

AAP (American Academy of Pediatrics) Committee on Bioethics. (2007). Guidelines on forgoing life-sustaining medical treatment. *Pediatrics, 119* (2), 405.

Austin, A. W. (2007). Medical decisions and children: How much voice should children have in their medical care? *Arizona Law Review, 49*, 143-169.

Braddock III, C. H. et al. (2008). Establishing the boundaries of informed consent. *American Medical Association Journal of Ethics, 10* (8), 483-537.

Canter, J. M. (2005). Non-judicial alternatives resolving end-of-life decisions for minors. *Family Court Review, 43*, 527-536.

Chen, J. E. (2007). Family conflicts: The role of religion in refusing medical treatment for minors. *Hastings Law Journal, 58*, 643-670.

Cohan, J. A. (2006). Judicial enforcement of lifesaving treatment for unwilling patients. *Creighton Law Review, 39* (4), 849-913.

Dickens, B. M., & Cook, R. J. (2005). Adolescents and consent to treatment. *International Journal on Gynecology & Obstetrics, 89*, 179-184.

English, A., & Kenney, K. E. (2003). *State minor consent laws: A summary* (2nd ed.). Chapel Hill, NC: Center for Adolescent Health & Law.

Ford, C. et al. (2004). Confidential health care for adolescents: Position paper for the society for adolescent medicine. *Journal on Adolescent Health, 35*, 160-167.

Kuther, T. L. (2003). Medical decision-making and minors: Issues of consent and assent. *Adolescence, 38*, 343-358.

Morreale, M. C. et al. (2004). Position paper of the Society for Adolescent Medicine: Access to health care for adolescents and young adults. *Journal on Adolescent Health, 35*, 342-344.

Paterick, T. J. (2008). Medical informed consent: General considerations for physicians. *Mayo Clinical Proceedings, 83* (3), 313-319.

Piaget, J. (2001). *Studies in reflecting abstraction.* Hove, UK: Psychology Press.

Schneider, B. A. (2003). Child welfare: Court may determine whether life-sustaining treatment should be withdrawn. *Journal on Law, Medicine & Ethics, 31,* 316.

Schwartz, P. H., & Meslin, E. M. (2008). The ethics of information: Absolute risk reduction and patient understanding of screening. *Journal on General Internal Medicine, 23* (6), 867-870.

Slonina, M. I. (2007). State v. physicians: Legal standards guiding the mature minor doctrine and the bioethical judgment of pediatricians in life-sustaining medical treatment. *Journal of Law & Medicine, 17*, 181-215.

Teaster, P. B. et al. (2007). Wards of the state: A national study of public guardianship. *Stetson Law Review, 37*, 193-241.

Towner, C. L. (2006). Case retrospective: Parents charged with kidnapping their own child: The Parker Jensen story. *Journal of Law & Family Studies, 8*, 191-202.

Vukadinovich, D. M. (2004). Minors' rights to consent to treatment: Navigating the complexity of state laws. *Journal of Health & Life Sciences Law, 37* (4), 667-691.

Watts, C. D. (2005). Asking adolescents: Does a mature minor have a right to participate in health care decisions? *Hastings Women's Law Journal, 16*, 221-250 (suggesting mature minors should have a voice in their well-being).

Wraith, J. E. et al. (2008). Mucopolysaccharidosis type II (Hunter syndrome): A clinical review and recommendations for treatment in the era of enzyme replacement therapy. *European Journal of Pediatrics, 167* (3), 267-277.

CHAPTER 30

CARE OF THE CRITICALLY ILL AND DYING

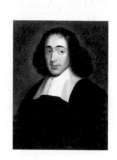

"It is impossible, that man should not be a part of nature, or that man should not follow nature's general order."

—BENEDICT DE SPINOZA (1632-1677), PORTUGUESE PHILOSOPHER

IN BRIEF

This chapter deals with the question of whether human beings have a right to die at a time and place of their own choosing. Answers to this question and the implications of palliative sedation (the induction of unconsciousness for the purpose of relieving intractable pain and distress) and assisted dying (self-administered medication for the purpose of hastening unconsciousness and death) are explained, as well as the distinction between the two acts.

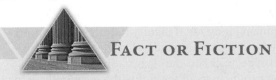

FACT OR FICTION

END-OF-LIFE CARE

When should you and your family plan end-of-life care?

Imagine that you are a college student with cancer. You undergo a year of chemotherapy and, after a brief return to normal life, you relapse. Your physician says chemotherapy and radiation therapy could be tried, but a bone marrow transplant (BMT) is your only chance for a real cure. He tells you and your parents complications from the transplant could cause your death but, without it, you may only live one year. You and your family discuss the alternatives and decide to have the transplant. You ask what will happen if the BMT fails, but your physician and family tell you to concentrate on getting better and avoid negative thoughts. You do not ask any more questions. The physician provides you with the consent form to read over. You briefly look at it and sign it.

The transplant preparation is worse than you had imagined and you experience painful side effects. You are fearful because you overheard through the hospital grapevine that some BMT patients went to the intensive care unit (ICU) and never came back. Still, you do not ask your family if these patients died and neither your family nor your physician ever inquires about your wishes in the event of your own need for intensive care.

One week after the BMT, before the new marrow has even taken hold in your body, you begin experiencing breathing difficulties. Over the next twenty-four hours, it becomes harder to breathe and difficult to speak more than two words at a time. You are frightened because you feel so hungry for air. As your family watches you struggle to breathe, they become frightened as well. A physician explains how you may soon need a ventilator, which requires a transfer to the ICU. You fear you will die there. You and your parents look to your physician, who is obviously worried. Your parents ask the physician to save you; he says the ventilator is your only chance.

You are transferred to the ICU and are put into a deep sleep, as the physician promised. You wake up enough to realize your fingers cannot move, your eyelids will not open, you cannot speak, and even a grimace is impossible. You are groggy most of the time. The voices of family members, of certain nurses that you come to recognize, occasional music, a light stroking on your arm, these become the highlights of your existence.

Time passes slowly and you lose track of the days. After some weeks, you notice you are more awake than before, yet you still cannot move. Nobody prepared you for the fact that you might be awake but unable to move a muscle. They had promised you would be asleep. The air goes into your lungs with so much force you feel like your lungs will burst. You choke on the tube in your windpipe. The ulcerations in your mouth and throat hurt continuously. Even worse than the pain and discomfort is the dawning realization that you are dying. You want to ask for more medicine to keep your discomfort and anxiety under better control. You want to say goodbye to your family and go home to die, but you cannot move or speak at all. You hear your family members whispering to each other. They tell you how much they love you, but you cannot respond to them. You die alone in the middle of the night; your last fleeting thought is that you wish you could have died surrounded by your family. They said you sighed before dying, but you were just trying to tell them not to die alone and totally helpless like you were just about to do. You know your death could have been different.

—Anonymous submission to a student nurse at Immaculata University; *see generally* Derish & Heuvel, 2000 (paraphrasing a similar scenario).

(See *Law Fact* at the end of this chapter for the answer.)

PRINCIPLES AND APPLICATIONS

The personal decision regarding how and when to die is one of the most intimate choices a person may make in a lifetime. *See Planned Parenthood of S.E. Pa. v. Casey*, 505 U.S. 833, 851 (U.S. Supreme Court 1992). During the past century, advances in health care have led to dramatic changes in the life expectancy and death processes of Americans. Social and legal conventions from earlier times have struggled to effectively respond to today's unprecedented and unforeseen medical advancements. The National Center for Health Statistics reports that since 1900, the average life span of Americans has increased by more than thirty years, to seventy-eight years. This chapter uses the more accurate and value-neutral term *assisted dying* rather than *physician-assisted suicide* or *assisted suicide* for physician-assisted death. Active opponents of this evolution in terminology are generally opponents of palliative sedation who continue to criticize the choice for assistance in dying (Tucker, 2008).

This increase in longevity is accompanied by the emergence of long-term, chronic disease as the major pattern of death (Dallner & Manning, 2004). At the beginning of the twentieth century, death was typically a relatively rapid process and could occur at any age; now, the U.S. Census Bureau reports that more than 80 percent of deaths in the U.S. result from a chronic, non-communicable illness. Unlike earlier times, most Americans will die slowly (Kass, 2004). Society and the legal system have struggled to respond to this shifting paradigm of dying; that we die is certain, while how we die is not.

RIGHT-TO-DIE

The U.S. Supreme Court speaks in terms of the right-to-die and the meaning of personal dignity in extremely individualized terms, analyzing both sides of the coin of death in individual and societal contexts. That dignity is individual suggests each individual may have their own definition of dignity; thus, recognizing individual dignity requires recognition of each person's uniqueness (Dallner & Manning, 2004). The "right-to-die" is broadly defined in this chapter to include all the rights the terminally ill may have in controlling the circumstances of their death. Thus, the right-to-die includes the right of the competent terminally ill to refuse life-sustaining medical treatment as well as the right to stop prolonging their death. Assisted dying is legal in Germany, the Netherlands, Switzerland, and the United Kingdom (Rode, 2007).

Challenges to the right-to-die have generally focused on the concept of bodily integrity. The legal notion of bodily integrity, which includes the freedom from battery, has its origin in the requirement that informed consent is generally required for medical treatment. *See Cruzan v. Director, Missouri Department of Health,* 497 U.S. 261 (U.S. Supreme Court 1990). This principle leads to the corollary that patients generally possess the right not to consent, that is, to refuse treatment. The informed consent principle and its corollary often lead to conflicts between patients asserting their right to be free from unwanted medical treatment, and health care professionals and families who want to provide treatment (McStay, 2003).

Important Legal Decisions and Legislation

- 1828—Earliest American law explicitly outlawing assisted dying is enacted in New York (Act of Dec. 10, 1828, ch. 20, § 4, 1828 N. Y. Laws 19)
- 1969—First living will is written by attorney Louis Kutner and his arguments for it appear in the *Indiana Law Journal* (Kutner, 1969)
- 1969—Daniel Callahan founds the Hastings Center and launches the discipline of bioethics
- 1972—U.S. Senate Special Commission on Aging, chaired by attorney and Senator Frank Church, holds the first national hearings on death with dignity
- 1973—American Medical Association adopts a Patient's Bill of Rights recognizing the right of patients to refuse medical treatment
- 1974—First American hospice opens in New Haven, Connecticut
- 1974—Society for the Right to Die is founded
- 1974—Federal funding is provided for hospice programs
- 1976—New Jersey Supreme Court allows parents of young woman in persistent vegetative state to remove her from a life-sustaining ventilator; Court authorized removal on the basis of a right to privacy[LN1] (*see Matter of Quinlan,* 355 A.2d 647 (New Jersey State Supreme Court 1976), *U.S. Supreme Court certiorari denied, Garger v. New Jersey,* 429 U.S. 922 (U.S. Supreme Court 1976))
- 1976—California Natural Death Act is passed; it is the nation's first aid-in-dying statute, giving legal standing to living wills and protecting physicians from being sued for failing to treat incurable illnesses (*see* California Probate Code § 4670 (2000); California Probate Code § 4740 (2000))
- 1976—Eight states (Arkansas, California, Idaho, Nevada, New Mexico, North Carolina, Oregon, and Texas) enact right-to-die laws recognizing the right to refuse life-sustaining medical treatment
- 1980—World Federation of Right to Die Societies is formed, numbering twenty-seven organizations from eighteen different countries

(continues)

(continued)

- 1983—Medicare Hospice Benefit: providing reimbursement for hospice programs caring for the terminally ill
- 1986—California Court of Appeals finds that a twenty-seven-year-old competent woman with severe cerebral palsy had the right to forgo life-sustaining treatment (*see Bouvia v. Superior Court of Los Angeles,* 179 Cal.App.3d 1127 (Court of Appeal, Second District, Division 2, California 1986))
- 1987—The California State Bar Conference passes a resolution to become the first public body to approve of physician aid in dying
- 1990—U.S. Supreme Court decides that states are free to adopt evidentiary standards to indicate when a family member can make end-of-life decisions for one unable to do so; five Justices recognize a constitutional right of competent people to refuse life-sustaining treatment[LN2] (*see Cruzan,* 497 U.S. 261)
- 1990—American Medical Association adopts the formal position that, with informed consent, a physician can withhold or withdraw treatment from a patient who is close to death, and may also discontinue life support of a patient in a permanent coma
- 1991—Patient Self Determination Act (PSDA) mandating that health care institutions receiving Medicare or Medicaid funding give patients written information about their right to participate in medical decision-making and write advance directives (*incorporated into* 42 U.S.C.A. 1395cc(f) (2008))
- 1993—Compassion in Dying is founded in Washington state to counsel the terminally ill and provide information about how to die without suffering
- 1997—U.S. Supreme Court finds there is no constitutional right to assisted dying; Court indicates the issue is one state legislatures should determine; several Justices' opinions establish that Americans have a right to palliative sedation (*see Washington v. Glucksberg,* 521 U.S. 702 (U.S. Supreme Court 1997) (holding there is no constitutionally protected interest in the right to die that prohibits states from enacting laws against assisted dying); *Vacco v. Quill,* 521 U.S. 793 (U.S. Supreme Court 1997) (holding state laws may distinguish between the withdrawal of life-sustaining treatment and assisted dying without violating the U.S. Constitution))
- 1997—Oregon voters legalize assisted dying; Oregonians reaffirm legalization of assisted dying through a second voter referendum, becoming the first state in the country where palliative care is legal (*see* Oregon Death with Dignity Act of 1997, Oregon Rev. Stat. §§ 127.800-127.897 (2003))
- 2001—Netherlands officially legalizes euthanasia
- 2005—U.S. Court of Appeals for the 11th Circuit upholds the trial court's decision finding that a clear and convincing standard of evidence was met and that termination of Terri Schiavo's life-sustaining treatment was appropriate (*see Schiavo ex rel. Schindler v. Schiavo,* 403 F.3d 1289 (U.S. Court of Appeals for the 11th Circuit 2005))
- 2006—U.S. Supreme Court holds that the Controlled Substances Act does not authorize the Attorney General to ban the use of controlled substances for assisted dying; Oregon's Death With Dignity Law is upheld (*see Gonzales v. Oregon,* 546 U.S. 243 (U.S. Supreme Court 2006))
- 2008—Washington voters legalize assisted dying referendum closely patterned after the Oregon Death with Dignity Act

Sources: Griffiths et al., 2008; Lynn et al., 2000; McStay, 2003; Straton, 2006; Warnock & Macdonald, 2008.

PALLIATIVE SEDATION

The term *palliative sedation* is used in this chapter, but the process is also called *palliative sedation to unconsciousness, terminal sedation, continuous deep sedation, primary deep continuous sedation,* or *pharmacological oblivion in end-of-life care.* When the U.S. Supreme Court endorsed palliative sedation as an alternative to assisted dying (termed *physician-assisted suicide* by the Court in 1997), it set the stage for another battle in the right-to-die controversy.

See Cruzan, 497 U.S. 261; *Glucksberg,* 521 U.S. 702; *Vacco,* 521 U.S. 793.

Most patients reach a point where the goals of medical care change from an emphasis on prolonging life and optimizing function to maximizing the quality of remaining life, and palliative care becomes a priority (VHA, 2007). Palliative sedation is a routine continuation of palliative care enabling patients to maintain a sense of self-control and strength in their final days and hours. Continued intimate involvement in each of the final stages of death is essential in palliative care. When palliative sedation is viewed as a continuum of effective medical care, it grants control to patients and their families under the principle of respect for personal autonomy (Griffiths et al., 2008).

Definition of Palliative Sedation

Palliative sedation is defined as the induction of an unconscious state to relieve otherwise intractable distress and pain, and is frequently accompanied by the withdrawal of any life-sustaining means (McStay, 2003). When less aggressive means fail for patients suffering from severe pain, dyspnea (difficulty in breathing), or other symptoms resistant to treatment, palliative sedation becomes a clinical option of last resort (VHA, 2007).

Palliative sedation was a palliative care option long before the U.S. Supreme Court considered the constitutional implications of assisted dying. Physicians have always used palliative sedation to:

- Alleviate physical discomfort and pain
- Produce an unconscious state before the withdrawal of nutrition and hydration
- Relieve non-physical suffering

There is currently no comprehensive data regarding the use of sedation for pain control among palliative care patients who, faced with the prospect of a horrible and painful death from a terminal illness, choose to end their lives instead in a peaceful and dignified manner (Tucker, 2008). Various hospice and other patient studies have reported that sedation, with or without medical intervention or the withdrawal of nutrition and hydration, is generally used for symptom control among terminally ill patients. The average time from sedation to death appears to be between two and ten days (McStay, 2003). Palliative sedation changes the timing of death in only a minor way, but adds control in a major and socially approved way (Tucker, 2008).

Doctrines Supporting Palliative Sedation

Palliative sedation is typically the combination of two distinct actions, the:

- Induction of unconsciousness
- Withholding or withdrawal of life-sustaining measures, such as nutrition and hydration

The implications of palliative sedation depend upon whether individuals view these acts separately or as a single action (McStay, 2003).

Double Effect Principle

Palliative sedation is justified by the double effect principle as an alternative to what otherwise could be a prolonged and painful death (Tucker, 2008). According to this principle, consequences that would be wrong if caused intentionally become acceptable, even when foreseen, if the actions creating those consequences are intended for a morally permissible purpose. Generally, reliance on the principle of double effect requires the presence of four conditions:

- Act creating the risk of adverse consequences should be good, or at least morally neutral
- Actor should intend the good effect and not the bad effect, although the bad effect may be foreseen
- Bad effect should not be a means to the good effect
- Good effect should outweigh the bad effect

(McStay, 2003)

Under this principle, drugs that may hasten death may be administered so long as the intent is solely to relieve suffering. In this scenario, the good effect of relief from suffering is intended, while death is merely foreseen. Criticism of the role of the double effect principle occurs on various grounds.

Overemphasis on Prohibition

Emphasis against intentionally causing death may encourage some health care professionals to be overly apprehensive in providing appropriate end-of-life care. This apprehension might lead to conflicts when patients wish to withdraw nutrition and hydration. Another risk is that pain medications may be underprescribed. Unfortunately, the likelihood of these situations arising is probably unavoidable, given the current state of the law.

Complexity of Determining Compassionate Intent

Although ascertaining intent is generally complex, the legal system regularly relies upon its ability to perform this function, particularly in the criminal justice context. While intent is difficult to judge, the law has developed a presumption in favor of compassionate intent in the context of end-of-life decisions, as opposed to intent to kill (Foley, 2004). Although the concept of compassionate intent is still undeveloped, the law will eventually take the complexity of this issue into account.

Lack of Unanimous Acceptability

While the absolute prohibition on intentionally causing death does not comport with all religious and cultural principles, it is consistent with the current state of the law (McStay, 2003). No state permits voluntary euthanasia, and only Oregon and Washington allow assisted dying. Voluntary euthanasia, where a lethal drug is administered by someone other than the patient, is prohibited in Oregon, but is legal in the Netherlands, Belgium, Columbia, and Japan, and is expected to become legal shortly in Luxembourg (Griffiths et al., 2008; Rode, 2007). Thus, the double effect principle represents a sound policy to the extent that it allows palliative sedation without engaging in illegal conduct.

The alternatives to the double effect principle are to:

- Accept the intent to cause death, or
- Forbid conduct with the foreseeable effect of hastening death

The former alternative directly contradicts the law of almost every state, and the latter alternative leaves some patients (those who are incapacitated before sedation, yet who have previously clearly stated their desire to hasten their death at some point) without the ability to obtain palliative sedation. Even with excellent pain and symptom management, a fraction of dying patients will still confront a dying process so prolonged and marked by such extreme suffering and deterioration, palliative sedation is the least-bad alternative (Tucker, 2008). Thus, as a matter of public policy, the double effect principle is arguably the most practical option.

Misplaced Emphasis on Personal Autonomy

Personal autonomy in medical decision-making, regardless of its merits, is of little value in end-of-life legal issues, since there is no constitutional right to state-sanctioned assisted dying. If states other than Oregon and Washington begin to permit assisted dying, then personal autonomy will become a more viable public policy to guide palliative sedation.

Moral Dilemmas

1. If personal autonomy extends to the time and manner of one's death in the states of Oregon and Washington, should this principle not also apply whenever people believe their death is better than continued life?

Foreseen and Unintended Consequences

The fact that both foreseen and unintended consequences are taken into account by the law does not necessarily mean that actions undertaken pursuant to the double effect principle is a basis for civil or criminal liability (McStay, 2003). None of the modern laws treat attempted suicide as a crime; moreover, even long ago when attempted suicide was a crime in the U.S., prosecutors only rarely filed charges for a suicide attempt that harmed no one but the attempter (LaFave, 2003). The reason for this suicide policy is obvious: criminal liability for foreseen consequences arises only upon unjustified actions.

Moral Dilemmas

1. If it is no longer criminal to attempt suicide, can it logically be criminal to assist someone in committing suicide?

Similarly, civil liability is based upon the objective, reasonable person standard. In the context of professional medical liability, the fact that palliative sedation is part of the standard continuum of palliative care should preclude liability. Thus, the fact that a patient's death is a foreseeable consequence of palliative sedation would only be one element for determining civil liability.

Moral Dilemmas

1. Why should the chronically ill have to endure pain, suffering, and indignity for a much longer time than the terminally ill (often defined as those with six months or less to live)?

Voluntary Refusal of Nutrition and Hydration

The voluntary refusal of nutrition and hydration takes two forms: patients refuse artificial nutrition and hydration or they simply refuse to eat and drink. Clinically, at the time of palliative sedation, most patients have generally already stopped eating and drinking. For patients who require artificial nutrition and hydration, the right to refuse is the same right as being free from unwanted medical intervention. The act of refusing artificial nutrition and hydration is like a medical intervention and, thus, the legal right to forego this treatment is more clearly established than the voluntary cessation of eating and drinking.

Voluntarily refusing to eat or drink has been likened to suicide by opponents of palliative sedation (without referencing the civil disobedience practiced by Mohandas Gandhi and other civil rights leaders). Despite the lack of judicial authority on this issue, courts are unlikely to intervene when competent dying patients voluntarily stop eating and drinking (McStay, 2003). A desire to die does not decide the final outcome of a refusal of medical intervention. As long as death is approached passively, palliative sedation is the same as withdrawal of life-sustaining medical treatment (*see* Douglas, 2007). Personal autonomy supports the refusal or withdrawal of life-sustaining medical care. Autonomy is not contingent upon whether the refusal is of artificial nutrition and hydration or whether the patient voluntarily elects to discontinue eating and drinking (McStay, 2003).

The Debate Over Palliative Sedation

The palliative sedation debate is often confused by focusing on whether palliative care constitutes euthanasia. There is a range of opinions, ranging from those inflexibly opposed to palliative sedation to advocates of the practice. Some critics of palliative sedation compare it to euthanasia, viewing the induction of unconsciousness and the withdrawal or refusal of life-sustaining intervention as continuous acts that cause death. Combining the induction of unconsciousness with the withdrawal of life-sustaining measures, however, confuses the legal issues raised by palliative sedation (McStay, 2003).

The induction of unconsciousness and the withdrawal of life-sustaining medical interventions are separate acts supported by different legal and ethical doctrines. The induction of unconsciousness relies upon long-standing and accepted palliative care (Griffiths et al., 2008); the withdrawal of life-sustaining interventions relies upon the principle of personal autonomy. Despite the U.S. Supreme Court's endorsement of palliative sedation, the debate continues. While many issues center on the principle of double effect, three general positions have emerged:

- Approval
- Conditional support
- Criticism

Approval of Palliative Sedation

Most Americans (Pew, 2006) and physicians (Lo & Rubenfeld, 2005) support palliative sedation based upon the principles of informed consent and double effect. The American Medical Association views palliative sedation as a medically proper way to assure a modicum of dignity at death. It is a form of patient affirmation and empowerment when properly understood (Tucker, 2008). Proponents of palliative sedation maintain the practice is best understood as a continuum of proper treatment to which every patient should be entitled; it validates personal autonomy and patient self-determination (*see generally* Battin et al., 2008).

Conditional Support for Palliative Sedation

Others conditionally support palliative sedation, depending upon the form it takes. While palliative sedation is clearly lawful, some people find the withholding of artificial nutrition and hydration to be problematic, particularly when it takes place at an earlier point in the dying process than the sedation. This viewpoint distinguishes three forms of palliative sedation:

- Accompanying the withdrawal of artificial nutrition and hydration

- At the end-stage of a dying process, where a patient has not been dependent upon artificial nutrition and hydration
- In a patient not dependent upon artificial nutrition and hydration and accompanied by palliative sedation

(McStay, 2003)

The first two forms of palliative sedation are justified under general principles of palliative care. The patient, or patient's surrogate, consents to the process and no less risky means of relief are available.

Simultaneous Request for Palliative Sedation and Refusal of Nutrition and Hydration

The troublesome scenario, for conditional supporters of palliative sedation, involves patients whose dependence on nutrition and hydration accompanies the sedation administered to relieve intractable symptoms during the dying process. There is resistance to scenarios in which patients address palliative sedation and the withholding of nutrition and hydration simultaneously. Awareness that the alternative is forcing patients to eat and drink against their will by physical restraints or any other means alters this calculus for some people. Others remain concerned that unlike patients who first elect to forego artificial nutrition and hydration, patients who simultaneously choose palliative sedation and the withdrawal of nutrition and hydration have no opportunity to reflect upon their decision and change course prior to the induction of unconsciousness (McStay, 2003).

Inconsequence of Timing

There is no logical distinction between palliative sedation administered following the withdrawal of nutrition and hydration and simultaneous sedation. Although a state's interests in the preservation of life may be implicated, palliative sedation has not relied upon the degree to which the patient's decision is irreversible in time (*see Cruzan*, 497 U.S. 261). The focus has always been on the need for, and right to, relief from pain and suffering when patients seek such relief. Assuming a state's procedural requirements with respect to the withdrawal of life-sustaining medical intervention are established, supporters of the process claim that patient decisions to forego artificial nutrition and hydration should not be subject to additional legal scrutiny based solely upon the timing of when this occurs. To do so would undermine the personal autonomy principle that grants patients this right in the first place (*see* Kamisar, 2008).

Criticism of Palliative Sedation

Criticism of palliative sedation often centers on its comparison to assisted dying. Unfortunately, empirical and anecdotal evidence indicates health care professionals are not always informing terminally ill patients of all legal options in the state in which patients receive their health care (Curlin et al., 2007). As a result, patients are not always given the opportunity to make fully informed decisions about palliative care at the end of their lives.

Imposing their view on unsuspecting patients, critics refuse to distinguish between withdrawal of medical treatment and euthanasia. Critics argue that the process of withholding nutrition and hydration to induce unconsciousness actively causes death. This refusal to distinguish underlying compassionate intent in end-of-life care is like the example U.S. Supreme Court Justice Oliver Wendell Holmes gave when he wrote about the need to distinguish between intentional conduct and irresponsible conduct. Over a hundred years ago, Holmes noted that even a dog distinguishes between being stumbled over and being kicked (Holmes, 1881).

Underlying Disease Distinctions

In rejecting all arguments that palliative sedation is an alternative to assisted dying, critics distinguish between death from palliative sedation and death resulting from the withdrawal of nutrition and hydration without the induction of unconsciousness. Critics claim that with palliative sedation, the induced state of unconsciousness is responsible for the inability to eat and drink, not the natural progression of the underlying disease. On the other hand, proponents claim the inability to eat and drink is a result of the underlying disease.

Validity of the Double Effect Doctrine

Critics of palliative sedation reject the doctrine of double effect. They maintain that because the doctrine of double effect justifies hastened death, it justifies only sedation; the withdrawal of nutrition and hydration does nothing to relieve pain, but serves only to bring about death. In contrast, proponents claim the withdrawing of life-sustaining medical treatment is premised on the doctrine of informed consent. Thus, the double effect principle should not be rejected simply because it offers only a partial justification.

Moral Dilemmas

1. Can anyone prove palliative care actually hastens death if there is no way of knowing whether the patient would have died naturally within the same timeframe?

Although viewing palliative sedation as a single act is not unreasonable, critics would reverse decades of case law related to personal autonomy. Whether palliative sedation is a superior alternative to assisted dying is a separate issue from whether it is a legal and appropriate continuation of palliative care.

Palliative Sedation Compared to Assisted Dying and Euthanasia

Critics often compare palliative sedation to assisted dying and euthanasia, concluding palliative sedation has become more problematic than assisted dying or euthanasia. Specifically, critics contend palliative sedation poses the same risks of abuse as euthanasia, and greater risks of abuse than assisted dying, while serving fewer purposes of the right-to-die than either alternative. The only right-to-die issues addressed by palliative sedation are those relating to pain and suffering. In contrast, assisted dying and euthanasia address concerns related to:

- Avoiding a death that compromises personal dignity
- Controlling the timing of one's death
- Pain and suffering

Similarly, all of the concerns related to assisted dying and euthanasia exist with palliative sedation:

- Danger that the lives of the terminally ill, elderly, and disabled may be undervalued
- Erosion of trust in the health care system as a result of health care professionals causing (euthanasia) or hastening death (assisted dying)

Critics contend that palliative sedation has more in common with euthanasia than with assisted dying because the death-causing act is more under the control of someone other than the patient. Finally, critics maintain palliative sedation offers no advantage over assisted dying. Blaming the underlying disease for creating the need for palliative sedation is equally applicable to assisted dying. Proponents dismiss all these contentions and maintain palliative sedation is not euthanasia; death results from the withdrawal of artificial nutrition and hydration, not the introduction of a fatal agent.

Intent to Cause Death or Alleviate Suffering

Critics claim that relying upon compassionate intent as a basis to justify palliative sedation fails because unlike the withdrawal of an unwanted medical treatment, the intent of palliative sedation is to induce death. Proponents who argue this characterization of palliative sedation is similar to euthanasia, however, do not take into account the legal distinction between the withdrawal of unwanted medical treatment and euthanasia. The withdrawal of unwanted treatment and the refusal of nutrition and hydration are related to the patient's liberty interest, not to intent. Regardless of whether clinical realities support personal autonomy, the law places this decision ultimately with the patient. Patients may elect to forego treatment or nutrition and hydration because of their:

- Liberty interest resulting from the principle of autonomy
- Right to be free from battery

Intent is irrelevant with respect to the refusal of or request for the withdrawal of a life-sustaining medical intervention. Intent is a legal factor only when there is an intervention to cause death. *See Vacco*, 521 U.S. at 802 (painkilling drugs may hasten death, but the intent is, or may be, only to ease pain and suffering). As a practical matter, intent is hard to discern when the same drugs used in both treatment of symptoms and in euthanasia, both end in the death of the patient (Battin et al., 2007; Pickett, 2009).

Justification for Palliative Sedation

Palliative sedation is justifiable palliative care, supported by established jurisprudence. The U.S. Supreme Court bases its reliance on the existence of palliative sedation upon long-standing principles arising from law and standards of clinical care. However, this conclusion does rely upon the double effect principle. Assuming the double effect principle is ethically sound, the legal justification is clear. As long as the compassionate intent is not to cause death, the risk of death is justifiable in end-of-life care. For instance, the double effect could be compared to ordering dinner at a fashionable restaurant, when diners do not intend to order the most expensive item on the menu, but when they order surf and turf, their selection is one and the same thing. Selecting the most expensive item on the menu is unacceptable; ordering surf and turf is an acceptable choice. Under the double effect principle, one may not justify an intended harm with good consequences, but may justify, with such consequences, a harm that is only foreseen (Ferzan, 2008).

The principle of double effect guides the provision of palliative care, and is not some fabrication to shield the truth, but rather a highly useful ethical construct guiding care at the bedside and reducing, but not eliminating, uncomfortable ambiguity in end-of-life care. Of course, licensed prescribers know the use of an opioid infusion, morphine drip, or other interventions may shorten life in those imminently dying from disease or illness. Under Justice Holmes's approach to the law, end-of-life law is not a science founded on abstract principles but a body of practices that responds to particular situations. This theme is announced in the famous quote at the beginning of his first lecture on the common law, "the life of the law has not been logic: it has been experience" (Holmes, 1881).

The debate surrounding palliative sedation revolves largely around the validity of the double effect principle as a viable ethical construct. Critics tend to view palliative sedation as one continuous act directed by health care professionals (Pew, 2006). Supporters, on the other hand, view palliative sedation as an extension of sound palliative care, fully justified by the double effect principle and the doctrine of informed consent. Logic and experience need not always be different in end-of-life debates.

End-of-life palliative care is challenging, presenting the potential for clinical ambiguities. Health care professionals should struggle with the conflicting imperatives they face. Nonetheless, struggling with concerns about hastened death is not the same as inaction. Palliative sedation is a topic almost everyone will eventually have to confront. The current alternative is the under-treatment of pain and discomfort, and the possibility of facing death alone in the middle of the night.

ASSISTED DYING

The American Academy of Hospice and Palliative Medicine and the American Public Health Association adopted the term *assisted death* to discuss the end-of-life choice made by a mentally competent, terminally ill patient to self-administer medication for the purpose of hastening death. The term *assisted suicide* has been rejected as too emotionally charged and less accurate.

A recent Gallup Poll commissioned by the National Hospice and Palliative Care Organization found that three out of four adults indicated that, if terminally ill, they would seek a hospice program until death occurred naturally. Only about one-third of the total polled indicated that they would ask their physician to assist them to end their life (NHPCO, 2008). Other studies have shown that hospice care is a meaningful alternative for terminally ill patients and is effective in reducing the demand for assisted death. Although the unease about assisted death has been tempered by a greater focus on palliative care principles to manage the treatment of patients with terminal and life-threatening illnesses, recent developments in the U.S. regarding end-of-life issues may indicate that closer attention will be paid to hospice care. Society is already actively discussing the intersection between medicine and technology, the issue that captivated the nation in the Terri Schiavo debate

(Lynn et al., 2000). At the corners of this intersection are the death-with-dignity discussions, health law, and the important court cases of *Quinlan*, 355 A.2d 647, *Cruzan*, 497 U.S. 261, and *Schiavo*, 403 F.3d 1289.

Assisted dying permits patients to actively choose to end their lives before their disease ends their lives (Straten, 2006). Since Oregon became the first state to enact an assisted dying law, there have been no reported instances of physician abuse and no successful wrongful death lawsuits under the Oregon law, while more than two hundred Oregonians have ended their lives pursuant to procedures approved by the state (Oregon DHS, 2008). One explanation for this very low number is the high quality of hospice care in Oregon; nine out of ten people who have used the Oregon Death with Dignity Act were enrolled in hospice (Jackson, 2008). At the same time, this compares to the Netherlands, where about 2 percent of all Dutch deaths are due to assisted dying or euthanasia; 2 percent of approximately 145,596 deaths per year in the Netherlands is about 2,912 annual requests (*see* CIA, 2009).

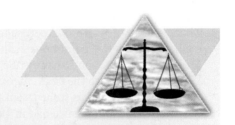

ASSISTED DYING

Gonzales v. Oregon
[U.S. Attorney General v. State of Oregon]
546 U.S. 243 (U.S. Supreme Court 2006)

FACTS: Voters approved a ballot initiative making Oregon the first state to legalize assisted dying. Three years later, voters affirmed the measure. The Oregon Death with Dignity Act exempts licensed prescribers who, in compliance with specific safeguards, prescribe a lethal dose of drugs upon the request of terminally ill patients, from civil or criminal liability. The law requires that patients seeking clinical assistance in committing suicide:

- Receive a diagnosis that they suffer from an incurable and irreversible disease that, within reasonable medical judgment, will cause death within six months
- Have two separate physicians review their request in order to determine it was made voluntarily and the decision was informed

The Oregon law, however, encountered resistance on the federal level from Attorney General John Ashcroft. The drugs used to assist patients with suicide are federally regulated under the federal Controlled Substances Act (CSA). Enacted in 1970, the CSA's main objectives are combating drug abuse and controlling the legitimate and illegitimate traffic of controlled substances. Drugs used in assisted dying are grouped under Schedule II, and the CSA requires that patients receive a written, non-refillable prescription before gaining access to Schedule II drugs.

The federal government grants licensed prescribers a registration subject to regulations from the U.S. Justice Department so Schedule II drugs can be lawfully prescribed. The CSA also provides that the federal government may deny, suspend, or revoke this registration if prescriber registrations are inconsistent with the public interest. One regulation under the CSA requires that prescribers acting in the usual course of their medical care issue prescriptions for a legitimate medical purpose. Ashcroft, an opponent of assisted dying, issued an interpretive rule declaring that the use of controlled substances in assisted dying was not legitimate medical care, thus making such prescriptions under the Oregon law a federal offense. Accordingly, anyone who prescribed a lethal dose of a controlled substance under the Oregon law would render their prescribing registration inconsistent with the public interest and could have their licenses suspended or revoked. Because prescribers could not prescribe controlled substances without a registration, the Ashcroft rule effectively blocked assisted dying. The state of Oregon, along with a physician, a pharmacist, and several terminally ill patients, sought declaratory and injunctive relief to prevent enforcement of the Ashcroft rule.

ISSUE: Does the federal government have the authority under the CSA to prohibit prescribing lethal doses of controlled substances under a state law decriminalizing assisted dying?

HOLDING AND DECISION: No, the CSA does not authorize the federal government to ban the use of controlled substances for assisted dying.

(continues)

(continued)

ANALYSIS: The U.S. Supreme Court held that the Ashcroft rule was not entitled to the deference to which administrative rules are generally entitled. Administrative rules may receive substantial deference if they interpret an issuing agency's own ambiguous regulation. Unlike regulations that give specificity to laws and reflect the expertise of the agency interpreting the regulations, the regulation the Ashcroft rule was interpreting merely restated the terms of the CSA in 1970. An agency does not acquire special authority to interpret its own words, when, instead of using its expertise to formulate a regulation, it merely paraphrases statutory language. Moreover, because the Ashcroft rule interpreted the 1984 amendments to the CSA, the Ashcroft rule could not be justified as some intent Congress or the U.S. Department of Justice had in 1970, fourteen years before adoption of the amendments.

Furthermore, the Court held that the Ashcroft rule was not entitled to deference as an interpretation of an ambiguous law. Rules interpreting an ambiguous law may receive substantial deference when Congress delegated authority to the agency to make rules carrying the force of law, and the agency interpretation was in the exercise of that authority. While the Court held the CSA term *legitimate medical purpose* was ambiguous, the federal government did not have the authority to declare state laws illegitimate; state law authorizes medical standards for patient care and treatment. According to the Court, Congress only delegated authority to the federal government to promulgate rules regarding the registration and control of the dispensing of controlled substances. The Ashcroft rule did not fall within the statutory definition of control, a term that was limited to adding drugs and other substances to regulatory schedules. Moreover, the Ashcroft rule did not fall within the registration authority of the U.S. Department of Justice. The Ashcroft rule was an interpretation of the federal requirements for valid prescriptions and went well beyond the federal government's power to register or deregister. Furthermore, the Court held the federal government was not entitled to define the substantive state standards of medical care as it did in promulgating the Ashcroft rule.

After finding that the Ashcroft rule did not deserve deference, the Court held that the federal government's interpretation of the CSA was not persuasive. From the CSA's text, the Court found Congress intended to regulate the medical care given by physicians insofar as it bars physicians from using their prescription-writing powers as a means to engage in illicit drug dealing and trafficking, but not to regulate medicine generally. The CSA presumes the regulation of medicine is a function of state police powers. In addition, the CSA specifically included a pre-emption provision stating the CSA should not be construed as congressional intent to occupy the medical field to the exclusion of any state law within the authority of a state. In the Court's analysis, the medical regime under the Oregon law was precisely the type of state regulation CSA had presupposed not to regulate. In the face of CSA's silence on palliative care and CSA's recognition of state regulation of the medical profession, the Court found it difficult to defend the federal government's declaration that the CSA criminalized state-sanctioned assisted dying.

The Court went on to address the federal government claim that the CSA's requirement to dispense every Schedule II drug pursuant to a prescription necessarily implies the substance is being made available to a patient for a legitimate medical purpose, thus requiring the federal government's judgment about the term *medical*. In turn, the federal government argued that *medical* refers to a healing art and cannot embrace the intentional causing of a patient's death. The Court, however, rejected the argument that the CSA's prescription requirement allowed the federal government to ban the prescription of controlled substances for state-sanctioned assisted dying. While the Court recognized the federal government's interpretation was reasonable, it held the CSA undermined this assertion of an expansive federal authority to regulate medicine. Regarding the remainder of the CSA, the prescription requirement is understood as a provision to ensure patients use controlled substances under the supervision of a physician and to prevent addiction and recreational abuse. This bars physicians from prescribing Schedule II drugs to patients who crave the drugs for prohibited uses. Read this way, the Court held the CSA did not support the federal government's interpretation.

RULE OF LAW: The regulation of licensed prescribing has traditionally been within the states' police power; it is unlikely the federal government has the authority to prohibit prescriptions of lethal doses of controlled substances under the CSA.

(See generally, Allen, 2006; Cass & Strauss, 2007; Gilman, 2007; Rutledge, 2005).

While this decision appears to clear the way for state measures to decriminalize assisted dying, the U.S. Supreme Court may not have settled the issue. The decision sparked some in Congress to attempt to pass legislation that would allow the federal government to prevent state-sanctioned assisted dying, but there was very little interest in any such restrictions. (Jackson, 2008; *see also* Warnock & Macdonald, 2008).

Several opponents of assisted suicide, the disability-rights organization Not Dead Yet, and the Catholic Church, are vocally seeking federal legislation to ban assisted dying or grant the federal government the specific authority the U.S. Supreme Court said it lacked (Battin et al., 2008). The Court did not say Congress could not act to block state laws authorizing assisted dying, although no such move is underway (Jackson, 2008).

More Compassionate Palliative Care

One of the unexpected, yet undeniable, consequences of Oregon and Washington permitting assisted dying is that many improvements in end-of-life care have occurred following implementation of each state's assisted dying legislation (*see* Tucker, 2008). Rather than becoming the brutal abattoir for unfortunate patients as some critics predicted, the states have become national leaders in providing compassionate palliative care (*see* Schneiderman, 2005). They have helped the nation create medical environments where end-of-life issues can be openly discussed (GAO, 2007).

Prescriptions for Controlled Substances

Specialists in palliative care have developed guidelines for the aggressive pharmacological management of intractable symptoms in dying patients, including sedation for those near death (VHA, 2007). Nonetheless, licensed prescribers may find their palliative care scrutinized for the prescription of legally controlled substances by opponents of palliative sedation and state-sanctioned assisted dying. At least two state medical boards have pursued physicians for over-prescribing pain medications (McStay, 2003).

Palliative sedation is more likely to alleviate concerns if safeguards exist to address opponents' concerns. Where assisted dying is already legal, there is no current evidence for the claim that legalized assisted suicide will have a disproportionate impact on patients in vulnerable groups (Battin et al., 2008). The most vulnerable patients often share three characteristics, they:

- Fear being a burden and adversely impacting their families
- Have misperceptions of what the last stages of life will be like
- Lack effective symptom control

(McStay, 2003)

Groups Considered Vulnerable to Assisted Dying
- Chronically ill
- Elderly
- Infants and minors
- Patients at the bottom of the economic pyramid
- Patients with psychiatric illnesses, including depression
- Physically disabled
- Uninsured and underinsured

Source: Battin et al., 2008.

Safeguards should be responsive to individual patients while being rigorous enough to protect vulnerable groups by:

- Ensuring the availability and effectiveness of palliative care
- Maintaining clarity with respect to the patient's disease state and anticipated life span
- Obtaining fully informed consent from patients
- Reaching a consensus with the patient's immediate family

(McStay, 2003; Starks et al., 2007)

The patient's terminal prognosis should be imminent. Patients should also be competent and fully informed, or incompetent with irreversible suffering and an ascertainable intent through an advanced health care directive or otherwise. When patients are incompetent, and a surrogate decision-maker is not available, caregivers should agree that no other acceptable means of palliative care is available (McStay, 2003). As a matter of informed consent, sedation should not occur until an agreement is reached that cardio-pulmonary resuscitation (CPR) will not be initiated. CPR is futile in this situation, and is inconsistent with the purpose of assisted dying (*see* GAO, 2007).

Moral Dilemmas

1. Is death always the least desirable option?

CONFRONTING THE END OF LIFE

This chapter and the preceding two chapters have looked at the debate over end-of-life issues, a topic that everyone is eventually forced to confront. As the U.S. Supreme Court has observed, controlling the time and manner of one's own death is the most evident way, the most profound way, to "define one's own concept of existence, of meaning, of the universe, and of the mystery of human life." *Casey*, 505 U.S. at 851.

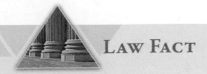

LAW FACT

END-OF-LIFE CARE

When should you and your family plan end-of-life care?

Today, everyone should plan and decide what health care they would like to receive at the end of their lives, who should make decisions on their behalf if they are dying and incapable of deciding when they have the right to die, and when they would consider, if ever, that their lives would not be worth saving because they were beyond their own definition of an acceptable quality of life.

—Anonymous submission to a student nurse at Immaculata University; *see generally* Derish & Heuvel, 2000 (paraphrasing a similar scenario).

CHAPTER SUMMARY

- The increase in Americans' life expectancies now means chronic disease is a common form of death, necessitating the reconsideration of how individuals approach and cope with death. Most patients reach a point where the goal of medical care changes from prolonging life and improving health to maximizing quality and comfort of remaining life.
- The U.S. Supreme Court has repeatedly leaned toward protecting personal dignity, bodily integrity, and autonomy in the right-to-die debate.
- Palliative sedation, endorsed by the U.S. Supreme Court, is an induced state of unconsciousness, usually accompanied by the withdrawal of life-sustaining medical care, such as artificial nutrition and hydration; it is not the same as physician-assisted suicide or euthanasia, as the physician does not actively or directly cause death, such as by administering a lethal drug cocktail.
- Long-accepted palliative care methods support the induction of unconsciousness, while the withdrawal of life-sustaining medical intervention is supported by the principle of personal autonomy.
- The double effect principle consists of two distinct actions viewed separately: one, the induction of unconsciousness, and two, the withholding or withdrawal of life-sustaining measures (such as artificial nutrition and hydration).
- Palliative sedation is justified by the double effect principle, which requires that the physician's actions leading to the consequence of death be intended for a morally permissible purpose (to relieve discomfort and pain).
- The double effect principle has been criticized by those who argue it may discourage physicians from palliative care, intent is difficult to ascertain, intentional death is not necessarily unacceptable, personal autonomy should take priority over the physician's intent, and physicians should be responsible for all consequences.
- Most Americans and physicians approve of palliative sedation; others conditionally approve of it depending on the form it takes; still others refuse to view it as anything other than euthanasia.
- Oregon and Washington are the first two states to decriminalize physician-assisted death, and thus far, the legislation appears to have had a positive effect in terms of providing compassionate end-of-life care.
- End-of-life legislation employs safeguards, such as ensuring that the patient is terminally ill and obtaining fully informed consent from the patient, or at least ascertainable intent, such as from an advanced directive.
- Americans can protect their end-of-life wishes by drafting an advance directive and health care power of attorney; yet more than 70 percent have failed to do so, despite their strong desire to exercise power over their own health care decisions.

LAW NOTES

1. In *Quinlan*, 355 A.2d 647, the New Jersey Supreme Court held that an incompetent patient in a persistent vegetative state has a constitutional right to privacy that overrides the state's interest in preserving the patient's life; the patient's surrogate may dictate that life-sustaining medical interventions be removed. While the states are split as to whether this right to refuse treatment is based solely on the doctrine of informed consent, or also in the federal and state constitutions, under either theory, the emphasis is on personal autonomy. Moreover, the right to forego unwanted medical treatment exists where the patient is neither terminal nor in a persistent vegetative state.

2. In *Cruzan*, 497 U.S. 261, the U.S. Supreme Court found that although patients may refuse life-sustaining treatment, states may establish rational procedures to ensure the patient's intent is accomplished. Focusing on common law doctrines supporting informed consent and against battery, the Court concluded that the corollary of the doctrine of informed consent is that patients generally possess the right not to consent; that is, they have the right to die. The Court inferred a competent person has a constitutionally protected liberty interest in refusing unwanted medical treatment. This inference was based on four prior decisions: *Washington v. Harper*, 494 U.S. 210 (U.S. Supreme Court 1990) (recognizing a significant liberty interest in avoiding the unwanted administration of antipsychotic drugs under the Due Process Clause of the Fourteenth Amendment); *Vitek v. Jones*, 445 U.S. 480 (U.S. Supreme Court 1980) (noting that transferring a patient to a mental hospital coupled with mandatory behavior modification treatment implicates liberty interests); *Parham v. J.R.*, 442 U.S. 584 (U.S. Supreme Court 1979) (recognizing a substantial liberty interest in not being confined unnecessarily for medical treatment); and *Jacobson v. Massachusetts*, 197 U.S. 11 (U.S. Supreme Court 1905) (balancing an individual's liberty interest in declining an unwanted smallpox vaccine against the state's interest in preventing the disease). Because of the consequences involved in refusal of life-sustaining treatment, the Court was willing to assume the Constitution would grant a competent person a constitutionally protected right to refuse nutrition and hydration.

CHAPTER BIBLIOGRAPHY

Allen, M. P. (2006). Justice O'Connor and the "right to die": Constitutional promises unfulfilled. *William & Mary Bill of Rights Journal, 14*, 821-840.

Battin, M. P. et al. (2008). Physician-assisted dying and the slippery slope: The challenge of empirical evidence. *Willamette Law Review, 45*, 91-136.

___. (2007). Legal physician-assisted dying in Oregon and the Netherlands: Evidence concerning the impact on patients in "vulnerable" groups. *Journal of Medical Ethics, 33*, 591-597.

Boucek, M. M. et al. (2008). Pediatric heart transplantation after declaration of cardiocirculatory death. *New England Journal of Medicine, 359* (7), 709-714.

Cass, R. A. & Strauss, P. L. (2007). The last word? The constitutional implications of presidential signing statements: The presidential signing statements controversy. *William & Mary Bill of Rights Journal, 16*, 11-25.

CIA (Central Intelligence Agency). (2009). *World Factbook: Netherlands*. Washington, DC.

Curlin, F. A. et al. (2007). Religion, conscience, and controversial clinical practices. *New England Journal of Medicine, 356*, 593-600.

Dallner, J. E., & Manning, D. S. (2004). Death with dignity in Montana. *Montana Law Review, 65*, 309-341.

Derish, M. T., & Heuvel, K. V. (2000). Mature minors should have the right to refuse life-sustaining medical treatment. *Journal of Law, Medicine & Ethics, 28*, 109-145.

Douglas, S. (2007). Conflict resolution at end-of-life relative to life support. *Ohio State Journal on Dispute Resolution, 23*, 89-103.

Ferzan, K. K. (2008). Beyond intention. *Cardozo Law Review, 29*, 1147-1190.

Foley, K. (2004). Compassionate care, not assisted suicide. In K. Foley & H. Hendin (Eds.), *The case against assisted suicide: For the right to end-of-life care* (pp. 293-310). Baltimore, MD: Johns Hopkins University Press.

GAO (Government Accountability Office). (2007). *End-of-life care: Key components provided by programs in four states*. Washington, DC: GAO.

Gilman, (2007). If at first you don't succeed, sign an executive order: President Bush and the expansion of charitable choice. *William & Mary Bill of Rights Journal, 15*, 1103-1172.

Griffiths, J. et al. (2008). *Euthanasia and law in Europe* (2nd ed.). Oxford, England: Hart Publishing.

Holmes, Jr., O. W. (1881). *The common law*. Boston, MA: Little, Brown, and Co.

Jackson, A. (2008, Fall). The inevitable death: Oregon's end-of-life choices. *Willamette Law Review, 45*, 137-160.

Kamisar, Y. (2008). Can *Glucksberg* survive *Lawrence*? Another look at the end of life and personal autonomy. *Issues in Law & Medicine, 24*, 95-119.

Kass, R. (2004). I will give no deadly drugs: Why doctors must not kill. In K. Foley & H. Hendin (Eds.). *The case against assisted suicide: For the right to end-of-life care* (pp. 17-40). Baltimore, MD: Johns Hopkins University Press (overviews the principles of compassion and patient autonomy).

Kutner, L. (1969). Due process of euthanasia: The living will: A proposal. *Indiana Law Journal, 44*, 539-554.

LaFave, W. R. (2003). *Criminal law* (4th ed.). San Francisco, CA: Thomson/West.

Lo, B., & Rubenfeld, G. (2005). Palliative sedation in dying patients. *Journal of the American Medical Association, 294*, 1810-1816.

Lynn, J. et al. (2000). *Improving care for the end of life: A sourcebook for health care managers and clinicians*. New York, NY: Oxford University Press.

McStay, R. (2003). Terminal sedation: Palliative care for intractable pain, post-*Glucksberg* and *Quill*. *American Journal of Law & Medicine, 29*, 45-76.

NHPCO (National Hospice and Palliative Care Organization). (2008, April 29). Press release: NHPCO responds to Medicare's proposal that will cut hospice rates. Alexandria, VA: NHPCO.

Oregon DHS (Oregon Department of Human Services). (2008). *Tenth annual report on Oregon's Death with Dignity Act*. Portland, OR: Oregon DHS Office of Disease Prevention & Epidemiology.

Pew (Pew Research Center for the People and the Press). (2006). *Strong public support for right to die*. Washington, DC: Pew.

Pickett, J. (2009). Can legalization improve end-of-life care? An empirical analysis of the results of the legalization of euthanasia and physician-assisted suicide in the Netherlands and Oregon. *Elder Law Journal, 16*, 333-373.

Rady, M. Y. et al. (2007). Non-heart-beating, or cardiac death, organ donation: Why we should care. *Journal of Hospital Medicine, 2* (5), 324-334.

Rode, S. (2007). End-of-life decision-making for patients in persistent vegetative states: A comparative analysis. *Hastings International & Comparative Law Review, 30* (3), 477-503.

Rutledge, P. B. (2005). Looking ahead: October term 2006. *Cato Supreme Court Review, 2005-2006*, 361-385.

Schneiderman, L. J. (2005), Physician-assisted dying. *Journal of the American Medical Association, 293*, 501.

Starks H. et al. (2007). Family member involvement in hastened death. *Death Studies, 31*, 105-130.

Steinbrook, R. (2007). Organ donation after cardiac death. *New England Journal of Medicine, 357* (3), 209-213.

Straton, J. B. (2006). Physician assistance with dying: Reframing the debate; restricting access. *Temple Political & Civil Rights Law Review, 15*, 475-482.

Truog, R. D., & Miller, F. G. (2008). The dead donor rule and organ transplantation. *New England Journal of Medicine, 359* (7), 674-675.

Tucker, K. L. (2008). In the laboratory of the states: The progress of *Glucksberg*'s invitation to states to address end-of-life choice. *Michigan Law Review, 106*, 1593-1611.

Van der Heide, A. et al. (2007). End-of-life practices in the Netherlands under the Euthanasia Act. *New England Journal of Medicine, 356* (19), 1957-1965.

Veatch, R. M. (2008). Donating hearts after cardiac death: Reversing the irreversible. *New England Journal of Medicine, 359* (7), 672-673.

VHA (Veterans Health Administration): National Ethics Committee. (2007). The ethics of palliative sedation as a therapy of last resort. *American Journal of Hospice & Palliative Care, 23* (6), 483-491.

Warnock, M., & Macdonald, E. (2008). *Easeful death: Is there a case for assisted dying?* New York, NY: Oxford University Press.

PART XI

OUR HEALTH CARE SYSTEM'S RESPONSE TO NEW TECHNOLOGIES

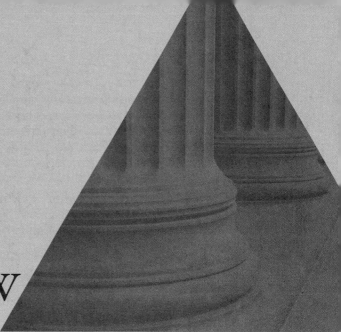

CHAPTER 31

STEM CELLS AND REGENERATIVE MEDICINE*

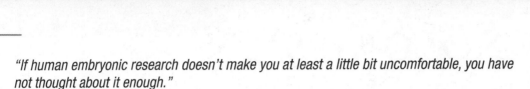

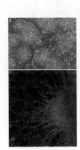

"If human embryonic research doesn't make you at least a little bit uncomfortable, you have not thought about it enough."

—DR. JAMES A. THOMSON, DIRECTOR OF REGENERATIVE BIOLOGY, MORGRIDGE INSTITUTE FOR RESEARCH, WHOSE GROUP ISOLATED THE FIRST HUMAN EMBRYONIC STEM CELL (hESC) LINES

IN BRIEF

This chapter starts with a tutorial, underscoring how the term *stem cell* can have different meanings. It then looks at the potential of stem cell therapy and the controversy surrounding the use of human embryonic stem cells (hESCs). This is the only topic in this textbook where an appreciation of the science is essential to understanding the political and ideological agendas dictating the direction of this controversial medical research.

While regenerative medicine focuses attention on hESCs, multipotent stem cells also typically give rise to the type of cells in the tissues in which they are found. With the promise of pluripotent and multipotent stem cells, studying the scientific, ethical, and legal aspects of this research will illustrate the possibilities of implementing innovative technologies and the infrastructure needed for such medical breakthroughs to flourish. Progress has been brisk since hESCs were first isolated in 1998.

Fact or Fiction

Research on Human Embryonic Stem Cells

Should the federal government provide funding for basic scientific research involving hESCs?

Mary Doe is a frozen human embryo in liquid nitrogen in a state of cryopreservation in which her life is presently suspended, at an unnamed *in vitro* fertilization (IVF) clinic. Mary Doe's name was given by the National Association for the Advancement of Preborn Children, an organization dedicated to advocating for equal humanity and personhood of preborn children, including children *in vitro*. In response to President Clinton's policy favoring research and permitting funding for stem cells from cadaveric fetal tissue and embryos remaining after infertility treatments, a lawsuit was filed on behalf of Mary, and all other frozen human embryos similarly situated. The lawsuit sought a permanent injunction against any and all plans to undertake hESC experimentation in the U.S.

—*Doe v. Shalala*, 122 Fed.Appx. 600 (U.S. Court of Appeals for the 4th Circuit 2004),

U.S. Supreme Court certiorari denied, 546 U.S. 822

(U.S. Supreme Court 2005).

(See *Law Fact* at the end of this chapter for the answer.)

Principles and Applications

The International Society for Stem Cell Research has called for the U.S. government to join the global community in funding all avenues of stem cell research, and to replace politics and ideology with dispassionate scientific investigation. An open letter from the Society noted that while reprogramming of multipotent stem cells has captured the imagination of scientists everywhere, research on hESCs should not be abandoned (ISSCR, 2008).

For more than a decade, the pharmaceutical industry has been using animal and human stem cells in its laboratories to help screen new drug compounds and identify safer and more effective medicines (Pfizer, 2009). In the past fifty years, many of the common human virus vaccines, such as measles, rubella, hepatitis A, rabies, and poliovirus, have been produced in cells derived from human embryos. Both hESCs and multipotent stem cell lines with the characteristics of hESCs are remarkable in drug discovery.

As illustrated in Figure 31-1, stem cells also help the medical products industry better understand personalized medicine, genetic development and control, and indentify important biomarkers. *Personalized medicine* is the anticipated use of a genotype or gene expression profile to tailor medical care to meet the needs of a specific patient, as distinct from medical care based on a patient's history and physical profile (derived from laboratory tests, imaging, and other medical tests); it also refers to drugs tailored to specific genotypes in terms of dosing, as distinct from drug dosing developed for a general disease population.

Stem Cells

Stem cells are primal cells that have the potential to develop into many different cell types in the body; they are not yet specialized or differentiated into any of over two hundred somatic cell types (NIH, 2008). Stem cells do not perform the tasks somatic body cells do. For instance, they do not deliver oxygen like the red blood cells do (Hayes et al., 2006). Rather, they act as the repair system for the body; theoretically they can divide without limit to replenish other cells. When a stem cell divides, each new daughter stem cell has the potential to remain a stem cell or become a more specialized cell, such as a red blood cell or a muscle cell (*see generally* Ramalho-Santos & Willenbring, 2007).

The National Institutes of Health reports over two thousand clinical trials for multipotent stem cells and seven for hESCs. Stem cell research could greatly facilitate the study of disease, drug development, and toxicology testing, and may allow the production of therapeutically useful immune-compatible hESCs. If developed to the point of scientific reliability, stem cell technologies could be a valuable research tool for the study of other aspects of human cell development and differentiation, including gene expression patterns, imprinting, and cell-cell signaling (Hurlbut, 2007).

Categories of Stem Cells

Many of the terms used to define stem cells depend on the behavior of the cells in the living organism, under specific laboratory conditions outside a

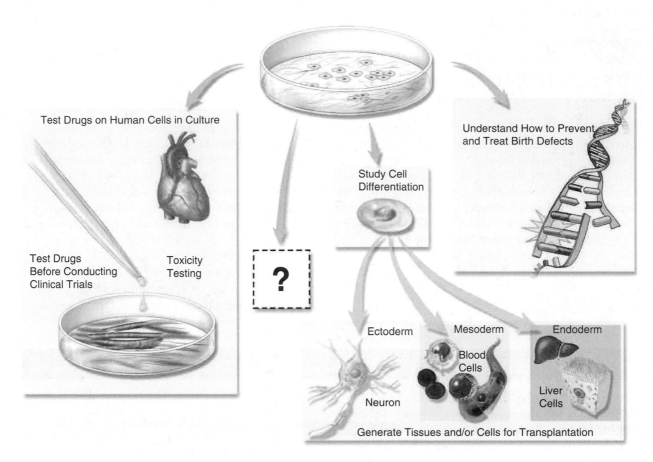

FIGURE 31-1: Potential Applications of Stem Cell Research

Source: NIH, 2008. © Terese Winslow (2008).

living organism (*in vitro*), or after transplantation into a living organism (*in vivo*) (Domen, 2006). By definition, embryonic stem cells are undifferentiated pluripotent cells that can indefinitely grow *in vitro* in a controlled environment (NIH, 2008a). Because of recent findings of alternative sources of hESCs and the techniques of preparing them that do not involve the use of embryo intermediates, the terms *pluripotent* and *multipotent* will be used in this chapter rather than *embryonic* and *adult stem cells*, which are better suited for *in vivo* discussions. As illustrated in Figure 31-2, there are four categories of stem cells based on their ability to differentiate:

- Totipotent
- Pluripotent
- Multipotent (or progenitor)
- Unipotent

Totipotent Stem Cells

Totipotent, from the Latin word *totus* meaning entire, stem cells' potential is total (NIH, 2008).

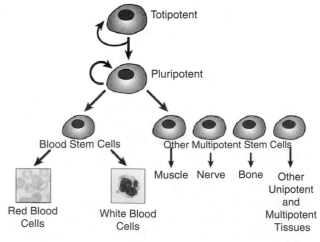

FIGURE 31-2: Hierarchy of Stem Cells

Source: NIH, 2008.

Totipotent stem cells are able to differentiate into an entire organism (Irish Council on Bioethics, 2008). A fertilized ovum is considered totipotent. An oocyte is a female germ cell in the process of development. The oocyte is produced in the ovary and gives rise to the ovum, which can be fertilized. For sake of simplicity, this chapter refers to the ovum rather than making a distinction between oocytes that develop into ovum.

Distinction Between *In Vivo* and *In Vitro* Embryos

In vivo, a fertilized ovum, also known as a zygote, undergoes cell division after it travels through the oviduct to the uterus where it may implant and may grow to an embryo. In this chapter, human organisms in the early stages of growth and differentiation, from fertilization to the beginning of the third month of pregnancy, are defined as embryos. Here, it is important to distinguish between the viability of an embryo *in vivo* and its viability *in vitro*. An *in vitro* embryo is not viable in terms of a living human organism outside the uterus. An *in vivo* embryo is not viable until week twenty-four or twenty-five following fertilization. To simplify understanding of stem cells, no distinction is made between embryos *in vivo* and *in vitro* in this chapter.

Continuous Processes

A range of positions are taken about fertilization as a continuous process and the moral status, if any, that defines the value accorded to this status. The moral status attributed to embryos is therefore likely to determine the level of legal protection granted to them. This is the core of the debate about stem cell research (Irish Council on Bioethics, 2008).

In general science terms, about three days after fertilization, the cells are totipotent, or capable of giving rise to an entire organism, including all the cell types in the human body, and all the cell types in the extra-embryonic supporting tissues, such as the placenta and the umbilical cord (Atala et al., 2007). The process of fertilization begins with the union of sperm and ovum and ends with the fusion of the maternal and paternal DNA creating a single cell, called a zygote (Irish Council on Bioethics, 2008). In this chapter, fertilization refers to the implantation of the newly developing embryo at five days after conception, or the blastocyte, into the wall of the uterus (NIH, 2008). Embryos develop from this cluster of blastocyte cells, which

are pluripotent embryonic stem cells and give rise to all of the different types of cells of the developing embryo. Implantation connects the embryo to the maternal blood supply, allowing it to continue developing and establishing pregnancy (*see generally* Black's, 2004; NAS, 2006). Embryonic stem cells can therefore be either totipotent or pluripotent, depending on the state of the development of the embryo from which they are isolated (Irish Council on Bioethics, 2008).

Pluripotent Stem Cells

While there is no standardized definition of *pluripotency* (NIH, 2007), pluripotent sten cells can give rise to any type of cell in the body except those needed to develop an embryo (NIH, 2008). Pluripotent stem cells are able to differentiate into all of the specialized cell types of the body, but cannot generate an entire organism on their own (Irish Council on Bioethics, 2008). Placenta and umbilical cord cells are extra-embryonic supporting tissues.

As illustrated in Figure 31-3, hESCs are derived from the inner cell mass (ICM) of early embryos. Because of their ability to differentiate into all three embryonic germ layers (mesoderm, endoderm, and ectoderm), the embryonic source of all cells of the body, and finally into specialized somatic cell types, hESCs are thought to have much greater developmental potential than multipotent stem cells. This means hESCs may be able to give rise to cells found in all tissues of the embryo except for germ cells (NIH, 2008).

The first differentiation event occurs in humans at approximately five days, when an outer layer of cells committed to becoming part of the placenta, or the trophectoderm, separates from the ICM. The ICM cells are pluripotent and have the potential to generate any cell type of the body. After implantation, they are quickly depleted as they differentiate into other specialized somatic cell types with more limited development potential, or multipotent and unipotent stem cells (Atala et al., 2007).

Multipotent Stem Cells

Stem cells that can give rise to a small number of different cell types are generally called multipotent (NIH, 2008a). Multipotent stem cells can only differentiate into a particular subset of specialized cell types (Irish Council on Bioethics, 2008). Found in very small numbers throughout the body, multipotent

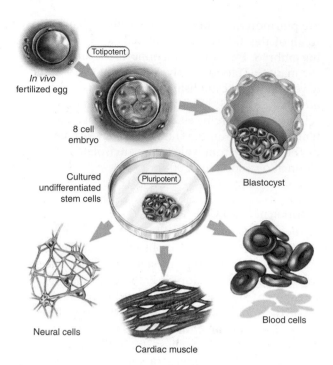

FIGURE 31-3: Pluripotent Stem Cells

Source: Wikimedia Commons (2009).

stem cells replenish and repair many of the cells of the body.

In vivo, they are believed to differentiate only into the types of cells near where they are located (Hayes et al., 2006). Multipotent stem cells are difficult to locate in the organs because there may be only one multipotent stem cell in the millions of cells making up an organ (Atala et al., 2007). In addition, multipotent stem cells are more challenging to culture in the lab than hESCs (Hayes et al., 2006).

Unipotent Stem Cells

Unipotent stem cells are usually cells in adult organisms that are capable of differentiating along only one lineage. Multipotent stem cells in many differentiated, undamaged tissues are typically unipotent and give rise to just one cell type under normal conditions; this process allows for a steady state of self-renewal for tissues and organs (Domen et al., 2006).

Sources of Human Stem Cells

The sources of human stem cells now include:

- hESCs (isolated from the inner mass of human embryos)
- Multipotent stem cells
- Stem cells from amniotic fluid
- Umbilical cord blood cells

Alternative Sources of Human Pluripotent Stem Cells

hESCs isolated from human embryos are a few days old (NIH 2008a). Initial hESCs are derived by removing the ICM from its normal embryonic environment and culturing the cells under appropriate conditions (Atala et al., 2007). Cells from these embryos can then be used to create pluripotent stem cell lines, as cell cultures can be grown indefinitely in the laboratory (NIH, 2008). These ICM-derived cells can continue to proliferate and replicate themselves indefinitely and still maintain the developmental potential to form any cell type of the human body (Battey et al., 2008). These pluripotent, ICM-derived cells are hESCs (Atala et al., 2007).

Stem cell lines grown in the lab provide scientists with the opportunity to engineer them for use in transplantation or treatment of diseases. For example, before scientists can use any type of tissue, organ, or cell for transplantation, they must overcome attempts by the immune system to reject the transplant. In the future, scientists may be able to modify hESC lines in the laboratory by using gene therapy or other techniques to overcome this immune rejection. Scientists might also be able to replace damaged genes or add new genes to hESCs in order to give them characteristics to ultimately treat or even cure diseases (Battey et al., 2008).

Techniques Involving Embryonic Intermediates

While hESCs usually come from surplus embryos from IVF clinics, hESCs can also be created from:

- Primordial germ cells
- Dead embryos
- Genetically abnormal embryos
- Single cell embryo biopsies
- Parthenogenesis
- Somatic cell nuclear transfers (SCNT)
- Altered nuclear transfers (ANT)

Traditional Techniques from Surplus Embryos

The University of Wisconsin-Madison generated the first hESC lines in 1998 from embryos obtained from an IVF clinic. These embryos were no longer wanted for reproductive purposes and donated with consent for research purposes. IVF embryos no longer wanted for reproductive purposes are generally incinerated as medical waste. The original hESC lines were prepared by removing the ICM from the donated blastocyst and placing those cells into a specialized culture medium (Battey et al., 2008). A blastocyst is a pre-implantation embryo that develops five days after the fertilization of an ovum by a sperm. It contains all the material necessary for a complete human being. It is smaller than the period at the end of a sentence (NAS, 2006).

hESC lines are extremely difficult to grow in culture. The cells require a highly specialized growth medium that contains essential ingredients critical to maintain the cell's self-renewing and pluripotent properties. Cultures require the support of cells either directly as a feeder cell layer or indirectly as a source of conditioned medium in feeder-free culture systems. The feeder cells secrete important nutrients and otherwise support stem cell growth, but are treated so they cannot divide (Battey et al., 2008).

Critically, until 2009, scientists were only permitted government funding to continue work on a handful of batches of stem cells already extracted from embryos. The number of viable batches varied, from about sixty to about twenty. Many of these embryos were created at IVF clinics and were either in indefinite frozen storage or destined to be discarded (Wharton, 2006). In addition, the culture medium used for the hESC lines approved by the federal government for research contained mouse cells and bovine serum. This made these approved lines unacceptable for therapy due to the risk that they may cause immune rejection and cancers.

Moral Dilemmas

1. Is the federal government's justification for freezing a fast-growing area of scientific inquiry acceptable in a democratic capitalist economy?

2. When should the Executive Orders of a president influence private/public funding balances and restrict scientists' freedom to conduct their research?

3. Should private/public funding balances be a legislative function rather than a function of the executive branch of government?

4. Should public funds be used for hESC research when there is political deadlock about its merits and morality?

From Primordial Germ Cells

Of all the cell types obtained from the differentiation of hESCs, primordial germ cells are arguably the most fascinating, as they represent the *in vitro* completion of the reproductive cycle of the organism from which the hESC line was derived (Marques-mari et al., 2009). Primordial germ cells are destined to become either ovum or sperm cells. The resulting cell lines are called germ cell lines and share many of the same properties as hESCs (Battey et al., 2008).

While scientists at Johns Hopkins Medical School first developed a technique for generating hESC lines in 1998 by culturing primordial germ cells from five- to seven-week-old embryos, it took a decade of European research to produce human primordial germ cells in useful numbers. Scientists at the University of Newcastle in England recently isolated two hESC lines from human primordial germ cells, which will significantly expand this research avenue (Torrisi, 2007).

From Dead Embryos

There is no legal criterion for determining when human embryos are dead. For developed humans, life is considered to end when the criteria for brain death are met, but corresponding criteria are lacking for human embryos (Landry, 2006).

In 2006, scientists at the University of Newcastle in England generated hESC lines from IVF embryos that had stopped dividing (Zhang, 2006). They derived the hESCs using traditional techniques from surplus blastocysts; the IVF embryo was simply considered dead because it had ceased to divide. Embryos that stop dividing are not suitable for implantation; they are considered nonviable because they are not capable of living or developing successfully.

The legal framework for justifying the use of this technique is similar to organ donation from a deceased donor who is declared brain dead. Embryos that die from natural causes cannot develop into fetuses. Since dead embryos are not preferentially selected for implantation in women undergoing fertility treatment, they can provide a source from which to derive hESCs without destroying a living embryo. Therefore, this source of hESCs should be morally acceptable and consequently legally acceptable to the federal government (Landry, 2006).[LN1]

To be useful for therapy, hESC lines derived from dead embryos should be carefully monitored for genetic abnormalities or other defects which may have caused the morula, which, in human development, is a four-day old embryo, or normal blastocyst not to develop.

From Genetically Abnormal Embryos

When a couple is concerned about producing a child with a genetic disorder, they may chose to conceive via IVF, using a technique known as pre-implantation genetic diagnosis (PGD) to determine whether the embryo carries the genetic disorder. The PGD technique involves the removal of a single cell from the embryo for testing. If the embryo is found to be positive for the genetic disorder it is generally discarded as medical waste.

Scientists at the University of New South Wales in Australia have derived hESC lines from genetically abnormal embryos to help understand genetically based disorders (Sidhu et al., 2008). Muscular dystrophy, Huntington's disease, thalessemia, fanconi's anemia, Marfan syndrome, adrenoleukodystrophy, and neurofibromatosis, as well as other genetic disorders, are being researched using this technique (Battey et al., 2008).

From Single Cell Blastocyst Biopsies

In 2006, scientists at Advanced Cell Technologies established hESC lines from single blastomeres taken from pre-implantation blastocysts (Chung et al., 2006). Biopsy of a single blastomere is similar to the technique used in PGD, which does not interfere with the development potential of the blastocyst (Klimanskaya et al., 2006). By growing a single blastomere, the resulting cells may be used for both genetic testing and stem cell derivation without affecting the clinical outcome of the procedure. The resulting stem cells derived from this biopsy technique retain the potential to form derivatives of all three embryonic germ layers, both *in vitro* and *in teratomas*, or noncancerous tumors.

Nevertheless, there is debate about the ethics of this technique. Proponents of this technique suggest that since it requires only one blastomere, the remaining blastomeres may yet be implanted and develop into a human being (Chung et al., 2006). The ability to create new stem cell lines and clinical therapies without destroying blastocysts should address any ethical concerns and allow the generation of matched tissue for children and siblings born from transferred blastocysts. Critics maintain the question is unanswered as to whether the single blastomere removed for the purposes of developing a stem cell line is itself totipotent and therefore capable of developing into an embryo. If this is the case, then its destruction is destruction of a potential embryo, which is no different than destruction of the blastocyst from which it was extracted (NIH, 2007).

Created via Parthenogenesis

In 2006, scientists at Kyoto University in Japan first showed that four genes inserted into the mature skin cell of a mouse were enough to return the cell to a primordial, embryonic-like state (Takahashi & Yamanaka, 2006). Several groups of scientists have since achieved the same result with human cells. Within a year, scientists at the University of Wisconsin-Madison and Kyoto University in Japan used parthenogenesis to derive hESCs (Yu et al., 2007). Parthenogenesis is the creation of a human embryo without fertilizing the ovum with a sperm. To achieve this feat, scientists tricked the ovum into believing it was fertilized, so it would begin to divide and form a blastocyst (Battey et al., 2008).

Essentially, human somatic cells are reprogrammed to become hESCs (Yu et al., 2007). This technique may lead to the ability to generate tissue-matched stem cells for transplantation to treat women who are willing to donate their own ova (Battey et al., 2008). Such induced hESC lines should also be useful in the production of new disease models and in drug development, as well as for other applications in transplantation medicine.

From Altered Nuclear Transfer

In 2006, scientists at the Massachusetts Institute of Technology (MIT) demonstrated that ANT can be carried out to produce hESCs (Meissner & Jaenisch, 2006). This method employs the techniques of SCNT; the nucleus of the host ovum is removed and replaced with the nucleus from a somatic cell, then stimulated to divide. In ANT, scientists turn off a gene needed for implantation in the uterus in the patient cell nucleus before it is transferred into the donor ovum (Battey et al., 2008). This alteration precludes the coordinated organization and developmental potential necessary for the resulting biological entity to be an embryo, but it still allows the entity to generate hESCs (Hurlbut, 2007). Abnormal nuclear transfer blastocysts are then created that are inherently unable to implant into the uterus, but which are capable of generating customized hESCs (Meissner & Jaenisch, 2006).

The derivation of hESCs by ANT holds great promise for research and therapy. In contrast to traditional techniques from surplus blastocysts, ANT could produce hESC lines with an unlimited range of specifically selected and controlled genotypes. ANT could also help define the boundaries that distinguish true organisms from "biological artifacts" and thereby provide moral precedent to guide future progress in developmental biology (Hurlbut, 2007).

From Somatic Cell Nuclear Transfers

As illustrated in Figure 31-4, this technique uses a genetically modified somatic cell as the source of a nucleus and genome for SCNTs into a human oocyte (NIH, 2007). In SCNT, human ova are collected from a volunteer donor who has taken drugs to stimulate the release of more than one ovum during the menstrual cycle. Scientists then remove the nucleus from the donated ovum and replace it with the nucleus from a somatic cell, a differentiated multipotent cell from elsewhere in the body. The ovum with the newly transferred nucleus is then stimulated to develop through parthenogenesis. The ovum may develop only if the transplanted nucleus is returned to the pluripotent

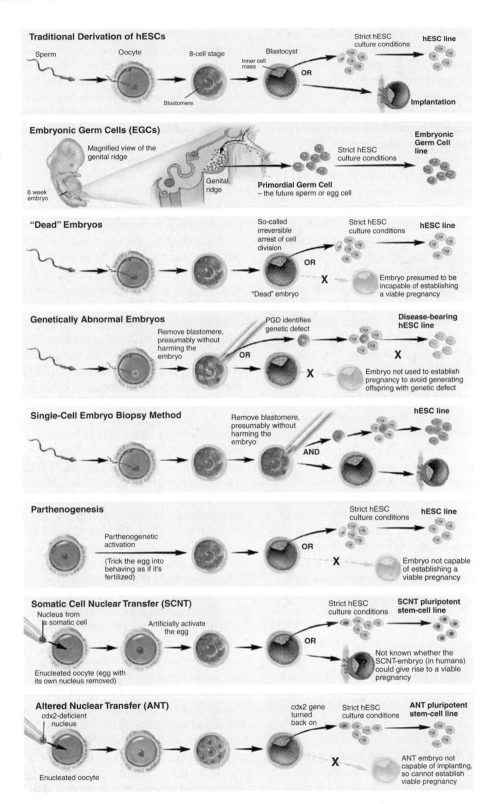

FIGURE 31-4: Creation of hESCs

state by factors present in the ovum cytoplasm. This alteration in the state of their mature nuclei is called nuclear reprogramming. When the parthenogenesis progresses to the blastocyst stage, the ICM is removed and placed into culture (Battey et al., 2008).

While traditional techniques involving embryonic intermediates may trigger the immune response when introduced into the body of another person, SCNT has the advantage of being made from a person's own body cells. Therefore, hESCs produced from SCNT should not illicit rejection on a primary genetic basis. SCNT-induced hESCs still may, however, have some chance of rejection because mitochondrial DNA from the ovum donor is still present when the nucleus is transferred. Most importantly, SCNT may be used to create a bank of stem cells from people who have a genetic disease; this will in turn help scientists learn more about genetic diseases and their progression. This type of second-generation cloning technique would lend itself to patient-tailored cell therapy in the future, bypassing the need for creating or destroying embryos (McCarthy, 2005).

Techniques Not Involving Embryonic Intermediates

For the past decade, since the original isolation of hESC lines at the University of Wisconsin-Madison and the isolation of embryonic germ cell lines at the Johns Hopkins Medical School, controversy has surrounded pluripotent cell lines. The most basic objection to hESC research is rooted in the fact that cell derivation deprives embryos of any further potential to develop into a complete human being (Chung et al., 2006). Therefore there is interest in two techniques for deriving stem cell lines that do not result from the controversial use of embryonic intermediates:

- Amniotic-fluid-derived stem cells (AFSC)
- Induced pluripotent stem cells (iPSC)

While these latest advances have spurred a rush to improve non-embryonic techniques, they have also given fresh ammunition to those who oppose research on hESCs, an alternative embryonic technique (Naik, 2009).

Amniotic Fluid-Derived Stem Cells

In 2007, scientists at Wake Forest University generated non-embryonic stem cell lines from amniotic fluid. AFSCs are unique and are in between pluripotent and multipotent cells in terms of plasticity, or the ability to permanently change into specialized cells, also referred to as differentiation (Atala et al., 2007).

AFSCs can produce cells from each of the three embryonic germ layers. While these self-renewing cells maintain the normal number of chromosomes after a prolonged period in culture like hESCs, undifferentiated AFSCs do not produce all of the proteins expected of pluripotent cells and cannot form teratoma (Battey et al., 2008). Nerve cells, liver cells, and bone-forming cells can be produced from AFSCs. Further experiments using the nerve, liver, and bone-forming cells have also shown they can produce proteins typical of specialized cells (Holden, 2007). The research opportunities for AFSCs are tremendous.

Induced Pluripotent Stem Cells

This new and exciting area of research has many advantages over the embryonic intermediate techniques, including the potential for patient-specific cell lines that could reduce immune rejections prevalent with many transplants. In 2007, scientists at the University of California-San Francisco and the University of Wisconsin-Madison concurrently detailed the creation of iPSCs through somatic cell reprogramming without going through an embryonic intermediate. iPSCs have all the defining criteria for pluripotency, with the exception that they are not derived from embryos. Several other groups have reported generating reprogrammed stem cells.

Although in its infancy, iPSC research is now showing results. Scientists at Harvard University produced iPSC lines for ten diseases by cultivating skin cells from patients suffering conditions ranging from diabetes to muscular dystrophy to Parkinson's disease (Hotz, 2008). The generation of iPSCs from an individual patient could enable the large-scale production of the cell types affected by that patient's disease. These cells could in turn be used for disease modeling, drug discovery, and eventually autologous cell replacement therapies.

Recent research at Harvard University has demonstrated successful stem cell reprogramming in patients with genetically-based amyotrophic lateral sclerosis (ALS). ALS, or Lou Gehrig's disease, is a neurodegenerative disorder in which motor neuron loss in the spinal cord and motor cortex leads to progressive paralysis and death (Dimos et al., 2008). Patient-specific iPSCs possessed pluripotency properties and were successfully directed to differentiate into motor neurons, the cell type destroyed in ALS (Dimos et al., 2008).

In addition, scientists at the University of California-Los Angeles generated iPSCs from human dermal fibroblasts. The resultant cell lines are morphologically indistinguishable from hESCs generated from the inner cell mass of human pre-implantation embryos. This is another important step toward manipulating somatic human cells to generate an unlimited supply of patient-specific cells (Lowry, 2008). The Dana Farber Cancer Institute also successfully replicated the generation of iPSCs from human dermal fibroblasts (Park et al., 2008; *see e.g.*, Borowia et al., 2009).

Since the iPSC technique does not use embryo intermediates, such research has the advantage of potentially being federally-funded. Nevertheless, iPSC is not without controversy. One goal of using the iPSC technique is for scientists to prepare stem cell lines that model diseases with no cures. Scientists must be careful, however, not to take unfair advantage of volunteer donors. Unlike stem cell research using IVF embryos, human iPSC research leaves a developed human donor behind who is the genetic source of an iPSC line; these donors are likely to suffer from grave medical conditions. Those who volunteer to donate somatic human cells for iPSC research may do so in the hopes of directly benefiting through downstream therapeutic applications of genetically matched stem cell lines (Hyun, 2008), an expectation that may not always be realistic or possible.

Transgenics   There are some issues around transgenics, or the mixing of animal genes into human genes to study what would happen. This may be too radical for many Americans and may alienate people to the point of thinking there is a risk of making chimera come to life (Wharton, 2006). Moreover, some scientists are using iPSCs in animal trials, including ones where the cells are implanted into animal brains. The fear of a chimera-like organism being related to a donor may not be something every stem cell donor is comfortable with, especially if it is done without the donor's knowledge. Rodent research is already underway at MIT, so this is no longer simply a theoretical concern.

Another controversial issue is that iPSCs might be used to derive gametes. Ovum and sperm could both be derived from iPSCs, for instance, and then be used in an IVF procedure. The result would not be an identical clone, but it could be dangerous (Cyranoski, 2008).

Cell Replacement Therapy   Several challenges must still be resolved before cell replacement therapy using iPSC technology can become a clinical reality (Dimos et al., 2008). Because the technique of preparing iPSCs uses a retrovirus and a gene known to cause cancer, the technique could not be used to prepare cells for clinical trials, but could be used to prepare cell lines for developing a better understanding of the mechanisms of diseases and to screen potential cures (Svendsen & Ebert, 2008). Among several safety issues, iPSC-derived neurons may not be suitable for transplantation until the oncogenic genes and retroviruses are replaced with more controlled techniques

of reprogramming (Dimos et al., 2008). Recently, scientists from Scripps Research Institute announced that they were able to generate murine iPSC using recombinant proteins rather than the viral vectors (Zhou et al., 2009).

Second, it likely will be necessary to understand and correct any intrinsic defects in the patient's neurons and glial cells before they can be used as a basis for cell therapy (Dimos et al., 2008). Nevertheless, iPSCs will be important tools for further studying mechanisms by which familial diseases arise.

Donation of Human Ova for Stem Cell Research

One of the drawbacks of the SCNT technique is the need for many ova from donors. The ethical controversy involves having a donor volunteer ova in the same manner as women go through IVF: hyper-stimulation of the ovary followed by surgery to remove the ova with all the risks associated with IVF, but without any of the benefits. It took Harvard two years and $100,000 in local advertising to secure a single ova donor for its attempt to model diseases. Although Harvard's highly publicized ova donation program received plenty of responses, many donors decided against volunteering to donate their ova for research when they were informed a fertility clinic would better compensate them for the same procedure ($5,000 compensation for research purposes versus $25,000 to more than $100,000 in compensation for reproduction purposes). Regulations for donation of human ova vary from state to state. Some states allow for reimbursement of lost wages, expenses, or child care during the procedure. Other countries, including England, allow compensation in different forms, such as offsetting the costs of fertility treatment in return for research material (Maher, 2008).

The National Research Council advises against indirect compensation (costs for other than reimbursement of expenses), and Massachusetts, Connecticut, Indiana, and Maryland all allow embryonic research but prohibit compensation to ova donors (NRC, 2005). The International Society for Stem Cell Research prohibits undue inducements, leaving open the possibility of compensation beyond direct expenses (Daley et al., 2007).

Supporters of the no-compensation rule contend allowing compensation would unduly influence donor decisions to provide their ova for research and the potentially large sums of money would induce low-income women to subject themselves to unnecessary risks. Critics argue withholding compensation is paternalistic, but concede large sums of money can be coercive (Davenport, 2005). While debate over whether women should be allowed to exploit themselves by choice continues, the current voluntary

Donation of Ova for Stem Cell Research

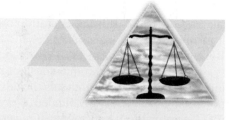

No Compensation Rule of 2006 California Stem Cell Research and Cures Act

Facts: California approved the nation's first no-compensation policies prohibiting payments to donors who donate their ova for private research. This policy does not affect compensation for ovum donations for *in vitro* fertilization for reproductive purposes.

Issue: Will a no-compensation rule protect ova donors, or will it slow the growth of the multimillion-dollar private research sector if donors' altruism fails to produce enough ovum donations?

Analysis: The California Institute of Regenerative Medicine (CIRM), the agency responsible for overseeing the state's stem cell research, passed ethical guidelines prohibiting compensation to ovum donors who donate for research purposes beyond the reimbursement of reasonable expenses for:

- Actual lost wages
- Child care
- Health insurance
- Housing
- Medical care
- Travel

guideline for IVF clinics is $5,000 if ova donations are for research.

Underlying the debates about the best way to preserve women's autonomy is the seriousness of the medical risks to the donors. As in live organ donations, the potential for harm is so severe, any inducements which might cloud the risk evaluation are forbidden. In contrast, when one donates bone marrow or other tissues for research, the risks are not as high and donors are generally reimbursed for their time and discomfort. Nevertheless, payments for time and discomfort are not allowed for ova donors (Guenin, 2003).

The risks and demands of ova donation are substantial, requiring significant investments of time, fifty-six hours by one estimate, plus several weeks of discomfort from the medications. It also involves a small but serious risk of ovarian hyper-stimulation syndrome. The long-term health risks remain unknown; some research suggests a link between the hormone treatments needed for ova retrieval and some cancers. Finally, there may be detrimental effects on future fertility and future offspring.

On the other hand, these risks are also cited as justification for fair compensation (Korobkin, 2007). However, if excessive payments exploit donors, so do low payments. Moreover, profit incentives are acceptable for the scientists, universities, biotechnology companies, pharmaceutical companies, state governments, lawyers, and health care providers profiting from research and regenerative medicine, while ova donors, without which the research cannot be done and new medical treatments cannot be developed, are singled out for remuneration prohibitions (Korobkin, 2007). This is largely similar to organ donation, where everyone except the donor is paid.

As a result of the no-compensation rule, there is a substantial risk of having an insufficient supply of ova for research (Steinbock, 2004). The use of SCNT to clone hESCs and create a viable stem cell line requires large numbers of donor ova. While stem cell lines can and have been created without SCNT, the use of ova is important for basic science research, it is the only technique thought to have the potential ability to create stem cells genetically matched to donors, which may then be used to develop replacement organs. In European countries with a no-compensation policy for both research and IVF, demand outstrips the supply (ISSCR, 2008). Massachusetts has similarly faced shortages in ova for research. Indeed, IVF compensation practices developed as demand exceeded supply. Further accentuating the potential shortage in California is that compensation for IVF ova donation remains unregulated. Donors interested in donating their ova have the choice between donating for no money and uncertain research goals and donating for money ($35,000 to $50,000). Thus, stem cell scientists not only need donors willing to make their ova available for free, but donors willing to forgo a substantial amount of money in the bargain (Gerber, 2008).

Pluripotent Stem Cell Therapies

Since this research area has been around for little more than a decade, there are no hESC therapies approved by the U.S. Food and Drug Administration (FDA) as of 2008. In early 2009, the FDA gave Geron Corporation the green light to begin the first human trials of hESC to treat spinal cord injuries (Alper, 2009). Currently two private biotechnology companies are dedicated to hESC research: Geron Corporation and Advance Cell Technology. Recently, GlaxoSmithKline, Roche, AstraZeneca, Novartis, and Pfizer have started new research divisions to focus on stem cell therapies.

Expectations are that a commercial market may develop within ten to fifteen years for transplantation of engineered organs (Wharton, 2007). There might also be a day when cell biologists are engineering the human genome (as the pharmaceutical industry currently does in plasmids, yeast, and bacteria genomes) to make anything in the human body from hESCs, including neurons, lung cells, and blood-forming cells (McCarthy, 2005).

Meanwhile, Geron, the company which funded the original derivation of stem cells at the University of Wisconsin-Madison, is still attempting to develop therapeutic products for cancer and degenerative diseases including spinal cord injury, heart failure, and diabetes. Following regulatory delays to begin the first clinical trial using hESCs, Geron recently relocated to Europe.

As the evidence mounts implicating stem cells with cancer treatments, the pharmaceutical industry is showing increasing interest in stem cell research. GlaxoSmithKline just formed a $1.4 billion strategic alliance with OncoMed of California to target cancer stem cells; clinical tests began in June of 2008. Meanwhile patents covering cancer stem cells doubled to seventy in 2007 and the number of companies dedicated to this sector has doubled to almost forty in the past year (Schmidt).

Multipotent Stem Cell Therapy

Although initially believed to be limited in plasticity, scientists are currently evaluating the trans-differentiation ability of multipotent stem cells. Though demonstrated only in mice so far, there are key achievements in the fledgling science of cellular reprogramming of multipotent cells. The hope is to create human, embryonic-like stem cells, which can be turned into all the other tissue types of the body, without using ovum or destroying embryos. Freshly derived tissue could then be transplanted into ill or diseased patients to treat various illnesses or diseases in which cells or tissues are damaged (Naik, 2009).

Cord Blood Therapies

One of the sources of human stem cells now includes umbilical cord blood cells. While the early patenting of stem cell processes remains a concern, it can be addressed case by case (Wharton, 2006). This case does demonstrate, however, the result of the federal government's policy not to fund hESC research. Based on this case, it is not clear whether the bar is being raised for patentability of medical products or whether excessively technical requirements that shield medical patents from invalidation claims are being reined in when patents are merely obvious modifications and combinations of prior art teachings (Beardsley, 2007). Patent questions like this are of critical importance since intellectual property regimes are the foundation of the profit structure for the medical industry involved in stem cells and regenerative medicine. Private entities will likely not fund stem cell research if they cannot be guaranteed the benefit of exclusive profits from their research.

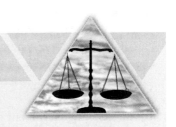

TRANSPLANTATION OF STEM CELLS IN UMBILICAL CORD BLOOD

PharmaStem Therapeutics, Inc. v. ViaCell, Inc.
[Inventor v. Competing Regenerative Medicine Companies]
491 F.3d 1342 (U.S. Court of Appeals for the Federal Circuit 2007)
U.S. Supreme Court certiorari denied 128 S.Ct. 1655 (U.S. Supreme Court 2008)

FACTS: Inventors alleged their competitors infringed two patents relating to a procedure for treating persons with compromised blood and immune systems. The two patents recite compositions and techniques relating to a transplantation procedure. The treatment is based on the discovery

(continues)

(continued)

that blood from a newborn infant's umbilical cord is a rich source of stem cells useful for rebuilding an individual's blood and immune system after the system has been compromised by disease or a medical treatment such as chemotherapy.

Stem cells are fundamental, immature cells from which specialized, mature cells derive. Hematopietic, or somatic, stem cells are ultimately responsible for producing the various specialized cells of the blood and immune system. Hematopietic stem cells produce progenitor cells and more hematopietic stem cells. The progenitor cells, which are less primitive than the stem cells, in turn give rise to the specialized cells constituting the blood and immune systems.

Although hematopietic, or somatic, stem cells are present in various types of human tissue, they are found in unusually high concentration and potency in umbilical cord blood. The patents in this case describe a process for collecting a new-born infant's umbilical cord blood at the time of birth, testing it for suitability for later use, preserving it through cryopreservation, and infusing it into an individual, either the donor or another person, whose hematopietic stem cells have been destroyed. The object of such transplantations is grafting. A successful graft results when the donor's stem cells migrate into the recipient's bone marrow, resulting in the renewed production of normal, specialized blood cells and ultimately the reconstitution of the recipient's entire blood and immune system.

Issue: Were the inventors' patents for a transplantation procedure intended for treating persons with compromised blood and immune systems infringed?

Holding and Decision: No, the inventors' patents for using cryopreserved umbilical cord stem cells for rebuilding a person's compromised blood and immune systems were an obvious

transplantation procedure, therefore the inventors' patents were invalid and not infringed.

Analysis: The issue of obviousness turns on whether the prior art gave a reasonable expectation of patent success when using cord blood in transplants for hematopoietic reconstitution. The court found the inventors had demonstrated only the presence of stem cells in cord blood, which was inferred by prior art.

While the inventors may have proved conclusively what was strongly suspected before, that umbilical cord blood is capable of hematopoietic reconstitution, and while their work may have significantly advanced the state of the science of hematopoietic transplantations by eliminating any doubt as to the presence of stem cells in cord blood, the conclusions drawn from their work were not inventive in nature. Instead, the inventors merely used routine research techniques to prove what was already believed to be the case.

Medical advances occurring in the ordinary course of research, without real innovation, retards progress; verification of new properties through testing does not satisfy the test for patentability. The inventors did not invent a new transplantation procedure or a new composition; instead, they simply provided experimental proof that umbilical cord blood may be used to effect hematopoietic reconstitution of mice and, by extrapolation, could be expected to work in humans as well. Such patents would deprive earlier innovations of their value.

Rule of Law: Scientific confirmation of what is already believed to be true does not give rise to a patentable medical invention.

(*See generally* Field, 2009).

The federal government is proposing development of a national cord blood stem cell bank network and registry to advance research in cord blood clinical therapies. The state of New Jersey created the nation's first public cord and placental blood bank for research in late 2005 (Svendsen & Ebert, 2008). With higher concentrations of multipotent stem cells in umbilical cord blood from the placenta, many parents are storing their newborn's cord blood for the possibility of use in future medical treatments.

Scientists at the University of Florida are conducting pediatric clinical trials to ameliorate and reverse the progression of Type I diabetes (Haller et al., 2008), while researchers successfully reversed Type I diabetes in adults at Northwestern University in Chicago (Burt, 2009). Stem cells derived from umbilical cord blood are also showing early potential in fighting Alzheimer's disease, while Yale University is looking at the possibilities of cord blood tissue engineering.

REGENERATIVE MEDICINE

Regenerative medicine has long been heralded as the new frontier of medicine (Caldwell, 2006). The business of regenerative medicine involves many facets, from harvesting stem cells, to creating good laboratory cultures and "scaffolding" to grow cells and tissues, to devising delivery techniques to get the final product back into patients. Scientists hope stem cells will be able to trigger the body to repair itself or alternatively to grow cells, tissues, and organs to replace those damaged or deteriorated due to injury, disease, or the aging process. Stem cell research could have unintended benefits for the field of regenerative medicine; scientists are apt to discover a biomarker or some other diagnostic tool having nothing directly to do with stem cells, but with the potential to revolutionize personalized medicine (*see generally* Wharton, 2008).

Stem Cell Therapies

In addition to repairing or replacing damaged or deteriorating body parts, scientists are trying to understand what factors influence a stem cell to rapidly multiply or become almost immortal. This area of research could lead to:

- Treatment techniques to control cancer and diabetes
- Screening potential pharmaceuticals for their potential risks or benefits toward disease
- Testing the toxicity or irritation of pharmaceutical products destined for market rather than using animal models

(Everts, 2007)

Hematopoietic (Somatic) Stem Cell Transplants

The most established stem cell therapies use hematopoietic (somatic) stem cells, or specialized stem cells that give rise to all blood cell types. Hematopoietic stem cell transplants treat patients with:

- Bone marrow damage
- Immunodeficiency
- Leukemia
- Metabolic disorders
- Sickle cell anemia
- Skin grafts for healing severe burns (skin contains stem cells immediately under its top layer)

Autologous Stem Cell Transplants

Autologous, or allogeneic, stem cell transplants are used to treat blood cancers and related diseases, diabetes, and developmental disorders. About fifteen thousand people have autologous stem cell transplants each year for:

- Leukemia
- Lymphoma
- Myeloma (Kahler's disease)
- Myleodysplastic syndrome
- Other blood cancers

(NAS, 2006)

Diabetics need replacement insulin-secreting beta cells that would not require immune suppressants, or alternatively, the ability to reactivate their own insulin-secreting beta cells. Scientists from the University of North Carolina at Chapel Hill have shown mature human skin cells can be reprogrammed into cells to produce insulin, the hormone used to treat diabetes (Naik, 2009). Recently, Northwestern University researchers announced that using autologous nonmyeloablative hematopoietic stem cells, they were able to reverse type 1 diabetes in twenty out of twenty-three patients. One patient remained insulin-free for more than four years (Voltarelli, 2008).

Stem cell therapies also offer a chance for diagnosis and prevention of early human developmental problems and treatment of infertility, miscarriages, and birth defects. Stem cells offer the potential to treat, cure, and understand the more complicated diseases that have so far eluded cure by simple molecules.

Neural Transplants

Early neural transplantation research with hESCs shows promising results in alleviating the symptoms of Parkinson's disease and other neurodegenerative disorders. According to scientists at Memorial Sloan Kettering Cancer Center, neural transplantation could also prove effective in a wide range of neurological disorders including amyotrophic lateral sclerosis and spinal muscular atrophyis.

StemCells, a clinical stage biotechnology company in Palo Alto, California, is targeting human neural stem cells derived from normal brain tissue derived from donated corpses (McGlynn, 2006). The company has FDA approval to begin transplanting the cells into children with Batten disease, a fatal, inherited neurodegenerative disorder (Wharton, 2007). This treatment offers the potential of using normal, non-genetically modified cells as cell-based clinical therapies.

Bone Marrow Transplants

In 1956, the first successful bone marrow transplant took place; today, more than forty thousand transplants are performed annually (NAS, 2006). A higher concentration of hematopoietic, or somatic, stem cells can be found in bone marrow which has led to their study for more than fifty years and clinical use for treating:

- Leukemia
- Lymphoma
- Patients undergoing high-dose chemotherapy
- Aplastic and sickle cell anemia

(Atala et al., 2007)

A leader in bone marrow transplantation is Neuronyx, a biopharmaceutical company in Malvern, Pennsylvania, which works with stem cells from adult human bone marrow to devise treatments for heart disease and other disorders (Webster, 2008). A sample of cells from a donor can be turned into a batch of cells that can be frozen and then thawed and administered as needed. The therapy has been characterized as little factories that secrete a potent cocktail of pro-regenerative cells. In animal models, the cells promote repair of damaged heart tissue. Neuronyx has applied to the FDA to begin testing the therapy in heart attack patients. While the technique may be on the cutting edge, it could also be cost-effective. A sample of cells from a single donor could be turned into six billion doses of therapy. It has the potential to keep the cost of regenerative clinical therapies reasonable in the future (*see generally* Wharton, 2007).

Autologous Organ Replacements

Regenerative medicine focuses on repairing and replacing cells, tissues, and organs (Atala et al., 2007). Animals such as starfish and salamanders have the innate ability to re-grow limbs; salamanders can also grow back their tails, parts of their hearts, and retinas and lenses in their eyes. Humans can regenerate their livers, muscles, and bones, but human regeneration is generally limited to single types of tissues. This regeneration can be achieved by administering stem cells, or specific cells derived from stem cells, or by administering drugs to coax stem cells already present in tissues and organs to more efficiently repair the damaged areas.

Tengion, a regenerative medicine company in King of Prussia, Pennsylvania, is growing replacement bladders using a patient's own cells (Nichtberger, 2008). The technology, which could replace surgery currently done, would be aimed initially at children with spina bifida or people with spinal cord injuries who lose bladder function. The technique involves doing a biopsy of the patient's bladder to collect progenitor cells, which are capable of regeneration. The cells are placed on a biodegradable scaffold in the shape of a bladder and given time to grow and mature. The neo-bladder is then implanted in the patient and becomes functional. Pfizer is backing EyeCyte, a startup in San Diego working on a treatment for retina damage using multipotent stem cells.

MORAL ISSUES AND PUBLIC SENSITIVITIES

Stem cells, autologous organs, and other technologies offer great promise, though scientific, business, and political challenges remain. Despite many advances in hESC technology, the ethical dilemma involving the destruction of a human embryo is one factor that has limited the development of stem cell-based clinical therapies (Kastenberg & Odorico, 2008).

> *Moral Dilemmas*
> 1. Are embryo-destructive experiments morally permissible?

The sensitive political issues raised by research must be acknowledged by both sides of the debate. Proper ethical safeguards should take into account both the moral issues and public sensitivities. For instance, the pharmaceutical industry and the states that are funding stem cell research adhere to the Guidelines developed by the National Academy of Sciences.

Why is stem cell research so controversial? When is the beginning of life? Fertilization? Implantation? Viability? How many cells does it take to be a human? What if there is a mixture of human and other animal cells? If an embryo is no longer wanted for reproduction and is considered medical waste, is it acceptable to use that embryo to help find a medical cure?

These ethical approaches start with the presumption of their application to humans by humans. When do organisms become a human? Is it when the ovum and sperm fuse to form a zygote? If a technique such as SCNT is used, would the zygote be considered human? "The two primary ethical dilemmas of research revolve around the assessment of when human life begins and the use of human embryos as research subjects (Nguyen, 2006). It involves a debate over potential people versus actual people (Wharton, 2008).

Pluripotent Versus Multipotent Stem Cells

Those who oppose hESC and SCNT argue AFS and iPSC cells show embryos are not needed for hESC research. Scientists, however, insist hESCs are the gold standard of pluripotency; the newer techniques must be tested against hESCs. Scientists also point out that since the iPSCs are made using genes known to promote cancer, the resulting cells can be used to study disease, but may not used as stem cell therapy.

Neither scientific assertion convinces critics of hESC research. Multipotent stem cells are viewed as being sufficient for research purposes and the direction research should take because they offer hope for real clinical applications with no loss of human life. Phrases such as "just because it is scientifically possible does not make something ethically right to pursue" and "the ends do not justify the means" are cited to justify this position. Research to promote iPSC cell production without these ontological promoters is under way.

Potential Versus Actual People

Backers of stem cell research believe hESCs hold the promise of some day curing diseases from Alzheimer's to Parkinson's. Unlike multipotent stem cells, which generally replicate the tissue of their origin, hESCs have the potential to develop into other cell types, offering the tantalizing potential of regenerating a variety of diseased or damaged tissues (Wharton, 2008). At this end of the spectrum, supporters of hESC research view the zygote as representing a potential for human life; it is not human until successfully implanted at the earliest. While *Roe v. Wade* granted the embryo some value, it does not have the same value or rights and legal status of an adult until it is viable (*see* 410 U.S. 113 (U.S. Supreme Court 1973)).

In addition, many persons with the potential for genetic disease wish to avoid passing disorders onto the next generation. They use IVF to prepare embryos and have them screened for genetic abnormalities, using PGD prior to implantation. Embryos found to have the genetic code causing the disease are discarded. The embryos slated to be discarded due to abnormality arguably have no potential for life since they will not be implanted. Moreover, women generally miscarry when they are carrying an embryo with a chromosomal abnormality. The argument is that these embryos should be used to benefit society by either using the hESCs to study the disease and hopefully provide a cure or by using the discarded embryos and replacing their nucleus with the nucleus of a cell that does not have the disease in order to prepare hESC lines for stem cell therapies for actual people.

Critics maintain the zygote is a human with unique DNA and inherent rights; therefore no technique to produce hESCs that uses an embryo is acceptable. They object to hESCs taken from embryos or aborted fetal tissue. This view disallows generating or creating embryos as disposable, destructible cells for research or stem cell therapies. Even though the hESCs come from IVF clinics that would otherwise destroy excess embryos, critics warn the process desecrates life. They suggest using stem cells taken from adults, umbilical cords, or placentas, though these cells are not as flexible in creating different organs or tissue (Wharton, 2006).

Private Versus Public Funding of Scientific Research

Yet another obstacle is the set of ethical questions raised by the debate over hESCs and whether the stem cell therapies will widen the rift between haves and have-nots. Critics of stem cell research claim venture capitalists and the pharmaceutical industry, rather than taxpayers, should pay for research and development costs. These cost arguments are used as another reason to limit hESC research. With many people not able to afford preventive medicine and care, critics argue resources are better distributed by using known cures and treatments for those who are presently suffering and can definitely have their suffering relieved by current medical treatments, but who lack the financial access to those treatments; diverting limited resources to research with no proven clinical therapies is a disservice to those who are in need of medical care and could benefit now. Supporters counter these cost arguments by asking critics how known cures were found to begin with.

Slippery Slope

Critics also fear this research tinkers with the very stuff of life and poses ethical risks. They claim it would be the first step on the slippery slope to human cloning (Wharton, 2008). Critics fearing hESC research will open the door a crack toward allowing human cloning are making a red herring argument. While one technique for hESC production involves duplicating embryos, state initiatives expressly bar efforts at reproductive human cloning.

FUNDING OF STEM CELL RESEARCH

The very process of government sponsorship of scientific research was under siege during the Bush Presidency (2001-2009). American political and ideological agendas dictated what stem cell research should be publicly funded. Forcing controversial areas of research to rely on the marketplace, however, proved to be an unsatisfactory solution to scientific advancement because the market wants returns and will take only a measurable risk of failure, and the risk of a lot of early scientific research cannot be measured (Wharton, 2008). Unless Congress passes legislation codifying the 2009 rules enacted under the Obama administration, making it harder for a future president to change them, the federal restrictions on basic scientific research could return again.

Important Legal Developments

1973—*Roe v. Wade* fetus acquires legal status when it is viable (*Roe v. Wade*, 410 U.S. 113 (U.S. Supreme Court 1973) (finding normal gestation of a human is forty weeks; present medical technology can help a child live who is born at twenty-four weeks of gestation))

1974—Congressional moratorium on federal funding of fetal research extended to embryos

1979—National Ethics Advisory Board recommends 1974 funding moratorium be overturned

1992—*Planned Parenthood v. Casey* reaffirms but weakens *Roe v. Wade* (*Planned Parenthood v. Casey*, 505 U.S. 833 (U.S. Supreme Court 1992))

1993—Congress eliminated the need for the National Ethics Advisory Board to approve embryo research

1993—National Institutes of Health (NIH) formed the National Embryo Research Panel to review federal funding of embryo research

1994—NIH recommended federal funding of embryo research

1994—President Clinton forbid the use of federal funding for embryo research in which embryos were created or destroyed; this left open the possibility for federal funding of hESC research using embryos created for reproductive purposes that would otherwise be discarded, in other words, excess IVF embryos

1995—President Clinton ordered a review of all research involving human subjects and created the National Bioethics Advisory Commission (Executive Order No. 12975 (42 U.S.C.S. § 6601 note), as amended by Executive Order Nos. 13018, 13046, and 13137, establishing the National Bioethics Advisory Commission)

1996—Congress prohibits federal funding for all embryo research (Dickey Amendment) (appropriations ban on human research on embryos: NOT-OD-07-050: NIH notice of legislative bans in effect)

1997—Dolly, the world's first cloned mammal, is born

1997—Executive Order forbids use of federal funding for human cloning

1997—President's Council on Bioethics recommends use of fetal cells or leftover embryos from IVF for research, but not somatic nuclear transfer to create stem cells

1998—hESCs and germinal cells are isolated

1999—Robb memo permits funding of hESCs since blastocyst is not a human embryo within the statutory definition

2001—Eighty Nobel Laureates urge federal government to support hESCs

2001—Presidential policy decision restricts federal funding of hESCs (Presidential policy decision (2001, August 9))

2004—New Jersey becomes the first state to fund hESC research

2005—President's Council on Bioethics endorses four techniques involving embryonic intermediates as potential sources of pluripotent stem cell lines: dead embryos, altered nuclear transfers, single cell embryo biopsy, and cellular reprogramming

2007—President Bush issues an Executive Order that expands four techniques for expanding stem cell lines endorsed by the President's Council on Bioethics (Executive Order No. 13435 (2007, June 20). *Expanding approved stem cell lines in ethically responsible ways*)

2007—*Gonzales v. Carhart* reaffirms but further weakens *Roe v. Wade* (*Gonzales v. Carhart*, 127 S.Ct. 426 (U.S. Supreme Court 2007))

2009—FDA approves the first clinical trial using embryonic stem cells to treat spinal cord injuries

2009—President Obama issues an Executive Order allowing federal funding of all stem cell research

Federal Restrictions on Stem Cell Research

For more than seven years (September 2001 to March 2009), federal restrictions prohibited the use of federal funds for the creation of human embryos for research purposes or research in which human embryos were destroyed, discarded, or knowingly subjected to risk of injury or death greater than that allowed for research on fetuses (over eight weeks in utero development) (Dolgin, 2004). NIH policy continued to permit federal funding for research using:

- Multipotent stem cells
- Animal stem cells
- Cord blood stem cells

(Executive Order No. 13435 (2007, June 20). *Expanding approved stem cell lines in ethically responsible ways*)

Now, hESCs derived from IVF embryos no longer needed for reproductive purposes can be used for research. Each embryo can yield one stem cell line, which can continue replicating indefinitely (Meckler, 2008).

Moving forward, researchers must have a stable regulatory framework based on dispassionate science in which to conduct their long-term research, rather than an unpredictable framework influenced by politics (Wharton, 2008). Debate is ongoing about the effect of U.S. scientists not having consistent federal funding for hESC research during the Bush Administration and why it is important they obtain basic research funds for unfettered research. At issue in this debate is how political controversy over federal funding affects scientists and funding of private medical research (ISSCR, 2008).

Restricted U.S. Competitiveness

Those supporting federal funding of hESC research contend stem cell science is so young it needs public funds to get off the ground and attract private capital (Akers, 2007). Typically in the U.S., the bulk of basic medical research is funded through the federal government; private funding is generally directed toward taking the government's basic research findings and converting them into commercial medical products. The rationale for public funding of hESC is that the U.S. should stay at the competitive forefront in this new frontier of medicine in the interests of economic stability. To remain competitive and help reduce its trade deficit, the U.S. should remain at or near the forefront of innovation and health care technology in the global marketplace.

The role of regulatory agencies and their potential impact on U.S. company competitiveness in regenerative medicine is therefore of vital importance (Snead, 2009). Unfortunately, when Geron, the U.S. company that funded generation of the first hESC lines at the University of Wisconsin-Madison, chose to relocate to Europe to overly burdensome U.S. regulatory restrictions, the U.S. lost its competitive edge in this marketplace (ISSCR, 2008). Political controversy that affects regulatory agencies eventually adversely affects U.S. global competitiveness in a fast-moving area of the health care industry.

Hindered Research Universities

The Bayh-Doyle Act allowed research universities to receive patents and grant licenses, including exclusive licenses on patents resulting from basic research

funded by the federal government. *See* Bayh-Doyle Act of 1980, 35 U.S.C.A. §§ 200 - 211 (2000). The hope was faster commercialization would mean the benefits of university research would reach the consumer more quickly (Raferty, 2008). Restriction of federal funding, however, actually made some things at research universities worse.

With stem cell science ready to rapidly expand, struggling biotechnology firms looking to break even, and pressure to provide cures for diseases, there was a great deal of pressure on research universities to obtain funding (Akers, 2007). With the restriction of federal funding on already prepared hESCs, all of the questions needing answers at the most basic level had to be met with private research funds to prepare stem cell lines so:

- Culture mediums can be improved
- Cell integrity can be assessed
- Genetic diversity can be obtained
- Cells based on appropriate diseases can be prepared

Federal restrictions meant scientists using private funds for hESC research had to work in separate facilities from scientists who were doing other medical research using federal funds. Otherwise, the portion of a university building each scientist used and the amount of time they used a piece of equipment had to be monitored and logged based on the source of their research funding. The resultant bureaucracy and application of such an accounting system was impractical; therefore separate laboratory facilities and equipment had to be built to protect scientists and staff who were not working on hESC research, but who were using federal funds for other medical research. Accounting violations could have resulted in a loss of federal funding by a university or federal prosecution for misuse of federal funds. Critics claimed duplicating university lab facilities and equipment was expensive, time consuming, and arguably wasteful (Leshner & Thomson, 2007).

Fostered Uncertainty in the Commercial Sector

A steady, generous source of money is the lifeline for stem cell scientists in a research sector with high capital requirement and long development time. Scientists can accept venture capital and go private with a small company, but this means leaving the research university, and many academic scientists do not want to leave academia. Moreover, most do not have the infrastructure to leave and continue their research. Also, proprietary and trade secret issues begin to intervene and a lot of scientists dedicated to academia are turned off by the trade secrecy required in private models of research (Wharton, 2006).

The federal restrictions also made it difficult for scientists to work in the stem cell field, since hESC scientists could not collaborate with other stem cell researchers (Hayes et al., 2006). Such limitations and controversy lead many scientists to choose other subject matters on which to expend their efforts. While one major bottleneck for research was funding restrictions, the most devastating one was the perception of the controversial nature of the hESC field (Nguyen, 2006).

Lack of a specific legal status in a controversial area also led to less private funding since venture capitalists wanted a return on their investment (Wharton, 2006). Controversial areas meant there could be pending laws restricting potential opportunities and therefore the potential return on investment. For instance, bills have been introduced to make therapeutic cloning, such as SCNT and ACT, a criminal offense. Other legislation proposes to protect SCNT, but prohibit reproductive cloning (Su & Chan, 2008).

State Initiatives for Stem Cell Research

State initiatives were intended to replace, in part, the federal National Institutes of Health funds that had been withheld (Wharton, 2006). Individual states circumvented the lack of federal funding on hESC lines by independently raising monetary support for the research (Beardsley, 2007). Forty-one states tried to create bioscience clusters.

It was legal to conduct research using blastocysts and to derive new cell lines in most states (NAS, 2006). Many state laws responding to the federal restrictions on research were enacted to address abortion and IVF. Varying laws restrict the use of hESCs from some or all sources, or specifically permit certain activities (NCSL, 2008). While most state laws encourage embryonic research:

- South Dakota strictly forbids research on embryos regardless of the source
- Louisiana specifically prohibits research on *in vivo* fertilized embryos
- Illinois and Michigan prohibit research on live embryos
- Arkansas, Indiana, Michigan, North Dakota, South Dakota, and Virginia prohibit research on cloned embryos
- California, Connecticut, Illinois, Iowa, Massachusetts, New Jersey, New York, and Rhode Island prohibit human cloning only for the purpose of initiating a pregnancy or reproductive cloning, but allow for hESC research

While states may serve as a national laboratory to develop optimal business models for scientific

experimentation on hESC research of the kind envisaged by former Supreme Court Justice Louis Brandeis, who believed one of the strengths of federalist structure is that each state can be a lab for social and institutional experimentation, there are dangers to this approach. Leaving hESC research to a handful of states risks fragmentation of the overall stem cell effort and raises the question of whether there will be enough resources to successfully fund stem cells and regenerative medicine long term (Wharton, 2006). Further, it is arguably inequitable for all of the states to benefit from the research funded by a few.

Moral Dilemmas

1. While research remains legal, should scientists working on this research be regulated by the government?

California Institute for Regenerative Medicine

The California Institute for Regenerative Medicine is the largest source of funding for hESC research in the U.S. Whether stem cell research ever leads to miracle cures, the California initiative is apt to shift the biotechnology research landscape in multiple and perhaps unpredictable ways. In the near future, it benefits the California biotechnology industry, because companies tend to locate where the research is. This will cement California's existing advantage (Wharton, 2006).

Some of the guidelines include:

- Time limits for obtaining cells, generally eight to twelve days after cell division begins
- Prohibiting compensation to research donors or participants, while permitting reimbursement of expenses
- hESCs may be derived from somatic cell nuclear transfer or from surplus products of IVF treatments when such products are donated under appropriate informed consent procedures; such excess cells from IVF treatments would otherwise be discarded if not utilized for medical research
- Requiring companies to which it gives money to offer any resulting therapies to state citizens at a discount
- Requiring academic institutions to license their CIRM-funded inventions only to persons who agree to have a plan in place at the time of commercialization to provide access to resultant clinical therapies and diagnostics for uninsured California patients

CIRM prohibits funding for:

- Human reproductive cloning (the practice of transferring the nucleus from a human cell into an ovum cell from which the nucleus has been removed for the purpose of implanting the resulting product in a uterus to initiate a pregnancy)
- *In vitro* culturing of any intact human embryo or any product of SCNT, parthenogenesis, or androgenesis after the appearance of the primitive streak or after twelve days
- Implantation of stem cells, whether human or nonhuman, into human embryos or nonhuman primate embryos
- Transfers of genetically modified human embryo into human uteruses

The actual spending on research is less than $300 million a year, which is significant, though in the normal course, the federal money would have been five times that amount. Despite the best hopes of the stem cell proposal's backers, California probably will not recoup its investment. Biotechnology companies tend to be relatively small operations. Even if California creates one hundred companies, which would be a lot, the state is unlikely to create enough jobs to cover its $3 billion investment over ten years. The calculations turn positive if the potential health care gains from finding new treatments for diseases, even years down the road, are factored in. Then the rest of the country is likely to get a free ride on California, the way much of the world gets free rides on medical advances coming out of the U.S. (Wharton, 2006).

INTELLECTUAL PROPERTY RIGHTS OF STEM CELLS

In addition to the laws governing the practice and funding of stem cell research at the state and federal level, scientists must legally protect their intellectual property.[LN2] Scientists need first-mover profit advantage in this competitive medical sector to obtain venture capital, especially in light of the federal funding restrictions, and to protect their ability to do their research.

At the same time, issues surrounding the intellectual property rights of stem cells, such as patent infringement and liability, create great uncertainty in stem cell research. The research community is already fractured by ideological agendas dictating the direction of scientific research, leading to a lack of cooperation among scientists and regenerative medicine companies so concerned about guarding their stem cell patents that they essentially divert

funds away from the primary goal of research and development for new therapies and toward legal fees instead (Gould, 2008). With the federal restrictions, there is not enough money for stem cell research as it stands, and diverting money to infringement issues, particularly when most of the activity is exempt anyway, is puzzling given the limited resources for this medical sector.

WARF Patent Litigation

In vivo stem cells are naturally occurring and cannot be patented. The process for obtaining, culturing, and the *in vitro* purified preparation of hESCs can be patented. The Wisconsin Alumni Research Foundation (WARF) obtained three patents on hESCs. In 2006, the Foundation for Taxpayers and Consumer Rights and Public Patent Foundation challenged the patents as overreaching and a barrier to promising stem cell research (Holden, 2006). The Patent and Trademark Office (PTO) reexamined the patents and in a preliminary ruling found prior literature references to work similar to the material claimed in the patents. The prior work was not applied in the original examination of the patent application. Therefore, the PTO rejected the patents on the basis of this previous work, concluding the patented material was not novel and was obvious to a person skilled in the field (Morrissey, 2007). WARF appealed the PTO ruling.

In early 2008, the PTO upheld the three WARF patents stating that given the unpredictability associated with both the isolation and long-term sustainability of hESCs, the present claims were not obvious. During the course of the patent examination, WARF eased up on the proprietary claims:

- Stopped demanding licensing fees from companies doing university-based research with its cells
- Narrowed its claims to apply only to hESCs derived from fertilized embryos and not hESCs from other sources such as clones or iPSC cells

(Holden, 2008)

Bayh-Dole Act

Congress understood the importance of enabling innovative technologies and medical sector infrastructure. In 1980, the Bayh-Dole Act made it much easier for universities to obtain patents from research funded by the federal government. The act provided incentives to universities to reduce basic research, which does not generate licensing fees, and increase applied research, which does generate patents and licensing fees. In addition, industry is more willing to fund university research and development projects because the results would now be easier to patent.

The federal government did not sponsor the basic research to derive human hESCs. The research was paid for by a private company, Geron Corp. In return, it received certain exclusive rights. If the federal government had funded the research, the Bayh-Dole Act would have applied, and we might have a much different situation nationally (Raferty, 2008).

European Patents for Stem Cells

In Europe, the first patents claiming unmodified stem cells have been denied based on a European Patent Convention rule excluding inventions involving the use of human embryos for industrial or commercial purposes. These denials include the WARF decisions (Atala et al., 2007). The European ruling applies to patenting embryos and any downstream product of embryos, but not necessarily to the isolated hESCs, which are available through legal importation in many European countries. One could infer Europe will allow patents on hESCs derived from techniques not involving an embryo, such as iPSC techniques.

MOVING FORWARD WITH INNOVATIVE MEDICAL TECHNOLOGIES

An understanding of stem cells provides an appreciation of regenerative medicine and the innovative medical technologies that are rapidly emerging in this medical sector. Scientists do not yet know which path this promising research will follow and want all pathways to remain open until they can scientifically determine the best paths to pursue with stem cells (Leshner & Thomson, 2007). Regenerative medicine is very much in the early days in terms of stem cell therapies, with the medical products industry essentially being in a race to the starting line. (*See* Clarke, 2008).

Americans are divided on when human life begins, but agree the zygote is more than just a cluster of cells. The spectrum of belief ranges from full human rights from fertilization to rights once the fetus is viable. The legal ramifications of determining the rights, if any, of a zygote through viability of the fetus have far-reaching implications and are the subject of political controversy, including two

presidential vetoes. Investors are concerned about funding research, given the:

- Political controversy
- Threat of regulatory changes
- Upheaval of intellectual property rights

Even more damaging to the controversial stem cell field may be the discouragement of scientists from entering regenerative medicine. To maintain U.S. competitiveness, states have begun to fill the funding gap federal restrictions have caused. Citing the insufficient federal funding of hESC research and expansion of stem cell research in other countries, states have strong economic motives to fund stem cell research.

Multipotent stem cells have already proved their use mainly in blood disorders utilizing the cord blood and bone marrow. One source of confusion seems to be the belief multipotent stem cells would not have an immune rejection problem; this is only true in cases where the patient's own stem cells can be used for the therapy. For genetic diseases where patients' stem cells would also carry the disease or are damaged, the use of their own stem cells without modification, which is not presently available, would not render a cure. In this case, patients would need to have a good match and immune suppressants to avoid immune rejection. As the cell sorting process improves, isolation of rare stem cells will open new research opportunities.

The low turnover numbers in cultivating multipotent stem cells relative to hESCs make them less attractive for research, while the current clinical use and lack of potential for producing teratomas make them more attractive for fighting disease. Multipotent stem cells cannot, however, further understanding of early embryo development stages that can contribute to birth defects and miscarriage.

Many scientists are excited about the recent pluripotency discovery of iPSC cells and AFS cells, which are easier to prepare and do not have the controversy of an embryo intermediate. Recent work using hESCs resulting in generating glucose-responsive, insulin-secreting cells may lead to a cure for diabetes (Kroon et al., 2008).

While significant confusion exists over what stem cells, autologous organs, and other technologies may someday offer, there are important roles for entrepreneurs in shaping regenerative medicine into an important health care sector (Seay, 2008). Backers of research believe hESCs hold the promise of curing diseases from Alzheimer's to Parkinson's and replacement of tissue and organs. Unlike multipotent stem cells, which generally replicate the tissue of their origin, hESCs have the potential to develop into other cell types, offering the exciting potential of regenerating a variety of diseased or damaged tissue (Wharton, 2008).

The key for most scientists is simply proceeding forward. Stem cell research and its resulting applications will unquestionably have a major impact on the American health care system. As Hans Keirstead, a University of California physician-scientist, was quoted as saying at a legislative hearing on the merits of providing public funding for stem cell research: "Maybe every one hundred years there is one major milestone, like the invention of penicillin. Stem cell research is such a thing."

Moral Dilemmas

1. How significant can stem cells actually become?

2. Are stem cells an area where there is more controversy than actual scientific potential?

3. Is hESC research morally different from research on the birth control pill and IVF, both of which developed in the U.S. without federal funds and in an environment of ambiguous legality?

4. Is the field of stem cells and regenerative medicine merely a collection of clever medical technologies, or does it have the potential for revolutionizing health care?

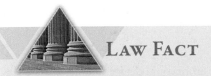 **LAW FACT**

RESEARCH ON HUMAN EMBRYONIC STEM CELLS

Should the federal government provide funding for basic scientific research involving hESCs?

In August 2001, while the lawsuit was pending, President Bush issued a presidential policy decision restricting federal funding for hESC research. No federal funds could be used to further scientific research involving the derivation of new stem cell lines from intact human embryos like Mary Doe; federal funding was limited to scientific research involving already-existing hESC lines from the University of Wisconsin-Madison. As a result, the court dismissed the case as moot because Mary Doe would no longer be threatened.

In March 2009, President Obama reversed the Bush policy decision. Some contend embryos like Mary Doe are now threatened, so cases like this may no longer be moot (Meckler, 2008).

—*Doe v. Shalala*, 122 Fed.Appx 600 (U.S. Court of Appeals for the 4th Circuit 2004),
U.S. Supreme Court certiorari denied, 546 U.S. 822
(U.S. Supreme Court 2005).

CHAPTER SUMMARY

- Pluripotent stem cells are cells that can develop into any of over two hundred kinds of specialized cells in the human body.
- The main focus of the current research is on pluripotent stem cells, which can develop into any kind of specialized cell other than those needed to create an embryo, and multipotent stem cells, which can develop into a limited number of kinds of specialized cells.
- Stem cells can be obtained from live embryos, primordial germ cells, dead embryos, genetically abnormal embryos, single cell blastocyst biopsies, parthenogenesis, animals, cord blood, altered nuclear transfer, somatic cell nuclear transfer, amniotic fluid, and inducement.
- Some states allow women to be reimbursed for ova donation, but donation regulations differ between states.
- Federal funding of stem cell research is extremely limited, and only a handful of private companies are conducting such research in the U.S.

- Stem cell research has the potential to result in organs and tissue engineered for transplantation and treatments for diseases such as cancer, diabetes, Alzheimer's, and Parkinson's.
- The ability to patent stem cell research findings is crucial to encourage such research; private companies are unlikely to fund such research if they cannot be guaranteed exclusive profits from it, necessary to recoup the costs of the initial research and development; it is currently difficult to tell whether the federal government will make such patents relatively accessible.
- Perhaps the majority of the controversy surrounding stem cell research centers on the derivation of hESCs that deprives human embryos of the potential to become a completely developed human.
- Human cloning is expressly prohibited in the U.S.
- Restricted federal funding for stem cell research has resulted in a limited number of stem cell lines available for research, the failure of the U.S. to keep pace with other countries' stem cell research developments, additional research expenses due to the need to build separate facilities for federally-funded and privately-funded research due to the need to address legal concerns, and a lack of collaboration between scientists.
- Limited federal funding has resulted in state funding initiatives; this creates the potential for all of the states to benefit from the research funded by a few.
- The California Institute for Regenerative Medicine is currently the largest source of funding for stem cell research in the U.S.; it provides guidelines that other states may in turn follow in developing their own initiatives.
- Stem cell research is the first major scientific endeavor the U.S. federal government has attempted to strictly regulate; the effects of this have dramatically altered scientific research in the U.S.

Law Notes

1. Scientists at Columbia University undertook a natural history study of embryonic death. Viable embryos were compared to nonviable embryos created for IVF, but not used for implantation. Many nonviable embryos had fewer cells than normal and lacked compaction. All of the dead embryos did not progress to compacted morula (in human development, a four-day-old embryo) or normal blastocyst (a five-day-old embryo). No criteria could be discerned for the diagnosis of death on the three-day-old embryo. The scientists therefore concluded that arrested development at the multi-cellular stage on embryonic day five indicates an irreversible loss of integrated organic function, and hence, the condition of death for the organism. Consequently, they proposed that the ethical framework currently used for obtaining essential organs from deceased persons for transplantation could be applied to the harvesting of live cells from dead human embryos for the creation of stem cells (Landry, 2006). Therefore, scientists should be able to ethically harvest cells from organismically dead human embryos in experimental efforts to generate hESC lines (NIH, 2007b).

2. A patent for an invention is the grant of a property right to the inventor, issued by the U.S. Patent and Trademark Office. Generally, the term of a new patent is twenty years from the date on which the application for the patent is filed, or, in special cases, from the date an earlier related application was filed, subject to the payment of maintenance fees. The right conferred by the patent is the right to exclude others from making, using, offering for sale, or selling the invention in the U.S., or importing the invention into the U.S. What is granted is not the right to make, use, offer for sale, sell, or import, but the right to exclude others from making, using, offering for sale, selling, or importing the invention. Once a patent is issued, the patentee must enforce the patent.

Chapter Bibliography

AAAS (American Association for the Advancement of Science). (2007). *AAAS policy brief: Stem cell research.* Washington, DC: AAAS.

Akers, M. A. (2007, October 17). Going against Bush, NIH director urges expanded research. *Washington Post,* p. A15.

Alper, J. (2009, March). Geron gets green light for human trial of ES cell-derived product. *Nature Biotechnology, 27* (3), 213-214.

Atala, A. et al. (2007). *Principles of regenerative medicine.* (3rd ed.). New York, NY: Academic Press (offering scientists in stem cell biology, bioengineering, and developmental biology an advanced understanding of the latest technologies in regenerative medicine).

Bailey, R. L. (2008). Pressing forward: Connecticut's approach to embryonic research. *Law & Inequality: A Journal of Theory & Practice, 26,* 133-170.

Battey, J. F. et al. (2008). Alternate methods for preparing pluripotent stem cells. In NIH (National Institutes of Health). *Regenerative Medicine* (pp. 58-76). Washington, DC: U.S. Department of Health & Human Services, NIH.

Baylis, F. (2008). Animal eggs for stem cell research: A path not worth taking. *American Journal of Bioethics, 8* (12), 18-32.

Beardsley, D. (2007). A two-front assault on the stem cell patents. *John Marshall Review of Intellectual Property Law, 6* (501), 513-524.

Ben-Shaanan, T. L. et al. (2008). Transplantation of neural progenitors enhances production of endogenous cells in the impaired brain. *Molecular Psychiatry, 13* (2), 222-231 (describing research at The Hebrew University of Jerusalem).

Black's (Black's Law Dictionary). (2004) (8th ed.). Eagan, MN: Thomson Reuters West Publishing Co.

Borowia, M. et al. (2009). Small molecules efficiently direct endodermal differentiation of mouse and human embryonic stem cells. *Cell Stem Cell, 4* (4), 348-358 (used small protein molecules to differentiate mouse and hESCs into endoderm).

Burt, R. K. of the Northwestern University Feinberg School of Medicine, Chicago. (2009, May 3). JAMA media briefing: Stem cell transplantation helps patients with diabetes become insulin free. Washington, DC: National Press Club.

Caldwell IV, W. M., chief executive officer, Advanced Cell Technology. (2006). Wharton Health Care Business Conference Entrepreneurship Panel: Stem cells and regenerative medicine-entrepreneurial opportunities and challenges. Philadelphia, PA.

Chung, Y. et al. (2006). Embryonic and extraembryonic stem cell lines derived from single mouse blastomeres. *Nature, 439* (7073), 216-219.

Clarke, J. (2006). Managing general partner at Cardinal Partners Venture Fund at the Wharton Health Care Business Conference Panel: Emerging technologies and the innovation of competitive advantage. Philadelphia, PA.

Cyranoski, D. (2008). Stem cells: Five things to know before jumping on the iPSC bandwagon. *Nature, 452*, 406-408.

Daley, D. Q. et al. (2007). International Society for Stem Cell Research (ISSCR) guidelines for human embryonic research. *Science, 2*, 603-604.

Davenport, R. J. (2005). Drumming up dollars for research, *Cell, 123* (7), 1169-1172 (when there were stringent U.S. restrictions on funding for human embryonic research, states struggled with the issue of whether and how to fund such research themselves).

Dimos, J. T. et al. (2008). Induced pluripotent stem cells generated from patients with ALS can be differentiated into motor neurons. *Science, 321* (5893), 1218-1221.

Dolgin, J. L. (2004). Embryonic discourse: Abortion, stem cells and cloning. *Issues in Law & Medicine, 19*, 203-261.

Dome, J. et al. (2006). Bone marrow (hematopoietic) stem cells. In NIH (National Institutes of Health). *Regenerative Medicine* (pp. 13-34). Washington, DC: U.S. Department of Health & Human Services, NIH.

Everts, S. (2007). Getting to the root of cancer: The dark side of stem cells is initiating a revolution in cancer research. *Chemical & Engineering News, 85* (3), 28-29.

Federal Register. (2000, August 25). *National Institutes of Health guidelines for research using hESCs.* 65 F.R.

51976-01 (providing for future research funding by NIH for stem cells derived from fetal tissue or from certain early embryos that are the products of IVF).

Field, T. L. (2009). Improving the federal circuit's approach to choice of law for procedural matters in patent cases. *George Mason Law Review, 16*, 643-699.

Gautam Naik, G. (2007, June 16). The devout doctor's prescription for stem-cell research. *Wall Street Journal*, p. A10.

Gerber, E. (2008). California limits egg donor compensation in privately-funded research. *Journal of Law, Medicine & Ethics, 35*, 220-223.

Gould, R., patent attorney with Philadelphia-based law firm Duane Morris. (2008). Wharton Health Care Business Conference Panel: Emerging technologies and the innovation of competitive advantage. Philadelphia, PA.

Guenin, L. (2003). *Resources on the ethics of human stem cell research*. Deerfield, IL: International Society for the Study of Stem Cell Research.

Haller, T. et al. (2008). Autologous umbilical cord blood infusion for type 1 diabetes. *Experimental Hematology, 36* (6), 710-715.

Hayashi, J. (2006). Primate embryonic stem cell-derived neuronal progenitors transplanted into ischemic brain. *Journal of Cerebral Blood Flow & Metabolism, 26* (7), 906-914.

Hayden, E. C. (2008). The 3-billion dollar question. *Nature, 453*, 18-21.

Hayes, R. et al. (2006). *Stem cells and public policy: The basics.* Unpublished manuscript, New York, NY: Century Foundation.

Holden, C. (2008). Canada-CIRM cancer deal. *Science, 320* (5884), 1709 (describing the collaboration agreement between the California Institute for Regenerative Medicine and Canada's Cancer Stem Cell Consortium).

___. (2007). Versatile stem cells without the ethical baggage? *Science, 315* (5809), 170 (explaining discovery of a new type of cell from amniotic fluid with many of the characteristics of hESCs).

___. (2006). Scientists object to Massachusetts rules. *Science, 313* (5792), 1372 (state legislature sanctioned medical research using hESC but regulations restricted the research).

Hotz, R. L. (2008, August 8). Stem cells' new sugar daddy. *Wall Street Journal*, p. A9.

Hurlbut, W. B. (2007). Ethics and embryonic research: Altered nuclear transfer as a way forward. *BioDrugs, 21* (2), 79-83.

Hyun, I. (2008). Stem cells from skin cells: The ethical questions. *Hastings Center Report, 38* (1), 20-22.

Irish Council on Bioethics. (2008). *Ethical scientific and legal issues concerning stem cell research*. Dublin, Ireland: Irish Council on Bioethics.

ISSCR (International Society for Stem Cell Research). (2008). *Guidelines for the clinical translation of stem cells*. Deerfield, IL: ISSCR.

Kastenberg, Z. J. & Odorico, J. S. (2008). Alternative sources of pluripotency: Science, ethics, and stem cells. *Transplant Reviews, 22* (3), 215-222.

Klimanskaya, I. et al. (2006). Human embryonic stem cell lines derived from single blastomeres. *Nature, 444*, 481-485.

Korobkin, R. (2007). Buying and selling human tissues for stem cell research. *Arizona Law Review, 42*, 49-67.

Kroon, E. et al. (2008). Pancreatic endoderm derived from human embryonic stem cells generates glucose-responsive insulin-secreting cells in vivo. *Nature Biotechnology, 26* (4), 443-452.

Landry, D. W. (2006). Hypocellularity and absence of compaction as criteria for embryonic death. *Regenerative Medicine, 1* (3), 367-371.

Leshner, A. I., & Thomson, J. A. (2007, December 3). Standing in the way of research. *Washington Post,* p. A17.

Lowry, W. E. (2008). Generation of human induced pluripotent stem cells from dermal fibroblasts. *Proceedings of the National Academy of Sciences, 105* (8), 2883-2888.

Maher, B. (2008, September 25). Ovum shortage hits race to clone human stem cells. *Nature, 453,* 828-829.

Marques-Mari, A. I. et al. (2009). Differentiation of germ cells and gametes from stem cells. *Human Reproduction Update, 15* (3), 379-391.

McCarthy, A. A. (2005). Advanced cell technology: Embryonic-stem-cell-based regenerative medicine. *Cell, 12* (6), 605-607.

McGlynn, M., president, chief executive officer, and director of StemCells. (2008). Wharton Health Care Business Conference Panel: Emerging technologies and the innovation of competitive advantage. Philadelphia, PA.

Meckler, L. (2008, March 7). Obama to reverse policy on stem cells. *Wall Street Journal,* p. A4.

Meissner A. & Jaenisch, R. (2006). Generation of nuclear transfer-derived pluripotent ES cells from cloned Cdx2-deficient blastocysts. *Nature, 439* (7073), 212-215.

Morrissey, S. R. (2007, January 15). Claims under fire: The future of embryonic research in the U.S. may hinge on the current review of key patents. *Chemical & Engineering News, 85* (3), 31-32.

Naik, G. (2009, April 24). Chemist cites advance in stem-cell field. *Wall Street Journal,* p. A4.

NAS (National Academies of Science). (2006). *Understanding stem cells: An overview of the science and issues from the National Academies.* Washington, DC: NAS.

NCSL (National Conference of State Legislators). Stem cell research. Washington, DC: NCSL.

Nguyen, L. T. (2006). The fate of stem cell research and a proposal for future legislative regulation. *Santa Clara Law Review, 46,* 419-449.

Nichtberger, S., president and chief executive officer, Tengion. (2008). Wharton Health Care Business Conference Panel: Emerging technologies and the innovation of competitive advantage. Philadelphia, PA.

NIH (National Institutes of Health). (2008). *Frequently asked questions (FAQs): In stem cell information.* Bethesda, MD: U.S. Department of Health & Human Services, NIH.

___. (2008a). *Stem cell basics.* Bethesda, MD: U.S. Department of Health & Human Services, NIH.

___. (2007). *Plan for implementation of Executive Order 13455: Expanding approved stem cell lines in ethically responsible ways.* Bethesda, MD: U.S. Department of Health & Human Services, NIH.

___. (2007a). *Information on eligibility criteria for federal funding of research on hESC cells.* Bethesda, MD: U.S. Department of Health & Human Services, NIH.

___. (2007b). *Stem cells and diseases.* Bethesda, MD: U.S. Department of Health & Human Services, NIH.

___. (2006). *Regenerative medicine.* Bethesda, MD: U.S. Department of Health & Human Services, NIH.

NRC (National Research Council). (2005). *Guidelines for human embryonic research.* Washington, DC: NRC Committee on Guidelines for *hESC* Research.

Okita, K. et al. (2007). Generation of germline-competent induced hESCs. *Nature, 446,* 313-317.

Park I. H. et al. (2008). Reprogramming of human somatic cells to pluripotency with defined factors. *Nature, 10* (451), 135-136.

PBAC (President's Bioethics Advisory Commission). (2005). *A white paper: Alternative sources of hESC.* Washington, DC: PBAC.

Pfizer (Pfizer's stem cell research policy). (2009). New York, NY.

Raferty, M. (2008). The Bayh-Dole Act and university research and development. *Medical Policy, 37,* 29-40.

Ramalho-Santos, M., & Willenbring, H. (2007). On the origin of the term "stem cell." *Cell: Stem Cell, 1* (1), 36-38.

Schmidt, C. (2008). Drug makers chase cancer stem cells. *Nature Biotechnology, 26* (4), 366-367.

Seay, N. (2008). Stem cells as a business: A pragmatic approach. *World Stem Cell Report 2008,* 145-148.

Sidhu, K. S. et al (2008). Derivation of a new hESC line, endeavour-1, and its clonal propagation. *Stem Cells Development, 1,* 41-51.

Silver, L. (2007, June 21). *George Orwell Bush: The latest stem cell veto.* New York, NY: American Council on Science & Health.

Snead, O. C. (2009). The George W. Bush administration: A retrospective: Public bioethics and the Bush presidency. *Harvard Journal of Law & Public Policy, 32,* 867-913.

Spar, D., & Harrington, A. (2007). Selling stem cell science: How markets drive law along the technological frontier. *American Journal of Law & Medicine, 33,* 541-565.

Steinbock, B. (2004). Payment for ovum donation and surrogacy. *Mount Sinai Journal of Medicine, 71,* 255-265.

Su, Y-C et al. (2008). Mary Doe's destiny: How the U.S. has banned human embryonic research in the absence of a direct prohibition. *Richmond Journal of Law & Technology, 14,* 12-78.

Svendsen. C. N. & Ebert, A. D. (2008). *Encyclopedia of stem cell research.* Thousand Oaks, CA: Sage Publication.

Takahashi, K. et al. (2007, November). Induction of pluripotent stem cells from adult human fibroblasts by defined factors. *Cell, 131* (5), 861-872.

___. & Yamanaka, S. (2006). Induction of hESCs from mouse embryonic and adult fibroblast cultures by defined factors. *Cell, 126,* 663-676.

Torrisi, C. P. (2007). Embryonic vs. adult: The history and future of the stem cell debate. *Journal of Health & Biomedical Law, 3,* 143-161.

Voltarelli, J. C. et al. (2008). Autologous *hematopoietic stem cell transplantation for type 1 diabetes. Annals* of the New York Academy of Sciences, 1150, 220-229.

Webster, S. W., president, chief executive officer, and director, Neuronyx. (2008). Wharton Health Care Business Conference Panel: Emerging technologies and the innovation of competitive advantage. Philadelphia, PA.

Wharton (Wharton School at the University of Pennsylvania). (2006). Industry leaders debate big pharma R&D (too little hope?) and stem cell research (too much hype?). *Knowledge@Wharton.*

___. (2004). Will Proposition 71 make California the Mecca of stem-cell research? *Knowledge@Wharton.*

___. (2002). Bettering ourselves through biotech: Greater productivity, sharper memories, hair feathers. *Knowledge@Wharton*.

Yamanaka, S. (2007). Strategies and new developments in the generation of patient-specific hESCs. *Cell, 127*, 39-49.

Yu, J. et al. (2007). Induced pluripotent stem cell lines derived from human somatic human cells. *Science, 318* (5858), 1917-1920.

Zhang, X. (2006). Derivation of human embryonic stem cells from developing and arrested embryos. *Stem Cells, 24* (12), 2669-2676.

Zhou, H. et al. (2009). Generation of induced pluripotent stem cells using recombinant proteins. *Cell: Stem Cell, 4*, 1-4.

NOTE

*Contributor: Cyndy Walton, MBA, PhD, Adjunct Faculty in the MBA Program in Biotechnology & Health Industry Management at Pennsylvania State University, Malvern, PA and Drexel University's LeBow College of Business, Philadelphia, PA.

CHAPTER 32

REPROGENICS AND ASSISTED REPRODUCTIVE TECHNOLOGY EXPERIMENTATION

> *Double, double toil and trouble; Fire burn, and caldron bubble. Fillet of a fenny snake,*
> *In the caldron boil and bake; Eye of newt, and toe of frog, Wool of bat, and tongue of*
> *dog, Adder's fork, and blind-worm's sting, Lizard's leg, and owlet's wing, For a charm of*
> *powerful trouble, Like a hell-broth boil and bubble.*
>
> —WILLIAM SHAKESPEARE (1564-1616), ENGLISH POET AND PLAYWRIGHT, FROM *MACBETH*

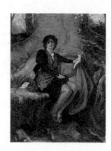

IN BRIEF

The technologies at the intersection of reproductive medicine and genetics have been termed *reprogenics*, which is distinct from eugenics. Reprogenic technologies are rapidly evolving into tools not only to customize and enhance children through assisted reproductive technologies (ART), but to develop wholly new genetic recipes derived from modification of the genome. A related emerging field approaching the same goals is synthetic biology. While also known as analytic biology, synbio, synthetic genomics, constructive biology, and systems biology, this chapter will use the term *synthetic biology* as most descriptive of the new area of biological research that combines science and engineering in order to design and build, or synthesize, novel biological functions and systems. Both approaches to genome modification are approaching the point of taking genetic techniques, ingredients, and diagnostic tools and engineering personalized medicines that have the potential to revolutionize the delivery of health care. Who will own the patent rights to the modified genomes underlying these new medicines is unknown.

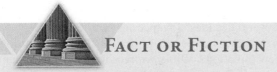

FACT OR FICTION

PATENTING "HUMANZEE"

*How many human gene sequences are needed for the U.S. Patent Trade Office (PTO)
to decide an organism is human?*

As part of the omnibus appropriations bills each year since 2004, Congress has enacted the Weldon Amendment, which bans the use of federal funds to issue patents on claims directed to or encompassing a human organism (Weldon Amendment to Consolidated Appropriations Act, Pub. L. 104-447 (2008); Consolidated Appropriations Act, 2006, Pub. L. No. 109-149, § 509, 119 Stat. 2833, 2880 (2006); Consolidated Appropriations Act, 2005, Pub. L. No. 108-447, § 626, 118 Stat. 2809, 2920 (2005); Consolidated Appropriations Act, 2004, Pub. L. No. 108-199, § 634 (2004)). This is distinct from the patenting of biotechnology derived from human beings, for instance, modified animals that include a few human genes so the animals can produce a human protein or antibody. The patent ban does not affect the patentability of human-animal chimeras. *See* 149 Cong. Rec. E2234-03 (daily ed. Nov. 5, 2003) (statement of Rep. Weldon). Chimeras are different from hybrids and genetic recombinant organisms.

In 1997, Stuart Newman, a developmental biologist at New York Medical College and founding member of the Council for Responsible Genetics, and Jeremy Rifkin, author-economist and president of the Foundation for Economic Trends, filed an application to patent a human-chimpanzee ("humanzee") and the various methods of creating it. The humanzee was purely theoretical. Newman and Rifkin did not file the application with the intention of creating the humanzee, but rather to secure the exclusive right to the technology after the patent was granted, or, if the patent was denied, to reduce the economic incentive for others to develop chimeras. The application specified the percentage of human DNA in the humanzee to be up to 50 percent, to force the PTO to grapple not only with whether human beings can be patentable subject matter, but also with how much human genetic material it takes to make a living organism human.

The PTO initially rejected the application in 1999 because it claimed the invention embraced a human being. When the PTO was asked to identify the legal basis for banning their patent, the PTO stated the patent would violate the Thirteenth Amendment, which forbids slavery and the ownership of human beings. After an appeal, the PTO issued its last rejection letter in early 2005. The PTO believed that the humanzee would be too closely related to a human to be patentable under the Weldon Amendment. The PTO stated that reaching this decision was not difficult, for the proposed technique was too crude to be able to fine-tune the percentage of human cells in the humanzee and therefore could have easily produced a creature that was more human than chimpanzee.

In 2009, ARTs makes such fine-tuning more feasible. The PTO will likely have to face the question of what is human again. Still, no one claims to know how to differentiate between humans and animals.

—The only case law applicable to chimeras pertains to the PTO's denial of patents on human life: Transaction History, U.S. Patent App. No. 08/993,564 (filed December 18, 1997); the PTO issued a final notice of abandonment for failure to respond to office action on March 1, 2005.

(See *Law Fact* at the end of this chapter for the answer.)

PRINCIPLES AND APPLICATIONS

A mathematical parrot, a Dutch-speaking orangutan, and a chimpanzee that can pass for a boy are the characters that anchor Michael Crichton's 2006 novel *Next*. Trained as a physician, Crichton's futuristic fiction takes scientific possibilities to their logical extremes. *Jurassic Park* (1990) explored the ethics of cloning by way of a theme park populated by genetically engineered dinosaurs (Wharton, 2007). In *Next*, Crichton examines reproductive medicine and genetics from the vantage point of the law.

Given the limited federal involvement in human pluripotent stem cell research, the U.S. National Academy of Sciences concedes that privately funded research has thus far been carried out under a patchwork of existing regulations, many of which were not designed with reprogenic research and advanced techniques from molecular biology, computer science, and engineering specifically in mind. *Next* weaves together several storylines in order to trace the complex interplay of scientific innovation, law, ethics, politics, and economic opportunity:

- Bounty hunters pursuing a child who has inherited an unusual cell from a grandfather who signed away the commercial rights to his tissues; the courts have agreed that the owners with the rights to the cell can forcibly harvest samples from the child
- A biotechnology company calculating how much money it could make with its patented maturity gene, after a scientist's drug-abusing brother accidently inhales a spray containing a retrovirus used to induce aging in rats and then suddenly matures into a responsible, sober adult
- After a scientist discovers he is the father of a transgenic humanzee, the product of an embryonic experiment he had assumed was abortive, the scientist adopts the half-human as his son and integrates him into his family and enrolls him in school
- The jilted husband who uses the threat of genetic testing to pressure his wife into giving up custody of their children
- A parrot whose conversational and mathematical abilities stem from an injection of human transgenes received as a chick

In *Next*, these fantasy plots take their place alongside published material on genetic engineering (Wharton, 2007). Today, there is not yet a public consensus on completely human subject research, such as human cloning and embryo research. However, with rapid developments in gene sequencing, Crichton's characters in *Next* are no longer solely products of science fiction. Rapid advances in genetics, cloning, and embryology have already resulted in the blurring of specie lines (Kopenski, 2003). While technically cloning involves one species and chimering involves two or more (DeCoux, 2007), recent advances in the sequencing of the genome and synthetic biology have led to the creation of a variety of recipes and ingredients with both human and animal components (Kopenski, 2003). Crichton's incredible plot in *Next* thus poses problems that have a significant basis in reality for the health care industry (Wharton. 2007).

CHIMERA TECHNOLOGY

The word *chimera* has its origin from a mythological creature that was part lion, part serpent, and part goat, slain by the hero of Greek mythology, Bellerophon, considered the greatest slayer of monsters (Hesiod, B.C.; Homer B.C.; Graves, 1993). Although scientists have been creating human-animal chimeras

for several decades, advances in synthetic biology, embryology, and cloning have pushed this technology in new directions. While unprecedented developments in reproductive medicine and genetics have generated public debate, most research involving early human life is unregulated. There are no federal laws regulating privately funded embryo research, and no significant restrictions on human cloning or the pursuit of inheritable genetic modifications (Kopinski, 2003).

Nonetheless, recent scientific advances have expanded the potential to blend species beyond the limits of traditional transplantation and genetic recombination techniques (Nguyen & Xu, 2008). Innovations in embryology and cloning enable the creation of modern chimeras, which increasingly blur the line between human and animal. Despite these scientific developments, no regulations address chimeras. The Food and Drug Administration (FDA) has not extended its regulatory reach to embryonic chimeras, although it has claimed jurisdiction over human cloning. Since regulation of new stem cell lines does not encompass chimera technology, chimeras are created with increasing quantities of human tissues and genetic materials without limitation (Kopinski, 2003).

Definition of Chimera

The definition of *chimera* is an organism with a mixture of cells from at least two different genetically distinct organisms, from the same or different species (Baylis & Fenton, 2007). Chimeras are generally created by mixing cells from one species with cells of another species, resulting in a combination of mismatched parts. Because the DNA from each species ordinarily does not combine in this process, any offspring of the chimera contains DNA from just one of the original species (Kopinski, 2003).

Moral Dilemmas

1. Could reprogenics and synthetic biology replace natural selection, thereby permanently altering the relationship between humans and their environment?

2. If evolution is similar to selection through competition, is it conceivable chimeras could evolve to compete with humans?

3. Could there be a time in the future when the reproductive process would be replaced by a manufacturing process?

Human-Human Chimeras

Chimeras are found in nature when fertilized ova fuse or when a fertilized ovum fuses with a sperm other than the one that fertilized the ovum (as opposed to the normal fusion of a female ovum with the male sperm that fertilized the ovum). An indeterminate number of people are born as natural human-to-human chimeras (Kopinski, 2003). Usually, a chimeric person was destined to be born a twin, but due to a developmental anomaly, cells from the twin become incorporated in the chimeric person's body in one of two ways:

• Either the twin was spontaneously aborted, leaving behind embryonic blood cells that became part of the chimeric person's bone marrow, or
• Cells of the twin failed to separate at the embryonic stage, so the chimeric person was born with some somatic cells containing DNA from the twin

These chimeric people possess two types of cells containing different sets of DNA as a result of a rare genetic anomaly that is seldom detected (Kopinski, 2003). There is no clear evidence the incidence of natural human-to-human chimeras is increasing as the use of *in vitro* fertilization (IVF) techniques expand, although this would be the expectation as multiple births are becoming more common in the U.S.

In contrast to animal-animal, the creation of human-human chimeras in the laboratory has been shunned. An experiment that combined male and female human embryos into a single hermaphroditic human-human chimera was severely criticized and viewed as an example of the inevitable product of years of under-regulation of the reproductive technology industry (Gleicher & Tang, 2003; Powledge, 2003).

Moral Dilemmas

1. Considering that not all humans have the same rights as other humans, should chimeras in which human brain cells are implanted or developed have different rights than other primates or chimeras?

Animal-Animal Chimeras

Scientists have already manipulated this developmental anomaly of embryonic mixing in animals. By combining embryos of two organisms at a very early stage, unnatural yet viable transgenic chimeras can be produced. It is important to note that chimeras are not hybrids, which are created as a result of sexual reproduction across species and contain recombined genes throughout their bodies (Baylis & Robert, 2007). The first successful experiment resulted in a goat-sheep chimera, or "geep," which exhibited attributes of both animals (Bennett, 2006).

Based on this success, scientists proposed injecting human cells into pigs to develop various types of tissues (Nguyen & Xu, 2008). The hypothesis was if the cells survived and became pluripotent, they would contribute to the formation of all of the chimera's tissues, including cells that could be used for germ line gene therapy. This theory was tested when scientists produced human-pig chimeras by injecting human stem cells into developing pig embryos. The developing pigs contained both human and pig cells, and some cells fused spontaneously to incorporate both human and pig DNA (Kopinski, 2003). This human-pig DNA can then be inserted into an individual's cells and tissues to treat a hereditary disease in which defective genes are replaced with functional ones.

On a non-embryonic level, the public generally accepts scientific practices involving the transfer of human material to animals, such as in the creation of transgenic pigs for routine supply of organs for xenotransplantation (Ballard, 2008). The creation of mice with human neurons in their brains received publicity at the Salk Institute for Biological Studies in California, but did not generate much disapproval (DeCoux, 2007). The mice were injected with a human gene that makes an insulin-like growth hormone that delayed symptoms in mice with a laboratory form of Lou Gehrig's disease; the mice did not otherwise manifest any human traits.

Moral Dilemmas

1. What kind of rights should chimeras have, considering animal rights vary from country to country, and in some countries, animal rights are totally nonexistent?

Traditional Technologies for Crossing Species Boundaries

Species boundaries have been crossed for decades by transferring specific genes and other materials from one species to another. Conventional technologies include:

• Animal breeding to produce hybrids, such as mules (the male donkey and female horse), geeps, ligers, and wolphins (Munzer, 2007)
• Genetic recombination techniques
• Interspecies organ donation (xenotransplantation)

Scientists hope that, in the future, specially bred animals will provide an abundant supply of organs for human recipients. Scientists are also modifying donor animals using genetic engineering techniques such as:

- Genetic recombination, which involves the transfer of genes from one species to another
- Recombinant DNA technology, which produces synthetic insulin for humans with diabetes from the pancreas of cows, pigs, and some fish species

(*See* Kopinski, 2003)

Subsequent innovations have allowed scientists to engineer uniquely human susceptibilities into mammals. For instance, scientists have refined recombinant DNA technology to create mice that expressed human proteins and mice that contained entire human immune systems (Kopinski, 2003). These innovations could potentially be used to:

- Raise organs for transplants
- Study embryonic development
- Test new drugs

Cloning to Produce Human-Animal Chimeras

A controversial research area is interspecies combinations, such as hybrids. The terms *hybrid* and *chimera* are often used interchangeably and confused; it is important to note that they are in fact distinguishable.

Hybrids are created when an ovum and a sperm from different but closely related species join to form a single zygote (Kopinski, 2003). In a hybrid, each species contributes half of the DNA contained within a single cell, resulting in a blending of the two species' characteristics, and every cell in the body has that same genome. Although scientists create hybrids in the laboratory by mixing the cells of two zygotes, they also combine material from different species into a single cell using cloning technology.

Cloning Technology

Cloning, a common procedure in molecular labs, involves enucleating a donor ovum (which is haploid). *Enucleating* means removing the entire nucleus, which contains all of the genetic material, and inserting the nucleus of a somatic cell from the human body (which are diploid). The transferred diploid genetic material when inserted into the haploid donor ovum then replicates the state of the ovum after fertilization, allowing normal development to occur. This also allows a perfect clone of the somatic cell donor to be grown up, theoretically to adulthood. Scientists use chemicals or electricity to stimulate cloned embryos to begin dividing as an ovum fertilized by a sperm would.

It is important to understand that joining a somatic cell nucleus from one species and an ovum cell from another species does not result in an organism containing the DNA of both species. This is

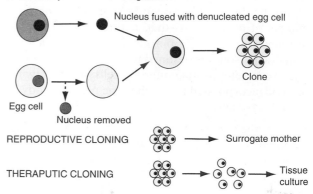

FIGURE 32-1: Cloning

Source: Figure derived from image drawn by/de: Quelle: Zeichner: Schorschski/Dr. Jürgen Groth, with text translated (Wikimedia Commons).

because an ovum cell is haploid, meaning it has only one copy of the entire set of chromosomes. Somatic cells are diploid; all cells in a human being are diploid except sperm cells and ovum cells. If the genetic material of both types of cells were combined, a triploid cell would be created, which is not viable (Kopinski, 2003). Opponents of cloning technology do not always understand the science illustrated in Figure 32-1; what they envision occurring is a scientific impossibility: a creature with human-animal DNA.

The FDA regards cloning as a form of gene therapy subject to biologics regulations, which govern the medical manipulation and reinsertion of human cells. The FDA suggested that it would regulate cloning for reproductive purposes but not necessarily cloning for biomedical research. The FDA further stated that cloning to produce children would require filing an investigational new drug application, but it was not prepared to grant such applications for cloning.

Nuclear Transfer Technology

Nuclear transfer means transferring the nucleus with its chromosomal DNA from one donor cell to another recipient cell. In cloning, the recipient is a human ovum cell and the donor cell can be any one of a number of different adult tissue cells. Three fascinating, but controversial areas of medical research involve the transfer of human cells to cows, rabbits, and sheep. There is much that is not known about the creation of these entities. As is often said, more research is needed.

Human-to-Cow Chimeras

In the first reported human-animal nuclear transfer in 1998, scientists at Advanced Cell Technology, a company in Massachusetts, fused the nuclei of human body cells with cow ovums from which the nuclei had been removed. Only one of the resulting embryos, which contained 99 percent human DNA from the transferred human nucleus and 1 percent cow DNA from the ovum's mitochondria, developed past the sixteen-cell stage (Hagen & Gittens, 2008).

The PHG Foundation, an international independent charity working to achieve evidence-based applications of science, and based in Cambridge, England, reports that three research teams from Newcastle University and Kings College in London and from Edinburgh University are pursuing the research first pioneered in the U.S. more than a decade ago. Approved in early 2008, human-to-cow chimeras are being used to create embryonic stem cells for medical research (Ballard, 2008).

Human-to-Rabbit Chimeras

Thereafter, in 2003, scientists at the Shanghai University in China removed the DNA from the nuclei of rabbit ovums and replaced it with DNA from human body cells. The scientists then allowed the embryos to develop for several days before destroying them (Kopenski, 2003). If this group of human-animal chimeras were allowed to mature, they would likely have exhibited some human and some animal characteristics, both internally and externally (DeCoux, 2007). If the human-rabbit chimeras had been allowed to grow to maturity, they would have become adults who, whatever their outward appearance, were both human and leporine (Chen et al., 2003). The emergence of these and other human-animal chimeras demonstrates the inadequacy of one of the law's most basic assumptions: that there is a sharp line of demarcation between humans and animals (DeCoux, 2007).

Human-to-Sheep Chimeras

Sheep at the University of Nevada have human liver cells. In 2007, human cells were injected around halfway through gestation of the sheep fetus, after the body plan for the fetus had formed but before the sheep fetus's immune system developed to reject the transplanted cells. Between 7 and 15 percent of all the cells in the sheep livers were human and a few human liver cells formed clusters, yielding functionally and fully human liver units available for transplantations as auxiliary organs (Ballard, 2008).

Geron's Cloning Technology

Geron, a California biotechnology firm attempting to develop therapeutic products for cancer and degenerative diseases, is at the forefront of cloning through a collaboration with the University of Edinburgh's Centre for Regenerative Medicine. Geron funded the two teams of researchers that isolated stem cells in 1998: James Thompson's team at the University of Wisconsin and John Gearhart's at John Hopkins (Spar & Harrington, 2009). Cloning could become a more potent technique than stem cell research alone in repairing or replacing human tissue (Wharton, 2006). Cloning could also develop animals that:

- Have modified organs for xenotransplantation to patients
- Produce humanized antibodies
- Secrete therapeutic proteins in their milk

Also known as nuclear transfer, cloning involves putting the nucleus of an adult animal cell into an unfertilized ovum cell. Cloning can create a genetically identical creature. Another strategy is to generate stem cells and use the stem cells to create healthy new tissue. That tissue could be implanted in the nucleus-donor, and it likely would be acceptable to the patient's immune system. Geron is working with scientists at Scotland's Roslin Institute, famous for cloning Dolly, to develop a nuclear transfer technique using regular cells rather than harvested ovum cells. Dolly, a domestic sheep, was the first mammal to be cloned from an adult somatic cell, using nuclear transfer technology. The company believes cloned tissue using only adult cells from a would-be transplant recipient would not trigger any immune system rejection (*see* Wharton, 2006).

Pluripotent Stem Cells for Human Transplantation

Scientists claim cloning techniques may yield pluripotent stem cells, from which they could produce cells and tissues for human transplantation (Kopinski, 2003). As exciting as this may be, the concern with this is that if these human-animal experiments are continued without regulatory oversight, it is possible they could lead to the development of human-animal beings as portrayed by Crichton in *Next*.

When the U.S. National Academy of Sciences published its amended 2008 Guidelines for Human Embryonic Stem Cell Research, one of the few research prohibitions in the guidelines concerned the creation of certain kinds of human-animal chimeras (Baylis & Fenton, 2007). At issue is whether this prohibition will remain in force, or whether it is even related to rescission of the federal restrictions on stem cell research. The aspects of procurement, derivation, banking, and use of pluripotent stem cell lines were given attention to ensure that every step of chimera research is done in a highly ethical and transparent manner.

Human-Animal Chimeras

Many non-embryonic cell transfers from animals to humans are widely accepted. For instance, an adult human-animal chimera resulted when humans with Parkinson's disease underwent a research procedure in which cells from the brains of pig embryos were injected into each human's brain at Boston Medical Center. Autopsies on the human research subjects (whose deaths were unrelated to the experiment) demonstrated viable porcine dopaminergic neuroids at the injection site (DeCoux, 2007). In other words, the pig brain cells had become part of the human brains.

In the area of xenotransplantation, the placing of pig heart valves in human beings caused some initial concern among recipients; however, after thirty years, this transplant procedure is now regulated and accepted. It seems the public does not object to the development of single organ transplants from animals into human beings (Greely, 2003; *see* Kopinski, 2003). Taking science one step further, creation of human-to-animal chimeras to produce human organs offers a chimerism-induced tolerance that would make these organs advantageous over xenotransplants in overcoming tissue rejection that currently hinders composite tissue allograft in clinical practice (Ballard, 2008). Yet, using animal parts as transplant organs has its limits.

If a human were to receive many organs from an animal, or if it were possible to transfer a single vital organ from a similar species (such as a primate brain) into a human, then concern might arise as to whether the resulting organism was really human. Thus, the President's Council on Bioethics raises concerns about chimeras made by moving animal parts into human beings when the transfer is significant enough to cast doubts on the humanity of the recipient, such as implanting human-animal chimera or hybrid embryos into women (PCB, 2004; *see* Kopinski, 2003). Placing monkey tails on humans might also raise concerns.

Moral Dilemmas

1. Could a sub-human species be produced to perform tasks humans refuse to do?

2. Is there less of an ethical issue to experiment on or destroy human-animal chimeras than there is to experiment on or destroy human life?

SYNTHETIC BIOLOGY

While many people have never heard of this emerging field, a growing number think synthetic biology represents a significant turning point in the life sciences (Kaebnick, 2008). In December 2008, medical device billionaire Hansjörg Wyss, chairman of Synthes, gave $125 million to Harvard University, which will expand an institute for biological engineering.

Synthetic biology takes genetic engineering techniques many steps forward. It approaches the goals of genetic engineering from the other end; instead of just modifying existing biological systems, it seeks to build new systems from the ground up. Earlier genome manipulations were largely confined to moving genes from one organism to another. Now, synthetic biology aims to create wholly new genetic recipes (and ingredients) that the older engineering simply could not cook up. (Kaebnick, 2008a) Today, synthetic biology uses techniques from:

- Computational biology
- Engineering
- High-throughput molecular biology
- Nanotechnology

Synthetic biology is seen as turning the same corner chemistry rounded about one hundred years ago, when chemists began to go beyond merely studying chemicals to designing and building them. Now, instead of just trying to figure out how living organisms work, analytic biologists will learn how to build them, either by making genetic changes to existing organisms or by creating essentially new kinds of organisms from scratch (Kaebnick, 2008). More effective targeted medicines and intelligent tumor-seeking bacteria are just a few of the hoped-for medical applications at the forefront of this revolution in personalized medicine (Hastings, 2008).

BAN ON PATENTING HUMAN ORGANISMS

In response to the public controversy over reprogenics, the Weldon Amendment prohibited the PTO from issuing patents on human organisms, including:

- Genetically engineered adult human organisms
- Fetal human organisms
- Embryonic human organisms

The ban, however, does not affect the patentability of biological products of human origin:

- Cell lines
- DNA sequences
- Stem cells
- Tissues
- Other biological products

Nor does the ban prevent scientists from seeking patents for processes to create biological products. The ban also allows the PTO to continue to address new claims, including chimeras. The PTO already grants patents on animals that have been modified to include a few human genes for the production of a human protein or antibody; however, it remains unclear which chimeras are so humanlike that they cannot be patented, such as the transgenic humanzee described by Crichton in *Next*, along with the chimera described in the Newman-Rifkin patent application. Since patents cannot be granted on claims encompassing human organisms at any stage of development, chimeras created from human stem cells may not qualify for patent protection (Kopinski, 2003).

Regulation of Genetically Modified Human Organisms

There is currently debate on whether chimera research should be further regulated. Multiple federal agencies currently regulate genetically modified animals. The Coordinated Framework for Regulation of Biotechnology ("Framework") formalized this decentralized approach. The agencies listed in the Framework are governed by almost a dozen federal statutes, regulations, and guidelines. No single agency, however, provides for the comprehensive regulation of genetically modified human organisms, and none of the federal agencies address modern chimera technology directly (Kopinski, 2003).

Under the Framework, the FDA, the Environmental Protection Agency, and the U.S. Department of Agriculture regulate the research, development, and approval of biotechnology products. The Framework regulates these products according to their composition and proposed uses, rather than by their method of production. As a result, biotechnology is subject to the same laws and policies that govern conventional medical products (Kopinski, 2003).

The FDA's Legal Mandate

The FDA has claimed authority over various forms of ART, although it has not added human-animal chimeras specifically to its jurisdiction. Jurisdiction has been claimed over:

- Human cloning
- Stem cell research
- Tissue transplants[LN1]

Chimeras could be regulated as biological products or drugs, or the procedures used to create chimeras could be medical devices. Either way, if the FDA decides it has jurisdiction, then it would have to approve investigative new drug applications before research could proceed.

President's Council on Bioethics

The President's Council on Bioethics has incorporated chimeras into its discussions of ARTs, as it examines the governance of biotechnologies that touch the beginnings of human life. Suggesting the need to overhaul existing regulations, the Council admits that it is unable to offer clear recommendations regarding major reforms. The Council has also examined ART and explored whether legislation could be tailored to include new technology such as chimeras. The only federal law currently in place to regulate ART is the Fertility Clinic Success Rate and Certification Act, which does not encompass chimeras directly. *See* Fertility Clinic Success Rate and Certification Act of 1992, 42 U.S.C.A. §§263a-1 through a-7 (1992); *see also* Kopinski, 2003.

Proposed Reproduction and Responsibility Act

The Council recognized the need to define the terms surrounding chimera and discussed the need to preserve a reasonable boundary between humans and animals during the early stages of life. Because no public institutions are responsible for setting appropriate limits for these rapidly advancing technologies, the President's Council urged Congress to adopt targeted restrictions on several well-defined activities. The Council recommended collecting these measures in a Reproduction and Responsibility Act, which would acknowledge the need for a moratorium on certain practices until the public and legislators had an opportunity to debate the appropriate governance of these medical technologies (Kopinski, 2003).

Human and Animal Tissues

Creation of human-animal chimeras raises unique challenges to the character of human reproduction. The President's Council distinguished various contexts in which scientists create chimeras, opining that there is nothing inherently objectionable about mixing human and animal tissues. In the context of therapy and preventative medicine, the President's Council endorsed:

- Animal-derived pharmaceuticals
- Insertion of animal genes into humans or human fetuses to prevent disease
- Xenotransplantation

The President's Council recommended two prohibitions:

- Production of hybrid human-animal embryo by fertilization of:
  - Human ovum by animal sperm
  - Animal ovum by human sperm
- Transfer, for any purpose, of any human embryo into the body of any member of an animal species, explaining that humans should be placed only in human wombs

The different combinations of human and animal ova and sperm, known as embryonic chimeras, was not prohibited (Kopinski, 2003).

Gene Patents

There is ongoing debate over which forms of life are patentable, particularly in the area of intellectual property law. The issue first arose when a genetically engineered bacterium was determined to be a patentable invention. *See Diamond v. Chakrabarty*, 447 U.S. 303 (U.S. Supreme Court 1980) (holding bacteria designed to consume oil is patentable subject matter); *see also* Kopinski, 2003. Since then, patentable subject matter has come to include anything under the sun made by man, excluding the ideas, laws (such as the law of gravity), and processes of nature (snow). The current debate involves those who believe no one should possess the exclusive rights to living organisms, and those who hope to secure patents on human and animal combinations for the generation of stem cells and tissues (Kopinski, 2003).

Patents exist to protect inventions; they permit scientists to publish their findings without suffering financial losses, and as such they are a means to encourage the free flow of scientific information (Wharton, 2007). They also encourage funding of innovation by protecting the innovators' exclusive right to profit from their innovations beyond simply recouping the costs of research and development. Patents allow for profitable transparency. Problems arise, however, when patents are granted to things that exist independent of an invention, such as gene patents (Wharton, 2007). The National Center for Biotechnology Information's database shows that more than three-fifths of the patents are assigned to private firms and that, of the top ten gene patent assignees, nine were based in the U.S. (Kane, 2007). The question is whether basic truths of nature should be owned.

If a company invents a new test, the company may patent it and sell it for as much as the market will permit. Companies can certainly own a test they have invented. However, should they own the disease itself, or the gene that causes the disease, or essential underlying facts about the disease (Wharton, 2007)? There are no consistent answers to patent questions like this in the U.S. or elsewhere in the world. Moreover, just because something is patentable in one country does not means it is patentable in another country.

Hepatitis C Genome

What is certain is that gene patents can impair scientific progress, making it prohibitively expensive for scientists to study certain diseases. Innogenetics is currently litigating the validity of the method for genotyping the Hepatitis C virus with Abbott Laboratories. *See Innogenetics, N.V. v. Abbott Laboratories*, 512 F.3d 1363 (U.S. Federal Circuit Court of Appeals 2008). While Innogenetics sought a permanent injunction against Abbott, its request for equitable relief was denied on the basis that Abbott's use of the genome was not in direct competition with Innogenetics' patent. With the denial of the injunction, the power and therefore the value of the Hepatitis C genome patent has been diminished. Although the full extent of the diminution is yet to be determined, it has impacted Innogenetics's entitlement to relief and it likely has impacted Innogenetics's ability, as the patent holder, to share its rights to the genome through a license.

Breast Cancer Genome

Gene patents can also price patients out of the health care market. Because of costly patents, a test for a breast cancer gene that should cost about $1,000 now costs three times that from Utah-based Myriad Genetics ("Myriad"), which monopolizes genetic testing for breast cancer in the U.S. This is not the case in Europe. In 2004, the European Patent Office revoked Myriad's patent on a breast cancer gene in order to facilitate cheaper and more widespread screening across the continent (Wharton, 2007). Europe objected to a single company essentially controlling breast cancer genetic research and testing for commercial gain (Institute Curie, 2005).

After a sixteen-year effort (1974-1990), Mary-Claire King of the Washington University School of Medicine identified the chromosome where the breast cancer genes were located, a breakthrough that induced a classic scientific race for the gene. Besides King, the European Breast Cancer Consortium and Myriad competed for this discovery. Myriad first sequenced the gene in 1994 and filed for a patent, claiming rights to the mutations of the gene and the nucleic acid probes that specifically hybridize to these mutations (Wang, 2008). *See* Linked Breast and Ovarian Cancer Susceptibility Gene, U.S. Patent No. 5,693,473 (filed June 7, 1995) (issued Dec. 2, 1997). Myraid also claimed a patent on a second breast cancer gene. *See* Genetic Markers for Breast, Ovarian, and Prostatic Cancer, U.S. Patent No. 5,622,829 (filed Apr. 19, 1995) (issued Apr. 22, 1997).

The Myriad patents cover the compounds for diagnostic purposes, including genetic tests for cancer and gene therapy (Kane, 2007). Although the unearthing of the breast cancer genes was achieved by King, Myriad controls the licensing for cancer screenings with at least eight patents and disallows all other genetic tests based on its inventions, including sequencing, except for those conducted in its own laboratories (Kane, 2007).

Myriad's restrictive licensing requires scientists to submit their cancer screening samples to its testing facility, where Myriad gains access to clinical information that takes other scientists decades to accumulate. Each sample enriches Myriad's collection of DNA and patient profiles, which allows the company to take even more control over the breast cancer genome (*see also* Wang, 2008).

Unfortunately, Myriad's licensing may have delayed the progress of studies about breast cancer (Wang, 2008). For instance, when researchers at the Hospital of the University of Pennsylvania (HUP) offered breast cancer testing to patients where breast cancer was apparently being passed down in families, HUP received cease and desist letters from Myriad, threatening litigation unless the University of Pennsylvania Health Care System licensed the Myriad patents (Wang, 2008). In one such case at HUP, the Myriad test came back negative, but because no other institution in the U.S. performed advanced research in this field, the family had to go to the Institute Curie in Paris to seek a second opinion. The Institute Curie confirmed the mother and the daughter both suffered from significant breast cancer gene deletions. Missing sections of DNA on these two genes were just coming to scientists' attention in the U.S., and thus were not detectable by the Myriad test. The delay for the deletion issue to come up in America would not have probably happened if more academic labs had been able to do this research (*see* Caulfield et al., 2006; *see also* Wang, 2008).

Myriad does not dominate breast cancer genetic testing in Europe as it does in the U.S. In fact, the European Parliament passed a resolution that opposed the issuance of breast cancer genome patents by the European Patent Office. *See* Resolution on the Patenting of (Breast Cancer) Genes, European Parliament Doc. (2001) (noting that a monopoly on breast cancer genetic testing "could seriously impede or even completely prevent the further use of existing cheaper and more effective tests for the breast cancer genes"). Congress could create a similar research exemption from infringement for research on genetic sequence information and an infringement exemption for genetic diagnostic testing (*Federal Register,* 2005; *see also* Kane, 2007).

DNA Patents

Patents on breast cancer genes implicate the larger issue of patenting DNA, which has been a controversial issue for years. As recently as 2005, the National Institutes of Health recommended careful consideration of where incentives are required and, therefore when genomic inventions should be patented; NIH recommended licensing practices to facilitate full access to DNA sequences (*Federal Register,* 2005). Nevertheless, nearly 20 percent of all protein-coding human genes have been patented, with the majority patented by private biotechnology companies (Jensen & Murray, 2005; *see also* Wang, 2008). Though it is now widely conceded that such patents violate the spirit of the law, the PTO continues to grant gene patents nevertheless (Wharton, 2007).

Patent Quandaries

The legal system that created and upholds gene patents is Crichton's real prey in *Next*. The courts do not realize how fast things are changing, a character observes. They do not:

- Understand that there is already a new world
- Get the new issues
- Comprehend what scientific procedures are done or not done

As science outpaces the law, coherent legal positions are being compromised, as shown by the instances of the Hepatitis C and breast cancer gene patents. In *Next*, Crichton crafts a novel around this argument as a way of developing his analysis. From an analytical viewpoint, while it may leave something to be desired, a novel offers Crichton something nonfiction does not: it provides him with a way to help readers use their imaginations to grasp the implications of the law as it now stands (Wharton, 2007).

Synthetic biology poses special problems for those seeking ownership of, or access to, what might become vast arrays of new medical technologies. Both patent thickets (the need to receive licenses from multiple patent holders) and the anti-commons (many patent owners blocking each other) are potential roadblocks to the use and distribution of these technologies. Besides patented genes, scientists also often hit roadblocks with therapeutic targets because a receptor has been patented. *See Merck KGaA v. Integra Lifesciences I, Ltd.*, 545 U.S. 193 (U.S. Supreme Court 2005). In order to work around this, they develop a test using a mutant receptor or a receptor from a different but similar species. This is particularly a problem in drug research and discovery when chemical compounds are restricted from use. This is an area that will need significant attention as the fields of reproductive medicine and generics develop. It is being studied by several groups within the academic legal community, such as the:

- Center for the Public Domain at Duke Law School
- Samuelson Clinic at the University of California Berkeley School of Law

The U.S. is at the juncture where it has to decide whether its patent practices should be aimed at maximizing profit or at maximizing the social benefit of academic research (Johnston, 2007).

Moral Dilemmas

1. Who should decide which genes should be kept and which altered, and what role should science play in this decision process?

THE FUTURE OF REPRODUCTIVE MEDICINE AND GENETICS

While there are a myriad of issues fueling the debate about the future of reprogenics, most would agree there is a need to ensure this branch of reproductive medicine and scientific inquiry about genetics is conducted responsibly (Parens et al., 2008). The policies under debate include:

- Advantages and disadvantages of patenting genes
- Scientific and medical use of human tissue
- Merits of banning certain biomedical research, such as human cloning
- Value of the Bayh-Dole amendments, which allow academic scientists to maximize profit by licensing their scientific discoveries to the commercial sector practices, versus maximizing the social benefit of academic research by granting open access to anyone interested

(Johnston, 2007)

Reprogenics begs questions about how we know what we know about our reality; indeed, it forces us to wonder whether we know anything at all about it (Wharton, 2007). For Crichton in *Next*, the limits of the real, the parameters of how life is understood, are systematically changed by science, while everyone remains secure in unfounded beliefs, such as:

- Human biology is a settled fact of nature
- Individual autonomy only resides within the human species
- Humans are a species separate and distinct from other species
- Humanity is not going to be altered or threatened anytime soon

(Bennett, 2006)

As Crichton's epigraph to *Next* announces: his novel is fiction, except for the parts that are not.

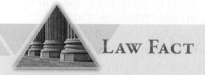

LAW FACT

PATENTING "HUMANZEE"

How many human gene sequences are needed for the U.S. Patent Trade Office (PTO) to decide an organism is human?

While there is no consensus in the scientific community on how many human cells scientists should be permitted to implant into animals (Sherringham, 2008), the PTO has maintained it will not grant patents on human life nor for the processes to create human life. In denying the Newman-Rifkin patent, however, the PTO did not explain why chimeras containing less than 50 percent human DNA encompass a human being and therefore are un-patentable. Hence, the question remains about the humanness of a chimera.

—The only case law applicable to chimeras pertains to the PTO's denial of patents on human life. Transaction History, U.S. Patent App. No. 08/993,564 (filed December 18, 1997); the PTO issued a final notice of abandonment for failure to respond to office action on March 1, 2005.

CHAPTER SUMMARY

- There is little federal regulation in the field of synthetic biology, particularly in regard to human subject research on embryos, cloning, or genetic modifications.
- The FDA has claimed jurisdiction over regulating cloning, stem cell research, and tissue transplants for reproductive purposes, but not necessarily for biomedical research purposes.
- The U.S. National Academy of Sciences published one of the few sets of guidelines to encourage ethical and transparent chimera research.
- The PTO is prohibited from issuing patents on human organisms, such as genetically engineered adult human organisms, fetal human organisms, and embryonic human organisms; however, biological products of

human origin, such as cell lines, DNA sequences, stem cells, and tissues, may be patented, as well as animals that have been modified to include human genes.

- The problem the PTO faces is how to define when something is too human or too much a basic part of nature to be patented.
- No single federal agency comprehensively regulates genetically modified organisms, and none of the agencies address modern chimera technology.
- Chimeras are organisms with cells from at least two genetically distinct organisms, whether from the same or different species; they can be animal-animal, human-human, or human-animal.
- Because current federal regulations do not encompass chimera technology, chimeras are created with increasing quantities of human tissues and genetic materials without limitation.
- Scientists have crossed species' boundaries for decades, by breeding hybrids, developing genetic recombination techniques, and conducting xenotransplantation.
- Benefits of this kind of technology include raising organs for transplants, studying embryonic development, and testing new drugs.
- The U.S. legal system must decide whether patents should be granted in order to maximize profit, which encourages research and development, or to maximize the social benefit of this research, which may pose problems with encouraging scientific innovation.
- Reprogenics forces us to question long-held, but perhaps unfounded beliefs, such as human biology being a settled fact of nature, humans being the only species to possess individual autonomy, humans being distinct from other species, and the lack of any threat to humanity.

LAW NOTES

1. Although the FDA declared jurisdiction over porcine heart valves, used in xenotransplantations as biological materials, the FDA did not extend its jurisdiction to human heart valves until many years later. The FDA acknowledged human tissues could be regulated as drugs, medical devices, or biotechnology products; however, it did not regulate tissues until concerns about the transmission of infectious diseases, such as HIV, from donors to transplant recipients compelled it to assert its regulatory authority (Appel, 2006).

CHAPTER BIBLIOGRAPHY

Appel, J. M. (2006). The monster's laws: A legal history of chimera research. *Genewatch: A Bulletin of the Committee for Responsible Genetics, 19* (2), 12-60.

Ballard, R. A. (2008). Animal/human hybrids and chimeras: What are they? Why are they being created? And what attempts have been made to regulate them? *Michigan State Journal of Medicine & Law, 12,* 297-319.

Baylis, F., & Fenton, A. (2007). Chimera research and stem cell therapies for human neurodegenerative disorders. *Cambridge Quarterly of Healthcare Ethics, 16* (1), 195-208.

Baylis, F., & Robert, J. S. (2007). Part-human chimeras: Worrying the facts, probing the ethics. *American Journal of Bioethics, 7* (5), 41-45.

Bennett, D. S. (2006). Chimera and the continuum of humanity: Erasing the line of constitutional personhood. *Emory Law Journal,* 55, 347-386.

Caruso, D. (2008). *Synthetic biology: An overview and recommendations for anticipating and addressing emerging risks.* Washington, DC: Center for American Progress.

Caulfield, T., et al. (2006). Evidence and anecdotes: An analysis of human gene patenting controversies. *Nature Biotechnology, 24,* 1091-1094.

Chen, Y., et al. (2003). Embryonic stem cells generated by nuclear transfer of human somatic nuclei into rabbit oocytes. *Cell Research, 13* (4), 251-263.

DeCoux, E. L. (2007). Pretenders to the throne: A First Amendment analysis of the property status of animals. *Fordham Environmental Law Review, 18,* 185-230.

FDA News. (2005, June 23). FDA Approves BiDil heart failure drug for black patients.

Garfinkel, M., et al. (2008). Synthetic biology. In M. Crowley (Ed.), *From birth to death and bench to clinic: The Hastings Center briefing book* (pp. 163-168). Garrison, NY: Hastings Center.

___. (2007). *Synthetic genomics: Options for governance.* Rockville, MD: J. Craig Venter Institute.

Gleicher, N., & Tang, Y. S., Center for Human Reproduction in Chicago and New York. (2003, July 1). Colloquium on blastomere transplantation as a possible treatment. Annual Meeting of the European Society of Human Reproduction & Embryology, Madrid, Spain.

Graves. R. (1993). *The Greek myths.* New York, NY: Penguin.

Greely, H. T. (2003). Defining chimeras and chimeric concerns, *American Journal of Bioethics, 3,* 17-20.

Hagen, G. R., & Gittens, S. A. (2008). Patenting part-human chimeras, transgenics and stem cells for transplantation in the U.S., Canada, and Europe. *Richmond Journal of Law & Technology, 14,* 11-87.

Hastings Center. (2008). *Alfred P. Sloan Foundation supports Hastings Center work on ethical issues in synthetic biology project will examine moral implications of a rapidly developing new technology.* New York, NY: Hastings Center.

Hesiod. (Greek original ca. late eighth century BC). *Theogony* (Richard S. Caldwell trans., Focus Information Group 1987).

Homer. (Greek original c. eighth century BC). *The Iliad* (Robert Fagles trans., Penguin 1990).

Institute Curie, Assistance Publique-Hopitaux de Paris & Institut Gustave-Roussy. (2005). *Joint press release: Another victory for opponents of patents held by Myriad Genetics: European Patent Office rejects the essential points of BRCA1 gene patents.*

Jensen, K., & Murray, F. (2005). Intellectual property landscape of the human genome. *Science, 310* (5746), 239-240 (referencing a study of 4,382 of the 23,688 genes in the National Center for Biotechnology Information's database that showed that 63 percent of the patents are assigned to private firms and that, of the top ten gene patent assignees, nine were based in the U.S.).

Johnston, J. (2007). Health-related academic technology transfer: Rethinking patenting and licensing practices. *International Journal of Biotechnology, 9* (2), 156-177.

Kaebnick, G. (2008). *Science and society: Taking control of biology.* New York, NY: Hastings Center.

___. et al. (2008a). *Ethical issues in synthetic biology: Toward clearer understanding and better policy principal investigators.* New York, NY: The Hastings Center.

Kane, E. M. (2007). Molecules and conflict: Cancer, patents, and women's health. *American University Journal of Gender, Social Policy & Law, 15*, 305-335.

Knowles, L. P., & Kaebnick, G. E. (Eds.). (2007). *Reprogenetics: Law, policy, and ethical issues.* Baltimore, MD: Johns Hopkins University Press.

Kopinski, N. E. (2003). Human-animal chimeras: A regulatory proposal on the blurring of species lines. *Boston College Law Review, 45*, 610-666.

Munzer, S. R. (2007). Human-animal chimeras in embryonic stem cell research. *Harvard Journal of Law & Technology, 21*, 123-178.

Nguyen, D., & Xu, T. (2008). The expanding role of mouse genetics for understanding human biology and disease. *DMM: Disease Models & Mechanisms, 1* (1), 56-66.

NRC (National Research Council) Committee on Guidelines for Human Embryonic Stem Cell Research. (2008). *Guidelines for human embryonic stem cell research: As amended.* Washington, DC: U.S. National Academy of Sciences.

Paradise, J. K. (2005). Lessons from the European Union: The need for a post-grant mechanism for third-party challenge to U.S. patents. *Minnesota Journal of Law, Science & Technology, 7* (1), 315-326.

Parens, E., et al. (2008). Do we need "synthetic bioethics"? *Science, 321* (5895), 1449.

Powledge, T. M. (2003). Mixed-sex embryo controversy: Scientific skepticism and ethical criticism of chimera research presented in Spain. *The Scientist, 4* (1), 708.

President's Council on Bioethics. (2004). *Reproduction and responsibility: The regulation of new biotechnologies.* Washington, DC: PCB.

___. (2002). *Human cloning and human dignity: An ethical inquiry.* Washington, DC: PCB.

Price II, W. N. (2007). Patenting race: The problems of ethnic genetic testing patents. *Columbia Science & Technology Law Review, 8*, 119-136.

Robert, J. S. (2006). The science and ethics of making part-human animals in stem cell biology. *Federation of American Societies for Experimental Biology Journal, 20*, 838-845.

Sherringham, T. (2008). Mice, men, and monsters: Opposition to chimera research and the scope of federal regulation. *California Law Review, 96*, 765-799.

Spar, D., & Harrington, A. M. (2009). Building a better baby business. *Minnesota Journal of Law, Science & Technology, 10*, 41-69.

Wang, R. L-D. (2008). Biomedical upstream patenting and scientific research: The case for compulsory licenses bearing reach-through royalties. *Yale Journal of Law & Technology, 10*, 251-330.

Wharton (Wharton School at the University of Pennsylvania). (2007). A novel on genetic research: It's "fiction, except for the parts that aren't." *Knowledge@Wharton.*

___. (2006). Lawton Burns on the critical, and costly, role of companies that make healthcare-related products. *Knowledge@Wharton.*

___. (2002). Bettering ourselves through biotech: Greater productivity, sharper memories, hair feathers. *Knowledge@Wharton.*

PART XII

ADDITIONAL PRESSING ISSUES FACING OUR HEALTH CARE SYSTEM

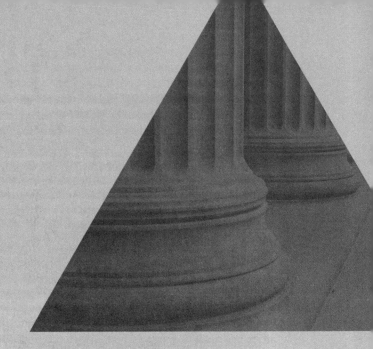

CHAPTER 33

GLOBAL PANDEMICS AND PUBLIC HEALTH EMERGENCY THREATS

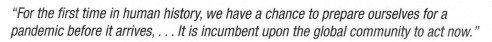

> *"For the first time in human history, we have a chance to prepare ourselves for a pandemic before it arrives, . . . It is incumbent upon the global community to act now."*
>
> —MARGARET CHAN, DIRECTOR-GENERAL OF THE WORLD HEALTH ORGANIZATION (WHO)

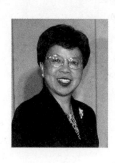

IN BRIEF

This chapter deals with the increasing focus on global health, specifically addressing community health and safety in the event of a global pandemic. It is suggested that the U.S. health care industry must put more emphasis on planning how to respond to the appearance of novel or previously controlled or eradicated infectious agents and biological toxins as part of a rethinking of its broader strategic plans for health emergency threats. New information about the avian and swine influenzas is discussed. While some view the H5N1 (avian flu) virus in a lackadaisical manner with the emergence of the H1N1 (swine flu) virus, as long as a virus remains active, it threatens to mutate into something more deadly.

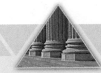

FACT OR FICTION

NATIONAL STRATEGY FOR PANDEMIC INFLUENZA

Could a disease outbreak threaten the political, social, and legal fabric holding society together at the height of a global pandemic responsible for over 250,000 deaths per day for a year?

The timeline begins in January with sporadic human cases of the H5N1 virus in the Nile Delta and Nigeria. By March, several family clusters are confirmed in Africa and Iraq, and by May the virus is suspected to have spread beyond families in scattered areas of China. In June and July, cases of human-to-human transmission of H5N1 appear in Europe and South America, killing one in twenty of those infected. The World Health Organization (WHO) declares a global pandemic is under way.

Five clusters appear in the U.S. and, soon after, are traced to illegal cockfights in Louisiana and New Mexico. They are initially controlled. In August, clusters emerge in Southern California. They spread despite control measures, and by the end of August, H5N1 has spread throughout the country. By mid-September, the global pandemic is very serious and getting worse. H5N1 has become resistant to oseltamivir and zanamavir, two antiviral drugs, so although the medicines are of some use, they are not as effective as hoped. By the end of September, forty-five million people have been infected, or 15 percent of the U.S. population. Outpatient care is provided to serve the needs of eighteen million Americans, and 314,000 are hospitalized. Hospitals and clinical staffs are making decisions as to whom to vaccinate. Eighty-nine thousand Americans have already died. The major impact is on young people with strong immune systems and anyone who did not receive the seasonal influenza vaccinations. The safety net for the uninsured is non-existent, as access to clinicians is invisibly rationed.

The U.S. planned to produce enough vaccine to inoculate all Americans within six months, but the country runs out of vaccines in early October, before the pandemic peaks. By November, an effective pandemic vaccine becomes available and a national vaccination campaign swings into action as an additional one hundred thousand die. The vaccine is not perfectly protective and deaths continue into December with mortality rates of 70 percent. Thirty-five percent of the population is now infected, or one hundred million people; 735,000 Americans are hospitalized. Many bodies remain in frozen storage, while the survivors of families organize funerals. Fear is paralyzing societal life and beginning to lead to panic and further distrust in governments and institutions. The economic burden is estimated at $167 billion. In January, a congressional commission is set up to investigate the country's management of the pandemic.

—Adaptation of Exercise Cruickshank in New Zealand based on scenario data from the U.S. Department of Defense.

(See *Law Fact* at the end of this chapter for the answer.)

PRINCIPLES AND APPLICATIONS

An infectious agent steadily gaining virulence in Southeast Asia or Mexico and making its way around the globe will combine with a highly resistant African strain of the HIV virus (scientists' worst nightmare), and develop into a global pandemic that will infect and kill millions, create mass chaos, and send the world economy into a tailspin. Or it will not. This uncertainty represents a colossal challenge for the health care industry and governments worldwide. No one knows what will happen regarding highly contagious infectious diseases in the coming years and decades. Will some novel disease mutate into a deadly strain where people readily infect others and sicken or kill untold numbers? Or will the concern fizzle out (Lossau, 2006)?

To plan for what could become a public health calamity, all health care providers must assess how their enterprises could be harmed by a global pandemic and take preventive measures to mitigate the damage and keep their enterprises operating (Wharton, 2007). Pandemics are like hurricanes and most natural disasters: they are one area of public health where predictions can be made beforehand (Ahle, 2007). Indeed, all health care systems, hospitals, and medical products companies should actually be planning for all sorts of risks and preparing for public health emergencies within their broader strategic plans.

POTENTIAL DANGERS TO PUBLIC HEALTH

Anyone seeking lessons about the value of emergency preparedness need not look far. A good place to begin is the U.S. Gulf Coast, still reeling from the devastation caused by Hurricane Katrina in 2005 (Rosenblum, 2006). The potential dangers of an ultra global pandemic could be catastrophic, potentially taxing federal and state governments to a higher degree than Katrina. While influenza pandemics generally infect from 15 to 40 percent of a population, the concern is not simply with people getting sick and dying (Barry, 2004). The greater concern is the disruptive force with the capability to cause a fairly substantial breakdown in the nation's infrastructure. If there is an ultra pandemic involving a highly infectious, lethal virus, people will be reluctant to leave their homes; that means disruptions in food supplies, supply chains, mass transit systems, and information technology systems (Wharton, 2007). What happens when infrastructure systems stop is simply indescribable.[LN1]

OPERATING IN A CONTEXT OF TURMOIL

The question, then, is how to manage in the context of turmoil. Each health care system, hospital, and medical products company must plan for a substantial breakdown in the physical and social infrastructure in the event of a global pandemic (Lossau, 2006). A supply chain breakdown could cause the health care industry to go into a tailspin since at the first sign of panic all medical products and supplies would disappear from supplier shelves. An example of this phenomenon is how Tamiflu (the medication used to treat seasonal flu) disappeared with the emergence of the 2009 swine flu, a relatively mild strain of the H1N1 virus, only proven thus far to be as lethal as the seasonal winter flu. In a pandemic, essential imported goods, such as raw materials, medicines, and certain foods, would also become suddenly unavailable (Wharton, 2007). How to ensure day-to-day medical care and treatment is the uncertainty that must be addressed.

Imagine just a few of the effects a pandemic would have on attendance at any number of venues (schools and colleges; workplaces, including manufacturing floors; and mass transit systems) as people stayed home, either because they were already sick or feared becoming ill. Absenteeism at work soared to over 50 percent during the 1918 Spanish flu global pandemic (Barry, 2004). Economic disruption would be immense, as large portions of the population stayed home and away from public places, known as social distancing.

Another significant problem would be a sharp drop in consumer demand; two-thirds of the U.S. economy is sustained by consumer spending, but buying a lot of items can be postponed indefinitely (Lossau, 2006).

Then there are venues for entertainment and tourism. If an infectious disease was highly transmissible from person to person, this could have a massive economic impact, as businesses would grind to a halt with forced quarantine of civilian populations, mandatory masking, and harsh restrictions on travel (Lossau, 2006). Foreign investment would be deterred as governments sealed their national borders to prevent spread of the disease, the effects of which could resonate for years after the disease had been contained. A global pandemic involving a highly virulent flu strain such as the Spanish flu of 1918 could cost the American economy anywhere from $675 billion (CBO, 2005) to $800 billion (Marsh Risk Consulting, 2004).

One example of how countries react to turmoil is the epidemic of Severe Acute Respiratory Syndrome (SARS) in 2003. Within days, international air travelers carried SARS from Hong Kong to Singapore, Hanoi, and Toronto. Within months, the disease had infected more than eight thousand people in thirty countries. In Singapore, each morning, companies made employees report their body temperatures (an indicator of whether they were infected with SARS) before being allowed into their offices to work; a buddy system was implemented nationwide under which one employee was required to take the temperature of a coworker to certify the buddy was not lying about the thermometer reading (Wharton, 2006). Infrared cameras were placed at airports and public venues to identify people with fevers. If someone had a fever, they were required to notify public health officials who would screen the individual for symptoms and, if the individual was sick, would quarantine the individual at home (Ahle, 2007). Toronto imposed two types of quarantines: one confined people to their homes; the other allowed some hospital employees to commute in their own cars from home to work but nowhere else (Cherney, 2003). With SARS causing such great damage to the economies, there was a national sense in Eastern Asia and Canada that everyone had to work together to quickly control the situation. The economic damage from SARS was $10 to $30 billion (Lee, 2004).

An example of how the U.S. reacted can be seen in the example of the Spanish flu pandemic of 1918. Draconian laws were instituted. Coughing or sneezing without covering one's face was punishable by a year in jail, since flu viruses are spread from person to person by coughing and sneezing, entering the body through the mucous membranes of the eyes, nose, and mouth (*see* Barry, 2004). However, the world has changed dramatically since 1918. With today's sharp rise in air travel and the steady increase in worldwide commerce, economic globalization has made the spread of new influenza viruses much more rapid.

Symptoms of the annual winter flu are recognizable to most people. Fever, headache, sore throat, cough, muscle aches, and fatigue typically last anywhere from twenty-four hours to seven days. Seasonal flu is attributed to three virus types: influenza A, B, and C. The influenza A virus causes widespread serious infections and affects animals and humans alike, while milder illnesses are attributed to influenza types B and C. Because both virus types A and B go through antigenic drift, or constant but relatively slight mutations, it is difficult to control the illness from one flu season to the next. Additionally, influenza viruses are constructed of ribonucleic acid (RNA). This is significant because when an RNA virus replicates itself from inside a human cell, its copying mechanism makes numerous small mutations in genetic translation. These slight mutations are the reason one year's seasonal flu vaccines do not protect against the following year's flu types (CDC, 2008).

The risk of a global pandemic is difficult to predict; there is much uncertainty. The consequence is that millions of people might lose their lives (Osterholm, 2005). If a pandemic mirrors the 1918 Spanish flu pandemic, there is no way to rationally consider the possibilities. Quarantine measures have not been implemented in the U.S. on a large scale since 1918-1919 (Daubert, 2007). The list of diseases for which quarantine is authorized in the U.S. includes cholera, diphtheria, infectious tuberculosis, plague, smallpox, yellow fever, viral hemorrhagic fevers, SARS, and influenza that either causes or has the potential to cause a global pandemic.

Moral Dilemmas

1. What U.S. health laws should apply if a global pandemic occurs, and what ethical standards should determine who receives limited hospital beds, ventilators, respirators, vaccines, or even the attention of overwhelmed hospital staff?

2. Who will determine why some people will receive medical treatments, as well as the more difficult to understand reason why some will be denied treatments?

THE BASICS ABOUT PUBLIC HEALTH EMERGENCY THREATS

Public health capabilities are deteriorating in some areas of the U.S. and virtually nonexistent in many developing nations (Choi, 2008). At the same time as many antimicrobial drugs are losing their effectiveness in treating diseases, deeply rooted social, economic, and environmental problems provide infectious diseases with fertile conditions to develop infectious viruses (Blum, 2004). In the U.S., as well as many parts of the world, but especially in Africa, a growing problem is the shortages of public availability of vaccines, antibiotics, antiviral drugs, and other medical technologies (WMA, 2006; *see* Smith, 2009).

Moral Dilemmas

1. What are the broader ethical issues defining the responsibility of the U.S. to, and its relationship with, the global community in a situation of a pandemic risk?

New and Re-Emerging Infectious Diseases

A large number of communicable diseases with the potential to turn into public health threats are either directly transmitted from animals to humans or are close ancestors of veterinary strains (Bolin, 2004). The term *communicable* is synonymous with *contagious* when emphasizing person-to-person transmission of infection and, by implication, excluding other infectious diseases. Infectious diseases include any disease transmitted to a human being from any source, whether human, animal, or environmental. Communicable or contagious diseases are a subcategory of infectious diseases only transmitted from one human to another. (Mariner, 2007) About 75 percent of the new and re-emerging infectious diseases affecting humans over the past twenty years have been caused by pathogens originating from an animal or from products of animal origin (Choi, 2008).

About one-third of the world's population is infected with tuberculosis bacilli (WHO, 2008). Cholera is becoming distressingly common in Iraq, several decades after it was assumed the disease had been eradicated. Africa, in particular, has seen an alarming increase in the scale and frequency of infectious disease outbreaks. In the past decade, there have been epidemic outbreaks of yellow fever in Burkina Faso and Côte d'Ivoire, Rift Valley fever in Madagascar, and Lassa fever in Sierra Leone (WHO, 2008a). However, it was not until the 2003 and 2009 outbreaks of SARS and swine flu revived fears of natural epidemics that world complacency began to change (*see* Mariner, 2007). The topic of infectious diseases now has some prominence on the global health agenda.

Swine Influenza (Swine Flu)

While not all the facts about swine influenza, or so-called swine flu, are yet known, three facts are noteworthy:

- Appeared at the end of a normal flu season
- Deaths are occurring in otherwise healthy young adults versus children and those with compromised immune systems (individuals with HIV/AIDS or receiving chemotherapy).
- Strain has mutated from pigs versus the previously feared mutating avian influenza

Avian Influenza (Avian Bird Flu)

Avian influenza, or so-called avian flu, is an infectious disease that has affected animals (usually birds, and less commonly pigs) for over one hundred years. Pigs are a common reservoir for emerging infectious diseases because they can be infected by both human and bird influenza viruses. Caused by type A strains of the influenza virus, it is particularly dangerous for domestic poultry. While transmission to humans is rare, there is cause for concern (Kaiser, 2008). Because type A strains can infect both animals and humans, there is a possibility that a novel A strain will develop, either through mutation or the mixing of different viruses from different species. A pandemic is triggered when a novel influenza A strain emerges in humans through recombination, or a major change in the virus's composition of human and animal antigens (swine or avian) causing serious illness, and then has sustained transmission from person to person.

In mid-2003, the largest and most severe avian flu outbreak in history began in Hong Kong, caused by a subtype of the influenza A virus, resulting in widespread transmission to poultry and some documented transmission to humans. Type A influenza viruses are subtyped according to surface proteins. There are sixteen different H proteins and nine different N proteins. All H and N proteins occur in birds. Human disease has traditionally been caused by three H subtypes (H1, H2, and H3). Recently, humans have become infected by three novel subtypes (H5, H7, and H9) from birds. The fear is one of these subtypes will emerge as the next influenza global pandemic, particularly H5N1. Transmission of H5N1 to humans is of particular concern because the virus mutates rapidly, and may therefore quickly change into a highly infectious form for humans, therefore becoming more highly contagious (Kaiser, 2008).

Unlike the normal seasonal influenza virus, H5N1 can cause severe disease in humans and is almost always fatal. Seasonal flu is caused by strains of influenza virus already circulating in the human population; people build up immunity either by having had prior contact with specific viruses or through vaccinations. A global pandemic flu, however, is a global outbreak caused by new strains of the influenza virus and, as such, no immunity exists in the population, making every individual highly susceptible to infection and serious illness (CDC, 2008).

Scientists disagree about the likelihood of a global pandemic arising from H5N1. Some public health officials view the data and believe a global pandemic will not occur because the avian flu has been around since 1997 without causing serious harm. Other officials view the same data and believe the world is much closer to a global pandemic. While not all H5N1 mutations lead to a global pandemic, the more times recombination occurs, the more likely the necessary mutations will occur to cause sustained human-to-human transmission. This is an ongoing debate, and no one really knows the correct answer (O'Leary, 2006). What is known is:

- Another global pandemic is overdue based solely on the evolution of influenza viruses; the mark for the longest interval between global pandemics was passed in 2008
- H5N1 mirrors the 1918-1919 Spanish flu virus
- There have been three influenza global pandemics in the twentieth century, the last one ending in 1969
- No one knows the origins of SARS, caused by a mutation of H5N1 in 2003

(Lee, 2004)

Twentieth Century Influenza Global Pandemics

The 1918-1919 Spanish flu:
- 40 to 50 percent of the world's population was infected
- 20 to 50 million died worldwide
- 500,000 died in the U.S.

The 1957-1958 Asian flu:
- Two million died worldwide
- 100,000 died in the U.S.

The 1968-1969 Hong Kong flu:
- One million died worldwide
- 70,000 died in the U.S.

Source: Sidorenko & McKibbin, 2005.

Other important facts about the avian flu include:

- More than two hundred million domestic and wild migratory birds in Asia, the Middle East, Europe, and Africa have died of the virus or been killed by authorities in an attempt to halt the virus's spread.

- Since 2003, less than three hundred cases of people dying from avian flu have been laboratory confirmed. At least another four hundred have confirmed infections. Young people with the strongest immune systems have been disproportionately affected by the disease.
- Since February 2006, eighty countries on five continents have reported their first outbreaks of avian flu in birds.
- More worrisome is that the disease in birds is out of control in more locations than ever, including places like the Nile Delta and Nigeria, where public health mechanisms are weak to nonexistent, increasing the chances of a mutation to allow human-to-human transmission. Despite this increased spread among birds, human infection with H5N1 remains relatively rare.

(Osterholm, 2005; WHO, 2007)

Sanofi-Aventis, GlaxoSmithKline, and Novartis are engaged in making vaccines to combat H5N1 and are stockpiling global supplies for the World Health Organization. The National Institutes of Health has ongoing clinical vaccine trials using new tissue-based technologies for quicker vaccine production. However, influenza viruses can rapidly become highly resistant, so available stockpiled vaccines may not always work. Generally, vaccines cannot be produced until a virus has emerged in the population, when it is already too late for prevention (CDC, 2007a). WHO implemented surveillance around the world in 1947 to detect prevalent and emerging types of the influenza virus, and this information is used annually in producing flu vaccines (*see generally* Wharton, 2007).

Some scientists suggest some of the flu medicines approved in the U.S. for seasonal human influenza should work in treating H5N1 infections in humans. H5N1, however, is resistant to amantadine and rimantadine, two antiviral medications commonly used for seasonal influenza. Two other antiviral medications, oseltamavir and zanamavir, might work to treat avian flu caused by H5N1, but additional studies must be conducted to confirm their effectiveness.

So far, few cases of H5N1 transmission from one human to another have been documented. If H5N1 is around and the regular human seasonal flu appears, the chances of H5N1 mutating into a strain easily transmittable to humans increases. For a global pandemic to occur, the H5N1 virus would have to mutate into a strain that could efficiently pass from person to person. In other words, to produce a global pandemic, there must be efficient human-to-human transmission, and this has not happened yet (WHO, 2007a).

Lest anyone think this could not happen, it must be remembered that highly pathogenic influenza global pandemics have occurred roughly two to three times per century. In addition, the prerequisites for a global pandemic have already emerged during the spread of H5N1 in Asia:

- Identification of a novel viral subtype in animal populations
- Viral replication causing disease and death in humans
- Sporadic human-to-human transmission

(Smolinski et al., 2003)

Most importantly, it should be realized that the 1918 influenza A virus appears to have jumped directly from birds to humans; the genetic changes that allowed it to do so are already beginning to appear in H5N1. Some scientists claim H5N1 has already acquired five of the ten genetic sequence changes associated with human-to-human transmission of the 1918 virus (CDC, 2008), while other scientists claim we simply do not know how many mutations are required to create global pandemic strains (WHO, 2007).

Cockfighting and the Spread of Avian Diseases

Spread of avian flu has been linked to live birds used for cockfighting (Sipress, 2005), a violent, high-stakes gambling activity where two gamecocks with razor-sharp pick implements strapped to their feet are entrapped in a ring to fight. Victorious gamecocks usually leave the ring with severe injuries, such as missing eyes, punctured lungs, and broken bones. Gamecock handlers often suck the blood out of their birds' wounds to alleviate the pain and pressure. This contact with the birds' blood and other bodily fluids puts the handlers at high risk for contracting avian flu and other infectious diseases. Spectators and children of gamecock handlers are also at risk of contracting the H5N1 virus if sprayed with the gamecocks' blood during the matches. A disproportionate number of children of gamecock handlers have already died from avian flu. Avian flu has not yet reached American soil, but the billion-dollar-a-year American cockfighting industry is a likely avenue for the disease to enter the country (Pacelle, 2007).

Gamecocks are illegally transported long distances both within and across international borders. Cockfighting is only legal in Louisiana and New Mexico, but matches regularly occur in several other states. Bans on cockfighting are routinely disregarded worldwide because the penalties for violations are so weak. Moreover, cockfighting has previously brought devastating diseases into the U.S. For instance, in 2003, California declared a state of emergency when illegally transported gamecocks contaminated the state's entire poultry population with the exotic and deadly Newcastle disease. At the time, there were over fifty thousand cockfight operators in Southern California alone. Consequently, the danger remains (Sipress, 2005).

EMERGENCY PREPAREDNESS PLANS

The possibility of a public health emergency, no matter how uncertain, has prompted health care systems, hospitals, and the medical products industry to think about how a global pandemic could affect their operations. The key is to identify potential surprises (Wharton, 2006). For example, major health care systems being called on to rapidly expand infrastructure capacity, or surge, beyond normal services to meet the increased demand for qualified personnel and medical care in the event suppliers refuse to deliver medicines and medical supplies and given that some health care professionals will decline to report to work because they are too afraid to leave their own families. To assist states and hospitals in bolstering medical preparedness, the federal government allocated $5 billion in grants over three years, but the money has been used toward other priorities.

Health Care Supply Chains

The health care supply chain is almost certain to break in the event of a global pandemic, which could cause manufacturers of medical products to close, leading to shortages of drugs and medical supplies, including shortages of drugs to treat the H5N1 virus itself. The very rules of capitalism, which make the U.S. an efficient marketplace, also make it exceptionally vulnerable in a global pandemic (Wysocki & Lueck, 2006). For example, many drugs are manufactured outside of the U.S. because of lower costs, while warehouses in the U.S. are generally kept nearly empty for efficiency reasons as well as the pharmaceutical industry's just-in-time manufacturing scheme. Many hospitals stock only thirty-day supplies of drugs because of costs and waste associated with stockpiling more (Wysocki & Lueck, 2006). Most, if not all, of the medical products industry, including protective device companies in the U.S., are operating almost at full capacity (Wysocki & Lueck, 2006a). Therefore, the reality is the health care supply chain operates with almost no surge capacity. If hospitals are to meet surge requirements in the event of a pandemic, clearly, this supply chain issue must be addressed.

Global Supply Chains

The most affected parts of the economy are likely to be those with worldwide operations, global supply chains, and international customers (Marsh Risk Consulting, 2004). Most large multinationals have emergency preparedness planning committees. Some have created task forces combining their strategic planning, operations-continuity procedures, human resources, and health services to adopt event-specific measures in anticipation of a public health emergency. Others, particularly those in the food industry, have prepared marketing campaigns aimed at allaying fears about the use of their products, and thus protecting their brands if a global pandemic should occur.

The federal government and some local and state governments have established emergency plans to curtail travel, close schools, quarantine individuals and communities, and ban public gatherings (HHS, 2005). Such social distancing steps were taken during the SARS epidemic, especially where the disease was most prevalent.

Despite the high degree of uncertainty over the future course of any public health emergency, there is little choice but to plan. Nearly everyone is myopic. It is difficult to think about the future in the long run. People often lack foresight and have difficulty taking steps today where the benefits occur over a number of years (Wharton, 2007). This means there is a need to rethink the "not in my term of office" philosophy and the resultant failure to maintain the nation's public health infrastructure. This conduct makes it more difficult to undertake long-range planning. For instance, most public health services exist at the state and local level, exactly where the economic crisis has hurt government the most. Just when substantial numbers of public health officials are being laid off, they may be needed. In most pandemics, more people die from official ineptitude than from the pandemic infections (Crosby, 2003).

BUSINESS CONTINUITY MANAGEMENT

Planning for a public health emergency is just one component of risk management. The question should not be how to prepare for a global pandemic alone, but how to take steps that could have planning benefits for any number of risks (Wharton, 2006). The focus should be on how planning for a public health emergency can help a health care provider on many different levels. This means planning for operations outside the silo structures of any one part of a health care system and taking a more comprehensive and sophisticated approach to management of risks. It also means planning for a number of risks that, when added together, appear very threatening, but in actuality are each driven by different factors. The chance of all hazards occurring at once, a perfect storm, would be small. Hence, it may be better not to hedge against all hazards all the time and focus instead on those high-impact risks that would be most catastrophic to the entire health care system or the community being served.

While it may seem counter-intuitive, *silo thinking* is how to think about planning for any public health emergency, global pandemic, bioterrorist attack, or natural disaster. For many regions of the U.S., this is the only way for community hospitals to adequately prepare for a global pandemic (IOM, 2006). Many of these community hospitals can barely handle a multiple car crash, let alone mass admissions from a pandemic (Landro, 2006). These community hospitals should prioritize pandemic preparedness efforts based on the type of events they are likely to face, rather than relying on all hazards programs outside their independent control.

National Biosurveillance Integration and Electronic Disease Surveillance Systems

Today, almost everyone is subject to public health surveillance for planning and management of health emergency threats. Like terrorism surveillance, the scope of government surveillance has significantly expanded beyond its contagious disease origins to include more than sixty human infectious diseases (McKibbin, 2007). The federal government's National Strategy for Pandemic Influenza has given the Department of Homeland Security the task of developing a National Biosurveillance Integration System (NBIS) to integrate this data. The Centers for Disease Control and Prevention, however, has already developed the National Electronic Disease Surveillance System (NEDSS), intended to bring all kinds of reporting systems into one national integrated electronic database. It can be assumed that, with NBIS and NEDSS, the U.S. is encouraging information sharing like Britain and Israel, while also ensuring competitive analysis of what the gathered intelligence really means (White House, 2005).

Moral Dilemmas

1. How does the U.S. retain public health surveillance for the common good without sacrificing the value of individual privacy?

Reactions of the Health Care Industry

The way in which health care industry providers react to the possibility of a global pandemic falls into two camps. Some providers spend a little time and money on planning, but believe global pandemic and bioterrorism fears are misplaced, overhyped phenomena that waste billions in resources planning and preparing for nonevents (Wharton, 2007).

Other providers take a more holistic approach. They realize there is the possibility of a global pandemic, and they look at these phenomena in a way that allows them to leverage whatever it is they do for other types of public health emergencies. These providers analyze a landscape of threats. They do not focus only on individual threats.

Independent of any specific threat, the outcome of public health emergencies affects four areas:

- People
- Technology and processing
- Physical environment
- Relationships

If providers understand their current risk mitigation and transfer strategy, and the extent to which their current strategy will protect them, they can model other catastrophic threats (Wharton, 2007). For instance, the operating margins of hospitals average only 3 percent. In a global pandemic, these hospitals would be forced to close clinics, cancel surgeries, and defer most money-making services to care for the volume of pandemic victims. Without strategies in place, many hospitals might be forced to close due to lack of staff and/or lack of revenue. They can get a sense of what sort of adjustments must be made in their risk management philosophy to deal with the potential of a global pandemic.

Moral Dilemmas

1. What should the health care industry do if a global pandemic strikes?

LOW PROBABILITY, HIGH IMPACT EVENTS

Health care providers who think about potential public health emergency scenarios will be better prepared for a global pandemic because they have thought about the scenarios ahead of time. Yet, it is very difficult to get health care systems, hospitals, and the medical products industry to do this. All health care systems conduct annual risk assessments to satisfy their auditors, but those risks are relatively routine, boilerplate topics, such as what would happen if the organization failed to keep pace with technology. Rarely do risk assessments go into low-probability events, even though these events can have a significant impact (Wharton, 2007).

If a vaccine is developed to prevent people from contracting the H1N1 or H5N1 strains, several thorny issues would arise. It is quite likely that if there is a vaccine, it will not be perfectly protective to keep people from getting this virus. It is obvious health professionals, rescue personnel, and so forth will be prioritized for receiving vaccinations. But among the general public, there could be hoarding and misallocations of vaccines (Katz, 2008). To avoid this "I-am-going-to-grab-mine" phenomenon, it is important to put emergency preparedness plans in place (*see generally* Wharton, 2007).

Moral Dilemmas

1. While U.S. health care professionals and some members of the military seem to be likely candidates to be vaccinated in the event of a pandemic, who should receive the second round of vaccines?

2. Would it be better to prepare and stockpile a vaccine in advance than to try to organize provisions of a vaccine if a global pandemic actually breaks out?

Moral Dilemmas

1. At what price should the U.S. be protected against a global pandemic? How does the U.S. accomplish this in such a way that developing nations, and those who cannot afford to take protection, be assisted?

2. What new policy outcomes could mitigate the impact of a global pandemic?

INTEGRATING PANDEMIC THREATS INTO BUSINESS STRATEGY

The biggest challenge presented by a global pandemic is still one of mobilizing the U.S. health care industry to act, and to act quickly, to help address infectious diseases worldwide. The industry, like most people, is myopic about threats from health emergencies outside its own back yard. Sufficient short-term returns are often required to justify the upfront costs of protection from a pandemic.

Estimated Impact of a Global Pandemic on the U.S.
The Lowy Institute for International Policy, based in Sydney, Australia, predicted:
- About forty-three million to one hundred million people, or 15 to 35 percent of the U.S. population, would be infected
- Outpatient medical care would be needed to serve the needs of eighteen million to forty-two million Americans
- Between 314,000 and 733,000 Americans would be hospitalized
- Approximately 89,000 to 207,000 would die
- Health related economic burden would be $71 billion to $166 billion

(Sidorenko & McKibbin, 2005; TFAH, 2007)

If a novel influenza virus does emerge, given modern travel patterns, it will likely spread even more rapidly before detection than it did in 1918. It may infect at least several hundred million, and probably more than a billion, people worldwide (Barry, 2004). As for the effects on business, a global pandemic would likely:
- Cut the global labor forces to different degrees in different countries due to a rise in mortality and illness
- Increase the cost of doing business
- Shift consumer preferences away from exposed sectors
- Cause a re-evaluation of country risk as investors observed the responses of governments

(McKibbin, 2007)

Impact of a Global Pandemic
Mild global pandemic (similar in scale to the 1968 flu)
- Deaths of 1.4 million worldwide
- Close to 0.8% of global GDP ($330 billion) in lost economic output globally
Ultra global pandemic (worse than the 1918 catastrophe)
- Deaths of 142 million worldwide
- GDP loss of $4.4 trillion or 12%
- Some country economies in the developing world could shrink by more than half

(McKibbin, 2007)

Decisions not to invest in risk-reducing measures in high-risk areas of the world are made because of a failure to understand the expected benefits from these actions. Benefits are likely to extend over many years. Expenditures to reduce or mitigate pandemic risks outside the U.S. are regularly justified by expecting to recoup investments within a two- or three-year period. There is also a tendency to procrastinate, waiting to make decisions on whether to incur the costs to prepare for a pandemic (Wharton, 2007).

The risk of a pandemic is global. One major feature of a global risk is the fact that the U.S.

health care industry cannot face a global pandemic alone (DeMaria, 2004). The world is now so interdependent, actions taken today five thousand miles away affect the U.S. health care industry tomorrow. Conventional wisdom holds that one health care system or one hospital cannot have the capacity and expertise to manage pandemic risks alone. In an increasingly interdependent world, the U.S. currently has neither the capacity nor the expertise to manage the risk of an ultra global pandemic that could suddenly threaten the public's health.

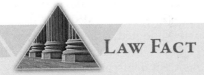

LAW FACT

NATIONAL STRATEGY FOR PANDEMIC INFLUENZA

Could a disease outbreak threaten the political, social, and legal fabric holding society together at the height of a global pandemic responsible for over 250,000 deaths per day for a year?

The congressional panel is asking whether it would have been better for the U.S. to have prepared and stockpiled a pandemic vaccine in advance (as has been done in Europe) rather than to have organized provisions of a vaccine once a global pandemic actually broke out. Investigations are also under way to determine why the U.S. and other developed economies did not help people in advance of a pandemic, which would have required public health subsidies to developing nations for infrastructure development, rather than waiting until after the pandemic occurred when the world was forced to provide large amounts of global assistance to developing economies at the bottom of the global economic pyramid. Indeed, economic globalization has created an environment for the evolution and more rapid spread of new strains of contagious diseases, such as influenza.

—Adaptation of Exercise Cruickshank in New Zealand based on scenario data from the U.S. Department of Defense.

CHAPTER SUMMARY

- Even though no one is sure when, or if, a global pandemic will strike, it is actually possible to predict in advance the effects it might have, and therefore to plan ahead in order to mitigate damage.
- Because a pandemic could infect a huge proportion of the population, the concerns go beyond just the number who fall ill or die; the concerns also include how society would continue to function if people were not available to operate mass transit, information technology systems, and manufacturing facilities, as well as how the global economy would recover from the damage.
- We cannot predict how the U.S. might be able to handle a modern pandemic, as it has been over ninety years since the U.S. had to implement quarantine or social distancing measures.
- Environmental, social, and economic problems, such as the shortage of public health care, create ideal conditions for infectious diseases to become pandemics.
- Tuberculosis, cholera, yellow fever, Rift Valley fever, Lassa fever, and SARS are recent examples of epidemics that have helped focus increased global attention on infectious diseases.
- Avian flu is perhaps the most pressing threat, as it easily mutates, is transmissible between humans and animals, is widespread, and is almost always fatal, even to young people with relatively strong immune systems.
- It is difficult to create vaccines because viruses can quickly become resistant and time is needed to manufacture the needed quantities, during which the virus continues spreading.
- One of the most important potential problems for the U.S. to address is its health care supply chain; the U.S. has little ability to surge production if necessary and does not have sufficient stockpiles.

- One reason for procrastinating on emergency preparedness is that it is difficult to justify spending large sums of money now for benefits that may never come later; however, the costs of the damage of a pandemic would likely far outweigh the costs to mitigate it in advance.
- Probably the most difficult thing to plan for in the event of a pandemic would be prioritizing who would receive limited vaccinations or treatments.
- The risk of a pandemic is global due to increased travel and countries' interdependence.

LAW NOTES

1. Following the 9/11 attacks on the World Trade Center and Pentagon, federal and state authorities turned great attention to the nation's health emergency preparedness. Many of the laws passed after 9/11 asserted greater influence by the federal government in matters that affect public health emergencies. A global pandemic, as a matter of national security, will now be subject to federal jurisdiction (Mariner, 2007). Two model acts developed subsequent to 9/11, the Model State Emergency Health Powers Act (MSEHPA) and the Model State Public Health Act, include provisions that all states have now adopted, either in whole or in part, to deal with health emergency threats like a global pandemic (CLPH, 2006). Both acts deal with health emergency powers, such as compulsory medical examinations, vaccinations, treatments, and quarantines combined with surveillance and travel restrictions.

   Despite considerable health emergency planning, the devastation caused by Hurricane Katrina to the U.S. Gulf Coast in 2005 provided vivid lessons about the nation's deficiencies in emergency preparedness and business continuity management. A global pandemic is likely to produce far more serious disruptions, casualties, and deaths than Hurricane Katrina, only this time, efforts will be directed not to getting people out but to keeping people in.

   Much additional planning, forethought, and funding needs to be implemented before a pandemic outbreak hits the U.S. The immediate medical needs of Americans and adequate resources to both treat pandemic victims and return to normal operations after the pandemic crisis has passed must be secured. The underpinnings of this new theoretical framework are the focus of this chapter.

CHAPTER BIBLIOGRAPHY

Ahle, H. R. (2007). Anticipating global pandemic avian influenza: Why the federal and state preparedness plans are for the birds. *DePaul Journal of Health Care Law, 10*, 213-250.

Arras, J. D. (2005). Rationing vaccine during an avian influenza pandemic: Why it won't be easy. *Yale Journal of Biology & Medicine , 78*, 287-300.

Barry, J. M. (2004). *The great influenza: The epic story of the deadliest plague in history*. New York, NY: Penguin Group (describing how the influenza virus mutates so fast, 99 percent of the one hundred thousand to one million new viruses that burst out of a cell in the reproduction process are too defective to infect another cell and reproduce again, but that still leaves between one and ten thousand viable viruses to infect another cell).

Blakeley, K. (2007, April 17). *Exercise Cruickshank*. Ministry of Health, New Zealand: Wellington Regional Civil Defence Emergency Management Group.

Blum, J. D. (2004). Law as development: Reshaping the global legal structures of public health. *Michigan State Journal of International Law, 12*, 207-228.

Bolin, C. et. al. (2004). Emerging zoonotic and water. In J. A. Contruvo et al. (Eds.). *Waterborne zoonoses: Identification, causes and control* (pp. 19-93). Geneva, Switzerland: World Health Organization (discussing the key factors to the complex emergence process of an infectious disease).

Brookings Institution. (2007). *Top ten global economic challenges: An assessment of global risks and priorities*. Washington, DC: Brookings Institution.

Brown, C. (2004). Emerging zoonoses and pathogens of public health significance - an overview. *Science & Technical Review, 23* (2), 435-442 (suggesting a recent stream of

new diseases has elevated the importance of understanding emerging zoonotic diseases).

CBO (Congressional Budget Office). (2005). *A potential influenza global pandemic: Possible macroeconomic effects and policy issues*. Washington, DC: CBO.

CLPH (Center for Law & the Public's Health). (2006). *The Model State Emergency Health Powers Act legislative surveillance table* (summarizing the extent to which the model provisions have been incorporated into each state's laws). Washington, DC: Georgetown University and Baltimore, MD: Johns Hopkins University.

CDC (Centers for Disease Control & Prevention). (2008). *How does seasonal flu differ from global pandemic flu?* Washington, DC: CDC.

____. (2007). *Interim pre-global pandemic planning guidance: Community strategy for global pandemic influenza mitigation in the U.S., early, targeted, layered use of non-pharmaceutical interventions*. Washington, DC: CDC.

____. (2005). *Fact sheet on isolation and quarantine*. Washington, DC: CDC.

Cherney, E. (2003, October 8). Canada hears call for disease center. *Wall Street Journal*, p. D7.

Choi, K. J. (2008). A journey of a thousand leagues: From quarantine to international health regulations and beyond. *University of Pennsylvania Journal of International Law, 29*, 989-1022.

Crosby, A. (2003). *America's forgotten global pandemic: The influenza of 1918*. New York, NY: Cambridge University Press.

Daubert, M. A. (2007). Global pandemic fears and contemporary quarantine: Protecting liberty through a continuum of due process rights. *Buffalo Law Review, 54*, 1299-1353.

DeMaria, A. (2004). The globalization of infectious diseases: Questions posed by the behavioral, social, economic and environmental context of emerging infections. *New England Journal of International & Comparative Law, 11*, 37-58.

DOD (U.S. Department of Defense). (2008). *Addendum to policy for release of the Department of Defense antiviral stockpile during an influenza pandemic.* Washington, DC: DOD.

___. (2006). *Implementation plan for pandemic influenza.* Washington, DC: DOD.

Gostin, L. O. (2004). Global pandemic influenza: Public health preparedness for the next global health emergency. *Journal of Law, Medicine & Ethics, 32*, 565-573 (analyzing awareness of the essential prerequisites for an influenza global pandemic and public health responses to such warning signs).

Greger, M. (2007). The human/animal interface: Emergence and resurgence of zoonotic infectious diseases. *Critical Reviews in Microbiology, 33* (4), 243-299.

HHS (U.S. Department of Health & Human Services). (2005). *HHS global pandemic influenza plan.* Washington, DC: HHS.

IOM (Institute of Medicine). (2006). *The future of emergency care in the U.S.* Washington, DC: IOM (describing overcrowded emergency departments and trauma centers and fragmented EMS systems in existence today).

Kaiser (Kaiser Family Foundation). (2008). *Avian influenza (H5N1).* Menlo Park, CA: Kaiser.

Katz, M. (2008). Current development 2007-2008: Bioterrorism and public law: The ethics of scarce medical resource allocation in mass casualty situations. *Georgetown Journal of Legal Ethics, 21*, 795-826.

Landro, L. (2006, September 6). Hospitals step up disaster-preparedness. *Wall Street Journal*, p. D4.

Lee, J-W. (2004). *Globalization and disease: The case of SARS.* Washington, DC: Brookings Institution.

Lossau, N., panel moderator. (2006, January 28). Panel: Preparing for a pandemic. World Economic Forum. Davos, Swizerland.

Lowry (Lowy Institute for International Policy). (2008). *The emerging global order.* Sydney, Australia: Lowry.

Mariner, W. K. (2007). Extraordinary powers in ordinary times, mission creep, public health surveillance and medical privacy. *Boston University Law Review, 87*, 347-395.

Marsh Risk Consulting. (2004). *Preparing for an avian flu pandemic.* New York, NY: Marsh.

McKibbin, W. J. (2007). The global costs of an influenza pandemic. *The Milken Institute Review, 9* (3), 18-27.

McKibbin, W. J., scholar, Lowy Institute for International Policy. (2006). Economic Studies, Global Economy & Development Briefing: Assessing the Impact of Pandemic Flu at the Brookings Institution, Washington, DC.

O'Leary, N. O. M. (2006). Cock-a-doodle-doo: Pandemic avian influenza and the legal preparation and consequences of an H5N1 influenza outbreak. *Journal of Law & Medicine, 16*, 511-551.

Osterholm, M. T. (2005). Preparing for the next global pandemic. *Foreign Affairs, 84*, 24-28.

Pacelle, president and CEO of the Humane Society of the U.S. (2007, February 6). *Animal Fighting Prohibition Act of 2007. Hearing before the U.S. House Subcommittee on Crime, Terrorism, & Homeland Security*, 110th Congress. Washington, DC.

Rosenbaum, S. (2006). U.S. health policy in the aftermath of Hurricane Katrina. *Journal of the American Medical Association, 295*, 437-440.

Sidorenko, A. A., & McKibbin, W. J. (2005). *Global macroeconomic consequences of pandemic influenza.* Sydney, Australia: Lowy Institute for International Policy.

Sipress, A. (2005, April 14). Bird flu adds new danger to bloody game; Cockfighting among Asian customs that put humans at risk. *Washington Post*, p. A16.

Smith II, G. P. (2009). Re-shaping the common good in times of public health emergencies: Validating medical triage. *Annals of Health Law, 18*, 1-34.

Smolinski, M. S. et al. (2003). *Microbial threats to health: Emergence, detection, and response.* Washington, DC: IOM.

TFAH (Trust for America's Health). (2007). *Pandemic flu and the potential for U.S. economic recession: A state-by-state analysis.* Washington, DC: TFAH (organization dedicated to making epidemics and disease prevention a national priority).

Wharton (Wharton School of the University of Pennsylvania). (2009). Has the response to swine flu been too feverish? *Knowledge@Wharton.*

___. (2007). When local risks become global risks, and how we can minimize them. *Knowledge@Wharton.*

___. (2006). Avian flu: What to expect and how companies can prepare for it. *Knowledge@Wharton.*

White House, The. (2006). *National strategy for pandemic influenza: Implementation plan.* Washington, DC: The White House Homeland Security Council.

___. (2005). *National strategy for global pandemic influenza.* Washington, DC: The White House Homeland Security Council.

WHO (World Health Organization). (2008). *Global tuberculosis control: Surveillance, planning, financing.* Geneva, Switzerland: WHO.

___. (2008a, September 10). Epidemic and pandemic alert and response: *Cholera in Iraq;* (2008, August 8). Geneva, Switzerland: WHO.

___. (2008b, August 8). *Yellow fever in Côte d'Ivoire.* Geneva, Switzerland: WHO.

___. (2008c, April 18). *Rift Valley fever in Madagascar.* Geneva, Switzerland: WHO.

___. (2007). *Avian influenza, including influenza A (H5N1), in humans: Interim infection control guideline for health care facilities.* Geneva, Switzerland: WHO.

___. (2007a). *Summary of the second WHO consultation on clinical aspects of human infection with avian influenza A (H5N1) virus.* Geneva, Switzerland: WHO.

___. (2006). *Project on addressing ethical issues in pandemic influenza planning: Draft paper for working group one: Equitable access to therapeutic and prophylactic measures.* Geneva, Switzerland: WHO.

___. (2006a). *Pandemic influenza: Draft protocol for rapid response and containment.* Geneva, Switzerland: WHO.

___. (2005, September 22). Epidemic and pandemic alert and response: *Yellow fever in Burkina Faso and Côte d'Ivoire.* Geneva, Switzerland: WHO.

___. (2004, May 18). Epidemic and pandemic alert and response: *China's latest SARS outbreak has been contained, but biosafety concerns remain.* Geneva, Switzerland: WHO.

___. (2004, April 20). *Lassa fever in Sierra Leone.* Geneva, Switzerland: WHO.

WMA (World Medical Association). (2006). *World Medical Association statement on medical ethics in the event of disasters.* Ferney-Voltaire, France: WMA.

Wysocki, B., & Lueck, S. (2006, January 12). Just-in-time inventories make U.S. vulnerable in a global pandemic. *Wall Street Journal*, p. A1.

___. (2006a, January 12). Global pandemic flu could cause breakdown of drug-supply chain. *Wall Street Journal*, p. A1.

CHAPTER 34

HEALTH CARE ISSUES FOR WOMEN

> *"If access to health care is considered a human right, who is considered human enough to have that right?"*
>
> —DR. PAUL FARMER, PROFESSOR OF SOCIAL MEDICINE IN THE DEPARTMENT
> OF GLOBAL HEALTH AND SOCIAL MEDICINE AT HARVARD MEDICAL SCHOOL
> AND A FOUNDING DIRECTOR OF PARTNERS IN HEALTH

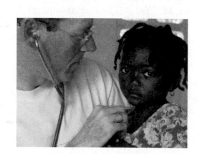

IN BRIEF

This chapter focuses on the disparate provision of medical care for procreation concerns, and addresses reproductive issues against the backdrop of how the newer forms of contraception and maternity care coverage are falling out of reach for more women in the U.S. While abortion is emphasized, with a focus on partial-birth abortions and state regulations that attempt to limit access, this chapter will also concentrate on related sexual privacy issues such as conscience clause legislation and Plan B, or morning-after-pill, provisions.

While gender disparities affecting health care are a major problem in the U.S., the economics of this disparity have not received much attention. Sexually transmitted diseases have become a critical issue in women's health care today as well. In addition, only recently has the health industry discovered that the same diseases and illnesses have different effects or symptoms in women. Adding to these concerns, prescription drugs often work differently for women (or not at all, or may even be harmful), and yet the health care industry has not studied this aspect of most drugs currently on the market. For too long, the industry has largely assumed that what goes for men also goes for women, and this basic assumption is now being called into question.

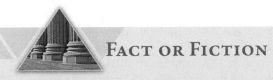

FACT OR FICTION

IN VITRO FERTILIZATION RESTRICTIONS

Who has the right to decide what to do with embryos created through in vitro *fertilization?*

The Georgia legislature has introduced legislation that would make illegal the fertilization procedures used in the high-profile case of a California mother who recently gave birth to octuplets. The bill is the first state legislation introduced in the wake of the case of Nadya Suleman, a thirty-three-year-old single woman who gave birth in January to eight babies through *in vitro* fertilization. Nadya had six frozen embryos left from prior *in vitro* treatments and asked that they all be implanted because she did not want them to be destroyed. Two of the embryos split, creating eight total embryos.

To make embryos, a physician injects a woman with hormones to produce eggs. These are then harvested in a surgical procedure. The eggs are mixed with sperm in the laboratory, and some of the developing embryos are transferred into the uterus. A single cycle with fresh embryos costs more than $15,000, often not covered by insurance. Subsequent attempts at pregnancy are less costly if frozen embryos are on hand, and the supply of extras spares a woman another round of hormones to produce eggs. About half the people who undergo *in vitro* fertilization end up with one or more frozen embryos, but no one can predict how many embryos will be produced and used (Roan, 2008).

The Georgia legislation would limit the number of embryos that may be implanted in a woman to a maximum of three for a woman age forty or older and two for a woman younger than that. The law would also limit the number of embryos created in one cycle to the number to be transferred. Supporters of the Georgia legislation oppose abortion and seek regulation that would treat embryos as human beings. To supporters, this is a human rights issue. Embryos deserve legal protection as living human beings rather than property.

Several *in vitro* fertilization experts and scientific organizations oppose the law, arguing that a successful pregnancy sometimes can only be achieved by implanting more than two or three embryos, and that the law would effectively prevent would-be mothers from freezing unused embryos for later implantation. Opponents maintain that it is the right of the women who have gone through this procedure to decide what they can do with those embryos, not their physicians and not the government.

The Reproductive Medicine Society's guidelines currently urge physicians to limit the transfer of embryos to two in a woman under age thirty-five years and to no more than five embryos for a woman over age forty. The guidelines are not mandatory and can vary according to a woman's individual diagnosis and the condition of the embryos.

—McKay, 2009.

(See *Law Fact* at the end of this chapter for the answer.)

PRINCIPLES AND APPLICATIONS

Women's health is jeopardized by limited access to health care, reproductive rights are under concerted attack, and women's health needs are often overlooked (NWLC, 2009). Still facing gender discrimination, the battle to maintain the rights women have won since passage of the civil rights act in the mid-1960s has shifted its form into attempts to carve out exceptions to women's rights. In this chapter, there are eight appellate decisions of first impression, or decisions where there was no prior binding legal authority existing on the matter presented to the highest state and federal courts. Most of the increased litigation pressure and most of the appellate cases of first impression affecting women's health have involved

disputes over attempts to restrict, rather than expand, application of anti-discrimination laws and the rights of women to health care.

During the last three decades, the U.S. Supreme Court has played a crucial role in prohibiting discrimination against women and in protecting women's health, safety, and welfare. Nevertheless, the legal rights that some have come to take for granted are not secure (NWLC, 2009). *See generally, Aetna Health Inc. v. Davila*, 542 U.S. 200 (U.S. Supreme Court 2004) (restricting patients' rights under the Employee Retirement Income Security Act); *Gonzaga University v. Doe*, 536 U.S. 273 (U.S. Supreme Court 2002) (limiting right to sue to enforce personal civil rights under federal statute); and *Stenberg v. Carhart,* 530 U.S. 914 (U.S. Supreme Court 2000) (state laws regulating banning partial-birth abortions, the most common form of abortion for second-trimester pregnancies, need not contain an exception for the mother's health).

HEALTH RISKS OF WOMEN AND CHILDREN

Women's health risks involve medical conditions that are:

- Conditions for which the risk factors might be different in women (HIV/AIDS and heart disease)
- More prevalent in women (lupus and other auto-immune disorders)
- More serious in women (consequences of sexually transmitted diseases)
- Unique to women (pregnancy and ovarian cancer)
- Different to treat (including all of the above)

(Wood, 2007)

More must be learned about the distinctions between men and women: when they exist and do not exist, and where there are differences and similarities. This knowledge will then help drive more appropriate interventions and health care.

Infant Mortality

According to the Centers for Disease Control, infant mortality (death of children less than one year of age, not including abortions) is one of the most important indicators of the health of a nation, as it is associated with a variety of factors:

- Maternal health
- Public health practices
- Quality and access to medical care
- Socioeconomic conditions

(MacDorman & Mathews, 2008)

There are more than 28,000 infant deaths each year in the U.S. (MacDorman & Mathews, 2008). The National Commission to Prevent Infant Mortality estimates that 10 percent of infant deaths in the U.S. could be prevented if all pregnancies were planned and the mothers had access to prenatal care so the babies could be carried to term. While the U.S. rate of infant mortality and morbidity is high compared to other industrialized countries, research indicates that these rates result because babies are born prematurely without proper prenatal care (Law, 2008). Each year, an alarming number of U.S. babies, almost 13 percent, are born preterm at less than nine months' gestation (ACOG, 2008; Behrman & Butler, 2007;

Petrini et al., 2005). In 2006, forty-one nations had lower infant mortality rates than the U.S., including virtually all European countries and many less developed countries such as Cuba (CIA, 2008).

Premature Births

This high rate of premature births in the U.S. constitutes a public health concern that costs society. The Institute of Medicine and the Centers for Disease Control estimate the cost of prematurity in the U.S. exceeds $26 billion (Behrman & Butler, 2007). The March of Dimes finds it costs, on average, about $2,800 to provide medical care to infants who are carried to term, compared to $41,600 for preterm babies. Prolonging pregnancy by weeks or even days can dramatically affect both health and cost. Moreover, the health consequences of prematurity can include cerebral palsy, intellectual disability, physical and neurodevelopment disabilities, respiratory distress syndrome, intracranial hemorrhage, and chronic illnesses, such as lung disease (Wolke, 2007).

17P Treatment Regimen

Yet, with proper prenatal care, most babies can be carried to term. For instance, there is persuasive evidence that a drug based on the hormone progesterone, also referred to as 17P (or alpha hydroxy-progesterone caproate), helps to prolong gestation and decrease the occurrence of prematurity (ACOG, 2008). The National Institute of Child Health and Human Development released reports showing that weekly injections of 17P reduces the chance of preterm birth by one-third and decreases the rate of neonatal morbidity (*see* Klebanoff et al., 2008; Meis et al., 2005; Northen et al., 2007; Sponge et al., 2005). The American College of Obstetricians and Gynecologists strongly endorses the 17P regimen, and has conducted research with the March of Dimes demonstrating its effectiveness (Petrini et al., 2005). Several state Medicaid programs cover this treatment regime for women, including New York, North Carolina, and Pennsylvania (NCSL, 2007).

REPRODUCTIVE HEALTH

The state of reproductive health in the U.S. is poor. The needs of women are not being met. Examples of this include:

- Nearly half of all pregnancies are unintended and nearly 40 percent of all unintended pregnancies end in abortion
- Women at the bottom of the economic pyramid are four times more likely to have an unintended pregnancy than more affluent women

- Many women still lack adequate access to the most effective birth control method for their circumstances and medical needs, especially women from low income families
- One in three sexually active adolescent girls becomes pregnant before twenty years of age, and 80 percent of these pregnancies are unintended
- Each year more than 750,000 teens become pregnant; the teen pregnancy rates are higher in the U.S. than any other developed country in the world, yet over the past decade, more than $1 billion has been spent by the federal government on abstinence programs

(Golub & Gartner, 2007; Kaiser & HRET, 2008; NWLC, 2009; Schwarz, 2007)

Emergency Contraception (Plan B Morning-After Pill)

The National Center for Health Statistics estimates 6 percent of American women have used emergency contraception pills (ECPs), also known as Plan B, or morning-after pills. ECPs are a concentrated dose of a hormone found in many regular birth control pills that can prevent pregnancy when taken shortly after unprotected sexual intercourse (most effectively, within twelve to twenty hours, but up to seventy-two hours) (Kaiser, 2009). ECPs are estimated to be 75 to 90 percent effective at preventing pregnancy.

ECPs were first approved as a form of emergency contraception for women in 1999. Over-the-counter use for women over eighteen years of age was approved in 2006, but women younger than eighteen still had to obtain a physician's prescription in order to receive ECPs, except in states that allowed a pharmacy provision. In these states, all women (including teens) could obtain ECPs directly from a pharmacist under a state-approved protocol, without obtaining a prescription in advance from a physician (Kaiser, 2008). Nine states allowed pharmacists to initiate ECP therapy if they were working in collaboration with a prescriber, a physician, or a nurse practitioner, after they completed a training program in emergency contraception: Alaska, California, Hawaii, Maine, Massachusetts, New Hampshire, New Mexico, Vermont, and Washington.

Then in 2009, the U.S. Food and Drug Administration (FDA) was directed to allow sales of ECPs to all women without a prescription, rolling back the age limit imposed in 2006. The federal court ruling came in response to a lawsuit filed in 2005 by the Center for Reproductive Rights, a women's health advocacy group. *See Tummino v. Torti*, 603 F.Supp.2d 519 (U.S. District Court for the Eastern District of New York 2009) (the court criticized current and former FDA officials for using "political considerations, delays and implausible justifications" to hold

up nonprescription sales of ECPs for several years). Opponents argue that teenagers are not able to make rational decisions about their reproductive health. The Family Research Council, a conservative advocacy group, claims expanded access jeopardizes girls' health and the ability of parents to care for their daughters' physical and emotional well-being (Mundy, 2009). In 2006, the FDA had announced it wanted more time to review the safety of Plan B, despite support for over-the-counter sales by the FDA's scientific experts (Mundy, 2009).

Pharmacists Conscience Legislation

As Americans increasingly integrate religion into their daily lives, conscience legislation is proliferating and influencing the conduct of health care professionals across the U.S. (Duvall, 2007). *See McCreary County v. ACLU*, 545 U.S. 844, 882 (U.S. Supreme Court 2005) (O'Connor, J., concurring) ("Americans attend their places of worship more often than do citizens of other developed nations, and describe religion as playing an especially important role in their lives."). Pharmacists are one of the latest groups to seek conscience protection.

Whether the *Tummino* trial court decision mandating over-the-counter sales of ECPs puts an end to the controversy as to whether women's need to obtain ECPs on a timely basis outweighs the rights of pharmacists licensed by the states remains to be seen. Most likely, it will result in further federal-state conflicts between the FDA and the states. Some pharmacists, whose religious beliefs prohibit abortion or the use of birth control, claim that dispensing ECPs to women is an infringement on their free exercise of religion since they view emergency contraception as a form of abortion (Kaiser, 2008a).

Pharmacist refusals began when the FDA approved ECPs in 1999 and intensified in 2006 after proponents for restrictions lost their battle for over-the-counter access. According to the National Women's Law Center, these refusals have occurred, regardless of state law and company policy, at outlets of large drugstore chains, such as Walgreens, Osco, K-Mart, CVS, and Eckerd, as well as at small independent pharmacies.

State laws restricting prescription access to ECPs include:

- At least eleven states are considering conscience clause laws that would permit pharmacists to refuse to fill certain prescriptions
- Four states have laws that specifically allow pharmacists to refuse to fill prescriptions that violate their beliefs, including ECPs (Arkansas, Georgia, Mississippi, and South Dakota)

- Arkansas and North Carolina exclude ECPs from their contraceptive coverage mandate
- Arkansas, Georgia, and South Dakota hope to strengthen existing laws so pharmacists would be able to refuse to transfer or refer prescriptions for contraceptives, including ECPs, to other pharmacies

(*See* Guttmacher Institute, 2009; Kaiser, 2009; NCSL, 2007)

Opponents object to conscience laws because they say that pharmacists have an obligation to fill all prescriptions and that refusing to fill them violates women's freedom of conscience (Kaiser, 2009). While state laws generally mandate that pharmacists dispense all safe, legal prescriptions and put the best interests of their customers ahead of their own (Duvall, 2007), California and New Jersey are the only states that explicitly require pharmacists to fill all prescriptions (Guttmacher Institute, 2009).

Moral Dilemmas

1. Should pharmacists who refuse to fill prescriptions for contraceptives or ECPs also refuse to fill prescriptions for Viagra or other male sexual enhancement drugs?

2. What considerations underlie the conflict between the rights of health care professionals to not provide certain health care services to women, such as filling of contraceptive prescriptions and the sale of over-the-counter morning-after pills, and the rights of women to receive these legal medical services?

Constitutional Arguments

The Free Exercise Clause of the First Amendment protects an absolute freedom of belief and an individual right to practice religion. One side of the pharmacist debate maintains that their religion prohibits the use of birth control or practice of abortion, and therefore they cannot freely exercise their religious beliefs if they are forced to dispense contraceptives. Since the First Amendment protects individual free exercise of religion, pharmacists claim they have a right to exercise their religion in the workplace (Kaiser, 2009). *See Cutter v. Wilkinson*, 544 U.S. 709, 719 (U.S. Supreme Court 2005) (defining free exercise of religion as government "respect for" and "noninterference with" citizens' religious beliefs and practices). The other side argues that since pharmacists are not required to take the drugs themselves, there is no free exercise issue.

In addition to the First Amendment arguments, the Fifth Amendment is used in the debate for and against conscience legislation. The Fifth Amendment protects property, and the prescription is the woman's property. The Fifth Amendment prohibits deprivation of personal liberty without due process. Opponents of conscience laws maintain that passing laws to allow individual pharmacists to refuse to fill prescriptions that offend the personal morals of some pharmacists deprives women of their liberty without due process (Kaiser, 2009; *see* Clark, 2003).

Moral Dilemmas

1. How are Congress, state legislatures, and the courts dealing with competing interests involving the sale of over-the-counter Plan B pills?

2. Should the federal government and states consider conscience clause legislation to balance competing interests for health care services to women? Is this the way this conflict should be resolved, and if so, will it not result in denial of needed medical care for women?

Coverage for Contraceptives

Having won the right to health insurance coverage for birth control, the debate has shifted to attempts to carve out exceptions to the mandate that health insurance plans must provide coverage for contraceptives. Health insurance plans and employers will continue to face increased litigation pressure as new legal theories based on the application of anti-discrimination laws continue to be unleashed.

Almost half the states have passed laws requiring health insurance plans to cover prescription contraception under most circumstances.[LN1] Several additional states are considering similar legislation, but the reach of the legislation is limited to state regulated plans, and most large employers are self-funded and not subject to state mandates. While studies have shown that state laws requiring insurance providers to cover contraception have significantly expanded access for women, it is not known whether the health insurers would remove birth control from their coverage plans if state mandates expired (Simon, 2008).

Mandated Pelvic Exams as a Condition of Access to Contraceptives

Federally funded family planning programs require women to undergo pelvic exams as a condition of access to oral contraceptives and sometimes other hormonal methods of birth control. *See* Title X (42 U.S.C.A. §§ 300 *et seq.* (2009) and 42 C.F.R.

Part 59 (2009)); Title XIX, Medicaid (42 U.S.C.A. § 1396 (2009); and block grants under Titles V (42 U.S.C.A. §§ 701-709 (2009)) and XX (42 U.S.C.A. § 1397 (2009)). There is vigorous debate on whether this invasive procedure infringes upon women's bodily privacy rights, especially since women seeking the same birth control from private providers are not subject to this mandate. Moreover, men seeking contraception or sexual-performance-enhancing drugs from publicly funded health clinics are not required to undergo invasive prostate exams, despite presenting the same opportunity for preventive health care as women seeking oral contraceptives (Dixon, 2004).

In areas of health care services other than women's reproductive care, it is not appropriate to withhold a prescription from someone who has been informed of the risks involved and chooses to forego screening for an unrelated condition. Yet for the past fifty years, annual pelvic exams have been required of

women seeking birth control at health clinics receiving federal funding. The justification for the government mandate is the FDA-approved package inserts accompanying oral contraceptives that recommend pelvic exams if women are using the pill. Oral contraceptives are dispensed over-the-counter without a prescription in Europe and much of the world (Dixon, 2004).

Exclusion of Contraception Coverage

Some states with mandated contraception coverage include exemptions for companies with religious affiliations that are opposed to birth control. These exempted companies have not yet been required to contribute additional taxes or assessments to state health and welfare funds due to the additional social and economic costs that states incur from unwanted pregnancies arising from women's lack of access to contraceptives.

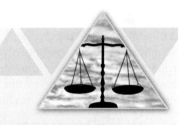

EXCLUSION OF CONTRACEPTION COVERAGE

Standridge v. Union Pacific Railroad Company
[Employee v. Employer]
479 F.3d 936 (U.S. Court of Appeals for the 8th Circuit 2007)

FACTS: Union Pacific Railroad Company provided health care insurance to its employees through several different health insurance plans. These plans provided coverage for services such as routine physician visits, tetanus shots, and drug and alcohol treatments. The plans excluded, for both males and females, prescription and non-prescription contraception unless the contraception was medically necessary for a non-contraceptive purpose, such as treating skin problems. Two Union Pacific female employees, Brandi Standridge and Kenya Phillips, brought suit against Union Pacific for gender discrimination under the federal Civil Rights Act Title VII as amended by the Pregnancy Discrimination Act (PDA) of 1978, 42 U.S.C.A. § 2000e(k) (1991). Standridge and Phillips claimed Union Pacific discriminated against its female employees by failing to cover prescription contraception.

Title VII provides that employers cannot discriminate against any person regarding their compensation, terms, conditions, or privileges of employment because of their gender. *See* 42 U.S.C.A. § 2000e-2(a)(1) (1991). After the U.S.

Supreme Court held that denial of pregnancy benefits did not violate Title VII (*General Electric Company v. Gilbert*, 429 U.S. 125 (U.S. Supreme Court 1976), *superseded by statute*), Congress enacted the PDA. The PDA mandates that women affected by pregnancy, childbirth, or related medical conditions must be treated the same, including receipt of health insurance plan benefits. *See* 42 U.S.C.A. § 2000e(k) (1991).

ISSUE: May employers exclude contraception coverage from their health insurance plans?

HOLDING AND DECISION: Yes, employers may exclude contraception coverage from their health insurance plans.

ANALYSIS: The Eighth Circuit distinguished between preventing conception and medical conditions that occur only after conception (*see Krauel v. Iowa Methodist Medical Center*, 95 F.3d 674 (U.S. Court of Appeals for the 8th Circuit 1996)). Applying this distinction, the court held the PDA does not apply to contraception because

(continues)

(continued)

contraception is a treatment used prior to pregnancy. Moreover, since contraception is a gender-neutral term that applies to men and women equally, health insurance plans that deny coverage for contraception do not violate Title VII.

The court also considered whether the health insurance plan discriminated on the basis of gender. Under a claim of disparate treatment under Title VII, female employees have to establish they were treated less favorably than similarly situated male employees. If pregnancy is a medical disease that only adversely affects women, then the issue is whether the coverage provided to male employees poses a lesser threat to employees' health than pregnancy does. The court declined to decide whether pregnancy was a disease. Instead,

the court held that the comparative of coverage provided by the health plan was too broad. The proper comparative was the medical benefit of contraception. Because the health plan did not cover men's contraception (condoms and vasectomies), the court held the plan did not treat men more favorably than women. Thus, the denial of contraception coverage did not discriminate against women.

RULE OF LAW: Since the PDA does not require employers to cover contraception as part of their health insurance plans, employers do not violate Title VII by excluding contraception as a benefit. (*See generally* Bapat, 2007; Law, 2008; Phillips, 2008; Pisoni, 2008; Pugh, 2007; Vartanian, 2009; Weins, 2008).

Union Pacific now provides contraception coverage, and announced it had no plans to drop coverage for prescription contraception notwithstanding the *Standridge* ruling. While *Standridge* allows employers to drop coverage for prescription contraception, the ruling is unlikely to have such an effect for a number of reasons:

- Contraceptive coverage has become standard practice for most employers
- It is less costly for employers to cover prescription contraceptives than to cover a pregnancy

- Most states already mandate contraception coverage in health insurance plans acquired from commercial insurers

(Golub & Gartner, 2007; Pugh, 2007)

Exceptions for Religious Employers

More and more, religious restrictions are limiting women's access to reproductive health care (NWLC, 2009). This is becoming a divisive issue for many states.

COVERAGE FOR CONTRACEPTIVES BY RELIGIOUS EMPLOYERS

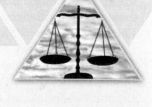

Catholic Charities of Sacramento, Inc. v. Superior Court of Sacramento County
[Religious-Affiliated Charities v. Local Municipality]
85 P.3d 67 (Supreme Court of California 2004),
U.S. Supreme Court certiorari denied, 543 U.S. 816 (U.S. Supreme Court 2004)

FACTS: The California legislature enacted the Women's Contraception Equity Act (WCEA) to eliminate gender discrimination in health care benefits (*see* California Health & Safety Code § 1367.25(b)(1)(A)-(D) (2003)). Evidence had shown that women spent a great deal more on health care costs during their reproductive years than did their male counterparts. The WCEA requires that

certain health care plans that include prescription drugs must cover prescription contraceptives. At the time, about 10 percent of California's commercially insured did not have coverage for prescription contraceptives.

Catholic Charities of Sacramento, a church-affiliated charity, challenged the constitutionality of the WCEA. In particular, Catholic Charities took

(continues)

CHAPTER 34: HEALTH CARE ISSUES FOR WOMEN

(continued)

issue with the WCEA's exception for religious employers. In order for a church-affiliated charity to meet the definition of a religious employer under California law, it must meet four criteria. The entity must:

- Have as its primary purpose, the inculcation of religious values
- Primarily employ persons who share the religious tenets of the entity
- Serve primarily persons who share the religious tenets of the entity
- Be a nonprofit organization

While acknowledging it did not meet any of the criteria for exemption as a religious employer, Catholic Charities maintained the WCEA was unconstitutional because it:

- Burdened the right to free exercise of religion
- Interfered with the autonomy of a church-affiliated charity
- Would fail both strict scrutiny and rational basis tests

Although the religious employer exemption does not apply to all charities affiliated with the Catholic Church, the lower trial court did not agree that this amounted to discrimination against the Church.

ISSUE: Must church-affiliated charities provide state-mandated coverage for contraceptives?

HOLDING AND DECISION: Yes, church-affiliated charities that are not exempt as religious employers must provide state-mandated coverage for contraceptives.

ANALYSIS: The California Supreme Court first analyzed whether the WCEA interfered with the religious autonomy of Catholic Charities. Courts must accept decisions made by the highest church judicatories regarding questions of discipline, faith, ecclesiastical rule, custom, or law. *See, e.g., Watson v. Jones*, 80 U.S. 679, 727 (U.S. Supreme Court 1871). Catholic Charities claimed that the WCEA interfered with matters of internal church governance. The court however, determined that the legislature had not decided any religious question in enacting the WCEA.

Catholic Charities also made the argument that the WCEA burdened the right to free exercise of religion. Specifically, Catholic Charities argued that the WCEA effectively coerced a violation of

religious beliefs. Regarding this argument, the general rule is that religious beliefs do not excuse compliance with otherwise valid laws regulating matters the state is free to regulate. *See Reynolds v. U.S.*, 98 U.S. 145, 166-167 (U.S. Supreme Court 1878). This standard removes the need for a law to be justified by compelling governmental interests if it is neutral and of general applicability, even when the law has the incidental effect of burdening a particular religious practice. The court found the WCEA applies to religious and non-religious employers equally, except for those employers that fall under the religious employer exemption. The religious employer exemption does not impose a burden on any employer; rather, it removes a possible burden from employers that meet the exemption criteria.

Catholic Charities additionally contended that the WCEA discriminated against the Catholic Church and other charities affiliated with the Church. The court did not agree with this contention since the Church had requested the religious employer exemption; the exemption was justified as an accommodation to the exercise of religion. Although the exemption does not apply to all charities affiliated with the Church, the court did not agree that this amounted to discrimination against the Church itself.

Finally, Catholic Charities argued that strict scrutiny should be applied to the WCEA and that it would fail such a test. The court again disagreed. While a decision was not made regarding whether strict scrutiny should apply, the court found that the WCEA would nevertheless pass under strict scrutiny standards. In reaching this conclusion, the court explained that the California legislature had shown that the law was meant to achieve a compelling interest and it was narrowly tailored to that purpose: the elimination of gender discrimination. Any narrowing of the WCEA would decrease the positive intended effect on female employees. Furthermore, because the WCEA does not require any church-affiliated charity to offer prescription benefit coverage, Catholic Charities is not compelled to offer coverage for contraceptives.

RULE OF LAW: The WCEA does not violate the Establishment or Free Exercise Clauses of the U.S. or California Constitutions.

(*See generally* Afif, 2005; Bailey, 2005; Brown, 2008; Colletta & Kapulina, 2007; Collins 2006; Dong, 2007; Duvall, 2006; Haff, 2006; Hudak, 2007; Kalscheur, 2006; Kuhn, 2007; Lumpkin, 2005; Magid & Prenkert, 2005; Pisoni, 2008; Spreng, 2008).

The outcome of this decision may have a negative impact on commercially insured Californians. Those entities that do not want to provide coverage for prescription contraceptives may elect to do away with prescription coverage benefits altogether as the only legal way of avoiding the WCEA's requirements.

Coverage for Newer Birth Control Alternatives

There is a new front in the continuing battle to have the health insurance industry pay for women's birth control. A number of contraceptive alternatives have arrived on the market (from hormone patches, rings, and injections, to new-generation IUDs and non-invasive sterilization techniques), offering women a broad range of choices beyond the birth control pill. However, many insurers and employer-provided health insurance plans refuse to cover the newer methods. Women's health advocates believe most state-mandate laws apply to all forms of contraception approved by the U.S. FDA (NWLC, 2009).

The most recent employer-based studies indicate three out of four employer-provided health insurance plans cover all methods of prescription contraception approved by the FDA (Kaiser & HRET, 2008). In recent years, most employers and health insurers have moved to cover birth control pills, but this still leaves out large numbers of women who cannot take the pill or who prefer other methods of contraception. The recent wave of birth control innovation offers women alternatives that have fewer side effects and can be simpler to manage.

The newer methods, however, often are far more expensive for the health insurance industry, which can negotiate discounted bulk rates for birth control pills from the many manufacturers competing for business. Insurers can pay at least ten times as much for the patch as they do for certain birth control pills (Golub & Gartmer, 2007). Moreover, if alternative methods are less popular, limiting access to them is a way to curtail health care costs without affecting large numbers of women.

Many health insurers will not cover a new, less invasive form of permanent sterilization called Essure, an alternative to tubal ligation. Other insurers cover birth control pills, the patch, and the vaginal ring, but will not cover IUDs or injectable forms of contraception, such as Depo-Provera. Many insurers will only cover birth control pills (Kaiser & HRET, 2008).

Gender Discrimination

Much of the effort to have health insurance coverage for alternative methods of birth control has centered on the issue of gender discrimination: if health insurance plans cover men's drugs, then they should cover contraception as well (Golub & Gartner, 2007).

Among the reasons insurers give for denying benefits is that the new contraception methods do not have enough safety and efficacy data behind them. Most new drugs, however, gain coverage shortly after they are approved by the FDA. Viagra and Cialis were added to most health insurance plans very quickly, yet FDA-approved contraceptive methods for women appear to be treated differently (NCSL, 2007).

When the U.S. Supreme Court first evaluated gender discrimination by the insurance industry, the Court held that there was no discrimination when plans denied benefits for pregnancy-related health issues. The primary rationale was that pregnancy exclusions did not adversely impact all women, just those who became pregnant. A secondary rationale was that the pregnancy exclusion was the same for men and women. *See General Electric Co. v. Gilbert*, 429 U.S. 125 (U.S. Supreme Court 1976). Shortly after *Gilbert,* the federal PDA was enacted, making pregnancy-related discrimination impermissible in employment situations. *See* 42 U.S.C.A. § 2000e(k) (1991). Subsequent court decisions that have followed have upheld women's right to contraceptives coverage; this area of law, however, is by no means settled, as only a few courts have addressed the issue (Dong, 2007).

Maternity Care Coverage

With approximately four million births in the U.S. each year, pregnancy- and childbirth-related conditions are the leading causes for hospital stays and account for almost 11 percent of the nation's hospitalizations (Law, 2008). Yet, maternity care coverage is increasingly falling out of reach for more women in the U.S. Women, including many with otherwise comprehensive health insurance, are finding themselves uncovered for one of their biggest medical costs: maternity care. Even women with no history of complicated births have a hard time getting maternity coverage in the U.S. By law, employers that offer a group health insurance plan must include maternity care (Fuhrmans, 2005).

Nevertheless, for one-fourth of the working-age women who do not have employer-provided health insurance benefits or Medicaid insurance coverage, there are few options (Law, 2008). While the PDA requires maternity care coverage if employers offer group health insurance as an employee benefit, there is no requirement that U.S. employers provide health insurance to their employees. Only one-third of the individual health insurance plans nationwide now provide some sort of maternity coverage, and usually at a high premium. In many states, only one or two plans include maternity coverage, usually limiting coverage or requiring waiting periods of up to twelve months (to avoid coverage of women who purchase health insurance coverage to cover the costs of their pregnancies only after discovering they are pregnant).

In many states, once a woman is pregnant, it is impossible to obtain individual health insurance. While most state insurance laws require unexpected complications during delivery (for instance an emergency Caesarean) to be covered by health insurance policies, even without explicit maternity care coverage, standard vaginal deliveries are not covered (Fuhrmans, 2005). While no research supports the correlation between the nation's failure to provide basic maternity care coverage to all women and the fact that the U.S. has the highest rates of Caesarean surgeries of any nation in the world, this may not be a coincidence (CIA, 2008).

Moral Dilemmas

1. As maternity care coverage falls out of reach for more American women, how should the U.S. health care system deal with the 25 percent of working-age women who do not have maternity care coverage or who do not qualify for Medicaid insurance?

Price Discrimination by the Health Insurance Industry

To keep health care costs down, health insurers actively steer women toward specific forms of birth control (Dong, 2007). For instance, the patch and the ring are often excluded from the list of covered drugs provided to physicians, making it more difficult for women to obtain these more expensive options.

Physicians may still prescribe methods not on the list, but they must explain their reasons. The insurers hope the additional hassle will encourage physicians to work with less expensive products before they try others. Physicians maintain there is coercion that goes on in medical practice (Drazen, 2007).

Lack of Federal Legislation

The reach of state laws is limited because they do not apply to companies that are self-insured and fund their own insurance plans. About half of all Americans with insurance through their employers are covered by self-insured plans (Kaiser & HRET, 2008). Those plans are regulated by the federal government, which has yet to pass legislation requiring companies to cover contraception.

WRONGFUL LIFE, BIRTH, AND PREGNANCY

Wrongful life actions are distinguishable from actions for wrongful birth and wrongful pregnancy:

- Wrongful birth: parent sues for failing to detect the defect that is present at birth
- Wrongful pregnancy: parent sues for an unplanned pregnancy, usually resulting from negligent sterilization or abortion procedures, or the negligent distribution or manufacture of contraceptives
- Wrongful life: child, born with natural defect, sues on their own behalf for negligence that deprived their parents of information during gestation that would have prompted them to terminate the pregnancy

(Beshara, 2005)

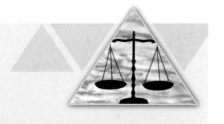

WRONGFUL LIFE

Willis v. Wu
[Mother on Behalf of Her Minor Disabled Son v. Physician]
607 S.E.2d 63 (Supreme Court of South Carolina 2004)

FACTS: Jennie Willis, on behalf of her minor son, Thomas Willis, brought an action for wrongful life against Dr. Donald Wu. Thomas Willis was born with maximal hydrocephalus and will not develop cognitive functions beyond those of an infant. Jennie Willis claimed Dr. Wu was negligent when he failed to detect this congenital defect during a prenatal ultrasound procedure. According to Willis, had she known about the defect, she would have terminated the pregnancy.

ISSUE: Should South Carolina recognize a common law cause of action for wrongful life brought on behalf of children born with congenital defects?

(continues)

(continued)

HOLDING AND DECISION: No, children cannot have a cause of action for wrongful life because being born does not constitute an injury.

ANALYSIS: Some courts reject wrongful life actions because physicians do not actually cause a congenital defect, which makes it improper under established tort principles to hold physicians liable for damages. The Supreme Court of South Carolina dispensed with this argument, however, since Willis did not claim Dr. Wu caused her son's defects. Instead, Willis claimed Dr. Wu's negligence deprived her of knowledge that would have led her to terminate the pregnancy.

In actions for wrongful life, children do not contend that they should have been born without defects, but rather, that they should not have been born at all. Thus, most courts that reject actions for wrongful life hold that being born is not a legally cognizable injury. The typical rationale for these holdings is that life, whether experienced with or without a major physical handicap, is more precious than non-life. These courts maintain that societal values serve as the foundation for this principle and that to recognize an action for wrongful life would contradict the widely held belief that all life has value.

Courts adjudicating actions for wrongful life also face the difficult task of assessing damages. Courts that refuse to recognize wrongful life actions need not reach the issue of damages, but many are willing to do so in order to expose what they believe to be a second fatal flaw in arguments for wrongful life. These courts hold that even if life may not always be preferable to non-life, it would be impossible to determine damages based on the difference in value between life in an impaired condition and non-life. The Supreme Court of South Carolina agreed, stating that the inability to determine a proper damage award should further preclude a cause of action for wrongful life.

The few courts that have recognized an action for wrongful life generally concede the impossibility of an accurate measure of damages. For instance, California recognizes wrongful life actions, but only allows damage awards for the extraordinary expenses associated with treating the child's condition. The few other jurisdictions that recognize actions for wrongful life also limit damage awards to such extraordinary expenses.

The South Carolina Supreme Court was unable to reconcile the inherent difficulties in recognizing an action for wrongful life. Instead, the court adopted the majority rationale that the prospect of a child arguing that he would have been better if he had never been born at all as untenable. The court further held that the impossibility of determining damages also precludes an action for wrongful life. In addition, the court claimed that those jurisdictions recognizing an action for wrongful life fail to properly address the issue of damages.

This case would have taken on a new dimension if Dr. Wu possessed knowledge or equipment that was capable of curing or at least ameliorating Willis's condition at the time of the failed diagnosis. Under such circumstances, Willis could bring a malpractice action against Dr. Wu for damages associated with his arguably preventable condition. However, since Willis did not present such evidence, the court could not discuss the issue.

RULE OF LAW: Being born does not constitute an injury for children with congenital defects.

(See generally Beshara, 2005; McEntire, 2007).

With this decision, the Supreme Court of South Carolina joined the majority of courts that refuse to recognize an action for wrongful life. While some courts have fashioned arguments that life may not always be preferable to non-life, they have not been able to determine damages. Thus, children seeking to bring an action for wrongful life in one of the twenty jurisdictions that have yet to decide the issue must establish that the severity of their condition would make non-existence preferable to life with their medical condition. Children must then argue that the impossibility of arriving at an accurate assessment of damages should not be a fatal defect. Instead, damages can be set at the extraordinary expenses associated with treating their condition. In the end, however, children pursuing a cause of action for wrongful life face a daunting task, especially when considering the mounting precedents set by courts refusing to recognize such actions (Beshara, 2005).

ABORTIONS

The National Women's Law Center reports that ten states are considering bans on abortion in anticipation that the U.S. Supreme Court may overrule *Roe v. Wade*, 410 U.S. 113 (U.S. Supreme Court 1973). Now that women have the right to an abortion, the debate is over defining that right and permissible abortion regulations. In the past two decades, no federal circuit court has found an abortion restriction to be unconstitutional simply because some women are unable to obtain an abortion. *See Cincinnati Women's Services, Inc. v. Taft,* 468 F.3d 361 (U.S. Court of Appeals for the 6th Circuit 2006) (noting the 1992 U.S. Supreme Court decision, *Planned Parenthood of Southeastern Pennsylvania v. Casey*, upheld an abortion regulation where some 47 percent of the women affected by the restriction would be unable to obtain an abortion).

The number of abortions in the U.S. has dropped steadily over the past two decades and now stands at about 1.2 million a year (Kaiser, 2008a). The Allan Guttmacher Institute estimates that the use of emergency contraception after unprotected sex or a contraceptive failure accounted for almost half of the total decline in abortions (Slaughter, 2007). Another reason for this decline is the state restrictions placed on access to abortions; more than one-third of American women live in counties with no medical professional who performs abortions (Simon, 2008).

Partial-Birth Abortions

While more than thirty states and the federal government have made it a crime to perform partial-birth abortions, the *Carhart* decision is the first time the U.S. Supreme Court has ever held that physicians can be prohibited from using a medical procedure deemed necessary by the physician to benefit a patient's health (Annas, 2007).

PARTIAL-BIRTH ABORTIONS

Gonzales v. Carhart
[Federal Government v. Physician]
550 U.S. 124 (U.S. Supreme Court 2007)

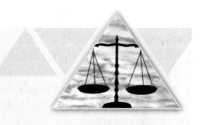

FACTS: States are prohibited from restricting abortion in any way before the fetus develops to the point where it could live independently of the mother, a period known as pre-viability (*see Planned Parenthood of Southeastern Pennsylvania v. Casey*, 550 U.S. 833 (U.S. Supreme Court 1992)). During pre-viability, states cannot impose an undue burden on women seeking to exercise their right to abortion. In the period after viability, known as post-viability, states may regulate abortion as long as the restrictions do not endanger the life or health of the mother.

After the U.S. Supreme Court struck down Nebraska's partial-birth abortion ban in 2000 (*see Stenberg v. Carhart*, 530 U.S. 914 (U.S. Supreme Court 2000)), Congress enacted a federal version of the Nebraska law. Congress had previously attempted to enact federal legislation banning partial-birth abortions, but President Clinton vetoed both efforts. Congress specifically banned intact dilation and extraction (D&X) procedures that are used in the second trimester of pregnancy. Most D&Xs involve partially delivering the fetus intact until part of it passes through the vagina, where it is then aborted, a procedure that Congress maintained is never medically necessary. The federal law includes an exception when the woman's life is in danger, but not an exception if the woman's health is merely at risk. The Partial-Birth Abortion Ban Act was signed into law in 2003 (*see* 18 U.S.C.A. § 1531 (2003)). The U.S. Courts of Appeal in the Eighth and Ninth Circuits upheld permanent injunctions that facially challenged the federal partial-birth abortion law and enjoined the federal government from enforcing the law.

ISSUE: Does the lack of a health exception in the federal partial abortion law banning D&Xs withstand constitutional scrutiny?

HOLDING AND DECISION: Yes, D&Xs are never medically necessary and women have alternatives to the banned procedure.

(continues)

(continued)

ANALYSIS: The majority found that in D&Xs, a health exception was unnecessary based on congressional findings that the procedure was never medically necessary. Additionally, because medical alternatives to the banned procedure exist that do not violate federal law, the Court found that there was no undue burden on pregnant women.

The Court also stated that facial challenges to the federal partial abortion law require a showing that the law would be unconstitutional in a large fraction of relevant cases. The Court held that relevant cases are comprised of situations in which physicians want to perform D&Xs and not merely when women are suffering from medical complications. It also held that the burden for the relevant cases had not been met. While an as-applied challenge to the federal law might lead to a different result, the Court noted that review was not needed when a woman's life was threatened because of the law's life exception.

The dissent emphasized the necessity of a health exception for the federal law to be constitutional. Since *Roe v. Wade*, the U.S. Supreme Court had never upheld a restriction on abortion that did not have a health exception. The dissent recalled the holding in *Stenberg v. Carhart*, that a health exception is required whenever there is substantial medical authority supporting the proposition that banning a particular abortion procedure could endanger women's health. Lower court findings were reviewed in detail by the dissent, and it was noted that substantial medical authority existed indicating that, in some cases, an intact D&X is the safest procedure.

The dissent also stated that the majority did not respect the difference between pre-viability and post-viability, a distinction that is crucial for determining the state's interest in the fetus. The majority stated that the federal law applies during both pre-viability and post-viability, because the law uses the term *fetus*, which does not specify viability, and the issue was not discussed further. Examining further inconsistencies with past precedent, the dissent declared that the majority abandoned the heightened constitutional scrutiny of *Planned Parenthood of Southeastern Pennsylvania v. Casey*, and instead applied a rational basis test to uphold the federal law. Finally, the dissent took issue with the majority's definition of the relevant group that ought to be examined under *Casey* for determining whether the restriction creates an undue burden. Under *Casey*, when examining whether an undue burden exists, the Court must consider the women who need the procedure to preserve their health as the relevant group and not a large fraction of women, as the majority maintained.

RULE OF LAW: Persons are prohibited from intentionally partially delivering a viable fetus and then performing an overt act that the person knows will kill the delivered fetus.

(*See generally* Bernwanger, 2009; Eisenman, 2009; Engelman, 2007; Fleming, 2008; Garrow, 2007; Ginsburg, 2008; Hamers, 2009; Hansen, 2008; Kessler, 2007; Mitchell, 2007; Perry, 2007; Sandstad, 2008; Stahle, 2007; Tai, 2009; Tobin, 2008; Vartanian, 2009; Wharton, 2009; Whitebread, 2007; Wilcox 2008).

Following this decision is the fear that it will prevent physicians from performing even legal abortion procedures out of fear that they might be investigated for criminal wrongdoing (Drazen, 2007). Additionally, *Carhart* creates uncertainty for practitioners because it resurrects many states' partial-birth abortion bans, which are now in the process of being modified with constitutionally ambiguous language (Charo, 2007). A professor of obstetrics and gynecology at Harvard University wrote that the ambiguity of the act's intent requirement will cause physicians to avoid similar legal medical procedures, possibly even when the mother's life is in jeopardy (Greene, 2007).

The impact of *Carhart* expands beyond the issue of abortion and intrudes into the practice of medicine. Legislative judgment was allowed to trump medical judgment by preventing physicians from performing a medical procedure they believe to be in the best interests of their patients (Annas, 2007). *Carhart* marks a significant change in the U.S. Supreme Court's abortion jurisprudence. Future cases will have to further define the state's power to restrict the right to abortion and the rights of physicians to treat their patients.

Parental Notification Prior to Abortion Regulations

Many states have parental notification requirements before abortions may be performed on unemancipated minors that generally require young women to wait at least forty-eight hours after written notice of the pending abortion has been delivered. There are often exceptions where a physician may perform an abortion on a minor child without parental notification.

PARENTAL NOTIFICATION FOR ABORTIONS

Ayotte v. Planned Parenthood of Northern New England
[New Hampshire v. Reproductive Clinic]
546 U.S. 320 (U.S. Supreme Court 2006)

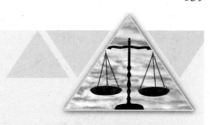

FACTS: New Hampshire enacted a parental notification law that mandated that abortions could not be performed upon an unemancipated minor until at least forty-eight hours after written notice of the pending abortion had been delivered to the minor's parents or guardian. *See* Parental Notification Prior to Abortion Act, N.H. Rev. Stat. Ann. §§ 132:24-132:28 (2003), *repealed* (2007). The law allowed for three exceptions where a physician could perform an abortion on a minor child without parental or guardian notification:

- Abortion is necessary to prevent the minor's death and there is insufficient time to provide the required notice
- Person or persons entitled to receive notice certify in writing that they have been notified
- Minor petitions a judge to authorize an abortion and the judge finds that the minor is mature and capable of giving her informed consent, or that an abortion without parental notification serves the minor's best interests

This judicial bypass measure is confidential and given precedence over other pending matters so that the court may reach a prompt decision. Additionally, the trial and appellate courts must rule on bypass petitions within seven days. Though the exceptions to parental notification are acknowledged prior to a minor's abortion, abortions may not be performed in a medical emergency without parental notification.

    Dr. Wayne Goldner, obstetrician and gynecologist, and three clinics including Planned Parenthood of Northern New England that offer reproductive health services and abortions for pregnant minors, brought this lawsuit claiming that New Hampshire's parental notification law was unconstitutional because it did not include an exception allowing a physician to perform an abortion on a minor in a medical emergency. The U.S. District Court declared the law unconstitutional because:

- It failed to meet the constitutional requirement that any law that restricts a woman's access to an abortion must provide an emergency health exception

- The judicial bypass provision would not operate quickly enough in medical emergencies
- It forced physicians to certify with impossible precision when abortion was medically necessary to avoid death

On appeal, the U.S. Court of Appeals for the First Circuit concluded that the law was unconstitutional notwithstanding the judicial bypass measure, because the judicial bypass was not an adequate substitute for an emergency health exception. The First Circuit affirmed the District Court's decision, declaring the law unconstitutional and permanently enjoining the law's enforcement and thereby invalidating it entirely.

ISSUE: What should the appropriate judicial relief be when a court is faced with a law that, in restricting access to abortion, may be applied in a manner that unconstitutionally harms a woman's health?

HOLDING AND DECISION: Remanded to determine whether the First Circuit could, consistent with New Hampshire's legislative intent, formulate a more narrow remedy than a permanent injunction against enforcement of the parental notification law in its entirety.

ANALYSIS: The opinion began by stating that the U.S. Supreme Court was not revisiting its abortion precedents, but rather addressing a question of remedy. The Court carefully sidestepped the opportunity to confront its controversial abortion precedents by phrasing the question around the issue of whether the lower courts erred by invalidating the New Hampshire parental notification law in its entirety because it failed to provide an emergency health exception. When confronted with a constitutional flaw in any law, the Court noted that the remedial preference would be to enjoin only the unconstitutional applications of a law while leaving other applications in force or to sever its problematic portions while leaving the remainder intact. The Court enumerated three

(continues)

(continued)

principles that should inform a court's approach to remedies:

- Courts must not invalidate any more of a legislature's work than is necessary, because invalidating an entire law as unconstitutional frustrates the intent of the people's elected representatives (*see Regan v. Time, Inc.*, 468 U.S. 641 (U.S. Supreme Court 1984)); a partial invalidation of the portions of the law that are unconstitutional is the correct response, while the rest of the law is left otherwise intact (*see Brockett v. Spokane Arcades, Inc.*, 472 U.S. 491 (U.S. Supreme Court 1985))
- Courts must avoid rewriting state law to conform to federal constitutional requirements, even while the courts attempt to salvage the law; making distinctions in murky constitutional contexts may involve an invasion of the legislature's field, and therefore courts should be hesitant to enter that domain (*see Virginia v. American Booksellers Association, Inc.*, 484 U.S. 383 (U.S. Supreme Court 1988))
- Courts cannot use their remedial powers to skirt the legislature's intent; once a court finds an application or portion of a law unconstitutional, the court must ask whether the legislature would prefer what is left of its law to no law at all (*see Califano v. Westcott*, 443 U.S. 76, 94 (U.S. Supreme Court 1979) (Powell, J., Stewart, C.J., and Rehnquist, J., concurring in part and dissenting in part))

In *Ayotte*, the Court found that the lower courts had chosen the most blunt remedy by invalidating the parental notification law in its entirety. The Court agreed with New Hampshire's position that such a wholesale invalidation of the parental notification law was unnecessary. Therefore, the Court concluded, as long as the lower courts remain faithful to legislative intent, the lower courts can issue a more narrowly drawn injunction preventing enforcement of only the law's unconstitutional applications while leaving the rest of the law in force. Or, if the lower courts find that they cannot issue an injunction preventing the unconstitutional applications of the law, then they could invalidate the law in its entirety as long as the courts find that such an action was within the state legislature's intent. The crucial question for the First Circuit to answer on remand was legislative intent: whether the state legislature would have preferred a law with an emergency exception for pregnant minors in medical emergencies, or no requirement for parental notification at all.

The Court vacated the First Circuit's decision and remanded the case to the lower court to determine whether a remedy exists that would correct the constitutional flaw without invalidating the entire law. Most significantly, the Court avoided addressing its controversial abortion precedents and decided *Ayotte* on the grounds of choice of remedy. Precedents include: *Stenberg*, 530 U.S. 914 (holding a Nebraska law prohibiting partial-birth abortions unconstitutional because it imposed an undue burden on a woman's right to choose abortion); *Planned Parenthood of Southeastern Pennsylvania*, 505 U.S. 833 (rejecting the trimester framework established in *Roe v. Wade* and establishing an undue burden test for when a state may regulate abortions while reaffirming *Roe's* central holding that a state may not prohibit any woman from making the decision to terminate her pregnancy before viability); and *Roe*, 410 U.S. 113 (holding a Texas law prohibiting abortions except for lifesaving procedures unconstitutional and establishing a trimester framework for when a state may regulate abortions).

RULE OF LAW: New Hampshire's parental notification law could be applied unconstitutionally in certain situations, such as when a pregnant minor's health is at risk, and thus required revision.

(*See generally* Barth, 2006; Fink, 2007; Willis, 2006).

In deciding *Ayotte*, the U.S. Supreme Court reaffirmed that state legislatures may require parental involvement in abortion decisions involving minors, but that restriction on abortions must have an emergency health exception (*see Planned Parenthood of Southeastern Pennsylvania*, 505 U.S. 833 and *Roe*, 410 U.S. 113). The decision broke little new ground on the abortion issue, as the Court declined to go beyond its established abortion precedents. The Court's limited decision merely addressed the question of what remedies a court may choose when faced with an unconstitutional application of an abortion law. Response to this ruling has been mixed. The ruling may remind state legislatures that an emergency health exception must be included in state abortion laws. The decision may also make courts less likely to invalidate entire abortion laws. Yet another consequence of the decision may be an increase in abortion litigation. What is certain is the status quo has been preserved in the abortion controversy (Law, 2008).

INFORMED CONSENT FOR ABORTION

Acuna v. Turkish
[Pregnant Woman v. Gynecologist]
930 A.2d 416 (Supreme Court of New Jersey 2007),
U.S. Supreme Court certiorari denied, 129 S.Ct. 44 (U.S. Supreme Court 2008)

FACTS: Rosa Acuna, a married mother of two young children, consulted her gynecologist of five years, Dr. Sheldon Turkish, about abdominal pains. After Turkish informed her that she was six to eight weeks pregnant, Acuna decided to terminate the pregnancy. Turkish performed the operation, but after complications relating to the abortion, Acuna was sent to a local hospital. When she asked a nurse why a further procedure had been performed, the nurse responded that Turkish had left parts of the baby inside of her. It was only at this point, Acuna claims, that she started to realize there was a baby inside her and not just blood. This realization led to a decline in her mental health and a diagnosis of post-traumatic stress disorder.

The facts of the information exchange prior to the decision to terminate were disputed. Acuna maintained that Turkish told her that due to a complication with her kidneys, she would have to terminate the pregnancy or die in three months. Acuna further claimed she asked Turkish if it was the baby in there, to which Turkish replied, it is only blood. Turkish, on the other hand, asserted that Acuna suggested the option of abortion and that he had never encouraged her to terminate her pregnancy to preserve her health. Turkish could not remember the conversation but believed he would have told her that a seven-week pregnancy is not a living human being, but merely tissue at that time.

Acuna filed a lawsuit alleging a lack of informed consent. She claimed that had Turkish provided her with the necessary medical and factual information surrounding the nature of abortion and the fact that her child was a complete, separate, and unique human being, she would not have had the abortion procedure.

ISSUE: Are physicians required to inform patients that their embryos are living human beings in order to properly obtain informed consent for abortion procedures?

HOLDING AND DECISION: No, physicians are not required to inform patients seeking abortions that the procedure will kill an actual existing human being.

ANALYSIS: The court dismissed Acuna's informed consent claim and ruled there was no common law duty for a physician to inform a patient seeking an abortion that the abortion would kill an actual existing human being. According to the court, the instructions sought were opinion and not medical fact; they were, therefore, a departure from the doctrine of informed consent. The court emphasized it would only compel physicians to provide medical information, not moral information. Negligence actions predicated on lack of informed consent must demonstrate that a physician withheld medical information that a reasonably prudent pregnant woman would have considered material before consenting to a termination of pregnancy. The knowledge Acuna sought cannot be compelled from a physician who may have a different scientific, moral, or philosophical viewpoint on the issue of when life begins.

Physicians might be required to convey information that reflects a consensus from the New Jersey medical community, the New Jersey legislature, or the New Jersey people. However, without such a consensus, instructions cannot be required that are not the medical norm.

The court also found the instructions were at odds with current state abortion law, suggesting that both the physician and the patient would be complicit in committing the equivalent of murder. This in turn would have contradicted the New Jersey legislature's choice to exclude a fetus from within the definition of a person in the Wrongful Death Act.

RULE OF LAW: While potential parents should be provided sufficient medical information to make an informed decision whether or not to continue a pregnancy to term, physicians have no duty to provide moral guidance as well.

(*See generally* Corbin, 2009; Shacker, 2008; Tobin, 2008).

Mandatory In-Person, Informed Consent Meetings

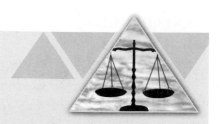

Judicial Bypass of Parental Consent Requirement and Mandatory In-Person, Informed Consent Meetings

Cincinnati Women's Services, Inc. v. Taft
[Reproductive Clinic v. Governor]
468 F.3d 361 (U.S. Court of Appeals for the 6th Circuit 2006)

Facts: Prior to 1998, Ohio law required that minors receive informed consent of a parent or guardian before receiving an abortion. The law, however, allowed minors to petition a juvenile court for a judicial bypass of the parental consent requirement so the court could decide whether the minor was sufficiently mature and well enough informed to decide whether to have an abortion or whether notification of her parents was not in her best interest. The law did not impose any limitations on the number of times a minor could petition a court for such a bypass.

Additionally, Ohio law mandated that women seeking an abortion receive information about the procedure from a physician at least twenty-four hours prior to the abortion (*see* Ohio Rev. Code Ann. § 2919.12(B)(1)(a)(i) (1995)). The informed consent provision required that a physician inform the pregnant woman, verbally or by other non-written means of communication, about the procedure. This was interpreted to mean that videotaped or audiotaped physician statements would be an adequate means of imparting the necessary information to those seeking abortions.

In 1998, the Ohio General Assembly amended the judicial bypass and informed consent provisions of Ohio's abortion regulations.

- Single petition rule: limited a minor to only one judicial bypass petition during the term of each pregnancy (*see* Ohio Rev. Code Ann. § 2919.121(c)(4) (1998) (providing that no juvenile court shall have jurisdiction to rehear a petition concerning the same pregnancy once a juvenile court has granted or denied the petition))
- In-person rule: required that the informed consent meeting take place in person (*see* Ohio Rev. Code Ann. § 2317.56(B)(1) (1999))

The U.S. Supreme Court has ruled such bypass procedures are required if a state wishes to enact a parental informed consent requirement (*see Lambert v. Wicklund*, 520 U.S. 292 (U.S. Supreme Court 1997) and *Bellotti v. Baird*, 443 U.S. 622 (U.S. Supreme Court 1979)). Cincinnati Women's Services (CWS), a health care provider that offers family planning services, brought a pre-enforcement facial attack against the single petition and in-person rules. CWS claimed the rules were unconstitutionally vague and invalid. The federal District Court upheld both provisions, noting that neither rule created an undue burden on minors seeking abortions. CWS appealed.

Issue: Can a state law limit minors to only one petition for judicial bypass of the parental consent requirement for an abortion and require minors to attend an in-person meeting with a physician at least twenty-four hours before receiving an abortion?

Holding and Decision: No, limiting minors to only one petition for judicial bypass of a parental consent requirement for an abortion was an unconstitutional undue burden and yes, minors may be required to attend an in-person meeting with a physician at least twenty-four hours prior to receiving an abortion.

Analysis: The Sixth Circuit began its analysis by determining that the proper standard to apply to facial challenges of abortion restrictions is the large fraction test (*see Planned Parenthood of Southeastern Pennsylvania*, 505 U.S. 833). The large fraction test requires a reviewing court to determine whether a large fraction of the women for whom the law is a restriction will be deterred from procuring an abortion as surely as if the government has outlawed abortion in all cases. The court explicitly rejected application of the more demanding "no set of circumstances test," noting that every federal circuit except one has opted instead to apply the large fraction test to facial challenges of abortion laws

(continues)

(continued)

(*see U.S. v. Salerno*, 481 U.S. 739 (U.S. Supreme Court 1987) (constitutional challenges to a law must establish that no set of circumstances exists under which the law would be valid)); the court recognized that its own practice of applying the large fraction test in similar situations made it the obvious choice for analyzing the two challenged provisions.

Applying the large fraction test to the single petition rule, the court held that the regulation created an unconstitutional undue burden to a large fraction of women who are initially refused a bypass but later experience changes entitling them to a bypass. The court reasoned that the single petition rule affected those women who were denied a bypass at first, but who would be bypass-eligible if they were to reapply because of changed circumstances in their life (for instance, increased maturity or discovery of medical anomalies with the fetus). The court concluded that because the single petition rule would form a substantial obstacle to obtaining an abortion for most women who had experienced changes in their circumstances, it was facially unconstitutional.

Next, the court sustained the in-person rule, holding that the number of abortion seekers likely to be frustrated by the regulation was not a large enough number of women to justify overturning the provision. In determining the number of women who would be unduly burdened by the in-person rule, the court noted that 25 percent of the women excused from the in-person meetings were in abusive relationships. Of this 25 percent, only half would be completely unable to obtain an abortion if they were forced to have a separate in-person meeting twenty-four hours prior to an abortion for reasons ranging from geographic and financial constraints to fear of repercussion given their abusive relationships. The court held that an undue burden on 12 percent was not enough to consider the law unconstitutional.

RULE OF LAW: In-person, informed consent meetings may be required before abortions may be performed.

(*See generally* Casey, 2008; Fink, 2007; Tobin, 2008; Wharton, 2009).

While this decision will not alter the abortion law battleground, it does suggest that legislative efforts to curtail bypass procedures will be reviewed carefully if challenged. The decision also reinforces the large fraction test, which has been criticized as being vague and subjective as the legislative and judicial branches struggle to identify groups for whom abortion laws are an impermissible restriction. Additionally, while the court acknowledged that the term *large fraction* is more of a concept than an algebraic application, what constitutes a large fraction remains unclear (Fink, 2007).

In refusing to clearly identify the boundaries for impermissible restrictions on abortions, the judicial branch is seeking at least the possibility of common ground with the legislative branch. The refusal by the courts to expand upon the large fraction test in the past twenty years acknowledges recognition of the fact that the two sides of the abortion issue will most likely never agree on the underlying question of whether abortion should be legal.

When there is a national recognition and acceptance of the fact that the nation's foundation is built on the diversity of its immigrant population, that the U.S. has always chosen to be a diverse nation, comprised of cultural differences by people who may not think precisely alike or believe in precisely the

same values, that is when the need to balance competing interests may be accepted and the laws on public controversies like abortion will be grounded in the consent of the governed. This does not mean that religious differences will no longer arise, but it does mean that differences of faith will be accepted in a diverse society. After all, the ultimate irony of faith is that it necessarily admits doubt (Meckler, 2009).

Moral Dilemmas

1. If a minor is not deemed sufficiently mature and well enough informed to decide whether to have an abortion without parental notice, can the minor logically be deemed sufficiently mature to raise a child?

One aspect of the current debate on abortion centers on the issue of whether minors have the maturity to independently make decisions about abortion. While it may be logically inconsistent to maintain minors lack the maturity to make decisions about abortion, while considering the same minors mature enough to raise children on their own, this part of the abortion debate may indicate some discussion is moving away from the focus on whether abortion should be legal to a more economic and practical discussion of whether minors are prepared to accept responsibility for raising children.

In Latin, *e pluribus unum* (one from the many) refers to the U.S. as one people out of many. There are many philosophies about raising one's children in the U.S. since the country is comprised of many families from many nations, yet the many families are one when it comes to the need to protect one's children. The abortion discussion may not be as logical or illogical when viewed through this legal set of lenses.

Per Se Medical Exceptions

In 2000, the FDA approved a medical abortion drug. Six years later, Ohio became the first state to restrict its use by physicians.

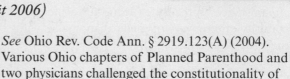

PER SE MEDICAL EXCEPTIONS

Planned Parenthood Cincinnati Region v. Taft
[Reproductive Clinic v. Governor]
444 F.3d 502 (U.S. Court of Appeals for the 6th Circuit 2006)

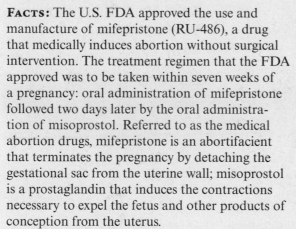

FACTS: The U.S. FDA approved the use and manufacture of mifepristone (RU-486), a drug that medically induces abortion without surgical intervention. The treatment regimen that the FDA approved was to be taken within seven weeks of a pregnancy: oral administration of mifepristone followed two days later by the oral administration of misoprostol. Referred to as the medical abortion drugs, mifepristone is an abortifacient that terminates the pregnancy by detaching the gestational sac from the uterine wall; misoprostol is a prostaglandin that induces the contractions necessary to expel the fetus and other products of conception from the uterus.

Generally, once the FDA has approved a drug, physicians have the legal authority to prescribe it for off-label uses, unless state regulations require otherwise. An off-label use of RU-486 was the so-called Schaff protocol (named after the physician whose research primarily led to its development), which allowed for the administration of RU-486 within up to nine weeks of a pregnancy. The Schaff protocol provided for the oral administration of mifepristone followed one to three days later by misoprostol administered vaginally. Off-label use does not violate federal law because the FDA regulates the marketing and distribution of drugs in the U.S., not the practice of medicine, which had always been the exclusive realm of individual states until 2007 (*compare Gonzales v. Carhart,* 550 U.S. 124 (U.S. Supreme Court 2007)).

The Ohio legislature enacted legislation that prohibited the off-label use of RU-486 in Ohio.

See Ohio Rev. Code Ann. § 2919.123(A) (2004). Various Ohio chapters of Planned Parenthood and two physicians challenged the constitutionality of this law.

ISSUE: Do all state laws regulating abortions need a per se medical exception?

HOLDING AND DECISION: No, not all state laws regulating abortions are required to contain a medical exception.

ANALYSIS: The Sixth Circuit first addressed and rejected the claim that all statutes regulating abortion must include an exception to preserve the life and health of the mother. The court found that medical exceptions are only required when a law regulating abortion poses a significant health risk to a woman. The court bolstered this conclusion by maintaining that a per se requirement of medical exceptions would preclude judicial review of whether regulations lacking such exceptions were unconstitutional. The court then undertook to summarize U.S. Supreme Court decisions to support its application of medical exception jurisprudence. *See Ayotte,* 546 U.S. 320 (state may not restrict access to abortions that are necessary for preservation of the life or health of the mother); *Stenberg,* 530 U.S. 914 (medical exceptions are required where it is necessary for the preservation of the life or health of the mother).

The court then described the standard for medical exceptions. Where substantial medical

(continues)

(continued)

authority supports that an abortion-regulating law could endanger women's health, a medical exception is required when the procedure is necessary for the preservation of the life or health of the mother. The court emphasized that medical exemptions are required when RU-486 is safer than available alternatives (surgery), but then partially closed the door on women by restricting the use of RU-486 to situations where alternative procedures posed a significant medical risk.

To determine whether the medical exception standard had been met, the court deferred to physician experts who established that the law would pose a significant risk to women's health in narrow circumstances. Specifically, the physicians claimed the seven-week time limit on RU-486 could potentially harm certain pregnant women to whom physicians administered RU-486 in accordance with the Schaff protocol, whose time limit is nine weeks. Without the Schaff protocol as an option, physicians risk the health of the pregnant women by prescribing or administering other more dangerous treatments, including surgical abortion or methotrexate, a cancer agent.

The final issue that the court decided was the severability of the law. The court here held that when evaluating the severability of an abortion law that lacks a constitutionally necessary medical exception, the court is to defer to legislative intent. The court should ask whether the legislature would prefer what is left of its law to no law at all. If the court answers in the affirmative, then the court should prohibit enforcement of the unconstitutional provisions and leave the balance of the law intact. If, however, the court answers in the negative, then the court may invalidate the entire law. The question of severability was remanded.

RULE OF LAW: Only state abortion regulations that pose a significant risk to a woman's health or life are required to have medical exceptions.

(*See generally* Harper 2006).

The implications of this decision are twofold: first, medical exceptions are not always required in abortion regulations, and second, states may restrict off-label uses of abortion-inducing drugs if a medical exception is included in the restriction. This decision could inhibit physician autonomy and medical innovation; now FDA regulations on marketing and labeling may become substantive law if a state legislature acts similarly to the Ohio legislature. Thus, state law may prevent physicians from prescribing FDA-approved abortion drugs off-label (*see generally* Bennett, 2004).

Moral Dilemmas

1. How does the nationwide scarcity of individual health insurance plans that provide some sort of maternity coverage impact the abortion and conscience clause controversies?

SEXUALLY TRANSMITTED INFECTIONS

Women are more likely than men to contract sexually transmitted infections (STIs) and suffer serious complications as a simple result of their biology. One in four teenage girls between the ages of fourteen and nineteen has an STI (NWLC, 2009). The burden is highest among young women ages twenty to twenty-four, with a prevalence rate approaching 50 percent for human papilliomavirus (HPV), the most common STI (Kaiser, 2008b).[LN2]

HPV Vaccines: Gardasil and Cervarix

In 2006, the FDA licensed Gardasil, a three-dose (zero, two, and six months) quadrivalent vaccine, for use in females ages nine to twenty-six for the prevention of cervical pre-cancers and cancers, vulvar and vaginal pre-cancers, and genital warts. Health care professionals may administer the vaccine to girls as young as age nine at their discretion (Villaet al., 2005).

Following FDA approval, the Advisory Committee on Immunization Practices (ACIP) recommended Gardasil for routine use with females ages eleven and twelve, with catch-up immunization for women ages thirteen to twenty-six who have not received the vaccine. ACIP consists of fifteen experts in fields associated with immunization who have been selected by the Secretary of the U. S. Department of Health and Human Services to provide advice and guidance on the most effective means to prevent vaccine-preventable diseases.

Of the twenty-seven states that took action to require HPV vaccination for school entry in 2007, only Virginia has enacted the requirement (ASHA, 2007). In 2009, GlaxoSmithKline obtained FDA approval for Cervarix, a competing vaccine to Merck's HPV vaccine. Cervarix induces a higher immune response in women against HPV than Gardasil (GSK, 2009).

Gender-Based HPV Vaccination Mandates

The approval of a vaccine against cancer-causing HPV is a significant public health advance (Javitt et al., 2008). The Centers for Disease Control and Prevention estimates 15 percent of the U.S. population, or twenty million Americans, are infected with HPV. The American Cancer Society suggests up to 80 percent of sexually active women will become HPV-infected at some point in their lives by the time they reach age fifty, with the highest prevalence of HPV infections among sexually active females aged fourteen to nineteen years (Saslow et al., 2007).

The attempt to mandate the HPV vaccine for only one gender presents concerns because it requires only girls to be vaccinated (CDC, 2006). While short-term clinical trials in thousands of young women did not reveal serious adverse effects, serious adverse events reported since the vaccine's approval (especially Guillain-Barre syndrome, a neurological illness resulting in muscle weakness and sometimes in paralysis) are a reminder that rare adverse events may surface as the vaccine is administered to millions of girls and young women (Javitt et al., 2008). When girls receiving the vaccine face a risk of potential adverse events as well as risk that the vaccine will not be completely protective, the gender-based vaccination mandates raise equal protection issues (Harper et al., 2006).

Laws that make gender-based distinctions are reviewed with heightened scrutiny: gender-based HPV vaccination mandates must serve an important state interest and the gender classification must substantially relate to serving that interest. While the goal of preventing cervical cancer is an important public health objective (and while cervix cancer is not a risk factor for males since they do not have cervixes, men can have HPV), the justification for burdening females with the risks of HPV vaccination, and not males, is unclear (Dunne et al., 2007). Males:

- Benefit from an aggressive vaccination program for females
- Contribute to HPV transmission
- May reduce their own risk of HPV infections and disease through HPV vaccination

(Javitt et al., 2008)

Admittedly, during clinical trials of the vaccine, significantly more males than females reported mild fevers after the HPV vaccination, which lends support for the implementation of gender-neutral HPV vaccination programs (Block et al., 2006). Whether a mild

fever would withstand a challenge for general-based mandates is debatable since the vaccine industry made this medical determination, not the government units who might mandate the coverage (Villa et al., 2005).

> *Moral Dilemmas*
>
> 1. Are females being burdened with the HPV vaccination simply because of the preponderance of women affected by the virus?
>
> 2. If so, do gender-based HPV vaccination mandates serve that interest in a nondiscriminatory manner?

MEDICAL PRODUCTS INDUSTRY

While women's health encompasses all different areas of medicine, the medical products industry has concentrated on disorders that affect the female reproductive system and other disorders where there is at least a 70 percent preponderance of women affected by the disorders:

- Autoimmune diseases (chronic fatigue syndrome, fibromyalgia, rheumatoid arthritis, scleroderma, sjogren's syndrome, systemic lupus erythematosus)
- Cancer (breast, cervical, endometrial, ovarian, vaginal)
- Gynecological and sexually transmitted diseases
- Hormones
- Osteoporosis
- Urinary disorders

(Kalorama Information, 2009)

Nearly two-thirds of women who gave birth from 1996 through 2000 took a medication during pregnancy, a large federally funded study found. Of those, nearly 40 percent took a drug whose safety in pregnancy is not established, and nearly 5 percent took a drug potentially risky to the fetus (Law, 2008). More pregnant women have taken new medicines for cancer, depression, and other problems. More than thirty drug registries now track outcomes of pregnant women on various drugs (Steinbrook, 2006).

Teratogen Isotretinoin (Accutane)

A classic example of a product that is contraindicated for a specific population is Accutane. Accutane is indicated for patients suffering severe acne but is specifically and expressly contraindicated for women who are pregnant or may become pregnant because of its potential teratogenic effects (Hall & Sobotka, 2007). To date, the FDA has approved nineteen therapeutic classes of drugs with warnings, concerning their risk in pregnancy (Fetterman et al., 2003). An issue of heated debate is whether and when medical treatments that may harm fetuses should be available on the market (Doshi, 2007).

Medications with Teratogenic Effects on Fetuses
Drugs known to be teratogens and therefore contraindicated in pregnancy:

- Androgens (testosterone replacement therapies)
- Anticonvulsants (migraine headaches)
- Antineoplastics (cancer treatment)
- Diethlystillbestol (acne)
- Etretinate (severe psoriasis)
- Iodides (thyroid disease and thyroid cancer)
- Isotretinoin (acne)
- Lithium (prevention of headaches or biopolar depression treatment)
- Live vaccines, including the seasonal flu vaccines
- Methimazole (hyperthyroidism)
- Penicillamine (rheumatoid arthritis)
- Tetracyclines (used in dentistry to prevent infections)
- Warfarin (anticoagulant medication)

Drugs suggested to be teratogens and therefore have warnings against use in pregnancy:

- Angiotension converting enzyme inhibitors (ACE-I) (heart and vascular disease)
- Benzodiazepines (sleep disorders, panic disorders, essential tremors)
- Estrogens (postmenopausal hormone replacement therapy)
- Oral hypoglycemic (oral health problems and diabetes)
- Progestogens (estrogen replacement therapy)
- Quinolones (urinary tract infections)

Source: Cleveland Clinic, 2008; Fetterman et al., 2003.

Accutane is a potent teratogen: it carries a significant (more than 25 percent) risk of miscarriage and major birth defects such as facial deformities, severe mental retardation, and lethal cardiac abnormalities (Noah, 2007). Women are required to have two negative pregnancy tests before initiating Accutane treatment and then monthly pregnancy tests for every month that therapy continues, along with monthly counseling on contraceptive use. Women have to also agree to use two methods of birth control. Given the U.S. Supreme Court's clear recognition of a right to privacy in the context of contraception, however, one has to wonder about FDA distribution restrictions

that require women to use two methods of birth control as a condition of access to Accutane (Noah, 2007). In contrast with the tight access requirements for isotretinoin (the chemical compound in Accutane) in this country, British regulators require that patients agree to undergo an immediate abortion if they become pregnant while using Accutane.

Over the last two decades, and parallel with the FDA's incremental approach to addressing Accutane's teratogenicity, users of Accutane have pursued tort litigation against Hoffmann-La Roche for birth defects. For the most part, courts have rejected inadequate warning claims with regards to birth defects. *See, e.g., Gerber v. Hoffmann-La Roche Inc.*, 392 F. Supp.2d 907, 916-920 (U.S. District Court, Southern District of Texas, Houston Division 2005) (holding that the 1983 warning was adequate as a matter of law notwithstanding the failure to recommend the use of more than one form of contraception). While Hoffmann-La Roche, motivated in part by a desire to avoid tort liability, has acted affirmatively and with approval of the FDA to increase warnings of risks associated with use of Accutane, mass tort litigation is currently ongoing over the adverse effects of the drug.

Moral Dilemmas

1. Does the FDA cross the line when it requires women to undergo periodic pregnancy testing and use contraceptives as a condition of access to drugs known to cause birth defects?

2. If access restrictions to teratogen drugs fails to reduce the number of birth defects, should the FDA require women to undergo a sterilization procedure if they wish to use such drugs, at least for chronic use?

3. Should the FDA insist that women who become pregnant while using a teratogen take an abortifacient drug?

4. Would requiring an immediate abortion if a woman becomes pregnant while using Accutane be ethically or constitutionally permissible?

Restrictive Enrollment Criteria in Clinical Trials

While women consume more prescription drugs than men and disproportionately suffer a greater number of side effects from these drugs (Korzec, 2007), many drugs on the market have never been clinically tested on women specifically. The reason for this is FDA regulatory restrictions.

The FDA excluded women of childbearing age from early phases of studies with investigational drugs until 1993 (Guideline for the Study and Evaluation of Gender Differences in the Clinical Evaluation of Drugs. 58 *Federal Register* 39,406-01 (July 22, 1993)). While today federal law explicitly calls for the FDA to develop appropriate guidance on the inclusion of women in clinical trials, the FDA still places restrictive enrollment criteria on women participating in clinical trials of investigational products (Investigational New Drug Applications; Amendment to Clinical Hold Regulations for Products Intended for Life-Threatening Diseases and Conditions, 65 *Federal Register* 34,963-01 (June 1, 2000)). [LN3] *See* 21 U.S.C.A. § 355 (2008). In contrast, the U.S. Department of Health and Human Services, the FDA's parent agency, encourages greater inclusion of women in clinical trials (Protection of human research subjects. 66 *Federal Register* 3878-01 (2001, January 17)). *See* 45 C.F.R. Part 46 (2009).

HHS indicates that the influence of menstrual status (whether women are pre- or post-menopausal) and menstrual cycle on the pharmacokinetics of investigational drugs should be explored, as should the effects of concomitant supplementary estrogen treatment or systemic contraceptives. Finally, HHS suggests that the influence of the investigational drug itself on the pharmacokinetics of selected oral contraceptives should be explored.

Even though the FDA is largely passive during the clinical trial stage of the research and development process, the FDA still grants an application for an investigational new drug (IND). So whenever there is an apparent conflict between the FDA and its parent, HHS, in enrollment criteria for women, private entities undertaking clinical trials of potential teratogens will generally go with the more restrictive requirements to help avoid liability in case an adverse event occurs. On the other hand, the National Institutes of Health have actively included women in their federally-funded clinical trials since the early 1990s.

Given the regulatory inconsistency in this area, private pharmaceutical companies and academic institutions generally require women to agree to undergo an abortion in the event of contraceptive failure when participating in clinical trials of potential teratogens. Experimental protocol restrictions must be approved by local institutional review boards (IRBs) before clinical trials get under way, but few demands have been made to counter this abortion policy. However, since neither private entities nor IRBs generally qualify as state actors, even if women objected to the restrictive enrollment criteria in privately-sponsored clinical trials, they probably could not invoke constitutional protections against discrimination. Moreover, there is no recognized right to participate in clinical trials.

Breast Cancer

Breast cancer is the most common cause of cancer death in U.S. women aged twenty to sixty years; more than 211,000 women develop breast cancer and 20 percent do so before the age of fifty. Approximately two in fifteen American women are expected to develop breast cancer in their lifetimes, and nearly 40,000 women die of the disease annually. During the past four decades, breast cancer rates have risen steadily, especially among younger women.

The association between oral contraceptives and risk of subsequent breast cancer has varied within the medical literature over time. While the Women's Health Initiative Clinical Trial reported that prolonged exposure to exogenous estrogens and progestins in hormone therapy increases a woman's risk of developing breast cancer, more recent studies have noted an increase in risk for women who use oral contraceptives four or more years before their first full-term pregnancy (Kahlenborn et al., 2006). Yet many of the newer, more expensive alternatives to oral contraceptives are not covered by health insurance, especially for young women covered by Medicaid insurance.

ECONOMIC IMPACT OF FAILING TO PRIORITIZE WOMEN'S HEALTH

As this chapter has demonstrated, it is necessary to distinguish women from men when addressing health care issues that affect women. Failing to prioritize women's health is costly to the nation's health care system. For instance, women's contraception has the potential to significantly reduce public health funding; for every one dollar spent on providing family planning services, an estimated four dollars are saved in Medicaid expenditures for unintended pregnancy-related and newborn care (Slaughter, 2007). This is one of those instances where spending one health care dollar saves four dollars.

Access to health care on an equal basis for men and women will also help eliminate discrimination against women as far as their education and workplace opportunities. Two issues discussed in this chapter, the refusal to grant young women over-the-counter access to emergency contraception and the requirements of parental consent or notification for an abortion, are just two examples of how young women's sexual and reproductive lives are shaped and limited by laws and public policies that constrict their education opportunities and subsequent ability to compete economically in the workplace. When so many adolescent girls have unintended pregnancies by the time they reach the age of twenty, the nation is unnecessarily disadvantaging a large segment of its working-age population. Americans should really ask themselves whether it is necessary to circumscribe the health care options available to young women who experience sexual desire or sexual violence in the name of protecting the young; is this really the right road to travel given the economic costs to society by this choice?

It has been almost fifty years since the U.S. Supreme Court stated women have the right to access contraception. Many American women, half a century later, still cannot choose when to become pregnant and how many children to have because they lack access to maternal health care. Contraception and abortion are about more than fighting economic inequalities. Women's rights and freedoms are limited by strict controls on unwanted pregnancies, while at the same time, little is done to ensure unintended pregnancies do not occur in the first place or to fund the consequences. It is necessary to begin effectively addressing the root causes of gender health disparities.

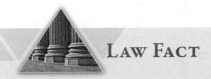

LAW FACT

IN VITRO FERTILIZATION RESTRICTIONS

Who has the right to decide what to do with embryos created through in vitro *fertilization?*

Like Nadya Suleman, many former infertility patients are grappling over the fate of embryos. Patients with leftover frozen embryos have four choices: discard them, donate to research, donate to another couple for pregnancy, or defer the decision and leave them in storage. An estimated 500,000 embryos are in cryopreservation in the U.S.

—McKay, 2009.

CHAPTER SUMMARY

- Although advancements in women's civil rights have been made since the 1960s, continued attempts are made to restrict and carve out exceptions to those rights, as evidenced by the sheer amount of litigation.
- The U.S. rate of infant mortality is high compared to other industrialized nations, perhaps because many babies are born prematurely without proper prenatal care.
- Reproductive health care needs are not adequately met in the U.S., as evidenced by the high rate of unintended pregnancies, high number of abortions, lack of access to birth control, and high rate of teen pregnancy.
- Plan B, the morning-after pill, is approved by the FDA, but women often face obstacles to obtaining it, such as hospitals and pharmacists refusing to dispense it.
- Not all health insurance plans are required to provide coverage for prescription contraceptives, but many do for the simple reason of economics: birth control costs are less than those of a pregnancy.
- Health insurance coverage for drugs related to males' reproductive systems appears to be granted more quickly and easily than it is for female drugs, particularly newer, less invasive forms of birth control.
- It is difficult for women to obtain maternity care coverage, as offerings are limited and often unaffordable or unattainable.
- Many suspect price discrimination within the health insurance industry, as it seems companies attempt to steer women toward less expensive forms of birth control and there is little or no state or federal legislation on this topic.
- Wrongful birth and wrongful pregnancy are two kinds of lawsuits that may be brought related to childbirth; wrongful life suits are much less commonly accepted by courts.
- Although the U.S. Supreme Court ruled that women have the right to an abortion in the 1973 landmark *Roe v. Wade* decision, litigation has steadfastly continued in various states in an attempt to regulate abortion to the point where it is nearly impossible for many women to obtain one, even when their health or life is at stake.

- Women are more likely than men to contract STIs and to suffer serious consequences from them, such as infertility or cancer.
- The safety of many drugs for use by pregnant woman, and even women in general, has not been thoroughly studied; it is often assumed that drugs work the same way for women as they do for men and that there are no different risks or side effects.

Law Notes

1. Arizona, Arkansas, California, Connecticut, Delaware, Georgia, Hawaii, Illinois, Iowa, Maine, Maryland, Massachusetts, Missouri, Nevada, New Hampshire, New Jersey, New Mexico, New York, North Carolina, Rhode Island, Vermont, Washington, and West Virginia have contraceptive equity laws or regulations. Texas and Virginia require that employers' group health insurance plans offer the option to include contraceptive coverage (NCSL, 2007). Individual plans and self-insured plans are not subject to mandates.

2. There are over one hundred strains of HPV, with over thirty types that can cause cervical cancer and genital warts. HPV is the major cause of cervical cancer (Dunne et al., 2007). Most sexually active adults (ages fifteen to forty-nine) will acquire HPV at some time in their lives and will never even know it since it usually has no symptoms, goes away on its own, and does not generally cause disease (AHSA, 2007). Some types of HPV can infect a woman's cervix and cause the cells to change; when HPV is gone, the cervix cells go back to normal. However, sometimes HPV does not go away; instead, it persists and continues to change the cells on a woman's cervix, which can lead to cancer over time if not treated (CDC, 2006).

3. *See* FDA, Investigational New Drug Applications; Amendment to Clinical Hold Regulations for Products Intended for Life-Threatening Diseases and Conditions, 65 *Federal Register* 34,963-01 (June 1, 2000). The agency has issued guidelines that address the inclusion of women who might become pregnant (FDA, 2000). *See* FDA, Guideline for the Study and Evaluation of Gender Differences in the Clinical Evaluation of Drugs, 58 *Federal Register* 39,406-01 (July 22, 1993) (discussing its 1977 policy that had called for the exclusion of women of childbearing age from early phases of studies with investigational drugs); *id.* at 39,410 (rescinding this policy); *id.* at 39,411 ("Clinical protocols should also include measures that will minimize the possibility of fetal exposure to the investigational drug. These would ordinarily include providing for the use of a reliable method of contraception (or abstinence) for the duration of drug exposure (which may exceed the length of the study)...."). The agency's guidelines have no binding effect, however. *See id.* at 39,408-39,409 ("The agency recognizes that this change in FDA's policy will not, by itself, cause drug companies or IRBs to alter restrictions they might impose on the participation of women of childbearing potential.").

Chapter Bibliography

Abel, R. (2006). General damages are incoherent, incalculable, incommensurable, and inegalitarian (but otherwise a great idea). *DePaul Law Review, 55,* 253-328.

ACOG (American College of Obstetricians & Gynecologists) Committee Opinion 419. (2008). *Use of progesterone to reduce preterm birth.* Washington, DC: ACOG.

Afif, M. T. (2005). Prescription ethics: Can states protect pharmacists who refuse to dispense contraceptive prescriptions? *Pace Law Review, 26,* 243-272.

Alvare, H. M. (2003). The case for regulating collaborative reproduction: A children's rights perspective. *Harvard Journal on Legislation, 40* (1), 1-63.

Annas, G. J. (2007, May 2). The Supreme Court and abortion rights. *New England Journal of Medicine, 356* (21), 2201-2207.

ASHA (American Social Health Association). (2007). *FAQs about cervical cancer/HPV vaccine access in the U.S.* Research Triangle Park, NC: ASHA.

Baciu, A. et al. (2007). *The future of drug safety: Promoting and protecting the public health* (pp. 119-121). Washington, DC: Institute of Medicine (discussing the model for risk management restrictions provided by those used for Accutane).

Bailey, M. K. (2005). Contraceptive insurance mandates and *Catholic Charities v. Superior Court of Sacramento*: Towards a new understanding of women's health. *Texas Review of Law & Policy, 9,* 367-388.

Bapat, S. (2007). Fighting collectively for contraceptive equity: Class action litigation and emerging labor union support for contraceptive coverage. *University of Pennsylvania Journal of Labor & Employment Law, 9,* 951-971.

Barth, A. S. (2007). Abortion: State statutes regulating abortion need not contain a per se exception for mother's health or safety: *Planned Parenthood Cincinnati Region v. Taft. American Journal of Law & Medicine, 32,* 405-408.

Behrman, R. E., & Butler, A. S. (2007). *Preterm birth: Causes, consequences, and prevention.* Washington, DC: Institute of Medicine.

Bennett, W. M. (2004, March 1). Off-label use of approved drugs: Therapeutic opportunity and challenges. *Journal of the*

American Society of Nephrology, 15 (3), 830-831 (listing examples of current treatments founded on off-label drug uses).

Bernwanger, B. (2009). Tenth annual review of gender and sexuality law: Health care law chapter: Health care access. *Georgetown Journal of Gender & the Law, 10,* 891-930.

Beshara, N. (2005). Wrongful life: An issue of first impression for the Supreme Court of South Carolina - *Willis v. Wu. Journal of Law, Medicine & Ethics, 33,* 616-617.

Block, S. L. et al. (2006). Comparison of the immunogenicity and reactogenicity of a prophylactic quadrivalent human papillomavirus (types 6, 11, 16, and 18) L1 virus-like particle vaccine in male and female adolescents and young adult women. *Pediatrics, 118* (5), 2135-2146.

Brinker, A. et al., (2005). Trends in adherence to a revised risk management program designed to decrease or eliminate Isotretinoin-exposed pregnancies. *Archives Dermatology 141,* 563-568.

Brown, J. R. (2008). The once and future First Amendment. *Cato Supreme Court Review, 2008,* 9-22.

Casey, P. M. (2008). Ninth annual review of gender and sexuality law: Abortion. *Georgetown Journal of Gender & the Law, 9,* 1097-1123.

CDC (Centers for Disease Control & Prevention). (2006, June 29). *Press release: CDC's Advisory Committee recommends human papillomavirus virus vaccination.* Atlanta, GA: CDC.

Charo, R. A. (2007, May 24). The partial death of abortion rights. *New England Journal of Medicine, 356* (21), 2125.

CIA (Central Intelligence Agency). (2008). *The world factbook, rank.* Washington, DC: CIA.

Colletta, K., & Kapulina, D. (2005). Employment discrimination and the First Amendment: Case analysis of Catholic Charities. *Hofstra Labor & Employment Law Journal, 23,* 189-233.

Collins, M. K. (2006). Conscience clauses and oral contraceptives: Conscientious objection or calculated obstruction? *Annals of Health Law, 15,* 37-60.

Corbin, C. M. (2009). The First Amendment right against compelled listening. *Boston University Law Review, 89,* 939-1016.

Clark, B. R. (2003). When free exercise exemptions undermine religious liberty and the liberty of conscience: A case study of the Catholic hospital conflict. *Oregon Law Review, 82,* 625-693.

Cleveland Clinic. (2008). *Current clinical medicine 2009.* Philadelphia, PA: Saunders Publishing.

Dailard, C. (2006). The public health promise and potential pitfalls of the world's first cervical cancer vaccine. *Guttmacher Policy Review, 9* (1), 6-9.

Dixon, H. S. (2004). Pelvic exam prerequisite to hormonal contraceptives: Unjustified infringement on constitutional rights, governmental coercion, and bad public policy. *Harvard Women's Law Journal, 27,* 177-233 (arguing that publicly funded family planning clinics cannot condition access to oral contraceptives on intrusive exams that serve only collateral purposes).

D'Orazio, P. (2006). Half of the family tree: A call for access to a full genetic history for children born by artificial insemination. *Journal of Health & Biomedical Law, 2,* 249-276.

Dong, A. (2007). Access to contraception. *Georgetown Journal of Gender &Law, 8,* 775-805.

Doshi, A. E. (2007). The cost of clear skin: Balancing the social and safety costs of iPLEDGE with the efficacy of Accutane (Isotretinoin). *Seton Hall Law Review, 37,* 625-660 (concluding that the FDA should withdraw approval).

Drazen, J. M. (2007, May 24). Government in medicine. *New England Journal of Medicine, 356* (21), 2195.

Dunne, E. et al. (2007, February 28). Prevalence of HPV infections among females in the U.S. *Journal of the American Medical Association, 297* (8), 813-819.

Duvall, M. (2007). Pharmacy conscience clause statutes: Constitutional religious "accommodations" or unconstitutional "substantial burdens" on women? *American University Law Review, 55,* 1485-1522.

Eisenman, N. S. (2009). Tenth annual review of gender and sexuality law: Abortion. *Georgetown Journal of Gender & the Law, 10,* 827-857.

Engelman, K. E. (2007). Fetal pain legislation: Protection against pain is not an undue burden. *Quinnipiac Health Law Journal, 10,* 279-316 (counterview by Stahle that fetal pain legislation is an undue burden).

Farmer, P., & Garrett, L. (2007). From "marvelous momentum" to health care for all: Success is possible with the right programs. *Foreign Affairs, 85* (4), 155-167.

FDA (U.S. Food and Drug Administration). (2001). *FDA scholarship in women's health program: Participation of females in clinical trials and gender analysis of data in biologic product applications.* Bethesda, MD: FDA.

___. (1995). *Executive summary: Gender studies in product development: Scientific issues and approaches.* Bethesda, MD: FDA.

Fetterman, J. E. et al. (2003). *A framework for pharmaceutical risk management.* Washington, DC: Food and Drug Law Institute.

Fink, D. K. (2007). Refining permissible abortion regulations: Mandatory in-person, informed-consent meetings held constitutional, but restriction on number of petitions by minors for judicial by-pass of parental-consent requirement overturned: *Cincinnati Women's Services, Inc. v. Taft. American Journal of Law & Medicine, 33,* 145-148.

Fleming, M. B. (2008). Feticide laws: Contemporary legal applications and constitutional inquiries. *Pace Law Review, 29,* 43-74.

Fuhrmans, V. (2005, April 5). Childbirth for bargain-hunters; pregnant women take lead in negotiating over prices amid cutbacks in coverage. *Wall Street Journal,* p. D1.

Garrow, D. J. (2007). Significant risks: *Gonzales v Carhart* and the future of abortion law. *Supreme Court Review, 2007,* 1-50.

Ginsberg, R. B. (2008). Dissent is an appeal for the future. *Alaska Bar Rag, 32,* 1-7.

Golub, D., & Gartner, E. C. (2007). *Equity in prescription insurance and contraceptive coverage.* Washington, DC: Planned Parenthood.

Greene, M. F. (2007). The intimidation of American physicians: Banning partial-birth abortion. *New England Journal of Medicine, 356* (21), 2128.

GSK (GlaxoSmithKline). (2009). *Press release: U.S. Department of Health & Human Services (HHS) purchases GSK's A (H1N1) influenza antigen and proprietary adjuvant system.* London, England & Philadelphia, PA: GSK.

Guttmacher Institute. (2009). *State policies in brief: Emergency contraception.* New York, NY: Guttmacher.

Haff, N. (2006). Health care coverage: Contraception and Viagra. *Georgetown Journal of Gender & the Law, 7*, 1185-1199.

Hall, R. F., & Sobotka, E. S. (2007). Inconsistent government policies: Why FDA off-label regulation cannot survive First Amendment review under Greater New Orleans. *Food & Drug Law Journal, 62*, 1-49.

Hamers, J. (2009). Reeling in the outlier: *Gonzales v. Carhart* and the end of facial challenges to abortion statutes. *Boston University Law Review, 89*, 1069-1101.

Hansen, A. (2008). Unqualified interests, definitive definitions: *Washington v. Glucksberg* and the definition of life. *Hastings Constitutional Law Quarterly, 36*, 163-189.

Harper, D. M., et al. (2006). Sustained efficacy up to 4.5 years of a bivalent L1 virus-like particle vaccine against human papillomavirus types 16 and 18: Follow-up from a randomized control trial. *Lancet, 367*, 1247-1255.

Harper, S. (2006). "The morning after": How far can states go to restrict access to emergency contraception? *Columbia Human Rights Law Review, 38*, 221-262.

Hudak, G. P. (2007). Group prescription plans must cover contraceptives: *Catholic Charities of the Diocese of Albany v. Serio*, 859 N.E.2d 459 (N.Y. 2006). *Rutgers Journal of Law & Religion, 8*, 16.

Javitt, G. et al. (2008). Assessing mandatory HPV vaccination: Who should call the shots? *Journal of Law, Medicine & Ethics, 36*, 384-393.

Kahlenborn, C. et al. (2006). Oral contraceptive use as a risk factor for premenopausal breast cancer: A meta-analysis. *Mayo Clinic Proceedings, 81*, 1290-1302 (review of original data from thirty-four research studies worldwide).

Kaiser (Kaiser Family Foundation). (2009). *Pharmacist provision of emergency contraception to women without a doctor's prescription*. Menlo Park, CA: Kaiser.

___. (2008). *Sexual health of adolescents and young adults in the U.S.* Menlo Park, CA: Kaiser.

___. (2008a). *Abortion in the U.S.: Utilization, financing and access*. Menlo Park, CA: Kaiser.

___. (2008b). *HPV vaccine: Implementation and financing policy in the U.S.* Menlo Park, CA: Kaiser.

___. & HRET (Health Research and Educational Trust). (2008). *Employer health benefits 2008 annual survey*. Menlo Park, CA: Kaiser & Chicago, IL: HRET.

Kalorama Information. (2009). *Women's health: Worldwide prescription drug markets*. New York, NY: Kalorama.

Kalscheur, G. (2006). Moral limits on morals legislation: Lessons for U.S. constitutional law from the Declaration on Religious Freedom. *Southern California Interdisciplinary Law Journal, 16*, 1-48.

Kessler, B. (2007). Abortion: Supreme Court upholds partial-birth abortion ban act against facial challenge: *Gonzales v. Carhart*. *American Journal of Law & Medicine, 33*, 523-526.

Klebanoff, M. A. et al. & National Institute of Child Health and Human Development Maternal-Fetal Medicine Units Network. (2008). Salivary progesterone and estriol among pregnant women treated with 17-a-hydroxyprogesterone caproate or placebo. *American Journal of Obstetrics & Gynecology, 199* (506), 1-7.

Korzec, R. (2007). Maryland tort damages: A form of sex-based discrimination. *University of Baltimore Law Forum, 37*, 97-118.

Kuhn, C. G. (2007). An EPICC oversight: Why the current battle for access to contraception will not help reduce unintended pregnancy in the U.S. *Health Matrix, 17*, 347-375 ("EPICC" refers to the proposed federal Equity in Prescription Insurance & Contraceptive Coverage Act).

Law, N. (2006). Supreme Court avoids disturbing abortion precedents by ruling on grounds of remedy: *Ayotte v. Planned Parenthood of Northern New England*. *Journal of Law, Medicine & Ethics, 23*, 469-471.

Law, S. A. (2008). Childbirth: An opportunity for choice that should be supported. *New York University Review of Law & Social Change, 32*, 345-380.

Lumpkin, C. A. (2005). Does a pharmacist have the right to refuse to fill a prescription for birth control? *University of Miami Law Review, 60*, 105-130.

MacDorman, M. F., & Mathews, T. J. (2008). *NCHS data brief: Recent trends in infant mortality in the U.S.* Washington, DC: National Center for Health Statistics.

Magid, J. M. & Prenkert, J. D. (2005). The religious and associational freedoms of business owners. *University of Pennsylvania Journal of Labor & Employment Law, 7*, 191-224.

Malinowski, M. (2006). Creating life? Examining the legal, ethical, and medical issues of assisted reproductive technologies: A law-policy proposal to know where babies come from during the reproductive revolution. *Journal of Gender, Race & Justice, 9*, 549-568.

Manning, P. J. (2004). Baby needs a new set of rules: Using adoption doctrine to regulate embryo donation. *Georgetown Journal of Gender & Law, 5* (2), 677-721.

McEntire, M. (2007). Compensating post-conception prenatal medical malpractice while respecting life: A recommendation to North Carolina Legislators. *Campbell Law Review, 29*, 761-797.

McKay, B. (2009, March 3). Georgia bill seeks a limit on embryos. *Wall Street Journal*, p. A3

Meckler, L. (2009, May 18). Obama confronts abortion debate. *Wall Street Journal*, p. A3.

Meis, P. J. et al. for the National Institute of Child Health & Human Development Maternal-Fetal Medicine Units Network. (2005). Does progesterone treatment influence risk factors for recurrent preterm delivery? *American Journal of Obstetrics & Gynecology, 106*, 557-561.

Mitchell, K. J. (2007). Guarding the threshold of birth. *Regent University Law Review, 20*, 257-299.

Mundy, A. (2009, March 24). Judge lowers bar for Plan B contraceptives. *Wall Street Journal*, p. A4.

NCSL (National Conference of State Legislatures). (2007). Fifty state summary of contraceptive laws. Washington, DC: NCSL.

Noah, L. (2007). Too high a price for some drugs?: The FDA burdens reproductive choice. *San Diego Law Review, 44*, 231-258.

Northen, A. T. et al. for the National Institute of Child Health and Human Development Maternal-Fetal Medicine Units Network. (2007). Follow-up of children exposed in-utero to 17-alpha hydroxyprogesterone caproate versus placebo. *American Journal of Obstetrics & Gynecology, 110*, 865-872.

NWLC (National Women's Law Center). (2009). *Fact sheet: Ensuring that the government helps women meet their reproductive health needs*. Washington, DC: NWLC.

Perry, J. E. (2007). Partial birth biopolitics. *DePaul Journal of Health Care Law, 11*, 247-257.

Petrini, J. R. et al. (2005). Estimated effect of 17- alpha hydroxyprogesterone caproate on preterm birth in the

U.S. *American College of Obstetricians & Gynecologists Journal, 105* (2), 267-272.

Phillips, K. (2008). Resurrecting Gilbert: Facial parity as unequal treatment in the Eighth Circuit's in *Re Union Pacific Railroad Employment Practices Litigation. Hamline Law Review, 31,* 309-350.

Pisoni, D. (2008). Ninth annual review of gender and sexuality law: Access to contraception. *Georgetown Journal of Gender & the Law, 9,* 1125-1151.

Pugh, C. (2007). Contraception coverage: Employers may exclude contraception coverage from their health insurance plans: *Standridge v. Union Pacific Railroad Company. American Journal of Law & Medicine, 33,* 530-533.

Roan, S. (2008, October 6). On the cusp of life, and of law; Half a million embryos sit in clinic freezers in the U.S., now infertility patients privately steer their fates, but that may change in some states. *Los Angeles Times,* p. A1.

Sandstad, N. C. (2008). Pregnant women and the Fourteenth Amendment: A feminist examination of the trend to eliminate women's rights during pregnancy. *Law & Inequality Journal, 26,* 171-201.

Saslow, D. et al. (2007). American Cancer Society guideline for human papillomavirus (HPV), vaccine use to prevent cervical cancer and its precursors. *Cancer, 57* (1), 7-28.

Scheib, J. E., & Cushing, R. A. (2007). Open-identity donor insemination in the U.S.: Is it on the rise? *Fertility & Sterility, 88* (1), 231-232.

Schiebinger, L. (2003). Women's health and clinical trials. *Journal of Clinical Investigation, 112,* 973 (describing historic underrepresentation of women in clinical trials).

Schwarz, A. (2007). Comprehensive sex education: Why America's youth deserve the truth about sex. *Hamline Journal of Public Law & Policy. 29,* 115-160.

Shacker, C. (2008). Assigning and empowering moral decision making: *Acuna v. Turkish* and wrongful birth and wrongful life jurisprudence in New Jersey. *Journal of Law, Medicine & Ethics, 36,* 193-196.

Simon, S. (2008, August 22). Rules let health workers deny abortions: Regulation's effect on contraception remains unclear. *Wall Street Journal,* p. A3.

Slaughter, L. M. (2007, February 5). Introduction of the Prevention-First Act to the 110th Congress. *Congressional Record, 110,* 259-260 (NY Representative to the House).

Spar, D. L. (2005). *The baby business: How money, science, and politics drive the commerce of conception.* Boston, MA: Harvard Business Press.

Spong, C. Y. et al. for the National Institute of Child Health & Human Development Maternal Fetal Medicine Units Network. (2005). Progesterone for prevention of recurrent preterm birth: Impact of gestational age at previous delivery. *American Journal of Obstetrics & Gynecology, 193,* 1056-1060.

Spreng, J. E. (2008). Pharmacists and the "duty" to dispense emergency contraceptives. *Issues in Law & Medicine, 23,* 215-277.

Stahl, H. (2007). Fetal pain legislation: Protection against pain is an undue burden. *Quinnipiac Health Law Journal, 10,* 251-278 (counterview by Engelman that fetal pain legislation is not an undue burden).

Steinbrook, R. (2006). The potential of human papillomavirus vaccines. *New England Journal of Medicine, 354* (11), 1109-1112.

Storrow, R. F. (2007). The bioethics of prospective parenthood: In pursuit of the proper standard for gate keeping in infertility clinics. *Cardozo Law Review, 28,* 2283-2320.

Sullivan, B. (2004). Naked fitzies and iron cages: Individual values, professional virtues, and the struggles for public space. *Tulsa Law Review, 78,* 1687-1717.

Tai, S. (2009). Uncertainty about uncertainty: The impact of judicial decisions on assessing scientific uncertainty. *University of Pennsylvania Journal of Constitutional Law. 11,* 671-727.

Tobin, H. J. (2008). Confronting misinformation on abortion: Informed consent, deference, and fetal pain laws. *Columbia Journal of Gender & Law, 17,* 111-152.

Vartanian, K. (2009). Tenth annual review of gender and sexuality law: Equal protection. *Georgetown Journal of Gender & the Law, 10,* 227-278.

Villa, L. L. et al. (2005). Prophylactic quadrivalent human papillomavirus (types 6, 11, 16, and 18) L1 virus-like particle vaccine in young women: A randomized double-blind placebo-controlled multicentre phase II efficacy trial. *Lancet Oncology, 6,* 271-278.

Weins, W. J. (2008). Employer funding of fertility awareness training: An acceptable alternative to mandated prescription contraceptive coverage in employee benefits. *Michigan State Journal of Medicine & Law, 12,* 321-339.

Wharton, L. J. (2009). *Roe* at thirty-six and beyond: Enhancing protection for abortion rights through state constitutions. *William & Mary Journal of Women & Law, 15,* 469-534.

Whitebread, C. H. (2007). New high court pronouncements on civil law. *Orange County Lawyer, 49,* 33-45.

Wilcox, M. C. (2008). Why the Equal Protection Clause cannot "fix" abortion law. *Ave Maria Law Review, 7,* 307-337.

Willis, A. R. (2006). The emergency exception in parental involvement laws and the necessity of post-emergency notification. *Ave Maria Law Review, 4,* 171-210.

Wolke, A. (2007). A shot in the arm to prevent preterm births. *State & Federal Issues, 28,* 500. Washington, DC: National Conference of State Legislatures.

Wood, S. F. (2007). The role of science in health policy decision-making: The case of emergency contraception. *Journal of Law & Medicine, 17,* 273-289.

Yuen, S. (2007). An information privacy approach to regulating the middlemen in the lucrative gamete market. *University of Pennsylvania Journal of International Law, 29* (2), 527-562.

CHAPTER 35
CLINICAL TRIALS

> *"The history of the last twenty years is one of crises with drugs and medical devices, many approved despite the objections of the FDA's own scientists."*
>
> —Sidney Wolfe, M.D., member, Drug Safety and Risk Management Committee, U.S. Food and Drug Administration; acting President of the advocacy organization Public Citizen; editor of the book and Web site, *Worst Pills, Best Pills*

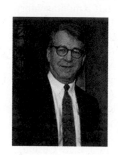

IN BRIEF

This chapter provides an overview of the complex multistage pathways of medical product research and development. The laws and regulations governing clinical trials are examined, including access to experimental drugs and devices, transparency and full disclosure in clinical testing, informed consent and participation of children in human subject research, conflicts of interest, and informed consent in general. The statistics involved in clinical trials and observational studies are generally outlined. In this chapter, the generic term *drugs* includes pharmaceuticals and biopharmaceuticals.

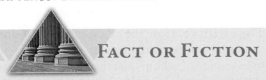

FACT OR FICTION

CLINICAL TRIALS IN DEVELOPING NATIONS

Should the medical products industry be liable in U.S. courts for violation of good clinical practice standards in international clinical trials?

She was ten years old and suffering from bacterial meningitis, a serious infectious disease that was sweeping through West Africa. Meningitis attacks the protective membranes covering the brain and spinal cord and can cause serious neurologic damage or even death. An effective treatment for this disease is intravenous antibiotics. Once the family arrived at the clinic in Kano, Nigeria, they met physicians who were offering free drugs. However, three days later, the girl died; she had not received the proven antibiotic therapy, but only an experimental drug called Trovan. The girl's family, along with many others, claimed that instead of receiving health care, they were unwittingly participating in clinical trials sponsored by Pfizer that led to the serious impairment or death of many children. After several weeks, and injuries and fatalities to some two hundred children resulting from the experimental drug treatment, Pfizer concluded its clinical trial and left without administering follow-up care.

—*Abdullahi v. Pfizer, Inc.*, 562 F.3d 163 (U.S. Court of Appeals for the 2nd Circuit 2009), *petition for U.S. Supreme Court certiorari filed*, 2009.

(See *Law Fact* at the end of this chapter for the answer.)

PRINCIPLES AND APPLICATIONS

Clinical trials are essential to understanding the efficacy of medical interventions (Wood, 2009). In 2007, the pharmaceutical and biopharmaceutical industries invested $59 billion in researching and developing new drugs, an increase of $2.7 billion over the previous year (PhRMA, 2008). This represents almost 19 percent of the total U.S. sales for the combined industries. This 19 percent commitment by the pharmaceutical and biopharmaceutical industries is almost five times the investment level of other U.S. manufacturers who invest on average about 4 percent of their sales into research and development (PhRMA, 2008). An additional $29 billion in basic research funding for development of drugs was provided by the National Institutes of Health (HHS, 2008). The result of this $88 billion investment is that over 2,700 compounds were in development in 2007, compared to 2,000 compounds in 2003 (*see* Adis, 2009).

RESEARCH AND DEVELOPMENT INVESTMENTS FUND A COMPLEX MULTISTAGE PATHWAY

Research and development funding for innovative medical products, not generic products, covers a complex, multistage pathway from discovery through approval of drugs for participants. Although clinical testing represents the greatest share of costs, each stage in the process is:

- Time-consuming: ten to fifteen years (Dickson & Gagnon, 2004)
- Expensive: $1.3 billion to bring a new pharmaceutical to market (Gotec & DiMasi, 2008); $1.2 billion for a new biopharmaceutical (Tufts Center, 2006)
- Risky: only two out of ten marketed drugs ever recover their research and development costs (Gotec & DiMasi, 2008)

Some major expenses are research materials, advanced computers, other highly sophisticated machines that support research activities, and salaries of scientists (PhRMA, 2008). Stage-specific activities include:

- Drug discovery
- Pre-clinical testing
- Clinical trials
- Approval by the U.S. Food and Drug Administration (FDA)
- Post-marketing surveillance

Drug Discovery

Researchers first identify a target for a new drug, such as a molecule believed to affect a particular disease. Then they use computers to screen or biotechnology to create thousands of compounds, identifying hundreds of potential drugs. While most will never be approved for use in participants, each one is evaluated to determine its potential value compared to existing therapies, complexity of large scale manufacturing, and other factors (PhRMA, 2008).

Pre-Clinical Testing

Candidate drugs from the discovery stage then receive one to three years of extensive testing in the laboratory and in animals to assess safety and show biological activity against a disease. In addition:

- Chemical tests establish a compound's purity, stability, and shelf life
- Manufacturing tests determine what will be involved in mass producing the drug
- Pharmaceutical development studies explore dosing, packaging, and formulation of the drug (capsule, inhaler, injection, tablet, etc.)

(PhRMA, 2008)

Clinical Trials

In the three phases of clinical trials, which can take anywhere from two to ten years, teams of research investigators test a new drug in participants to learn if it is safe and effective. For drugs in various stages of development, the odds for reaching the market are well known (PhRMA, 2008). There is a significant drop-off during each of the three phases of clinical trials before submission of a new drug application (NDA).

- 20% for Phase I: twenty to eighty healthy participants are generally tested at low dosage levels, if the FDA approves human testing to determine safety, safe dose range, and mechanism of action (*see* 21 C.F.R. § 312.21(a) (2005))
- 30% for Phase II: one hundred to three hundred participants who have the disease are tested to look for efficacy, side effects, and determine optimal dose strength and schedule (*see* 21 C.F.R. § 312.21(b) (2005))
- 60% for Phase III: one thousand to five thousand participants are tested to determine effectiveness and monitor adverse reactions to long-term use (*see* 21 C.F.R. § 312.21(c) (2005))
- 80% for NDAs

In Phase I clinical trials, researchers find the best way to administer a new treatment and how much they can safely give. Healthy humans are used, if the FDA allows it, especially if there are no animal models for the disease or condition. All testing is done first in animals to determine if it is safe to be tested in humans (*see* 21 C.F.R. § 312.21 (2005)).

These trials compare the experiences of randomly selected groups of participants with similar characteristics, some of whom take the new drug being tested while others take a placebo (PhRMA, 2008). By taking part in a clinical trial, participants who have the disease can try a new treatment that may or may not be better than those that already exist. In addition, participants are generally paid $100 to $200 per day; if travel to a trial site is required, travel expenses are covered for participants, including international travel. In comparison, egg donors receive $5,000 to $8,000 per cycle and sperm donors receive $50 to $100 per contribution; prices vary by site.

While Phase I to III studies are taking place, research investigators are also:

- Conducting toxicity tests and other long-term safety evaluations
- Evaluating dosage forms
- Planning for mass production
- Designing packaging
- Preparing the extensive application required for FDA approval

Even with this complex process, only one out of five drugs that enter clinical testing is ever approved by the FDA (PhRMA, 2008).

Moral Dilemmas

1. Should sponsors have a duty to test for off-label related risks?

Approval by the U.S. Food and Drug Administration

The NDA is the vehicle through which the pharmaceutical and biopharmaceutical industries formally propose that the FDA approve a new drug for sale and marketing in the U.S. The data gathered during the animal studies and human clinical trials becomes part of the NDA (Smith, 2008). The FDA's goal is to review 90 percent of NDAs within ten months. FDA scientists and sometimes advisory committees review all clinical trial results and the company's application and decide whether the data justifies approval for patient use (PhRMA, 2008).

According to the FDA, the documentation required in an NDA is supposed to tell the drug's whole story as illustrated in Figure 35-1, including:

- What happened during the clinical trial tests
- What the ingredients of the drug are
- Results of the pre-clinical animal studies

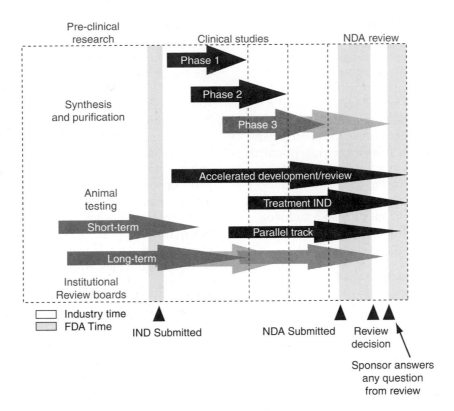

FIGURE 35-1: Clinical Trial Process

Delmar/Cengage Learning

- How the drug behaves in the human body
- How the drug is manufactured, processed, and packaged

(FDA, 2007a)

Post-Marketing Surveillance

Phase IV studies are generally ongoing for years. These studies continue to evaluate safety and generate more data about how the drug affects particular groups of participants, such as children or the elderly. In addition to these targeted post-marketing surveillance studies, companies continue to monitor all approved drugs for long-term safety and regularly report results to the FDA (PhRMA, 2008).

It is important to note that clinical trials cannot always detect risks that are relatively rare, have long latency periods, or affect vulnerable sub-populations. In addition, clinical trials cannot detect risks involved in patients that take multiple prescribed drugs, over-the-counter drugs, vitamins, and nutritional supplements at the same time. For these reasons, most serious adverse effects do not become evident until a drug is used in larger population groups for periods in excess of one year (Vladeck, 2008). The Health Research Group at Public Citizen, a nonprofit critic of the medical products industry, advocates the ultraconservative rule of seven: consumers should

only take approved drugs that have been on the market for at least seven years without adverse effects (Wolfe et al., 2005).

CLINICAL TRIALS OF GENERIC DRUGS

In contrast to the billion-dollar, ten- to fifteen-year investment that branded, innovative drugs undergo, approval for generics only requires clinical trials of one hundred patients at an average cost of $100,000. Congress lessened the standards for generic drug product market entry, favoring economic advantages over detailed scientific evaluation of drugs. *See* Drug Price Competition and Patent Term Restoration Act of 1984, 21 U.S.C.A. § 355(j) (2008) (allowing the filing of, and stating the requirements for, an abbreviated application for the approval of a new drug).

Branded generics are becoming a very important part of the pharmaceutical industry (Gorsky, 2005). They enable very large, underserved population segments to access important drugs. In addition, branded generics ensure that innovation truly takes place in the marketplace (Wharton, 2006). With truly innovative pharmaceutical companies that are continually producing new and innovative products, when generics enter the market following patent expiration, it frees up resources to license off-patent drugs and invest in new breakthrough products. More innovative approaches are starting to appear in the larger pharmaceutical companies with the expanded use of branded generics. The line between brand name and branded generic drugs is beginning to blur within the industry, just as the line between the pharmaceutical and biotechnology industries is blurring. Branded generics are evolving both as an opportunity to get access to drugs as well as an emerging business model for the brand-name pharmaceuticals (Wharton, 2006). The companies of the future may have a breadth of businesses across biotechnology, pharmaceutical, and branded generics (*see generally* Chang, 2009).

Distinction Between Bioequivalent and Biotherapeutic

Generic versions of branded drugs need not demonstrate their scientific merits by controlled human clinical trials and other testing the brand pharmaceutical companies conducted (*see* 21 U.S.C.A. § 355(j) (2)(A)(ii)-(iv) (2008); *see also* 21 U.S. CA. § 355(j)(8) (b) (2008)). Moreover, while generics may be more or less efficacious in delivering the active ingredient to the target condition in the human body, generics are labeled bioequivalent as long as the active ingredient's rate of absorption is similar (or bioequivalent) to the delivery of the active ingredient in the branded drug (*see* 21 C.F.R. § 320.23 (1999)).

By definition, generics may be up to 45 percent less or 25 percent more efficacious than branded drugs, yet still meet the legal definition of being bioequivalent. This is because of how the term *bioequivalent* is defined (Berndt et al., 2007). The relative mean of the generic formulation should be within 80 percent to 125 percent of the brand formulation, which is the basis for stating generics may be more or less efficacious than branded drugs. For instance, the response that a drug elicits in individual patients can be significantly different for generics that are deemed bioequivalent; slight changes in the chemical composition can affect the molecular degradability of the generic and be responsible for widely varying responses (Zain, 2007). A critical distinction between generics and branded drugs is the difference between being bioequivalent and biotherapeutic. Bioequivalence concerns the dose and rate of absorption. A generic drug is considered a bioequivalent to the branded drug if the rate and extent of absorption of the drug is not significantly different than that of the branded drug at the same dosage when taken in the prescribed amount. *See* 21 U.S.C.A. § 355(j)(7)(B) (2008); *see generally* Jaquette, 2007.

While the active ingredient in generic drugs is required to be therapeutically the same as branded drugs, generics do not have to treat the disease in the same way as branded drugs as long as they are absorbed by the body in a similar manner, up to 20 percent less metabolism of the active ingredient to 20 percent more is deemed bioequivalent (Jaquette, 2007). Generic drugs may have side effects, may be absorbed differently by the human body, and yet still be defined as bioequivalent to the branded drug. Most importantly, and this cannot be emphasized enough, generics are not required to provide independent proof of their safety and efficacy to be labeled bioequivalent (*see* 21 U.S.C.A. § 355(j)(2)(A) (2008)). Generics may be safe and efficacious, but no evidence is required that they are, or that they are not.

Distinction Between Branded Generics and Generics

The pharmaceutical industry also markets authorized branded generics, which are branded drugs that have lost their patent status but are labeled and marketed as generics (Berndt et al., 2007). Off-patent branded drugs are available as authorized generics; sometimes the same drug is sold as a branded drug and an authorized generic drug at the same time by the same firm. Since the early 1990s, numerous authorized generics have been marketed by pharmaceutical companies holding the original patent or their licensee.

As the practice of branded generics has grown in recent years, the generic industry has met the competition by turning to the FTC and Congress about the competitive effects of this practice. The pharmaceutical industry has challenged the generic industry's argument against it by maintaining branded generics are simply bringing competition to the generic industry. Both empirical and theoretical studies evince that generic entry is inversely related to price (Zain, 2007). The greater the number of generics, the lower the price. So far, the pharmaceutical industry appears to be winning the battle against the generic industry; no court has found branded generics to be unlawful, and the FDA and the Federal Trade Commission have expressed favorable opinions on the practice. Moreover, no government regulator or enforcement agency has publicly condemned or challenged the practice of introducing branded generics to the market (Zain, 2007).

HEALTH RISK ASSESSMENTS

The ethical foundation of clinical trials involving human subjects is codified in the Belmont Report and the Declaration of Helsinki (FDA, 1979; WMA, 2006). These documents require that the results of trials be publicly available to inform medical practice as well as future research. In addition, basic principles of evidence-based medicine require the analysis of all data on a given topic (Wood, 2009). Recent debate has evolved around the practice of publishing only some results of clinical trials, but not others. Industry critics claim this undermines the health industry's collective ability to make rational decisions about health care.

Information on Post-Phase I Clinical Trials

Congress expanded the requirements for all sponsors and research investigators to share information about post-Phase I clinical trials, including selected aspects of trial results, on the U.S. government Web site, ClinicalTrials.gov. The International Committee of Medical Journal Editors and the World Health Organization require the registration of all clinical trials on human subjects regardless of phase. This site has more than 67,000 registered trials for drugs, devices, surgical interventions, and procedural interventions from about 160 countries (Wood, 2009). These expanded requirements apply no matter what the source of funding is for the clinical trials and include, for the first time, penalties for noncompliance, including the loss of funding from the National Institutes of Health and civil penalties of up to $10,000 per day. *See* Food and Drug Administration Amendments Act of 2007, 21 U.S.C.A. § 350f *et seq.* (2009).

Balancing Risks and Benefits

Proper health risk assessment is critical for new drug product treatments. Patients and physicians often weigh the pros and cons of one treatment versus another; the FDA also wrestles with the trade-offs between health risks and benefits (Wharton, 2007). There are eleven thousand FDA-regulated drug products on the market (including both prescription and over-the-counter drug products), with nearly one hundred more approved each year (FDA, 2007). The reality is that the FDA does not have the resources to perform the Herculean task of monitoring comprehensively the performance of every drug product on the market (Kessler & Vladeck, 2008). An ongoing issue is whether the FDA should do more to ensure the safety of new drug products and expose potential side effects before a drug product comes into widespread use (FDA, 2008). Patients who have life-threatening illnesses for which there is no effective treatment, however, are generally willing to assume the health risk of taking a drug product that has not been studied for very long if it offers them the possibility of a cure or at least less suffering (Wharton, 2007).

There is a tug of war between the two mind sets. In the European model, decisions cannot be based only on clinical or medical knowledge, but also depend in part on patient preferences. The question is which, or whose, preferences should dominate. Virtually any drug will be too risky for the most risk-averse patients, but virtually any delay is too long for many more patients willing to take a chance for much better outcomes. Also in the equation are industry interests, which want the FDA to approve new drugs as quickly as possible so they will begin getting a return on the money they spent on research and development (Wharton, 2007).

Participants with advanced cancer are now arguing for something closer to the European model when it comes to approval of new drug products. They are willing to accept the health risk of side effects from investigational treatments because they attach more value to the possibility of good outcomes and less value to the possibility of side effects. The FDA and its expert panels, on the other hand, place more weight on the health risk of side effects (Wharton, 2007; *see* Wolf et al., 2008).

Moral Dilemmas

1. Has patient protectionism translated into ever-longer clinical trials and administrative delays, with the real risk being that too few drugs now reach the market rather than too many?

EXPANDED ACCESS PROTOCOLS

Human use of investigational new drugs takes place in controlled clinical trials. Data from the trials serves as the basis for the NDA. Sometimes, however, patients do not qualify for these carefully controlled trials because of other health problems, age, or other factors. For patients who may benefit from the drug but do not qualify for the clinical trials, FDA regulations enable manufacturers to provide for expanded access to the drug during the trial stage before being approved to market.

An investigational new drug (IND) application, or treatment protocol, is a relatively unrestricted study. The primary intent of an IND is to authorize shipment of an unapproved drug product into interstate commerce. A much less common purpose is to provide for access to the new drug for patients with a life-threatening or serious disease for which there is no alternative treatment, which comprises about 2 percent of the IND shipments. Another secondary purpose, which comprises about 1 percent of the purpose for an IND, is to generate additional information about the drug, especially its safety. INDs can be undertaken only if clinical research investigators are actively studying the experimental treatment in clinical trials, or all trials have been completed. In addition, there must be evidence the drug may be an effective treatment in patients like those to be treated by the IND. Furthermore, the drug cannot expose patients to unreasonable risks given the severity of the disease to be treated (NLM, 2008).

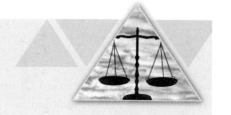

RIGHT TO LIFESAVING EXPERIMENTAL DRUGS

Abigail Alliance v. von Eschenbach
[Patients v. FDA]

495 F.3d 695 (U.S. Court of Appeals for the District of Columbia Circuit 2007),

U.S. Supreme Court certiorari denied, 128 S.Ct. 1069 (U.S. Supreme Court 2008)

FACTS: In 2006, the Abigail Alliance for Better Access to Developmental Drugs appeared to have won a victory when a divided panel of the Court of Appeals for the District of Columbia Circuit ruled that terminally ill, mentally competent adult patients had a constitutionally protected right to access experimental drugs that have not reached Phase II clinical trials (*see Abigail Alliance v. von Eschenbach,* 445 F.3d 470 (U.S. Court of Appeals for the District of Columbia Circuit 2006)). This victory was short lived, however. In 2007, the D.C. Circuit sitting *en banc* reversed this earlier decision, marking a setback in the campaign for removal of the regulatory barriers that currently prevent terminally ill patients from gaining early access to experimental drugs.

The *en banc* reversal represents the latest act in a drama that began in June of 2003, when Abigail filed a citizen petition with the FDA (*see* 21 C.F.R. § 10.30 (2000)). Abigail's petition proposed adding an early approval regime for experimental drugs, a scheme Abigail called "Tier 1 Initial Approval" that would allow terminally ill participants to gain earlier access to those experimental drugs. Although many other advocacy groups and advisory committees wrote to the FDA either in support of or in opposition to Abigail's Tier 1 Initial Approval concept, the FDA failed to respond to Abigail's proposal, thus prompting the Alliance to proceed to judicial challenge.

ISSUE: Does a fundamental right exist under the Fifth Amendment, which contains the Due Process Clause, that provides terminally ill patients access to potentially lifesaving experimental drugs?

HOLDING AND DECISION: No, terminally ill patients do not have a fundamental right to access experimental drugs under the Due Process Clause of the Fifth Amendment. Thus, there was no constitutional deficiency in the existing FDA regulations regarding experimental drugs, and because those regulations had a rational basis, the court could not disturb them. The dissent argued that terminally ill patients do have a fundamental right to access potentially lifesaving experimental drugs.

ANALYSIS: Whether an asserted right in a particular case constitutes a fundamental right and liberty interest is extremely important in constitutional litigation. If the state wishes to restrict a fundamental right, then the state must prove that it has a compelling governmental interest justifying the restriction, and that the restriction is narrowly tailored to serve that interest. The restriction is subject to the strict scrutiny standard (*see Skinner v. Oklahoma ex rel. Williamson,* 316 U.S. 535 (U.S. Supreme Court 1942)). If the restricted right is not a fundamental right, however, then the state can justify its intervention by showing that there is a rational basis for the restriction, an easier standard to meet than strict scrutiny for fundamental rights.

What, then, are the fundamental rights and liberty interests protected by the Due Process Clause? Since such rights are not explicitly enumerated in the U.S. Constitution, the U.S. Supreme Court has established a two-pronged analysis, known as the substantive due process analysis, to determine if the asserted right is a fundamental one (*see Washington v. Glucksberg,* 521 U.S. 702 (U.S. Supreme Court 1997)). This analysis requires proponents of a proposed fundamental right to do the following:

- Provide a careful description of the asserted fundamental liberty interest

(continues)

(continued)

- Show that the asserted right is deeply rooted in the nation's history and tradition and implicit in the concept of ordered liberty, such that neither liberty nor justice would exist if it were sacrificed

The first prong of the substantive due process analysis, the description of the asserted right, is very important: too broad and a right becomes all-encompassing and impossible to evaluate; too narrow and a right appears trivial.

RULE OF LAW: The majority opinion described Abigail's asserted right as terminally ill patients' right to access experimental drugs and found it not to be a fundamental right. The dissenting opinion cast it as the right to attempt to preserve one's life and found it to be a fundamental right.

(*See generally* Harper, 2008; Lee, 2008; Madara, 2009; Marcee, 2008; O'Reilly, 2008; Pedersen, 2008; Plionis, 2008; Rossen, 2009; Saver, 2009; Winniford, 2009; Winter, 2008).

The key question, if the U.S. Supreme Court had heard this case, would have been how the rights asserted by Abigail would have been described. Given that the majority and dissent in this decision each came up with substantially different rights, it will be interesting to see if future cases provide a more principled manner of extracting the fundamental rights to be analyzed. If future cases choose to define Abigail's asserted right narrowly, whether courts will infer a narrow right from a broader, established fundamental right will be noteworthy. This has been done in the past, for instance, the specific rights to:

- Determine extended family living arrangements has been inferred from broader constitutional protections for the sanctity of the family (*see Moore v. City of East Cleveland*, 431 U.S. 494 (U.S. Supreme Court 1977))
- Terminate a pregnancy from a broader right to privacy (*see Roe v. Wade*, 410 U.S. 113 (U.S. Supreme Court 1973))
- Use contraception from a general right to be free from intrusion into the sacred precincts of marital bedrooms (*see Griswold v. State of Connecticut*, 381 U.S. 479 (U.S. Supreme Court 1965))

Abigail Alliance's Two-Tier Approval Proposal

The issue of access to lifesaving experimental treatments and medical products continues to present itself. If Congress were to permit terminally ill patients to access experimental medical products, then the FDA would have to create a system to allow that access. The Abigail Alliance's Tier 1 Approval proposal represents one legislative possibility for addressing this problem for drug products. The proposal would involve:

- Granting terminally ill patients who have exhausted all FDA-approved therapies the autonomy of selecting post-Phase I experimental medical products with their physicians

- Lifting the current prohibition of charging any price higher than the cost for experimental products

The second feature of the Abigail Alliance's proposal, allowing commercialization, or charging a price higher than the cost of experimental products, would safeguard clinical trials. The intention of this feature is to create incentives for the medical products industry to actively distribute its experimental products, rather than merely impose cost recovery under the current FDA regulation. Sufficiently high price may act as a barrier to some patients seeking access to experimental products, thus forcing them to participate in free clinical trials, while creating disparities in access based on economics (Lee et al., 2008).

Balancing Patient Rights:

Access v. Autonomy

Determining the safeguards for access to clinical trials is an economic decision, as opposed to the question of patient autonomy. In a sense, the right to autonomy affects individual interests in obtaining investigational medical treatments and medical products, while the right to access pertains to the public's interests in filtering safe and efficacious products through clinical trials. It will be more difficult to find a rational basis in preventing investigational access if an alternative regulation like the Abigail Alliance's proposal can manage to preserve the public's interests while also promoting individual interests. (Lee et al., 2008) Congress may be better suited to decide the proper balance between the risks and benefits of medical technology. The individual autonomy of terminally ill individuals, if not a constitutional right, is still a policy issue that Congress can endorse.

TERMINATION OF CLINICAL TRIALS

Regardless of the reason for termination of a clinical trial, the high cost of bringing a medical product to market presents a valid reason for halting a clinical investigation

(Cerino, 2008). Clinical trials usually get halted for one of two reasons:

- New drug shows overwhelming promise and it would not be fair to delay its release
- Results suggest great risk

(Biliak, 2006)

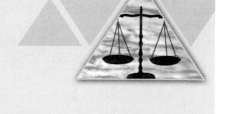

OBLIGATIONS TO PROVIDE EXPERIMENTAL DRUGS TO CLINICAL TRIAL PARTICIPANTS

Abney v. Amgen, Inc.
[Clinical Trial Participants v. Pharmaceutical Company]
443 F.3d 540 (U.S. Court of Appeals for the 6th Circuit 2006)

FACTS: Amgen sought to evaluate a method of delivering a potential breakthrough drug for Parkinson's disease, glial-cell-line-derived neutrotropic factor (GDNF), to dopamine-producing neurons in the brain. Two open label studies where all participants received GDNF, and a Phase II trial that later converted to a third open label study, were conducted by Amgen. The delivery method, known as bilateral intraputaminal (IPu) administration, required research investigators to implant into a participant's abdomen a drug reservoir and pump, drill a hole in the participant's skull, and run an attached catheter from the pump through the participant's neck, cheek, and skull, and into the brain, where the GDNF from the reservoir was delivered by the pump via the catheter.

Amgen supported its first open label trial involving five participants suffering from Parkinson's disease in the United Kingdom, which yielded favorable results. Desiring further support, Amgen sponsored a second open label trial that showed improvement in ten participants at the University of Kentucky Medical Center. Lacking control groups to validate these positive results in the open label studies, Amgen next sponsored a multi-center Phase II, randomized, double-blind, placebo-controlled study of GDNF's efficacy. Amgen selected eight sites to carry out the Phase II clinical trials.

A protocol is a study plan on which a clinical trial is based. The plan is designed to safeguard the health of the participants as well as answer specific research questions. A protocol describes:

- Who may participate in a clinical trial
- Schedule of tests, procedures, and investigational drugs
- Length of the study

While in a clinical trial, participants following a protocol are seen regularly by the clinical trial research investigators to monitor their health and to determine the safety and effectiveness of their experimental treatment.

Amgen's protocol, approved by the Institutional Review Boards (IRBs) at the study centers agreeing to follow it, provided that after an initial study period, participants could elect to continue treatment for up to an additional two years. Amgen and the research investigators signed a clinical trial agreement, but Amgen did not sign the consent forms signed by the participants that explained the risks of the trial. The consent forms provided the option to continue receiving GDNF for two years after the trial, and further reserved the right to end the trial if investigators found that its risks outweighed its benefits, or if Amgen decided to prematurely terminate the trial.

Amgen hoped to see increases in the motor scores of participants receiving GDNF 25 percent greater than those of the placebo, or control group. Research investigators observed that motor scores increased by only 10 percent in the GDNF group and 5 percent in the placebo group. Seven of the thirty-four Phase II trial participants demonstrated dramatic improvement, but four of the seven were receiving the placebo. Amgen responded by continuing the trial, but converted it into an open label study, providing all participants with GDNF.

After receiving the FDA's authorization, Amgen decided to terminate all clinical use of GDNF after several study participants developed neutralizing antibodies, which could neutralize the drug's effect and could attack GDNF occurring naturally in the body, and primates receiving GDFN via IPu during

(continues)

(continued)

a long-term toxicology study developed cerebellar lesions. Cerebellar lesions could affect cognitive functions in humans and lead to muscular weakness. The participants claimed Amgen stopped providing GDNF regardless of markedly improved physical, cognitive, and emotional states among all participants. They maintained Amgen terminated the trial for financial reasons.

Despite the FDA's permission to permit compassionate use of GDNF after the termination, Amgen denied such use. The participants responded by filing this lawsuit against Amgen.

Issue: Are pharmaceutical companies obligated to continue providing experimental drugs to clinical trial participants after the trials are terminated?

Holding and Decision: No, sponsoring pharmaceutical companies are not obligated to continue providing experimental drugs to participants after termination of clinical trials.

Analysis: After filing the lawsuit, the participants moved for a preliminary injunction, which would have required Amgen to provide GDNF to research investigators and to allow them to fill the participants' pumps with the drug. The court denied the motion, finding no contract bound Amgen to continue supplying GDNF to the participants. The consent form signed by the participants and the principal investigators did not directly bind Amgen because neither Amgen nor any agent of Amgen signed the consent forms. Although the principal investigators promised to act in the participants' best interest, and to continue administering GDNF if it proved safe and effective, no such promises were ever made by Amgen.

While acts of the research investigators participating in the clinical trials might have bound Amgen, there was nothing that led the participants to believe the principal investigators were agents of Amgen. The court found the participants could probably not prove Amgen undertook a fiduciary duty, through the principal investigators, to treat their disease with the best drug available. No evidence suggested a fiduciary relationship was established; neither Amgen nor the participants understood that benefiting the participants would be the primary reason for Amgen's sponsorship of the clinical trials. While a special relationship between investigators and participants normally creates duties enforceable in tort for negligence, this duty was never characterized as fiduciary. Furthermore, Amgen designed its protocol to comply with FDA regulations. While the clinical sites and investigators conducted the GDNF trial, recruited the participants, and obtained their consent, Amgen did not. Thus, there was no breach of fiduciary duty by Amgen.

The court suggested the participants might be more likely to succeed in establishing a contract between themselves and either the IRBs, or the research investigators involved in the clinical trial, noting that the consent forms constituted a contract that obligated the clinical sites to continue providing GDNF, and that the FDA's regulations charge IRBs, not the medical products industry, with ensuring the rights and welfare of participants in clinical trials. The court also noted that IRBs could possibly avoid similar suits by clearly disclosing in consent forms the terms for terminating the participants' access to investigational drugs and experimental treatments.

The court next held that the desired injunction would not serve the public interest. While the participants claimed research investigators, not Amgen, should decide whether to administer experimental drugs, and that denying the injunction would cause unnecessary suffering and deter others from participating in clinical trials, the court found that granting the injunction could deter Amgen from sponsoring future clinical trials. In addition, the claim that the investigators should be the sole arbiter of patient care wholly undermines the purpose and value of the FDA. The public has a strong interest in ensuring the FDA decides what drugs are safe and efficacious.

Rule of Law: Amgen was not required to continue supplying an experimental drug because:

- Amgen undertook no fiduciary duties with respect to the participants
- The research investigators lacked agency status or apparent authority to bind Amgen and the participants to a contract or quasi-contract
- There was no contract between Amgen and the participants

(*See generally* Barth, 2007; Leonard 2009; Saver, 2009; Talbott, 2007; Winter, 2008).

This decision may leave injured participants, who have had invasive procedures to participate in clinical trials (like the abdominal implants with internal catheters into the brain in the Amgen trials), with limited recourse for damages from the medical products industry when participating in clinical trials that are terminated. The trial protocol that participants sign at the onset of their participation in any clinical trial defines participant rights to recovery, if any, with regard to termination of a trial in which they choose to participate. There is an ethical obligation to participants injured in a clinical trial, but causality of injuries is legally difficult to determine, often impossible. The necessary relationship between participation in a clinical trial (the claimed cause of an injury) and the alleged injury (the effect) must be the direct consequence of participation. IRBs fearing liability may respond by more clearly explaining the risks and consequences of participating in clinical trials. The medical products industry will likely avoid fiduciary status and binding agreements with respect to clinical trial participants by:

- Designing sponsor protocols to comply with FDA regulations
- Forgoing control over clinical studies
- Outsourcing clinical trial design and administration

Clinical trial sponsors as a rule usually reimburse participants for the necessary medical expenses incurred for the treatment of any injuries. The exceptions to this general rule are if the trial research investigator failed to follow the trial protocol, was negligent, or there was willful misconduct. The right to recover, if any, generally survives termination of a clinical trial.

Monitoring Board Decisions

This section on the statistical analysis of clinical trials draws on the "Numbers Guy" column by Carl Biliak of the *Wall Street Journal.* Pfizer rattled the health industry when it abandoned a potential blockbuster cholesterol drug, Lipitor-plus, called torcetrapib, after some participants died during clinical trials. While each clinical trial is different, for many trials, monitoring boards set numerical thresholds for bad outcomes before the trial begins. When the thresholds are crossed, the trials are stopped.

Often, the decisions seem hasty. In this instance, the Pfizer clinical trial involved over fifteen thousand participants at high risk for cardiovascular disease. Some eighty-two people taking the new drug died, while fifty-one people in a control group also died. The issue is why such a small difference was enough to justify a decision to walk away from a drug Pfizer had spent over $1 billion developing. A closer look at the numbers and an understanding of the roles

statistics plays in clinical trials shows why this small difference had such an impact at Pfizer.

Participant pools are generally divided down the middle in clinical trials. In this clinical trial, half the control group took the cholesterol-lowering drug Lipitor and the other half took Lipitor-plus. On a straight percentage basis, about 0.7 percent of those in the Lipitor group died, while 1.1 percent of people taking Lipitor-plus died. This is a difference of only 0.4 of a percentage point.

Relative Risks

What is more important, however, is the relative risk facing the two groups. The relative risk is that participants taking the Lipitor-plus were 60 percent more likely to die. This statistic suggests why Pfizer might have wanted to stop the trial. To understand why Pfizer chose to stop the testing when it did, statistical boundaries have to be examined. As in most clinical trials, the difference between stopping and proceeding comes down to just a few deaths.

Statistical Boundaries

When an imbalance in deaths crosses the statistical boundary set before the trial begins, clinical trials are automatically halted. This statistical boundary is not some arbitrary figure, but rather a single number that is calculated as part of the trial protocol.

The magic number is called a *p value.* Generally, p measures the probability that a particular result, in this case, the difference in the rates of death between the two drug groups, can be a statistical anomaly. In simple terms, a p value of 0.01 means that there is a one in one hundred chance that the results are due to some statistical quirk. Put another way: if a different fifteen thousand participants had been selected to participate in the Pfizer clinical trial, would the outcome have been the same? The lower the p value, the more certain it is that the deaths are not due to some anomaly.

Calculating p in this case is complex, and takes into account several factors, including the number of participants in the clinical trial. The threshold for the Pfizer study was set at 0.01, meaning that once research investigators computed a p that fell below that number, they would know that the results were significant, and not something that would be likely to change by evaluating a different pool of participants. Investigators calculated p monthly; given the deaths, any number below 0.01 would mean immediately halting the trial. Indeed, the study was halted when new data produced a p that crossed the threshold.

Statistical Significance

Thresholds are usually set at 0.05 for statistical significance. Using such a value, the Pfizer study could have been halted even sooner. However, thresholds are set higher when there are frequent measurements of *p*, to make sure that too much weight is not given to any single reading (Biliak, 2006).

While one anecdote does not drive the decision to halt a clinical trial, subjective clinical expertise does determine these thresholds before the clinical trial starts. If a new drug could cure cancer or another incurable disease when there is no other investigational treatment, more risk is tolerated before a trial is terminated. Where the new drug is a lifestyle drug or one where there are other safe drugs available, less risk is tolerated. In this instance, the purpose of the drug was to reduce the chance of death, and since Lipitor-plus increased the death rate, there was no reason to pursue it further. This Pfizer analysis shows how sensitive outcomes are to small numbers. Just two fewer deaths among those taking Lipitor-plus, or eighty instead of eighty-two, would have led to a *p* value just above the threshold (Biliak, 2006).

With Lipitor coming off patent in 2011 and accounting for about one-quarter of Pfizer's sales, this decision to terminate the clinical trial for Lipitor-plus received little attention outside the health industry. While it was the right clinical decision and an ethical decision, industry critics ignored the merits of the decision.

With a different drug approval strategy, Pfizer could have sought initial approval for a narrow use by adjusting inclusion and exclusion criteria in a clinical trial so that participants included only those patients most likely to benefit from Lipitor-plus without adverse events. Once the narrow use was approved by the FDA and Pfizer had more definitive data on Lipitor-plus, Pfizer could have adjusted its inclusion and exclusion criteria before running a subsequent trial for general use.

> *Moral Dilemmas*
> 1. What are the merits of seeking a narrow use for new medical products until a sponsor has definitive clinical data on a product and then adjusting the inclusion and exclusion criteria before running a clinical trial for general use?

OBSERVATIONAL STUDIES

Can eating breakfast cereal determine the sex of a baby (Mathews et al., 2008)? A debate over this question shows why observational studies, which

are not experiments with control groups, should be considered with a grain of salt. In this instance, faculty research at Exeter and Oxford Universities found breakfast cereals eaten before conception were the most significant food linked with baby boys. Researchers asked 740 pregnant women to record what they ate just before their pregnancy; 56 percent of women who consumed the most calories before conception gave birth to boys, compared with 45 percent of those who consumed the least; of 132 individual foods tracked, breakfast cereal was the most significantly linked with baby boys (Beck, 2009).

Statisticians claim these findings were simply a false association that can occur by chance in a large set of data. In observational studies, it is impossible to prove that some other underlying factor is not causing what has been observed (Beck, 2009). For instance, some myths have been observed for generations: meat and other high-protein foods, as well as foods rich in potassium, vitamins, and salt, produce baby boys; for other families, it is beans, peas, and salty foods. While the best research appears to support practices in a variety of diverse anatomical positions for three to seven months, the gender results appear inconclusive and deserving of additional research. A bewildering number of hormones and growth factors are involved in sex determination differentiation beyond the traditional sex chromosomes, or karyotype (*see* Gilbert, 2006).

Regardless, following health news reporting observational studies is like watching a ping-pong match: reports linking lattes or alcohol with various illnesses one week often get contradicted the next. Such findings come from observational studies that are not as precise as randomized, controlled trials. Many experts think they should not be published at all until they have been confirmed with repeat studies (Beck, 2009).

Nature of Nontrivial Chance

Behind the cereal debate is the divide between statisticians and epidemiologists about the nature of nontrivial chance in observational studies where research investigators track participants' habits and look for associations with their health, but do not intervene at all. Statisticians say random associations are widespread in observational studies, which is why so many have contradictory findings. To prove the point, research investigators in Ontario studied the astrological signs of hospital patients and found that Sagittarians are susceptible to fractures and Pisces are prone to heart failure (Austin et al., 2006). The links met the traditional mathematical standard for statistical significance but were completely random, and disappeared when the study was repeated with a different sample (*see* Beck, 2009).

Validation

Some statisticians argue for validation, that a tougher standard of proof should be required when research investigators are fishing in large data sets. One method, a Bonferroni adjustment, requires dividing the usual mathematical formula by the number of variables; if one hundred foods are studied, the link must be one hundred times as strong as usual to be considered significant. Otherwise, statisticians say only strict clinical trials with a control group and a test group and one variable can truly prove a cause and effect association.

Epidemiologists argue that a Bonferroni adjustment throws out many legitimate findings, and that it is irrelevant how many other factors are studied simultaneously. They also note that controlled clinical trials are costly, time-consuming, and sometimes unethical. So does breakfast cereal affect a baby's gender? A good rule is to wait and see if an observation association appears when the study is repeated several times.

INTERNATIONAL CLINICAL TRIALS

Most clinical late-stage human trials are now done at sites outside the U.S., where results can be obtained cheaper and faster. Researchers at Duke University found that more than half the sites being used for trials sponsored by the largest pharmaceutical companies (Amgen, AstraZeneca, Bayer, Boehringer Ingelhelm, Bristol-Myers Squibb, Eli Lilly, GlaxoSmithKline, Johnson & Johnson, Merck, Novartis, Pfizer-Wyeth, and Roche) were international; the number of countries conducting trials has doubled over the past ten years (Glickman, 2009). Over the past three years, the percentage of trials conducted in low- and middle-income countries has increased from 40 percent to 55 percent (Schipper & Weyzig, 2008). This change has raised concerns about the treatment of participants and the integrity of the research data produced in today's clinical trials (Glickman, 2009).

Moral Dilemmas

1. Is enough being done to ensure the safety of participants in international clinical trials?

Fifty Percent Cost Savings

Late-stage clinical trials in lower-income countries cost less than half the cost in the U.S. and Europe because of lower salaries for physicians and clinical research personnel (Glickman, 2009). Moreover, patient recruitment is faster in countries such as India, China, and in Eastern Europe, where:

- Competition for patients is less intense
- Participants are far less likely to be taking other medicines, which is important for trials requiring "drug-naive" patients; drug-naive patients are sought because it is easier to show that experimental treatments are better than placebos, rather than trying to show an improvement over currently available drugs
- Patient populations are larger
- Patients are more willing to enroll in studies because of lack of alternative treatment options

(Hathaway et al., 2008)

Good Clinical Practices

In 2008, the FDA adopted standards used by many countries and organizations known as "good clinical practices" that:

- Encourage post-market medication access to be discussed during protocol design
- Mandate that studies be reviewed by international ethics committees
- Permit placebo-controlled trials only under certain circumstances
- Require informed consent from all participants

(Kipnis, et al. 2006)[LN1]

Good clinical practices are meant to assure quality clinical trials worldwide. The regulatory hurdles and administrative requirements in the U.S. are partly responsible for making going abroad so attractive. In the U.S., each site seeking to conduct a study must have its ethics board approve it. However, many studies these days are considered multisite, where one sponsor runs the same trial at different centers and pools the data. The U.S. review process means redundant effort and costs for multisite studies.

If a trial sponsor, research investigator, or monitor fails to follow the standards on how clinical trials should be conducted, approval of the investigational drug will be delayed or may never obtain FDA approval. Documentation of adherence to good clinical practices is part of every NDA.

Inconsistent Oversight and Informed Consent

Research suggests oversight and adequate informed consent for participants in clinical trials is inconsistent in developing countries (Glickman, 2009; OIG,

2007; Schipper & Weyzig, 2008). In one clinical trial, only half of the sites had been approved by ethics boards or health officials. In another clinical trial, less than one out five participants was informed about the study before being enrolled (Kent et al., 2004). While the medical products industry generally uses the same protocol regardless of where its clinical trials occur, international sites are not routinely monitored and not all research investigators have experience conducting clinical trials (OIG, 2007). Regulatory approval is not always sought in each nation in which clinical trials are conducted and participants do not always have access to the products or a suitable alternative after the trials end (Glickman, 2009).

INFORMED CONSENT IN GENERAL

At the beginning of the twentieth century, Justice Benjamin N. Cardozo, later an Associate Justice of the U.S. Supreme Court, stated that "Every human being of adult years and sound mind had a right to determine what shall be done with his own body." *Schloendorff v. Society of New York Hospital*, 105 N.E. 92 (Court of Appeals of New York 1914) (later abrogated on other grounds). The doctrine of informed consent has evolved from simply telling clinical trial participants how they were going to be treated, to disclosing alternatives and risks, to letting participants make the decision. Informed consent protects individual autonomy and the participant's status as a human being. It also helps:

- Avoid charges of fraud or duress against clinical trial sites
- Encourage research investigators to carefully consider their clinical decisions
- Foster rational decision-making by the participants
- Involve the public generally in medicine

Participants have the right to consent based on all of the information available. A physician must disclose all material risks and major acceptable alternatives. A material risk is one that would cause participants to change their minds about participation in a study or procedure. A risk that is too small to be material need not be disclosed. In other words, the physician should disclose what a reasonable participant would need to know in order to make an informed decision. Medical custom dictates that a physician should disclose what would be under the circumstances. Disclosure may include:

- Diagnosis
- Nature and purpose of the proposed treatment
- Risks of the treatment
- Legitimate treatment alternatives, including doing nothing

Federal regulations govern clinical research protocols, define human subjects that are covered, and define what information is required to obtain informed consent:

- Major legitimate and acceptable alternative courses of treatment
- Circumstances under which the study might be terminated
- Compensation
- Details of the research
- Foreseeable benefits to the subjects
- No penalty to withdraw
- Material risks of the treatment
- Voluntary participation

(45 C.F.R. Part 46 (2009))

Placebos

Placebos may be used in order to test the rate of success. IRBs must continually review the research and determine that the:

- Confidentiality is maintained
- Data collected is monitored
- Informed consent was obtained
- Risks are minimized and reasonable in relation to the anticipated benefits
- Selection of volunteer subjects is equitable

IRBs have the authority to suspend or terminate approval of research, and have the responsibility to satisfy federal requirements in order to use federal funds for research. Informed consent should be ongoing.

Declaration of Helsinki

The Declaration of Helsinki sets forth the international ethical principles for medical research involving human subjects. Research on human subjects who cannot give consent is only permissible if the condition that prevents consent from being given is what is being tested or researched. Other forms of consent may still be required, however, and placebos may not be used if there is a treatment available.

Battery Claims

Courts usually do not consider whether a patient comprehended the information disclosed during the risk discussion. If there was no consent given at all, participants may have a battery claim, which simply requires a showing that there was unconsented-to contact. Participants need not prove the contact caused injury and expert testimony is not required. There are few defenses against a battery claim.

Informed Consent Claims

If there was insufficient consent, participants may have an informed consent claim, which is pursued under a theory of negligence. It is very difficult to win a negligence-based informed consent case because it is almost impossible to show that participants would have chosen otherwise if fully informed of all the details and risks.

Consent forms are presumptively valid consent to the treatment, with the burden to rebut such consent being on the patient. The researcher is responsible to obtain informed consent for the record when the therapy is experimental. However, informed consent forms are not generally an important part in a patient's decision-making process because they are treated as a formality.

Emergency Research Rule

Something few Americans realize is that they may receive experimental drugs, devices, or surgical and procedural interventions in emergency situations. Clinical trial research may be conducted on unconscious people or shock patients experiencing life-threatening conditions, such as cardiac arrest, stroke, or traumatic injury, without obtaining informed consent.

In 2006, draft guidelines on exceptions from informed consent requirements were issued (FDA, 2006). Since then, there has been a substantial increase in the use of the Emergency Research Rule, with most of this increase related to studies supported by the National Institutes of Health. *See Federal Register,* 1996. Currently, NIH is funding emergency research studies, which consider consent waived after hospital IRBs sign off on each clinical trial, if:

- A physician and an IRB agree that a patient's life is in danger
- Proven treatments will not work
- Clinical research is necessary to determine what intervention is best
- Research could not be done otherwise

The procedural interventions must also be related to the emergency. Emergency situations are pre-defined in clinical trial protocols approved by hospital IRBs. For instance, unconscious trauma patients may be transfused with experimental artificial blood products; they will not, however, receive new artificial breast implants. Patients will not be transfused with experimental artificial blood products in non-emergency situations without their informed consent.

The studies seek to enroll more than thirty-six thousand non-consenting patients with life-threatening conditions, with an unspecified additional number of patients to be enrolled in studies currently in planning stages. With the increasing frequency of research studies entailing waived informed consent, it is important to understand this aspect of clinical trial research.

It is widely argued that the benefits and burdens of clinical trial research must be fairly distributed (FDA, 1979). One criticism is that NIH emergency research is occurring primarily in poor urban areas of the U.S. (Gillenwater, 2008). One such instance is the patient study involving over seven hundred trauma patients by Northfield Laboratories of Chicago (Burton, 2006). Thirty-one inner city hospitals in eighteen states participated in a clinical trial for the blood substitute PolyHeme. Half the patients got PolyHeme both in the ambulance and the hospital, while the other half got saline solution in the ambulance followed by donor blood in the hospital. The study was conducted under the Emergency Research Rule based on the belief that a blood substitute could potentially be a lifesaving therapy, especially for the military.[LN2] While participating hospitals received $10,000 for each patient that participated in the clinical trial, most patients never learned of their participation (Burton, 2006f). A concern raised by many ethicists with this clinical trial protocol was that the Emergency Research Rule requires that standard treatment (in this case, the use of donor blood) be unproven or unsatisfactory; giving donor blood to trauma patients was neither unproven nor unsatisfactory (Kipnis et al., 2006; *see generally* Burton, 2006a-f).

Moral Dilemmas

1. What standards should regulate clinical trials conducted on participants experiencing life-threatening conditions without informed consent?

Informed Consent and Participation of Children in Human Subject Research

Children in general are considered vulnerable research subjects (HHS, 2008). Federal regulations establish specific protections for clinical trials involving children and limit the level of risk permitted. IRBs can approve pediatric research only in three risk-benefit categories:

- Minimal risk (category 404)
- Greater than minimal risk but with a prospect of direct benefit (category 405)
- Minor increase over minimal risk without a prospect of direct benefit (category 406)

(45 C.F.R. §§ 46.404-407 (2001))

Research that exceeds these risk levels (category 407) can in some cases be approved by special review (*see* Varma & Wendler, 2008).

Approximately half of the children in the U.S. known to have HIV/AIDS are in foster care. New York City's Administration for Children's Services made the controversial decision to enroll foster children in HIV/AIDS clinical trials sponsored by NIH, beginning in the late 1980s and early 1990s. At least seven states (Illinois, Louisiana, Maryland, New York, North Carolina, Colorado, and Texas) followed New York City's lead and are involved in almost fifty different NIH clinical trials. North Carolina does not have policies of any kind regarding the enrollment of foster children in clinical trials. Thirteen additional states lack policies: Alaska, Georgia, Kansas, Minnesota, Missouri, Nevada, New Hampshire, New Jersey, North Dakota, Pennsylvania, South Carolina, West Virginia, and Wisconsin (HHS, 2008). The foster children range from infants to teenagers. The NIH trials were most widespread through the 1990s as foster care agencies sought treatments for HIV-infected children that were not yet available in the marketplace.

While the practice ensures that foster children, mostly poor, receive care from researchers at government expense, it also exposes a vulnerable population to the risks of experimental drugs that are known to have serious side effects in adults and for which the safety for children is completely unknown (FDA, 2007b). For foster children, access to health care without sufficient protections is, perhaps, worse than no access at all (Buske, 2007). For instance, the Vera Institute, an independent research organization commissioned by New York City to independently monitor this situation, finds continuing violations of clinical trial review, enrollment policies, and federal regulations for human subjects for foster children in the City:

- One in five foster children is enrolled in clinical trials without informed consent
- Foster children are enrolled in unapproved clinical trials
- Medical records are unavailable or incomplete for almost one-third of the children
- Foster children are being enrolled in Phase I clinical trials
- Foster children receive unapproved experimental drugs for HIV/AIDS

(Ross & Lifflander, 2009)

In addition, child advocates express concerns that not all foster children receiving HIV/AIDS drugs and vaccines in clinical trials have been properly diagnosed with the disease (Buske, 2007; Ross & Lifflander, 2009).

While foster children are covered by the same regulations as other children and while foster children should arguably have the same access to clinical trials as other children, current federal regulations are not always strictly enforced to adequately protect foster children in trials (APA, 2005). Foster children generally have no real advocate to protect their interests and ensure that regulations designed to protect children are enforced for them, especially when the government agencies charged with protecting the interests of foster children are seeking to enroll them in trials for free drugs or compensation is paid to the agency responsible for their care rather than the child research subjects.

Child advocates should be appointed for all foster children participating in pediatric clinical trials, and children should be afforded additional protections if they are wards of the state. For instance, additional regulations could require that significant compensation for participation in clinical trials be held in trust for foster children, a mandate that could be easily implemented through the regulations of individual child protection agencies. Furthermore, IRB oversight of pediatric clinical trials is particularly weak when government agencies seek enrollment of foster children; few IRBs have child welfare experts reviewing pediatric trials (HHS, 2008; Buske, 2007).

TRANSPARENCY AND FULL DISCLOSURE IN CLINICAL TESTING

A major shortcoming of the full disclosure requirement, also referred to as the § 801 requirement, is that the results of older clinical trials of drugs that were approved before the disclosure requirement became law in 2007 do not need to be made public, and such drugs constitute the vast majority of the drugs currently used by patients. *See* Food and Drug Administration Amendments Act of 2007, 21 U.S.C.A. § 350f, *et seq.* (2009). Likewise, there is no requirement for posting the results of trials of drugs that were never approved (Zarin & Tse, 2008; *see also* Wood, 2009).

FINANCIAL CONFLICTS OF INTEREST

It is tempting to think of the lack of transparency and full disclosure in clinical testing in terms of unethical people doing unethical things. The conflicts of interest problem is, however, more complex than that. The increase in financial conflicts of interest is likely a result of the change in federal policy that was designed to expedite the progress of research results from the laboratory to patients. This occurred primarily as a result of the Bayh-Dole Act, which transferred the property rights in the products of federally funded research to the research investigators and their institutions, thereby relieving the federal government of the task of patenting results.

Confidence in clinical trials has been undermined by the conflicts of interest on the part of the research investigators and the medical products industry. The concern mainly centers on financial conflicts of interest, particularly regarding the relationship between academic and industry interests. While research organizations are in the best position resource-wise to assess and manage conflicts of interest, they should also make use of independent, external methods of evaluating potential conflicts. Perhaps more important than instituting or reforming legal mechanisms of governing conflicts of interest is that the health industry cultivate an ethical research culture.

The Institute of Medicine suggests that the health care providers' IRBs review the ethics of clinical trials. While financial interests should not affect the scientific foundation of clinical trials, the potential for conflicts is expanding, both in terms of frequency and complexity, as the convergence of many health care sectors is rapidly changing the laws governing provider competition and regulation.

A process for analyzing such potential conflicts is critical to public confidence in the health industry. For example, during the 1970s, 80 percent of the public had confidence in the FDA; in 2000, 61 percent reported confidence in the FDA; by 2006, the percentage of the public having confidence in the FDA dropped to 36 percent (FDA, 2007). So, the issue is how the health industry and the FDA, as well as other regulatory agencies, should help restore public confidence in the nation's health care system.

Commitment to the Life Sciences

First and foremost, the health industry and the government must renew their commitment to science. The ability to reach this goal depends heavily upon strict adherence to scientifically motivated decision-making. Scientists should be insulated from financial and political pressures when making decisions about which medical treatments and products warrant approval to enter the marketplace and about which measures are appropriate when addressing unforeseen risks to patients. In short, financial and political decisions by the industry and government agencies should be separate from science.

Affirmative Support of the Life Sciences

In addition, an affirmative case for the merits of the life sciences must be made to the public. Too often, there has been leadership voids in the health industry and the government. Neither party consistently defends the life sciences in the court of public opinion. This reticence has contributed to an adverse effect on public health, and consequently has eroded public confidence in the health industry and the government. Industry and regulatory mishaps, especially highly publicized ones, occupy the public's attention but obscure the full story of the overall performance of the nation's health care system. For the most part, the health industry and the government do a remarkable job keeping the nation's medical treatments and products safe and effective. The American public should judge the nation's health care system on its excellent track record, but those many successes are often overshadowed by public outcry over isolated, but highly publicized failures.

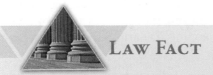

LAW FACT

CLINICAL TRIALS IN DEVELOPING NATIONS

Should the medical products industry be liable in U.S. courts for violation of good clinical practice standards in international clinical trials?

Yes, the prohibition in customary international law against nonconsensual human medical experimentation can be enforced through the Alien Tort Statute.[LN3]
    —*Abdullahi v. Pfizer, Inc.*, 562 F.3d 163 (U.S. Court of Appeals for the 2nd Circuit 2009), *petition for U.S. Supreme Court certiorari filed, 2009.*

CHAPTER SUMMARY

- The pharmaceutical and biopharmaceutical industries spend billions of dollars on clinical trials each year.
- Research and development of new medical products is complex, time-consuming, expensive, and risky.
- The stages of research and development include drug discovery, pre-clinical testing, clinical trials, FDA approval, and post-marketing surveillance; the clinical trial stage alone involves three phases.
- Even the most thorough clinical trial cannot detect all negatives, such as rare risks, risks that take an exceedingly long time to manifest, risks that only affect vulnerable sub-populations, and risks for patients who take other drugs and supplements.
- In contrast to the requirements for new medical products to obtain FDA approval, the standards for generic versions are much lower, reflecting Congress's decision to prioritize financial advantages over therapeutic advantages.
- There is ongoing debate over how much influence patients' preferences should have in drug approval; some patients, especially the terminally ill, are willing to accept a much higher risk than others.
- Clinical trials may be halted if a new drug shows such promise that it would be unethical to delay its release or if the new drug presents risks not outweighing the potential benefits.
- Before a clinical trial begins, a numerical threshold for bad outcomes is determined that, if crossed, will halt the trial; although the threshold may seem arbitrarily low in some cases, the statistic it represents is significant because it represents whether the bad outcomes are simply an anomaly or whether they represent a real risk to participants.
- Clinical trial research may be conducted without obtaining informed consent on people who are experiencing a life-threatening condition.
- An ongoing controversy in clinical trials involves research conducted outside the boundaries of the U.S.; the integrity of the research is called into question because it is more difficult to regulate, good clinical practices may not be observed, and informed consent may not be obtained.
- Observational studies and results that have not been validated may not be as reliable as other studies.
- Many argue that the results of all clinical trials, including older clinical trials and unsuccessful clinical trials, should be fully disclosed.
- Informed consent allows participants to protect their autonomy and make an informed decision as to whether or not to participate in the research based upon its predicted nature, purpose, risks, benefits, and alternatives, including doing nothing; obtaining informed consent from children, and particularly foster children, is replete with problems.
- Conflicts of interest, especially financial, call the integrity of clinical trials into question, and do not necessarily result from intentional unethical conduct.

LAW NOTES

1. ICH is the *International Conference on Harmonisation of Technical Requirements for Registration of Pharmaceuticals for Human Use*, a joint initiative involving both regulators and research-based industry representatives of the European Union, Japan, and the U.S. in scientific and technical discussions of the clinical testing procedures required to assess and ensure the safety, quality, and efficacy of drugs. The ICH Observers are the European Free Trade Association (represented by Swissmedic (Swiss Agency for Therapeutic Products)), Health Canada, and the World Health Organization.

2. Scientists have been searching for a blood substitute for more than half a century. Unlike donated human blood, artificial blood may reduce the risk of hepatitis or HIV infection. It also eliminates the need to match blood types of donor and recipient, and has a longer shelf life without refrigeration. One use for artificial blood is in the military. Blood needs to be refrigerated and usually cannot be carried into combat. It goes bad after more than a month, whereas PolyHeme lasts a year or more. Soldiers who would otherwise bleed to death on the battlefield might be saved if they could quickly be infused with an oxygen-carrying blood substitute. *See* Burton 2006.

3. The military dictatorship that was in power during the Trovan clinical trial at the start of this chapter was subsequently replaced by a democratically elected civilian government. In 2006, the *Washington Post* ran an exposé about Pfizer's clinical trial that prompted Abdullahi's lawsuit and a Nigerian government investigation into what happened to children at the clinic in Kano, Nigeria (Stephens, 2006). A government report,

authored in 2001, had concluded that Pfizer conducted an illegal drug trial that exploited those who did not clearly know that their children were participating in a clinical trial and that the government never gave authorization for this trial. However, for unidentified reasons, the Nigerian government suppressed this report for over five years. One of the authors of the report allegedly received death threats in connection with producing the document. It was only through an anonymous leak to the *Washington Post* that this report became public five years later in 2006. As a result of the leaked report, Nigeria filed criminal charges against Pfizer and sought almost $7 billion in a separate civil lawsuit for the children injured in Pfizer's clinical trial (Khan, 2008). In March 2009, Pfizer settled the multibillion-dollar damages case with two hundred alleged victims in Kano, Nigeria (*see* Bray & Wang, 2009).

Chapter Bibliography

Adis R&D Insight Development Database (2009, February). Bridgewater, NJ: Wolters Kluwer Pharma Solutions.

APA (American Academy of Pediatrics) Task Force on Health Care for Children in Foster Care. (2005). Fostering health: Health care for children and adolescents in foster care. New York, NY: APA District II.

Austin, P. C. et al. (2006). Testing multiple statistical hypotheses resulted in spurious associations: A study of astrological signs and health. *Journal of Clinical Epidemiology, 59*, 964-969.

Barth, A. S. (2007). Clinical research: Pharmaceutical manufacturer sponsoring terminated clinical trial not obligated to continue providing drug to volunteers. *American Journal of Law & Medicine, 32*, 405-408.

Beck, M. (2009, January 27). Does bran make the man? What statistics really tell us. *Wall Street Journal*, p. D1.

Berndt, E. et al. (2007). Authorized generic drugs, price competition and consumers' welfare. *Health Affairs, 26* (3), 790-799.

Biliak, C. (2006, December 6). Relatively small number of deaths have big impact in Pfizer drug trial. *Wall Street Journal*, p. D1.

Bray, C., & Wang, S. S. (2009, January 30). Court revives cases against Pfizer. *Wall Street Journal*, p. B1.

Burton, T. M. (2006, July 11). FDA to weigh test of blood substitute out of public view. *Wall Street Journal*, p. D3.

___. (2006a, July 6). FDA to weigh using fake blood in trauma trial. *Wall Street Journal*, p. B1.

___. (2006b, March 20). Use of substitution for blood draws ethics challenge. *Wall Street Journal*, p. A2.

___. (2006c, March 17). SEC begins probe of Northfield Labs over blood studies. *Wall Street Journal*, p. A2.

___. (2006d, March 14). Grassley accuses FDA of laxity in study of blood substitute. *Wall Street Journal*, p. D5.

___. (2006e, March 10), Blood-substitute study is criticized by U.S. agency. *Wall Street Journal*, p. A3.

___. (2006f, February 22). Red flags: Amid alarm bells, a blood substitute keeps pumping: Ten in trial have heart attacks, but data aren't published; FDA allows a new study; Doctors' pleas are ignored. *Wall Street Journal*, p. A1.

Buske, S. L. (2007). Foster children and pediatric clinical trials: Access without protection is not enough. *Virginia Journal of Social Policy & Law, 14*, 253-307.

Cerino, J. R. (2008). The statutory limits of compassion: Can treatment INDs provide meaningful access to investigational drugs for the terminally ill? *Temple Journal of Science, Technology & Environmental Law, 27*, 79-95.

Chang, N., chairman and managing director, Asia Orbmed. (2009). Wharton Health Care Business Conference: Catalyzing: Pharma-biotech panel: The blurring line between pharma and biotech. Philadelphia, PA.

Danzon, P. M. et al. (2005). Productivity in pharmaceutical-biotechnology R&D: The role of experience and alliances. *Journal of Health Economics, 24*, 317-339.

Dickson, M., & Gagnon, J. R. (2004). Key factors in the rising cost of new drug discovery and development. *Nature Reviews: Drug Discovery, 3*, 417-429.

FDA (U.S. Food & Drug Administration). (2008). *FY 2009 budget in brief*. Bethesda, MD: FDA.

___. (2007). *FDA science and mission at risk*. Science Board Report of the Subcommittee on Science & Technology. Bethesda, MD: FDA (extensive report of blue ribbon panel commissioned by the FDA that concludes that the FDA is in a precarious position: the agency suffers from scientific deficiencies and is not positioned to meet current or emerging regulatory responsibilities).

___. (2007a). *New drug application (NDA) process*. Center for Drug Evaluation & Research. Bethesda, MD: FDA.

___. (2007b). *The future of drug safety: promoting and protecting the health of the public: FDA's response to the Institute of Medicine's 2006 report*. Bethesda, MD: FDA.

___. (2006). *Draft guidance for institutional review boards, clinical research investigators, and sponsors: Exception from informed consent requirements for emergency research*. Good Clinical Practice Program, Center for Devices & Radiological Health, Center for Biologics Evaluation & Research, Center for Drug Evaluation & Research, Center for Devices & Radiological Health, Office of Regulatory Affairs, FDA. Bethesda, MD: FDA.

___. (1979). *Belmont report: Ethical principles and guidelines for the protection of human subjects of research*. Bethesda, MD: FDA.

Federal Register. (1996, October 2). Informed consent and waiver of informed consent requirements in certain emergency research, 61 F.R. 51,498-01, 51,528 (codified at 21 C.F.R. § 50.24 (2001)).

Gilbert, S. F. (2006). *Developmental biology* (8th ed.). Sunderland, MA: Sinauer Associates Inc. (explaining chromosomal sex, sperm-egg attraction and binding by presence or absence of the testis determining factor, and the effects of maternal nutrition on gene expression).

Gillenwater, G. E. (2008). Analyzing the laws, regulations, and policies affecting FDA-regulated products: FDA's emergency research rule: An inch given, a yard taken. *Food & Drug Law Journal, 63*, 217-254.

Glickman, S. W. (2009). Ethical and scientific implications of the globalization of clinical research. *New England Journal of Medicine, 360* (8), 816-823.

Gorsky, A., chief executive officer, Novartis Pharmaceuticals. (2005, September 14). New Jersey Wharton Club Executive Forum Series. Novartis Pharmaceuticals, East Hanover, NJ.

Gotec, J. V., & DiMasi, J. (2008). Drug development costs when financial risk is measured using the Fama-French Three Factor Model. Unpublished working paper. Philadelphia, PA: Wharton School at the University of Pennsylvania.

Harper, R. M. (2008). A matter of life and death: Affording terminally-ill patients access to post-phase I investigational new drugs. *Michigan State Journal of Medicine & Law, 12,* 265-295.

Hathaway, C. R. et al. (2008). Looking abroad: Clinical drug trials. *Food & Drug Law Journal, 63,* 673-682.

HHS (U.S. Department of Health & Human Services). (2008). *Survey of states on the participation of foster children in clinical drug trials.* Washington, DC: HHS.

Jaquette, I. (2007). *Merck KGaA v. Integra Lifesciences I, Ltd:* Implications of the Supreme Court's decision for the people who matter most . . . the consumer. *American Journal of Law & Medicine, 33,* 97-117.

Kent, D. M. et al. (2004). Clinical trials in Sub-Saharan Africa and established standards of care: A systematic review of HIV, tuberculosis, and malaria trials. *Journal of the American Medical Association, 292* (2), 237-242.

Kesselheim, A. S., & Mello, M. M. (2007). Confidentiality laws and secrecy in medical research: Improving public access to data on drug safety. *Health Affairs, 26,* 483-491.

Kessler, D. A., & Vladeck, D. C. (2008). Health regulation and governance: A critical examination of the FDA's efforts to preempt failure-to-warn claims. *Georgetown Law Journal, 96,* 461-495.

Khan, F. (2008). The human factor: Globalizing ethical standards in drug trials through market exclusion. *DePaul Law Review, 57,* 877-915.

Kipnis, K. et al. (2006). Trials and errors: Barriers to oversight of research conducted under the emergency research consent waiver. *IRB, 28* (2), 16-20.

Lee, W. B. et al. (2008). *Abigail Alliance v. von Eschenbach:* Constitutional rights of terminally ill patients reconsidered. *Journal of Law, Medicine & Ethics, 36,* 191-193.

Leonard, E. W. (2009). Right to experimental treatment: FDA new drug approval, constitutional rights, and the public's health. *Journal of Law, Medicine & Ethics, 37,* 269-275.

Madara, M. R. (2009). Sacrificing the good of the few for the good of the many: Denying the terminally ill access to experimental medication. *Western New England Law Review, 31,* 535-580.

Marcee, A. K. (2008). Expanded access to phase II clinical trials in oncology: A step toward increasing scientific validity and compassion. *Food & Drug Law Journal, 63,* 439-457.

Mathews, F. et al. (2008). You are what your mother eats: Evidence for maternal preconception diet influencing foetal sex in humans. *Proceedings of the Royal Society of Biological Sciences, 275* (1643), 1661-1668.

NIH (National Institutes of Health). (2007). *Understanding clinical trials.* Washington, DC: NIH.

NLM (National Library of Medicine). (2008). *Clinical research FAQ.* Washington, DC: NLM.

OIG (Office of Inspector General). (2007). *The Food and Drug Administration's oversight of clinical trials.* Washington, DC: U.S. Department of Health & Human Services, OIG (recommending improvements to FDA research monitoring).

O'Reilly, J. T. (2008). Losing deference in the FDA's second century: Judicial review, politics, and a diminished legacy of expertise. *Cornell Law Review, 93,* 939-979 (describing the historical reputation of the Agency).

Pedersen, S. L. (2008). When Congress practices medicine: How congressional legislation of medical judgment may infringe a fundamental right. *Touro Law Review, 24,* 791-848.

PhRMA (Pharmaceutical Research & Manufacturing Association). (2008). *Biotechnology drugs in development: Biotechnology research continues to bolster arsenal against disease with 633 drugs in development.* Washington, DC: PhRMA.

Plionis, N. J. (2008). The right to access experimental drugs: Why the FDA should not deprive the terminally ill of a chance to live. *William & Mary Bill of Rights Journal, 16,* 901-933.

Ross, T., & Lifflander, A. (2009). *The experiences of New York City foster children in HIV/AIDS clinical trials.* New York, NY: Vera Institute.

Rossen, B. R. (2009). FDA's proposed regulations to expand access to investigational drugs for treatment use: The status quo in the guise of reform. *Food & Drug Law Journal, 64,* 183-223.

Saver, R. S. (2009). At the end of the clinical trial: Does access to investigational technology end as well? *Western New England Law Review, 31,* 411-451.

Schipper, I. & Weyzig, F. (2008). *Ethics for drugs testing in low and middle income countries.* Amsterdam, Netherlands: Centre for Research on Multinational Corporations.

Smith, W. T. (2008). FDA requires foreign clinical studies be in accordance with good clinical practices to better protect human subjects. *ABA Health eSource, 5* (2), 1-3.

Stephens, J. (2006, May 7). Panel faults Pfizer in '96 clinical trials in Nigeria. *Washington Post,* p. A1.

Talbott, M. K. (2007). Currents in contemporary ethics: The implications of expanding access to unapproved drugs. *Journal of Law, Medicine & Ethics, 35,* 316-318.

Tufts Center for the Study of Drug Development. (2006). *Average cost to develop a new biotechnology product is $1.2 billion, according to the Tufts Center for the Study of Drug Development.* Boston, MA: Tufts University.

Varma, S., & Wendler, D. (2008). Research involving wards of the state: Protecting particularly vulnerable children. *Journal of Pediatrics, 152* (1), 9-14.

Vladeck, D. C. (2008). The FDA and deference lost: A self-inflicted wound or the product of a wounded agency? A response to Professor O'Reilly. *Cornell Law Review, 93,* 981-1002.

Wang, S. S. (2009, February 19). Most clinical trials done abroad. *Wall Street Journal,* p. D3.

___. et al. (2008, December 1). Scrutiny grows of drug trials abroad. *Wall Street Journal,* p. B1.

Wharton (Wharton School at the University of Pennsylvania). (2007). A prescription for healthier medical care decisions: Begin by defining health risk. *Knowledge@Wharton.*

___. (2006). Novartis's Alex Gorsky: Ensuring that patients get access to the medicines they need. *Knowledge@Wharton.*

Winniford, A. (2009). Expanding access to investigational drugs for treatment use: A policy analysis and legislative proposal. *Health Matrix, 19*, 205-246.

Winter, J. D. (2008). Is it time to abandon FDA's no release from liability regulation for clinical studies? *Food & Drug Law Journal, 63*, 525-536.

WMA (World Medical Association). (2006). *Declaration of Helsinki: Ethical principles for medical research involving human subjects, as amended by the 48th World Medical Assembly, Somerset West, Republic of South Africa.* France: Ferney-Voltaire.

Wolf, S. M. et al. (2008). Incidental findings in human subjects research: From imaging to genomics: Managing incidental findings in human subjects research: Analysis and recommendations. *Journal of Law, Medicine & Ethics, 36*, 219-243,

Wolfe, S. et al. (2005). *Worst pills, best pills.* New York, NY: Simon & Schuster, Pocket.

Wood, A. J. (2009). Progress and deficiencies in the registration of clinical trials. *New England Journal of Medicine, 360* (8), 824.

Zain, S. (2007). Sword or shield? An overview and competitive analysis of the marketing of authorized generics. *Food & Drug Law Journal, 62*, 739-777.

Zarin, D., & Tse, T. (2008). Closing a loophole in the FDA Amendments Act. *Science, 322*, 44-46.

"*Tell me what kind of food you eat, and I will tell you what kind of person you are.*"

—JEAN ANTHELME BRILLAT-SAVARIN (1755-1826), FRENCH LAWYER
AND POLITICIAN WHO STUDIED THE RELATIONSHIP BETWEEN CULTURE
AND FOOD, FROM "THE PHYSIOLOGY OF TASTE" (1825)

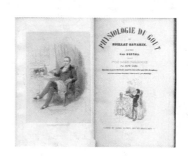

IN BRIEF

This chapter examines the debate between the food industry and public health advocates over junk food, advertising, and food safety in general. What this food fight means to already strained health care systems struggling to battle diabetes, high blood pressure, heart disease, and other weight- and diet-related illnesses is addressed. Also reviewed are federal legislation from the Personal Responsibility in Food Consumption Act that would protect the food industry from obesity lawsuits, similar so-called cheeseburger bills on the state level, and citizen groups like the Alliance for American Advertising that persuade legislators not to introduce bills that would restrict food advertising targeted to children.

FACT OR FICTION

FOOD LABELING

Should the producers and sellers of milk be required to warn consumers of the risks of sickness from lactose intolerance on their packaging?

A group of lactose-intolerant consumers purchased milk in Washington, D.C., and suffered the consequences of its consumption. Before they were aware of their lactose intolerance, they suffered temporary flatulence, bloating, cramps, and diarrhea as a result of drinking milk. They filed suit claiming the producers and sellers breached their duty of reasonable care; in other words, dairy processors and grocery store retailers that sold milk knew about lactose intolerance but failed to warn consumers about those effects. The lactose-intolerant individuals sought damages and a permanent injunction requiring the milk producers and sellers to include warnings on their packaging.

—*Mills v. Giant of Maryland*, 508 F.3d 11 (U.S. Court of Appeals for the District of Columbia Circuit 2007).

(See *Law Fact* at the end of this chapter for the answer.)

PRINCIPLES AND APPLICATIONS

Faced with a President saying the current food safety system is a "hazard to public health" and the possibility of civil as well as regulatory actions, members of the food industry are seeking to demonstrate that they are concerned about consumer health (Zhang, 2009). Consider just a few, some would say confusing, developments resulting from the political debate over junk food, advertising, and food safety:

- The Institute of Medicine points to the large-scale consumption of sugar-laden fruit juice by preschool children as the likely culprit in the recent rise in childhood obesity. U.S. dietary guidelines suggest parents give their children fresh fruit, water, or milk instead (IOM, 2007).
- When Kraft Foods (sister company of Philip Morris, the tobacco giant, now a veteran of class action lawsuits) was accused of misleading advertising about the fat content of its Oreo cookies from consumers who mistook them as health food, it tried to forestall a lawsuit by promoting its commitment to healthy foods and announced it was taking steps to reduce obesity by reducing the portion sizes of some products and introducing various healthier products with reduced fat content (Kraft Foods, 2005). Kraft then eliminated its extensive in-school marketing programs and banned its popular Weinermobiles from schoolyards. While some claim this was all designed to ward off government regulation after its "snack attack," Kraft's moves were made in part to reduce the risk of legal action, although dismissed as

frivolous. Even as fat is reduced in Dairylea and Angel Delight, Kraft fears food could be the new tobacco. Kraft knows that by producing nutritionally good foods and marketing them in a responsible way, there is no real case against the company.

- After pressure from consumer groups, Kellogg decided to phase out food advertising aimed at children under twelve. Not to be outdone, Kraft agreed to stop advertising Oreos, Chips Ahoy cookies, Kool-Aid, and other non-nutritional snack foods on television to children under twelve (AHG, 2006; Zhang, 2005).
- General Mills replaced refined grains with whole grains in many of its cereals. Then, it launched a new Berry Lucky Charms brand with brightly colored marbits, the artificially flavored marshmallows laden with sugar and corn syrup.
- Soft drink companies voluntarily pulled sugary sodas and other high-calorie drinks out of schools when research showed that American children on average were drinking three twelve-ounce cans per day. Pepsi said it would eliminate trans-fats from Doritos, Tostitos, and Cheetos, and promised to broaden its portfolio of reduced-fat and low-calorie products (AHG, 2006a).
- Ever since Nestle was attacked for promoting powdered milk to mothers in emerging economies, it is more sensitive than ever and invests heavily to make sure that its foods avoid controversy. Pick up a Nestle Crunch or a Baby Ruth and see that Nestle puts health warnings on most of its chocolate bars to remind consumers of the importance of exercise.

- Cadbury Schweppes began emphasizing its move into natural products after analysts at JPMorgan predicted the company faced the highest risk of being sued because of the predominance of unhealthy products in its portfolio (Wharton, 2005).
- When the *Super Size Me* documentary exposed the health risks of eating a McDonald's-only diet (Gilbert, 2004), the company advised French consumers to eat in its restaurants only once per week. Meanwhile, McDonald's now buys about fifty-four million pounds of fresh apples per year, up from zero several years ago, making the company the largest global wholesale purchaser of apples. Apples now show up on the McDonald's menu in salads and desserts, alongside the double quarter-pounders with cheese, chicken selects premium breast strips with sauce, deluxe McGriddles breakfasts, large French fries, and chocolate triple-thick shakes.

(*See generally* Wharton, 2005)

Research food safety, and it is likely the only common point of agreement is that the problem is critical (Wharton, 2005). Consumer health is a problem that has long occupied the brightest minds in the food industry. Every company involved in food is looking at its complete product portfolio and looking to develop lower-calorie, lower-fat, and more natural products. By using different ingredients and careful marketing, the food industry likely hopes a legal time bomb of consumer litigation can be diffused.

State governments have successfully sued the tobacco industry for billions in health care costs. Food companies may be next as a result of the fat, sugar, and cholesterol content in many of their products (Roller et al., 2006). Many consumers are trying to find a scapegoat, even though the increasingly sedentary lifestyle of many Americans has contributed to the increasing level of weight-related chronic illnesses (Frazier, 2007). If exposés of the fast food and meatpacking sectors, like turn-of-the-twentieth-century *Fast Food Nation* (Schlosser, 2001) and turn-of-the-nineteenth-century *The Jungle* (Sinclair, 1906), continue to remain bestsellers, the food industry may have to become more accountable and go further than it has already gone in addressing food safety and nutrition (Ausness, 2005).

DISTINCTION OR SIMILARITY BETWEEN THE FOOD AND TOBACCO INDUSTRIES

A major difference between tobacco- and food-related litigation is in the products themselves. Cigarettes are extremely hazardous to health. The only way to completely eliminate the hazard is to eliminate the commodity. With food, the obesity-promoting characteristics involve not just product content but marketing, packaging, labeling, consumers' lifestyles, and genetics. Foods are not harmful when used in moderation, whereas cigarettes are. Moreover, while it may be possible to prove that smoking caused a particular lung cancer, and even to identify the company that sold it, it may be difficult to determine how much of a role obesity played in a heart attack death, and impossible to specify the responsibility of the sources of high-fat and high-calorie foods. Most important, the actions of the tobacco industry have no counterpart with the food industry. While food advertising usually does not stress the dangers of overeating, tobacco companies went far beyond a mere failure to disclose by deliberately lying and actively concealing evidence (McMenamin & Tiglio, 2006).

Under the federal Nutrition Labeling and Education Act (NLEA) some foods are exempt from nutrition labeling. *See* Nutrition Labeling and Education Act (NLEA) of 1990, 21 U.S.C.A. § 343-1 (2006). These include:

- Food served for immediate consumption, such as that served in cafeterias and that sold by food service vendors
- Ready-to-eat food not for immediate consumption but prepared primarily on site (bakery)
- Food shipped in bulk, as long as it is not for sale in bulk form to consumers
- Medical foods, such as those used to address the nutritional needs of patients with certain diseases
- Plain coffee and tea and some spices
- Foods containing no significant amounts of any nutrients or dietary supplements in the product (insignificant nutrients, calories, cholesterol, or fiber)

HEALTHY VERSUS UNHEALTHY FOODS

Food safety is routinely described as a global problem affecting children and adults, not only in the U.S. and Western Europe, but also in emerging economies (Filippi, 2005). Public health officials warn of a coming health crisis in already struggling health care systems soon to be hit by even more patients with diabetes, high blood pressure, heart disease, and other chronic illnesses directly attributable to obesity and weight-related conditions (Wharton, 2005). Statistics from the National Health and Nutrition Examination Survey, a nationally representative sample of the U.S. population, are disturbing. Almost 40 percent of America's preschoolers are overweight or are at risk of being overweight (Nelson et al., 2006). Obesity rates for elementary school students have tripled since the 1980s and Type 2 diabetes has become so common in children that it is no longer called adult-onset diabetes. In addition, about one-third of American adults are considered obese, meaning they are at least thirty pounds overweight (Ogden et al., 2006). Obesity and related illnesses are now costing America $97 billion a year and causing 300,000 premature deaths; obesity may soon be responsible for as many deaths as cigarette smoking (Surgeon General, 2001).

America's sudden explosion of chronic illnesses due to obesity and weight-related conditions cannot be attributed simply to genetics. Further, there is no evidence American consumers have suddenly become less responsible about their health over the past fifteen years. Rather, what has changed is that Americans are now eating one-third of their calories outside the home; nowadays, high-calorie fast food and chain restaurant meals are consumed at a higher level than ever before (Frank, 2006). Today, only about 5 percent of the meals eaten inside the home consist of fresh food (Kysar, 2004). At the same time, Americans are eating more than half of their daily dietary intake from highly processed, prepackaged, and prepared meals high in carbohydrates and sodium (Merrill & Francer, 2000). The U.S. Department of Agriculture finds that frozen prepared meals have been one of the fastest growing categories of food in American supermarkets every year over the past decade.

The question is whether this change in consumer eating is contributing to weight-related chronic illnesses (Frank, 2006). One research organization, the National Bureau of Economic Research, says 65 percent of America's obesity is due to fast foods and ready-prepared meals (Chou et al., 2005). If this is so, who exactly is responsible for this nutritional state of affairs?

- The fast food sector, with its high-calorie menus and advertising that seems to be everywhere at once?
- Parents, who relinquish their responsibilities to provide healthy, nutritional meals and promote exercise?
- Schools that fail to offer healthy eating alternatives in cafeterias and vending machines?
- Cereal and juice manufacturers that add sugar to their products?
- Government agencies that publish dietary guidelines but take no regulatory action to limit junk food advertising targeted at children (*see* 7 U.S.C.A. §§ 5301, *et seq.* (2009); the *Dietary Guidelines for Americans* are a joint effort of the U.S. Department of Health and Human Services (HHS) and the U.S. Department of Agriculture (USDA))?
- Powerful lobbies that have kept the federal sugar subsidy program in place since the Great Depression in the 1920s?

- Overweight and obese individuals who keep spooning the food into their bodies, one bite at a time?
- All of the above?

These are very challenging public health concerns, with weight-related illnesses very much an issue for the U.S. health care system in particular.

Moral Dilemmas

1. How should the U.S. food industry that manufactures, sells, and advertises high-calorie foods respond to food safety and nutrition concerns?

2. Should the marketing strategies for food products continue to be self-regulated?

3. Should the food industry be obligated to promote healthier products, and reduce or eliminate less healthy foods and beverages, regardless of consumer demand?

4. Who is responsible for what American children and adults eat?

5. Are overweight and obesity conditions an individual and family responsibility, or do government and public health agencies have a role?

For example, the American Sugar Alliance is a trade association that represents domestic producers, processors, and refiners of sugar. It has ensured that the sugar industry has long been one of the most protected sectors in American agriculture. Government support to some of the wealthiest Americans includes special loans to producers and a program designed to prop up prices by controlling the amount of sugar put on the market through import limits and production allotments granted to farmers with gross incomes up to $2.5 million (Hitt, 2008).

In some ways, the food industry is faced with a choice between two adverse and contrary alternatives toward nutrition. Consumers say they want healthier foods, but if you look at consumer behavior, many consumers choose unhealthy foods over healthy ones. Indeed, fast food and restaurant chains that have tried to reduce the size of their meal portions and reduce prices have been criticized and often reinstate their original serving sizes and return to their original pricing in response to consumer demand (Wharton, 2005). When restaurant chain Ruby Tuesday tried to reduce the size of its portions, consumers soundly criticized the move and the company quickly reinstated original serving sizes (Wharton, 2007). At the same time, consumers say they want healthy options that are just as fast and cheap as the unhealthy ones. How does the food industry navigate its way through this nutritional maze? The food industry in general wants to offer healthier alternatives, in part because of all the dire warnings about the relationship between food safety and health; it simply does not have many other choices.

The food industry maintains it is always looking to lower fat levels and sugar levels, but it is not always possible to get ingredients to the recommended levels. It is impossible to make chocolate without more than 30 percent of the calories coming from fat, which is the recommended dietary amount. It would not be chocolate anymore! It is possible that altering the composition of chocolate could lead to litigation to restore it, given its immense, unwavering popularity.

In response to attacks on chocolate, and over the years, some chocolate manufacturers and sellers have responded by putting health warnings on their chocolate bars to remind consumers of the need to exercise or to include chocolate as part of a balanced diet. Nevertheless, more is required of the food industry than quick-fix changes to its packaging and labeling.

> *Moral Dilemmas*
> 1. Should advice about food safety and protection from unhealthy foods by the food industry or government ever give way to individual choice and personal responsibility?

FRAGMENTED REGULATORY SYSTEM

Food safety in the U.S. is fragmented; some health care advocates even characterize the regulatory fragmentation as broken. More than a dozen expert panels inside and outside the government have called for the consolidation of the federal agencies that exercise and share food safety responsibility (Merrill & Francer, 2000). Apart from the U.S. Food and Drug Administration (FDA) and the U.S. Department of Agriculture, about ten more federal agencies have some food safety responsibility under some thirty-five federal statutes. This federal oversight is in addition to the fifty separate state agricultural agencies and fifty intersecting state environmental protection agencies, with all their overlapping state statutes and related agencies. Some agencies and statutes have similar regulations, others are contradictory, but all have the common mandate of food security and consumer protection.

FOOD MARKETING AND ADVERTISING

The decision by Kraft and Kellogg's to stop advertising to children has caused concern within the food industry (Wharton, 2005). When advertising to children is stopped in response to demands from public health advocates, it implies an acknowledgment that there is something wrong with that advertising (Kunkel et al., 2004). Does this suggest culpability, or did Kraft and Kellogg's act responsibly?

It is not easy to change food products or to predict what the effect of such changes will be. There is always the risk of altering a product and then losing customers because of the change. Coke faced this peril when it attempted to introduce a new Coca-Cola and was forced to return to the original formula in less than three months in the mid-1980s. The "New Coke" with high-fructose corn syrup was withdrawn and the sugar-sweetened "Coca Cola Classic" returned to shelves post-haste following a public outcry for the original product (Hays, 2004).

The food industry has changed the word "super-size" because the meaning has changed in popular culture from denoting something positive to denoting something negative (Wharton, 2005). When McDonald's dropped the word, it substituted the words "deluxe" and "premium" in its menu; the marketing association, however, remained the same: excessive and extremely large. One could ask whether this word choice is designed to move product or whether it has different meanings.

Beyond marketing, there is a distinction between giving consumers what they want and saying, in essence, "We know what you want, but we know it is not healthy, and we are not willing to offer it" (Making, 2005). There may be a joint responsibility between the food industry and consumers. If so, this makes it harder to determine what should be done. It is always much easier for the food industry to go through a systematic, rigorous process of segmentation, targeting, and positioning, a long-standing approach to marketing, than it is to really know what consumers want and why they want it. If the food industry simply makes projections based on what it thinks is healthy based on its own experience and intuition, it may deliver one type of food product. However, simply because the food industry thinks one type of food is not healthy does not mean everybody else will think it is unhealthy. The industry's assumption may not be true.

When healthy food becomes a tough sell, it is because consumers have obvious objections to it. The goal of marketing, therefore, is to frame an offer to do away with the objection. For example, it may be as simple as consumers wanting healthy food that is as fast, cheap, and readily available as traditional fast food.

The food industry goes after consumer value, which includes offering products consumers are willing to pay for. The industry is not making consumers eat unhealthy foods (Wharton, 2005). The industry argues it is just delivering foods consumers want. The counterargument to this contention is that consumers never knew they wanted Ben & Jerry's ice cream or McDonald's French fries until they existed and everyone found out about them. Consumers are always ready to indulge themselves when marketers are able to get their message through. Food products are not about what is needed, but about wants and desires.

In the case of McDonald's, some customers would be more satisfied with the menu offerings if they did not cause weight gain. So McDonald's keeps some fast food customers by offering healthier choices like the Fruit 'n Yogurt Parfait and salads. Still, there are other customers who do not care if they gain weight, at least some of the time, and some marketers aim to appeal to that segment. Marketing, as the term itself implies, responds to the free market to increase responses from its intended audiences.

FUNCTIONAL FOODS

The marketing spin in the food industry hides a deeper concern about increasing levels of fat. The food industry is remarketing its products in light of health fears. The issue of healthy food is at the top of the food industry's agendas. The food industry realizes it takes more than simply tinkering around with products; a completely new way of thinking is needed.

Strategy has changed in the food industry; by offering more fruits and salads, business is increasing. Functional foods, or foods that provide health benefits beyond basic nutrition, are being marketed by drug and consumer goods companies. Grocery aisles are stacked with rows of whole-grain breakfast cereals, enhanced salad dressings, and fortified snacks and drinks that promise to fight heart disease, osteoporosis, and other ailments. In some cases, products with dietary supplements are billed as alternatives to medicine. Consumers like these healthy options. Moreover, by having options, the food industry avoids dictating to consumers (Smith, 2006).

FOOD LABELING LAWS

This raises the question of whether consumers have enough information about the foods they choose to eat. While federal legislation requires easy-to-read Nutrition Facts labels on almost all packaged foods,

the U.S. FDA drug labeling rules focus solely on format (Mathews, 2006). *See* Nutrition Labeling and Education Act of 1990, 21 U.S.C.A. § 343-1 (2006). There is an ongoing policy debate as to whether consumers have the right information to decide what to eat at fast food restaurants like McDonald's or what to drink at Starbucks.

The good news is that Dasani Water is now on McDonald's menu with no calories, and Starbucks offers skim milk in its lattes and asks whether whipped cream should be added. One fact is certain: many consumers do not know how much to eat. They do not eat to satisfy hunger. Most adults do not stop eating when they are no longer hungry. The same is not true for children. When children are not hungry, they will not eat. They will stop in the middle of a bite. Somehow, adults have "unlearned" this skill (Wharton, 2005). What adults eat is largely dictated by environmental cues, not internal cues. The notion is that it is not hunger driving how much adults eat; it is perceptual cues, like portion amounts, plate size, or the sense of variety (Wharton, 2007). Adults do not always eat for fullness. They often unconsciously eat for these other rules. Weight Watchers has developed a business model that encourages its clients to stop eating when they are satisfied rather than full, but this alone does not help the fact that overweight and obese people often ignore satiety signals anyway, giving in instead to emotional triggers or social pressures to eat. Therefore, Weight Watchers also attempts to teach its clients to handle the psychological and environmental contributors to weight problems.

Moreover, many adults are not aware of how many calories they consume (Wharton, 2005). Researchers note that when it comes to a plethora of food choices, the problem is not simply that consumers make bad choices. The sheer amount of available choices actually drives individuals to eat more. Other research shows that simply labeling a food as healthy makes the item unappealing. Just the mind-set that something is going to be healthy turns off consumers. Consumers taste what they think; they believe if it is healthy, it is not going to be as good. To complicate matters even more, consumers who think they are eating healthy actually tend to reward themselves with more food (Wharton, 2007). This concept is called "calorie compensation and reward" in restaurant studies (Wansink, 2007).

As consumers become more cognizant of how much they are eating, and realize they could be satisfied with less, there may be a "downsizing of the supersizing." The move toward downsizing or changing eating habits in the U.S. in general suggests Americans may be willing to assume personal responsibility for their actions. This is another predominant issue in the food safety debate (Wharton, 2005).

The restaurant chain T.G.I. Friday's offers a "right portion, right price" menu with smaller portions at lower prices for select dishes. This seemingly consumer-health driven effort, however, has a headline over the downsized entrees on its Web site that promises, "Smaller Portions Allow More Room for Dessert," a higher-profit-margin item. This may be T.G.I. Friday's application of the "calorie compensation and reward" concept. This concept might explain why there has been a sharp rise in sales of low-fat foods as obesity levels have soared.

Ideally, consumers should be responsible for making their own life decisions. What the food industry tries to do is provide choices so that consumers can make the right decisions based on their own needs, including price, portability, and convenience. If consumers do not buy the choices offered, then these items are pulled from the marketplace (Wharton, 2005). For instance, there are veggie burgers in some markets, but they do not sell as well as other meat burger products.

Almost every decision the food industry makes is based on what consumers indicate they want to eat. In the early nineties, McDonald's had the McLean deluxe burger, but it did not stay on the menu for long. Salads have been on McDonald's menu since 1984. McDonald's even tried a salad shaker in a drink cup that could be eaten on the run, but the product failed. Milk was sold for years, but when low-fat milk was put in a Ronald McDonald re-useable plastic container, sales increased dramatically. Wendy's offers chili, a baked potato, a side salad, or a Caesar side salad with its classic sandwiches, which have become popular menu options instead of French fries. Despite the consequences, research shows that when consumers go to a fast food restaurant, they want to splurge.

McLawsuits and Cheeseburger Legislation

Others in the food fight, however, contend that personal responsibility only goes so far. Two teenagers filed a lawsuit in 2002 blaming McDonald's food and advertising for causing obesity. After being tossed out twice, the case was reinstated on a technicality. Although many consider the lawsuit frivolous, it raises the specter of additional suits against other fast food chains on similar grounds (Wharton, 2005). Public health advocates maintain most restaurant chain food is misleadingly advertised as healthy; the chains say the advocates' view is based on incomplete information and outdated material (Richardson, 2005).

LIABILITY FOR WEIGHT-RELATED ILLNESSES

Pelman v. McDonald's Corp.

[Minor Consumer v. Fast Food Chain]

237 F.Supp.2d 512 (U.S. District Court for the Southern District of New York 2003)

FACTS: Two New York City teenagers sought to hold McDonald's liable for their obesity and obesity-related illnesses. McDonald's advertises its food as nutritious and part of a healthy lifestyle, while failing to warn its consumers of the health-related risks and adverse health effects associated with consumption of foods high in cholesterol, fat, salt, sugar, and other additives. They claimed McDonald's persuaded its consumers to ingest unhealthy quantities of fattening, highly processed food substantially less healthy than represented in advertisements. In addition, McDonald's represents it provides nutritional information in all of its stores, when in fact such beneficial information is often not available. The teenagers claimed McDonald's engaged in deceptive marketing that enticed them to eat unhealthy food with substantial frequency. Therefore, they now face a higher likelihood of developing diabetes, heart disease, and a host of obesity-related conditions as a direct result of eating at McDonald's. For example, they pointed to advertising that sodium was reduced across the McDonald's menu, and then cited products whose sodium content had not been reduced in years.

ISSUE: Should McDonald's be responsible for the obesity-related illnesses of its consumers?

HOLDING AND DECISION: No, if consumers know, or should know that eating McDonald's supersized food orders is unhealthy and may result in weight gain, it is not the place of the law to protect them from their own excesses.

(continues)

(continued)

ANALYSIS: The Federal District Court rejected the argument that McDonald's should have warned its consumers about the adverse health effects associated with foods high in fat, salt, and sugar, reasoning that such information is well known to the average consumer. Nothing suggests McDonald's food is any less nutritious than the average consumer expects it to be. In addition, the court did not find any specific advertisements or public statements by McDonald's to be deceptive. The court also found that McDonald's failure to provide nutritional information could not be considered deceptive because consumers could reasonably obtain such information. Additionally, there was no causal link between McDonald's food and the obesity-related illnesses of its consumers. The court noted that heredity, sedentary lifestyles, and other health-related factors must be eliminated to show McDonald's food is a substantial factor in consumers' weight gain.

The court did not find consumers were addicted to McDonald's food, and no causal link was established between the consumption of McDonald's food and obesity. The court conceded a discrepancy existed between the advertising around McDonald's use of 100 percent vegetable oil and the fact that beef tallow was also used, but dismissed this disparity as irrelevant to the obesity-related illnesses of its consumers. The court found the plaintiffs did not allege the beef tallow contained cholesterol, and thus there was no evidence to support the claim that McDonald's acted deceptively in stating its fries were cholesterol-free. The fact that the vegetable oil contained "trans-fatty acids responsible for raising detrimental blood cholesterol levels" (LDL) was deemed irrelevant because the contents of food and the effects of food are different. In dismissing the case with prejudice, the court indicated the claims could not be re-filed.

RULE OF LAW: There are substantial obstacles to tort liability for obesity-related illnesses allegedly brought on by consumption of fast food.

(*See generally* Adams, et al., 2009; Andrews, 2004; Choi, 2008; Courtney, 2006; Ellender, 2006; Frazier, 2007; Luna, 2004; McMenamin & Tiglio, 2006; Munger, 2004; Pennel, 2009; Reich, 2006; Ritter, 2003; Roller, et al., 2006; Romero, 2004; Vladeck, 2004).

In another separate lawsuit four years after the *Pelman* decision, another court did find a discrepancy between the advertising around McDonald's use of 100 percent vegetable oil and the fact that beef tallow was also used. McDonald's publicly apologized and reached a $10 million settlement on behalf of vegetarians and other individuals opposed to eating beef products (Burnett, 2007). In an effort to ridicule the litigation against fast food companies, a restaurant in Seattle created the most fattening and delicious dessert imaginable. In order to indulge in the restaurant's "delectable deep fried, ice cream anointed banana," consumers had to sign a waiver that read, in part: "I will not impose any sort of obesity-related lawsuits against the 5 Spot or consider any similar type of frivolous legislation created by a hungry trial lawyer" (Harden, 2003). Unfortunately, some attorneys, rather than bringing lawsuits that clients demand, engage in a complex game of legal arbitrage in order to force the health industry (as well as other industries) to negotiate immediate settlements with them without the risk of litigation. It is debatable whether this behavior by attorneys should be tolerated, since it hampers investment and stifles innovation in the nation's health care system.

Meanwhile, the food industry claims eating smaller portions and healthier foods will do more to counter the spread of weight-related illnesses than novel "McLawsuits" aimed at the fast food industry. Food can hold only part of the blame for the growing levels of obesity. Food is an important factor, but not the only factor.

Still, the food industry's fear of McLawsuits is one reason why Congress is debating the Personal Responsibility in Food Consumption Act, federal legislation that would protect food industry manufacturers from McLawsuits whose products are in compliance with existing laws and regulations.[LN1] Similar so-called *cheeseburger bills* (or commonsense consumption bills) have been introduced on the state level as well. Such bills aim to remove responsibility from food manufacturers and place it back on the consumer. Passage of such legislation is a legislative priority and industry proponents are expected to keep pushing for their passage. Others disagree and claim that eliminating the threat of litigation against the food industry also eliminates one point of pressure encouraging the industry to take responsibility for its role in combating obesity and weight-related illnesses (Walker, 2006).

Moral Dilemmas

1. If Congress passes a personal responsibility statute regarding fast food consumption, should it go on to pass personal responsibility statutes aimed at unwed mothers, smokers with lung cancer, high school dropouts on welfare, people who purchase on credit what they cannot afford, etc.?

FOOD ADVERTISING TO CHILDREN

In addition to forestalling litigation, the Alliance for American Advertising (consisting of the American Advertising Federation, the American Association of Advertising Agencies, the Association of National Advertising, and the Grocery Manufacturers Association) was established to persuade legislators not to introduce legislation restricting food advertising targeted to children. The group maintains the issue is a First Amendment concern because attempts to restrict advertising violate the right to free speech. Others differ and point to current bans on cigarette and alcohol advertising (Wharton, 2005).

Critics of the food industry's push to sell unhealthy foods find as much to criticize in the advertisements as in the products themselves. Advertising is not only on television, but increasingly on the Internet, in video games, and on cell phones. Many nutritionists already claim there is ample evidence linking advertising to childhood obesity. One case against McDonald's argued the company should warn consumers that Chicken McNuggets contain more fat than burgers. Some commentators claim the food industry spends more effort warning consumers not to let their children choke on the plastic toys they give away than they do on warning of the dangers of eating too much sugar or fat.

Members of the fast food sector claim healthy options are on their menus and that they provide nutritional information about consumer items, all in order to inform consumers about what is available. They say they are not in the business of taking away consumer choice and point to the fact that fat levels in food have declined since the 1970s. They argue there is increased pressure on marketers to compete on calorie content when advertising is not restricted; food ad restrictions inhibit such competition (Zywicki et al., 2004).

The trouble is, though, that many advertisements for food products are targeted at children. As soon as cartoon characters are used and products are tied

in with children's movies and so forth, the question becomes whether consumers really make fully informed choices or whether they are flooded with marketing material that alters their behavior. The food industry's response to this is that children do not make the purchasing decisions; it is their parents. Nevertheless, children can be persuasive. In fact, many of the McLawsuits against the fast food industry have been brought by parents of minors because of the health effects on their children and because children often cannot make educated food decisions. Also, there has been a big push to ensure schools contain healthy snacks in their vending machines and fewer calorie-laden beverages (Plemmons, 2004).

Fast food restaurants and school systems are rethinking ways in which they can influence the debate about food (Wharton, 2005). Some will sell only water, certain fruit juices, and low-fat or fat-free milk in schools, with diet or low-calorie sodas, teas, and sports drinks for sale only in high schools. Portion sizes in school cafeterias are also being tailored to each age group.

McDonald's promotes the idea that it is cool to be active through, for example, associations with Olympic athletes and sports celebrities. Healthy eating versus unhealthy eating information is placed on McDonald's tray liners, on store posters, and its packaging. Kraft, for its part, advertises sugar-free Crystal Light and whole-grain Triscuits, and labels foods and beverages that meet federal nutritional guidelines (Fishman & Hagerty, 2003).

There are many marketing vehicles to communicate these kinds of healthy messages, beyond paid advertising (Wharton, 2005). The Institute of Medicine maintains the food industry should not walk away from advertising to children, but instead be a part of the solution (IOM, 2005).

HEALTHY OPTIONS AND NUTRACEUTICAL ADVERTISING

There is also the issue of advertising seemingly healthy options that are actually worse for consumers. Salads can be drowned in dressing with cheese and bacon bits. This contributes to consumers' confusion and lack of knowledge about what they are eating. They are choosing the salad, but overlooking the things added to make it appetizing. A lot of packaged goods are guilty of this as well by trying to make products seem healthier than they really are (Wharton, 2005).

In addition, nutraceuticals and nutritional supplements are added to products, such as calcium to chocolate syrup and Vitamin C to soda, to make foods more appealing to health-conscious consumers. *See* FDA's Food Fortification Policy, 21 C.F.R.

§ 104.20 (1998). Makers of children's food are rolling out yogurt and soy milk products enhanced with DHA omega-3 fatty acid, which Beech-Nut and Dannon say can aid in brain and vision development, but pediatricians question their benefit (Muñoz, 2008). Coca-Cola and PepsiCo have carbonated drinks fortified with vitamins and minerals. Milk, breads, cereals, and other products have been nutrient-fortified for years. Nutritionists maintain fortified junk food is still junk food. Adding supplements does not address the larger issue of how to encourage changes in eating habits (Wharton, 2005).

McDonald's response to the *Super Size Me* documentary (Gilbert, 2004), which is that the company is not suggesting consumers eat at McDonald's every day, ignores the fact that the company advertises with an "all day every day" theme and tries to create demand at every meal. There is clearly some inherent tension between the food industry and its critics. Hardee's sells a Loaded Breakfast Burrito, a menu item consisting of eggs, diced ham, bacon bits, and a sausage patty with shredded cheddar cheese and salsa. If Hardee's is responding to demand for such a product, that is one thing. However, if Hardee's is creating a demand, and if consumers would not otherwise be eating 780 calories and 51 grams of fat for breakfast, then this is a gray area and may call for changes in the way the company should operate.

The Center for Science in the Public Interest claims the food industry tries to create demand for its products, often at the expense of healthier options. A number of companies claim marketing is intended to simply move customers from one brand to another, but this is not always the case (Wharton, 2005). For instance, fruit snacks are a whole new category of product not in existence years ago. Food companies compete not only with other similar products, but with real fruit. So a parent may pack fruit gummies in a child's lunchbox instead of an apple or bag of grapes. When a child wants to go to McDonald's for dinner, that choice is competing not only with Wendy's or Burger King, but with a meal cooked at home. Marketing works. That is why the food industry does it and why health advocates are concerned about it.

The food industry is very concerned about being blamed for the rising obesity rate, and it should be, because many of its products and practices are significant contributors (Wharton, 2005). The industry is also nervous about new regulations, legislation, and lawsuits, and is moving to head these off (Frank, 2006). Kraft's decision to limit certain kinds of advertising is a meaningful step forward. PepsiCo is trying to add healthier versions of its products in schools, although it still markets and sells a lot of soda.[LN2] All the fast food restaurants have fruit options: Wendy's has mandarin oranges, Burger King has applesauce, and McDonald's

has apples in its salads and desserts. However, in most cases, an overwhelming number of the entrees remain unhealthy. Red Lobster offers a Lighthouse menu advertising seafood with less than five hundred calories, but each dish is surrounded by high-calorie accompaniments, sides, and dipping sauces not included in the nutritional content advertisements. Indeed, hamburgers and French fries will continue to be at the core of fast food menus for the long term, although salads and deli-style sandwiches are being added.

Moral Dilemmas

1. Are fast food and chain restaurant meals, served without any readily available nutrition information, contributing to weight-related chronic illnesses in the U.S.?

VOLUNTARY MARKETING GUIDELINES

The Center for Science in the Public Interest developed guidelines for responsible food marketing, calling on the food industry to use its power to create and market healthy foods consumers will ask for and enjoy. The industry wants to respond to consumer demand, but this does not happen in a vacuum. Many interested in consumer protection believe marketers have the power to influence wants and needs as much as they respond to wants and needs (Wharton, 2005). The assumption is marketers could determine that the food industry is making American consumers unhealthy and that there are costs for the U.S.

Why not influence consumer preferences in ways that favor healthy choices? For example, when marketers began advertising the link between fiber in cereals and the reduced risk of cancer in the mid-eighties, there was a consumer shift to high-fiber diets. Such changes in food labeling rules could play an important role in bringing information to consumers and adding to food industry incentives to focus on the calorie profiles of their foods. Another such change could be decreased portion sizes; portion sizes today almost always greatly exceed those offered twenty to thirty years earlier (Zywicki et al., 2004).

FOOD INDUSTRY AND PUBLIC HEALTH SECTOR VIEWPOINTS

On one hand, members of the food industry should not be expected to change their practices unless it is profitable to do so. They can accomplish profitability by, for example, retraining consumers to be proactive and encouraging them to gravitate toward healthy foods. Healthy as well as non-healthy foods should be offered. Food retailers should offer consumers options, rather than erode or dictate choices, and give consumers more information on nutrition. Consumers are not aware of the calories and fat in food (Wharton, 2005).

The bigger challenge is developing a concerted effort across disciplines and across fields. The public health sector is skeptical that the food industry is trying to promote healthy foods when its major concern is profits. The food industry views public health advocates as unaware of how businesses operate. To complicate the issue, the available evidence to support any proffered link between food advertising and obesity is quite limited and often contrary to the thesis. Although many European companies have limited advertising to children, evidence suggests advertising does not appear to be a significant factor in the rise of childhood obesity; this does not, however, mean that advertising, marketing, and government policies cannot be part of the solution to the problem of obesity (Zywicki et al., 2004).

Consumers are a large part of the problem as well, in terms of purchasing patterns and parental responsibility. A multi-domain effort is required across the public and private sectors (Wharton, 2005). Public health scholars and practitioners in several countries have called for a broad system of taxes on unhealthy foods, possibly combined with subsidies for certain healthy foods (Strnad, 2005). The World Health Organization (WHO) recommends limits on sugar consumption and advertising targeted to children. WHO also encourages governments to discourage advertising that promotes the consumption of unhealthy foods by children. The European Union has threatened to restrict advertising aimed at children if the food industry fails to take action on its own (Sealing, 2007).

Moral Dilemmas

1. Is government advertising about the risks of obesity more politically feasible than direct regulation of food or food consumption, given the anti-paternalistic sentiments of the American public?

REGULATION OF TRANS-FATS

There are two types of trans-fatty acids. The food processing industry switched from animal fats to mixing vegetable fat with hydrogen, believing that this cheaper raw material might be healthier.

Hydrogenated fat, used in many biscuits, chocolate, and other products, has now proven to be just as bad as animal fats for clogging arteries (Spivey, 2007).

The most dramatic new regulatory change for the food industry occurred when the FDA issued a rule requiring food labels to list the amount of trans-fatty acids, or trans-fats, in their products (Atwell, 2007). Food labels and packaging must reveal how much trans-fat they contain. *See* Nutrition Labeling of Dietary Supplements, 21 C.F.R. § 101.36(b)(2)(i) (2006); Food Labeling, 21 C.F.R. Part 101 (2009).

In the realm of dietary dangers, hydrogenated trans-fats rank very high (Abboud, 2003). The FDA estimates that merely revealing trans-fat content on labels could save between 2,000 and 5,600 lives a year. Still, trans-fats are responsible for an estimated 30,000 early deaths per year in the U.S. Worldwide, the toll of premature deaths is in the millions.

Though trans-fats are found naturally in meats and some dairy products, Americans ingest far greater amounts of them through the chemical process of hydrogenation of oils found in crackers, cookies, chips, and other snack foods. Hydrogenation is a chemical process used to solidify oils, vegetable shortenings, and margarines, to increase the shelf life and flavor stability of foods, and it creates hydrogenated trans-fats. Nearly all fried and baked goods have hydrogenated trans-fats, including food labeled as low fat. Nutritionists claim trans-fats are so harmful, no level is entirely safe. Not only do trans-fats raise bad cholesterol, but they also lower good cholesterol helpful in reducing the risk of clogged arteries.

The new FDA requirements force the food industry to add nutrition labels showing how many grams of trans-fats are included in each serving. Beyond requiring that some labels list the amount of trans-fats in food, the FDA also defined the term *trans-fat free* and limited use of certain nutrient or health claims related to fat content, such as lean and low saturated fat.

Together, these regulations could affect the food industry as well as consumer eating habits, just as requiring warning labels on cigarettes in the sixties led some consumers to give up smoking and resulted in the tobacco industry developing lower-nicotine products. New York City became the first major American city to enact a nearly complete ban on trans-fats (Leuck & Severson, 2006). There are ways to reduce trans-fats while keeping the familiar taste and texture in popular food products.

Reducing Trans-Fats
- Avoid foods containing partially hydrogenated oils that sound healthy, like soybean oil
- Select foods low in saturated fats; trans-fats and saturated fats act similarly in the body and generally come together
- Use olive or canola oil
- Avoid all deep-fried foods, which are prime culprits in purveying trans-fats

GENETICALLY MODIFIED FOODS

In the U.S., over three hundred million consumers have spent more than a decade consuming genetically modified foods, without any adverse effects (Wharton, 2004). The first genetically modified (GM) food, a genetically engineered tomato, was sold in the U.S. market in 1995 (Strauss, 2006). Since then, agricultural biotechnology has received both unproven praise and unproven attacks. Myths on both sides of the issue of GM foods need to be debunked (Marden, 2003). The U.S. policy is that GM foods, derived from genetically engineered plants and animals, should be permitted to flourish in the absence of proven hazards (Moyer & Anway, 2007).

Genetically engineered plants used in industrial agriculture isolate specific genes from virtually any organism and insert them into the genetic material of crops. On one hand, this offers tremendous benefits with increased crop yields and reduction in the use of dangerous pesticides. On the other hand, the engineering process must be monitored because the process has the potential to create foods containing new toxins and previously unknown allergens. Two human health risks associated with GM foods are potential allergies to novel proteins that appear in GM food and the risk that antibiotic resistance could be spread through genetically engineered organisms (Zurek, 2007). In addition, genetically engineered crops protected from insects and herbicides may have unforeseen adverse impacts on wildlife and plants.

The U.S. has not established GM-specific requirements; rather, modified foods are regulated under the existing framework of the FDA, the Environmental Protection Agency, and the U.S. Department of Agriculture. Currently, the regulatory process on what constitutes genetic engineering in plants is voluntary (Galant, 2005). The existing regulatory scheme has led to widespread consumer demand for the labeling of GM foods. The issue reached the Federal Circuit in *Alliance for Bio-Integrity v. Shalala*.

LABELING OF GENETICALLY MODIFIED FOODS

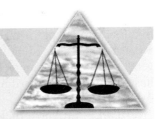

Alliance for Bio-Integrity v. Shalala
[Coalition Concerned About GM Foods v. FDA]
116 F.Supp.2d 166 (U.S. District Court for the District of Columbia 2000)

FACTS: The FDA presumes that foods produced through recombinant deoxyribonucleic acid (rDNA) technology are generally recognized as safe. *See* Statement of Policy: Foods Derived From New Plant Varieties, 57 *Federal Register* 22,984-01 (May 29, 1992). Therefore, labeling of rDNA-developed foods is not required. The Alliance for Bio-Integrity filed suit to invalidate this FDA policy based on two concerns: first, that new breeds of GM foods contain unexpected allergens and toxins and second, that some religions forbid consumption of foods produced by rDNA technology.

ISSUE: Is labeling of genetically modified organisms (GMOs) in food required?

HOLDING AND DECISION: No, scientific applications of FDA policies that do not require labeling of GMOs will not be second-guessed by the courts.

ANALYSIS: The Alliance challenged the FDA policy on grounds that the policy was not subjected to notice-and-comment procedures as required by the Administrative Procedure Act; the FDA violated the National Environmental Protection Act by not performing an Environmental Assessment or an Environmental Impact Statement in conjunction with the policy; the presumption that GMOs are generally accepted as safe was arbitrary and capricious; and the policy failed to require labeling of GMOs in violation of the Food, Drug,

(continues)

(continued)

and Cosmetic Act (FDCA), the Free Exercise Clause of the U.S. Constitution, and the Religious Freedom Restoration Act.

The court rejected each of the Alliance's arguments and granted a motion for summary judgment in favor of the FDA. The FDA was not required to conduct notice-and-comment procedures because the policy merely created a presumption rather than a substantive rule. In addition, the FDA did not violate the National Environmental Protection Act because the policy was not a major federal action and, therefore, was neither subject to an Environmental Assessment nor an Environmental Impact Statement. Finally, the court determined that scientific applications of statutory law were within the expertise of the FDA and that principles of administrative law prevented the court from overriding the FDA.

The court also deferred to the FDA's decision not to require the labeling of GMOs. The FDCA provides that the FDA shall take action for the misbranding of food. The FDA may only consider consumer demand for labeling if GMO food differs materially from unmodified food. Because the FDA had concluded that genetic modification of a food was not a material change in the food, the court deferred to that conclusion.

The court concluded its analysis by noting that the failure of the FDA to require labeling violated neither the Free Exercise Clause nor the Religious Freedom Restoration Act. In support of this conclusion, the court reasoned that the FDA policy was neutral and did not substantially burden religious practices.

RULE OF LAW: GMO food is not materially different from unmodified food; therefore, labeling is not required.

(*See generally* Farquhar & Meyer, 2007; Lawrence, 2007; McCabe, 2008; Mindrup, 2007; Moyer & Anway, 2007; Murphy, 2008; Noah, 2006; Strauss, 2006).

The Alliance for Bio-Integrity remains one of the first reported opinions to address the safety concerns associated with GMOs, mainly that biotechnology allows scientists to manipulate a variety of factors in our environment through genetic engineering. Nevertheless, the food industry expects additional genetics-related litigation (Filippi, 2005). Litigation has already begun regarding genetically engineered seeds by Monsanto.

In addition, most of Europe refuses to import any meat from the U.S. containing hormones used to promote growth in cattle, creating a major dispute within the World Trade Organization. Europe takes the position that where potential health effects are serious and the relevant science is inadequate to draw a conclusion, a ban is warranted until definitive research is performed (Shapiro, 2007).

Moral Dilemmas

1. Should genetically engineered crops be subjected to a mandatory approval process that would ensure such food is safe to eat, rather than assuming food is generally recognized as safe unless a hazard is proven to exist?

FOOD ADDITIVES AND CONTAMINANTS

Over the past several decades, Congress and the FDA have increasingly turned to disclosure regulations on food safety (Dalley, 2007). Beginning in the 1980s, the FDA banned sulfite preservatives from fresh fruits and vegetables and required better, more informative labeling on packaged foods. Sodium nitrites, dyes, and other chemicals are more clearly labeled or more restricted than ever (CFSAN, 2006).

Still, other harmful levels of additives remain in processed foods without monitoring for potential long-term chemical toxicity (Waldman, 2005), albeit with warnings:

- Acrylamide (probable carcinogen found in many processed foods that forms in carbohydrate-containing foods baked, fried, or broiled, like breads, cereals, potato chips, and coffee)
- Olestra (fat substitute that can cause diarrhea and stomach cramps)
- Quorn (fungus-based meat substitute that can cause severe vomiting and anaphylactic reactions)
- Sorbitol (sugar substitute added to diet drinks and ice cream)

Four additives recognized by the Institute of Medicine (IOM, 2006), the U.S. Pharmacopeia (USP), FDA, and international food regulatory authorities as being generally recognized as safe are excluded from this list, even though some public health advocates maintain they are harmful and question their long-term safety:

- Artificial sweetener acesulfame-k
- Aspartame (artificial sweetener also sold under the brand names NutraSweet and Equal)
- Saccharin (artificial sweetener used in diet drinks, fruit juices, and alcoholic beverages)
- Potassium bromate (used in bread)

In several large European studies conducted at the European Mamazzini Foundation in Italy, researchers found that feeding rats aspartame, at simulated doses at or below levels considered safe for humans, increased the rats' risk of leukemia, lymphoma, and breast cancer (Soffritti et al., 2006). In April 2008, the U.S. Environmental Protection Agency affirmed the European research and called for the government to urgently reevaluate its guidelines on the use of aspartame (Caldwell, 2008). The oldest artificial sweetener, saccharin, was almost banned in 1977 after studies in rats linked it to cancer. But research in humans largely failed to turn up that risk, with the possible exception found in one study of people consuming six or more servings a day. In 2000, the government's National Toxicology Program delisted saccharin as a possible carcinogen.

EMERGING ISSUES

A report by the Pew Charitable Trusts and Johns Hopkins Bloomberg School of Public Health calls for broader regulation of industrial livestock and poultry farming, including restrictions on using antibiotics for growth promotion (Halden & Schwab, 2008). A public consensus appears to be requiring much stronger protection of the U.S. meat and poultry sectors, which have had an extraordinary number of recent food safety recalls (Williamson, 2008).

Voluntary Identification and Tracking Systems

Specifically, the U.S. does not have a mandatory animal identification system. For instance, mad cow disease can jump to humans who eat contaminated meat and can cause rare, but always fatal brain damage. At this time, public health officials cannot trace infected cattle back to originating farms so other herd cattle can be tested; they have to rely on voluntary recalls by the industry (Halden & Schwab, 2008; Zahn, 2008).

For example, government inspections of U.S. slaughterhouses routinely find significant problems with *E. coli* contamination and the treatment of cattle at the largest beef processors. Audits at Westland/Hallmark Meat Co. in California in early 2008 led to the largest beef recall in American history.

About 150 million pounds of beef were recalled. If this quantity is difficult to imagine, picture it as the equivalent of about forty continuous miles of livestock trailers filled with cattle. This would be enough beef to supply every McDonald's in the country with hamburgers for two months. Westland, a major supplier of ground beef to the National School Lunch Program, was closed indefinitely after the National Humane Society videotaped slaughterhouse workers shoving and kicking sick, crippled cattle, and forcing them to stand using electric prods, forklifts, and water hoses (AP, 2008). The stunning of cattle by air injection rifles as they are driven from holding pens is now prohibited. This was a common practice that was contaminating meat with potentially infective brain tissue until just recently. Until the practice was prohibited in mid-2009, electrical stun guns were used to pull cattle through restrainers to be shackled, hung, and bled. The issue here was the fact that downer cows presented a higher risk of bovine spongiform encephalopathy (or mad cow disease) and related phenomena before they were slaughtered and entered the nation's food supply. Both General Mills and Nestle were forced to recall products after using Westland meat. Investigation of Westland is ongoing, while two videotaped slaughterhouse workers are facing criminal charges. *See generally* Zahn, 2008.

Federal Inspections

Another concern is that the federal meat and poultry inspection agency is so understaffed that some inspectors are assigned to as many as twenty-four plants or facilities in a geographic region too large to traverse for the required daily inspections. A 2007 survey by the National Joint Council of Food Inspection Local Unions found that 75 percent of inspectors did not visit their plants daily, as required, and when they did, the processing lines often moved so quickly that contamination was difficult to detect (Zhang, 2008). The National Joint Council of Food Inspection Local Unions claims that inspectors who blow the whistle on slaughterhouse violations often find themselves targets of retaliation within the federal Food Safety and Inspection Service. In addition, inspectors are told not to record violations, giving companies time to fix problems instead (Zhang, 2008).

Private Sector Standards

What this means for U.S. food safety is another emerging question. Amid growing fears about food safety and impatience with lack of or slow government response, standards set by the private sector are starting to emerge in the U.S. In a key move, Wal-Mart, McDonald's, and Wegmans Food Markets are now buying produce, meat, and seafood only from suppliers accredited by private inspection offices (Miller, 2008). The largest private regulator, GlobalGAP, which stands for "Global Good Agricultural Practice," is based in Germany. At the same time, many sellers, including grocery store chains, have established their own certification programs that go beyond the standards set by the FDA and U.S. Department of Agriculture.

The table appears set to make changes in U.S. food safety. After all, as Jean-Anthelme Brillat-Savarin implied at the beginning of this chapter, we are what we eat.

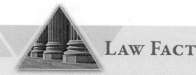

LAW FACT

FOOD LABELING

Should the producers and sellers of milk be required to warn consumers of the risks of sickness from lactose intolerance on their packaging?

Tort law does not provide protection from obvious and widely known risks of consuming particular foods. Milk producers are not required to warn consumers of the risks of sickness from lactose intolerance on their packaging. The risk that milk may cause temporary flatulence and related stomach discomfort is well known, even if lactose intolerance as the cause may not be known to everyone who experiences a brief fit of indigestion.

—*Mills v. Giant of Maryland*, 508 F.3d 11 (U.S. Court of Appeals for the District of Columbia Circuit 2007).

CHAPTER SUMMARY

- The recent increase in weight-related chronic illnesses in the U.S. coincides with the change in American eating habits, with dietary intake consisting mostly of highly processed, prepackaged, and ready-made meals high in carbohydrates and sodium content.
- Fully one-third of the daily calories Americans eat are eaten outside the home at high-calorie fast food and chain restaurants.
- Federal legislation requires easy-to-read Nutrition Facts labels on almost all packaged foods, with few exceptions.
- Proposed federal and state legislation would protect the food industry from lawsuits when products are in compliance with existing laws and regulations.
- Marketers in the food industry have the power to influence wants and needs as much as they respond to wants and needs.
- Food labeling rules could play an important role in bringing information to consumers and adding to food industry incentives to focus on the nutritional profiles of its foods.
- The most dramatic new regulatory change for the food industry occurred when the FDA required the amount of trans-fatty acids or trans-fats to be listed on almost all food labels and packaging.
- Though trans-fats are found naturally in meats and some dairy products, far greater amounts are ingested as hydrogenated oils added to food to increase shelf life and flavor stability.
- Nutritionists claim trans-fats are so harmful in raising bad cholesterol and lowering good cholesterol, which reduces the risk of clogged arteries, that no level is entirely safe.
- Nearly all fried and baked goods have hydrogenated trans-fats, including foods labeled as low fat.
- Over three hundred million U.S. consumers have spent more than a decade consuming genetically modified foods without any known adverse effects.
- Genetically modified foods, derived from genetically engineered plants and animals, are permitted in the U.S. in the absence of proven health hazards.
- Potentially harmful levels of additives are in many highly processed, prepackaged foods in the U.S., albeit with warnings.

LAW NOTES

1. The National Restaurant Association reports that twenty-three states have enacted legislation which blocks 'McLawsuits' by mandating dismissal at the summary judgment stage: Arizona, Colorado, Florida, Georgia, Idaho, Illinois, Indiana, Kansas, Kentucky, Louisiana, Maine, Michigan, Missouri, North Dakota, Ohio, Oregon, South Dakota, Tennessee, Texas, Utah, Washington, Wisconsin, and Wyoming. Similar legislation is pending in eight states: Alabama, Minnesota, Nebraska, New York, New Jersey, Oklahoma, Pennsylvania, and South Carolina (Miller, 2008).

2. The question always arises: which is preferable, diet or regular beverages? An eight-ounce individual serving of Coca-Cola classic packs ninety-seven calories while a Pepsi has one hundred calories, compared to zero calories for a Diet Coke or a Diet Pepsi. So, less calories, but what about the artificial sweeteners? Ever since 1982, when the government first approved aspartame for use in diet sodas, debate has raged about its possible long-term health risks. Whether aspartame, one of the most contentiously debated substances ever added to beverages, contributes to cancer is proving to be very controversial in the U.S. and Europe (Warner, 2006). So the jury is out with regards to the safety of today's diet sodas. Even if proven safe, some research has pointed to the theory that consumption of diet beverages tricks consumers' brains into craving real sugar, leading consumers to consume even more calories than they would have had they chosen the regular beverage.

CHAPTER BIBLIOGRAPHY

Abboud, L. (2003, July 10). The truth about trans-fats: Coming to a label near you, FDA orders more disclosure; A new excuse to eat Cheerios. *Wall Street Journal*, p. A3.

Adams, D. C. et al. (2009). Deja moo: Is the return to public sale of raw milk udder nonsense? *Drake Journal of Agricultural Law, 13*, 305-346.

AHG (Alliance for a Healthier Generation). (2006, October 6). Press release, statement from AHG & Centers for Disease Control and Prevention (CDC) concerning agreement by five U.S. food companies to meet nutritional guidelines for food sold in schools. Washington, DC: AHG.

___. (2006a, May 3). Press release, Clinton Foundation and American Heart Association and industry leaders set healthy school beverage guidelines for U.S. schools. Washington, DC: AHG.

Andrews, F. L. (2004). Small bites: Obesity lawsuits prepare to take on the fast food industry. *Albany Law Journal of Science & Technology, 15*, 153-182.

AP (Associated Press). (2008, April 30). U.S. beef processors cited for humane violations. *Wall Street Journal*, p. B1.

Atwell, B. L. (2007). Obesity, public health, and the food supply. *Indiana Health Law Review, 4*, 1-27.

Ausness, R. C. (2005). Tell me what you eat, and I will tell you whom to sue: Big problems ahead for "big food"? *Georgia Law Review, 39*, 839-868 (discussing possible future legal claims against the food industry).

Burnett, D. (2007). Fast-food lawsuits and the cheeseburger bill: Critiquing Congress's response to the obesity epidemic. *Virginia Journal of Social Policy & the Law, 14*, 357-417.

Caldwell, J. C. (2008). Environmental and molecular mutagenesis: Evaluation of evidence for infection as a mode of action for induction of rat lymphoma. *Environmental & Molecular Mutagenesis, 49* (2), 155-164.

Catlin, G. M. (2007). A more palatable solution? Comparing the viability of smart growth statutes to other legislative methods of controlling the obesity epidemic. *Wisconsin Law Review, 2007*, 1092-1121.

CFSAN (Center for Food Safety & Applied Nutrition) & U.S. Food & Drug Administration. (2006). *Approaches to establish thresholds for major food allergens and gluten in food.*

Rockville, MD: CFSAN (describing factors to consider in setting thresholds and the problem of serious reactions to very low doses of allergens).

Choi, E. (2008). Trans fat regulation: A legislative remedy for America's heartache. *Southern California Interdisciplinary Law Journal, 17*, 507-542.

Chou, S. et al. (2005). *Fast-food restaurant advertising on television and its influence on childhood obesity.* New York, NY: National Bureau of Economic Research.

Courtney, B. (2006). Is obesity really the next tobacco? Lessons learned from tobacco for obesity litigation. *Annals of Health Law, 15*, 61-106.

Dalley, P. J. (2007). The use and misuse of disclosure as a regulatory system. *Florida State University Law Review, 34*, 1089-1131.

Ellender. D. (2006). A class-action lawsuit against aspartame manufacturers: A realistic possibility or just a sweet dream for tort lawyers? *Regent University Law Review, 18*, 179-208.

Farquhar, D. & Meyer, L. (2007). State authority to regulate biotechnology under the federal coordinated framework. *Drake Journal of Agricultural Law, 12*, 439-474.

Filippi, I. (2005). Food safety in the WTO: Where do we stand? *International Trade Law & Regulation, 11*, 71-77.

Fishman, M. J., & Hagerty, K. M. (2003). Mandatory versus voluntary disclosure in markets with informed and uninformed consumers. *Journal of Law, Economics & Organization, 19*, 45-50.

Frank, T. (2006). A taxonomy of obesity litigation. *University of Arkansas at Little Rock Law Review, 28*, 429-441 (contrasting tort claims for injuries from otherwise safe foods with social crusader lawsuits against the food industry).

Frazier, D. A. (2007). The link between fast food and the obesity epidemic. *Health Matrix, 17*, 291-317 (raises the issue of whether fat, sugar, and cholesterol have addictive qualities similar to the drug nicotine).

Galant, C. R. (2005). Labeling limbo: Why genetically modified foods continue to duck mandatory disclosure. *Houston Law Review, 42*, 125-164.

Gilbert, A. (2004). Super size me. *Cineaste, 29* (4), 47-50.

Halden, R. U., & Schwab, K. J. (2008). *Report: Environmental impact of industrial farm animal production*. Baltimore, MD: Pew Commission on Industrial Farm Animal Production at the Johns Hopkins Bloomberg School of Public Health.

Harden, B. (2003, September 20). Eatery joins battle with "the bulge"; Obesity lawsuits spur dessert protest. *Washington Post*, p. A3.

Hays, C. (2004). *The real thing: Truth and power at the Coca-Cola Company*. New York, NY: Random House.

Hitt, G. (2008, May 5). Farm bill stuck on sugar-support proposal. *Wall Street Journal*, p. A3 (describing the five-year-long, $300 billion federal farm bill for 2009-2014).

IOM (Institute of Medicine). (2007). *Nutrition standards for foods in schools: Leading the way toward healthier youth.* Washington, DC: IOM.

___. (2006). *Food chemicals codex: First supplement* (5th ed.). Washington, DC: IOM (accepted standard for defining the quality and purity of food chemicals by the FDA and international food regulatory authorities).

___. (2005). *Food marketing to children and youth: Threat or opportunity?* Washington, DC: IOM.

Kraft Foods. (2005, December 20). Press release, Kraft Foods reformulates hundreds of U.S. products as part of voluntary trans-fat reduction efforts. Northfield, IL: Kraft.

Kunkel, D. et al. (2004). *Report of the American Psychological Association (APA) Task Force on Advertising and Children.* Washington, DC: APA.

Kysar, D. A. (2004). Preferences for processes: The process-product distinction and the regulation of consumer choice. *Harvard Law Review, 18*, 526-642.

Lawrence, S. (2007). What would you do with a fluorescent green pig? How novel transgenic products reveal flaws in the foundational assumptions for the regulation of biotechnology. *Ecology Law Quarterly, 34*, 201-290.

Luce, P. (2007). *Monsanto Co. v. Scruggs*: Has Federal Circuit biotechnology patent scope jurisprudence gone to seed? *Tulane Journal of Technology & Intellectual Property, 9*, 385-393.

Lueck, T. J., & Severson, K. (2006, December 6). New York bans most trans-fats in restaurants. *New York Times*, p. A1.

Luna, G. T. (2004). The new deal and food insecurity in the "midst of plenty." *Drake Journal of Agricultural Law, 9*, 213-253.

Making, D. (2005). The elephant in the room: Evolution, behavioralism, and counter-advertising in the coming war against obesity. *Harvard Law Review, 116*, 1161-1184 (discussing FDA's failed efforts to ensure a useful format for nutrition labels).

Marden, E. (2003). Risk and regulation: U.S. regulatory policy on genetically modified food and agriculture. *Boston College Law Review, 44*, 733-787.

Martin, R. et al. (2008, April 28). *Putting meat on the table: Industrial farm animal production in America.* Baltimore, MD: Pew Commission on Industrial Farm Animal Production at the Johns Hopkins Bloomberg School of Public Health.

Mathews, A. W. (2006, January 19). FDA issues new rules for drug labels. *Wall Street Journal*, p. D1 (describing FDA drug labeling rules aimed at physicians).

Mayo Clinic. (2007). *Counting calories: Getting back to weight-loss basics.* Rochester, MN: Mayo Foundation for Medical Education & Research.

McCabe, M. S. (2008). Got controversy? Milk does. *Drake Journal of Agricultural Law, 13*, 475-495.

McMenamin, J. P., & Tiglio, A. D. (2006). Not the next tobacco: Defenses to obesity claims. *Food & Drug Law Journal, 61*, 453-486 (presenting a comprehensive explanation of the causes of obesity).

Merrill, R. A., & Francer, J. K. (2000). Organizing federal food safety regulation. *Seton Hall Law Review, 31*, 61-173.

Miller, J. (2008, March 11). Private food standards gain favor, Wal-Mart, McDonald's adopt European safety guidelines. *Wall Street Journal*, p. B1.

Mindrup, J. J. (2007). Transgenic crops in the age of human rights: Moral uncertainty and rational risk policy. *Chapman Law Review, 11*, 213-241.

Moyer, T. J., & Anway, S. P. (2007). Biotechnology and the bar: A response to the growing divide between science and the legal environment. *Berkeley Technology Law Journal, 22*, 671-731.

Munger, L. J. (2004). Is Ronald McDonald the next Joe Camel? Regulating fast food advertisements that target children in light of the American overweight and obesity epidemic. *Connecticut Public Interest Law Journal, 3*, 390-413.

Muñoz, S. S. (2008, March 27). Fortified yogurt, soy milk. *Wall Street Journal*, p. D2.

Murphy, J. F. (2008). Analyzing the laws, regulations, and policies affecting FDA-regulated products: Mandatory labeling of food made from cloned animals: Grappling with moral objections to the production of safe products. *Food & Drug Law Journal, 63*, 131-150.

Nelson, J. et al. (2006, April). Diet, activity, and overweight among preschool-age children enrolled in the special supplemental nutrition program for women, infants, and children (WIC). *Preventing Chronic Disease, 3* (2), 1-12.

Noah, L. (2006). Managing biotechnology's revolution: Has guarded enthusiasm become benign neglect? *Virginia Journal of Law & Technology, 11*, 4-63.

Ogden, C. L. et al. (2006, April 5). Prevalence of overweight and obesity in the U.S. *Journal of the American Medical Association, 295* (13), 1549-1555.

Pennel, J. L. (2009). Big food's trip down tobacco road: What tobacco's past can indicate about food's future. *Buffalo Public Interest Law Journal, 27*, 101-130.

Plemmons, K. L. (2004). The national school lunch program and USDA dietary guidelines: Is there room for reconciliation? *Journal of Law & Education, 33*, 181-212.

Reich, J. B. (2006). Getting the skinny: Fast food fat-based litigation is not a legal threat to business, but it should be. *Hofstra Labor & Employment Law Journal, 23*, 345-371.

Richardson, D. R. (2005). "Want fries with that?" A critical analysis of fast food litigation. *West Virginia Law Review, 107*, 575-601.

Ritter, L. et al. (2003). Fast food fighters fall flat: Plaintiffs fail to establish that McDonald's should be liable for obesity-related illnesses. *Journal of Law, Medicine & Ethics, 31*, 725-728.

Roller, S. T. et al. (2006). Obesity, food marketing and consumer litigation: Threat or opportunity? *Food & Drug Law Journal, 61*, 419-444 (providing an historical overview of governmental food regulation).

Romero, S. J. (2004). Obesity liability: A super-sized problem or a small fry in the inevitable development of product liability? *Chapman Law Review, 7*, 239-278.

Schlosser, E. (2001). *Fast-food nation: The dark side of the all-American meal*. New York, NY: Houghton Mifflin (compares and makes various references to Upton Sinclair's *The Jungle*).

Sealing, K. E. (2007). From hand to mouth, via the lab and the legislature: International and domestic regulations to secure the food supply. *Vanderbilt Journal of Transnational Law, 40*, 1015-1037.

Shapiro, H. S. (2007). The rules that swallowed the exceptions: The WTO SPS Agreement and its relationship to GATT articles XX and XXI: The threat of the EU-GMO dispute. *Arizona Journal of International & Comparative Law, 24*, 199-233.

Sinclair, U. (2006). *The jungle*. New York, NY: Penguin Classics (original work published 1906) (classic novel on food safety that led to the passage of the Meat Inspection Act and the Pure Food & Drug Act of 1906, which established the FDA).

Smith, J. A. (2006). Setting the stage for public health: The role of litigation in controlling obesity. *University of Arkansas at Little Rock Law Review, 28*, 443-455.

Soffritti, N. et al (2006). First experimental demonstration of multipotential carcinogenic effects of aspartame administered in the feed to Sprague-Dawley rats. *Environmental Health Perspectives, 114* (3), 379-385 (NIH peer-reviewed research calling for an urgent reevaluation of the guidelines on the use of Aspartame).

Spivey, E. Y. (2007). Trans-fat: Can New York City save its citizens from this metabolic poison? *Georgia Law Review, 42*, 273-306.

Strauss, D. W. (2006). The international regulation of genetically modified organisms: Importing caution into the U.S. food supply. *Food & Drug Law Journal, 61*, 167-196.

Strnad, J. (2005). Conceptualizing the "fat tax": The role of food taxes in developed economies. *Southern California Law Review, 78*, 1221-1326.

Surgeon General's Call to Action to Prevent and Decrease Overweight and Obesity. (2001). Rockville, MD: Public Health Service.

USP (U.S. Pharmacopeia). (2008). *Food chemicals codex* (6th ed.). Rockville, MD: USP Convention.

Vladeck, D. et al. (2004). Commercial speech and the public's health: Regulating advertisements of tobacco, alcohol, high fat foods and other potentially hazardous products. *Journal of Law, Medicine & Ethics, 32*, 32-34.

Waldman, P. (2005, July 25). Toxic traces: New questions about old chemicals. *Wall Street Journal*, p. A1 (describing new research casting doubt on much that is currently believed about chemical toxicity).

Walker, M. (2006). Low-fat foods or big fat lies? *Georgia State University Law Review, 22*, 689-710.

Wansink, B. (2007). *Mindless eating: Why we eat more than we think*. New York, NY: Bantam.

Warner, M. (2006, February 13). Not so sweet anymore: Aspartame under fire; Study reignites dispute over cancer risk. *International Herald Tribune*, p. 14.

Wharton (Wharton School of the University of Pennsylvania). (2007). Serving up smaller restaurant portions: Will consumers bite? *Knowledge@Wharton*.

___. (2005). Food fight: Obesity raises difficult marketing questions. *Knowledge@Wharton*.

___. (2004). Biotechnology in Chile: Looking for a boost from copper and fruits. *Universia Knowledge@Wharton*.

Williamson, E. (2008, April 30). Farming critics fault industry's influence. *Wall Street Journal*, p. A4.

Zhang, J. (2009, May 16). Obama sets steps to toughen food safety regulation. *Wall Street Journal*, p. D1.

___. (2008, April 18). Meat inspectors can't keep up, official says. *Wall Street Journal*, p. A3 (describing congressional testimony by the Joint Council of Food Inspection Local Unions before the House Committee on Oversight and Government Reform's domestic policy panel).

___. (2005, October 13). How much soy lecithin is in that cookie? *Wall Street Journal*, p. D1.

Zurek, L. (2007). The European community's biotech dispute: How the WTO fails to consider cultural factors in the genetically modified food debate. *Texas International Law Journal, 42*, 345-368.

Zywicki, T. et al. (2004). Working paper series: Obesity and advertising policy. *George Mason University School of Law, 3*, 2-75.

CHAPTER 37

ENVIRONMENTAL SAFETY

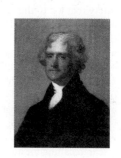

"A strong body makes the mind strong. As to the species of exercises, I advise the gun. While this gives moderate exercise to the body, it gives boldness, enterprise and independence to the mind. Games played with the ball, and others of that nature, are too violent for the body and stamp no character on the mind. Let your gun therefore be your constant companion of your walks."

—THOMAS JEFFERSON (1743-1826), THIRD PRESIDENT OF THE UNITED STATES,
TO HIS NEPHEW PETER CARR

IN BRIEF

This chapter addresses one aspect of the quandary of the modern U.S. health care system: while it is the most expensive heath care system in the world, Americans are neither healthier nor do they live longer than citizens in other countries. The environmental safety issues stemming from firearms homicides and suicides are highlighted based on the medical and financial impact of guns on American society. The focus of this chapter is on the data and research on decreased life expectancy as a result of gun violence and how this information might be used in Second Amendment jurisprudence.

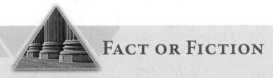

Fact or Fiction

Gun Violence

How can the risk of gun violence be reduced on college and university campuses?

On April 16, 2007, one university student, senior Seung Hui Cho, murdered thirty-two and injured twenty-five students and faculty in two related incidents on the campus of Virginia Tech before committing suicide himself. Cho used high-powered handguns with high-capacity ammunition clips for the mass murder, despite the fact that it was unlawful for him to have a handgun at all due to having been diagnosed as mentally deficient some four months earlier.

—*Mass shootings at Virginia Tech*, 2007.
(See *Law Fact* at the end of this chapter for the answer.)

Principles and Applications

The emotions surrounding the gun debate are volatile. This chapter attempts to rationally depict what each side has in common by discussing facts one cannot reasonably disagree with. Most of the data presented in this chapter are for the period 2005-2007, and are from the:

- Federal Bureau of Investigation's Supplementary Homicide Reports and its Uniform Crime Reporting Program (one-year time lag on crimes data)
- Center for Disease Control's National Vital Statistics System at the National Bureau for Health Statistics (more than a thirty-month time lag on deaths)
- Bureau of Justice Statistics National Crime Victimization Survey in the U.S. Department of Justice (two-year time lag)

Background and Context

Despite its status as an advanced, high-income country, the U.S. has some remarkable characteristics. For instance, while the U.S. is considered among the safest countries in the world in terms of avoiding personal harm or injury, deaths from gunshot wounds are astoundingly high (Wharton, 2005).

Data from the National Vital Statistics System, a public health data system that collects relevant vital statistics from death certificates, reveals that the number of children and teens killed by guns in the U.S. every year is more than the total number of American service men and women who have died in combat in Iraq and Afghanistan since those wars began in 2003; it is more than the total number of people killed in the 9/11 attacks in New York, Pennsylvania, and Washington, D.C. (CDF, 2007).

Estimates are that at least four to five times as many people suffer from firearms injuries as are killed by firearms, both from homicides and suicides, in the U.S. (CDF, 2007). The Consumer Product Safety Commission's National Electronic Injury Surveillance System (NEISS) is used to collect hospital emergency data on non-fatal firearm injuries, firearm assaults, and firearm suicides (NEISS Coding Manual, 2009).[LN1]

Since the U.S. first collected national data in 1979, gun violence has killed over 101,000 children and teens under the age of eighteen (NCHS, 2007). These 101,000 children and teens could fill over four thousand school classrooms. The 101,000 child and teen gun deaths total is more than the total number of American fatalities in all wars since World War II ended, including the Korean, Vietnam, Iraq, and Afghanistan conflicts (CDF, 2007).

America's large cities are experiencing an alarming number of homicides, mostly committed with firearms (Macinko & Marinho de Souza, 2006). The debate surrounds how to address these facts. One city, New York City (NYC), decided to attack the so-called iron pipeline of illegal guns by holding gun manufacturers, distributors, and dealers liable for crimes with illegal guns. This illegal gun litigation was pursued on the basis of the community's environmental safety.

ILLEGAL GUN SALES

City of New York v. A-1 Jewelry & Pawn, Inc. (A-1 Jewelry III)
[New York City v. Gun Dealer]
252 F.R.D. 130 (U.S. District Court for the Eastern District of New York 2008)

FACTS: In 2006, NYC sued twenty-seven gun dealers in Georgia, South Carolina, Virginia, Pennsylvania, and Ohio, claiming their lax screening practices and illegal gun sales created a public nuisance in the city.

ISSUE: Does gun violence constitute a public nuisance? If so, does such a public nuisance exist in NYC, and may gun dealers be held responsible for this nuisance as a result of illegal gun sales?

HOLDING AND DECISION: There is enough evidence to go forward with the case.

ANALYSIS: Twenty-six dealers settled with NYC and agreed to court appointment of a federal monitor to oversee gun sales at their stores. The twenty-seventh dealer moved for summary judgment, but this motion was denied in part because extensive discovery revealed at least seventy-two guns sold by this dealer were recovered in connection with criminal activity. A subsequent piece of the litigation found "A public nuisance exists in the City of New York, in the form of large numbers of illegally possessed firearms. Illegally possessed guns interfere with the health and safety of a large number of persons within the City." *See* 2008 WL 4298501 (U.S. District Court for the Eastern District of New York 2008).

RULE OF LAW: The exercise of personal jurisdiction over out-of-state dealers is appropriate and the sales practices of dealers can be considered a public nuisance.

The early evidence indicates this illegal gun litigation is having a positive effect on gun violence in NYC. At the same time, Congress passed the Protection of Lawful Commerce in Arms Act (PLCAA), 15 U.S.C.A. §§ 7901-7903 (2005), in response to NYC's threat of litigation with regards to illegal guns. PLCAA shields gun manufacturers, distributors, and dealers from civil liabilities arising from gun violence. *See A-1 Jewelry II*, 247 F.R.D. 296, 349-354 (U.S. District Court for the Eastern District of New York 2007) (denying a motion to dismiss on the grounds that this lawsuit was prohibited by the PLCAA).

A court filing in the *A-1 Jewelry III* case shows a 75 percent drop in illegal guns coming from a sample of the dealers sued. Between 2006 and 2007, there was a 16 percent drop in the number of guns used in crimes in NYC traced to any dealers in the states where the sued dealers were located. NYC's success may provide a model for other jurisdictions and may serve to influence Second Amendment jurisprudence.

Since 2003, Congress has blocked access to a federal database from the Bureau of Alcohol, Tobacco, Firearms, and Explosives (BATFE) that traces guns used in crimes back to particular dealers. *See* PL 110-161, 2007 HR 2764 (2007). NYC was able to file the Jewelry civil lawsuit using trace data collected before the ban. As time passes, that data will become less and less useful,

making it harder to stop gun dealers whose conduct results in gun violence. While there is concern that the Tiahrt Amendment restricts information needed by state and local authorities to control gun violence in their communities, the legislation has not been repealed.

Moral Dilemmas

1. Should Congress be permitted to use its appropriation strategies to restrict the collection of and access to federal databases used in injury prevention research and environmental safety litigation?

SECOND AMENDMENT JURISPRUDENCE

The flashpoint in the long running political debate over regulation of firearms is the Second Amendment to the U.S. Constitution, which states: "A well regulated militia, being necessary to the security of a free state, the right of the people to keep and bear arms shall not be infringed." Gun control proponents read the amendment as permitting regulation of firearms possession;

advocates of gun rights read it as enshrining in law an individual's unfettered right to own guns (Wharton, 2005). Although the right to own guns is not absolute, there are ways to achieve common goals without sacrificing the Second Amendment. There is not an absolute trade-off between gun control and gun rights.

In 2007, the U.S. Court of Appeals for the District of Columbia entered this debate and made history as the first federal appeals court to strike down a strict gun ban as a violation of the Second Amendment. The U.S. Supreme Court agreed to review this appellate decision on gun ban regulations.

The ruling by the U.S. Supreme Court in *Heller* further explained and made clear that individuals bore arms before the Second Amendment was ever adopted (NRA, 2008). This right to be armed pre-existed, like all individual rights in the Bill of Rights, except the Tenth Amendment. The Tenth Amendment speaks explicitly about the allocation

of governmental power. It reads as follows: "The powers not delegated to the United States by the Constitution, nor prohibited by it to the states, are reserved to the states respectively, or to the people." The ruling in *Heller* may help move the gun violence debate forward. If the nation as a whole should ultimately decide an individual right to be armed is ill advised, it can then amend the U.S. Constitution (Mocsary, 2003).

While the concept of the public good is often used to justify gun control, political trade-offs involving Second Amendment rights, indeed involving any of the people's rights, are rarely simple. Gun control laws remain controversial. While the assertion of an absolute right to guns often creates political deadlock, this stalemate changed slightly in favor of gun rights advocates with the U.S. Supreme Court decision in *Heller*. Gun rights adherents rely on the fact that the Second Amendment mentions "people," while those espousing gun control rely on the presence of "militia" to limit individual rights (Mocsary,

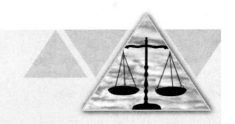

REGULATION OF FIREARMS

District of Columbia et al. v. Heller
[Nation's Capitol v. Special Police Officer]
128 S.Ct. 2783 (U.S. Supreme Court 2008)

FACTS: A District gun ban prohibits ownership of guns without a license and requires all registered firearms to be kept in an inoperable condition. Dick Heller, a special police officer, was denied a license to keep a handgun at his home based on the District's gun ban. He claimed he had a Second Amendment right to possess guns for self-defense in his home.

ISSUE: Did the District's gun ban violate the Second Amendment right of individuals who wish to keep guns for private use in their homes?

HOLDING AND DECISION: Yes, the District's gun ban violated the rights bestowed on individuals under the Second Amendment.

ANALYSIS: Heller, who had no association with any militia, challenged the District's gun ban; he did not assert a right to carry weapons outside his home, nor did he challenge the District's authority to require the registration of firearms. As a special police officer, he was authorized to carry a handgun

while on duty, but he also wanted to keep a gun in his home for self-defense purposes.

The Court extensively analyzed the precedent, text, and history of the Second Amendment and held that the amendment granted an individual right to bear arms, subject to reasonable restrictions. The District gun ban was struck down as unconstitutional. The District ban reduced some modern-day categories of guns to the point of being useless, and unconstitutionally prohibited the lawful use of guns for self-defense.

RULE OF LAW: General gun bans on private possession of handguns for self-defense violate the Second Amendment. However, gun control laws prohibiting felons or the mentally ill from possessing firearms, prohibiting possession in sensitive areas such as schools and government buildings, and regulating sales of firearms remain permissible.

(*See generally* Borgmann, 2009; Burkett, 2008; Card 2009; Chemerinsky, 2009; Kaufman, 2009; Kessler, 2009; Neily, 2008; Tushnet, 2008; Weisselberg, 2007).

2003). As the gun violence in America, with its attendant costs of health care, continues to escalate, Americans may ultimately decide their individual right to be armed should be balanced against the costs to society arising from near-unfettered exercise of that right.

In an earlier case, a divided U.S. Supreme Court declared the Gun-Free School Zones law unconstitutional. The Court held that Congress had overstepped its Commerce Clause power in passing the law. In so doing, a nationwide debate between gun rights and gun control advocates began that continues to this day.

ENFORCEMENT OF EXISTING GUN CONTROL LAWS

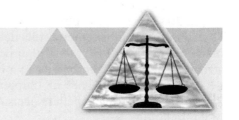

United States v. Lopez
[U.S. Government v. High School Student]
514 U.S. 549 (U.S. Supreme Court 1995)

FACTS: Alfonso Lopez, Jr., a senior high school student from Texas, was convicted of violating the federal Gun-Free School Zones law after carrying a concealed handgun and bullets to school.

ISSUE: Can Congress make a federal crime out of handgun possession in the vicinity of a school?

HOLDING AND DECISION: No, the federal Gun-Free School Zones law was beyond the scope of the commerce power.

ANALYSIS: The Court started its analysis by tracing the constitutional history of the Commerce Clause. While acknowledging the power of Congress had been expanded under the Commerce Clause, the Court noted this power was still subject to limits. The Court then identified three broad activities Congress may regulate under its commerce power:

- Use of the channels of interstate commerce
- Protection of the instrumentalities of interstate commerce, or persons in interstate commerce, even though that threat may come only from intrastate activities
- Activities substantially related to or substantially affecting interstate commerce

While the Court stated that the Gun-Free School Zones law could only be upheld as a regulation of an activity in the third category, it found the law had nothing to do with commerce or any other economic activity. Therefore, the law was not a legitimate regulation of commercial transactions affecting interstate commerce. The Court further found the possession of a handgun in a local school zone was not an economic activity that might substantially affect any sort of interstate commerce.

The Court pointed out that the legislative history of the Gun-Free School Zones law did not contain any legislative findings regarding the economic effects of handgun possession in a local school zone. Such findings are considered part of the Court's independent evaluation of the constitutionality of legislation enacted under the Commerce Clause. Future gun regulations, containing such findings, might convince the Court that gun possession substantially affects interstate commerce.

The Court held that the interstate effects of the costs of crime could not justify the Gun-Free School Zones law; otherwise, Congress could regulate not only all violent crimes, but all activities that might lead to violent crime. Nor could the law be upheld on a national productivity theory that guns in schools pose threats to the educational process, and thus lead to a less productive citizenry. If such a finding could justify a wielding of the commerce power, the Court held that Congress could then directly regulate any activity found to be related to the economic productivity of individuals. The Court could not accept these arguments, stating it would be hard pressed to posit any activity Congress was without power to regulate under this line of reasoning.

The Court ultimately found the Gun-Free School Zones law to be inconsistent with the federalist structure of the U.S. Constitution. To expand the commerce power of Congress to enact the law would require the Court to conclude there will never be a distinction between what is truly national and what is truly local. This it was unwilling to do.

RULE OF LAW: Congress cannot federalize prosecution of local and state firearms offenses.

(*See generally* Laughlin, 2005).

The question is whether the current Court will permit local governments to place reasonable restrictions on the individual right to bear arms within the zone of possibilities left open by *Lopez*. Environmental safety researchers (and cynics alike) note federal databases from the BATFE, the CDC, and the NEISS subsequent to this decision suddenly became severely restricted (GAO, 2008). The recent U.S. Supreme Court ruling in *Heller* left the door open for accepting reasonable gun control legislation, especially if supported by findings of fact regarding the epidemiology of gun violence. Debates about this epidemiology are just beginning to emerge in the lower courts.

THE EPIDEMIOLOGY OF GUN VIOLENCE

Research studies of gun violence in the U.S. come at this subject from a number of health care perspectives, including the costs of health care (AMA, 2007). Yet, other costs are more difficult to quantify (Lemaire, 2005), including:

- Lost productivity of victims and changes in the quality of life
- Cost of public resources devoted to law enforcement
- Private investment by individuals in protection and avoidance
- Limits on freedom to live or work in certain places
- Restrictions on residential and commercial location decisions
- Limitations in hours of operation of retail establishments
- Emotional costs to the forced adaptation to increased risk
- Cost of pain and fear

(Lemaire, 2005)

The aggregate cost of gun violence in the U.S. is estimated at approximately $100 billion annually, or approximately $360 per capita (Wharton, 2005). This is the same aggregate cost as smoking, obesity, and other preventable behaviors and conditions (Thorpe et al., 2007). Put another way, the equivalent of $720 per American is spent each year that could be avoided, with healthier lifestyle choices as a society.

Reduced Life Expectancy

Life expectancy is considered one of the best measures of quality of life when evaluating health care decisions. This measure summarizes in a single number all individual and external damages affecting a person (Lemaire, 2005). Life expectancy is affected by numerous individual and external factors, for instance, unhealthy nutrition, high-risk sexual behavior, defective family genes, accident history, limited access to high-quality health care, proximity to environmental degradation, poor social-economic status, civic violence, and wars. In addition, the life expectancy measure is not affected by age distribution, so it is an appropriate epidemiological tool for comparing different populations with dissimilar age structures. The question is how Americans compare to other countries in terms of life expectancy. The unfortunate answer is that Americans do not measure up very well.

In 2006, the life expectancy of Americans was seventy-eight years, or two years less than other similar, high-income countries around the world (WHO, 2008). From a country with the world's highest expenditures on health care ($6,037 annual per capita, the U.S. ranks twenty-eighth in life expectancy (Thorpe et al., 2007).

Key 2006 Statistics: Global Life Expectancies
- Japan: eighty-three years, the world's highest life expectancy and considered the safest country in the world
- Andorra, Australia, Belgium, Monoraco, San Marino, and Switzerland: eighty-two years
- Canada, France, Iceland, Israel, Italy, Spain, Sweden, and the United Kingdom: eighty-one years
- Cyprus, Germany, Greece, Ireland, Luxemburg, Netherlands, New Zealand, Norway, and Singapore: eighty years
- Belgium, Denmark, Finland, Portugal, South Korea: seventy-nine years
- Chile, Costa Rica, Cuba, Kuwait, Slovenia, United Arab Emirates, U.S.: seventy-eight years

(WHO, 2008)

One might ask what the U.S. has in common with Slovenia, Kuwait, United Arab Emirates, and Chile (four countries that have experienced civil war, domestic terrorism, and/or civil unrest during this generation). Each country spends significantly less on health care than the U.S., so similar health care expenditures on a per capita basis does not appear to be the right response (WHO, 2008).

Firearms are not used uniformly in the U.S. Evidence of this can be derived from the striking data on the life expectancy of African American males in the U.S. (Krieger et al., 2005). African American males live eleven years less than most Americans, or sixty-seven years versus seventy-eight years (Kung, 2008). This begs the question: what creates this difference in life expectancies?

Is there the possibility that environmental safety influences life expectancy in the U.S.? Several respected research studies at Harvard University and the University of Pennsylvania have analyzed the impact on typical American life expectancy due to violent behavior, specifically violence from firearms.

Availability of Firearms in Relationship to Life Expectancy

The Public Health Disparities Geocoding Project at Harvard University found both life expectancies and firearm deaths to be unevenly dispersed throughout the U.S. population. The disparity in firearm deaths for African American males, however, was prominent (Krieger et al., 2005).

A research study at the Insurance and Risk Management Department at The Wharton School of the University of Pennsylvania found both firearm homicides and suicides reduce life expectancy by an average of 104 days. Broken down by race and gender, however, there are notable gaps in how various groups fare (Lemaire, 2005).

African American men face almost four times the rate of death from gun violence as other groups of Americans, or thirty-seven deaths per 100,000 compared to ten deaths per 100,000:

- African American men lose more than twice as many days of life from gun violence as white men: 361 v. 151 days of life
- African American men lose more than ten times the days lost by white women from gun violence: 361 v. 3 days of life

In addition, firearm homicides and suicides kill mostly young people:

- African American males are killed by guns at a younger average age than white males
- African American men on average are twenty-eight years of age at their death from firearm homicides, as compared to thirty-two for white males
- African American males commit suicide, on average, when they are thirty-seven years of age, as compared to forty-nine for white males

To put these statistics into context among all fatal injuries, only motor vehicle accidents have a greater effect on life expectancy than firearm deaths (Lemaire, 2005).

The same Wharton research study analyzed how much more Americans pay for their health benefit plans as a result of the reduced life expectancy from gun violence. Victims of gun violence are more likely to need medical treatment requiring high payouts from the insurance industry; this, in turn, raises the costs of the state risk pools,[LN2] thereby raising costs for everyone participating in the pools. The annual

medical costs ascribed to gun-related injuries are $2 billion to $2.3 billion (Lemaire, 2005). The average cost per gunshot victim, excluding rehabilitative and long-term care, is $45,000 (CDF, 2007). This means the state risk pools must therefore add an additional $2 billion to $2.3 billion to cover the anticipated costs of treating victims of gun violence. About half of this is borne by taxpayers (CDF, 2007).

An additional $2.4 billion in estimated costs is needed for administering the criminal justice system due to gun deaths, including incarceration costs for the perpetrators of gun violence (Lemaire, 2005). In short, this means the total direct cost of gun violence in the U.S. is between $4.4 and $4.7 billion each year.

Moral Dilemmas

1. Can regulation and control of firearms be an effective strategy in reducing health care costs in the U.S.?

The Substitution Effect

One objection to the idea that reducing firearm deaths would increase life expectancy and reduce health care costs is the argument that guns are simply a means to an end. In other words, people who are intent on violence, either toward themselves or others, will find a way to achieve that objective with whatever tools are available. This is called the substitution effect (Wharton, 2005). The question then becomes whether Americans are necessarily more violent than the Japanese or the Europeans. Certainly history shows violence is not unique to Americans.

While Japan generated more than its fair share of violence in the twentieth century, today it is among the safest countries in the world and has some of the world's strictest gun control restrictions. With few handguns in Japan, crimes committed with firearms are low. Japan also has an extremely low rate of thefts and burglaries (Ajdacic-Gross et al., 2006). This is a counterweight to the gun rights adherents' substitution effect argument that guns at home reduce property crimes. The failure of the substitution effect is apparent in Japan and might also be in the U.S.; at least, there is no obvious reason why it should not be.

Of course, some skeptics will argue it is the cultural differences in these two affluent democracies accounting for the difference in violence between Japan and the U.S., not simply the lack of accessibility to guns in Japan. Japan is very much a paternalistic, collective society and American society is more individualistic with a deeply ingrained sense of a right to self-defense and duty to protect property.

No gun control policies are going to change this cultural difference.

The question remains, however, what cultural factors explain the cross-country differences in violence between the U.S. and Japan? There is empirical support for many economic and social factors (demographics, ethnic diversity, education, income, inequality, deterrence, and the like), but it is not clear why such cultural factors would explain the large difference in violence between the U.S. and Japan, nor is it clear how these factors can explain the existing patterns of gun availability, gun control, and violence (Ajdacic-Gross et al., 2006).

The Substitution Effect Does Not Affect Firearm Homicides

Moreover, a number of research studies show that, in the area of homicides, there is little or no substitution effect (Wharton, 2005). There is a positive correlation between the rate of household gun ownership and the national rate of homicides, as well as the proportion of homicides committed with a gun (Lemaire, 2005). One study, by the University of Washington's Department of Surgery, contrasted two cities with nearly identical climates, populations, unemployment levels, and average income: Seattle, Washington, with relaxed gun control laws, and Vancouver, British Columbia, with strict gun controls. As a result of far stricter gun laws in Canada:

- Gun ownership by residents: 12 percent in Vancouver compared to 41 percent in Seattle
- Burglary, robbery, homicide, and assault rates without a gun: same
- Assault rates with a firearm: Seattle is seven times higher than in Vancouver
- Homicide rates with a handgun: Seattle is almost five times higher

(Sloan et al., 1988)

The conclusions of this research study were threefold:

- The availability of handguns in Seattle increased the assault and homicide rates with a gun
- The availability of handguns does not decrease the rate of crimes without guns
- Restrictive handgun laws reduced the homicide rate in Vancouver

(Sloan et al., 1988; *see also* Wharton, 2005)

A Swiss study from the University of Lausanne compared gun ownership in eleven European countries, Australia, Canada, and the U.S., and suggested gun ownership increases the likelihood of homicides, but found little or no substitution effect in the area of homicides. The research study concluded:

- High correlation between gun ownership rates and homicide rates, as well as the proportions of homicides committed with handguns
- Little or no correlation between guns and the rates of homicide committed by other means
- Other means were not used in homicides to compensate for the absence of guns in countries with a lower rate of gun ownership

(Killias, 1993)

A third comparative study by the Pacific Institute for Research and Evaluation in California also found the substitution effect does not affect firearm crimes. Firearms were involved in 50 percent of the assaults in the U.S., compared to only 8 percent in New Zealand, where there is strict regulation of guns (Spicer, 2005).

Finally, researchers at the Firearm and Injury Center at the University of Pennsylvania's Department of Surgery found gun violence generally declines after implementation of strict gun control laws (Macinko & Marinho de Souza, 2007). When the Center researchers looked at evidence from Brazil, a country with even greater levels of gun violence than the U.S. before Brazil strictly regulated handguns, they found that:

- A significant portion of the declines in firearm-related deaths and hospitalizations in Brazil were reasonably attributed to measures reducing the availability of firearms
- Strengthening the capacity of local law enforcement to enforce gun control measures affected the decline in gun violence

Recent gun legislation and other handgun reduction policies in Brazil reduced gun violence. Moreover, these improvements were not offset by homicides committed using other weapons. In late 2005, Brazilians voted to reject a complete ban on firearms. Thus, Brazil may serve as an important example of how the U.S. might address pervasive gun violence while maintaining private ownership of firearms.

Evidence of a Substitution Effect for Suicides

In the case of suicides, there is greater evidence of a substitution effect. The reduced availability of one method of suicide prompts an increase in other methods. The reduced availability of handguns prompted an increase in suicides by poisoning, suffocation, cuts, crashes, and jumps (Killias, 1993).

Indeed, in places like Japan and Hong Kong, suicide rates exceed the U.S. suicide rate, despite strictly limited access to firearms. Less than 1 percent of suicides in Japan and Hong Kong are committed with a firearm, whereas more than half the suicides in the U.S. are committed with a firearm. In addition, Norway, the United Kingdom, Canada, Australia, and New Zealand all experienced a decline in firearm suicides since the 1980s as the level of gun ownership continued to decline with stricter gun controls in place (Ajdacic-Gross et al., 2006).

The Substitution Effect Does Not Affect Life Expectancy

The substitution effect hardly changes the number of life expectancy days lost due to guns in the U.S. The average American loses from 96 to 104 days of life expectancy due to guns (Lemaire, 2005). At the same time, the U.S. health care industry spends billions to extend lives, often for medical treatments that sometimes offer Americans less than 96 to 104 extra days of life. Most Americans are willing to pay a lot for this extra life expectancy; many are willing to pay anything. When debates about extending life expectancy center on the costs of gun violence, however, emotional debates about the Second Amendment keep Americans from seeking common ground on the question of how to best address this public health problem.

Regardless, the evidence on life expectancies should stimulate further debate over whether regulation of firearms can be an effective strategy in reducing gun violence in the U.S. The estimate is that there are more than 220 million guns in America (Wellford et al., 2004); thus, it is extremely unlikely anyone will move to confiscate guns, nor should the U.S. necessarily ban guns. Therefore, the question for public health officials is how the U.S. can best reasonably and responsibly regulate and control the use of all these guns.

PREMIUM ADJUSTMENTS IN HEALTH BENEFIT PLANS

There may be potential opportunities in how the insurance industry can better price, and perhaps more equitably distribute, the cost of the risks associated with guns. Just owning a handgun significantly increases the chance of dying from gun violence, even when neighborhood variables are controlled. One logical thread to pursue is the risk calculations the insurance industry makes in pricing health benefits. Demographics and lifestyle choices are the bread and butter of risk calculations, but gun ownership is not yet a factor (Wharton, 2005). Yet, gun violence in the U.S.:

- Kills about 44,000 adults and children every year (121 deaths per day)
- Results in 135,000 to 168,000 non-fatal firearm injuries each year (nineteen injuries every hour)
- Shortens the life expectancy of an average American by 96 to 104 days (151 days for white males and 362 days for African American males)

(WISQARS, 2009)

The increased insurance premiums paid by Americans as a result of gun violence are probably on the same order of magnitude as the increased tax dollars collected to cover the total medical costs due to gunshots or the increased costs of administering the criminal justice system due to gun crime (Lemaire, 2005).

The Second Amendment right to bear arms comes with a price; someone must pay the multibillion-dollar cost of gun violence. The question is how to best balance this cost in the controversy between gun rights adherents and gun control proponents within the national debate on health care reform. Gun violence is a public health issue that can be resolved; the question is how. This is one national debate that will ideally continue until it is satisfactorily resolved.

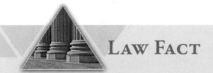

LAW FACT

GUN VIOLENCE

How can the risk of gun violence be reduced on college and university campuses?

The introduction of a gun into any act of aggression makes the resulting violence potentially lethal regardless of what gun control laws are in place. Government has a responsibility to its citizens to enforce the gun control laws preventing the purchase of handguns by those suffering from mental illness; only twenty-two states report any mental health information to the FBI's National Instant Check System (NICS) for firearms transactions (Flannery, 2008).

—Mass shootings at Virginia Tech, 2007.

CHAPTER SUMMARY

- The individual practice of bearing arms pre-existed long before the right to be armed was (arguably) made explicit in the Second Amendment of the U.S. Constitution.
- Whereas the Second Amendment right to own guns is not absolute, gun rights adherents read the Amendment as enshrining an individual's right to own guns, while gun control proponents read it as permitting the regulation of firearms possession, and neither side of the debate identifies or acknowledges goals in common with the other side.
- The cost of gun violence in the U.S. is approximately $100 billion annually, while smoking, obesity, and other preventable behaviors and conditions cost another $100 billion annually; these are expenditures that could be avoided simply by healthier lifestyle choices.
- Life expectancy is one of the best epidemiological measures of quality of life when evaluating health care decisions; it measures all the individual and external damages affecting a person.
- Although the U.S. spends more on health care than any other country in the world, Americans rank twenty-eighth in life expectancy at seventy-eight years.
- If the average American has the same life expectancy as people in Chile, Kuwait, Slovenia, and the United Arab Emirates (four countries who have experienced civil war, domestic terrorism, and/or civil unrest during this generation), then gun violence in the U.S. may possibly explain some of this similarity in life expectancies.
- Life expectancies and firearm deaths are unevenly distributed throughout the U.S. population; however, the disparity in firearm deaths for African American males is striking, with African American males living, on average, eleven years less than other groups of Americans.
- African American men are four times more likely to die from gun violence than other groups of Americans, at the rate of thirty-seven deaths per one hundred thousand, compared to the U.S. average of ten.
- Firearm homicides and suicides reduce life expectancy in the U.S. by an average of 104 days.
- There are notable gaps in how various groups fare when comparing life expectancies, with firearm homicides and suicides killing mostly young people; only motor vehicle accidents have a stronger effect on life expectancy than firearm deaths.
- Americans pay about $2 billion in additional costs for their health benefits as a result of reduced life expectancy from gun violence; victims of gun violence are more likely to need medical treatment requiring high payouts from the insurance industry, which in turn raises the costs of the risk pool, thereby raising costs for everyone in the pool.
- One objection to the suggestion that reducing gun violence would increase life expectancy, which would reduce the costs of health benefits, is the argument that guns are simply a means to an end; people intent on violence will achieve their objective with or without firearms, a phenomenon called the substitution effect.
- One counterweight to the substitution effect argument that fewer guns reduce property crimes is Japan's tight gun restrictions and its extremely low rate of thefts and burglaries.
- Rates of household gun ownership are proportional to the rates of homicides and the proportion of homicides committed with a gun.
- There is some evidence of a substitution effect on suicides; the reduced availability of handguns prompts an increase in suicides by other methods.
- The substitution effect hardly changes the number of life expectancy days lost due to guns in the U.S., with Americans losing from 96 to 104 days of life expectancy due to guns.
- While it is extremely unlikely anyone will move to confiscate all 220 million guns in America, nor should the U.S. necessarily ban guns, the question is, how can all these guns be best regulated and controlled?

LAW NOTES

1. During the Bush presidency, national data was severely restricted on non-fatal injuries resulting from gun violence (Schwab et al., 2007). The federal Consumer Product Safety Commission advised hospital emergency rooms to discontinue collecting data on non-fatal firearm injuries, firearm assaults, and attempted suicides with firearms. At the same time, the 2008 NEISS Coding Manual advised hospitals the CDC would be collecting this information. The CDC, however, only collected this data on children under the age of eighteen. The 2009 NEISS Coding Manual returned to collecting this gun violence information. It should be noted, however, that following failed attempts to eliminate the CDC's National Center for Injury Prevention and Control, Congress effectively gagged the CDC from pursuing any injury-prevention research for years

(Wellford et al., 2004). Similar appropriation strategies also restricted access to data on access and use of gun crime trace data and federal firearms licenses from the BATFE during the Bush presidency (GAO, 2008).

2. Risk pools are special programs created by most state legislatures to provide a safety net for the medically uninsurable population. Victims of gun violence are often denied health insurance coverage because of their pre-existing gun-related injuries or can only access private health insurance coverage that is restricted or has extremely high rates. Some state-owned nonprofit associations assess all health insurance carriers, HMOs, and other health insurance providers to cover their costs; others provide an appropriation from state general tax revenue; some states share funding of loss subsidies with the health insurance industry, using an assessment, and providing them a tax credit for the assessment; while other states have a special funding source, such as a tobacco tax or a hospital or health care provider surcharge. For the sixteen states without risk pools, the medically uninsured are part of the uninsured population facing financial devastation in the event of catastrophic injuries.

Chapter Bibliography

Ajdacic-Gross, V. et al. (2006). Changing times: A longitudinal analysis of international firearm suicide data. *American Journal of Public Health, 96* (10), 1752-1755 (updating the Swedish research with Killias as co-author).

AMA (American Medical Association). (2007). *Report of the Council on Science and Public Health.* Chicago, IL: AMA.

Borgmann, C. E. (2009). Holding legislatures constitutionally accountable through facial challenges. *Hastings Constitutional Law Quarterly, 36,* 563-610.

Brady Campaign to Prevent Gun Violence, et al. (2008, February 15). *Joint press release: Statement of national gun violence prevention organizations in wake of Northern Illinois University shooting.* Washington, DC: Brady, Coalition to Stop Gun Violence and Violence Policy Center.

Burkett, M. (2008). Much ado about . . . something else: *D.C. v. Heller,* the racialized mythology of the Second Amendment, and gun policy reform. *Journal of Gender, Race & Justice, 12,* 57-105.

Card, R. L. (2009). An opinion without standards: The Supreme Court's refusal to adopt a standard of constitutional review in *District of Columbia v. Heller* will likely cause headaches for future judicial review of gun-control regulations. *Brigham Young University Journal of Public Law, 23,* 259-287 (review of opposing federal circuit decisions leading up to the *Heller* decision by the U.S. Supreme Court).

CDF (Children's Defense Fund). (2007). *Protect children, not guns.* Washington, DC: CDF.

Chemerinsky, E. (2009), The Second Amendment and gun control. *Touro Law Review, 25,* 695-702.

Christoffel, K. K. et al. (2000, March 1). Youth violence prevention: The physician's role. *Journal of the American Medical Association, 283* (9), 1202-1203.

Engel, B. (2003). HIPAA: Regulation of theft from healthcare programs is within Congress's Commerce Clause authority: *United States vs. Whited. American Journal of Law & Medicine, 29,* 139-141.

Flannery, John P. (2008). Students died at Virginia Tech because our government failed to act! *George Mason University Civil Rights Law Journal, 18,* 285-304.

Fox, J. A. (2007). *Homicide trends in the U.S.* Washington, DC: U.S. Department of Justice, Bureau of Justice Statistics.

GAO (U.S. Government Accounting Office). (2008). *Centers for Disease Control and Prevention: Changes in obligations and activities before and after fiscal year 2005 budget reorganization.* Washington, DC: GAO.

Healy, G. (2003, May 1). Project safe neighborhoods and fair-weather federalism: "Saving" the Second Amendment by undermining the Tenth. *Engage, 4* (1), 40-43.

HHS (U.S. Department of Health & Human Services). (2007). *Report to the President on issues raised by the Virginia Tech tragedy presented to President George W. Bush.* Washington, DC: HHS.

Kaufman, E. (2009). The Second Amendment: An Analysis of *District of Columbia v. Heller. Tuoro Law Review, 25,* 703-724.

Kessler, D. K. (2009). Free to leave? An empirical look at the Fourth Amendment's seizure standard, *Journal of Criminal Law & Criminology, 99,* 51-88.

Killias, M. (1993). International correlations between gun ownership and rates of homicide and suicide. *Canadian Medical Association Journal, 148* (10), 1721-1725.

Krieger, N. et al. (2005). Painting a truer picture of U.S. socioeconomic and racial/ethnic health inequalities: The Public Health Disparities Geocoding Project. *American Journal of Public Health, 95,* 312-323.

Kung, H-C. (2008). *56* (10), 1-121. Atlanta, GA: Centers for Disease Control.

Laughlin, C. (2005). Recent developments in health law: U.S. Supreme Court hears oral arguments in *Ashcroft v. Raich* background. *Journal of Law, Medicine & Ethics , 33,* 396-399.

Lemaire, J. (2005). The cost of firearm deaths in the U.S.: Reduced life expectancies and increased insurance costs. *Journal of Risk & Insurance, 72* (3), 359-374.

Macinko, J., & Marinho de Souza, M. (2007). Reducing firearm injury: Lessons from Brazil. *Leonard Davis Institute Issue Brief, 12* (7), 1-4. Philadelphia, PA:. Wharton School at the University of Pennsylvania.

Mass shootings at Virginia Tech: Report of the review panel presented to Governor Timothy M. Kaine, Commonwealth of Virginia. (2007, August). Richmond, VA.

McNamara, N. K., & Findling, R. L. (2008). Guns, adolescents, and mental illness. *American Journal of Psychiatry, 165,* 190-194.

Mocsary, G. A. (2003). Explaining away the obvious: The infeasibility of characterizing the Second Amendment as a non-individual right. *Fordham Law Review, 76,* 2113-2175.

___. (2007, October 15). *State "emergency powers" vs. the right-to-arms.* Fairfax, VA: NRA.

NCIS (National Center for Health Statistics). (2009). *Health statistics for the U.S. population: National Health Interview Survey*. Atlanta, GA: Centers for Disease Control: NCIS.

Neily, C. (2008). *District of Columbia v. Heller*: The Second Amendment is back, baby. *Cato Supreme Court Review, 2008,* 127-159.

NEISS (National Electronic Injury Surveillance System). (2008). *Coding manual*. Washington, DC: Consumer Product Safety Commission.

NRA (National Rifle Association. (2008, May 6). *Right-to-carry-2008 fact sheet*. Fairfax, VA: NRA.

Schwab, C. W. et al. (2007). Censored: Data, research, action. *FICP Quarterly, 3* (2). Philadelphia, PA: Firearm & Injury Center at the University of Pennsylvania.

Sloan, J. H. et al. (1988). Handgun regulations, crime assaults and homicide: A tale of two cities. *New England Journal of Medicine, 319,* 1256-1262.

Spicer, R. (2005). Comparison of injury case fatality rates in the U.S. and New Zealand. *Injury Prevention, 11* (2), 71-76.

Thorpe, K. E. et al. (2007). Differences in disease prevalence as a source of the U.S.-European health care spending gap. *Health Affairs, 26* (6), 678-686.

Tushnet, M. (2008). *Heller* and the critique of judgment. *Supreme Court Review, 2009,* 61-86.

U.S. Surgeon General's Report. (2001). *Youth violence*. Washington, DC: U.S. Department of Health & Human Services.

Weiner, J. et al. (2007). Reducing firearm violence: A research agenda. *Injury Prevention, 13,* 80-84.

Weisselberg, C. D. (2007). Selected criminal law cases in the Supreme Court's 2007-2008 term, and a look ahead. *Court Review, 44,* 90-95.

Wellford, C. F. et al. (2004). *Firearms and violence: A critical review*. Washington, DC: Committee on Law & Justice, National Research Council of the National Academies.

Wharton School at the University of Pennsylvania. (2005). Insurance, life expectancy and the cost of firearm deaths in the U.S. *Knowledge@Wharton*.

WHO (World Health Organization). (2008). *Violence and injury prevention*. Geneva, Switzerland: WHO.

WISQARS (Web-based Injury Statistics Query and Reporting System). (2009, June). Special Data Request. Atlanta, GA: Centers for Disease Control & Prevention National Center for Injury Prevention & Control.

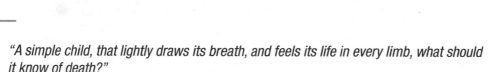

CHAPTER 38

PREVENTION OF CHILD ABUSE AND NEGLECT

> "A simple child, that lightly draws its breath, and feels its life in every limb, what should it know of death?"
>
> — WILLIAM WORDSWORTH (1770-1850), BRITISH POET LAUREATE

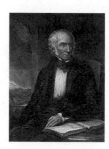

IN BRIEF

Child abuse and neglect are complex problems with no simple solutions. This chapter starts by examining survival-threatening physical abuse, psychological maltreatment, and sexual abuse of children from a clinical perspective, rather than from the management perspective that the rest of this textbook adopts. Particular attention is directed to neglect, specifically medical neglect.

While anyone who suspects child abuse or neglect arguably has a moral duty to report it, all fifty states have mandatory reporting laws requiring reporters (such as physicians, dentists, and employees working in the health care sector) to officially report suspected abuse and neglect of children to child welfare officials. There is no discretion or other options about reporting maltreatment for mandatory reporters; immediate reporting is obligatory. In many jurisdictions, mandatory reporters can be liable for a child's survival-threatening injuries or death when abuse and neglect should have been suspected but was implicit.

Protection of children is paramount for anyone working in health care, with mandatory reporters being held to a higher standard of understanding the expressions of a battered and neglected child; there is a duty to understand the unspoken, to not merely rely on overt statements by children and involved adults. For health care professionals, it is important to be familiar with the clinical issues in this chapter and have the awareness to suspect and report child abuse or neglect when appropriate.

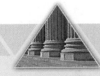

FACT OR FICTION

MEDICAL NEGLECT

Who gets to decide between competing Western medicine and alternative medical options for minor children in need of diagnostic care?

A sixteen-year-old high school student suffered from menorrhagia for two years before presenting herself to Children's Hospital for treatment. Recurring iron deficiency, or anemia, caused various symptoms, including shortness of breath, rapid heart rate, hair loss, fatigue, lightheadedness, and headaches. The parents provided her with iron supplementation and other alternative medical therapies, but had never before sought care from the Western medical establishment.

At Children's Hospital, it was recommended the student undergo blood tests and an ultrasound scan to properly diagnosis her condition. Controversy ensued when the child missed her follow-up appointment and the Children's Hospital determined the child's health was at risk without a proper diagnosis. At this point, there was disagreement between the parents and Children's Hospital over the most effective course of action needed to treat their daughter. The parents refused to consent to diagnostic testing. Children's Hospital charged the parents with child abuse and neglect, and child protective services began a complete investigation of the family, temporarily removing the child to foster care. The parents then applied to the courts to regain custody of their daughter and control over her medical treatment, asserting their parental prerogative to care for their daughter in accordance with their cultural traditions and their ability to pay for Western medical care.

Both parents were subsequently charged with medical neglect. The parents challenged the charges against them on multiple grounds, including a claim that criminal laws could not constitutionally punish them for choosing alternative methods of treatment for their daughter on non-religious grounds. The parents maintained they always sought their daughter's best interests and shared the goal with Children's Hospital of pursuing the treatment most likely to return her to health.

—Hypothetical case synopsis.
(See *Law Fact* at the end of this chapter for the answer.)

PRINCIPLES AND APPLICATIONS

Reported instances of child abuse are increasing dramatically in the U.S; there are many indications the rate of sexual abuse of children is growing as well. *See Kennedy v. Louisiana*, 128 S.Ct. 2641, 2669-70 (U.S. Supreme Court 2008) (Justice Alito, with whom Chief Justice Roberts, Justice Scalia, and Justice Thomas join dissenting). The children who most desperately need help are the ones whose very lives are at stake because of the lethal severity of their abuse. The repetitive nature of child abuse predetermines that if a child is not fully protected the first time survival-threatening maltreatment occurs, the abuse and neglect will not only continue but will become more severe.

Use of the term *survival-threatening* reflects the reality that even if the initial injury is not life-threatening, it may nonetheless be survival-threatening, since the abuse is almost certain to escalate in the future. Thus, if society does not act to protect a child at the time abuse begins, there may not be a second

chance. In fact, the only way to ensure the future protection of a child who suffers the first incidence of survival-threatening abuse is to remove the child immediately and perhaps permanently from the home environment (Sege & Flaherty, 2008).

INCIDENCE OF MALTREATMENT

The true incidence of child abuse and neglect in the U.S. is unknown (Jenny & Isaac, 2006). According to the most recent data from the National Child Abuse and Neglect Data System, approximately one million children are victims of serious child abuse or neglect each year, as measured by verified cases reported to state child protective agencies. The true incidence is probably closer to over eleven million children (*e.g.* Crume et al., 2002; Schnitzer et al., 2008). In addition, approximately 7 percent of all abused children suffer serious psychological maltreatment, while some form of neglect is found in approximately

80 percent of all child abuse cases. Moreover, more than three million children are traumatized as indirect victims of domestic abuse by witnessing the physical violence perpetrated against their siblings or between their parents (APA, 2005). In this chapter, the term *parents* is generically used, but the term is understood to include step-parents, guardians, live-in friends of a parent, or any other adult caregiver in a child's household.

The health care system does not adequately assess the circumstances surrounding child fatalities. Anywhere from half (Crume et al., 2002) to 90 percent (Schnitzer et al., 2008) of the children dying from maltreatment are not reported by health care professionals familiar and in touch with the families before a child's life-threatening injuries or death occurs. Child death review teams found most maltreatment fatalities were misidentified in emergency rooms and physician offices as attributable to accidents, natural causes, or other unknown causes. Children in medical settings are not being protected from abuse and neglect as required by the law of all fifty states. Mandatory reports are not being made to child welfare services for investigation of suspected abuse and neglect of children when their families seek medical care. Instead, many health care professionals are implicitly enabling abuse to be hidden; rather than intervening and advocating for the children they are medically treating, providers are helping to conceal the symptoms of abuse and neglect that is generally out of sight to others.

Ten years ago, approximately six hundred children were identified as being killed by their parents (ACF, 2004). By 2006, the estimate exceeded 1,500 child fatalities per year (ACF, 2008). Since stress, derived from economic hardship and conflict between parents, leads to increased maltreatment, these numbers can only be expected to increase (Moore et al., 2007). Assuming the research by Crume (et al., 2002) and Schnitzer (et al., 2008) is correct; eight to thirty-six children are actually killed each day by their parents. According to the National Child Abuse and Neglect Data System, over three-quarters of these children were under four years of age and almost one-half had not reached their first birthday. Eighty-four percent of children who died were abused by only one of their parents, while 17 percent suffered abuse at the hands of both parents (APA, 2005).

The U.S. Supreme Court also noted underreporting is a common problem with respect to child sexual abuse, finding most female rape victims under the age of eighteen did not disclose their abuse to authorities (*see Kennedy*, 128 S.Ct. at 2663). The most commonly cited reasons for nondisclosure were loyalty, emotional bond, and fear of negative consequences

for the rapist, especially where the rapist was a family member (Goodman-Brown, et al., 2003).

Child abuse may involve repeated abuse over a period of time (battered child syndrome), or it may involve a single, impulsive incident (Maikovich et al., 2008). More than three-fourths of all child abuse perpetrators were the parents of the child victim. *The Handbook of Clinical Child Psychology* describes parents beating, biting, squeezing, lacerating, binding, burning, suffocating, poisoning, or exposing their children to excess heat or cold (Gross & Hersen, 2008). Unfortunately, children who have been victims in the past are more likely to be victimized again unless the cycle of violence is broken.

CHARACTERISTICS OF CHILD ABUSE AND NEGLECT

Providing protection for abused and neglected children is a relatively recent endeavor in the U.S. Not until the early nineteenth century did the U.S. begin to actively prevent cruelty to children and then only on the basis that children were entitled to the same protection accorded family pets, such as cats and dogs.

Studies over the last century reveal several threshold characteristics of abuse and neglect:

- The repetitive nature of battering and neglect
- Often, only one child in a family may be targeted for physical abuse
- Mistreatment intensifies over time absent an intervention
- Physical abuse often results in life-threatening injuries

Parental assaults are not isolated, atypical events, but rather are part of a pattern of beatings and abuse that will not only continue, but will become more severe unless an intervention takes place. The repetitive nature of abuse explains why it is almost certain the abuse will be far more severe the second, third, and fourth time, until the child suffers permanent injuries or death. The phenomenon of the target child makes it clear a particular child can be singled out for survival-threatening abuse, even if other children in the home are well cared for and not abused.

Target Children

In the majority of physically abusive families, a particular child is singled out as the recipient of the abuse. Researchers theorize the target child has become a symbol of some kind to the parents, such as a financial burden or an unwanted interruption of life plans (Wright & Wright, 2007). Periodically, the parents' anger explodes against this symbol, leading to physical and psychological maltreatment.

The abuse is seldom provoked by the child's own behavior or, if it is, the punishment is grossly inappropriate and excessive for the child's misconduct. The verbal and psychological maltreatment, in the form of unremitting criticism and rebuke, usually extends over the life of the target child. Often, the batterer orders the target child out of the family home.

If the target child is removed from the family home, a sibling will sometimes be singled out as the new target child. However, the abuse of one child is generally not sufficient to remove other children in the household to ensure their safety.

Sadly, non-abused children in the family suffer emotional trauma from witnessing the abuse inflicted on their siblings. There is little doubt non-abused children frequently witness the abuse of the target child. In one study, almost two-thirds of the other children residing in the home were present at the time the abuse of the target child occurred (Moore et al., 2007). In fact, increasing evidence shows children who witness physical abuse of their siblings, as well as domestic violence between their parents, suffer as much as children who are abused directly (Wright & Wright, 2007). Child witnesses share the same combination of love and fear of the abuser as the target child does. Non-abused children, upon seeing the physical and verbal abuse of their sibling or other domestic violence, remain afraid of misbehaving because they see what happens when the battering parent goes into an uncontrolled rage and abuses other family members.

Child Battering Profile

The vast majority of physically abused children are battered by one or both of their parents. Most children who die from physical abuse are killed by their parents. Nearly half of all abused children are only abused by their mothers (Schnitzer et al., 2008). Predictably, the abuse increases when the mother is socially isolated or unemployed.

Fathers are more apt to abuse their sons, whereas mothers are more apt to abuse their daughters. Injuries inflicted by fathers, however, are often more serious and involve more fatalities than those inflicted by mothers.

A national survey of hospitals revealed other general characteristics of physically abusive parents. The study found many parents who inflict abuse on their children were of low or marginal intelligence. While educational achievement varied among abusing parents, most of the abusers were between twenty-one and thirty years of age when they began abusing their child. Abuse is often triggered following childbirth; approximately half of all battering mothers were either unmarried or newly married when they gave birth to the target child (ACF, 2008).

Active Batterers vs. Passive Acceptors

Often, one parent is the active batterer while the other parent passively accepts the action. In most circumstances, non-battering parents feel too weak and inadequate to interfere with the abuse for fear of being abused if they step in. Non-battering parents are often worried their interference will only escalate the violence. Passive parents may also suffer from feelings of apathy and be unable to respond emotionally.

Unique Profile of Immigrant Families

Federal immigration law clearly provides for removal of convicted child abusers or batterers who are lawful permanent resident aliens, or non-citizens with a green card. *See* 8 U.S.C.A. § 1227 (2008); *see also Nicanor-Romero v. Mukasey*, 523 F.3d 992 (U.S. Court of Appeals for the 9th Circuit 2008); *Nguyen v. Chertoff*, 501 F.3d 107 (U.S. Court of Appeals for the 2nd Circuit 2007). Individuals convicted of neglect will also be deported. Unfortunately, this further isolates immigrant families where chronic and enduring abuse occurs; there is a wall of family silence, and abused children are repeatedly admonished not to rely on outsiders because only their parents truly care for them.

Risk Factors: Abusers and Batterers

Some parents are at an increased risk of abusing their children. Abusive parents share one or more similar characteristics:

- Were themselves physically abused and the victims of excessive corporal punishment
- Are actively engaged in domestic violence and battering of the other parent
- Are substance abusers unable to control their emotions
- Are socially isolated and/or unemployed
- Have unrealistic expectations for their children, especially the target child

(*See* Oklahoma Senate, 2006; Wright & Wright, 2007)

Batterering parents are unable to handle their emotions in a socially acceptable fashion. Frequent, unprovoked outbursts of temper by the battering parent result in the recurring abuse. Often, the family is in a stressful economic and domestic situation, and the batterer is subject to loss of temper when added stress is presented (Moore et al., 2007). The more risk factors present in the battering parent, the more the target child is at risk of facing survival-threatening injuries and unintended death.

Victims of Abuse and Excessive Corporal Punishment Themselves

The one characteristic of almost all abusive parents is their own maltreatment as children at the hands of their own parents. Numerous studies demonstrate that parents who were themselves abused physically are far more likely than non-abused parents to pattern the abusive behavior, including the use of excessive corporal punishment learned from their parents. Most batterers were victims of harsh punishment themselves as they were growing up, which is the pattern they repeat in adulthood. An abused child's chances of becoming an abusive adult are a thousand times greater than those of a non-abused child (Wright & Wright, 2007). As many as 90 percent of child abusers were themselves physically abused or were the victims of corporal punishment as children (Davis, 2006).

Domestic Violence

There is a high correlation between child abuse and domestic violence; three out of four batterers who abuse their spouse also beat their children (Quester, 2007). Domestic violence is also an important predictor of future child abuse; in most cases where there is domestic violence among the parents, a child ultimately is abused as well.

Substance Abusers

Parents who are also substance abusers are at increased risk of abusing their children when their inhibitions are released while under the influence of drugs or alcohol or both. Former substance abusers are also at increased risk of abusing their children, especially parents who never completed treatment for their addictions. Untreated addicts never learn not to behave spontaneously and cannot control their emotions; *dry drunk* is the pejorative term given to their uninhibited abusive behavior.

Substance abuse by the batterer is also a high risk factor for domestic violence among parents. The alcoholic or drug-addicted parent has reduced inhibitions and distorted perceptions, increasing the likelihood battering will occur. It is estimated more than half the battering spouses have or at one time had addiction problems; 40 percent of children from homes where a parent was battered believe a parent had a drinking or drug problem and were more abusive when they were inebriated or high. Unfortunately, most batterers do not have the cognitive, emotional, or financial resources to change their life situation and break the cycle of violence (Wright & Wright, 2007).

Socially Isolated

The incidence of abuse and neglect is often attributed to changes in the nature of family life in the U.S. Contemporary family life is characterized by the:

- Social isolation of families
- Diminished or deteriorating community and personal support

- Increasing divorce rates
- Increasing rate of childbearing outside of marriage
- Increasing coupling of single adults isolated from support systems that have historically aided in child rearing

(Kelly, 2007)

Unemployed

The link between unemployment and risk for abuse or neglect is well supported. Losing a job correlates with increased abuse of children and violence within families (Gershuny, 2006).

As unemployment humiliates parents, they tend to degrade and abuse their children. Job losses have been directly related to increases in rates of child abuse, presumably perpetrated by feelings of rejection experienced by the unemployed parent. Large-scale epidemiological child abuse studies find unemployed parents report significantly more conflict with their children and indicate they were more likely to hit, slap, or spank their children when compared with families where parents were both employed (Gershuny, 2006). Health care professionals should be attentive to the fact that child abuse and neglect often involve complex cycles of psychological trauma within families, cycles frequently aggravated by chronic unemployment (Richardson, 2007).

Research suggests greater numbers of abused children's parents, especially fathers, are unemployed, compared to the population at large. In an analysis of over twenty thousand cases by the National Research Council's Panel on Child Abuse and Neglect, half of the abusive fathers were unemployed during the year they perpetrated abuse, and 12 percent were unemployed at the actual time of the abuse. In general, male unemployment rates account for two-thirds of the variance in total abuse and neglect rates (Gershuny, 2006). Mothers' long-term unemployment has also been linked to child abuse, although at lower and more variable correlations (Mapp, 2006).

Unrealistic Expectations for Their Children

Abusive parents also tend to have unrealistic expectations of their children, which may put the children at risk of harsh punishment when they do not, or cannot, live up to their parent's demands. Frequently, these unrealistic expectations involve toilet training or bed wetting in young children and involve academic achievements in school-aged children. It is not uncommon for abusive parents to restrict the target child to the home under the guise of studying in their attempt to totally control the child's behavior (literally, house arrest). Sometimes the punishment involves demeaning abuse, and punishment is almost always erratic.

Indicators of Intentional Abuse

Health care professionals should be cognizant of the behaviors of abusive and battering parents that generally indicate they are abusing their children. Certain behaviors of physically abused children should also put treating providers on the alert.

Abusive and Battering Parents

The failure of parents to provide a satisfactory explanation for their child's injury should alert treating health care professionals to the possibility of physical abuse. Intentional physical abuse should be suspected if the parents' explanation of how the child's injuries occurred is either extremely unlikely or simply cannot account for the nature of the injuries. Sometimes, abusive parents display unusual anger and may become overly defensive. In addition, they may seem uncaring about a diagnosis of serious injury.

In fact, serious injuries in infants, especially if they result in the death of the child, are rarely unintentional, nor are infants likely to induce accidents by themselves. Many abusive parents try to deny or minimize the child's medical problems. Often, injuries will often be found in a physical examination or skeletal survey of the child that were never reported by the parents.

Physically Abused Children

The behavior of physically abused children can also indicate to treating health care professionals that intentional abuse has occurred. In addition to sharing many demographic traits, abused children often display similar emotions, which parallel those suffered by a battered spouse. Oftentimes, abused children will:

- Appear extremely passive and submissive
- Lack spontaneity and have exceptionally constrained behavior
- Seem very fearful, timid, nervous, and easily frightened
- Flinch whenever someone lays a hand on them or casually touches them

Like abusive parents, battered children also may display abnormal behavior in dealing with their presented injuries. Abused children may be very non-communicative and reluctant to talk about their injury because of fear or embarrassment. This is in marked contrast to the behavior of non-abused children who usually talk freely about the nature of an injury.

Children who survive the battering and grow up in physically abusive homes often display markedly similar emotional attributes.[LN1] Abused children, as well as non-abused children who witness the abuse of the target child, are frequently withdrawn and suffer from depression and feelings of hopelessness. Having endured abuse, many target children blame themselves for their situations and are potentially suicidal (Reardon & Noblet, 2008).

SURVIVAL-THREATENING SYNDROMES AND INJURIES

Abused children who are most at risk of permanent disability or death suffer from certain syndromes and injuries. There are four syndromes regarded as survival-threatening per se because victims of these syndromes frequently suffer permanent disability or death without outside intervention:

- Battered child syndrome (BCS)
- Shaken baby syndrome (SBS)
- Medical abuse syndrome
- Non-organic failure to thrive (FTT) syndrome

A specific term describes the physiological and psychological effects of child abuse in a medical environment. This chapter simply uses the term *medical abuse* to reflect the notion this phenomenon is just another form of child abuse. This syndrome once referred to a psychological diagnosis for describing parents who abused their children in a medical environment. Sometimes this parental behavior is still identified as Munchausen's Syndrome by Proxy (MSBP), a parental disorder that manifests itself in child abuse (DSM-IV, 1994). FTT is sometimes referred to as parental neglect syndrome. Victims of BCS and SBS frequently suffer three types of specific injuries sufficiently serious to be categorized as survival-threatening per se:

- Head injuries, including subdural hematomas
- Multiple bone fractures at various stages of healings
- Severe abdominal trauma

Poisoning and asphyxiation are two far less frequent, but equally lethal, means of child abuse also included in the survival-threatening per se category. These two methods of abuse are commonly seen in children suffering from medical abuse where children are given toxic doses of various substances or are partially strangled or smothered by a parent who is attempting to get attention for themselves in a medical environment.

Finally, physical starvation and dehydration combined with psychological lack of attention are included in the survival-threatening per se category. Extreme physical and psychological neglect results in a failure to thrive; there is no organic basis for the medical condition of the children.

Battered Child Syndrome

Originally developed as a physical diagnosis for describing child abuse, BCS has come to describe both the physiological and psychological effects of a prolonged pattern of verbal, emotional, and physical abuse. The Supreme Court of Washington was one of the first states to recognize BCS in the early 1990s. *See State v. Janes*, 850 P.2d 495 (Supreme Court of Washington 1993) (describing one of the first uses of battered child syndrome as a defense for murder of the abusing parent or batterer). In trying to develop ways of dealing with ongoing abuse, children frequently manifest some of the same emotional characteristics as a battered spouse, including:

- Hyper-vigilance
- Learned helplessness

Hyper-Vigilance

The Supreme Court of Washington noted BCS children, unlike children who are not abused, live in a family environment where verbal, emotional, and physical abuse is commonplace and may occur at anytime with or without warning. BCS children display hyper-vigilance by picking up low-level cues of tension that un-traumatized people would never notice. Hyper-vigilant children are acutely aware of their environment and remain on alert for any signs of stress. The history of abusive encounters with a battering parent leads them to be overly cautious and to perceive subtle changes in the parent's expressions or mannerisms that generally precede an abusive incident. Such hyper-monitoring behavior means BCS children become overly sensitized to subtle changes in stress levels and constantly monitor their environment for signals of stress, and particularly for any signs of tension from the abuser (*see Janes,* 850 P.2d 495).

Learned Helplessness

Another key characteristic of BCS is known as learned helplessness. Like a battered spouse, BCS children often suffer from learned helplessness, resulting from feeling trapped in a situation from which they cannot escape. Although an abused child might be expected to seek outside help, there are compelling emotional reasons that make seeking and getting help the rare exception rather than the norm. The prolonged exposure to abuse results in feelings of powerlessness, embarrassment, fear of reprisal, and low self-esteem. These emotions often prevent a child from seeking help from anyone outside the family.

Ironically, despite the abuse they endure, BCS children frequently have strong emotional bonds with their abusive parents. As the *Janes* court noted, children are dependent on their parents for emotional and financial support; they are extremely vulnerable and tend to place great trust in their parents. Abusive parents sometimes exercise almost obsessive control over their children, regarding them as chattels to satisfy the parents' needs rather than as individuals in their own right.

These family bonds often make running away an emotionally unrealistic option. Moreover, BCS children often fear running away will only result in greater abuse should they return. Informing anyone of the abuse often is avoided for the same reason. Oftentimes, BCS children will have sought outside help without gaining any satisfactory outcome.

Shaken Baby Syndrome (Rotational Cranial Injuries)

A triad of rotational cranial injuries traditionally leads to a diagnosis of SBS, but not always. While the medical community is suggesting the triad should not be called SBS at all, but rather "infantile encephalopathy with subdural and retinal bleeding" (Geddes, 2003), this chapter uses the traditional and accepted term of SBS to describe this shaking phenomenon. The triad consists of:

- Brain hemorrhaging: bleeding between the dura mater (outermost membrane of the brain) and the arachnoid (the middle layer) or between the arachnoid layer and the pia mater (the innermost membrane)
- Brain swelling
- Retinal hemorrhaging (bleeding in the back of the eyes)

(Gena, 2007)

A debate in the medical community is emerging pointing to the possibility that the triad may sometimes have causes other than abusive shaking (Geddes, 2003). Consequently, incidents of suspected SBS should be evaluated case-by-case and collaboration sought to substantiate the medical findings.

SBS frequently causes permanent injury or death in infants and young children. Although SBS is survival-threatening, the severe permanent damage associated with SBS usually does not occur with the initial incident. Infants who survive SBS generally suffer from one or more of the following conditions: permanent vegetative state, permanent brain damage, paralysis, cerebral palsy, epilepsy, blindness, deafness, learning disabilities, behavioral disorders, and/or developmental delays. One study showed most survivors of SBS experienced speech and language problems, motor deficits, behavior problems, and/or visual disabilities. One in five had epilepsy or a related seizure disorder.

When a child is shaken aggressively or slammed against a surface, the forceful motion often causes extreme rotational cranial acceleration, meaning the infant's brain bounces around, repeatedly impacting the skull. Ironically, the violent shaking often leaves no outward signs of abuse, despite causing massive internal brain injuries and retinal hemorrhages that can lead to blindness (Wright & Wright, 2007). Nondepressed linear skull fractures are ordinarily detectable only by radiological examination. If a child dies from the shaking, an autopsy may reveal impact sites on the scalp of the head. However, even if the autopsy does not reveal any impact injuries, this does not eliminate the possibility that the child was slammed against a soft surface such as a mattress or stuffed furniture.

The National Center on Shaken Baby Syndrome estimates children are shaken violently or slammed into something approximately 1,500 times each year, meaning three children suffer from SBS every day.

Children are slammed into bed mattresses, changing tables, and upholstered furniture as well as against hard surfaces like walls and floors. Most of the children who suffer from SBS are under the age of four, with many under two years of age and often under one year of age. Approximately one-third of the infants do not survive the shaking.

The shaking usually is done by grasping the child by the trunk or arms (which accounts for any fractures or bruises) and violently shaking the child back and forth so the child's chin impacts the chest and then whip-saws to impact the upper back. SBS involves such significant shaking, the child's head is forcefully bounced from the chest and then all the way back to hit against the back and then the chest again, and so forth (Bandak, 2005). This movement of the head causes the veins connecting the brain to the skull to tear, leading to loss of oxygen to the brain and significant brain swelling (Gena, 2007).

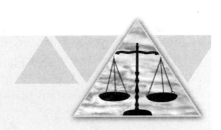

DEPRAVED INDIFFERENCE

Maddox v. State

[Child Abuser v. State]

31 A.D.3d 970 (Supreme Court of New York 2006)

FACTS: Maddox faced a jury trial after his live-in girlfriend's four-month-old infant, who had been under his care, died from SBS. Maddox struck the infant in the head and vigorously shook her before throwing her head-first into a bassinet within hours of her death. During the shaking, the rotational forces tore the bridging veins surrounding the infant's brain, causing subdural hematoma. In addition, the shaking tore the infant's brain tissue. This trauma caused the brain to swell, resulting in pressure on the brainstem, which, in turn, controls vital functions like heart rate and respiration. This led to a decrease in oxygen to the infant's brain, permanent brain damage, and eventually death.

When the mother notified Maddox the infant was not responsive, Maddox failed to call an ambulance and told her the infant accidentally fell on the floor. Expert medical evidence revealed the infant's injuries were not consistent with Maddox's version of events and reflected a pattern of abuse. For instance, when an infant is picked up and shaken, the repeated oscillations back and forth cause the skull (which is one density) and the brain (of a different density) to vary how fast they go back and forth. At one given moment, the brain will be going

one way and the skull will be going the opposite way. Specifically, autopsy reports showed multiple healing bone fractures and brain and spinal injuries. At the same time, other medical proof showed hemorrhaging and bruising on the scalp and face. The recurring violent shaking caused the blood vessels in the infant's retina to tear and bleed, resulting in retinal hemorrhages around the optic nerve. Widespread, multi-layered retinal hemorrhages identify SBS because they only occur from rotational head trauma and blunt force trauma.

ISSUE: Did the triad of symptoms established by medical evidence prove Maddox acted recklessly and under circumstances evincing a depraved indifference to the infant's life?

HOLDING AND DECISION: Yes, depraved indifference murder is an unintentional homicide requiring proof Maddox recklessly engaged in conduct that created a grave risk of serious physical injury or death to the infant.

ANALYSIS: Under New York State child homicide laws, the act of killing a child through protracted physical abuse can be punished as murder even if

(continues)

(continued)

the intent to kill cannot be proven. Such laws ease the difficulty of proving a more serious homicide offense by replacing the traditional mental state element for the crime of murder with either proof of the intent attached to the underlying felony or proof of recklessness or extreme indifference to human life. Many states, including New York, use the concept of depraved indifference to create statutes designed specifically to punish child abusers. The Model Penal Code uses extreme indifference language. *See* Model Penal Code § 210.2(1)(b) (1981).

RULE OF LAW: Following a jury trial, Maddox was convicted of depraved indifference murder and reckless endangerment and was sentenced to a prison term of eighteen years to life.

(*See generally* Maylor, 2007).

Infants are more vulnerable to brain injury from shaking than older children since an infant's head constitutes approximately 10 percent of the infant's total weight, versus only about 2 percent of the total weight of the brain of older children. Moreover, an infant's head is about one-quarter of the infant's body length, whereas, with older children, the head length is about an eighth of the body length. In addition, the consistency of an infant's brain is less developed than an older child's brain; it is soft rather than firm, which means that it is injured much more easily.

Survival-Threatening Injuries Common to Battered Child and Shaken Baby Syndromes

Physical abuse of children is an underreported and often unnoticed problem (O'Keefe, 2007). In addition to the injuries comprising BCS and SBS, children who are being physically abused often exhibit:

- Multiple intentional bone fractures in various stages of healing
- Intra-abdominal injuries
- Head trauma

Multiple Unexplained Bone Fractures

Although a single broken bone, in and of itself, is not usually a survival-threatening injury, even a single fracture may indicate a child is being abused intentionally (Wright & Wright, 2007). Victims of BCS and SBS frequently sustain multiple bone fractures, often along with other serious injuries. Any child with multiple intentional fractures in various stages of healing should be regarded as being at extreme risk of permanent injury or death (Kempe et al., 1984).

When the *Journal of the American Medical Association* first described BCS, physical abuse was characterized as repetitive. Abused children are shaken and jerked in such a manner as to break bones when a parent is angry, resulting in chip fractures, posterior rib fractures, skull fractures, and spiral fractures (Wright & Wright, 2007):

- Chip fractures in the joints result from an abuser twisting the child's limbs
- Rib fractures often occur when infants and small children are held by the abdomen and squeezed while being shaken
- Skull fractures can occur when children are slammed into objects
- Spiral fractures occur when a child's bones are forcefully twisted apart

(Kempe et al., 1984)

Intra-Abdominal Injuries

Intra-abdominal injuries are suffered frequently by victims of BCS and SBS and are survival-threatening. Bleeding and functional impairment of an intra-abdominal organ must be diagnosed early and dealt with immediately. In fact, abdominal trauma ranks as the second most common cause of death in physically abused children (ACF, 2008).

Contrary to the claims of some abusive parents, children do not usually fall with sufficient force to produce abdominal injuries (Wright & Wright, 2007), although such injuries could arise in children from seatbelt use in motor vehicle collisions. Abdominal trauma generally requires an external striking or compressive force of some sort applied to the abdomen. Despite the lethal nature of the abuse, some children who suffer, or even die from, blows to their abdomens do not show any external evidence of the abdominal trauma. There are, of course, many cases where children with severe intra-abdominal injuries do have external evidence of the abuse.

Head Trauma

Treating health care professionals need to be particularly vigilant in assuring the safety of children who are victims of head trauma. Not only can head injuries be survival-threatening in themselves but, if they have been inflicted by violent shaking, they are also markers for BCS and SBS.

Head injuries are the leading cause of death and disability in children under the age of five (ACF, 2008). What may not be as obvious, however, is that the majority of head injuries sustained by infants or young children are caused intentionally.

According to a study by the American Academy of Pediatrics, 64 percent of all head injuries in infants were caused by child abuse and, if uncomplicated skull fractures were excluded, the study estimated 95 percent of serious intracranial injuries were inflicted intentionally. Infants often suffer serious head injuries but do not suffer fractures of the skull because their skull bones are very pliable. For this reason, infants and young children suffer internal bleeding more often than skull fractures. The worst head injury, in terms of serious aftereffects or death, is a subdural hematoma, a very rapid collection of blood on the surface of the brain that causes an increase in intracranial pressure, compressing and damaging delicate brain tissue.

Medical Abuse (Munchausen's Syndrome By Proxy)

Abusive parents sometimes asphyxiate and poison their children. MSBP describes parents who purposefully harm their child(ren) in order to gain medical attention. Today, this parental behavior is generally recognized for what it is: physical child abuse (Roesler & Jenny, 2008). In addition, parents who harm their children abuse the medical system; thus the term *medical abuse.*

Children are betrayed in the medical environment when they are repeatedly presented for medical treatment for apparent acute illnesses based on plausible and dramatic, yet false, histories provided by parents (Wright & Wright, 2007). Children are then forced to undergo unnecessary and often harmful medical care for symptoms induced by their parents in an attempt to diagnose the nonexistent illness.

Still, this parental behavior is sometimes characterized by a type of mental disorder manifesting as child abuse (DSM-IV, 1994), described as the intentional faking of symptoms in another person who is under the individual's care for the purpose of indirectly assuming the sick role (DSM-IV, 1994). While some abusive parents will dissimulate by avoiding medical treatment to the point where a child's minor medical problem becomes serious, there

are several key elements that typically characterize medical abuse:

- Target child suffers from a false illness induced by physical abuse
- Parent exaggerates the child's medical problems and repeatedly requests medical evaluations and treatments for the child
- Parent inducing the illness denies having any knowledge as to the cause of the mysterious illness
- Parent aggravates the child's injuries caused by physical abuse (for instance, by manipulating a wound so it does not heal)
- Symptoms cease when the abusive parent is separated from the child
- Unexplained deaths or near-deaths of children in the same family

(Sweet, 2008)

The number of children being presented to the health care system each year by medically abusive parents is a complex phenomenon and is increasing dramatically (ACF, 2008). Medical abuse comprises both physical abuse and medical neglect and is also a form of psychological maltreatment (Stirling & Committee on Child Abuse and Neglect, 2007). Upwards of one thousand children are medically abused each year (Sweet, 2008).

Treating health care professionals should always be concerned by truly ill children with baffling symptoms who may be misdiagnosed as being abused and, therefore, denied appropriate medical care. To complicate matters, treating health care professionals sometimes raise suspicions about the treatment of abused children, and abusive parents are supported by those who want to limit the authority of state public health officials to intervene in family matters. *See Bush v. State*, 809 So.2d 107 (Court of Appeal of Florida, Fourth District 2002).

Poisoning

Although poisoning is a fairly unusual form of child abuse, it does occur (Wright & Wright, 2007). This abuse is generally perpetrated by mothers, especially those with a history of mental illness. Abusive mothers often induce illness in their children by poisoning them with a variety of toxic substances, including arsenic, aspirin, codeine, insulin, ipecac (a vomit inducer), laxatives, lye, oral and fecal matter, pebbles, psychotropic and barbiturate drugs, and salt. The intentional poisoning causes the children to suffer from anorexia, bleeding, diarrhea, pain, seizures, and vomiting (Roesler & Jenny, 2008).

One of the more serious cases of medical abuse by poisoning occurred in Florida and involved a mother who was a spokesperson and lobbyist for chronically ill children.

MEDICAL ABUSE

Bush v. State
[Abusive Mother v. State of Florida]
809 So.2d 107 (Court of Appeal of Florida, Fourth District 2002)

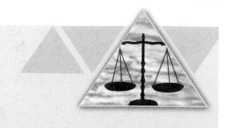

FACTS: By the time Jennifer Bush was nine years old, she had spent nearly two full years of her life in hospitals. She had been admitted to the hospital over two hundred times, had undergone over forty surgeries (including the removal of her gallbladder, appendix, and part of her intestines), and had undergone over eighteen hundred non-surgical treatments, many of which were serious. Digestive problems required surgically implanted feeding tubes in her stomach and intestines, and she required another tube near her heart for introducing medications. Finally, after nine years of medical abuse, hospital nurses noticed the child's condition would deteriorate after visits from her mother, Kathleen Bush. Toxic levels of drugs and fecal material were subsequently found in Jennifer's body.

After being removed from her mother's care and placed into foster care, Jennifer exhibited a full recovery and was not hospitalized once while in foster care. Medicaid paid over $2.0 million to physicians and Coral Springs Medical Center and Hollywood Memorial Hospital to compensate for Jennifer's medical bills and Jennifer became a national poster child for health care reform.

ISSUE: Is MSBP a recognized motive for prosecution of medical abuse, or a defense for diminished capacity?

HOLDING AND DECISION: Neither; testimony on MSBP cannot be presented by the prosecution as a motive for medical abuse or as a defense for diminished capacity.

ANALYSIS: After a four-month trial, Kathleen Bush was found guilty of aggravated child abuse for poisoning and infecting her daughter from the time she was five months old until her torture was discovered nine years later. She was also found guilty of organized fraud against Medicaid and sentenced to concurrent terms of imprisonment and probation for five years. No attempt was made to recover taxpayer funds.

RULE OF LAW: MSRP is inherently unreliable as a medical diagnosis; medical experts disagree about the syndrome and how to diagnose it. Therefore, it cannot be used as a defense.

Asphyxiation

Abusive parents also asphyxiate their children by:

- Suffocation
- Strangulation
- Smothering

Abused children often suffer from survival-threatening asphyxiation until they are rendered unconscious (when the body cells either fail to receive or are unable to utilize oxygen). The brain, which uses about 20 percent of the body's oxygen supply, is particularly susceptible to asphyxiation (Roesler & Jenny, 2008).

Of the three types of asphyxiation, suffocation is the one most commonly used by abusive parents. Parents suffocate their children with their hands or by blocking their airways, such as by ramming a gag into their mouth. Less frequently, abused children suffer from asphyxiation at the hands of their parents by strangulation, which involves cutting off oxygen by putting pressure on the neck. Children have been strangled by their parents forcefully tightening cords

or ropes around their necks or by using their hands or forearms or other implements, like a flashlight or crowbar, to occlude the neck vessels. Parental abusers also have smothered their children by obstructing the children's noses and mouths using a variety of implements, such as hands, clothes, pillows, blankets, plastic wrap, scarves, tape, or plastic bags (Wright & Wright, 2007).

Even very brief periods of asphyxiation can lead to devastating results in children. Asphyxiating for a minute can cause seizures, between one and two minutes can cause brain damage, and over two minutes can cause death. Physical abuse involving any of these forms of asphyxiation is usually very hard to diagnose because there are often few exterior signs of the abuse. Children suffering from asphyxiation at the hands of an abusive parent frequently experience medically unexplainable apnea, cyanotic episodes in which they involuntarily hold their breath until unconsciousness occurs, or cardiopulmonary arrest (Roesler & Jenny, 2008).

Other Manifestations of Survival-Threatening Injuries

In addition to BCS, SBS, and medical abuse, many children who endure physical abuse also suffer from parental neglect of their basic needs, such as:

- Sufficient food and water
- Appropriate clothing
- Safe home environment free of domestic violence
- Necessary medical and dental care

Starvation and Dehydration

Although usually not survival-threatening, in some cases severe parental neglect does result in children suffering from starvation or dehydration. Since malnutrition can depress the immune system, children whose basic needs for food are not met also frequently suffer from potentially survival-threatening secondary diseases. These illnesses can include tuberculosis, pneumonia, urinary tract infections, skin infections, ear infections, meningitis, and intracranial abscesses (Roesler & Jenny, 2008). In some cases, the immediate cause of the child's death may be one of these diseases, but the underlying cause would be the physical neglect. Once children are mobile, they can sometimes obtain sufficient food and drink to survive; consequently, most victims of lethal starvation or dehydration are under the age of one year (Spivack, 2006).

Non-Organic Failure to Thrive Syndrome

While extreme physical neglect can lead to dehydration and starvation, when combined with severe emotional neglect, a deadly condition known as non-organic failure to thrive can arise, which is survival-threatening. Children's height, weight, and motor development are significantly delayed with no medical explanation (Dixon, 2005).

In fact, inadequate nutrition and disturbed social interactions contribute to poor weight gain, delayed development, and abnormal behavior (Block et al., 2005). FTT develops in a significant number of children as a consequence of child neglect and often results from the failure of children to receive adequate nutrition. In its more extreme form and secondary to neglect, FTT may result in death.

The fundamental cause of FTT is nutritional deficiency. Often the mother of FTT children is depressed, with inadequate adaptive and social skills. Parental depression, stress, marital strife, and domestic violence are risk factors often linked to neglect as the cause of FTT (Moore et al., 2007).

This multifaceted term describes children whose weight is persistently below the third percentile for their age on standardized growth charts, or less than 85 percent of the ideal weight for their age. This causes poor muscle tone, decreased verbalization, weight loss, lack of growth, and listlessness. The condition can even result in catatonic states as a result of malnourishment (Wright & Wright, 2007).

Imprint Burns and Bite Marks

Burns and bites are commonly sustained by physically abused children. Parents who burn their children foreshadow survival-threatening injuries in the future (Wright & Wright, 2007). Parents employ an extensive variety of implements to inflict burns on their children; the most common type of burn is inflicted by a lit cigarette, forming distinctive circular, punched out areas of lesions, usually on the palms of the child's hands or soles of the child's feet. In addition to cigarettes, parents use other tools to cause burns leaving distinctive marks, such as branding irons, electric stove coils, grills of heaters, and steam irons, all of which leave exact imprints on children's skin.

Bite marks in various stages of healing may also indicate physical abuse. While abusive parents often blame the family pet for the marks on their children from biting, the Academy of Pediatrics notes bites produced by dogs and other animals tend to tear flesh, whereas human bites compress flesh. Human biting can cause abrasions, contusions, and lacerations but rarely tearing of tissue (Kellogg & Committee on Child Abuse and Neglect, 2007).

Extensive Bruises and Abrasions

Bruises and abrasions are the most common intentionally inflicted injuries sustained by abused children. Bruises are especially likely to indicate abuse in any infant under three months of age. Even if they are sustained as a result of misguided parental discipline, they can lead to serious harm.

Due to the primary beating, battered children may also suffer secondary injuries. For example, beaten children frequently suffer eye damage including impaired vision, acute hyphema (hemorrhage in the anterior chamber of the eye between the cornea and pupil), dislocated lens, and detached retina. There may also be general evidence of trauma, such as hematuria (the presence of blood in the urine), shock, vomiting, and/or or ataxia.

Abusive parents frequently batter their children by hitting them with their fists, slapping them, or kicking them. Parents employ an astonishing variety of techniques to cause their children's bruises and abrasions. Battering parents have beaten their children with extension cords, boards, rubber hoses, broomsticks, and shovels. Hand and finger marks are made by slapping a child, while handprints around a child's neck are indicative of choking. Bald spots or bruising on the scalp of a child often indicate the child's hair has been pulled out.

Bruises also vary in color depending on when they were inflicted. The color can be used to show the bruises were inflicted at different times and to determine approximately when each injury occurred. The location of the bruises can also help in determining whether the injuries were inflicted intentionally.

For example, 70 percent of all non-accidental injuries occur in what is sometimes referred to as the *Target Zone*, the base of the neck to the back of the knees and from fingertips to fingertips. Bruises on the back are especially suspect because most of the injuries sustained by a child during play occur on the front. Bruises on the inner thighs usually are not caused accidentally. Bruises on the arms or hands sometimes occur when children try to protect themselves from their abusers. Moreover, in school-aged children, injuries frequently are sustained in areas normally covered by clothes, such as the arms or the legs, making detection very difficult.

Sexual Abuse

Long-term studies show sexual abuse is grossly intrusive in the lives of children and is harmful to their normal psychological, emotional, and sexual development (*Kennedy*, 128 S.Ct. at 2677). Alarmingly, nearly 30 percent of child sexual abuse victims are between the ages of four and seven (*id.* at 2671 n.2).

The deep problems afflicting child-rape victims often become society's problems. There are correlations between childhood sexual abuse and later problems, such as substance abuse, dangerous sexual behaviors or dysfunction, inability to relate to others on an interpersonal level, and psychiatric illness. Victims of child rape are nearly five times more likely than non-victims to be arrested for sex crimes and nearly thirty times more likely to be arrested for prostitution (*id.* at 2677).

Rape of a Minor

Kennedy v. Louisiana
[Stepfather v. State]
128 S.Ct. 2641 (U.S. Supreme Court 2008)

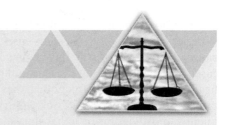

Facts: Louisiana charged Kennedy with the aggravated rape of his then-eight-year-old stepdaughter in the child's bedroom. An expert in pediatric forensic medicine testified the child's injuries were the most severe he had ever seen from a sexual assault. A laceration to the left wall of the vagina had separated her cervix from the back of her vagina, causing her rectum to protrude into the vaginal structure. Her entire perineum was torn from the posterior fourchette to the anus. The child's injuries required emergency surgery. The stepfather was subsequently convicted and sentenced to death.

Issue: Since children are a class in need of special protection from harm, is child rape deserving of death?

Holding and Decision: No, the U.S. Supreme Court determined there is a national consensus against capital punishment for the crime of child rape.

Analysis: In a split decision, the Court found the death penalty disproportionate to the crime where the rape did not result in the child's death.

Under federal law, rapists are death-eligible only when the sexual abuse or exploitation results in the victim's death. *See* 18 U.S.C.A. § 2245 (2006). This rationale was partially based on two facts: only six states authorize death for child rape and no individual has been executed for rape since 1964. Moreover, the Court believed the death penalty could add to the risk of non-reporting of child rapes out of fear of negative consequences for the perpetrator, especially if the rapist was a family member. Further, by in effect making the punishment for child rape and murder equivalent, the Court feared a strong incentive for the rapist not to kill his victim might be removed. In contrast, where a child abuse case results in death, courts have no difficulty in concluding capital punishment is proportionate to the crime. *See, e.g., Branstetter v. State*, 57 S.W.3d 105 (Supreme Court of Arkansas 2001).

Rule of Law: States are barred from imposing the death penalty for the rape of a child where the crime did not result, and was not intended to result, in the victim's death.

(*See generally* McLaine, 2008).

The strongly worded dissent in the *Kennedy* decision led to calls for Congress to adopt the second look doctrine. Canada, Britain, and Israel permit legislative majorities to adopt clear statutes to override erroneous high court rulings or suspend them from taking effect. In this instance, however, Congress could easily pass a federal law making child rapists death-eligible. On remand from the U.S. Supreme Court, the Supreme Court of Louisiana sentenced Kennedy to life imprisonment and hard labor without benefit of parole, probation, or suspension of sentence (*State v. Kennedy*, 994 So.2d 1287 (Supreme Court of Louisiana 2008)).

Five years after eleven-year-old Jacob Wetterling was abducted at gunpoint while riding his bicycle with his brother and a friend, Congress enacted the Jacob Wetterling Act requiring states to establish registration systems for convicted sex offenders and to notify the public about persons convicted of the sexual abuse of minors (*see* 42 U.S.C.A. § 14071 (2006) (Jacob's fate remains unknown)). All fifty states now have state registries.[LN2] In addition, about half the states permit the involuntary commitment of sexual predators,[LN3] and at least twelve states have residency restrictions for sex offenders.[LN4] Undeniably, there is a national consensus to seriously control the behavior of predators who sexually abuse children.

Psychological Maltreatment

Physically abused children frequently suffer from psychological maltreatment. About half of seven- to thirteen-year-old sexual assault victims are considered seriously disturbed; emotional problems include sudden school failure, unprovoked crying, dissociation, depression, insomnia, sleep disturbances, nightmares, feelings of guilt and inferiority, and self-destructive behavior, including an increased incidence of suicide. *See Kennedy*, 128 S.Ct. at 2677.

Often severe verbal aggression is directed at the target child. The American Academy of Pediatrics identifies the following behaviors as constituting psychological maltreatment if they are repetitive and sustained over a period of time:

- Spurning (belittling, degrading, shaming, or ridiculing the target child; singling the child out to criticize or punish)
- Isolating (confining, placing unreasonable limitations on freedom of movement and social interactions)
- Terrorizing (setting unrealistic expectations with threat of punishment and abandonment if they are not met; and threatening to and/or destroying the target child's possessions)
- Unreliable or inconsistent parenting (contradictory and ambivalent demands)
- Neglecting medical, dental, educational, and basic needs (ignoring, preventing, or failing to provide for the basic needs of the target child, including appropriate clothing and school materials)
- Witnessing domestic violence
- Denying emotional responsiveness (sporadically ignoring the target child or failing to consistently express affection, caring, and love for the child)
- Rejecting (avoiding or pushing the child away)
- Exploiting or corrupting the child by encouraging the child to develop inappropriate behaviors (encouraging or coercing abandonment of developmentally appropriate autonomy and independence; restricting or interfering with cognitive development)

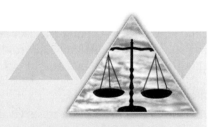

PSYCHOLOGICAL MALTREATMENT

U.S. v. Castillo-Villagomez
[Government on Behalf of Minor Daughter v. Father]
316 Fed.Appx. 874 (U.S. Court of Appeals for the Eleventh Circuit 2008)

FACTS: Father repeatedly threatened to hit his daughter, saying he hated her, and told her he would not give her money anymore.

ISSUE: Can psychological maltreatment constitute cruel and excessive mental pain?

HOLDING AND DECISION: Yes, although a non-physical offense, threats made to a child under the age of eighteen were nonetheless a felony involving a substantial risk physical force might be used.

ANALYSIS: The Court looked at the clear meaning of the offense of cruelty to children, as follows:

- "A parent . . . commits the offense of cruelty to children in the first degree when such

(continues)

(continued)

person willfully deprives the child of necessary sustenance to the extent that the child's health or well-being is jeopardized."
- "Any person commits the offense of cruelty to children in the first degree when such person maliciously causes a child under the age of eighteen cruel or excessive physical or mental pain."
- "Any person commits the offense of cruelty to children in the second degree when such person with criminal negligence causes a child under the age of eighteen cruel or excessive physical or mental pain."
- "Any person commits the offense of cruelty to children in the third degree when: Such

person, who is the primary aggressor, intentionally allows a child under the age of eighteen to witness the commission of a forcible felony, battery, or family violence battery; or Such person, who is the primary aggressor, having knowledge that a child under the age of eighteen is present and sees or hears the act, commits a forcible felony, battery, or family violence battery."

(Official Code of Georgia Annotated § 16-5-70(a-d) (2009)).

RULE OF LAW: Proof of physical force is not required to prove psychological maltreatment.

It is not uncommon for the verbally and emotionally abusive batterer to demand submission and an eagerness to follow the batterer's every order or wish. In the batterer's eyes, children can never be eager enough to obey them. Any resistance to the verbal and emotional battering only results in more physical abuse or harsh punishment. Generally, the non-abuser offers no protection while children are being abused and punished by the batterer. The non-abuser often remains emotionally detached and does nothing to stop the battering.

SURVIVAL-THREATENING NEGLECT

Neglect is three times more common than physical abuse of children. Recent estimates indicate some form of neglect is found in approximately 80 percent of all child abuse cases. Although neglect may simply result in a subnormal state of general health, it can also place children in situations that are survival-threatening.

Neglect of Basic Needs

As mentioned, in addition to survival-threatening syndromes (BCS, SBS, and medical abuse) and injuries, many children who endure physical abuse also suffer from parental neglect of their basic needs, such as:

- Sufficient nutrition
- Appropriate clothing
- Safe home environment free of domestic violence
- Proper care (locking the target child out of the house for extended periods of time)
- Needed medical and dental care
- Education

Parents who physically abuse their children often willfully neglect them by failing to provide for their basic

needs. Often the target child is completely neglected while other children in the household are provided the minimum basic needs.

Neglected children can die from hypo- or hyperthermia, caused, for example, by being left in an unheated house in the cold of winter or being locked in a car in the heat of summer. Improper supervision, combined with parental drug use, can result in the death of a child who accidentally consumes illegal drugs, the classic example being homes used as methamphetamine labs. Moreover, neglect frequently causes children to be very unhealthy, which can become survival-threatening if it means they are less able to recover from other forms of physical and sexual abuse.

Medical Neglect

Parents must provide medical treatment for their children. There are some religious exceptions to this general rule. For example, parents may exercise discretion regarding medical treatment when treatment decisions are tied to religious beliefs; however, they may not expose their children to the risk of death. *See, e.g., Prince v. Massachusetts*, 321 U.S. 158 (U.S. Supreme Court 1944). While several states distinguish between failure to provide medical care based on the financial inability to do so and the failure to provide it for no apparent financial reason, courts no longer accept excuses of financial inability for parents' failure to provide for medical care for their children. If parents do not provide medical care and thus put their child's health at risk, they can be found guilty of child abuse. Overall, more than nine out of ten American children are eligible for health insurance coverage in the U.S., with expanded access to public programs such as SCHIP and Medicaid widely available for children (HHS, 2005).

States vary as to their definitions of medical neglect, but all states have laws defining medical neglect as a form of child abuse. If parents refuse to provide their children with necessary medical care, thereby damaging the child's health, they can be found guilty of physical abuse. When parents refuse to promptly follow-up with medical orders for laboratory and radiological testing to properly diagnose a child's physical and emotional symptoms, judicial intervention is often necessary to protect the child's interests.

Of course, it is not for the courts to determine the most effective treatment when the parents have chosen among reasonable alternatives; but parents may not deny children treatment for medical conditions that may threaten their lives. The cases of children who bleed to death because of their parents' refusal to authorize blood transfusions present the classic example.

Medical neglect occurs when parents decline to provide their children with essential medical care. When treating health care professionals cannot persuade parents to provide treatment, a report of medical neglect is generally filed with child protective services. When a report is filed, social workers investigate and, in appropriate circumstances, file a petition in juvenile court seeking an order overriding the parents' refusal of medical care.

The law in all states authorizes court intervention in medical neglect cases. The issue is not whether states have authority to override parental medical decisions, but whether circumstances exist under which such intervention should occur. When medical treatment is essential to save a child's life, and is likely to be effective and without serious side effects, the treatment is usually required. On the other hand, if the treatment needed to save a child's life is experimental, or if the treatment has a relatively low probability of curing the child's condition, courts often defer to parents. When medical treatment is important, but not essential, to preserving life, outcomes are unpredictable. The result turns on the facts of the case. In non-life-threatening cases, the seriousness of the medical condition and the likelihood proposed treatment will be effective are taken into consideration.

A Different Problem: Adolescent Cosmetic Surgery

The number of adolescent girls undergoing serious cosmetic surgery in the U.S. is increasing. In 2007, more than thirty-four thousand cosmetic procedures

were performed on patients eighteen years of age or younger. About six thousand of those procedures involved breast augmentation and reductions, liposuction, tummy tucks, and nose reshaping (ASPS, 2008).

Since parents must give consent for all surgeries performed on minors, including plastic surgeries, a controversy is arising as to whether this consent constitutes abuse. The legal treatment of this issue is still practically nonexistent (Chiu, 2008).

Breast Augmentations on Adolescent Girls

While the official position of the American Society of Plastic Surgeons and American Society for Aesthetic Plastic Surgeons is that breast augmentations should not be performed on girls younger than eighteen years, nearly four thousand major surgeries are performed each year on minors, often as a high school graduation gift from parents to their daughters. These numbers have increased since 2006, when the FDA ended a fourteen-year moratorium on silicone breast implants and approved implants for general use for women twenty-two years of age and over (*see* ASAPS, 2008); however, it is legal to perform breast augmentations for anyone under eighteen as an off-label use. Off-label use in this instance means use for an age group different than the one that has been approved by the FDA.

The side effects of breast augmentations are serious because the bodies of adolescent girls are still developing. Most patients report, in studies done by implant manufacturers, at least one serious complication within the first three years of their breast surgery. Potential complications include breast pain, hardening of the breast, loss of sensation in the nipple area, reduction in ability to produce sufficient breast milk, significant interference with the detection of breast tumors, and possible infection leading to toxic shock syndrome, amputation, or death. Moreover, because breast implants only last an average of ten years, adolescents will need many future surgeries in their lifetime. In clinical trials of breast implant manufacturers, approximately one of every three patients requires follow-up surgeries for repositioning of implants, biopsies, and removal of implants within four to five years (none of which are covered by health insurance). General fee structures gathered from the Internet are:

- $7,000 to $10,000 for breast augmentation (silicone is more expensive than saline)
- $4,000 to $5,000 removal of implants
- $7,500 and upwards for replacement of old implants

There is little long-term research on the impact of breast augmentations on adolescent girls (Singer, 2008). For instance, the Food and Drug Administration (FDA) did not require clinical studies with time horizons beyond ten years before approving the new-generation silicone implants.

Parental Autonomy to Consent

Breast augmentations are a way to attain beauty, as measured by the dominant culture. Not only is it important for adolescent identity, but many parents believe it will help their daughters attain self-esteem and confidence (Singer, 2008). Finally, breast augmentations are regarded as insurance one's daughter will marry, or at least find a mate, because others will be more attracted to her due to her physical transformation (Chiu, 2008).

Breast augmentation involves the invasion of the minor's body, as authorized by the parents for non-medical reasons. It presents the risk of serious side effects. Essentially, parents decide whether it is in the best interest of their daughter to get breast implants. While the U.S. Supreme Court has acknowledged cosmetic surgery for medical reasons is within the right of parental autonomy, does this autonomy attach to major surgeries for nonmedical reasons? *See Parham v. J.R.*, 442 U.S. 584, 603-04 (U. S. Supreme Court 1979) (in analyzing the discretion of parents to admit their children into mental health facilities, the Court used the example of cosmetic surgery to conclude that parents are the medical decision-makers for children because children are usually not competent to make such decisions for themselves).

Moral Dilemmas

1. When determining the custody of children, should biological connections to children outweigh the best interests of children?

TERMINATION OF PARENTAL RIGHTS

Parental rights may be terminated on a voluntary or involuntary basis when children are abused and neglected. When children are removed from the home, some families can start on the road to recovery. Studies have shown that with appropriate intervention, the abusive parent can learn new attitudes and new ways to resolve conflict. Medical treatment for clinical depression generally works. Counseling can aim to confront parents about their

level of responsibility for their child abuse and neglect. Battering and abusive parents can learn to address the underlying attitudes that supported their battering and violence and begin to examine and change their beliefs about relationships and how to effectively deal with everyday stressful situations. Children can be temporarily placed with relatives, neighbors, or in foster care with regular parental visitation until the family can be restored to health (*see* Allison, 2005).

Moral Dilemmas

1. Based on prior adjudication of older children as abused and neglected in the same household, should a newborn be adjudicated as derivatively neglected?

2. Should relatives or other interested third parties be permitted to intervene and obtain custody of abused and neglected children without permission of the parents?

3. Given the high level of maltreatment of American children, plus limited taxpayer resources to deal with this sharply escalating problem, should consideration be given to returning to sterilization and castration procedures for abusive and neglectful parents who have numerous children in the foster care system or have forfeited their parental rights to other children?

4. Do birth families have the right to continued contact with children after the termination of their parental rights?

CHILD ABUSE REPORTING LAWS

For over two centuries, society has attempted to protect children from abuse. It was not until the American Medical Association publicly described injuries resulting from BCS, however, that the U.S. began to seriously address the problem (Kempe et al., 1984). Today, all fifty states have enacted child abuse reporting laws and the federal Child Abuse Prevention and Treatment Act provides states funding to promote programs to prevent children from being abused (*see* 42 U.S.C.A. §§ 5101-5107, 5116, 5118-5118(e) (2009)). Children subjected to child abuse and neglect generally have independent legal representation, and children involved in abuse and neglect proceedings in family court have

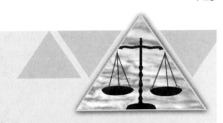

LIABILITY FOR FAILURE TO REPORT SUSPECTED CHILD ABUSE

Cooper Clinic, P.A. v. Barnes
[Medical Facility v. Estate of Abused Child]
237 S.W.3d 87 (Supreme Court of Arkansas 2006)

FACTS: Trenton McMillan, a three-year-old, was brought by his father to the Cooper Clinic for treatment of a head wound. The father claimed another child had accidentally hit Trenton in the head. The examining physician noted the child's body was covered in bruises and his teeth were chipped and decaying, but the physician did not report the suspected abuse. Instead, the physician relied on the father's assertions that Trenton's mother had abused Trenton and that he would promptly report the abuse to the police. The father subsequently brought Trenton back into the clinic to undergo a blood glucose test because he had been experiencing stomach pains, nausea, vomiting, and mood swings. The same attending physician saw Trenton, but did not ask the father if he had reported the abuse and, once again, failed to report the abuse. Approximately ten months after Trenton's first visit to the Cooper Clinic, Trenton died from blunt force trauma to his abdomen.

Trenton's father and stepmother were convicted of the negligent homicide of Trenton.

Subsequently, the estate of Trenton filed a wrongful death action against Cooper Clinic and its staff for their failure to report the child abuse.

ISSUE: Are hospitals and clinics liable for the failure of mandated reporters to report suspected child abuse?

HOLDING AND DECISION: No, only the individuals named in state mandatory reporting laws are liable.

ANALYSIS: A jury awarded Trenton's estate $500,000 against Cooper Clinic and the clinic appealed to the Supreme Court of Arkansas. The Supreme Court held the treating health care professionals' duty was an individual one; the duty did not extend to the clinic as a whole.

RULE OF LAW: Hospitals and clinics are not liable for failure to report suspected child abuse unless specifically listed as mandatory reporters in a state's child abuse reporting law.

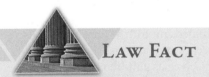

LAW FACT

MEDICAL NEGLECT

Who gets to decide between competing Western medicine and alternative medical options for minor children in need of diagnostic care?

While parents have a fundamental right to raise their children in their own traditions, the state has the power and responsibility to ensure children are not endangered by inadequate medical care. Parents who refuse diagnostic care for their children, when needed, are deemed neglectful.

In a similar real-life case, child protective services discovered survival-threatening physical abuse and psychological maltreatment of a sixteen-year-old when they conducted their investigation of the family's medical neglect, as well as a history of domestic violence that had been hidden for a decade. The younger child suffered from a failure to thrive, having spent much of her childhood witnessing the battering and abuse of her older sibling. However, it took months of appeals of decisions by child protective services before any action was taken to protect the children. It was not until a court-ordered physical examination of the oldest child took place that the extent of her physical injuries and medical neglect became evident and authorities began to take notice of what she had endured.

—Hypothetical case synopsis.

court-appointed guardians ad litem as long as the court's jurisdiction continues, which is often until the abused child is eighteen years of age.

States have both permissive and mandatory reporting laws. Permissive reporting laws define permissive reporters as anyone who may voluntarily report suspected child abuse but is not obligated to do so; parents are seldom included in this category (Kinter, 2005). Immunity is provided to permissive reporters making a report in good faith, even if their report turns out to be wrong. The standard to determine whether a permissive reporter acted in good faith is the objective reasonable person standard, or whether a reasonable person would have suspected abuse. *See* 43 C.J.S. Infants § 116 (2006). If permissive reporters choose not to act, they are not liable for failing to act, even if the individuals had direct knowledge of the abuse (CWIF, 2005).

State mandatory reporting laws define a mandatory reporter as anyone who is required to make a report of child maltreatment (CWIF, 2008). Most mandatory reporting laws only expressly place a duty to report on health care professionals and other child-related professionals, like teachers. Twelve states place an affirmative duty on everyone to report suspected child abuse.[LN5] Arizona is the only state that expressly includes parents, step-parents, and guardians as mandatory reporters of suspected child abuse. *See* Arizona Rev. Stat. Ann. § 13-3620 (2003).

Most states do not list health care institutions, such as clinics and hospitals, as mandated reporters; rather, they list treating health care professionals in their individual capacity.[LN6] Though most states do not require institutions to report child abuse, some require those employed by hospitals and clinics to report suspected child abuse to their supervisors, who are then required to make the official report.[LN7] Therefore, those institutions are indirectly required to report.

Chapter Summary

- Reported instances of child abuse, including sexual abuse, are on the rise in the U.S.; the true number of abuse and neglect cases is unknown because not every case is reported.
- Because life-threatening child abuse is rarely limited to one, isolated incident, if the child is not immediately removed from the situation, the child may suffer more severe forms of abuse, possibly resulting in permanent injury or death.
- Children often do not report their own abuse out of loyalty to the abuser (especially if the abuser is a family member), fear of negative consequences, or doubt that reporting the abuse will satisfactorily resolve the problem.
- In three-quarters of the reported cases, parents were the perpetrators of the abuse or neglect; often one parent is the active abuser while the other passively allows it to occur.
- Often, while only one child in the family, known as the *target child*, is singled out for the abuse, the abused child's siblings also suffer from the trauma of witnessing the violence perpetrated against the target child.
- Abusive parents share similar characteristics, such as being abused themselves as children, engaging in domestic violence with the other parent, abusing drugs and/or alcohol, being socially isolated and/or unemployed, and having unrealistic expectations for their children.
- Indicators health care professionals can use to determine whether a child's injuries were intentionally inflicted include both the parent's and child's conduct and explanations of the injury or injuries.
- Four common survival-threatening conditions are battered child syndrome, shaken baby syndrome, medical abuse syndrome, and non-organic failure to thrive syndrome.
- Other forms of abuse and neglect include asphyxiation, starvation and dehydration, burns and bites, and excessive bruises and abrasions.
- "Depraved indifference murder" is an easier crime to prove than regular murder because it replaces the traditional "evil intent" mental state element required to prove murder with either proof of the underlying death itself or proof of recklessness or extreme indifference to human life instead.
- Childhood sexual abuse is truly a societal problem, as sexually abused children are more likely to abuse drugs and/or alcohol, exhibit dangerous sexual behaviors and/or sexual dysfunction, be unable to relate to others on an interpersonal level, suffer from psychiatric illness, commit sex crimes, and/or engage in prostitution.
- The U.S. Supreme Court recently banned the death penalty as punishment for child rape where the rape did not result, and was not intended to result, in the victim's death.
- The Jacob Wetterling Act requires all states to establish registration systems for convicted sex offenders and to notify the public about offenders convicted of sexually abusing children; all fifty states have complied.

- In addition to physical abuse, children can also suffer from psychological abuse such as spurning, isolating, terrorizing, improper parenting, basic neglect, witnessing domestic violence, lack of emotional responsiveness, rejecting, exploiting, and/or corrupting; proof of physical harm is not necessarily required to prove psychological harm.
- Forms of neglect involve denial of basic needs such as sufficient nutrition, appropriate clothing, safe home environment, proper care, medical care, and education.
- All states have laws regarding medical neglect as a form of child abuse, but they differ on what exactly constitutes such neglect; one debate in particular involves whether parents consenting to cosmetic surgery for their children constitutes abuse.
- All states have laws regarding reporting of child abuse, but they differ on what is mandatory or permissive reporting.

LAW NOTES

1. Because physically abused children have seen only violence used to solve problems in their home, they are often unaware of other problem-solving methods. It is not surprising that research shows a high correlation between physical abuse as a child and violent behavior in youth and adults. For instance, there is a high correlation between child abuse and deviant behavior among violent juvenile delinquents, adults who commit violent crimes, and assassins (Reardon & Noblet, 2008). Most juvenile delinquents were bruised, lacerated, or fractured by their parents within months of their arrest; almost half had been rendered unconscious by a battering parent on several sporadic occasions (Wright & Wright, 2007). The cliché, "violence breeds violence" is supported by the finding that most violent criminals were abused and treated violently as children (Menninger, 2007).

   In addition, most of the death row inmates with frontal lobe damage sustained their brain damage from physical abuse in their infancy (Redding, 2007). One of the most compelling stories to arise at the intersection of child abuse and death row inmates is that of Johnny Paul Penry, a convicted rapist and murderer who has lived on death row in Texas since 1986. A survivor of brutal, long-term child abuse causing brain damage resulting in the intellectual functioning of a seven-year-old child, Penry is a central character in one of the legal dramas of the late twentieth century, that is, the debate over the justifiability of executing adult survivors of child abuse who are mentally retarded (Hall, 2002). The U.S. Supreme Court has twice heard Penry's appeal from his death sentence, and has twice found the procedures used by the State of Texas in imposing his sentence to be incompatible with the protections offered by the U.S. Constitution. *See Penry v. Texas*, 492 U.S. 302 (U.S. Supreme Court 1989); *but see, Zimmerman v. Cockrell*, 69 Fed.Appx. 658 (U.S. Court of Appeals for the 5th Circuit 2003), *U.S. Supreme Court certiorari denied, Zimmerman v. Dretke*, 540 U.S. 1076 (U.S. Supreme Court 2003) (denying death row inmate's appeal based on mental illness arising from physical child abuse).

2. All fifty states have state registries for convicted sex offenders who sexually abused a minor. *See* Alabama Code §§ 13A-11-200 to 13A-11-203, 1181 (1994); Alaska Stat §§ 1.56.840, 12.63.010-100, 18.65.087, 28.05.048, 33.30.035 (1994, 1995, and 1995 Cum. Supp.); Arizona Rev. Stat. Ann. §§ 13-3821 to -3825 (1989 and Supp. 1995); Arkansas Code Ann. §§ 12-12-901 to -909 (1995); California Penal Code Ann. §§ 290 to 290.4 (West Supp. 1996); Colorado Rev. Stat. Ann. § 18-3-412.5 (Supp. 1996); Connecticut Gen. Stat. Ann. §§ 54-102a to 54-102r (Supp. 1995); Delaware Code Ann. Tit. 11, § 4120 (1995); Florida Stat. Ann. §§ 775.13, 775.22 (1992 and Supp. 1994); Georgia Code Ann. § 42-9-44.1 (1994); 1995 Hawaii Sess. Laws No. 160 (enacted June 14, 1995); Idaho Code §§ 9-340(11)(f), 18-8301 to 18-8311 (Supp. 1995); Illinois Comp. Stat. Ann., ch. 730, §§ 150/1 to 150/10 (2002); Indiana Code §§ 5-2-12-1 to 5-2-12-13 (West Supp. 1995); 1995 Iowa Legis. Serv. 146 (enacted May 3, 1995); Kansas Stat. Ann. §§ 22-4901 to 22-4910 (1995); Kentucky Rev. Stat. Ann. §§ 17.500 to 17.540 (West Supp. 1994); Louisiana Stat. Ann. §§ 15:540 to 15:549 (West Supp. 1995); Maine Rev. Stat. Ann., Tit. 34-A, §§ 11001 to 11004 (West Supp. 1995); 1995 Maryland Laws p. 142 (enacted May 9, 1995); Massachusetts Gen. Laws Ann., ch. 6, § 178D; 1994 Michigan Pub. Acts p. 295 (enacted July 13, 1994); Minnesota Stat. § 243.166 (1992 and Supp. 1995); Mississippi. Code Ann. §§ 45-33-1 to 45-33-19 (Supp. 1995); Montana Rev. Stat. §§ 566.600 to 566.625 (Supp. 1996); Montana Code Ann. §§ 46-23-501 to 46-23-507 (1994); Nebraska Rev. Stat. §§ 4001 to 4014; Nevada Rev. Stat. §§ 207.080, 207.151 to 207.157 (1992 and Supp. 1995); N. H. Rev. Stat. Ann. §§ 632-A:11 to 632-A:19 (Supp. 1995); New Jersey Stat. Ann. §§ 2C:7-1 to 2C:7-11 (1995); New Mexico Stat. Ann. §§ 29-11A-1 to 29-11A-8 (Supp. 1995); New York Correct. Law Ann. §§ 168 to 168-v (West Supp. 1996); North Carolina Gen. Stat. Ann. §§ 14-208.5-10 (Lexis Supp. 1995);

North Dakota Cent. Code § 12.1-32-15 (Lexis Supp. 1995); Ohio Rev. Code Ann. §§ 2950.01-.08 (Baldwin 1997); Oklahoma Stat., Tit. 57, §§ 582-584 (2003 Supp.); Oregon Rev. Stat. §§ 181.507 to 181.519 (1993); 1995 Pennsylvania Laws p. 24 (enacted Oct. 24, 1995); Rhode Island Gen. Laws § 11-37-16 (1994); South Carolina Code Ann. § 23-3-430; South Dakota Codified Laws §§ 22-22-30 to 22-22-41 (Supp. 1995) Tennessee Code Ann. §§ 40-39-101 to 40-39-108 (2003); Texas Rev. Civ. Stat. Ann., Art. 6252-13c.1 (Vernon Supp. 1996); Utah Code Ann. §§ 53-5-212.5, 77-27-21.5 (Lexis Supp. 1995); Vermont Stat. Ann., Tit. 13, § 5402; Virginia Code Ann. §§ 19.2-298.1 to 19.2-390.1 (Lexis 1995); Washington Rev. Code §§ 4.24.550, 9A.44.130, 9A.44.140, 10.01.200, 70.48.470, 72.09.330 (1992 and Supp. 1996); W. Va. Code §§ 61-8F-1 to 61-8F-8 (Lexis Supp. 1995); Wisconsin Stat. § 175.45 (Supp. 1995); Wyoming Stat. Ann. §§ 7-19-301 to 7-19-306 (1995)

3. Almost half the states permit the involuntary commitment of sexual predators: Arizona, California, Connecticut, the District of Columbia, Florida, Illinois, Iowa, Kansas, Kentucky, Massachusetts, Minnesota, Missouri, Nebraska, New Jersey, North Dakota, Oregon, Pennsylvania, South Carolina, Texas, Virginia, Washington, and Wisconsin permit the involuntary commitment of sexual predators. *See* Arizona. Rev. Stat. §§ 36-3701 to 36-3713 (West 2003 and Supp. 2007); California Welf. & Inst. Code Ann. §§ 6600 to 6609.3 (West 1998 and Supp. 2008); Connecticut Gen. Stat. § 17a-566 (1998); District of Columbia Code §§ 22-3803 to 22-3811 (2001); Florida Stat. §§ 394.910 to 394.931 (West 2002 and Supp. 2005); Illinois Comp. Stat., ch. 725, §§ 207/1 to 207/99 (2002); Iowa Code §§ 229A.1-.16 (Supp. 2005); Kansas Stat. Ann. § 59-29a02 (2004 and Supp. 2005); Kentucky Rev. Stat. Ann. § 202A.051 (West); Massachusetts Gen. Laws, ch. 123A (1989); Minnesota Stat. § 253B.02 (1992); Montana Ann. Stat. §§ 632.480 to 632.513 (West 2000 and Supp. 2006); Nebraska Rev. Stat. §§ 83-174 to 83-174.05 (2007); New Jersey Stat. Ann. §§ 30:4-27.24 to 30:4-27.38 (West Supp. 2004); North Dakota Cent. Code Ann. § 25-03.3-01 (Lexis 2002); Oregon Rev. Stat. § 426.005 (1998); Pa. Stat. Ann., Tit. 42, §§ 9791 to 9799.9 (2007); South Carolina Code Ann. §§ 44-48-10 to 44-48-170 (2002 and Supp. 2007); Texas Health & Safety Code Ann. §§ 841.001 to 841.147 (West 2003); Virginia Code Ann. §§ 37.2-900 to 37.2-920 (2006 and Supp. 2007); Washington Rev. Code § 71.09.010 (West 1992 and Supp. 2002); Wisconsin Stat. § 980.01-13 (2005)

4. Alabama, Arkansas, California, Florida, Georgia, Illinois, Kentucky, Louisiana, Ohio, Oklahoma, Oregon, and Tennessee have residency restrictions for sex offenders. *See* Alabama Code § 15-20-26 (Supp. 2000) (restricts sex offenders from residing or accepting employment within two thousand feet of school or childcare facility); Arkansas Code Ann. § 5-14-128 (Supp. 2007) (unlawful for level three or four sex offenders to reside within two thousand feet of school or daycare center); California Penal Code Ann. § 3003 (West Supp. 2008) (parolees may not live within thirty-five miles of victim or witnesses, and certain sex offenders on parole may not live within a quarter mile from a primary school); Florida Stat. § 947.1405(7)(a)(2) (2001) (released sex offender with victim under eighteen prohibited from living within one thousand feet of a school, daycare center, park, playground, or other place where children regularly congregate); Georgia Code Ann. § 42-1-13 (Supp. 2007) (sex offenders required to register shall not reside within one thousand feet of any childcare facility, school, or area where minors congregate); Illinois Comp. Stat., ch. 720, § 5/11-9.3(b-5) (Supp. 2008) (child sex offenders prohibited from knowingly residing within five hundred feet of schools); Kentucky Rev. Stat. Ann. § 17.495 (West 2000) (registered sex offenders on supervised release shall not reside within one thousand feet of school or childcare facility); Louisiana Rev. Stat. Ann. § 14:91.1 (West Supp. 2004) (sexually violent predators shall not reside within one thousand feet of schools unless permission is given by school superintendent); Ohio Rev. Code Ann. § 2950.031 (Lexis 2003) (sex offenders prohibited from residing within one thousand feet of school); Oklahoma Stat., Tit. 57, § 590 (West 2003) (prohibits sex offenders from residing within two thousand feet of schools or educational institutions); Oregon Rev. Stat. §§ 144.642, 144.643 (1999) (incorporates general prohibition on supervised sex offenders living near places where children reside); Tennessee Code Ann. § 40-39-111 (2006) (repealed by Acts 2004, ch. 921, § 4, effective Aug. 1, 2004) (sex offenders prohibited from establishing residence within one thousand feet of school, childcare facility, or victim).

5. Everyone in Florida, Idaho, Indiana, Maine, Missouri, New Hampshire, New Jersey, New Mexico, Oklahoma, Tennessee, Texas, and Utah has an affirmative duty to report suspected child abuse. *See* Florida Stat. Ann. § 39.201(1)(a) (West 2006); Idaho Code Ann. § 16-1605(1) (West 2006); Indiana Code Ann. § 31-33-5-1 (West 2006); Maine Rev. Stat. Ann. tit. 22, § 4011-A (2006), amended by Legis. 139, 123 Leg., 1st Reg. Sess. (Me. 2007); Montana Ann. Stat. § 210.115(1) (West 2006); New Hampshire Rev. Stat. Ann. § 169-C:29 (2006); New Jersey Stat. Ann. § 9:6-8.10 (West 2006); New Mexico Stat. Ann. § 32A-4-3(A) (West 2006); Oklahoma Stat. Ann. tit. 10, § 7103(A)(1)(d) (West 2006); Tennessee Code Ann. § 37-1-403(a)(2) (West 2006); Texas Fam. Code Ann. § 261.101(a) (Vernon 2006); Utah Code Ann. § 62A-4a-403(1) (West 2006).

6. Most states list treating health care professionals as mandated reporters in their individual capacity. *See* Alaska Stat. § 47.17.020 (Supp. 2006); Arizona Rev. Stat. Ann. § 13-3620 (Supp. 2006); California Penal Code § 11166 (Supp. 2007); Colorado Rev. Stat. § 19-3-304 (Supp. 2005); Connecticut Gen. Stat. § 17A-101 (Supp. 2007); District of Columbia Code § 4-1321.02 (Supp. 2007); Delaware Code Ann. tit. 16 § 903 (2003); Florida. Stat. Ann. § 39.201(Supp. 2007); Georgia Code Ann. § 19-7-5 (Supp. 2007); Hawaii Rev. Stat. § 350-1.1 (Supp. 2006); Idaho Code Ann. § 16-1605 (amend. 2005); 325 Illinois Comp. Stat. 5/4 (Supp. 2007); Indiana Code Ann. § 31-33-1-1 (amend. 2005); Iowa Code Ann. § 232.69 (amend. 2005); Kansas Stat. Ann. § 38-1507 (amend. 2004); Louisiana Child Code Ann. art. 603 (Supp. 2007); Maine Rev. Stat. tit. 22, § 4011-A (Supp. 2006); Maryland Code Ann. [Fam. Law], § 5-704 (2006); Massachusetts Gen. Laws ch. 119 § 51A (Supp. 2007); Michigan Comp. Laws Ann. § 722.623 (Supp. 2007); Minnesota Stat. Ann. § 626.556 (Supp. 2007); Mississippi Code Ann. § 43-21-353 (Supp. 2007); Montana Rev. Stat. § 210.115 (Supp. 2007); Montana Code Ann. § 41-3-201 (amend. 2007); Nebraska Rev. Stat. § 28-711 (amend. 2005); Nevada Rev. Stat. § 432B.220 (amend. 2005); New Hampshire Rev. Stat. Ann. § 169-C:29 (2002); New Jersey Stat. Ann. 9:6-8.10 (Supp. 2007); New Mexico Stat. § 32A-4-3 (1999); New York Soc. Serv. Law § 413 (Supp. 2007); North Dakota Cent. Code § 50-25.1-03 (Supp. 2007); Ohio Rev. Code Ann. § 2151.421 (2007); Oklahoma Stat. tit. 10, § 7103 (Supp. 2007); Oregon Rev. Stat. § 419B.010 (2003); 23 Pennsylvania Cons. Stat. § 6115 (Supp. 2007); Rhode Island Gen. Laws § 40-11-3 (2006); South Carolina Code Ann. § 20-7-510 (Supp. 2006); South Dakota Codified Laws § 26-8A-3 (Supp. 2007); Tennessee Code Ann. § 37-1-403 (Supp. 2006); Texas Fam. Code Ann. § 261.101 (Supp. 2005); Utah Code Ann. § 62A-4a-403 (2006); Vermont Stat. Ann. tit. 33 § 4913 (Supp. 2006); Virginia Code Ann. § 63.2-1509 (2002); Washington Rev. Code § 26.44.030 (Supp. 2007); West Virginia Code § 49-6A-2 (Supp. 2006); Wisconsin Stat. 48.981 (Supp. 2006); Wyoming Stat. Ann § 14-3-205 (amend. 2005).

7. The District of Columbia and Georgia require those employed by hospitals and clinics to report suspected child abuse to their supervisors, who are then required to make the official report. *See* District of Columbia Code § 4-1321.02 (2008) and Georgia Code Ann. § 19-7-5 (2006).

CHAPTER BIBLIOGRAPHY

ACF (Administration for Children & Families). (2008). *Child maltreatment.* Washington, DC: U.S. Department of Health & Human Services, ACF.

Allison, D. (2005). *Bastard out of Carolina.* New York, NY: Plume (award-winning novel that was developed into a Showtime movie about child abuse).

APA (American Psychological Association). (2005). *Violence and the family: Report of the APA Presidential Task Force on Violence and the Family.* Washington, DC: APA.

ASPS (American Society of Plastic Surgeons). (2008). *Teenage plastic surgery.* Arlington Heights, IL: ASPS.

(ASAPS) American Society for Aesthetic Plastic Surgery. (2008, October). Cosmetic Surgery National Data Bank Statistics. New York, NY: ASAPS.

Bandak, F. A. (2005). Shaken baby syndrome: A biomechanics analysis of injury mechanisms. *Forensic Science International, 151* (1), 71-79.

Block, R. W., Krebs, N. F., & Committee on Child Abuse & Neglect and the Committee on Nutrition. (2005). Failure to thrive as a manifestation of child neglect. *Pediatrics, 116* (5), 1234-1237.

Chiu, E. M. (2008). The culture differential in parental autonomy. *University of California Davis Law Review, 41,* 1773-1828.

Crume, T. et al. (2002). Under-ascertainment of child maltreatment fatalities by death certificates, *Pediatrics, 110* (2), 1-6.

CWIF (Child Welfare Information Gateway). (2008). *State statutes series: Mandatory reporters of child abuse and neglect.* Washington, DC: U.S. Department of Health & Human Services, Administration for Children and Families.

___. (2007). *State statutes series: Infant safe haven laws.* Washington, DC: U.S. Department of Health & Human Services, ACF.

___. (2006). *State statutes series: Parental drug use as child abuse.* Washington, DC: U.S. Department of Health & Human Services, ACF.

___. (2005). *State statutes series: Immunity for reporters of child abuse and neglect.* Washington, DC: U.S. Department of Health & Human Services, ACF.

Davis, W. of the Beaumont Police Department. (2006). Keynote address at the 24th Annual Conference on Prevention of Child Abuse: Child abuse a national epidemic in Dallas, Texas.

Dixon, C. (2005). Best practices in the response to child abuse. *Mississippi College Law Review, 25,* 73-96.

DSM-IV (*Diagnostic and statistical manual of mental disorders*). (1994). (4th ed.). Washington, DC: American Psychiatric Association.

Dudley, S. H. (2004). Medical treatment for Asian immigrant children: Does mother know best? *Georgetown Law Journal, 92,* 1287-1307.

Geddes, J. F., et al. (2003). Dural haemorrhage in non-traumatic infant deaths: Does it explain the bleeding in shaken baby syndrome? *Neuropathology & Applied Neuropathology, 29,* 14-22.

Gena, M. (2007). Shaken baby syndrome: Medical uncertainty casts doubt on convictions. *Wisconsin Law Review,* 701-727.

Gershuny, P. (2006). Family values first when federal laws collide: A proposal to create a public policy exception to the employment-at-will doctrine based upon mandatory parenting duty. *Wisconsin Women's Law Journal, 21*, 195-222.

Goodman-Brown, T. B. et al. (2003). Why children tell: A model of children's disclosure of sexual abuse. *Child Abuse and Neglect, 27*, 525-540 (cited by the 2008 U.S. Supreme Court in *Kennedy v. Louisiana*).

Gross, A. M., & Hersen, A. M. (2008). *Handbook of clinical psychology, children and adolescents.* New York, NY: Wiley.

Hall, T. S. (2002). Legal fictions and moral reasoning: Capital punishment and the mentally retarded defendant after *Penry v. Johnson. Akron Law Review, 35*, 327-370 (summarizing the long-term child abuse of a death row inmate whose case went before the U.S. Supreme Court twice).

HHS (U.S. Department of Health & Human Services). (2005). *The national survey of children's health.* Rockville, MD: HHS, Health Resources & Services Administration, Maternal & Child Health Bureau.

Jenny, C., & Isaac, R. (2006). The relation between child death and child maltreatment. *Archives of Disease in Childhood, 91* (3), 265-269.

Kellogg, N. D. (2007). Evaluation of suspected child physical abuse. *Pediatrics, 119* (6), 1232-1241.

Kelly, R. (2007). Childhood neglect and its effects on neurodevelopment: Suggestions for future law and policy. *Houston Journal of Health Law and Policy, 8*, 133-160.

Kempe, C. H. et al. (1984). Landmark article: July 7, 1962: The battered-child syndrome. *Journal of the American Medical Association, 251* (24), 3295-3300.

Kinter, B. (2005). The other victims: Can we hold parents liable for failing to protect their children from harms of domestic violence? *New England Journal of Criminal & Civil Confinement, 31*, 271-297.

Lens, V. (2006). Work sanctions under welfare reform: Are they helping women achieve self-sufficiency? *Duke Journal of Gender Law & Policy, 13*, 255-284.

Maikovich, A. K. et al. (2008). Effects of family violence on psychopathology symptoms in children previously exposed to maltreatment. *Child Development, 79* (5), 1498-1544.

Mapp, S. C. (2006). The effects of sexual abuse as a child on the risk of mothers physically abusing their children: A path analysis using systems theory. *Child Abuse & Neglect, 30* (11), 1293-1310.

Maylor, C. L. (2007). Recalibrating depravity in a Feingold regime: Why New York courts should maintain register's approach to depraved indifference in cases of murder by abuse. *Cardozo Law Review, 29*, 405-441.

McLaine, M. (2008). Supreme Court 2007-2008 review. *Champion: National Association of Criminal Defense Lawyers, 32*, 28-35.

Menninger, K. (2007). *The crime of punishment.* Bloomington, IN: AuthorHouse (classic text originally published in 1966 addressing crime in America).

Moore, C. G. et al. (2007). The prevalence of violent disagreements in U.S. families: Effects of residence, race/ethnicity, and parental stress. *Pediatrics, 119*, S68-S76 (reviewing the National Survey of Children's Health).

Morey, M. (2006). The civil commitment of state-dependent minors resonating discourse that leave her heterosexuality and his homosexuality vulnerable to scrutiny. *New York Law Review, 81*, 2129-2156.

Myers, J. E. B. (2006). Decisions and families: A symposium on polygamy, same-sex marriage, and medical decision making: Neglect of children's health, too many irons in the fire. *Journal of Law & Family Studies, 8*, 317-324.

Nicholls, S. M. (2007). Responding to the cries of the innocent: Holding non-offending parents criminally responsible for failing to protect the abused child. *Thomas Jefferson Law Review, 30*, 309-343.

O'Keefe, L. (2007). Uncovering child abuse: Physical abuse is an underreported and often unnoticed problem. A new clinical report outlines the critical components of the medical assessment. *American Academy of Pediatric News, 28* (6), 9-10.

Oklahoma Senate News Release. (2006). *Senator Nichols targets child predators with death penalty.* Tulsa, OK: Oklahoma State Senate.

Quester, N. M. (2007). The Supreme Court's decision in *Town of Castle Rock v. Gonzales* continues to deny domestic violence victims meaningful recourse. *Akron Law Review, 40*, 391-433.

Reardon, K. K., & Noblet, C. (2008). *Childhood denied: Ending the nightmare of child abuse and neglect.* New York, NY: Sage Press (practical and journalistic exposé of child abuse and neglect in the U.S.).

Redding, R. E. (2007). The brain-disordered defendant: Neuroscience and legal insanity in the twenty-first century. *American University Law Review, 56*, 51-123 (noting brain damage arising from physical child abuse as the most prevalent type of brain injury among repeatedly violent individuals).

Richardson, E. (2007). Lawyers were children once: An ethical approach to strengthening child abuse and neglect legislation. *Journal of the Legal Profession, 31*, 357-369.

Roesler, T. A., & Jenny, C. (2008). *Medical child abuse: Beyond Munchausen Syndrome by Proxy.* Elk Grove Village, IL: American Academy of Pediatrics.

Schnitzer, P. G. et al. (2008). Public health surveillance of fatal child maltreatment: Analysis of three state programs. *American Journal of Public Health, 98* (2), 296-303.

Sege, R. D., & Flaherty, E. G. (2008, October 1). Forty years later: Inconsistencies in reporting of child abuse. *Archives of Disease in Childhood, 93* (10), 822-824.

Singer, N. (2008). Do my breast implants have a warranty? *New York Times,* p. G1.

Spivack, B. (2006). Recognizing intentional childhood starvation. *American Academy of Pediatrics: AAP Grand Rounds, 15*, 34-35.

Stirling, J. (2007). Beyond Munchausen Syndrome by Proxy: Identification and treatment of child abuse in a medical setting. *Pediatrics, 119*, 1026-1030.

Sweet, K. L. (2008). Munchausen Syndrome by Proxy: Treatment in the courts. *Buffalo Women's Law Journal, 16*, 89-102.

Towner, C. L. (2006). Parents charged with kidnapping their own child: The Parker Jensen story. *Journal of Law & Family Studies, 8*, 191-202.

Wright, N., & Wright, E. (2007). SOS (safeguard our survival): Understanding and alleviating the lethal legacy of survival-threatening child abuse. *American University Journal of Gender, Social Policy & the Law, 16*, 1-114.

PART XIII

CONCLUSION

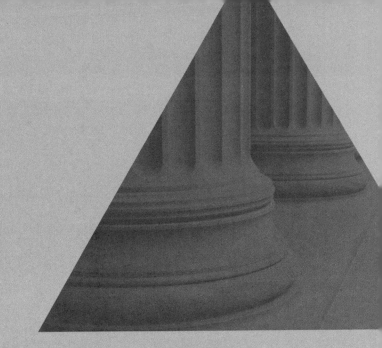

CHAPTER 39

FUTURE PROSPECTS: HEALTH CARE MANAGEMENT AND THE LAW

> "We will restore science to its rightful place and wield technology's wonders to raise health care's quality and lower its cost . . . . All this we can do. All this we will do."
>
> —INAUGURAL ADDRESS TO THE NATION BY PRESIDENT BARACK OBAMA, 44TH PRESIDENT OF THE UNITED STATES (JANUARY 20, 2009)

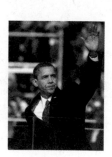

IN BRIEF

This last chapter is comprised of two parts concerning how our health care system may be revised and refurbished, which is one of the most important issues the U.S. is confronting in terms of politics, economics, law, and ethics. The first part summarizes Chapters 1 through 38, with an emphasis on today's most challenging management issues and topical health law concerns. The second part provides an overview of the shifts required to develop policy frameworks for instituting changes in health care management and the law in each of the major health care sectors: life sciences, health care delivery, and medical products.

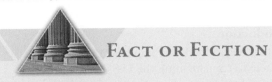

FACT OR FICTION

HEALTH CARE REFORM

Can public nonprofit health insurance exchanges compete with private health insurers?

There are various points of view about how to reform the nation's insurance system, but there are basically two views on competition in the health insurance sector. One view claims equal competition between public insurance exchange plans and private health insurance plans would be impossible; the public plans would inevitably crowd out private plans, leading to a single-payer system. Another view claims that public insurance exchanges could achieve significant savings in administrative costs and prevent excessive profits and multimillion-dollar compensation packages by private insurers.

The health insurance industry claims that a significant proportion of its administrative costs is incurred for creating and maintaining provider networks, and for monitoring reimbursements. There is an incentive to spend a dollar as long as the expected savings is at least a dollar. The challenge is for public insurance exchanges to have comparable incentives.

While profits are needed to earn normal returns on the capital the health insurance industry invests to back the sale of coverage, insurance profits have not been excessive compared with other industries. Public health insurance exchanges, on the other hand, would not have to hold amounts of capital comparable to private plans; the exchanges would be backed by the federal or state governments. Similarly, the public exchanges would not be subject to the same taxes that the insurance industry pays, including those on investment returns from holding capital. Competition on this level could only be possible with reform of the private for-profit sector and a commitment to addressing excessive executive compensation in an industry where the federal government funded 54 percent of the total health care spending in 2008 (CBO, 2008).

Equal competition in reimbursing health care providers and professionals is another area of debate. One proposal is for the public insurance exchanges to pay Medicare rates. But because Medicare reimbursements involve substantial cost-shifting to private health insurance plans, any expansion of Medicare rates would further shift costs to private plans and accelerate their crowd-out. Whether rate markups by Medicare could resolve this cost-shifting is debatable.

The alternatives to having private plans reimburse health care providers and professionals at Medicare rates would require significantly higher Medicare reimbursements. This approach would most likely produce universal price controls on health care services and raise the obvious question: why bother with private plans?

Having the public insurance exchanges instead pay private plan rates could challenge a major objective of health care reform: reducing costs. This approach would need to address complex design and administrative challenges to benchmark reimbursement rates negotiated between thousands of health care providers and professionals and numerous private health plans.

—Congressional Budget Office, 2009;
Council of Economic Advisors, 2009; MEDPAC, 2009.
(See *Law Fact* at the end of this chapter for the answer.)

PRINCIPLES AND APPLICATIONS

The many forces that can advance health care delivery, such as innovative practices among providers that effectively restrain prices while improving quality care, have been presented in this text. This chapter concludes by asking whether the real problem with U.S. health care is market distortions of the foundation underlying the equitable delivery of health care amidst competition for limited financial and human resources in each of the health care sectors. The question may not be whether any intrinsic market failure could be fixed by more regulation, but whether a more just and comprehensive system of regulation is required to ensure access to affordable health care for all U.S. residents.

THE HEALTH CARE CRISIS WITHIN THE U.S.'S LEGAL FRAMEWORK

The nation's health care laws and regulations must be reworked in order to create a system that works as intended, especially as the many health care industry sectors are rapidly converging and therefore defying the laws and regulations already in place. This is true as:

- Medically necessary health care is increasingly seen as a right for all U.S. residents
- Health care corporations from different sectors merge
- New medical products and technologies emerge that do not fall under any existing regulatory scheme

This progress is spurred by advancements in medical information technology that are requiring the American legal system to expand the boundaries of health care law to encompass the essential and best components of the U.S. health care system.

Some of this health care progress fits within established legal principles and rules of law, or the principles and rules can be adapted to include it. However, health care law and regulations are becoming so complex and nuanced that health care organizations are shifting their legal strategies away from complying with them and toward finding ways to evade them. In the past, Americans have resisted any limits on health care. However, going forward, as health care costs continue to increase, particularly regarding life-prolonging and end-of-life care, some Americans question whether health care law can be used to set limits on available health care. This is especially true as Americans continue to struggle with the question of whether everyone should be entitled to health care, and if so, how much care and how to fund it.

OUR APPROACH

This text summarized the current practices and advances in health care with attention directed to the moral dilemmas facing today's health care professionals. Basic legal principles were reviewed and practical applications of the law in health care delivery and practice were presented. The focus was on both the meaning and the effects of the law, so that the ethical implications of judicial decisions and their effect on the evolution of the law were understood. How current reforms of the U.S. health care system are evolving around the principles of distributive justice was highlighted throughout the text.

Introduction

The text began by describing how the greatest obstacle to transforming the U.S. health care system may be the nation's collective thinking. How the nation's mental models may create and limit opportunities was explained. This section also described how the U.S. legal system functions through the separation of governmental powers that is central to the U.S. Constitution. The role of "the People" and the agencies the federal government uses to administer and enforce U.S. health laws were reviewed, along with crucial public health issues currently facing relevant federal agencies.

Overview of Specific Health Laws

This section described common health care legal issues. Health care compliance programs focusing on corporate fraud and abuse were reviewed. This was the only topic in the textbook where an appreciation of specific policy regulations was essential to understanding the political and ideological agendas dictating the direction and enforcement of health care activities. The most effective fraud and abuse prevention and compliance programs were examined, including whether they actually encourage higher ethical standards. Antitrust rules and regulations were described, and whether they impede or improve the health care industry's ability to compete was questioned.

Access to Health Care

This section focused on developments in managed care and government care programs. The challenge of finding a way to provide access to basic health care for all U.S. residents was described. Legislative experiments such as "pay-or-play" laws and tax credits were discussed. In particular, the challenge of providing access to health care for those at the bottom of the economic pyramid was examined, including whether their constitutional rights are violated when they cannot access health care through government insurance programs. The challenge of reforming Medicare was also presented.

Affordable Health Care

This section described why affordable health care is so difficult to come by. The need for nonprofit hospitals to offer affordable or free health care in return for tax exemptions, and why it is difficult for them to do so, was summarized. The feasibility of providing basic health insurance for all U.S. residents was examined in the context of patient rights. Tort reform and reducing the occurrence and cost of medical malpractice was underscored.

Staffing of Health Care Systems

This section focused on health care providers. Human resources departments are an essential partner in building many of the legal infrastructures covered in this text, from compliance and ethics programs to policies that ensure the health industry adheres to its social missions. The idea of human resources departments within health care organizations serving as strategic partners rather than in their traditional administrative role was emphasized. Ways to lower employers' health care costs were examined, with particular focus on smoking- and weight-related health care costs. Labor relations within health care organizations were examined, including unionization and workload management.

Strategic Health Care Restructurings

This section explained the pressures on the health care and insurance industries to provide less restricted care. The multi-tiered model of the U.S. health care system, where the uninsured receive little care, if any, and the wealthy are able to access tomorrow's technology, was described. Mergers and acquisitions and bankruptcies within the industry were looked at. The current trend of business process outsourcing was also addressed.

Producers of Medical Products

This section focused on a critical aspect of the health care industry responsible for 25 percent of the U.S. economy: producers of medical products. Particular attention was paid to pharmaceutical corporations, regarding the high prices of drugs, the risks of lengthy product development, and the importance of vaccines. The emerging field of biotechnology, with its near unlimited potential for medical breakthroughs, was described. Also described was the rapid advancement in the field of medical devices due to changes in the population. The impact and possibilities of health information technology were presented.

Improving the Quality of Health Care

This section described four areas where there is broad agreement on how to lower costs and improve quality of medical treatment. The demand for greater physician treatment decision transparency as well as the demand for information technology to support better treatment decisions was discussed. Evidence-based medicine and its potential for improving the industry was presented. Programs targeting patient safety and aimed at preventing medical errors were reviewed. The practices of the nation's best hospitals were emphasized.

Our Health Care System's Response to Illness

This section took a systematic look at the dimensions of serious disease and disability in the U.S. Both the illicit and legitimate human body parts industries were described. Organ procurement and transplantation, a subset of the body parts industries, was detailed. The devastating HIV/AIDS epidemic and the global fight against it were addressed. The magnitude of the effect of mental illness on the U.S. health care system was also addressed.

End-of-Life Health Care

This section detailed the "right-to-die" controversy. It questioned how far the government should be permitted to intrude into personal health care. The economic advantages of hospice care were presented. Particular attention was paid to end-of-life issues for minors. The legal implications of assisted death and advanced directives were examined.

Our Health Care System's Response to New Technologies

This section questioned whether the U.S. health care system will be able to afford the new technologies that could change the direction of health care. Advances in stem cells and regenerative medicine were described, as well as advances in reprogenics and assisted reproductive medicine.

Additional Pressing Issues Facing Our Health Care System

This section focused on issues health care professionals may be most likely to confront in practice. The government's ability to respond to public health emergencies, such as pandemics or bioterrorist attacks, was discussed. The particular health care challenges women face, especially regarding reproductive care, were presented. The impact of the food industry on health care was examined. The fact that although the U.S. has the most expensive health care system in the world, Americans are neither healthier nor likely to live longer than others, was highlighted. The effects of child abuse and neglect on the health care system and society in general were also presented.

OUR FUTURE: PERSONALIZED HEALTH CARE

Today, with improved medical technology, it is becoming easier than ever to identify better response strategies for personalized health care. Health care providers and professionals are able to compare medical options quickly and cost-effectively, obtain detailed health information on experiences from elsewhere, and will soon be able to determine which personalized interventions will be most successful (Wilensky, 2005). Medical decisions can now be made using more data-driven and analytically rigorous underpinnings.

Across-the-Board Regulatory Reform

Despite the advances in medicine, there are escalating calls for new regulatory scrutiny of health care. One might ask why. One reason may be that America spends more than any other developed nation on health care: $2.4 trillion in 2008 alone according to the National Coalition on Health Care. This disparity in expenditures between America and other similarly developed nations cannot be attributed to Americans having access to the latest medical innovations with higher price tags for treatment; it also cannot be attributed to universal coverage, since millions of Americans remain uninsured and without access to basic health care. Furthermore, of the Americans who are insured, at least 125 million suffer from preventable health conditions that needlessly developed into chronic illnesses and diseases, costing more than $500 billion annually as a result (Landro, 2004).

Today, after decades of cat-and-mouse games between the regulated parts of the health industry and the regulators, a dramatic overhaul of the U.S. health care system may be possible. A depression-era-like reform of the complete health care regulatory system is needed, much like the nation experienced from the Roosevelt era's New Deal; rather than the incremental reforms of the past seventy years, reform of every government agency involved in health care is needed across the board. Any meaningful reform will be enormously complex and require long and careful consideration by all stakeholders, including the:

- Health care providers: physicians and other licensed health care professionals
- Delivery systems: hospitals, home health care providers, nursing, and long-term care facilities
- Health insurers: private insurance providers and public insurance programs (Medicare, Medicaid, military entitlement programs (TRICARE), the Civilian Health and Medical Program of the Department of Veteran Affairs (CHAMPVA), and other public hospital/physician coverage programs)
- Providers of medical products: pharmaceuticals, biotechnology, medical devices, and health information technology companies
- Consumers of health care of all socioeconomic backgrounds

Comprehensive Review of the Federal Food, Drug, and Cosmetic Act

For seventy years, Congress has sought to patch, rather than cure, a fractured regulatory system (Starr, 1983). The Food, Drug, and Cosmetic Act of 1938 (FDCA) replaced the earlier Pure Food and Drug Act of 1906 in response to a mass poisoning that resulted in more than one hundred children dying from an error in formulating a medicine. The so-called Elixir Sulfanilamide disaster involved the sulfanilamide medication where diethylene glycol, a solvent related to radiator antifreeze, was used to dissolve the drug and make a liquid form (Starr, 1983). At the time, medical quackery was the major concern of Congress, including proprietary medicines mixed by homeopathic and allopathic physicians for individual patients.

Since 1938, Congress has amended the FDCA several hundred times, word by word, provision by provision, to the point where the complexity of the law has resulted in inconsistencies in both its terms and scope.[LN1] Despite these regulatory inconsistencies and legal contradictions affecting virtually every provider of health care, the federal agency charged with implementing the FDCA has seen the significance of its role in the U.S. economy continue to expand; today, the U.S. Food and Drug Administration (FDA) regulates:

- More than 25 percent of the total U.S. economy
- Almost $3.5 trillion ($3,500,000,000,000.00) in U.S. economic activities
- About 80 percent of the U.S. food supply

(Emmanuel, 2008)

While the FDCA was largely successful, the U.S. pharmaceutical industry has evolved from 1938 into a $300 billion regulated industry today. The evolution of medicine over the past seventy years demands new approaches and a legal overhaul of its regulatory regime.[LN2] For instance, although the pharmaceutical industry is the most regulated industry in the U.S. (Golec & DiMasi, 2008), parts of the rapidly developing biotechnology industry remain virtually unregulated. In addition, any reform should likely include regulation of genomics, much of which until now has been relatively free of government oversight, including stem cell research and reprogenics.

Review of Federal Health Insurance Entitlement Programs

The U.S. is the only industrialized nation in the world that does not guarantee basic health care to all of its citizens (Daschle & Lambrew, 2008). While skeptics claim the U.S. cannot afford to provide health insurance coverage for everyone, almost everyone else maintains the nation cannot afford not to. The uninsured and the nation's fast-rising health care costs impede U.S. economic competitiveness (Emmanuel & Fuchs, 2008).

Moreover, the total cost of health care has grown steadily at an average rate of 7 percent for the past five years, or at twice the annualized five-year growth rate of the nation's gross national product (Kaiser, 2007). This growth rate in health care spending is simply unsustainable in the long term (Geithner, 2009).

Balancing Transparency and Protections for Consumers of Health Care with Medical Innovations

Americans want a better health care system than currently exists. It may not be a pure single-payer government-run system, nor will it probably be a free market private industry program, but it may be a hybrid. Only time will tell what kind of hybrid it may be. One principle is, however, inviolate: any new health regulations should balance the need to provide transparency and protections for consumers of health care, while also allowing the health industry to continue to innovate and generate the capital required for economic growth (*see* Relman, 2007).

The American public ranks health care reform as one of the nation's top priorities, according to a December 2008 national survey conducted by the Kaiser Family Foundation and the Harvard School of Public Health. For many Americans, the health care crisis is grave. Clearly the delivery mechanisms have broken down to the extent that the nation must seriously consider access to and affordability of health care.

Consolidated Health Care System

With the rate of health care costs rapidly outpacing the nation's gross domestic product, Americans can no longer afford to maintain the nation's fragmented delivery of care (Wilensky, 2005). The health industry's current posture, however, often puts it at odds with health care consumers. Perhaps the medical products industry should begin to align itself more closely with the patients who take its drugs and use its medical device products. This, after all, is the natural "sweet spot" of the pharmaceutical, biotechnology, and medical devices sectors where the industry achieves its profits.

Patient-Centered Model

Encouraging wellness could be one way to create alliances in a consolidated health care system. One possibility would be to link the medical products and health insurance industries. Medical products companies could offer lifetime health insurance packages to individuals who guaranteed they would follow lifelong wellness regimes, including drugs for chronic illnesses and diseases, abstaining from smoking, and controlling health with regular exercise and a well-balanced diet. Enrollees could be accepted into the lifelong health insurance program during their college years, at ages nineteen to twenty-four, and monitored for their lifetimes.

Skeptics state the industry has not moved toward this patient-centered model because the old one has created entrenched stakeholders. But strong and innovative leadership could take the medical products and insurance industries down a new path. The change must, however, amount to a new business model for the medical products and insurance industries, not just an offshoot of marketing operations.

Federal Health Board

One possible model might be a consolidated system in which health care providers, health insurers, and regulators are closely aligned, similar to that of the United Kingdom (Relman, 2007). A Federal Health Board could be created, similar to the Federal Reserve System and similar to the British National Institute for Health and Clinical Excellence (NICE), whose structure, functions, and enforcement capability would be largely insulated from politics. Like President Roosevelt did on monetary policy with the creation of the Federal Reserve System in 1913, decision-making on the immensely complex topics of health care policy and health care delivery reform could be delegated to a presidentially appointed panel of experts and consumers of health care (Dashle & Lambrew, 2008; Emmanuel, 2008).

A Federal Health Board could be structured with a central board and several regional boards. As an independent body, it could recommend coverage under government-run insurance plans for only those medications, treatments, and procedures backed by medical evidence, not marketing. The Board would determine what treatment services would be covered by public insurance programs based on evidence-based practices. Exactly how the Board would be organized, including how it would control costs, ensure universal, equal access, and guarantee quality of care is standardized, monitored, evaluated, and improved across the nation would have to be determined. The idea of creating a Board to regulate health care policy would allow an impartial group of experts to improve health care at the federal policy level without political biases (*see generally* Fuchs, 1998).

Unintended Consequences of Regulation

Often, enacted health care regulations create more problems than they solve. The nation could easily adopt regulations that would create a more orderly health care system, but those changes could also stifle innovation. Any change should occur in a carefully considered way; reforms should be more likely to have an impact over the long term, rather than dousing the multiple fires that are now burning.

There are many examples of how the health industry and regulators have been engaged in a dance, with the largest providers leading and regulators one step behind. Today's fragmented regulatory environment often allows shrewd industry players to choose an oversight venue where government agencies are more likely to approach their role with a narrow focus that prevents them from considering larger trends shaping the U.S. health care system.

For example, the convergence of many health care sectors is rapidly changing the laws governing provider competition and regulation. Pharmaceutical conglomerates are coupling with biotechnology corporations, while emerging biopharmaceutical products are developing that do not fit into any existing regulatory schemes. Separate regulatory schemes made sense when drugs were pharmaceuticals and the biotechnology industry was practically nonexistent. Today, providers of health care products learn how to package a product and choose its regulators, which means that neither actually regulates or controls what is going on. Similarly, the Federal Trade Commission regulates hospital and medical products matters, while the Justice Department handles health insurance issues. Again, all sorts of improper things can take place.

Redefine the Mission of the U.S. Department of Health and Human Services

The number one cause for bankruptcy in the U.S., medical bills, cannot be reflective of a good system of health care (Collins et al., 2006). Within the U.S. Department of Health and Human Services, the mission of the two agencies with the most direct impact on the health care industry should be redefined: the FDA and the Centers for Medicare and Medicaid Services (CMS).

U.S. Food and Drug Administration

The original mission of the FDA is no longer in line with the realities of the market. The FDA was created in 1938 to protect individual consumers of health care from unsafe drugs (Starr, 1983). Now, large institutional health care consumers dominate the market, but the FDA's structure remains geared toward individual health care consumers. The FDA is not as effective as it could be in regulating institutional problems.

Any framework for new forms of health regulation will need to address the role of the FDA, whose primary mission has been to manage the pharmaceutical industry and, to a lesser degree, the medical

devices and biotechnology industries. However, a sole dedication to ensuring the safety, efficacy, and security of medical products may leave out important considerations, leading to harsh consequences for the health care system when those issues are not comprehensively addressed, such as with drug pricing.

While it would have to be determined what levers directly affect the U.S. health care system, this does not mean the FDA could not have an opinion that is not necessarily consequential. For instance, a new regulatory system could include research and discussion of conditions in the health care system as part of open committee meetings, without the FDA taking any actions in response. This could be modeled after the Federal Open Market Committee meetings on raising or lowering interest rates by the Federal Reserve.

Centers for Medicare and Medicaid Services

While the recent expansion of Medicaid is to be applauded, public insurance provides amongst the lowest reimbursements for providers (Dashle & Lambrew, 2008). Many treatments and procedures simply cannot be performed at the Medicaid reimbursement level, such that major academic centers with federal support take a loss when doing business with these patients. In fairness, any expansion of Medicaid should increase government reimbursement rates so that institutions may recoup the actual costs of providing health care, rather than operating at a loss. One proposed possibility is to expand the Federal Employees Health Benefits Plan. This expansion would ensure access to health insurance for those unable to get employer-provided or public insurance programs.

Risk Adjusted Insurance

The concept of risk adjustment has merit, providing it can be used without encouraging unhealthy behavior. Under risk adjustment, and for those who joined health plans, Medicare/Medicaid would pay more for predictably sicker people than for predictably healthier people.

The difficulty is operational; the problem is how to define sicker individuals for coverage purposes. Under current law, Medicare payment adjustments are based upon certain hospitalizations in the preceding year. The concern is how individuals with coverage can be defined as sick or healthy only in terms of a previous year's hospitalization(s); this policy could encourage hospitalizations and penalize providers that attempt to reduce hospitalizations.

Partial Capitation

Partial capitation is another health care reform with merit. For instance, under partial capitation, fixed payments for Medicare/Medicaid insured services could be replaced by combining a fixed payment with a payment that reflects actual use of services (Wilensky, 2005). The relative weights attached to the fixed payment versus the variable payment to health care providers would be a policy judgment. The advantage of a partial capitation measure would be twofold:

- Acknowledges the important ability to measure health risk
- Eliminates incentives to withhold treatment by paying more for people who use more services

Reorganize Congressional Oversight

The FDA is probably skilled at knowing if a filing for drug approval is appropriate or not, but its track record of preventing big problems is not impressive (DiMasi & Faden, 2009). There should be some consolidation in oversight of the U.S. health care system, but it will take a great deal of thought on how to do this. Politically, it will be very difficult to consolidate because power in congressional committees is at stake. Health regulation remains fragmented because separate committees in Congress control different regulatory bodies, and no congressional committee is likely to give up power easily (Dashle & Lambrew, 2007).

Three-Tiered Approach to Regulatory Reform

The U.S. may have to start from scratch and think about how health care should be regulated while allowing it to thrive and not taking any undue risks for which society as a whole must pay. It would be a balancing act to achieve this goal and would require everything be put on the table. One way to start might be to adopt a three-tiered approach to regulatory reform:

- Issues that clearly require addressing
- Issues that are a major departure from current practices, but have strong cases
- Fundamental questions

Issues That Clearly Require Addressing

The first tier would consist of issues that clearly require addressing. For instance, most agree that the number of uninsured Americans who do not have access to basic health care is an issue requiring immediate attention.

Issues That are a Major Departure from Current Practices, But Have Strong Cases

The second tier would address issues in ways that seem like a major departure from current practices, but have strong cases. One example is excessive executive compensation in an industry subsidized by public funds, particularly at tax-exempt health care systems and within the health insurance industry. It is difficult to understand why presidents and chief executive officers in health care systems are allowed to earn multimillion-dollar performance bonuses when almost half of the three million aides are working for poverty wages, as are one in four of their support staff (BLS, 2009).

Moreover, it is debatable whether executive compensation in the health care industry should be based on a single year's results, when it is so easy for executives to take actions that enhance their performance one year, but may harm the delivery of health care for years into the future. Now, however, executive compensation is viewed as a corporate governance issue rather than a regulatory issue. It is not clear whether executive compensation in the health care industry requires attention in a regulatory fashion at some point.

Fundamental Questions

A third tier would address the more fundamental question of balancing the benefits of medical innovation against the risk of creating new products within the federal regulatory structure. Great enthusiasm is expressed for generic drugs, which in retrospect may not always be in the best interest of the consumers of health care (Grabowski & Kyle, 2007).

Redefine the Balance Between Regulation and Medical Innovations

If the U.S. wants to reap the fruits of medical innovation, Americans must support the policies that encourage investment in the providers of medical products where it costs more than $1.2 billion to develop a pharmaceutical drug (DiMasi & Grabowski, 2007) and $1.3 billion to develop a biopharmaceutical drug (Tufts Center, 2006) over ten to fifteen years (DiMasi, 2003).

In recent years, the balance between regulation and medical innovation has shifted toward regulation. Burrill & Company, a San Francisco-based venture fund and merchant bank, estimates the pharmaceutical industry is expending some $59 billion on research and development each year, and yet only twenty-three new drugs were approved by the FDA in 2007 (Silverman, 2008).

The nation may need to better understand the benefits of preventative care and begin to think more about the social stakes involved in providing access to basic health care and affordable, necessary care to every resident in the U.S. (*see* Golec & DiMasi, 2008).

Moreover, the FDA must redefine how it regulates the providers of medical products that are among the nation's most important industries.

For instance, with fifteen hundred public and private biotechnology companies employing tens of thousands of highly trained people, the U.S. is universally considered to be the global leader in biopharmaceuticals (NSB, 2009). Yet, in 2007, only seven biopharmaceuticals were approved by the FDA and only four ever saw the market (Silverman, 2008a). The question that begs asking is whether any of these numbers are acceptable to anyone. Alternatively, is it acceptable for regulation to replace medical innovation?

Comprehensive Regulatory Infrastructure

A careful approach must be taken to new health regulations as the nation decides how to go about setting up a better health care system. The current regulatory infrastructure was created in piecemeal fashion. In the wake of the current demand to take action, perhaps there is a need to start over with a comprehensive approach. In the end, the most pressing thing that nearly everyone agrees on is that the time to make changes in the U.S. health care system is now.

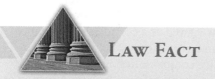

LAW FACT

HEALTH CARE REFORM

Can public nonprofit health insurance exchanges compete with private health insurers?

With or without public insurance exchanges, health care reform is almost certain to substantially change the dimensions on which health insurance plans compete. Given the need to control the costs of health care, there will probably be constraints on risk pools, benefit design, marketing, and perhaps profitability of the insurance industry.

—Congressional Budget Office, 2009;
Council of Economic Advisors, 2009; MEDPAC, 2009.

CHAPTER SUMMARY

- The real problem with health care may be the conflict between theoretical ideals and market limitations, thereby requiring the development of a more equitable system with the financial resources available.
- Intrinsic in the reform of health care is the reform of the nation's health care laws and regulations, which are complex, exceedingly nuanced, and incomplete.
- The future of the American health care system likely involves increasingly personalized care.
- One reason comprehensive regulatory reform is clearly needed is because Americans spend more on health care than any other developed nation, yet they are neither healthier nor likely to live longer. Further, the U.S. is the only industrialized nation that does not provide basic health care for all of its citizens, impeding its economic competitiveness.
- The current regulatory scheme encourages evasion and avoidance rather than compliance.
- Reform will require cooperation between health care providers, delivery systems, health insurers, medical product manufacturers, and consumers of health care; it will also require more transparency and protection for consumers, while allowing for innovation and capital generation.
- One method of partial reform would reward patients who take the initiative for their own wellness, thereby decreasing their health care costs.
- Another suggested method of reform would be the creation of a Federal Health Board responsible for determining what government-run insurance programs would cover and would be insulated from politics.
- The mission of the U.S. Department of Health and Human Services must be redefined, including reforming the role of the FDA away from individual consumers and toward institutional problems, as well as the role of the Centers for Medicare and Medicaid in reimbursing providers.
- The U.S. could take a three-tiered approach to regulatory reform, addressing issues that require immediate attention, issues that depart from current practices, and fundamental questions.
- The balance between regulation and innovation must be examined so that the U.S. can remain competitive in the global health care arena.

LAW NOTES

1. Twenty-two amendments have been incorporated into the FDCA since 1980. Note that many of the following Acts are not independent laws; rather they amend other, already existing laws, and thus the citations provided are to the laws they amend:
   - Animal Drug Availability Act of 1996, 21 U.S.C.A. § 354 (2004)
   - Animal Drug User Fee Act of 2003, 21 U.S.C.A. §§ 379j-11, 379j-12 (2008)
   - Best Pharmaceuticals for Children Act, 21 U.S.C.A. § 393a (2007); 21 U.S.C.A. § 355b (2003); 42 U.S.C.A. § 284m (2007)
   - Dietary Supplement and Nonprescription Drug Consumer Protection Act of 2006, 21 U.S.C.A. §§ 379aa, 379aa-1 (2006)
   - Drug Price Competition and Patent Term Restoration Act of 1984 ("Hatch-Waxman Act"), 35 U.S.C.A. § 156 (2002)
   - FDA Export Reform and Enhancement Act of 1996, 21 U.S.C.A. § 382 (1997)
   - Food Allergen Labeling and Consumer Protection Act of 2004, 21 U.S.C.A. § 374a (2004)
   - Food and Drug Administration Amendments Act of 2007, 21 U.S.C.A. §§ 350f *et seq.* (2009); 42 U.S.C.A. § 247d-5a (2007)
   - Food and Drug Administration Modernization Act of 1997, 21 U.S.C.A. §§ 343-3 *et seq.* (2009); 42 U.S.C.A. §§ 247b-8, 299a-3 (2009)
   - Food Quality Protection Act of 1996, 7 U.S.C.A. §§ 136 *et seq.* (2009); 21 U.S.C.A. §§ 321 *et seq.* (2009)
   - Generic Animal Drug and Patent Term Restoration Act of 1988, 21 U.S.C.A. §§ 321 *et seq.* (2009); 28 U.S.C.A. § 2201 (1993); 35 U.S.C.A. § 156 (2002); 35 U.S.C.A. § 271 (2003)
   - Infant Formula Act of 1980, 21 U.S.C.A. §§ 321 *et seq.* (2009)
   - Medical Device Amendments of 1992, 21 U.S.C.A. §§ 321 *et seq.* (2009); 42 U.S.C.A. § 262 (2008)
   - Medical Device User Fee and Modernization Act of 2002, 21 U.S.C.A. §§ 379i, 379j (2007); 42 U.S.C.A. § 289g-3 (2002)
   - Minor Use and Minor Species Animal Health Act of 2004, 21 U.S.C.A. §§ 360ccc *et seq.* (2004)
   - Nutrition Labeling and Education Act of 1990, 21 U.S.C.A. § 343-1 (2006)
   - Orphan Drug Act of 1983, 21 U.S.C.A. §§ 360aa-360ee (2009); 26 U.S.C.A. § 28 (1996); 35 U.S.C.A. § 155 (2002); 42 U.S.C.A. §§ 236, 255, 298b-4 (2009)
   - Pediatric Research Equity Act of 2003, 21 U.S.C.A. § 355c (2007)
   - Prescription Drug Amendments of 1992, 21 U.S.C.A. §§ 333 *et seq.* (2009)
   - Prescription Drug Marketing Act of 1987, 21 U.S.C.A. §§ 331 *et seq.* (2009)
   - Prescription Drug User Fee Act of 1992, 21 U.S.C.A. §§ 379g, 379h (2007)
   - Safe Medical Devices Act of 1990, 21 U.S.C.A. §§ 383, 3601 (2009)
   (FDA, 2008)

2. In addition to the FDCA, twenty-one other federal laws affect the FDA:
   - Bioterrorism Bill of 2002, 7 U.S.C.A. §§ 3353 *et seq.* (2002); 21 U.S.C.A. §§ 350c *et seq.* (2002); 29 U.S.C.A. § 669a (2002); 42 U.S.C.A. §§ 244 *et seq.* (2009)
   - Controlled Substances Act of 1970, 21 U.S.C.A. §§ 801 *et seq.* (2009)
   - Controlled Substances Import and Export Act of 1970, 21 U.S.C.A. §§ 951 *et seq.* (2009)
   - Egg Products Inspection Act of 1970, 21 U.S.C.A. §§ 1031-1056 (2009)
   - Fair Packaging and Labeling Act of 1966, 15 U.S.C.A. §§ 1451-1461 (2009)
   - Federal Advisory Committee Act of 1972, 5 U.S.C.A. App. 2 §§ 1-15 (2009)
   - Federal Anti-Tampering Act of 1983, 18 U.S.C.A. § 1365 (2002); 35 U.S.C.A. § 155A (2002)
   - Federal Meat Inspection Act of 1907, 21 U.S.C.A. §§ 601 *et seq.* (2009)
   - Federal Trade Commission Act of 1914, 15 U.S.C.A. §§ 41-58 (2009)
   - Filled Milk Act of 1923, 21 U.S.C.A. §§ 61-64 (2009)
   - Government in the Sunshine Act of 1976, 5 U.S.C.A. § 552b (1995)
   - Import Milk Act of 1927, 21 U.S.C.A. §§ 141-149 (2009)
   - Lead-Based Paint Poisoning Prevention Act of 1971, 42 U.S.C.A. §§ 4821 *et seq.* (2009)
   - Mammography Quality Standards Act of 1992, 42 U.S.C.A. § 263b (2004)
   - National Environmental Policy Act of 1969, 42 U.S.C.A. §§ 4321 *et seq.* (2009)
   - Poultry Products Inspection Act of 1957, 21 U.S.C.A. §§ 451-472 (2009)
   - Project BioShield Act of 2004, 6 U.S.C.A. § 320 (2007); 42 U.S.C.A. §§ 247d-6a *et seq.* (2009)

- Public Health Service Act of 1944, 42 U.S.C.A. §§ 201 *et seq.* (2009) (containing over one thousand sections of law)
- Reorganization Plan No. 1 of 1953, 5 U.S.C.A. App. 1 REORG. PLAN 1 1953 (1967)
- Sanitary Food Transportation Act of 1990, 21 U.S.C.A. § 350e (2005)
- Trademark Act of 1946 ("Lanham Act"), 15 U.S.C.A. §§ 1051 *et seq.* (2009)

(FDA, 2008)

CHAPTER BIBLIOGRAPHY

BLS (Bureau of Labor Statistics). (2009). *Occupational outlook handbook: Registered nurses.* Washington, DC: U.S. Department of Labor, BLS.

Collins, S. R. et al. (2006). *Squeezed: Why rising exposure to health care costs threatens the health and financial well-being of American families.* New York, NY: Commonwealth Fund.

Congressional Budget Office. (2009). *The budgetary treatment of proposals to change the nation's health insurance system.* Washington, DC: CBO.

___. (2008). *Key issues in analyzing major health insurance proposals.* Washington, DC: CBO.

Council of Economic Advisors. (2009). *The economic case for health care reform.* Washington, DC: The White House, CEA.

Daschle, T., & Lambrew, J. (2008). *Critical: What we can do about the health-care crisis.* New York, NY: Macmillan: Thomas Dunne Books.

DiMasi, D. J., & Faden, L. (2009). Factors associated with multiple FDA review cycles and approval phase times. *Drug Information Journal, 43* (2), 201-226.

___. & Grabowski, H. G. (2007). The cost of biopharmaceutical R&D: Is biotech different? *Managerial & Decision Economics, 28,* 469-479.

___. (2003). The price of innovation: New estimates of drug development costs. *Journal of Health Economics, 22,* 151-185.

Emmanuel, E. (2008). *Healthcare guaranteed: A simple, secure solution for America.* New York, NY: Perseus Books Group, PublicAffairs.

___. & Fuchs, V. (2008). Who really pays for health care? The myth of shared responsibility. *Journal of the American Medical Association, 299* (9), 1057-1059.

FDA (U.S. Food & Drug Administration). (2008). *Laws enforced by the FDA and related statutes.* Bethesda, MD: FDA.

Fuchs, V. (1998). *Who shall live? Health, economics, and social choice.* (expanded ed.) Hackensack, NJ: World Scientific Publishing Co. (classic by Stanford University Nobel Laureate in Economics).

Geithner, T., U.S. Treasury Secretary. (2009, January 21). Hearing before the U.S. Senate Finance Committee, 111th Congress. Washington, DC.

Golec, V. J., & DiMasi, J. (2008). Drug development costs when financial risk is measured using the Fama-French three factor model. Unpublished paper, Tufts University, Boston, MA.

Grabowski, H., & Kyle, M. (2007). Generic competition and market exclusivity periods in pharmaceuticals. *Managerial & Decision Economics, 28,* 491-502.

Kaiser (Kaiser Family Foundation). (2009). *The public's health care agenda for the new president and Congress.* Menlo Park, CA: Kaiser.

___. (2007). *Health care spending in the United States and OECD countries.* Menlo Park, CA: Kaiser.

Landro, L. (2004, February 12). Preventive medicine gets more aggressive. *Wall Street Journal,* p. D1.

MEDPAC (Medicare Payment Advisory Commission). (2009). *Report to the 111th Congress: Improving incentives in the Medicare program.* Washington, DC: MEDPAC.

Medtap International. (2003). *The value of investment in health care: Better care, better lives.* Bethesda, MD: Medtap.

NSB (National Science Board). (2009). *Research and development: Essential foundation for U.S. competitiveness in a global economy.* Washington, DC: NSB.

Relman, A. (2007). *A second opinion: Rescuing America's health care.* New York, NY: Perseus Books Group, PublicAffairs.

Silverman, B. (2008, January 14). FDA first-cycle approval rates in silver lining in cloud of low NME (new molecule entity) count. *The Pink Sheet, 70,* p. 2.

___. (2008a, January 21). Year in review: New biologics in total seven in 2007, but only four will see market. *The Pink Sheet, 70,* p. 3.

Starr, P. (1983). *The social transformation of American medicine.* New York, NY: Basic Books (classic by Princeton University Pulitzer Prize and Bancroft Prize Laureate in American History).

Tufts Center for the Study of Drug Development. (2006). *Average cost to develop a new biotechnology product is $1.2 billion.* Boston, MA: Tufts.

Wilensky, G., senior fellow at Project Hope and chair of the Medicare Payment Advisory Commission. (2005, March 3). Leonard Davis Institute Health Policy Seminar Series at the Wharton School at the University of Pennsylvania, Philadelphia, PA.

APPENDIX A

THE DECLARATION OF INDEPENDENCE

In CONGRESS, July 4, 1776

The unanimous Declaration of the thirteen united States of America

When in the Course of human events it becomes necessary for one people to dissolve the political bands which have connected them with another and to assume among the powers of the earth, the separate and equal station to which the Laws of Nature and of Nature's God entitle them, a decent respect to the opinions of mankind requires that they should declare the causes which impel them to the separation.

We hold these truths to be self-evident, that all men are created equal, that they are endowed by their Creator with certain unalienable Rights, that among these are Life, Liberty and the pursuit of Happiness.— That to secure these rights, Governments are instituted among Men, deriving their just powers from the consent of the governed, — That whenever any Form of Government becomes destructive of these ends, it is the Right of the People to alter or to abolish it, and to institute new Government, laying its foundation on such principles and organizing its powers in such form, as to them shall seem most likely to effect their Safety and Happiness. Prudence, indeed, will dictate that Governments long established should not be changed for light and transient causes; and accordingly all experience hath shewn that mankind are more disposed to suffer, while evils are sufferable than to right themselves by abolishing the forms to which they are accustomed. But when a long train of abuses and usurpations, pursuing invariably the same Object evinces a design to reduce them under absolute Despotism, it is their right, it is their duty, to throw off such Government, and to provide new Guards for their future security. — Such has been the patient sufferance of these Colonies; and such is now the necessity which constrains them to alter their former Systems of Government. The history of the present

King of Great Britain is a history of repeated injuries and usurpations, all having in direct object the establishment of an absolute Tyranny over these States. To prove this, let Facts be submitted to a candid world.

He has refused his Assent to Laws, the most wholesome and necessary for the public good.

He has forbidden his Governors to pass Laws of immediate and pressing importance, unless suspended in their operation till his Assent should be obtained; and when so suspended, he has utterly neglected to attend to them.

He has refused to pass other Laws for the accommodation of large districts of people, unless those people would relinquish the right of Representation in the Legislature, a right inestimable to them and formidable to tyrants only.

He has called together legislative bodies at places unusual, uncomfortable, and distant from the depository of their Public Records, for the sole purpose of fatiguing them into compliance with his measures.

He has dissolved Representative Houses repeatedly, for opposing with manly firmness his invasions on the rights of the people.

He has refused for a long time, after such dissolutions, to cause others to be elected, whereby the Legislative Powers, incapable of Annihilation, have returned to the People at large for their exercise; the State remaining in the mean time exposed to all the dangers of invasion from without, and convulsions within.

He has endeavoured to prevent the population of these States; for that purpose obstructing the Laws for Naturalization of Foreigners; refusing to pass others to encourage their migrations hither, and raising the conditions of new Appropriations of Lands.

He has obstructed the Administration of Justice by refusing his Assent to Laws for establishing Judiciary Powers.

He has made Judges dependent on his Will alone for the tenure of their offices, and the amount and payment of their salaries.

He has erected a multitude of New Offices, and sent hither swarms of Officers to harass our people and eat out their substance.

He has kept among us, in times of peace, Standing Armies without the Consent of our legislatures.

He has affected to render the Military independent of and superior to the Civil Power.

He has combined with others to subject us to a jurisdiction foreign to our constitution, and unacknowledged by our laws; giving his Assent to their Acts of pretended Legislation:

For quartering large bodies of armed troops among us:

For protecting them, by a mock Trial from punishment for any Murders which they should commit on the Inhabitants of these States:

For cutting off our Trade with all parts of the world:

For imposing Taxes on us without our Consent:

For depriving us in many cases, of the benefit of Trial by Jury:

For transporting us beyond Seas to be tried for pretended offences:

For abolishing the free System of English Laws in a neighbouring Province, establishing therein an Arbitrary government, and enlarging its Boundaries so as to render it at once an example and fit instrument for introducing the same absolute rule into these Colonies

For taking away our Charters, abolishing our most valuable Laws and altering fundamentally the Forms of our Governments:

For suspending our own Legislatures, and declaring themselves invested with power to legislate for us in all cases whatsoever.

He has abdicated Government here, by declaring us out of his Protection and waging War against us.

He has plundered our seas, ravaged our coasts, burnt our towns, and destroyed the lives of our people.

He is at this time transporting large Armies of foreign Mercenaries to compleat the works of death, desolation, and tyranny, already begun with circumstances of Cruelty & Perfidy scarcely paralleled in the most barbarous ages, and totally unworthy the Head of a civilized nation.

He has constrained our fellow Citizens taken Captive on the high Seas to bear Arms against their Country, to become the executioners of their friends and Brethren, or to fall themselves by their Hands.

He has excited domestic insurrections amongst us, and has endeavoured to bring on the inhabitants of our frontiers, the merciless Indian Savages whose known rule of warfare, is an undistinguished destruction of all ages, sexes and conditions.

In every stage of these Oppressions We have Petitioned for Redress in the most humble terms: Our repeated Petitions have been answered only by repeated injury. A Prince, whose character is thus marked by every act which may define a Tyrant, is unfit to be the ruler of a free people.

Nor have We been wanting in attentions to our British brethren. We have warned them from time to time of attempts by their legislature to extend an unwarrantable jurisdiction over us. We have reminded them of the circumstances of our emigration and settlement here. We have appealed to their native justice and magnanimity, and we have conjured them by the ties of our common kindred to disavow these usurpations, which would inevitably interrupt our connections and correspondence. They too have been deaf to the voice of justice and of consanguinity. We must, therefore, acquiesce in the necessity, which denounces our Separation, and hold them, as we hold the rest of mankind, Enemies in War, in Peace Friends.

We, therefore, the Representatives of the united States of America, in General Congress, Assembled, appealing to the Supreme Judge of the world for the rectitude of our intentions, do, in the Name, and by Authority of the good People of these Colonies, solemnly publish and declare, That these united Colonies are, and of Right ought to be Free and Independent States, that they are Absolved from all Allegiance to the British Crown, and that all political connection between them and the State of Great Britain, is and ought to be totally dissolved; and that as Free and Independent States, they have full Power to levy War, conclude Peace, contract Alliances, establish Commerce, and to do all other Acts and Things which Independent States may of right do.

— And for the support of this Declaration, with a firm reliance on the protection of Divine Providence, we mutually pledge to each other our Lives, our Fortunes, and our sacred Honor.

— John Hancock

New Hampshire:
Josiah Bartlett, William Whipple, Matthew Thornton

Massachusetts:
John Hancock, Samuel Adams, John Adams, Robert Treat Paine, Elbridge Gerry

Rhode Island:
Stephen Hopkins, William Ellery

Connecticut:
Roger Sherman, Samuel Huntington, William Williams, Oliver Wolcott

New York:
William Floyd, Philip Livingston, Francis Lewis, Lewis Morris

New Jersey:
Richard Stockton, John Witherspoon, Francis Hopkinson, John Hart, Abraham Clark

Pennsylvania:
Robert Morris, Benjamin Rush, Benjamin Franklin, John Morton, George Clymer, James Smith, George Taylor, James Wilson, George Ross

Delaware:
Caesar Rodney, George Read, Thomas McKean

Maryland:
Samuel Chase, William Paca, Thomas Stone, Charles Carroll of Carrollton

Virginia:
George Wythe, Richard Henry Lee, Thomas Jefferson, Benjamin Harrison, Thomas Nelson, Jr., Francis Lightfoot Lee, Carter Braxton

North Carolina:
William Hooper, Joseph Hewes, John Penn

South Carolina:
Edward Rutledge, Thomas Heyward, Jr., Thomas Lynch, Jr., Arthur Middleton

Georgia:
Button Gwinnett, Lyman Hall, George Walton

THE CONSTITUTION OF THE UNITED STATES

PREAMBLE

We the People of the United States, in Order to form a more perfect Union, establish Justice, insure domestic Tranquility, provide for the common defence, promote the general Welfare, and secure the Blessings of Liberty to ourselves and our Posterity, do ordain and establish this Constitution for the United States of America.

ARTICLES OF THE CONSTITUTION

Article I - The Legislative Branch

Section 1 – The Legislature

All legislative Powers herein granted shall be vested in a Congress of the United States, which shall consist of a Senate and House of Representatives.

Section 2 – The House

The House of Representatives shall be composed of Members chosen every second Year by the People of the several States, and the Electors in each State shall have the Qualifications requisite for Electors of the most numerous Branch of the State Legislature.

No Person shall be a Representative who shall not have attained to the Age of twenty five Years, and been seven Years a Citizen of the United States, and who shall not, when elected, be an Inhabitant of that State in which he shall be chosen.

(Representatives and direct Taxes shall be apportioned among the several States which may be included within this Union, according to their respective Numbers, which shall be determined by adding to the whole Number of free Persons, including those bound to Service for a Term of Years, and excluding Indians not taxed, three fifths of all other Persons.) **(The previous sentence in parentheses was modified by the 14th Amendment, section 2.)** The actual Enumeration shall be made within three Years after the first Meeting of the Congress of the United States, and within every subsequent Term of ten Years, in such Manner as they shall by Law direct. The Number of Representatives shall not exceed one for every thirty Thousand, but each State shall have at Least one Representative; and until such enumeration shall be made, the State of New Hampshire shall be entitled to [choose] three, Massachusetts eight, Rhode Island and Providence Plantations one, Connecticut five, New York six, New Jersey four, Pennsylvania eight, Delaware one, Maryland six, Virginia ten, North Carolina five, South Carolina five and Georgia three.

When vacancies happen in the Representation from any State, the Executive Authority thereof shall issue Writs of Election to fill such Vacancies.

The House of Representatives shall [choose] their speaker and other Officers; and shall have the sole Power of Impeachment.

Section 3 – The Senate

The Senate of the United States shall be composed of two Senators from each State, *(chosen by the Legislature thereof,)* **(The preceding words in parentheses superseded by 17th Amendment, section 1.)** for six Years; and each Senator shall have one Vote.

Immediately after they shall be assembled in Consequence of the first Election, they shall be divided as equally as may be into three Classes. The Seats of the Senators of the first Class shall be vacated at the Expiration of the second Year, of the second Class at the Expiration of the fourth Year, and of the third Class at the Expiration of the sixth Year, so that one third may be chosen every second Year; *(and if Vacancies happen by Resignation, or otherwise, during the Recess of the Legislature of any State, the Executive thereof may make temporary Appointments until the next Meeting of the Legislature, which shall then fill such Vacancies.)* **(The preceding words in parentheses were superseded by the 17th Amendment, section 2.)**

No Person shall be a Senator who shall not have attained to the Age of thirty Years, and been nine Years a Citizen of the United States, and who shall not, when elected, be an Inhabitant of that State for which he shall be chosen.

The Vice President of the United States shall be President of the Senate, but shall have no Vote, unless they be equally divided.

The Senate shall [choose] their other Officers, and also a President pro tempore, in the absence of the Vice President, or when he shall exercise the Office of President of the United States.

The Senate shall have the sole Power to try all Impeachments. When sitting for that Purpose, they shall be on Oath or Affirmation. When the President of the United States is tried, the Chief Justice shall preside: And no Person shall be convicted without the Concurrence of two thirds of the Members present.

Judgment in Cases of Impeachment shall not extend further than to removal from Office, and dis-qualification to hold and enjoy any Office of honor, Trust or Profit under the United States: but the Party convicted shall nevertheless be liable and subject to Indictment, Trial, Judgment and Punishment, accord-ing to Law.

Section 4 – Elections, Meetings

The Times, Places and Manner of holding Elections for Senators and Representatives, shall be prescribed in each State by the Legislature thereof; but the Congress may at any time by Law make or alter such Regulations, except as to the Place of [choosing] Senators.

The Congress shall assemble at least once in every Year, and such Meeting shall *(be on the first Monday in December,)* **(The preceding words in parenthe-ses were superseded by the 20th Amendment, section 2.)** unless they shall by Law appoint a different Day.

Section 5 – Membership, Rules, Journals, Adjournment

Each House shall be the Judge of the Elections, Returns and Qualifications of its own Members, and a Majority of each shall constitute a Quorum to do Business; but a smaller number may adjourn from day to day, and may be authorized to compel the Attendance of absent Members, in such Manner, and under such Penalties as each House may provide.

Each House may determine the Rules of its Pro-ceedings, punish its Members for disorderly Behavior,

and, with the Concurrence of two-thirds, expel a Member.

Each House shall keep a Journal of its Proceed-ings, and from time to time publish the same, except-ing such Parts as may in their Judgment require Secrecy; and the Yeas and Nays of the Members of either House on any question shall, at the Desire of one fifth of those Present, be entered on the Journal.

Neither House, during the Session of Congress, shall, without the Consent of the other, adjourn for more than three days, nor to any other Place than that in which the two Houses shall be sitting.

Section 6 - Compensation

(The Senators and Representatives shall receive a Compensation for their Services, to be ascertained by Law, and paid out of the Treasury of the United States.) **(The preceding words in parentheses were modified by the 27th Amendment.)** They shall in all Cases, except Treason, Felony and Breach of the Peace, be privileged from Arrest during their Atten-dance at the Session of their respective Houses, and in going to and returning from the same; and for any Speech or Debate in either House, they shall not be questioned in any other Place.

No Senator or Representative shall, during the Time for which he was elected, be appointed to any civil Office under the Authority of the United States which shall have been created, or the Emoluments whereof shall have been increased during such time; and no Person holding any Office under the United States, shall be a Member of either House during his Continuance in Office.

Section 7 – Revenue Bills, Legislative Process, Presidential Veto

All bills for raising Revenue shall originate in the House of Representatives; but the Senate may pro-pose or concur with Amendments as on other Bills.

Every Bill which shall have passed the House of Representatives and the Senate, shall, before it become a Law, be presented to the President of the United States; If he approve he shall sign it, but if not he shall return it, with his Objections to that House in which it shall have originated, who shall enter the Objections at large on their Journal, and proceed to reconsider it. If after such Reconsideration two thirds of that House shall agree to pass the Bill, it shall be sent, together with the Objections, to the other House, by which it shall likewise be reconsidered, and if approved by two thirds of that House, it shall become a Law. But in all such Cases the Votes of both Houses shall be determined by Yeas and Nays, and the Names of the Persons voting for and against the Bill shall be entered on the Journal of each House respectively. If any Bill shall not be returned by the President within ten Days (Sundays excepted) after it shall have been presented to him, the Same shall be a Law, in like Manner as if he had signed it, unless the Congress by their Adjournment prevent its Return, in which Case it shall not be a Law.

Every Order, Resolution, or Vote to which the Concurrence of the Senate and House of Representatives may be necessary (except on a question of Adjournment) shall be presented to the President of the United States; and before the Same shall take Effect, shall be approved by him, or being disapproved by him, shall be repassed by two thirds of the Senate and House of Representatives, according to the Rules and Limitations prescribed in the Case of a Bill.

Section 8 – Powers of Congress

The Congress shall have Power To lay and collect Taxes, Duties, Imposts and Excises, to pay the Debts and provide for the common Defense and general Welfare of the United States; but all Duties, Imposts and Excises shall be uniform throughout the United States;

To borrow Money on the credit of the United States;

To regulate Commerce with foreign Nations, and among the several States, and with the Indian Tribes;

To establish a uniform Rule of Naturalization, and uniform Laws on the subject of Bankruptcies throughout the United States;

To coin Money, regulate the Value thereof, and of foreign Coin, and fix the Standard of Weights and Measures;

To provide for the Punishment of counterfeiting the Securities and current Coin of the United States;

To establish Post Offices and Post Roads;

To promote the Progress of Science and useful Arts, by securing for limited Times to Authors and Inventors the exclusive Right to their respective Writings and Discoveries;

To constitute Tribunals inferior to the supreme Court;

To define and punish Piracies and Felonies committed on the high Seas, and Offenses against the Law of Nations;

To declare War, grant Letters of Marque and Reprisal, and make rules concerning Captures on Land and Water;

To raise and support Armies, but no Appropriation of Money to that Use shall be for a longer Term than two Years;

To provide and maintain a Navy;

To make Rules for the Government and Regulation of the land and naval Forces;

To provide for calling forth the Militia to execute the Laws of the Union, suppress Insurrections and repel Invasions;

To provide for organizing, arming, and disciplining the Militia, and for governing such Part of them as may be employed in the Service of the United States, reserving to the States respectively, the Appointment of the Officers, and the Authority of training the Militia according to the discipline prescribed by Congress;

To exercise exclusive Legislation in all Cases whatsoever, over such District (not exceeding ten Miles square) as may, by Cession of particular States, and the acceptance of Congress, become the Seat of the Government of the United States, and to exercise like Authority over all Places purchased by the Consent of the Legislature of the State in which the Same shall be, for the Erection of Forts, Magazines, Arsenals, dock-Yards, and other needful Buildings; And

To make all Laws which shall be necessary and proper for carrying into Execution the foregoing Powers, and all other Powers vested by this Constitution in the Government of the United States, or in any Department or Officer thereof.

Section 9 – Limits on Congress

The Migration or Importation of such Persons as any of the States now existing shall think proper to admit, shall not be prohibited by the Congress prior to the Year one thousand eight hundred and eight, but a tax or duty may be imposed on such Importation, not exceeding ten dollars for each Person.

The privilege of the Writ of Habeas Corpus shall not be suspended, unless when in Cases of Rebellion or Invasion the public Safety may require it.

No Bill of Attainder or ex post facto Law shall be passed.

(No capitation, or other direct, Tax shall be laid, unless in Proportion to the Census or Enumeration herein before directed to be taken.) **(Section in parentheses clarified by the 16th Amendment.)**

No Tax or Duty shall be laid on Articles exported from any State.

No Preference shall be given by any Regulation of Commerce or Revenue to the Ports of one State over those of another: nor shall Vessels bound to, or from, one State, be obliged to enter, clear, or pay Duties in another.

No Money shall be drawn from the Treasury, but in Consequence of Appropriations made by Law; and a regular Statement and Account of the Receipts and Expenditures of all public Money shall be published from time to time.

No Title of Nobility shall be granted by the United States: And no Person holding any Office of Profit or Trust under them, shall, without the Consent of the Congress, accept of any present, Emolument, Office, or Title, of any kind whatever, from any King, Prince, or foreign State.

Section 10 – Powers prohibited of States

No State shall enter into any Treaty, Alliance, or Confederation; grant Letters of Marque and Reprisal; coin Money; emit Bills of Credit; make any Thing but gold and silver Coin a Tender in Payment of Debts; pass any Bill of Attainder, ex post facto Law, or Law impairing the Obligation of Contracts, or grant any Title of Nobility.

No State shall, without the Consent of the Congress, lay any Imposts or Duties on Imports or Exports, except what may be absolutely necessary for executing [its] inspection Laws: and the net Produce of all Duties and Imposts, laid by any State on Imports or Exports, shall be for the Use of the Treasury of the United States; and all such Laws shall be subject to the Revision and [Control] of the Congress.

No State shall, without the Consent of Congress, lay any Duty of Tonnage, keep Troops, or Ships of War in time of Peace, enter into any Agreement or Compact with another State, or with a foreign Power, or engage in War, unless actually invaded, or in such imminent Danger as will not admit of delay.

Article II – The Executive Branch

Section 1 – The President

The executive Power shall be vested in a President of the United States of America. He shall hold his Office during the Term of four Years, and, together with the Vice President, chosen for the same Term, be elected, as follows:

Each State shall appoint, in such Manner as the Legislature thereof may direct, a Number of Electors, equal to the whole Number of Senators and Representatives to which the State may be entitled in the Congress: but no Senator or Representative, or Person holding an Office of Trust or Profit under the United States, shall be appointed an Elector.

(The Electors shall meet in their respective States, and vote by Ballot for two persons, of whom one at least shall not lie an Inhabitant of the same State with themselves. And they shall make a List of all the Persons voted for, and of the Number of Votes for each; which List they shall sign and certify, and transmit sealed to the Seat of the Government of the United States, directed to the President of the Senate. The President of the Senate shall, in the Presence of the Senate and House of Representatives, open all the Certificates, and the Votes shall then be counted. The Person having the greatest Number of Votes shall be the President, if such Number be a Majority of the whole Number of Electors appointed; and if there be more than one who have such Majority, and have an equal Number of Votes, then the House of Representatives shall immediately [choose] by Ballot one of them for President; and if no Person have a Majority, then from the five highest on the List the said House shall in like Manner [choose] the President. But in [choosing] the President, the Votes shall be taken by States, the Representation from each State having one Vote; a quorum for this Purpose shall consist of a Member or Members from two-thirds of the States, and a Majority of all the States shall be necessary to a Choice. In every Case, after the Choice of the President, the Person having the greatest Number of Votes of the Electors shall be the Vice President. But if there should remain two or more who have equal Votes, the Senate shall [choose] from them by Ballot the Vice-President.)* **(This clause in parentheses was superseded by the 12th Amendment.)**

The Congress may determine the Time of [choosing] the Electors, and the Day on which they shall give their Votes; which Day shall be the same throughout the United States.

No Person except a natural born Citizen, or a Citizen of the United States, at the time of the Adoption of this Constitution, shall be eligible to the Office of President; neither shall any Person be eligible to that Office who shall not have attained to the Age of thirty-five Years, and been fourteen Years a Resident within the United States.

(In Case of the Removal of the President from Office, or of his Death, Resignation, or Inability to discharge the Powers and Duties of the said Office, the same shall devolve on the Vice President, and the Congress may by Law provide for the Case of Removal, Death, Resignation or Inability, both of the President and Vice President, declaring what Officer shall then act as President, and such Officer shall act accordingly, until the Disability be removed, or a President shall be elected.) **(This clause in parentheses has been modified by the 20th and 25th Amendments.)**

The President shall, at stated Times, receive for his Services, a Compensation, which shall neither be increased nor diminished during the Period for which he shall have been elected, and he shall not receive within that Period any other Emolument from the United States, or any of them.

Before he enter on the Execution of his Office, he shall take the following Oath or Affirmation:

"I do solemnly swear (or affirm) that I will faithfully execute the Office of President of the United States, and will to the best of my Ability, preserve, protect and defend the Constitution of the United States.'"

Section 2 – Civilian Power over Military, Cabinet, Pardon Power, Appointments

The President shall be Commander in Chief of the Army and Navy of the United States, and of the Militia of the several States, when called into the actual Service of the United States; he may require the Opinion, in writing, of the principal Officer in each of the executive Departments, upon any Subject relating to the Duties of their respective Offices, and he shall have Power to grant Reprieves and Pardons for Offenses against the United States, except in Cases of Impeachment.

He shall have Power, by and with the Advice and Consent of the Senate, to make Treaties, provided two thirds of the Senators present concur; and he shall nominate, and by and with the Advice and Consent of the Senate, shall appoint Ambassadors, other public Ministers and Consuls, Judges of the supreme Court, and all other Officers of the United States, whose Appointments are not herein otherwise provided for, and which shall be established by Law: but the Congress may by Law vest the Appointment of such inferior Officers, as they think proper, in the President alone, in the Courts of Law, or in the Heads of Departments.

The President shall have Power to fill up all Vacancies that may happen during the Recess of the Senate, by granting Commissions which shall expire at the End of their next Session.

Section 3 – State of the Union, Convening Congress

He shall from time to time give to the Congress Information of the State of the Union, and recommend to their Consideration such Measures as he shall judge necessary and expedient; he may, on extraordinary Occasions, convene both Houses, or either of them, and in Case of Disagreement between them, with Respect to the Time of Adjournment, he may adjourn them to such Time as he shall think proper; he shall receive Ambassadors and other public Ministers; he shall take Care that the Laws be faithfully executed, and shall Commission all the Officers of the United States

Section 4 - Disqualification

The President, Vice President and all civil Officers of the United States, shall be removed from Office on Impeachment for, and Conviction of, Treason, Bribery, or other high Crimes and Misdemeanors.

Article III – The Judicial Branch

Section 1 – Judicial powers

The judicial Power of the United States, shall be vested in one supreme Court, and in such inferior Courts as the Congress may from time to time ordain and establish. The Judges, both of the supreme and inferior Courts, shall hold their Offices during good Behavior, and shall, at stated Times, receive for their Services a Compensation, which shall not be diminished during their Continuance in Office.

Section 2 – Trial by Jury, Original Jurisdiction, Jury Trials

(The judicial Power shall extend to all Cases, in Law and Equity, arising under this Constitution, the Laws of the United States, and Treaties made, or which shall be made, under their Authority; to all Cases affecting Ambassadors, other public Ministers and Consuls; to all Cases of admiralty and maritime Jurisdiction; to Controversies to which the United States shall be a Party; to Controversies between two or more States; between a State and Citizens of another State; between Citizens of different States; between Citizens of the same State claiming Lands under Grants of different States, and between a State, or the Citizens thereof, and foreign States, Citizens or Subjects.)
(This section in parentheses is modified by the 11th Amendment.)

In all Cases affecting Ambassadors, other public Ministers and Consuls, and those in which a State shall be Party, the supreme Court shall have original Jurisdiction. In all the other Cases before mentioned, the supreme Court shall have appellate Jurisdiction, both as to Law and Fact, with such Exceptions, and under such Regulations as the Congress shall make.

The Trial of all Crimes, except in Cases of Impeachment, shall be by Jury; and such Trial shall be held in the State where the said Crimes shall have been committed; but when not committed within any State, the Trial shall be at such Place or Places as the Congress may by Law have directed.

Section 3 - Treason

Treason against the United States, shall consist only in levying War against them, or in adhering to their Enemies, giving them Aid and Comfort. No Person shall be convicted of Treason unless on the Testimony of two Witnesses to the same overt Act, or on Confession in open Court.

The Congress shall have power to declare the Punishment of Treason, but no Attainder of Treason shall work Corruption of Blood, or Forfeiture except during the Life of the Person attainted.

Article IV – The States

Section 1 – Each State to Honor all others [Full Faith and Credit Clause]

Full Faith and Credit shall be given in each State to the public Acts, Records, and judicial Proceedings of every other State. And the Congress may by general Laws prescribe the Manner in which such Acts, Records and Proceedings shall be proved, and the Effect thereof.

Section 2 - State citizens, Extradition [Privileges and Immunities Clause]

The Citizens of each State shall be entitled to all Privileges and Immunities of Citizens in the several States.

A Person charged in any State with Treason, Felony, or other Crime, who shall flee from Justice, and be found in another State, shall on demand of the executive Authority of the State from which he fled, be delivered up, to be removed to the State having Jurisdiction of the Crime.

(No Person held to Service or [Labor] in one State, under the Laws thereof, escaping into another, shall, in Consequence of any Law or Regulation therein, be discharged from such Service or [Labor], But shall be delivered up on Claim of the Party to whom such Service or [Labor] may be due.) **(This clause in parentheses is superseded by the 13th Amendment.)**

Section 3 – New States [Territorial Clause]

New States may be admitted by the Congress into this Union; but no new States shall be formed or erected within the Jurisdiction of any other State; nor any State be formed by the Junction of two or more States, or Parts of States, without the Consent of the Legislatures of the States concerned as well as of the Congress.

The Congress shall have Power to dispose of and make all needful Rules and Regulations respecting the Territory or other Property belonging to the United States; and nothing in this Constitution shall be so construed as to Prejudice any Claims of the United States, or of any particular State.

Section 4 – Republican government [Right to Direct Democracy Clause]

The United States shall guarantee to every State in this Union a Republican Form of Government, and shall protect each of them against Invasion; and on Application of the Legislature, or of the Executive (when the Legislature cannot be convened) against domestic Violence.

Article V – Amendment

The Congress, whenever two thirds of both Houses shall deem it necessary, shall propose Amendments to this Constitution, or, on the Application of the Legislatures of two thirds of the several States, shall call a Convention for proposing Amendments, which, in either Case, shall be valid to all Intents and Purposes, as part of this Constitution, when ratified by the Legislatures of three fourths of the several States, or by Conventions in three fourths thereof, as the one or the other Mode of Ratification may be proposed by the Congress; Provided that no Amendment which may be made prior to the Year One thousand eight hundred and eight shall in any Manner affect the first and fourth Clauses in the Ninth Section of the first Article; and that no State, without its Consent, shall be deprived of its equal Suffrage in the Senate.

Article VI – Debts, Supremacy, Oaths

All Debts contracted and Engagements entered into, before the Adoption of this Constitution, shall be as valid against the United States under this Constitution, as under the Confederation.

[Supremacy Clause] This Constitution, and the Laws of the United States which shall be made in Pursuance thereof; and all Treaties made, or which shall be made, under the Authority of the United States, shall be the supreme Law of the Land; and the Judges in every State shall be bound thereby, any Thing in the Constitution or Laws of any State to the Contrary notwithstanding.

The Senators and Representatives before mentioned, and the Members of the several State Legislatures, and all executive and judicial Officers, both of the United States and of the several States, shall be bound by Oath or Affirmation, to support this Constitution; but no religious Test shall ever be required as a Qualification to any Office or public Trust under the United States.

Article VII – Ratification

The Ratification of the Conventions of nine States, shall be sufficient for the Establishment of this Constitution between the States so ratifying the Same.

Done in Convention by the Unanimous Consent of the States present the Seventeenth Day of September in the Year of our Lord one thousand seven hundred and Eighty seven and of the Independence of the United States of America the Twelfth. In Witness whereof We have hereunto subscribed our Names.

Go Washington - President and deputy from Virginia
New Hampshire - John Langdon, Nicholas Gilman

Massachusetts - Nathaniel Gorham, Rufus King
Connecticut - Wm Saml Johnson, Roger Sherman
New York - Alexander Hamilton
New Jersey - Wil Livingston, David Brearley, Wm
  Paterson, Jona. Dayton
Pennsylvania - B Franklin, Thomas Mifflin, Robt
  Morris, Geo. Clymer, Thos FitzSimons, Jared Inger-
  soll, James Wilson, Gouv Morris
Delaware - Geo. Read, Gunning Bedford jun, John
  Dickinson, Richard Bassett, Jaco. Broom
Maryland - James McHenry, Dan of St Tho Jenifer,
  Danl Carroll
Virginia - John Blair, James Madison Jr.
North Carolina - Wm Blount, Richd Dobbs Spaight,
  Hu Williamson
South Carolina - J. Rutledge, Charles Cotesworth
  Pinckney, Charles Pinckney, Pierce Butler
Georgia - William Few, Abr Baldwin
Attest: William Jackson, Secretary

Bill of Rights

The first ten Amendments to the Constitution
collectively are commonly known as the Bill
of Rights.

Amendment 1 – Freedom of Religion, Press, Expression

Congress shall make no law respecting an establishment of religion, or prohibiting the free exercise
thereof; or abridging the freedom of speech, or of the
press; or the right of the people peaceably to assemble, and to petition the Government for a redress of
grievances.

Amendment 2 – Right to Bear Arms

A well regulated Militia, being necessary to the security of a free State, the right of the people to keep and
bear Arms, shall not be infringed.

Amendment 3 – Quartering of Soldiers

No Soldier shall, in time of peace be quartered
in any house, without the consent of the Owner,
nor in time of war, but in a manner to be prescribed
by law.

Amendment 4 – Search and Seizure

The right of the people to be secure in their persons,
houses, papers, and effects, against unreasonable
searches and seizures, shall not be violated, and
no Warrants shall issue, but upon probable cause,
supported by Oath or affirmation, and particularly
describing the place to be searched, and the persons
or things to be seized.

Amendment 5 – Trial and Punishment, Compensation for Takings [Double Jeopardy, Self-Incrimination, Due Process, Eminent Domain Clauses]

No person shall be held to answer for a capital, or
otherwise infamous crime, unless on a presentment
or indictment of a Grand Jury, except in cases arising
in the land or naval forces, or in the Militia, when
in actual service in time of War or public danger;
nor shall any person be subject for the same offense
to be twice put in jeopardy of life or limb; nor shall
be compelled in any criminal case to be a witness
against himself, nor be deprived of life, liberty, or
property, without due process of law; nor shall
private property be taken for public use, without just
compensation.

Amendment 6 Right to Speedy Trial, Confrontation of Witnesses

In all criminal prosecutions, the accused shall enjoy
the right to a speedy and public trial, by an impartial
jury of the State and district wherein the crime shall
have been committed, which district shall have been
previously ascertained by law, and to be informed
of the nature and cause of the accusation; to be
confronted with the witnesses against him; to have
compulsory process for obtaining witnesses in his
favor, and to have the Assistance of Counsel for his
[defense].

Amendment 7 – Trial by Jury in Civil Cases

In Suits at common law, where the value in controversy shall exceed twenty dollars, the right of trial
by jury shall be preserved, and no fact tried by a
jury, shall be otherwise re-examined in any Court of
the United States, than according to the rules of the
common law.

Amendment 8 – Cruel and Unusual Punishment

Excessive bail shall not be required, nor excessive
fines imposed, nor cruel and unusual punishments
inflicted.

Amendment 9 – Construction of Constitution [Rights of the People]

The enumeration in the Constitution, of certain
rights, shall not be construed to deny or disparage
others retained by the people.

Amendment 10 – Powers of the States and People [Federalism]

The powers not delegated to the United States by the
Constitution, nor prohibited by it to the States, are
reserved to the States respectively, or to the people.

SUBSEQUENT AMENDMENTS

Amendment 11 – Judicial Limits [Sovereign Immunity]

The Judicial power of the United States shall not be construed to extend to any suit in law or equity, commenced or prosecuted against one of the United States by Citizens of another State, or by Citizens or Subjects of any Foreign State.

Amendment 12 – Choosing the President, Vice-President [Electoral College]

The Electors shall meet in their respective states, and vote by ballot for President and Vice-President, one of whom, at least, shall not be an inhabitant of the same state with themselves; they shall name in their ballots the person voted for as President, and in distinct ballots the person voted for as Vice-President, and they shall make distinct lists of all persons voted for as President, and of all persons voted for as Vice-President and of the number of votes for each, which lists they shall sign and certify, and transmit sealed to the seat of the government of the United States, directed to the President of the Senate;

The President of the Senate shall, in the presence of the Senate and House of Representatives, open all the certificates and the votes shall then be counted;

The person having the greatest Number of votes for President, shall be the President, if such number be a majority of the whole number of Electors appointed; and if no person have such majority, then from the persons having the highest numbers not exceeding three on the list of those voted for as President, the House of Representatives shall choose immediately, by ballot, the President. But in choosing the President, the votes shall be taken by states, the representation from each state having one vote; a quorum for this purpose shall consist of a member or members from two-thirds of the states, and a majority of all the states shall be necessary to a choice. And if the House of Representatives shall not choose a President whenever the right of choice shall devolve upon them, before the fourth day of March next following, then the Vice-President shall act as President, as in the case of the death or other constitutional disability of the President.

The person having the greatest number of votes as Vice-President, shall be the Vice-President, if such number be a majority of the whole number of Electors appointed, and if no person have a majority, then from the two highest numbers on the list, the Senate shall choose the Vice-President; a quorum for the purpose shall consist of two-thirds of the whole number of Senators, and a majority of the whole number shall be necessary to a choice. But no person constitutionally ineligible to the office of President shall be eligible to that of Vice-President of the United States.

Amendment 13 – Slavery Abolished

1. Neither slavery nor involuntary servitude, except as a punishment for crime whereof the party shall have been duly convicted, shall exist within the United States, or any place subject to their jurisdiction.
2. Congress shall have power to enforce this article by appropriate legislation.

Amendment 14 – Citizenship Rights

1. All persons born or naturalized in the United States, and subject to the jurisdiction thereof, are citizens of the United States and of the State wherein they reside. No State shall make or enforce any law which shall abridge the privileges or immunities of citizens of the United States; nor shall any State deprive any person of life, liberty, or property, without due process of law; nor deny to any person within its jurisdiction the equal protection of the laws.
2. Representatives shall be apportioned among the several States according to their respective numbers, counting the whole number of persons in each State, excluding Indians not taxed. But when the right to vote at any election for the choice of electors for President and Vice-President of the United States, Representatives in Congress, the Executive and Judicial officers of a State, or the members of the Legislature thereof, is denied to any of the male inhabitants of such State, being twenty-one years of age, and citizens of the United States, or in any way abridged, except for participation in rebellion, or other crime, the basis of representation therein shall be reduced in the proportion which the number of such male citizens shall bear to the whole number of male citizens twenty-one years of age in such State.
3. No person shall be a Senator or Representative in Congress, or elector of President and Vice-President, or hold any office, civil or military, under the United States, or under any State, who, having previously taken an oath, as a member of Congress, or as an officer of the United States, or as a member of any State legislature, or as an executive or judicial officer of any State, to support the Constitution of the United States, shall have engaged in insurrection or rebellion against the same, or given aid or comfort to the enemies thereof. But Congress may by a vote of two-thirds of each House, remove such disability.

4. The validity of the public debt of the United States, authorized by law, including debts incurred for payment of pensions and bounties for services in suppressing insurrection or rebellion, shall not be questioned. But neither the United States nor any State shall assume or pay any debt or obligation incurred in aid of insurrection or rebellion against the United States, or any claim for the loss or emancipation of any slave; but all such debts, obligations and claims shall be held illegal and void.

5. The Congress shall have power to enforce, by appropriate legislation, the provisions of this article.

Amendment 15 – Race No Bar to Vote

1. The right of citizens of the United States to vote shall not be denied or abridged by the United States or by any State on account of race, color, or previous condition of servitude.

2. The Congress shall have power to enforce this article by appropriate legislation.

Amendment 16 – Status of Income Tax Clarified

The Congress shall have power to lay and collect taxes on incomes, from whatever source derived, without apportionment among the several States, and without regard to any census or enumeration.

Amendment 17 – Senators Elected by Popular Vote

The Senate of the United States shall be composed of two Senators from each State, elected by the people thereof, for six years; and each Senator shall have one vote. The electors in each State shall have the qualifications requisite for electors of the most numerous branch of the State legislatures.

When vacancies happen in the representation of any State in the Senate, the executive authority of such State shall issue writs of election to fill such vacancies: Provided, That the legislature of any State may empower the executive thereof to make temporary appointments until the people fill the vacancies by election as the legislature may direct.

This amendment shall not be so construed as to affect the election or term of any Senator chosen before it becomes valid as part of the Constitution.

Amendment 18 – Liquor Abolished (Repealed by Amendment 21)

1. After one year from the ratification of this article the manufacture, sale, or transportation of intoxicating liquors within, the importation thereof into, or the exportation thereof from the United States and all territory subject to the jurisdiction thereof for beverage purposes is hereby prohibited.

2. The Congress and the several States shall have concurrent power to enforce this article by appropriate legislation.

3. This article shall be inoperative unless it shall have been ratified as an amendment to the Constitution by the legislatures of the several States, as provided in the Constitution, within seven years from the date of the submission hereof to the States by the Congress.

Amendment 19 – Women's Suffrage

The right of citizens of the United States to vote shall not be denied or abridged by the United States or by any State on account of sex.

Congress shall have power to enforce this article by appropriate legislation.

Amendment 20 – Presidential, Congressional Terms

1. The terms of the President and Vice President shall end at noon on the 20th day of January, and the terms of Senators and Representatives at noon on the 3d day of January, of the years in which such terms would have ended if this article had not been ratified; and the terms of their successors shall then begin.

2. The Congress shall assemble at least once in every year, and such meeting shall begin at noon on the 3d day of January, unless they shall by law appoint a different day.

3. If, at the time fixed for the beginning of the term of the President, the President elect shall have died, the Vice President elect shall become President. If a President shall not have been chosen before the time fixed for the beginning of his term, or if the President elect shall have failed to qualify, then the Vice President elect shall act as President until a President shall have qualified; and the Congress may by law provide for the case wherein neither a President elect nor a Vice President elect shall have qualified, declaring who shall then act as President, or the manner in which one who is to act shall be selected, and such person shall act accordingly until a President or Vice President shall have qualified.

4. The Congress may by law provide for the case of the death of any of the persons from whom the House of Representatives may choose a President whenever the right of choice shall have

devolved upon them, and for the case of the death of any of the persons from whom the Senate may choose a Vice President whenever the right of choice shall have devolved upon them.

5. Sections 1 and 2 shall take effect on the 15th day of October following the ratification of this article.

6. This article shall be inoperative unless it shall have been ratified as an amendment to the Constitution by the legislatures of three-fourths of the several States within seven years from the date of its submission.

Amendment 21 – Amendment 18 Repealed

1. The eighteenth article of amendment to the Constitution of the United States is hereby repealed.

2. The transportation or importation into any State, Territory, or possession of the United States for delivery or use therein of intoxicating liquors, in violation of the laws thereof, is hereby prohibited.

3. The article shall be inoperative unless it shall have been ratified as an amendment to the Constitution by conventions in the several States, as provided in the Constitution, within seven years from the date of the submission hereof to the States by the Congress.

Amendment 22 – Presidential Term Limits

1. No person shall be elected to the office of the President more than twice, and no person who has held the office of President, or acted as President, for more than two years of a term to which some other person was elected President shall be elected to the office of the President more than once. But this Article shall not apply to any person holding the office of President, when this Article was proposed by the Congress, and shall not prevent any person who may be holding the office of President, or acting as President, during the term within which this Article becomes operative from holding the office of President or acting as President during the remainder of such term.

2. This article shall be inoperative unless it shall have been ratified as an amendment to the Constitution by the legislatures of three-fourths of the several States within seven years from the date of its submission to the States by the Congress.

Amendment 23 – Presidential Vote for District of Columbia

1. The District constituting the seat of Government of the United States shall appoint in such manner as the Congress may direct: A number of electors of President and Vice President equal to the whole number of Senators and Representatives in Congress to which the District would be entitled if it were a State, but in no event more than the least populous State; they shall be in addition to those appointed by the States, but they shall be considered, for the purposes of the election of President and Vice President, to be electors appointed by a State; and they shall meet in the District and perform such duties as provided by the twelfth article of amendment.

2. The Congress shall have power to enforce this article by appropriate legislation.

Amendment 24 – Poll Tax Barred

1. The right of citizens of the United States to vote in any primary or other election for President or Vice President, for electors for President or Vice President, or for Senator or Representative in Congress, shall not be denied or abridged by the United States or any State by reason of failure to pay any poll tax or other tax.

2. The Congress shall have power to enforce this article by appropriate legislation.

Amendment 25 – Presidential Disability and Succession

1. In case of the removal of the President from office or of his death or resignation, the Vice President shall become President.

2. Whenever there is a vacancy in the office of the Vice President, the President shall nominate a Vice President who shall take office upon confirmation by a majority vote of both Houses of Congress.

3. Whenever the President transmits to the President pro tempore of the Senate and the Speaker of the House of Representatives his written declaration that he is unable to discharge the powers and duties of his office, and until he transmits to them a written declaration to the contrary, such powers and duties shall be discharged by the Vice President as Acting President.

4. Whenever the Vice President and a majority of either the principal officers of the executive departments or of such other body as Congress

may by law provide, transmit to the President pro tempore of the Senate and the Speaker of the House of Representatives their written declaration that the President is unable to discharge the powers and duties of his office, the Vice President shall immediately assume the powers and duties of the office as Acting President.

Thereafter, when the President transmits to the President pro tempore of the Senate and the Speaker of the House of Representatives his written declaration that no inability exists, he shall resume the powers and duties of his office unless the Vice President and a majority of either the principal officers of the executive department or of such other body as Congress may by law provide, transmit within four days to the President pro tempore of the Senate and the Speaker of the House of Representatives their written declaration that the President is unable to discharge the powers and duties of his office. Thereupon Congress shall decide the issue, assembling within forty eight hours for that purpose if not in session. If the Congress, within twenty one days after receipt of the latter written declaration, or, if

Congress is not in session, within twenty one days after Congress is required to assemble, determines by two thirds vote of both Houses that the President is unable to discharge the powers and duties of his office, the Vice President shall continue to discharge the same as Acting President; otherwise, the President shall resume the powers and duties of his office.

Amendment 26 – Voting Act Set to 18 Years

1. The right of citizens of the United States, who are eighteen years of age or older, to vote shall not be denied or abridged by the United States or by any State on account of age.
2. The Congress shall have power to enforce this article by appropriate legislation.

Amendment 27 – Limiting Congressional Pay Increases

No law, varying the compensation for the services of the Senators and Representatives, shall take effect, until an election of Representatives shall have intervened.

APPENDIX C

ABBREVIATIONS AND ACRONYMS

510(k): Premarket Notification

AAP: American Academy of Pediatrics
ACC: American College of Cardiology
ACHRE: Advisory Committee on Human Radiation Experiments
AHRQ: Agency for Health Research and Quality
AMA: American Medical Association
AMC: Academic Medical Center
ATF: Bureau of Alcohol, Tobacco, Firearms, and Explosives

CBER: Center for Biologics Evaluation and Research
CBO: Congressional Budget Office
CDC: Centers for Disease Control and Prevention
CDER: Center for Drug Evaluation and Research
CDRH: Center for Devices and Radiological Health
CERT: Centers for Education and Research on Therapeutics
CFR: Code of Federal Regulations
CHCA: Child Health Corporation of America
CMS: Centers for Medicare and Medicaid Services
CONSORT: Consolidated Standard of Reporting Trials
CRO: Contract Research Organization
CRS: Congressional Research Service
CSR: Center for Scientific Review (HHS)
CSREES: Cooperative State Research, Education, and Extension Service
CT: Computer-Assisted Tomography

DEA: Drug Enforcement Administration
DOL: Department of Labor
DSaRM: Drug Safety and Risk Management Advisory Committee

ECLS: Extracorporeal Life Support
ECMO: Extracorporeal Membrane Oxygenation
EO: Executive Order
EP&R: Emergency Preparedness and Response Directorate
EPA: Environmental Protection Agency
ESA: Employee Standards Administration (Labor)
EU: European Union

FBI: Federal Bureau of Investigation
FDA: U.S. Food and Drug Administration
FEMA: Federal Emergency Management Agency
FNS: Food and Nutrition Service
FOIA: Freedom of Information Act
FR: Federal Register
FSIS: Food Safety and Inspection Service

GAO: Government Accountability Office (formerly General Accounting Office)
GHTF: Global Harmonization Task Force
GMDN: Global Medical Device Nomenclature
GMP: Good Manufacturing Practices

HDE: Humanitarian Device Exemption
HHS: Department of Health and Human Services
HIPAA: Health Insurance Portability and Accountability Act of 1996
HIV/AIDS: Human Immunodeficiency Virus/Acquired Immunodeficiency Syndrome
HRSA: Health Resources and Services Administration
HUD: Humanitarian Use Device

ICD: International Classification of Diseases
ICH: International Conference on Harmonisation
IDE: Investigational Device Exemption
IOM: Institute of Medicine
IRB: Institutional Review Board
IRS: Internal Revenue Service
ISO: International Organization for Standardization
ISPE: International Society for Pharmacoepidemiology
IT: Information Technology

JCAHO: Joint Commission on the Accreditation of Healthcare Organizations

LVAD: Left Ventricular Assist Device

M-DEN: Medical Device Engineering Network
MDR: Medical Device Reporting
MedSun: Medical Product Surveillance Network
MRI: Magnetic Resonance Imaging

NACHRI: National Association of Children's Hospitals and Related Institutions
NAS: National Academy of Sciences
NEISS: National Electronic Injury Surveillance System
NGO: Non-Governmental Organization
NHLBI: National Heart Lung and Blood Institute
NICHD: National Institute for Child Health and Human Development
NIH: National Institutes of Health
NIST: National Institute of Standards and Technology
NLRB: National Labor Relations Board
NRC: National Research Council
NSF: National Science Foundation
NYPORTS: New York Patients Occurrence and Tracking System

ODEP: Office of Disability Employment Policy (Labor)
OIG: Office of Inspector General
OMB: Office of Management and Budget
OSC: Office of Special Counsel

PBGC: Pension Benefit Guaranty Corporation
PDP: Product Development Protocol

PHARMGKB: Pharmacogenetics and Pharmacogenomics Knowledge Base
PHTS: Pediatric Heart Transplant Study
PMA: Premarket Approval Application
PTO: U.S. Patent and Trademark Office

QuIC: Quality Interagency Coordination Task Force

SAMHSA: Substance Abuse and Mental Health Services Administration (HHS)
SEC: Securities and Exchange Commission
SSA: Social Security Administration
STAMP: Systematic Technical Assessment of Medical Products
STROBE: Strengthening the Reporting of Observational Studies in Epidemiology

TTB: Alcohol and Tobacco Tax and Trade Bureau

USC: United States Code
UMDNS: Universal Medical Device Nomenclature System

VAERS: Vaccine Adverse Event Reporting System

WIC: Special Supplemental Food Program for Women, Infants, and Children

GLOSSARY

501(k): section of the Food, Drug and Cosmetic Act that requires device manufacturers to register and/or notify the FDA at least ninety days in advance of their intent to market a new or significantly modified medical device. Also called "premarket notification ("PMN")."

Abuse: departure from legal or reasonable use; misuse; physical or mental maltreatment, often resulting in mental, emotional, sexual, or physical injury; intentional or neglectful harm.

Acquired condition: a condition or injury which occurs during the provision of health care services and which could reasonably have been prevented through application of evidence-based guidelines.

Acquisition: gaining of possession or control over something. *See also* "corporate acquisition."

Active surveillance: close and continuous observation or testing; the FDA's regular periodic collection of reports from health care providers or facilities in order to identify patterns of adverse events that may be related to specific drugs and which may not be identified through passive surveillance. *Compare* "passive surveillance."

Acute: sudden, brief, and extremely severe; treatment for a brief but severe episode of illness; direct cause of symptoms or death.

Adaptive disconnects: the different rates at which people, organizations, and societies change their thinking as some embrace new ideas and others resist them.

Adolescent: a young person who has undergone puberty but who has not yet reached full maturity; the end of adolescence and the beginning of adulthood varies by entity and function; within a single state or country there may be different ages at which an individual is considered an adolescent.

Advance directive: a document that takes effect upon one's incompetency and designates a surrogate decision-maker who makes decisions in accordance with one's relevant instructions or best interests for health care matters, and which ceases to be effective once one regains capacity. Also called "power of attorney for health care," "health care proxy," "medical directive," "physician's directive," or "written directive." *Compare* "living will."

Adverse event: an instance of harm during patient care or research or within a pre-specified time afterward that is not the result of the individual's disease or medical condition; can include events that have the potential to cause harm but did not; FDA maintains a database for reporting of adverse events called the Manufacturer and User Facility Device Experience Database which is open to the public.

Adverse selection: health insurers strive to maintain risk pools whose health, on average, is the same as the general population. Adverse selection arises when less healthy people disproportionately enroll in a risk pool.

Advisory opinion: a nonbinding statement by a court of its interpretation of the law on a matter submitted for that purpose; a written statement issued by an administrator of an employee benefit plan which applies to a specific factual situation and upon which only the parties named in the request for the opinion may rely.

Affidavit: a voluntary written, sworn declaration of facts; may be used to submit evidence.

Affiliate: a corporation that is related to another corporation by shareholdings or other means of control; a subsidiary, parent, or sibling corporation; one who controls, is controlled by, or is under common control with an issuer of a security.

Allogeneic stem cell transplant: stem cells that are collected from an individual and then given to another individual with a closely matched immune system, such as a brother or sister. *Compare* "autologous stem cell transplant."

Allopathic medicine: treatment which combats symptoms or disease by use of remedies which produce effects different from or incompatible with those produced by the ailment being treated; a system of medical practice which makes use of all measures with proven value in treatment of the ailment. Also called "conventional medicine" or "Western medicine." *Compare* "homeopathic medicine."

Allotransplantation: an organ or tissue transferred between genetically different individuals of the same species. *Compare* "autotransplantation."

Alternative dispute resolution: a means for settling a dispute other than by litigation, such as negotiation, arbitration, or mediation.

Alternative therapy: any healing practice which does not fall within the realm of conventional medicine and which may be used instead of or as a complement to conventional medicine; such therapies are usually not evidence-based or scientifically proven to be effective.

Anticompetitive: an act that harms or seeks to harm the market or process of competition among businesses and which has no legitimate business purpose.

Antigen: any substance foreign to the body that evokes an immune response either alone or after forming a complex with a larger molecule, such as a protein, and that is capable of binding with a product of the immune response, such as an antibody or T cell.

Antigenic drift: mutations in the genes of a virus that change the antigens of the virus and which help the virus evade the immune system, overcome immunity, or defy vaccination.

Antitrust: a body of law designed to protect the market from restraints, monopolies, price-fixing, and price discrimination; its goal is the maintenance of competition.

Antiviral: a class of medication used for treating viral infections; unlike antibiotics, they do not destroy the virus, but rather inhibit its development in order to limit the impact of some symptoms and reduce the potential for serious complications.

Approval: authorization to market a drug or device after submission of a premarket approval application and FDA review of safety and effectiveness.

Arbitrage: simultaneous buying and selling of identical securities in different markets, with the hope of profiting from the price difference between the markets.

Arbitration: a method of dispute resolution through one or more neutral third parties whose decision is usually binding.

Artificial nutrition and hydration: supplements or replaces ordinary eating and drinking by giving a chemically balanced mix of nutrients and fluids through a tube placed directly into the stomach, upper intestine, or a vein.

Assisted dying: end of life choice made by a mentally competent person to end life in as painless and dignified a manner as possible; in this text, it is the voluntary cessation of eating and drinking or termination of artificial nutrition and hydration, followed by the administration of pain-relieving medication which may also, but is not intended to, result in death. *Compare* "euthanasia."

Autologous stem cell transplant: stem cells that are collected from an individual and then given back to that same individual. Also called "autografts." *Compare* "allogeneic stem cell transplant."

Autotransplantation: transplantation of tissue from one part of the body to another in the same individual. *Compare* "allotransplantation."

Avian influenza: subtype of Influenza A virus which can cause illness in humans and many other animal species, in particular, the H5N1 strain, which is highly pathogenic and has the potential to mutate into a strain capable of efficient human-to-human transmission. Also called "avian flu" or "bird flu."

Baby boomer: a person born post-World War II; the exact years are debated, but are generally recognized as 1946-1964; they currently comprise about thirty percent of the U.S. population.

Bacteria: one-celled microorganisms, various species of which are involved in fermentation, putrefaction, and infectious diseases; most found in the human body are harmless, a few are beneficial, and some are pathogenic; used in pharmaceutical and biotechnology formulations and manufacturing.

Bankrupt: indebted beyond the means of payment; insolvent.

Battery: an intentional and unconsented-to touching of another without lawful justification; in criminal law, it is the use of force against another, resulting in harmful or offensive contact.

Benefit: advantage, privilege, profit, or gain; financial assistance that is received from an employer, insurance, or public program in time of sickness or disability.

Best practices: technique, method, process, activity, incentive, or reward that is more effective at delivering a particular outcome with fewer problems and unforeseen complications than any other; the most efficient and effective way of accomplishing a task based on repeatable procedures that have proven themselves over time for large numbers of people; in business, the process of developing and following a standard way of doing things that multiple organizations can use for management and policy.

Beyond a reasonable doubt: standard used by a judge or jury to determine whether a criminal defendant is guilty, starting with the presumption that the defendant is innocent; because everything relating to human affairs is subject to possible doubt, it must go beyond such possible doubt to rise to the sort of proof of such a convincing character that a person would reasonably rely upon it in conducting their own important affairs; it does not, however, rise to the level of absolute certainty. *Compare* "clear and convincing evidence" and "preponderance of the evidence."

Bicameralism: the practice of having two legislative entities with the goal of using checks and balances to avoid passing poor legislation; in the U.S., it is the Senate and the House of Representatives, which together comprise Congress.

Biobanking: collecting, storing, processing, and distributing biological materials and data associated with those materials for research, criminal investigation, human identification, or other purposes.

Bioequivalent: the condition in which different formulations of the same drug or chemical are equally absorbed when taken into the body; a value indicating the rate at which a substance enters the bloodstream and becomes available to the body. Compare therapeutic equivalence and generic equivalence.

Biogeneric: refers to any biopharmaceutical considered generic and not the innovator or patented brand-name product. Also called "biocomparable."

Bioinformatics: application of information technology to the field of molecular biology; using computers to create information databases that permit analyses of genomes, protein sequences, biomolecules, and other organic matter; common applications include mapping and analyzing DNA and protein sequences.

Biologic: a substance derived from animal products or other biological sources that is used to treat or prevent disease; a regulatory term related to FDA approval for biopharmaceuticals and associated products; includes all but the simplest biopharmaceuticals regulated as drugs by FDA. *Compare* "Drug."

Biomarker: distinctive biological or biologically-derived indicator of a process, event, or condition, such as aging, disease, or exposure to a toxic substance.

Biometric: statistical analysis of biological observations and phenomena; measurement of physical characteristics for use in verifying the identity of individuals. Also called "biostatistics."

Biopharmaceutical: a pharmaceutical product that is manufactured using live organisms and has an active ingredient that is biological in nature; does not include small molecules which are inherently chemical in their nature and manufacture.

Bioscience: any of several branches of science which deal with the biological aspects of living organisms and their organization, life processes, and relationships to each other and their environment, such as biology, medicine, anthropology, or ecology.

Biosimilar: new versions of brand-name innovator biopharmaceutical products officially approved following patent expiration of the innovator product.

Biotechnology: any technological application that uses biological systems, living organisms, or derivatives thereof, to make or modify products or processes; medical products industry which engineers drugs and devices from living cells instead of chemicals and inorganic materials.

Biotherapeutic: a therapeutic material produced using biological means, including recombinant DNA technology; a living microorganism administered to promote the health of the host by treating or preventing infections owing to pathogens.

Blastocyst: a pre-implantation embryo consisting of a varying number of cells depending on its age; consists of an outer layer that participates in the development of the placenta and an inner layer of cells which develops into the embryo proper.

Blastomere: a type of cell produced by division of the egg immediately after fertilization and prior to implantation.

Blockbuster drug: a drug generating more than one billion dollars per year in revenue for its patent owner; blockbuster drugs consist of approximately one hundred products which comprise approximately one-third of the pharmaceutical market.

Bone marrow transplant: a medical procedure to replenish the soft tissue within bones that produces new blood cells; necessary when marrow has been destroyed by drug or radiation therapy for cancer, often leukemia; bone marrow donors are usually a close relative of the patient.

Branded generic: a generic version of a brand-name drug introduced to the market by the brand-name drug's producer just prior to the expiration of the brand-name drug's patent, thereby mitigating the loss of sales to other generic producers.

Burden of proof: a party's duty to prove a disputed assertion or charge; the party with the burden of proof will lose if its evidence does not convince the jury, or the judge in a nonjury trial.

Bureaucratic: arbitrary and routine; rigidly devoted to the details of administrative procedure.

Business process outsourcing: a form of outsourcing which involves the contracting of specific business functions to a third party provider, such as accounting, claims processing (health insurance), clinical trials, and administrative functions traditionally performed by human resources departments.

Cafeteria approach: set up to allow a variety of choices; in health insurance plans, when each employee is allocated a dollar amount or number of credits based on salary, seniority, and/or age that the employee may use to choose from among a variety of benefit options.

Cartel: a group formed, particularly to regulate prices and output in a field of business, and sometimes to obtain a monopoly; a coalition of political or special-interest groups having a common cause, such as to encourage the passing of legislation.

Catastrophic illness or injury: severe illness or injury requiring prolonged hospitalization or recovery time and usually involving high costs for medical care.

Centers-of-excellence: a network of health care facilities selected for specific services based on criteria such as experience, outcomes, quality, efficiency, and effectiveness.

Certiorari: Latin, translating to "to be more fully informed"; today it is when a higher court directs a lower court to certify the record of the lower court's proceedings for purposes of the higher court's review; an extraordinary direction issued by a higher court, at its discretion, directing a lower court to deliver the case record for the higher court's review. Also called "writ of certiorari" and "cert." for short.

Channel stuffing: an illegal business practice used to temporarily inflate sales and earnings figures by sending health care providers more product than they are able to use in order to fraudulently raise the value of stock, and then accepting the excess items back from providers instead of cash.

Chattel: a moveable or transferable article of personal property capable of manual delivery.

Chemical: a substance with a distinct molecular composition produced by or used in the science that deals with the composition and properties of substances and various elementary forms of matter; a drug.

Chemical compound: a substance consisting of two or more different molecules or pure elements chemically bonded together in a fixed proportion.

Chemical equivalence: the idea that a certain measure of one substance is in some chemical sense equal to a different amount of a second substance; also referred to as pharmaceutical equivalence.

Child: a person under the age of majority; as defined by the FDA in connection with drugs, devices, and biologics, an individual from infancy to sixteen years of age.

Chimera: an organism composed of two or more genetically distinct tissues, such as an organism that is partly male and partly female, or an artificially produced individual having tissues of several species.

Chromosome: threadlike strands of DNA that carry genes in a linear order and serve to transmit hereditary information.

Chronic disease: a disease of long duration.

Circumstantial evidence: evidence based on inference and not on personal knowledge or observation.

Civil action: a proceeding in a court of justice by which one party seeks to enforce or protect a right, or to redress or prevent a wrong, and which results in a judgment or decree; a suit stating a legal cause of action and seeking only a legal remedy; noncriminal litigation.

Civil rights: rights to personal liberty established by the Thirteenth and Fourteenth Amendments to the U.S. Constitution and certain Congressional acts, particularly as applied to individuals or minority groups; the rights to full legal, social, and economic equality extended to African Americans; rights belonging to an individual by virtue of citizenship, including civil liberties, due process, equal protection of the laws, and freedom from discrimination; broad range of fundamental freedoms guaranteed to all individuals, such as rights of free expression and action, right to enter into contracts, own property, and initiate lawsuits, opportunities in education and work, freedom to live, travel, and use public facilities, and the right to participate in the democratic political system.

Class action: a lawsuit in which the court authorizes a single person of a small group of people to represent the interests of a larger group of similarly situated persons; generally, the class must be so large that individual suits would be impracticable, there must be legal or factual questions common to the class, the claims of the representative individual or group must be typical of those of the class, and the representative individual or group must adequately protect the interests of the class; occasionally, a member of the class must affirmatively opt-in or opt-out of the class action or risk being included or excluded by default.

Clawback: money taken back; the retrieval or recovery of tax allowances by additional forms of taxation.

Clear and convincing evidence: evidence indicating that the thing to be proved is highly probable or reasonably certain; this is the medium level of evidence and is the standard applied in most civil trials. *Compare* "beyond a reasonable doubt" and "preponderance of the evidence," the highest and lowest standards of evidence required, respectively.

Clearance: FDA authorization to market a medical device based on a review of evidence of ability to satisfy label claims, safety, and/or equivalence to previously marketed devices.

Clinical trial: scientific investigation of a new drug, device, biologic, diagnostic test or other medical product that has shown some benefit in animal or laboratory studies, but that has not yet been proven effective in humans.

Cloning: the process of making copies of a specific piece of DNA, usually a gene; when geneticists speak of cloning, they do not mean the process of making genetically identical copies of an entire organism.

Cognitive neuroscience: branch of neuroscience that studies the biological foundations of mental phenomena.

Cognitive science: the study of the precise nature of different mental tasks and the operations of the brain that enable them to be performed.

Coinsurance: a co-sharing agreement between the insured and the insurer which provides that the insured will cover a set percentage of the covered costs after the deductible has been paid.

Collateral source rule: the doctrine that if an injured party receives compensation from a source other than the wrongdoer, that payment should not be deducted from the amount that the wrongdoer must pay; insurance proceeds are the most common collateral source.

Combination device: a device comprised of two or more regulated components (drug/device, biologic/device, drug/biologic, or drug/device/biologic), that are physically, chemically, or otherwise combined or mixed and produced as a single entity.

Common law: the body of law derived from judicial decisions, rather than from statutes or constitutions. Also called "caselaw."

Communicable disease: any disease transmitted from one person or animal to another. Also called "contagious."

Comparability: refers to similarities, regulatory acceptability and supplemental approvals of products incorporating a change in the manufacturing process by the product's current manufacturer or contractors.

Comparative efficacy: comparing two or more treatments for a given condition; comparative efficacy evaluations may focus only on the relative medical benefits and risks of each option, or they may also weigh the costs. Also called "comparative effectiveness."

Compassionate use: a mechanism for securing FDA permission for the use with an individual patient of a drug, medical device, or biologic that has not been approved or cleared for marketing in general commerce.

Competitive medical plan: permission given by the federal government allowing an organization to write a Medicare risk contract; alternative health care delivery mechanisms such as preferred provider organizations or prepaid plans that meet Medicare qualifications for a risk-sharing contract.

Composite tissue allograft: a transplant involving several different types of tissue (bones, nerves, blood vessels, and muscle), such as a hand transplant.

Comprehensive health care: coordinated delivery of the total health care required or requested by the patient.

Computational biology: the application of computer science, applied mathematics, and statistics techniques to biological problems; addresses scientific research topics without a laboratory.

Computer physician order entry: electronic entry of medical instructions for the treatment of patients, particularly hospitalized patients, communicated over a computer network to the medical staff or departments responsible for fulfilling the order.

Computerized axial tomography scan: medical imaging method that generates a three-dimensional image of the inside of an object from a large series of two-dimensional x-ray images taken around a single axis of rotation. Also called "CAT scan" or "CT scan."

Computerized decision support system: the application of evidence-based clinical guidelines to a patient's electronic medical data to help flag potentially serious clinical errors or deviations from accepted best practices, identify clinical interventions, issue clinical recommendations, lower costs, and improve quality of medical care.

Condition-of-approval study: a study to be conducted after approval of a device to address issues of safety and effectiveness not sufficiently evaluated by studies submitted in support of a premarket approval application, such as long term effects and effects in populations not yet studied; the manufacturer agrees to perform these studies as a condition of approval.

Confidential commercial information: valuable data or information that is used in business and is of a type customarily held in strict confidence or regarded as privileged and not disclosed to any member of the public by the person to whom it belongs.

Conflict of interest: an incompatibility between one's private interests and one's public or fiduciary duties; when one's personal interests might benefit from one's official actions or influence; when one activity or interest can be advanced only at the expense of another.

Congenital condition: defects or damage to a developing fetus resulting from genetic abnormalities, the intrauterine environment, infection, errors in development, or chromosomal abnormality; physical condition recognizable at birth and significant enough to be considered a problem.

Congress: the legislative body of the federal government created by the U.S. Constitution and consisting of the Senate and the House of Representatives.

Consent decree: a court decision, similar to a judgment that all parties agree to.

Conspiracy: an agreement by two or more persons to commit an unlawful act.

Constitutional right: a right guaranteed by the U.S. Constitution or by a state constitution.

Consumer-directed health care plan: health care plans that combine high deductibles with a tax-advantaged health savings account or health reimbursement arrangement, designed to give patients greater control over health expenditures; the rationale for such plans is that patients will be more prudent in their consumption of health care if they must pay for it out of their own pockets.

Contraceptive: a device, drug, or chemical agent that prevents conception, or pregnancy.

Contract: an agreement between two or more parties creating obligations that are enforceable or recognizable at law; the writing that sets forth such an agreement.

Controlled substance: any drug whose possession and use is regulated by law, whether prescription or illegal.

Cooperative hospital service organization: an organization formed by two or more tax exempt hospitals to provide specifically enumerated services, such as purchasing, billing, or clinical services, solely for the benefit of its patron hospitals; these entities are required to distribute net earnings to patron hospitals on the basis of services performed.

Copayment: a contributory payment by an employer, usually matching that of an employee, toward the payment of health care or life insurance premiums, a pension fund, etc.

Corporate acquisition: takeover of one corporation by another, if both retain their legal existence after the transaction. *Compare* "merger."

Correction: a type of recall that involves an on-site repair, adjustment, labeling change, destruction, or inspection of a medical product.

Corrective action: action to eliminate the cause(s) of an existing defect or similar product or quality problem in order to prevent recurrence.

Cosmeceutical: a cosmetic that has or is purported to have medicinal properties; combination cosmetic and pharmaceutical product.

Cost-sharing: ways employers require employees to share costs of health care benefits, such as annual deductibles, annual out-of-pocket expense maximums, lifetime maximums, and coinsurance.

Criminal action: legal action instituted by the government to punish offenses against the public.

Cybersurgery: a surgical procedure in which the operative field is accessed and manipulated with a digital interface controlled at a distance, usually with joy sticks.

Dangerous mental disorder: a condition which causes a person to be a danger to themselves or others, usually warranting confinement in a secure facility.

Deductible: the amount for which the insured is liable for each treatment before an insurance company will make a payment.

Defensive medicine: practice of ordering many tests or consultations as a means of protection against charges of malpractice in the event of an unfavorable outcome of treatment.

Deferred prosecution agreement: when a business entity agrees to admit wrongdoing and enact reform policies in exchange for a promise by the U.S. Justice Department not to seek an indictment as long as the business lives up to its agreement.

Democracy: government by the people; a form of government in which the supreme power is vested in the people and exercised directly by them or by their elected agents under a free electoral system; a state of society characterized by formal equality of rights and privileges; political or social equality.

Device design controls: procedures to control the design of a medical device in order to ensure that specified design requirements are met; equivalent to pharmaceutical current good manufacturing practices.

Device distributor: anyone who furthers the distribution of a medical device from the original place of manufacture to the person who makes delivery or sale to the ultimate user, but who does not repackage or otherwise change the container, wrapper, or labeling of the device or device package; a device distributor may create kits for specific procedures.

Device failure: the failure of a medical device to perform or function as intended, including any deviations from the device's performance specifications or intended use.

Device malfunction: the failure of a medical device to meet its performance specifications or otherwise perform as intended; performance specifications include all claims made in the labeling for the device; the intended performance of a device refers to the intended use for which the device is labeled or marketed.

Diagnostic: serving to identify or characterize; being a precise indication; a device or substance used for the analysis or detection of diseases or other medical conditions.

Differential pricing: method in which a product has different prices based on the type of customer, quantity ordered, delivery time, payment terms, etc. Also called "discriminatory pricing" or "multiple pricing."

Diploid: having two similar complements of chromosomes; an organism or cell having double the basic haploid number of chromosomes; having a pair of each type of chromosome so that the basic chromosome number is doubled.

Direct benefit: a tangible positive outcome of a treatment event or medical action; sometimes justifies exposure to more than minimal risk.

Disability: the inability to perform some function; an objectively measurable condition of impairment, physical or mental; an incapacity caused by a physical defect or infirmity, or by bodily imperfection or mental weakness.

Disability-adjusted life-year: a measure of overall disease burden designed to quantify the impact of premature death and disability on a population; one disability-adjusted life-year is equal to one year of healthy life lost.

Discounted drug program: resource to help physicians, advocates, and patients access free or discounted medications through pharmaceutical company patient assistant programs.

Disease management: a system of coordinated health care interventions and communications for populations with conditions in which patient self-care efforts are significant; the process of reducing health care costs and improving quality of life for individuals by preventing or minimizing effects of a disease, usually a chronic condition, through integrative care.

Disgorge: to unwillingly surrender or yield something illicitly obtained on request, under pressure, or by court order in order to prevent unjust enrichment.

Distributive justice: principles designed to guide the allocation of the benefits and burdens of economic activity; concerns what is just or right with respect to the allocation of goods or services in a society, such as the idea that everyone in a society should receive equitable access to basic health care needs for living.

Divest: dispossess; to sell off or otherwise dispose of a subsidiary company or an investment.

DNA: the main component of chromosomes and the material that transfers genetic characteristics in all life forms; constructed of two strands coiled around each other in a ladderlike arrangement; the genetic information of DNA is transcribed as the strands unwind and replicate; a nucleic acid that carries the cell's genetic information and is capable of self-replication; it determines individual hereditary characteristics. Also called "deoxyribonucleic acid."

DNA sequencing: determining the exact order of the base pairs in a segment of DNA.

Double effect principle: a set of ethical criteria for evaluating the permissibility of acting when one's otherwise legitimate act will also cause an effect one would normally be obliged to avoid; this set of criteria states that an action having foreseen harmful effects practically inseparable from the good effect is justifiable if the nature of the act is itself good or at least morally neutral, the agent intends the good effect and not the bad effect either as a means to the good effect or as an end itself, the good effect outweighs the bad effect in circumstances sufficiently grave to justify causing the bad effect, and the agent exercises due diligence to minimize the harm.

Drug: a chemical substance used in the treatment, cure, prevention, or diagnosis of disease or used to otherwise enhance physical or mental wellbeing; includes the vast majority of pharmaceuticals. *Compare* "Biologic."

Due process: the conduct of legal proceedings according to established rules and principles for the protection and enforcement of private rights, including notice and the right to a fair hearing before a tribunal with the right to decide the case.

Durable medical equipment: medical equipment used in the home to aid in a better quality of living; devices which are resistant to wear and may be used over a long period of time, such as wheelchairs and artificial limbs.

Economy of scale: the decrease in average unit cost of a product or service resulting from large scale operations such as mass production; the increase in efficiency of production as the number of goods being produced increases.

Ectoderm: the outermost of the three primary germ layers of an embryo, from which the epidermis, nervous tissue, and sensory organs develop.

Effectiveness: the achievement of desired treatment results in actual clinical practice; producing the intended or expected result.

Efficacy: the achievement of desired treatment results in controlled clinical studies; capacity for producing a desired result or effect.

Electronic health records: an individual patient's medical record in digital format; may be made up of records from many locations or sources; believed to increase quality of care, improve physician efficiency, reduce costs, and promote standardization of care.

Embryo: in humans, the prefetal product of conception from implantation through the eighth week of development, at which point it is referred to as a fetus.

Embryology: the science dealing with the formation, development, structure, and functional activities of embryos; the origin, growth, and development of an embryo.

Embryonic germ layers: the three initial tissue layers arising in the embryo, the endoderm, mesoderm, and ectoderm, from which all other somatic tissues develop.

Embryonic stem cell: primitive, undifferentiated cells derived from the inner cell mass of the embryo that have the potential to become a wide variety of specialized cell types.

Employer mandate: a state or federal measure requiring that large employers provide health insurance benefits to their employees.

Employer-sponsored insurance: health insurance coverage employers may offer to employees as a benefit, usually with conditions attached, offering a broader scope of benefits than typically available under individually purchased coverage; employees may choose to enroll or forgo enrollment; the leading source of health insurance in America.

En banc: Latin meaning with all judges present and participating; in full court.

Endocrinology: the study of the glands and hormones of the body and their related disorders.

Endoderm: the innermost of three primary germ layers of an animal embryo, developing into the gastrointestinal tract, the lungs, and associated structures.

Enteral: of, relating to, or being within the intestine.

Enucleate: to remove the nucleus; to remove from an enveloping cover.

Epidemic: affecting many persons at the same time and spreading from person to person in a locality where the disease is not permanently prevalent; extremely prevalent, widespread.

Epidemiology: the branch of medicine dealing with the incidence and prevalence of disease in large populations and with detection of the source and cause of epidemics of infectious disease.

Equal access: equivalent availability, physical accessibility, and quality of medical services to the public; the non-discriminatory acceptability of different cultures, sexes, and age groups into the health care system; accessibility deals with non-discrimination, physical accessibility, economic accessibility, and information accessibility; the idea that all persons have the right to health services of all types and that each service should be within reach for all members of the population no matter what economic status, physical location, or nationality that a particular resident embodies.

Equitable: just; consistent with principles of justice and right.

Equity: fairness; impartiality; evenhanded dealing; the body of principles constituting what is fair and right; the recourse to principles of justice to correct or supplement the law as applied to particular circumstances; an ownership interest in property.

Estoppel: a bar that prevents one from asserting a claim or right that contradicts what one has said or done before or what has been legally established as true; a bar that prevents the relitigation of issues; an affirmative defense alleging good faith reliance on a misleading representation and an injury or detrimental change in position resulting from that reliance.

Et seq.: Latin meaning those pages or sections that follow.

Eugenics: the study of the possibility of improving the qualities of the human species or a human population, especially by such means as discouraging reproduction by persons having genetic defects or presumed to have inheritable undesirable traits or encouraging reproduction by persons presumed to have inheritable desirable traits.

Euthanasia: the act or practice of killing or bringing about the death of a person who suffers from an incurable disease or condition, especially a painful one, for reasons of mercy. *Compare* "assisted dying."

Evidence-based medicine: practice of applying evidence gained from the scientific method to certain parts of medicine; it seeks to assess the quality of evidence relevant to the risks and benefits of treatments, including lack of treatment; the conscientious, explicit, and judicious use of current best evidence in making decisions about the care of individual patients; recognizes that many aspects of medical care depend on individual factors such as quality- and value-of-life judgments, which are only partially subject to scientific methods; seeks to clarify those parts of medical practice that are subject to scientific methods to ensure the best prediction of outcomes in medical treatment, even as debate about which outcomes are desirable continues.

Exclusive dealing: an agreement requiring a buyer to purchase all needed goods from one seller.

Executive Order: an order issued by or on behalf of the President, usually intended to direct or instruct the actions of executive agencies or government officials, or to set policies for the executive branch to follow.

Expected utility maximization model: the combination of utility and objective probability, which model has been called into doubt as the existence of objective probability has been questioned by statisticians; alternatively, the combination of utility and subjective probability; because this is the basis upon which most people make decisions, most current work in formal decision theory and research occurs within the context of this more subjective model.

Experience rating: a quantitative measure used by an insurance company to determine how much a given policy should cost, calculated using historical data to determine the risk of future claims.

Experimental medical treatment: medical therapies intended or claimed to treat a condition by improving on, supplementing, or replacing existing conventional methods; often not covered by health insurers.

Federalism: the relationship and distribution of power between the national and regional governments within a federal system of government.

Fetus: a developing human from two months after conception until birth.

Fiduciary: one who owes to another the duties of good faith, trust, confidence, and candor; one who must exercise a high standard of care in managing another's money or property.

Follow-on biologic: comparable versions of biotechnology products marketed after expiration of patents which are claimed to have similar properties to existing biologic products; often used to describe a later biopharmaceutical, often involving a more technologically advanced version, but not necessarily improved version, of an innovator product. Also called "biosimilar." *Compare* "later generation."

Follow-on protein: protein and peptide products that are intended to be sufficiently similar to a product already approved or licensed to permit the applicant to rely for approval on certain existing scientific knowledge about the safety and effectiveness of the approved protein product; may be produced through biotechnology or derived from natural sources.

Formulary: formulas for making medicinal preparations; a book containing a list of pharmaceutical substances along with their formulas, uses, and methods of preparation.

Fundamental right: a right derived from natural or fundamental law; a significant component of liberty, encroachments of which are rigorously tested by courts to ascertain the soundness of purported governmental justifications; such rights include voting, interstate travel, and various aspects of privacy, such as marriage and contraception rights.

Futile medical care: the belief that in cases where there is no hope for improvement of an incapacitating condition, that no course of treatment is called for; withholding such care does not encourage nor speed the natural onset of death; it may be impossible to define this term because it depends upon universal agreement about the point at which there is no further benefit to intervention, which different involved parties may disagree upon.

Gene: a functional unit of heredity that is a segment of DNA located in a specific site on a chromosome which directs the formation of an enzyme or other protein.

Gene mapping: determining the relative positions of genes on a chromosome and the distance between them in order to understand genetic diseases.

Gene therapy: the application of genetic engineering to the transplantation of genes into human cells in order to cure a disease caused by a genetic defect, such as a missing enzyme.

General causation: the causing or producing of an effect; concerns the question of whether something can physically possibly cause the effect, not necessarily whether it actually did.

General controls: FDA requirements that all classes of drugs, medical devices, and biologics must meet to be lawfully marketed.

Generic: not protected by a trademark; any product sold without a brand name; common or descriptive, nonproprietary.

Genetic engineering: the development and application of scientific methods, procedures, and technologies that permit direct manipulation of genetic material in order to alter the hereditary traits of a cell, organism, or population; scientific alteration of genetic material; the manipulation of DNA to produce new types of organisms by inserting or deleting genes.

Genetic recombination: breaking a strand of genetic material and joining it to a different DNA molecule, such as during reproduction.

Genome: the genetic material in the chromosomes of an organism; the total gene complement of a set of chromosomes.

Genomics: the study of genomes, including gene mapping, which involves figuring out the positions of genes on a DNA molecule, in order to use that information to develop improved medicines as well as answer scientific questions.

Genotype: genetic constitution of an organism or a group of organisms, with reference to a trait, trait set, or all traits; a group or class having the same genetic constitution; genetic makeup as distinguished from physical characteristics.

Germ line gene therapy: introducing genes to reproductive cells in order to prevent defective genes being transmitted to a subsequent generation or to transmit desirable genes to a subsequent generation; currently this technology involves an unknown level of risk and is thus not yet widely applied to humans.

Gestation: the entire length of time in utero, from conception until birth.

Glial cell: cells that provide support and nutrition, maintain homeostasis, form myelin, and participate in signal transmission in the nervous system.

Global burden of disease study: numerical indicator of the impact of all forms of illness and disability on the expectancy of remaining years of healthy life in the population of a country, or in other segments of the population; calculated using nationally available data on life expectancy and major varieties of disability; time-based measure combining years of life lost due to premature mortality and years of life lost due to time lived in states of less than full health.

Governance: the relationship between the shareholders, directors, and management of a company as defined by the corporate charter, bylaws, formal policy, and rule of law; the ways in which the rights and responsibilities are shared between various corporate participants.

Gross domestic product: total market value of all the goods and services produced within the borders of a nation during a specified period; perhaps the best indicator of the economic health of a country.

Group practice: practice of medicine by an association of doctors and other health professionals who work together and share resources.

Group purchasing organization: an entity created to leverage the purchasing power of a group of businesses to obtain discounts from vendors.

Group-sponsored health plans: a health insurance plan that covers a group of people, such as the employees of a business or members of an organization; usually the employer or organization pays the majority of the coverage amount and the employees or members contribute a smaller amount.

Guaranteed access program: acceptance into insurance coverage plan for all applicants, including those with pre-existing conditions and higher than average medical costs

Guaranteed issue: legal requirement that all health insurance plans sold to small groups, such as a small business, cannot turn down any group based on its health status.

Guardian ad litem: a person, usually a lawyer, appointed by the court to appear in a lawsuit on behalf of an incompetent or minor party.

H5N1: The scientific name for a subtype of the avian influenza (bird flu) virus that has spread from birds to humans. The scientific names for these subtypes are classified by different proteins on the virus. New subtypes naturally occur when the proteins change.

Haploid: single; pertaining to a single set of chromosomes; an organism or cell having only one complete set of chromosomes, ordinarily half of the normal diploid number; 23 in humans.

Harm: a hurtful or adverse outcome of a treatment action or medical event, whether temporary or permanent; physical injury or mental damage.

Hazard: unavoidable danger or risk, even though foreseeable; lack of predictability; possible source of danger.

Health economist: one who studies the functioning of the health care system and private and social causes of health-affecting behaviors.

Health information technology: system where medical professionals store the information usually contained in a patient chart on a computer, rather than on paper, in order to improve the efficiency and quality of health care that patients receive.

Health management organization: a type of managed care organization that provides a form of health care coverage fulfilled through hospitals, doctors, and other providers with which the health management organization has a contract; the organization only covers care rendered by health professionals who have agreed to treat patients in accordance with its guidelines and restrictions in exchange for a steady stream of customers. Also called "health maintenance organization."

Health professional: a person trained to work in any field of physical or mental health; a person who delivers proper health care in a systematic way.

Health provider: the organization, system, or institution that delivers or provides health care services by health professionals, such as the insurer or government.

Health risk: any physical, behavioral, psychosocial, spiritual, intellectual, developmental, or environmental factor that increases the vulnerability of a person to illness or accident.

Health savings account: a tax-advantaged medical savings account available to U.S. taxpayers enrolled in high deductible health plans; not subject to federal tax liability and can accumulate from year to year if not spent. Also called "medical savings account."

Hermaphrodite: an individual or organism in which reproductive organs of both sexes are present.

High throughput molecular biology: shifts the focus of biological research from experimental science to information science; powerful computation methods applied to very large amounts of apparently incoherent data coming from biomedical research.

Hippocratic Oath: an oath embodying the duties and obligations of physicians, usually taken by those about to enter upon the practice of medicine; an oath of ethical professional behavior sworn to by new physicians.

Homeopathic medicine: a form of alternative medicine which attempts to treat illness with preparations thought to cause effects similar to the illness's symptoms, based upon the belief that illness is the result of imbalance within the body, rather than a separate thing or invading, foreign entity.

Hospice: health care facility for the terminally ill that emphasizes pain control and emotional support for the patient and family, typically refraining from taking extraordinary measures to prolong life; similar program of care and support for the terminally ill undertaken at home.

House of Representatives: lower chamber of the U.S. Congress, composed of 435 members apportioned among the states on the basis of population who are elected to two-year terms; the lower house of a state legislature.

Human factors: how people use scientific and medical technology; the interaction of human abilities, expectations, and limitations, with work environments and system design; physical or cognitive property of an individual or social behavior which is specific to humans and influences functioning of technological systems as well as human-environment equilibriums.

Humanitarian device exemption application: an application that is similar to a premarket approval application but is exempt from its effectiveness requirements; the application must contain information on the targeted medical condition, indication for the device's use, and rationale for the application including the risks and benefits of currently available alternatives in the U.S. and the lack of comparable devices for the medical condition.

Humanitarian use device: a medical device that is intended to benefit patients suffering from a disease or condition that affects fewer than four thousand individuals in the U.S. per year.

Hybrid: the offspring of two animals or plants of different breeds, varieties, or species, especially as produced through human manipulation for specific genetic characteristics.

Hypothesis: proposition set forth as an explanation for the occurrence of some specified group of phenomena, either to guide investigation or to be accepted as highly probable in light of established facts; tentative explanation for an observation or scientific problem that can be tested by further investigation.

Id.: Latin meaning referring to the authority cited immediately before.

Immunization: the fact or process of becoming resistant to a disease.

Implant: a device that is placed into a surgically or naturally formed cavity of the human body if it is intended to remain there for a period of time to continuously assist, restore, or replace the function of an organ system or structure of the human body throughout the useful life of the device.

Importer: one who imports a medical product into the U.S. and who furthers the marketing of a drug, device, or biologic from the original place of manufacture to the person who makes final delivery or sale to the ultimate user; does not include those who repackage or otherwise change the container, wrapper, or labeling of the product package.

In vitro: the union of an egg and sperm, where the event takes place outside the body and in an artificial environment; Latin meaning in glass.

In vivo: a biological process occurring or made to occur within a living organism or natural setting; Latin meaning in life.

Incapacity: lack of physical or mental capabilities; lack of ability to have certain legal consequences attach to one's actions.

Incompetent: lack of legal ability in some respect, especially to stand trial or to testify; state or fact of being unable or unqualified to do something.

Indemnity: a duty to make good any loss, damage, or liability incurred by another; the right of an injured party to claim reimbursement for its loss, damage, or liability from an entity that has such a duty.

Indictment: the formal written accusation of a crime, made by a grand jury and presented to a court for prosecution against the accused person.

Individual health insurance: health coverage purchased on an individual basis on the private market rather than through a group and not tied to workplace benefits.

Infant: a child during the earliest period of its life, especially before he or she can walk, sometimes extended to age seven.

Infectious disease: any disease caused by the entrance, growth, and multiplication of bacteria or protozoans in the body; it may not be contagious; it may be spread by germs carried in the air or water.

Infirm: feeble or weak in body or health, especially because of age or ailment.

Influenza: an acute, commonly epidemic disease, occurring in several forms and caused by numerous, rapidly mutating viral strains; characterized by respiratory symptoms and general prostration. Also called "flu."

Informed consent: a person's agreement to allow something to happen, made with full knowledge of the risks involved and the alternatives; a patient's knowing choice about a medical treatment or procedure, made after a health care professional discloses whatever information a reasonably prudent health care professional would give to a patient regarding the risks involved in the proposed care.

Injunction: a court order commanding or prohibiting an action; to get an injunction, the claimant must show that irreparable injury will result unless it is granted.

Innovator: refers to original products, usually the first to receive approvals, and associated companies; such products are presumed to have involved original and extensive research and development and full (not abbreviated) Phase III-type safety and efficacy testing.

Inpatient: the receipt of medical care or treatment while staying in a hospital for at least one night.

Isolated: to keep an infected person away from contact with noninfected persons; quarantine; in chemistry, to separate a substance in pure form from a combined mixture; in microbiology, to separate a pure strain from a mixed bacterial or fungal culture.

Insolvent: the condition of not being able to pay debts as they come due or in the usual course of business.

Insource: to keep within a corporation tasks that were previously outsourced.

Institutional review board: a group of qualified individuals charged under federal regulation with protecting the rights and welfare of patients involved in human research in accord with federal regulations; these boards review and approve plans for research involving humans.

Insurance: a method for managing medical risk by spreading the risk over a group of individuals through pooled premiums that cover the costs of unanticipated illnesses or injuries.

Insurance risk pool: the group of individuals who enroll in an insurance plan; when insurers sell an insurance plan to a group, they do not look at the information of any one particular member, but rather the medical experiences of the group as a whole and the total premium collected from and medical claims paid out on behalf of that insurance pool as a whole.

Integrated care: medical care provided by a team of health care professionals working together to provide complementary alternative and conventional health care, particularly beneficial for patients whose complex conditions require continuing care from multiple professionals in multiple settings.

Intellectual property rights: a category of intangible rights protecting commercially valuable products of the human intellect; primarily trademark, copyright, patent, trade-secret, publicity, and moral rights, as well as rights against unfair competition.

Intellectually disabled: an individual with below-average intelligence, ranging from mild to profound, and limitations in the ability to function in areas of daily life, such as communication, self-care, and social situations. Also called "cognitively disabled."

Intermediate scrutiny: a standard lying between strict scrutiny and rational basis review; under this standard, if a statute contains a quasi-suspect classification, such as gender, the classification must be substantially related to the achievement of an important governmental objective. *Compare* "strict scrutiny" and "rational basis test."

Intractable symptoms: hard to treat, alleviate, relieve, or cure; symptoms insufficiently controlled by symptom-specific therapies.

Investigational biologic: a biologic undergoing clinical studies to statistically determine whether it is efficacious for the target indication.

Investigational device: a medical device that is the object of a clinical investigation or human research involving one or more patients to determine safety or effectiveness of the device.

Joint and several liability: liability that may be apportioned either among two or more parties or to only one or a few select members of the group at the adversary's discretion.

Joint venture: a business undertaking by two or more persons engaged in a single, defined project; the necessary elements are an agreement, a common purpose intended to be carried out, shared profits and losses, and each member's equal voice in controlling the project.

Jurisdiction: a government's general power to exercise authority over all persons and things within its territory; a court's power to decide a case or issue a decree; the geographic area within which political or judicial authority may be exercised.

Jurisprudence: the study of the general or fundamental elements of a particular legal system, as opposed to its practical and concrete details; the study of legal systems in general; judicial precedents considered collectively; a system, body, or division of law.

Karyotype: the chromosome characteristics of an individual cell or cell line, usually presented as a systemized array of pairs in descending order of size.

Kickback: a return of a portion of a monetary sum received, especially as a result of coercion or a secret agreement. Also called "illegal remunerations."

Label: a display of written, printed, or graphic matter on the immediate container of a medical product; sn informative logo, title, or similar marking affixed to a manufactured product.

Latent: concealed; dormant or inactive; present, but not visible, apparent, or actualized; existing as potential.

Later generation: a biopharmaceutical similar to another prior product; the product often involves technological advances or other modifications such that it may not actually be similar to prior innovator product(s). *Compare* "follow-on biologic" and "follow-on protein."

Leverage: risky use of credit or borrowed funds to improve one's speculative capacity and increase the rate of return from an investment, control a larger investment, or reduce one's own liability for any loss.

License: revocable permission to commit some act that would otherwise be unlawful; the certificate or document evidencing such permission.

Litigation: the process of carrying on a lawsuit; a lawsuit itself.

Living will: an instrument signed in accordance with statutory requirements by which a person directs that his or her life not be artificially prolonged by extraordinary measures when there is no reasonable expectation of recovery from extreme physical or mental disability.

Magnetic resonance imaging: use of machinery to produce electronic images of internal organs and tissues; it work by putting the patient inside a magnet, then using radio waves to locate atoms, which a computer uses to produce an image.

Malfunction: the failure of a medical product to meet its performance specifications or to perform as intended.

Malpractice: an instance of negligence or incompetence on the part of a professional. Also called "professional negligence."

Managed care: comprehensive health insurance plans provided to participating members of a health care organization; organized into a network of providers and professionals including doctors and hospitals.

Manufacturer: any person, including any importer, re-packer, re-labeler, or specifications developer who manufactures, prepares, propagates, compounds, assembles, or processes a drug, device, or biologic.

Market withdrawal of medical device: a manufacturer's removal or correction of a distributed medical device which involves a minor violation that would not be subject to legal action by the FDA or which involves no violation, such as normal stock rotation practices, routine device adjustments, and repairs.

Mediation: method of nonbinding dispute resolution involving a neutral third party who tries to help the disputing parties reach a mutually agreeable solution.

Medical device: an instrument, apparatus, implement, machine, contrivance, implant, in vitro reagent, or other similar or related article, including a component, part, or accessory, which is recognized in the official National Formulary, or the United States Pharmacopoeia, intended for use in the cure, mitigation, treatment, or prevention of disease or intended to affect the structure or any function of the human body, and which does not achieve any of its primary intended purposes through chemical action within or on the human body and which is not dependent upon being metabolized for the achievement of its primary intended purposes; classified into Class I (low risk), II, or III (high risk).

Medical intervention: treatment undertaken to interfere or intercede with the intent of modifying an outcome, usually to treat or cure a condition.

Medicaid: U.S. government program, financed by federal, state, and local funds, providing health insurance for people within certain income limits.

Medical neglect: a form of child neglect; when a child's parent, guardian, or legal custodian neglects, refuses, or is unable, for reasons other than poverty, to provide medical or dental care so as to seriously endanger the physical health of the child.

Medical review panel: reviews the evidence in a case and renders an opinion as to whether the evidence supports the view that the defendant did or did not comply with the appropriate standard of care and whether the care in question was related to any harm suffered by the plaintiff; its opinion is admissible as evidence in the case, but is not legally binding; comprised of individuals such as attorneys and health professionals.

Medical tourism: traveling across international borders in order to obtain health care.

Medically necessary health care: treatments with proven value for use in the general population, usually have final government approval, are evidence-based, improve net health outcome, are as beneficial as established alternatives, demonstrate improvement outside of clinical trials, and are not experimental or investigational.

Medically underserved area: a geographic area or population designated as having too few primary care providers; a region that has a relative or absolute deficiency of health care resources, such as hospital beds, equipment, and medical personnel.

Medicare: program of health care for the aged and disabled established by the Social Security Act.

Mega-trend: major trend or movement; large-scale change in circumstances.

Mens rea: Latin meaning guilty mind; the state of mind that the prosecution, to secure a conviction, must prove that a defendant had while committing a crime; criminal intent or recklessness.

Mental disorder: mental condition marked by sufficient disorganization of personality, mind, and emotions which impairs the normal psychological functioning of the individual.

Mental health: psychological well-being and satisfactory adjustment to society and to the ordinary demands of life; the field of medicine concerned with the maintenance or achievement of such well-being and adjustment; the absence of mental disorder or illness.

Mental illness: any of various conditions characterized by impairment of an individual's normal cognitive, emotional, or behavioral functioning, and caused by social, psychological, biochemical, genetic, or other factors, such as infection or head trauma.

Mental model: an explanation in an individual's thought process for how something works in the world; representation of the surrounding world, the relationships between its various parts, and the individual's intuitive perception about their own acts and consequences; mental models shape behavior and define approaches to solving problems and carrying out tasks.

Merger: the absorption of one company which ceases to exist into another which retains its own name and identity and acquires the assets and liabilities of the former.

Mesoderm: middle embryonic germ layer, lying between the ectoderm and endoderm, from which connective tissue, muscle, bone, and urogenital and circulatory systems develop.

Metabolism: sum of the physical and chemical processes in an organism by which its material substance is produced, maintained, and destroyed, and by which energy is made available; any basic process of organic functioning or operating; processing of a specific substance within the living body.

Metric: pertaining to measurement; standard of measurement.

Microbe: microorganism, especially a pathogenic bacterium; minute, microscopic life form.

Microfluidics: performing engineering tasks such as optically analyzing DNA sequences by taking advantage of the chemical properties of liquids and gases and the electrical properties of semiconductors, and combining them on a single microchip.

Micro-trend: small trends that go unnoticed or ignored; small, under-the-radar patterns of behavior which take on real power when propelled by modern communications and an increasingly independent-minded population.

Minor: under the legal age of full responsibility.

Misbranded: a medical product failing to meet any one of several requirements, for example, if its labeling is false or misleading or if it was made in a manufacturing site not registered in accordance with FDA regulations.

Monopoly: control or advantage obtained by one supplier or producer over the commercial market within a given region; the market condition existing when only one economic entity produces a particular product or provides a particular service; not illegal if obtained through valid competition.

Morbidity: the proportion of sickness or of a specific disease in a geographical locality; the rate of incidence or prevalence of a disease.

Mortality: being subject to death; relative frequency of deaths in a specific population; death rate.

Multiplier effect: an economic effect in which an increase in spending produces an increase in national income and consumption greater than the initial amount spent; money used to create more money.

Multipotent stem cell: a cell that can produce two or more different types of differentiated cells; adult stem cells are multipotent.

Mutual health insurance plan: type of insurance where those protected by the insurance also have ownership rights in the organization consisting of the ability to elect the management of the organization and to participate in distribution of any net assets or surplus should the organization cease operating.

Nanodevice: any manufactured device whose scale is measured in nanometers (one billionth of a meter); such devices have enormous health care potential.

Nanoscale technologies: manipulation of matter at the level of atoms and molecules.

Nanotechnology: science of building devices, such as drug delivery systems, from single atoms and molecules.

National health information network: U.S. goal of personal electronic health care records and a uniform architecture for health care information that can be used throughout a patient's lifetime; currently four groups of health care and health information technology organizations are challenged to design a prototype network for secure information sharing among hospitals, laboratories, pharmacies, and physicians.

Neglect: the omission of proper attention to a person or thing, whether inadvertent, negligent, or willful; the act or condition of disregarding.

Negligence: failure to exercise the standard of care that a reasonably prudent person would have exercised in a similar situation; any conduct that falls below the standard established by law to protect others against unreasonable risk of harm; does not include conduct that intentionally, wantonly, or willfully disregards the rights of others.

Neuron: a specialized, impulse-conducting cell that is the functional unit of the nervous system, which includes the brain, spinal column, and nerves.

No-compete agreement: a promise not to engage in the same type of business for a stated time in the same market as the buyer, partner, or employer; generally disfavored as restraints of trade; must be reasonable for courts to enforce them.

Non-economic damages: damages that cannot be measured in money; damages that cannot be easily ascertained because there is no fixed monetary standard of measurement, such as damages for pain and suffering.

Nonprofit: a corporation organized for a purpose other than making a profit and usually afforded special tax treatment. Also called "not-for-profit corporation."

Nonsignificant risk device: a medical device that does not pose a significant risk to human research subjects; studies involving such devices require institutional review board approval and informed consent. *Compare* "significant risk device."

Nutraceutical: a food or supplement thought to have a beneficial effect on human health in addition to its basic nutritional value.

Occupational therapy: form of therapy in which patients are encouraged to engage in vocational tasks or expressive activities, usually in a social setting; the use of productive or creative activity in the treatment, rehabilitation, or recovery of physically or emotionally disabled people.

Off-label use: practice of prescribing drugs for a purpose outside the scope of the drug's approved label, most often concerning the drug's indicated use.

Ombuds: an official charged with representing the interests of the public or of employees of a corporation by investigating and addressing complaints reported by individuals; designated neutral party who aids with dispute resolution, tracks problem areas, and makes recommendations for changes to policies or procedures.

Open-label study: a type of clinical trial in which both the researchers and participants know which treatment is being administered.

Opportunistic infection: an infection by a microorganism that normally does not cause disease but becomes pathogenic when the body's immune system is impaired and unable to fight off infection.

Ordinary care: conformity to the reasonable business standards that prevail in a particular area for a particular business; care than an ordinarily reasonable and prudent person would use under the same or similar circumstances.

Orphan disease: a disease that is relatively rare, for which the development of drugs, without incentives, is considered commercially nonviable.

Orphan drug: a drug that remains undeveloped or untested or is otherwise neglected because of limited potential for commercial gain; incentives are available to develop such drugs to treat orphan diseases.

Orthotic: a device or support used to relieve or correct an orthopedic problem; specialized mechanical devices to support or supplement weakened or abnormal joints, limbs, or muscles.

Outpatient: when treatment is provided in a facility where room and board charges are not incurred, such as a doctor's office.

Outsource: to contract out jobs or services to an outside supplier or source; to obtain goods or services from an outside source; to send work out to an outside provider or manufacturer in order to cut costs.

Over-the-counter drug: drug sold without a prescription.

Palliative care: any form of medical care or treatment the concentrates on reducing the severity of disease symptoms, rather than halting, delaying, or reversing the progression of the disease itself or providing a cure; the goal is to improve quality of life for patients facing serious, complex illness.

Palliative sedation: practice of relieving distress in a terminally ill person in the last hours or days of the person's life, usually by means of continuous infusion of a sedative drug.

Pandemic: an outbreak of a disease that affects large numbers of people throughout a country, a continent, or the whole world; epidemic over a large area; general, widespread, or universal.

Parasite: an organism that lives on or in an organism of another species, known as the host, from the body of which it obtains nutriment, while contributing nothing to the survival of its host.

Parens patriae: state regarded as a sovereign; the state in its capacity as provider of protection to those unable to care for themselves; the doctrine by which a government has standing to prosecute a lawsuit on behalf of a citizen.

Parenteral: taken into the body in a manner other than through the digestive canal; not intestinal.

Parthenogenesis: a form of reproduction in which an unfertilized egg develops into a new individual; the process of inducing an unfertilized egg to initiate cell division.

Passive surveillance: FDA's program that receives reports of adverse events submitted by manufacturers, health care professionals, or patients. *Compare* "active surveillance."

Patent: the governmental grant of a right, privilege, or authority; exclusive right to make, use, or sell an invention for a specified period of time granted by the federal government to the inventor if the device or process is novel, useful, and nonobvious.

Pathogen: any disease-producing agent, especially a virus, bacterium, fungus, or other microorganism.

Pathology: science or study of the origin, nature, course, and consequences of diseases; conditions and processes of a disease; any deviation from a healthy, normal, or efficient condition.

Patient assistance program: assistance provided by pharmaceutical companies to supply free or reduced-cost medications to people who cannot afford them.

Pay or play: health care legislation requiring employers to either play by providing health insurance to employees, or pay into a public insurance fund.

Pediatric population: may refer to all children or a subgroup of children who share the same characteristics.

Per curiam: Latin meaning by the court as a whole; an opinion rendered by an appellate court without identifying the individual judge who wrote it.

Per se: Latin meaning of, in, or by itself; standing alone, without reference to additional facts.

Permanently implantable medical device: an implantable device is a device that is intended to be placed into a surgically or naturally formed cavity of the human body for more than one year to continuously assist, restore, or replace the function of an organ system or structure of the human body throughout the useful life of the device.

Persistent vegetative state: a condition of patients with severe brain damage who were in a coma, but progressed to a state of wakefulness without detectable awareness for more than four weeks; becomes a permanent vegetative state after approximately one year.

Personal health record: a health record that is initiated and maintained by an individual; ideally it provides a complete and accurate summary of the health and medical history of an individual by gathering data from many sources and makes the information available electronically to anyone with the necessary credentials to view it.

Personalized medicine: the concept that managing a patient's health should be based on the individual patient's specific characteristics, including age, gender, height, weight, diet, environment, etc.; the combination of comprehensive genetic testing with proactive, personalized preventative medicine.

Pharmaceutical: any medicinal product, particularly those with therapeutic or in vivo uses; two major subsets are drugs and biopharmaceuticals.

Pharmacoeconomics: scientific discipline that compares the value of one pharmaceutical drug or drug therapy to another; evaluates the monetary cost and effects on enhanced quality of life of a pharmaceutical product.

Pharmacogenetics and pharmacogenomics knowledge base: integrated resource containing information about how variation in human genetics leads to variation in response to drugs; funded by the National Institutes of Health; the database contains information on almost four hundred drugs and various gene-drugs, gene-diseases, and gene-drug-disease associations, and describes the evidence available to support these associations.

Pharmacokinetics: branch of pharmacology that studies the fate of pharmacological substances within the body, such as their absorption, distribution, metabolism, and elimination.

Pharmacy benefit manager: third party administrator of prescription drug programs; primarily responsible for processing and paying prescription drug claims.

Physical therapy: treatment or management of physical disability, malfunction, or pain by exercise, massage, hydrotherapy, etc., without the use of medicines, surgery, or radiation; intended to restore or facilitate normal function or development. Also called "physiotherapy."

Placebo: substance having no pharmacological effect but given merely to satisfy a patient who supposes it to be medicine or administered as a control in experimental or clinical testing of the efficacy of an active preparation.

Pluripotent cell: a cell that can produce all the cell types of the developing body; embryonic stem cells as well as the inner cell mass cells of the blastocyst are pluripotent.

Police power: inherent, fundamental, and plenary power of a sovereign to make all laws necessary and proper to protect the public security, order, health, morality, and justice.

Post-amendment medical device: a medical device available to consumers after the enactment of the Medical Device Amendments of 1976.

Postmarket: processes including evaluations, activities, and decisions that occur after FDA regulatory approval, clearance, or registration of a medical product for marketing.

Postmarket study commitments: refers collectively to condition-of-approval studies and Section 522 postmarket surveillance studies.

Postmarket surveillance: programs that seek to protect public health by systematically collecting, analyzing, and communicating information about medical events involving or potentially involving legally marketed medical products.

Postmarket surveillance study: required postmarket activity that may be ordered after the approval or clearance of certain Class II or Class III medical devices. Also called a "Section 522" study.

Poverty threshold: minimum level of income deemed necessary to achieve an adequate standard of living in a given country. Also called the "poverty line."

Power of attorney: instrument granting someone authority to act as an agent or attorney-in-fact for the grantor; a medical power of attorney is a legal mechanism that empowers a designated person to make medical decisions for a patient should the patient be unable to make the decisions due to incapacitation.

Preamendment device: a medical device available to patients before enactment of the Medical Device Amendments of 1976.

Predicate device: a medical device that was legally marketed in the U.S. prior to May 28, 1976, reclassified from Class III to Class II or I, and found to be substantially equivalent through the premarket notification 510(k) process.

Pre-emption: the principle that a federal law can supersede or supplant any inconsistent state law or regulation.

Preferred provider organization: a network of doctors, caregivers, and medical facilities that agree to provide health care services to plan members at less than their usual service fees so that members save money using the network; members may seek care outside of the network, but reduced benefits and higher out-of-pocket expenses may result.

Premarket: processes including evaluations, decisions, and other activities that occur prior to the FDA marketing approval of a medical product.

Premarket notification 510(k) process: process for securing FDA clearance to market medical devices that are substantially equivalent to devices marketed prior to May 28, 1976; 510(k) refers to the relevant section of the Federal Food, Drug, and Cosmetic Act.

Premium: the amount of money paid for a health insurance policy; the charge for insurance protection.

Prepaid health insurer: insurance plan in which health care professionals contract to provide a wide range of preventative, diagnostic, and treatment services to a group of enrolled participants.

Preponderance of the evidence: the greater weight of the evidence; superior evidentiary weight that, though not sufficient to free the mind wholly from all reasonable doubt, is still sufficient to incline a fair and impartial mind to one side of the issue rather than the other; this is the burden of proof in most civil trials, in which the jury is instructed to find for the side that on the whole has the stronger evidence, however slight the edge may be. *Compare* "beyond a reasonable doubt" and "clear and convincing evidence."

Presentment: act of presenting or laying before a court or other tribunal a formal statement about a matter to be dealt with legally; formal production of a negotiable instrument for acceptance or payment.

Preventable medical condition: adverse medical event or state of health directly resulting from a failure to follow recognized, evidence-based best practices or guidelines at the individual or provider level. Also called "preventable behavior" or "preventable condition."

Preventative care: health care that emphasizes health maintenance and the prevention of disease, early detection, and early treatment, thereby reducing the costs of health care in the long run.

Price discrimination: practice of offering identical goods or services to different buyers at different prices, when the cost of producing the goods or services are the same.

Price fixing: artificial setting or maintenance of prices at a certain level, contrary to the workings of the free market.

Prima facie: Latin meaning at first sight; sufficient to establish a fact or raise a presumption unless disproved or rebutted.

Primary care: basic level of health care provided by the physician with whom an individual has an ongoing relationship and who knows the patient's medical history; primary care services emphasis a patient's general health needs, such as preventative services, treatment of minor ailments, and identification of problems that require specialists.

Primary insurer: the insurer who pays the first medical claim.

Primordial germ cell: the earliest recognizable precursor of a germ cell in the embryo; develop into stem cells that in an adult generate the reproductive gametes.

Private insurance: insurance provided through an entity either for profit or not for profit and other than the federal or state government.

Procedural due process: the minimal requirements of notice and a hearing guaranteed by the Bill of Rights, especially if the deprivation of a significant life, liberty, or property interest may occur.

Profit margin: net profit after taxes divided by sales for a given year, expressed as a percentage; the percentage that profit constitutes of total sales.

Prosecution: commencement and carrying out of any action or scheme; criminal proceeding in which an accused person is tried.

Prosthetic: a device, either external or implanted, that substitutes for or supplements a missing or defective part of the body.

Protein therapy: mechanism that causes cells to be manipulated by the proteins in order to shift the balance of cell dynamics toward that of a healthy or productive cell; promising because it targets only cells affected by disease, avoiding collateral cell damage and surgery.

Proteomics: the cataloguing and analysis of proteins in cells and tissue; analysis of the expression, localizations, functions, and interactions of the proteins.

Protocol: the plan for carrying out a scientific study or a patient's treatment regimen.

Provider: any licensed institution that provides health care services.

Proximate cause: cause that is legally sufficient to result in liability; an act or omission that is considered in law to result in a consequence so that liability can be imposed on the actor; a cause that directly produces an event and without which the event would not have occurred.

Proxy: one who is authorized to act as a substitute for another, especially in corporate law; a health care proxy allows a person to make medical decisions on another's behalf.

Public health notification: an important message from the FDA to the health care community describing a risk associated with the use of a medical device and providing recommendations to avoid or reduce the risk.

Purchasing power parity per capita: method of measuring the relative purchasing power of different countries' currencies over the same types of goods and services; to compare economic statistics across countries, the data must first be converted into a common currency which allows rates of exchange to account for price differences between countries.

Quality-adjusted life-year: common measure of health status or treatment outcome used in cost-utility analysis; combines morbidity and mortality data.

Quality systems regulation: general control requirements that cover methods, facilities, and controls related to medical products design prior to actual production, manufacture, packing, storage, and installation; these regulations include Good Manufacturing Practices and seek to prevent safety problems related to system deficiencies and ensure that products consistently meet applicable requirements and specifications.

Quarantine: isolation of a person or animal afflicted with a communicable disease or the prevention of such person or animal from coming into a particular area, the purpose being to prevent the spread of disease.

Qui tam: Latin meaning in the name of the King; legal mechanism that allows a person, known as a whistleblower, to sue those committing health care fraud on behalf of the government.

Rare condition: a condition that affects or causes symptoms in fewer than four thousand individuals in the U.S. per year. Also called a "rare disease" or "orphan diease."

Rational basis test: principle whereby a court will uphold a law as valid under the Equal Protection Clause or Due Process Clause if it bears a reasonable relationship to the attainment of some legitimate governmental objective. *Compare* "intermediate scrutiny" and "strict scrutiny."

Recall: a device manufacturer's voluntary or directed removal or correction of a marketed device that the FDA considers to be in violation of the laws and regulations it administers and against which the agency would initiate legal action and seizure; does not include a market withdrawal or a stock recovery; Class I recalls involve dangerous or defective devices that have a reasonable probability of causing serious health problems or death; Class II recalls involve devices that might be expected to cause a temporary health problem or that pose only a slight threat of a serious nature; Class III recalls involve devices that are unlikely to cause any adverse health reaction, but that violate FDA labeling or manufacturing regulations.

Recombination: formation of new combinations of genes, either naturally, by crossing over or independent assortment, or in the laboratory by direct manipulation of genetic material.

Red herring: an irrelevant legal or factual issue intended to divert attention from the real problem or matter at hand.

Registry: a system for collecting information about a group of patients who have in common a disease, injury, condition, medical procedure or product, or similar characteristic; sometimes used narrowly to refer to the database itself and sometimes more broadly to refer to analyses and studies based on registry information.

Rehabilitation: restorative process through which an individual develops and maintains self-sufficient functioning consistent with her or his capability; the return to a recognized, acceptable, and attainable physical, mental, emotional, social, and economic usefulness for employment.

Re-import: import back into the country of exportation, particularly pharmaceutical products.

Reinsurance: contract by which an insurer procures a third party to insure it against loss or liability by reason of such original insurance; the practice of health insurers of purchasing insurance from another company to protect themselves from all or part of the losses incurred in the process of honoring the claims of policyholders.

Remote clinical management system: the use of medical devices to transmit secure patient data to health care professionals monitoring the patient in order to limit a patient's health risk, increase her or his level of comfort, and reduce the number and length of hospitalizations.

Reprogenics: term referring to the merging of reproductive and genetic technologies expected to happen in the near future as techniques become more available and more powerful. Also called "reprogenetics."

Restitution: return or restoration of some specific thing to its rightful owner or status; compensation for benefits derived from a wrong done to another.

Restructure: to change, alter, or restore the structure of; to effect a fundamental change in an organization or system; reorganize a company's operations.

Risk: a potential harm or the potential of a treatment action or medical event to cause harm.

Risk management: measuring, identifying, and controlling potential adverse outcomes; a systematic application of policies, procedures, and practices to the analysis, evaluation, and control of risks; key component of quality management systems.

Risk segmentation: the tendency of health plans to attract enrollees with higher or lower than average health costs; existence of uneven risk distributions between or among risk pools.

RNA interference: manipulation of ribonucleic acid (the genetic messengers of a cell) to interfere with, or silence, targeted genes in order to prevent the formation of disease-causing proteins; the basis for the 2006 Nobel Prize in medicine with the potential to produce treatments for diseases including cancer, blindness, and AIDS. Also called "RNAi."

RNA interference therapy: use of RNAi with a therapeutic objective, such as silencing a gene associated with the production of cholesterol.

Safe medical device: relative term meaning reasonable assurance that a device is safe once it can be determined, based upon valid scientific evidence, that the probable benefits to health from use of the device for its intended uses and conditions of use, when accompanied by adequate directions and warnings against unsafe use, outweigh any probable risks.

Safe harbor: acceptable payment practice that does not violate the Stark Amendments, fraud and abuse laws, or office of inspector general health insurance payment regulations.

Safety alert: issued by the FDA in situations where a medical device may present an unreasonable risk of substantial harm.

Safety signal: reported information on a possible causal relationship between an adverse event and a drug; further investigation is generally warranted to determine whether an actual connection exists.

Secondary disease: a disease that follows and results from an earlier disease, injury, or event

Secondary injury: an indirect result of the trauma which caused the primary injury; it occurs in the hours or days following the primary injury and may be a result of complications from the primary injury, such as brain damage from head trauma.

Secondary insurer: assumes responsibility for payment of charges not covered by the primary insurer.

Senate: upper chamber of a bicameral legislature; upper house of the U.S. Congress composed of one hundred members, two from each state, who are elected to six-year terms.

Serious adverse health consequence: any significant adverse experience related to a drug, device, or biologic, including events which are life threatening or which involve permanent or long term injury or illness.

Serious injury: an injury or illness that is life threatening, results in permanent impairment of a body function or permanent damage to body structure, or requires medical or surgical intervention to preclude permanent impairment or damage.

Severe mental illness: those from which psychosis is likely to occur; psychosis is the medical term used to identify symptoms where the individual experiences a loss of a sense of reality, where they cease to see and respond appropriately to the everyday world they are used to.

Shareholder: one who owns or holds a share or shares in a company or corporation.

Significant risk device: a medical device that cannot undergo tests in humans without institutional review board approval and FDA approval of an application for an Investigational Device Exemption; such a device presents a potential for serious risk to the health, safety, or welfare of patients and is intended as an implant, purported or represented to be for a use in supporting or sustaining human life, and for a use of substantial importance in diagnosing, curing, mitigating, or treating disease, or otherwise preventing impairment of human health.

Social distancing: a disease prevention strategy in which a community imposes limits on social face-to-face interaction to reduce exposure to and transmission of a disease; these limitations could include, but are not limited to, school and work closures, cancellation of public gatherings, and halted or limited mass transportation.

Somatic cell: any cell in the body other than an egg or sperm cell.

Special controls: requirements for Class II medical devices that are intended to ensure safety and effectiveness; unlike general controls, special controls may vary for different types of devices; special controls include performance standards, guidelines, patient registries, and postmarket surveillance.

Specific causation: the action or agent which definitely produces the disease or condition in question.

Spillover effect: externalities of economic activity; secondary effect which follows from a primary effect, and may be far removed from the event that caused the primary effect; effects on remaining drugs within the same therapeutic class after a prescription drug has been withdrawn from the market; can be positive or negative.

Stakeholder: disinterested third party who holds money or property, the right to which is disputed between two or more parties; a person who has an interest or concern in a business or enterprise, though not necessarily as an owner.

Standing: a party's right to make a legal claim or seek judicial enforcement of a duty or right; third party standing is the standing held by someone claiming to protect the rights of others.

State Child Health Insurance Program (SCHIP): program administered the U.S. federal government that provides matching funds to states for health insurance to families with children; designed to cover uninsured children in families with modest incomes, but that are too high to qualify for Medicaid.

Statute of limitations: a statute establishing a time limit for suing in a civil case, based on the date when the claim accrued, such as when the injury occurred or was discovered; the purpose of such a statute is to require diligent prosecution of known claims, thereby providing finality and predictability in legal affairs and ensuring that claims will be resolved while evidence is still reasonably available and fresh; a statute establishing a time limit for prosecuting a crime based on the date when the offense occurred.

Stem cells: undifferentiated multipotent precursor cells that are capable both of perpetuating themselves as stem cells and of undergoing differentiation into one or more specialized types of cells.

Strict scrutiny: standard applied to suspect classifications, such as race, in equal protection analysis and to fundamental rights in due process analysis; under strict scrutiny, a state must establish that it has a compelling interest that justifies and necessitates the law in question. *Compare* "intermediate scrutiny" and "rational basis test."

Subsidiary: a company whose voting stock is more than fifty percent controlled by another company, usually referred to as the parent company.

Subsidy: a grant, usually made by the government, to an enterprise whose promotion is considered to be in the public interest; a specific financial contribution by a foreign government or public entity conferring a benefit on exporters to the U.S.

Substantially equivalent medical device: when a medical device has the same intended use and has the same technological characteristics as a predicate device, or has the same intended use but different technological characteristics if these differences do not raise different questions of safety and effectiveness and if information is provided to show that the device is as safe and effective as a legally marketed device.

Substantive due process: the requirements of the Bill of Rights that legislation be fair and reasonable in content and be enacted to further a legitimate governmental objective.

Substitution effect: the theory that people who are intent on violence, either toward themselves or others, will find a way to achieve that objective with whatever tools are available; the economic theory that as prices rise, consumers will substitute away from higher priced goods and services, choosing less costly alternatives in order to maintain their standard of living.

Supplemental health insurance: type of insurance policy designed to cover the gaps that one's primary health insurance may have due to deductibles and co-payments; covers additional expenses that primary insurance does not cover, such as lost income and living expenses.

Supplier: entity that furnishes or provides something desired or required.

Surveillance: the ongoing, systematic collection, analysis, interpretation, and dissemination of data about a health-related event for use in public health action to reduce morbidity and mortality and to improve health.

Survival-threatening: ongoing abuse which potentially threatens survival whether through the physical risk of death from the abuse or the risk of developing a condition or disorder that threatens survival, such as severe depression.

Synthetic biology: an emerging field of medical research focused on developing new biologicals that have never existed before in nature; microscopic creatures, devices, and systems engineered for specific commercial jobs, such as growth of new human bones or tissue; advances in nanoscale technologies are contributing to advances in synthetic biology.

Target child: a child who is made the subject of domestic abuse over and above other siblings.

Tax credit: an amount subtracted directly from one's total tax liability, dollar for dollar, rather than a deduction from gross income.

Tax-exempt: not legally subject to taxation.

Tax subsidy: any form of subsidy where the recipients receive the benefit through the tax system, usually through the income tax, profit tax, or consumption tax systems.

Telemedicine: the diagnosis and treatment of patients in remote areas using medical information transmitted over long distances, especially by satellite.

Telemetry: the complete measuring, transmitting, and receiving apparatus for indicating, recording, or integrating at a distance, by electrical translating means, the value of a quantity; the science and technology of automatic measurement and transmission of data by wire, radio, or other means from remote sources to receiving stations for recording and analysis.

Teleradiology: radiology concerned with the transmission of digitized medical images over electronic networks and with the interpretation of the transmitted images for diagnostic purposes.

Telomere biology: the study of the segments of DNA that occur at the ends of chromosomes, particularly as it applies to aging in humans.

Teratogenic: a drug or other substance capable of interfering with the development of a fetus, causing birth defects.

Teratoma: a tumor consisting of different type of tissue, as of skin, hair, and muscle, caused by the development of independent germ cells.

Terminally ill: when a person is not expected to live more than twelve months.

Tertiary care: the aspect of in-patient care dealing with illnesses or conditions requiring specialized techniques; any medical treatment administered at a health care facility by highly specialized providers and often involving high-technology resources.

Therapeutic: of or pertaining to the treating or curing of disease; curative; having or exhibiting healing powers.

Thereapeutic equivalence: different drugs that control a symptom or illness exactly the same as other drugs used to control that symptom or illness; pharmaceutical equivalents that can be expected to have the same clinical effect and safety.

Third party beneficiary: a person who, though not a party to a contract, stands to benefit from the contract's performance.

Third party payer: an organization other than the patient (first party) or health care provider (second party) involved in the financing of personal health services.

Tort: a civil wrong for which a remedy may be obtained, usually in the form of damages; a breach of a duty that the law imposes on everyone in the same relation to one another as those involved in a given transaction.

Totipotent cell: a cell that can give rise to the entire organism, including the extra-embryonic membranes; the fertilized egg or zygote is totipotent.

Tracking: a process that allows manufacturers of medical products to provide certain critical information about the location of drugs, Class II or III medical devices, or biologics so they can promptly remove the product from the marketplace when required by the FDA.

Trade secret: information that may consist of any commercially valuable plan, formula, process, or product that is used for the making, preparing, compounding, or processing of trade commodities and that can be said to be the end product of either innovation or substantial effort; there must be a direct relationship between the trade secret and the productive process.

Trans-fat: a type of unsaturated fat; not essential to humans and do not promote good health.

Transfusion: direct transferring of blood, plasma, or the like into a blood vessel; transfer of whole blood or blood products from one individual to another.

Transgenic: of, pertaining to, or containing a gene or genes transferred from another species.

Transgenic chimera: an organism whose genome has been altered by the transfer of a gene or genes from another species or breed.

Transplant: to transfer an organ or tissue from one part of the body to another or from one person or animal to another.

Treatable medical condition: health ailment which can be cured, relieved, or controlled with medical intervention or lifestyle changes.

Treble damages: damages awarded in an amount three times higher than the amount for which the trier of fact finds the wrongdoer liable; treble damages are recoverable where authorized by statute and usually imposed as punishment.

Tying arrangement: an agreement by a party to sell one product but only on the condition that the buyer also purchases a different product or at least agrees that he or she will not purchase that product from any other supplier.

Ultrasound: application of ultrasonic waves for diagnostic or therapeutic purposes, specifically to image an internal body structure, monitor a developing fetus, or generate localized deep heat to the tissues; method of diagnosing illness or viewing internal body images by bouncing high frequency sound waves off internal organs and tissues from outside the body.

Underinsured: to insure for an amount less than the true or replacement value; to insure under a policy that provides inadequate benefits.

Underwrite: classifying applicants for insurance according to their degrees of insurability so that the appropriate premium rates may be charged.

Uniform Act: acts that the federal government drafts but does not actually enact as federal law; states are then free to modify the federal government's suggested draft before enacting it; law drafted with the intention that it will be adopted by all or most of the states.

Uninsured: not covered by insurance.

Union: persons or entities joined or associated together for some common purpose; an organization of workers.

Universal insurance: health care coverage for all eligible residents of a political region which covers medical, dental, and mental health care; typically, costs are paid by a single payer; implemented in all industrialized countries with the exception of the United States; the trend in health care worldwide. Also called "social insurance system."

Unlabeled use: use of a drug, medical device, or biologic for a purpose, patient group, or other use that is not specifically approved by the FDA; such use by physicians is considered part of the practice of medicine, which the FDA does not regulate.

Upcoding: misuse of standardized reimbursement codes in order to obtain more monetary reimbursement for a medical treatment than is allowed by law.

User facility: a hospital, ambulatory surgical facility, nursing home, outpatient diagnostic facility, or outpatient treatment facility that is not a physician's office; an outpatient treatment facility includes home health care groups, ambulance providers, and rescue services.

Vaccine: an injection, usually of an innocuous (weak or killed) form of the virus that stimulates the production of antibodies by the immune system to help prevent or create resistance to an infection; usually given as a preventive measure.

Vicarious liability: liability that a supervisory party such as an employer bears for the actionable conduct of a subordinate or associate such as an employee because of the relationship between the two parties. Also called "enterprise liability," "agency," and "respondeat superior."

Virus: ultramicroscopic, metabolically inert, infectious agent that replicates only within the cells of living hosts and often causing disease.

Withdrawal of FDA approval: an order withdrawing approval of a premarket approval if the FDA determines that certain requirements were not fulfilled.

Writ of mandamus: Latin meaning we command; an order issued by a superior court to compel a lower court or a government officer to perform mandatory or ministerial duties correctly.

Write-off: cancellation from the accounts as a loss; an uncollectable account; reduction in book value; depreciation.

Xenograft: a transplant of cells, tissues or organs taken from a donor of one species and implanted into a recipient of another species.

Xenotransplantation: transplant of tissue from an animal of one species to an animal of another species.

Xenozoonose: disease that can be passed from animals to humans.

Zygote: produced by a fertilization event between two haploid cells, an egg cell from a female and a sperm cell from a male, which combine to form a single diploid cell which precedes the blastocyst.

INDEX